Histopathology of the Liver

Histopathology of the Liver

Volume I

THE LATE
GERALD KLATSKIN, M.D.
David Paige Smith Professor of Medicine, Emeritus
Staff Member, Department of Pathology
Yale University School of Medicine
New Haven, Connecticut

HAROLD O. CONN, M.D.
Professor of Medicine, Emeritus
Yale University School of Medicine
New Haven, Connecticut
and
Department of Veterans Affairs Medical Center
West Haven, Connecticut

New York   Oxford
OXFORD UNIVERSITY PRESS
1993

Oxford University Press

Oxford   New York   Toronto
Delhi   Bombay   Calcutta   Madras   Karachi
Kuala Lumpur   Singapore   Hong Kong   Tokyo
Nairobi   Dar es Salaam   Cape Town
Melbourne   Auckland   Madrid

and associated companies in
Berlin   Ibadan

Published by Oxford University Press, Inc.,
200 Madison Avenue, New York, New York 10016

Oxford is a registered trademark of Oxford University Press

Library of Congress Cataloging-in-Publication Data
Klatskin, Gerald.
Histopathology of the liver /
Gerald Klatskin, Harold O. Conn.
p.   cm.   V. 2 contains illustrations.
Includes bibliographical references.   ISBN 0-19-504393-6 (set :)
1. Liver—Biopsy.   2. Liver—Histopathology.
I. Conn, Harold O., 1925–   .   II. Title.
[DNLM: 1. Liver—pathology.   2. Liver—pathology—atlases.
3. Liver Diseases—pathology.   4. Liver Diseases—pathology—atlases.
WI 700 K63h]   RC847.5.B56B57   1993   616.3′620758—dc20
DNLM/DLC   for Library of Congress   91-37259

2 4 6 8 9 7 5 3 1

Printed in the United States of America
on acid-free paper

To the forty-seven postdoctoral fellows
who collected the data and performed the biopsies,
to Hazel Hubbel,
who created the beautiful slides,
and to Ethelyn Henry Klatskin and Marilyn Barr Conn
who sustained the authors

Preface

The preparation of this book was a labor of love for both authors. It was the dream of Gerald Klatskin, who directed the Liver Study Unit at Yale from its creation in 1946 until his retirement in 1980, to write a textbook-atlas of hepatology, illustrated by color photomicrographs of the livers of patients seen on his own service, that would be useful for pathologists and clinicians involved in the interpretation of liver biopsies. Many alterations in hepatic structure can be caused by systemic diseases which affect other organs primarily, so that the appreciation of such hepatic lesions may provide clues to the identification of other nonhepatic disorders. Furthermore, the reactions of the liver to injury are limited, so that many of the lesions encountered on biopsy are not pathognomonic. Taken together with clinical and laboratory features, the histologic findings frequently are diagnostic or, at least useful in decreasing the number of diagnostic possibilities under consideration. Collaboration between the pathologist and the clinician is essential. In addition to contributing at the time of biopsy, clinicians are often able to confirm the accuracy of the diagnosis and to assess the prognostic significance of the lesions encountered. Clinicians who work closely with pathologists soon recognize the pitfalls of sampling errors and the need to obtain adequate biopsy specimens. Indeed, we are convinced that lack of experience is a much less serious handicap for pathologists than having to interpret sections that are too small or fragmented or poorly prepared. Pathologists faced with problems in biopsy interpretation soon discover that the available written material on hepatic histopathology is relatively sparse and that illustrations are usually limited to classic lesions, rarely showing atypical variants or unusual morphologic features that puzzle the pathologist. Moreover, with few exceptions, the illustrations are reproduced in black and white and are surprisingly different from the colored images seen in the microscope. This volume provides the opportunity to present in depth, and in color, a broad spectrum of the hepatic lesions seen in both hepatic and nonhepatic disorders. As his reputation as a hepatic pathologist spread, Dr. Klatskin was sent slides of confusing lesions for histologic consultations and slides of unusual lesions to enhance his collection.

The biopsies were performed by his postdoctoral fellows, who worked in the Unit and whose names appear in the listing on p. ix. To analyze the clinical, laboratory, and histologic details of these patients and their biopsies, Dr. Klatskin, known variously as Gerry, GK, or The Klat, developed a punch card from which most of the data could be recorded and easily retrieved by the "knitting needle" method (Fig. 1). For each patient, before the biopsy was performed, one of the fellows prepared a punch card with the biopsy and patient numbers and the provisional diagnosis. The completed card was left on GK's desk next to his microscope. After the biopsy, when the slides had

been stained—usually the same afternoon or the next day—Hazel Hubbel, Gerry's personal histology technician, placed them—one H & E, one Masson, and one iron stain—on top of the punch card.

Each patient was presented in detail by the fellow to Gerry, who examined the patient completely and made additions and corrections to the history and laboratory data on the punch card. Gerry read each biopsy and pointed out the important features to the fellow. In the beginning he did this by locating the pertinent field through the binocular microscope and then moved aside to allow the fellow to look through the scope. Later, use of a two-headed microscope made it possible for both to view the field at the same time. Dr. Klatskin wrote his interpretation of the biopsy, including his histologic diagnosis, in long hand on the back of the biopsy card (Fig. 2). After any missing historical and laboratory information had been obtained and additional histologic sections were cut and stained, GK added the supplemental information and entered the final diagnosis on the front of the card. He then personally punched all the data on the cards. Typed copies of each card were prepared in duplicate, one for alphabetical filing by the patient's last name and one by diagnosis. The original biopsy card was filed chronologically.

Gerry made 35 mm color transparencies of each biopsy on Kodachrome 25A or 40A film, using a Zeiss photomicroscope fitted with Planapochromat lenses, a light-blue filter and, occasionally, attachments for polarization or fluorescent microscopy. He recorded all notable aspects of each biopsy, including unusual or unrecognized lesions, which he filed for subsequent assessment. The lesion under scrutiny was often examined using different fixatives and/or stains. He took from 5 to 50 exposures of each biopsy and made careful notes about the appearance, stain, magnification, and the purpose of each photograph. Most of the sections illustrated were fixed in Carnoy's solution and stained with a modification of Masson's stain, a combination which we have found superior to others for demonstrating histologic detail. Since Carnoy's fixative cannot be used for fixing large specimens, most of the surgical wedge biopsies and postmortem specimens were fixed in 10% buffered neutral formalin.

When the transparencies were returned from the developer he entered all of this information, along with the patient's name, biopsy number, history, and diagnosis on the white edges of the cardboard mounts. If all the data did not fit on the upper edge, he would continue on the bottom and sides of the transparency (Fig. 3), and even on the back. No one who ever attended one of The Klat's weekly slide sessions will ever forget Gerry, sitting in the dark behind the projector, holding up a slide to a chink of light from the projector and squinting to read his micronotations. He then inserted the transparency into the

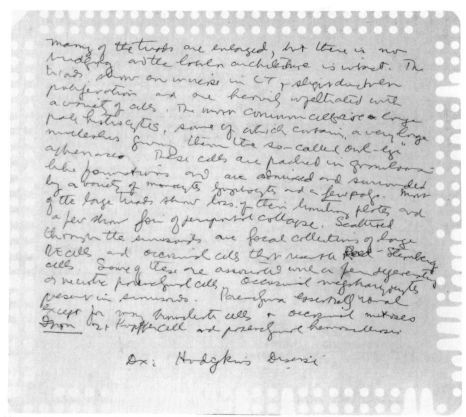

Klatskin liver biopsy data card (front side). All clinical and laboratory data are entered on the card and punched into the margins of the card for easy computer retrieval.

Klatskin liver biopsy data card (back side). The histologic interpretation by G. Klatskin is written in long hand.

The forty-seven postdoctoral fellows who studied with Gerald Klatskin.

Richard D. Aach
Waddell Barnes
Victorino S. Barreto
Michael Bayer
Gordon D. Benson
Joseph R. Bloomer
Herbert L. Bonkowsky
James L. Boyer
A. Russell Brenneman
Luitgard Bungards
Termchai Chainuvati
Beng Keng Chew
Robert Cimis
Harold O. Conn
Donald L. Davidson
Harold J. Fallon
L. Frederick Fenster
Cameron N. Ghent
Michael S. Gold
Peter B. Gregory
Philip S. Guzelian
Brunildo A. Herrero
Herbert Kaplan
Marshall M. Kaplan
Knut Kirkeby
Douglas R. Labrecque
Patricia S. Latham
Robert A. Levine
Willis C. Maddrey
Denis J. Miller
James V. Miller
David Molander
James P. Nolan
Masuyo Nomora
Leroy A. Pesch
William J. Powell, Jr.
Oscar M. Reinmuth
Caroline A. Riely
F. Joseph Roll
Shozo Saito
Robert L. Scheig
Jerome B. Simon
Marc J. Taylor
William A. Tisdale
Anthony S. Tornay, Jr.
Ralph Wright
David Young

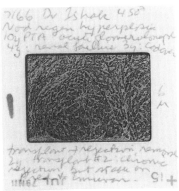

Photomicrograph of slide of patient 5158 with diagnosis, history, and laboratory data inscribed on the margins of the cardboard mount, front (top) and back (bottom).

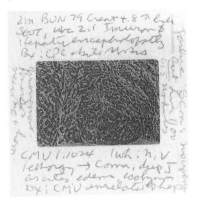

projector, and presented the complete, well-organized history, followed by his histologic interpretation of the biopsy. Those were magnificent teaching sessions.

Almost 300 biopsies were performed each year, so his experience and his slide collection were derived from some 9000 biopsies and about 45,000 transparencies. In addition to material from his patients and consultations, biopsies were contributed by skilled histopathologist friends, including Kamal Ishak, Peter Scheuer, and Luigi Bianchi, who sent slides of

lesions that GK himself had not seen. In completing this book, I have supplemented Gerry's slides with transparencies provided by histopathologists who have described new disorders or specific lesions not recorded by GK. Most are hepatic lesions that were first described during his terminal illness or after his death. All of these pathologists graciously gave their permission to include these slides, and they provided clinical, laboratory, and histologic information about their patients. The physicians who contributed slides are listed in the Acknowledgments.

Gerry wrote a detailed proposal for a book, which he submitted to Oxford University Press in 1977. He looked forward to his retirement years as a time to write it. When he retired, however, he accepted the assignment of reading liver biopsies for the Surgical Pathology Section at Yale, so progress on the book was slow.

A series of serious health problems ensued. In 1982 he had a severe myocardial infarction and, shortly thereafter lymphadenopathy appeared, which was subsequently shown to be a malignant lymphoma. In early 1984 he underwent coronary bypass surgery. This was followed by a devastating catastrophe. He abruptly lost foveal vision bilaterally, and his writing was virtually halted. (No cause for the bilateral macular degeneration was ever found.) By this time he had completed the first 18 of the planned 25 chapters. Members of the Liver Unit, including Caroline Riely, Jim Boyer, Dennis Miller, Adrian Reuben, and I worked with him, but progress was agonizingly slow.

In the summer of 1984 Gerry and Lyn Klatskin formally invited me to join him as co-author, to help him finish his "damned book," as Lyn called it. In the process he enumerated my virtues for the role. In his opinion (1) I was one of his first fellows; actually, I was the second, but the first to be formally appointed a postdoctoral fellow; (2) he had trained me in liver biopsy interpretation; (3) I had modeled my Liver Service at the West Haven VA Hospital after his and, indeed, used the Klatskin liver biopsy needle, biopsy technique, punch card system, and staining methods; (4) we had discussed interesting and problem biopsies at least once a week for about 30 years. He added that I had achieved an international reputation of my own in liver disease and wrote well, albeit in a style different from his. I jokingly said that it appeared that I had spent my whole life in preparation for this project. He seriously replied that it seemed so.

Many years before, Gerry had taught me by example that occasions would occur when one was asked to do an important favor that one could not refuse, and in such instances he said that one should agree graciously and promptly. I did so. He said that, of course, he wanted me to be his co-author in all that co-authorship implied. "You mean that I have all the "rights, honors, privileges and responsibilities," I asked, quoting the famous Yale litany.

"Yes," he said.

At this point Marilyn, my wife, broke in and warned me and Gerry that I was already overcommitted as Chief of the Liver Service, the director of a busy, productive research program, a faculty member with many teaching duties, one of the editors of *Hepatology,* the infant journal of the American Association for the Study of Liver Diseases, a busy speaker with commitments stretching two years into the future, a writer with other major writing commitments, and a husband and father of three, who already didn't have sufficient time to sleep. We all agreed that the going would be very slow, but under the circumstances it was the only reasonable choice. That evening in the privacy of our bedroom my wife asked me to tell Gerry that it really wasn't possible or practical for me to take on such a monumental task. I said that I didn't think I had that option. Progress throughout has been much slower than even she had predicted.

Gerry and I immediately started working, usually each morning for several hours in his office when he was able to get there. We followed his outline, and he suggested references from his reprint files. After he left I would locate the reprints in the files and take them home, where each evening I would write out the two or three pages we had produced. In the morning I would read aloud to him what I had written. He would suggest rewording, additions, deletions, and alterations, always gently and patiently. Then he suggested slides to illustrate that section, often remembering the patient's name. Finding them, however, usually involved my looking through the diagnostic biopsy files and reading all his pertinent biopsy interpretations on that topic. Finally, I described to him what I saw on the transparencies and we then chose the most appropriate illustrations. Then came preparation of the legends, assignment of figure numbers and labeling the slides by figure number, the primary histologic feature illustrated, and the stain and magnification. It was tedious, time-consuming, meticulous work, but it was a great education.

As we gradually moved ahead we also worked in reverse. Gerry suggested that we read together what had already been written, so that I had the opportunity to make any modifications. This was done usually at his home when he couldn't come to the office. Marilyn with one copy and I with another would alternate reading, and Gerry and I would make suggestions. Each session started only after Gerry had asked us about each of our children and we had asked about his. When I raised questions about content, concepts, or clarity, Gerry would pa-

tiently explain. Periodically he would ask Marilyn, "Is that clear?" and if it was not, he proceeded to explain, as if we had all the time in the world. Throughout this process he never rushed or compromised his meticulous attention to detail or his role as my preceptor.

On several occasions Gerry suggested the inclusion of new pertinent articles that he had read using a magnifying optical reader. These painstakingly slow readings of a few select journals suggested to us that the completed chapters would have to be brought up to date. He was greatly relieved when I assured him that I would incorporate any new publications of significance. Neither of us realized that we were standing on the brink of an explosion of hepatologic knowledge.

During all of this time my only basic criticism of the book was that there were subjects, such as tropical diseases, for which we had no illustrations. I felt that we should omit or abbreviate such sections or that we should attempt to obtain slides from experts to illustrate these areas. He was reluctant to do so, but he agreed that if I felt a specific omission was sufficiently important, we could consider obtaining excellent outside slides to illustrate the issue in question. Part of his reluctance, I am sure, was that he was unable to see and approve slides taken from sources outside his own collection.

Our work was frequently interrupted by hospitalizations for diagnostic investigations of his advancing lymphoma, and, thereafter, for a series of courses of chemotherapy. We continued to work as best we could, both at his home and during his hospitalizations at the Veterans Administration Hospital, where he always insisted on being admitted.

We discussed the possibility that he and I might not be able to finish the book together. He said simply that we would continue working as long as we were able, and that if we didn't finish it in time, he was confident that I would complete it. He indicated at that time that he had accumulated some funds from his histologic consultations that were to be used as needed to finish the book. By the time he died in March 1986, we had completed 20 chapters and portions of several others.

After Gerry died a number of problems plagued the project and delayed its completion. Aside from the shock of losing a close friend and coworker, his secretary was assigned to other departmental duties and for practical purposes was no longer available to me. In an attempt to have my secretary do the typing we learned that every word had been typed using a Xerox 850 word processor which was no longer available to us. When we tried to convert the tapes to either the Commodore computer, which we were using at that time, or to the IBM system we were frustrated to learn that neither Xerox, IBM, Commodore or the Yale Computer Center were able to convert the 3000 typed pages to a system with which we could work. Furthermore, none of these four institutions could tell us how or where to have the discs transformed. It seemed inconceivable that we would have to retype all these pages. After eight months of searching, and after we had just begun the tedious retyping process, we discovered a small firm in New York that could transpose the tapes from Xerox to another system and then to the IBM system. We had wasted a year before we had the tapes transcribed and had purchased word processing equipment with which we could proceed. In any event about 10% of the transcripts appeared to be printed in Sanskrit and had to be retyped, anyhow.

At this point I turned to the five unwritten chapters. It was much slower to write without GK's broad knowledge of medicine, his fabulous memory for references, his recollection of specific biopsies, and with my need to review every biopsy report and every transparency in the areas dealing with these chapters. These chapters are entitled, "Circulatory Disorders of the Liver," "Hepatic Granulomas," "Hepatic Injury in Infection," "Hepatic Lesions in Systemic Diseases" (this chapter alone included amyloidosis, collagen vascular diseases, hematology, gastroenterology, endocrinology and metabolism, pregnancy, and more), and "Neoplasms of the Liver and Intrahepatic Bile Ducts."

I realized that liver transplantation did not exist, for practical purposes, when GK had planned the book, and AIDS had not yet been described. Both of these topics would require new, unanticipated chapters. It was disheartening to realize that at this stage in mid-1988 every chapter would require up-dating. Consequently, chapter by chapter, page by page, and reference by reference, the whole tome had to be revised. Furthermore, to avoid heterogeneity, the new chapters and the revisions were all written by me, trying to emulate GK's characteristic writing style rather than my own, which is quite different.

In the process of making these revisions almost 200 new photomicrographs that illustrated newly described disorders or important lesions that had been omitted were added to the text. Oxford University Press required, properly I believe, that these extra figures be incorporated into the numbering system without using suffixes, e.g. Fig 35*A*, 78*A* and 78*B* etc. This required that *all* the figures be reassigned new consecutive numbers and that the new numbers be used throughout the text and legends. This was a complex undertaking that necessitated about 9000 individual transactions since every figure had been cited in the book, on average, seven times. This number-changing process itself required almost six months, since every transparency had to be reexamined each time it was cited and confirmed, and this arduous duty could not be delegated. Finally, during proof-reading of the galleys a few new photomicrographs were incorporated, but these were entered using letter suffixes, rather than repeating the whole tortuous renumbering process.

I describe these "Perils of Pauline" in detail because it is difficult without doing so even for me to understand why it took so long to complete this book. Without this background it would be impossible for Gerry's family and many colleagues, who have impatiently awaited its publication, to appreciate how this "simple" task could have taken nine years.

This magnum opus is by far the biggest task with which I have ever been involved. It is with awe that I contemplate Gerry Klatskin's bequest to me of his magnificent, uncompleted manuscript and his monumental collection of color transparencies. In fact, one of the lessons I learned most emphatically in completing this work is the unrelenting pace of progress. The appearance of new hepatic diseases and hepatic lesions and endless variations on these themes requires constant revision and updating. The major frustration in preparing a volume such as this is determining when, if ever, one can stop. The corollary, of course, is when does one start on the next edition.

I am honored by Gerry Klatskin's confidence in offering me the opportunity to complete his dream. I have done it to the best of my ability and in the way that I think he would have wanted it done. I am personally very proud of what has been accomplished and believe that The Klat would have been pleased too.

New Haven, Connecticut   H. O. C.
June 1992

Acknowledgments

First and foremost, I acknowledge my enormous debt to Gerald Klatskin. We met in 1951 over a patient with complicated liver disease, shortly after I had come to Yale as a fresh assistant resident from Johns Hopkins Hospital. He gently tolerated my unconventional, nonunitarian diagnosis of parenchymal, hemolytic, and obstructive jaundice all in the same patient, and he seemed surprised, but pleased, when the diagnosis was confirmed. Shortly thereafter he invited me to learn about the liver with him. He led me along the path of hepatic righteousness and taught me, by example, immense amounts about history-taking, physical examination, and clinical observation. Each was closely correlated with the histopathology of the liver. Each, he felt, could be standardized and made reproducible.

His implacable curiosity was contagious, and I learned the joys of making a difficult diagnosis, of searching the literature, and of feeling a previously unfelt liver or hearing an unheard murmur. It was the "sink-or-swim" school of learning at the feet of the master. There were few frills: see the patients, read the literature, look at the biopsies. We looked at biopsies endlessly. He often saw, photographed, and recorded new, variant, and unrecognized hepatic lesions. He felt it was important to record such lesions so that they could be retrieved when it was ultimately determined what they actually were. I was amazed years later when I realized that he had continually recorded α_1-antitrypsin cytoplasmic inclusion bodies long before α_1-antitrypsin deficiency had been described. I embraced his academic approach to the liver. Even his trademark—abstracting on 5 × 8 inch index cards every hepatic paper he read—became my way of life, too.

As an amateur photographer I admired both his black-and-white prints and his color histopathologic slides. He was a fine photographer. In addition to selecting each shot for content and clarity, his photomicrographs were well composed. Indeed, several artists, including one who arranged to have the whole collection duplicated, commented that many of the photomicrographs were works of art in their own right. Perhaps we may one day see some of them from a different point of view.

The hard work was leavened by good people. The cream of the faculty and the students and house staff took advantage of Gerry Klatskin's open-door policy. They were joined by hepatologists from all over the world who were passing through New Haven. The postdoctoral fellows, themselves, were a very special, immensely talented group. Their collective accomplishments were listed by Jim Boyer at the time Gerry received the Julius Friedenwald Medal in 1983 (*Gastroenterology* 1983; 85:1235). In addition, each November he took a few of the fellows to the annual meeting of the American Association for the Study of Liver Disease (AASLD) in Chicago. There they convened in Hans Popper's office at the Hecktoen Institute with the founders of the AASLD for an informal session before the meeting started. "The Klat" proudly introduced each fellow present to these liver legends.

In retrospect, his approach to teaching the liver was pure serendipity. He helped us prepare our minds, and presumably we were to keep our eyes open for *chance*. I will never forget the spontaneous get-together of a half-dozen of his fellows in a bar at the Drake Hotel after he had been elected President of the AASLD in 1958. The fellows were arguing about how important it was to one's career to present papers in person at the AASLD meeting. During a lull in the conversation Gerry quietly said that he himself had never presented a paper at the annual meeting and that he believed it was much more meaningful and efficient to publish carefully reasoned, well-written, peer-reviewed articles in the best journals. I can never thank him enough for his paying me the supreme compliment of asking me to help him finish this book.

I must acknowledge, again, the contributions of the Fabulous Forty-seven Fellows (or should I say the "other 46"), to whom this book is dedicated. He was proud of each one and maintained contact with each of them throughout his life. Although most were Americans, they came from ten different countries. G. K. was generous with his time, both professionally and socially, and the fellows became members of his extended family, joined together by the common bonds of Klatskin and the liver.

The contributions of Hazel Hubbell, his histology technician par excellence, cannot be overestimated. She left the Surgical Pathology Section at Yale to join Gerry, and for almost 20 years processed all the biopsies performed in his Liver Study Unit. Her knowledge, skill, and professionalism in her field were equal to Gerry's in his. She introduced him to Carnoy's fixative and the Masson trichrome stain, two techniques that helped make Yale hepatic histology sections at least the equal of any in the world. Dr. Klatskin felt that the demanding fixation process was fully justified by its accentuation of the colors of Masson staining. Until her death, Hazel remained a dedicated colleague and close friend who personally created the slides from which most of the photomicrographs in this book were made.

More than 100 colleagues around the world have graciously contributed tissue blocks or photomicrographs for inclusion in this volume. Their names appear in the accompanying list. I especially appreciate the generous offer of Dr. Lawrence Brandt and the late Dr. Gerald Bezahler who proffered many slides from their splendid collection of the hepatic lesions of AIDS. As Dr. Bezahler said, when I asked him how to acknowledge their contribution, "Brandt provided Bezahler; Bezahler provided the slides."

Several Yale pathologists were of ongoing assistance in reviewing slides, in locating specific histologic lesions, and in

We are indebted to the many physicians who graciously donated color transparencies of hepatic lesions for inclusion in this book.

W. Robert Anderson
H. O. Appelman
Victorino S. Barreto
Thomas W. Bauer
A. L. Beaudet
Michel Beaugrand
Gerald H. Bezahler
Luigi Bianchi
Herbert L. Bonkovsky
Kent Bottles
Sylvia S. Bottomly
Kevin S. Bove
Lawrence J. Brandt
J. P. Callard
Francesco Callea
John P. Cello
John R. Craig
James M. Crawford
Carol A. Czapar
Peggy M. Dalahoussaye
Gary L. Davis
Thomas DeBrito
A. Jake Demetris
Valeer S. Desmet
Hong P. Dienes
D. Droz
Paul H. Duray
Margaret E. Elmes
Rosa Enrichez
G. P. Everett
L. Frederick Fenster
M. J. Finegold
P. M. Girard
Gary L. Gitnick
Douglas R. Gnepp
Michael S. Gold
Sidney Goldfischer
Sigantha Govindarajan
I. S. Grimm
Phillip S. Guzelian
Oscar Haluszka
Krister Höckenstedt
Jay H. Hoofnagle
R. Horiuchi
Kamal G. Ishak
Anna-Marie Jezequel
Gary C. Kanel
Marshall M. Kaplan

Edward C. Klatt
K. M. Klein
Raymond Koff
H. Kojiro
A. Kondo
Jay H. Lefkowitch
Robert A. Levine
Klaus Lewin
Karen Lindsay
Jurgen Ludwig
Roderick N. M. MacSween
F. A. Mitros
Alberto Moreno
Milton G. Mutchnick
Yasuni Nakanuma
Francesco Negro
Steven J. Norris
K. Okuda
Barbara M. Osborne
Toshiaki Osuga
M. James Phillips
Hans Popper
Bernard C. Portmann
Thomas G. Pretlow
Emanuel Rubin
Adrian Reuben
Caroline A. Riely
Fenton Schaffner
Peter Scheuer
T. Shikata
Maria H. Sjogren
J. P. Sloane
Dale C. Snover
Richard E. Sobonya
Tadashi Terada
Swan N. Thung
T. Uchida
Wilma Veira
John M. Veirling
Dominique Vuitton
Ian R. Wanless
A. Brian West
Russell H. Wiesner
W. C. Winn, Jr.
C. L. Witzleben
Hideaki Yasui
Jonathan H. Yau
Raymond Yesner
Elie S. Zafrani

We apologize to any contributor whose name was inadvertently omitted or whose slide is not included.

We acknowledge the invaluable assistance of many friends, colleagues, and former postdoctoral fellows of the Yale Liver Study Unit who critically reviewed chapters and contributed many important ideas and suggestions.

Richard D. Aach
Irwin M. Arias
Gordon D. Benson
Gerald H. Bezahler
Joseph R. Bloomer
Herbert L. Bonkovsky
James L. Boyer
Lawrence J. Brandt
Termchai Chainuvati
John R. Craig
Robert M. Donaldson
Harold J. Fallon
L. Frederick Fenster
Cameron N. Ghent
Norman D. Grace
Philip S. Guzelian
Marshall M. Kaplan

Jay H. Lefkowitch
Robert A. Levine
Marc I. Lorber
Willis C. Maddrey
James P. Nolan
Adrian Reuben
Caroline A. Riely
John Ryan
Robert L. Scheig
Jerome B. Simon
Swan N. Thung
Ian R. Wanless
Kenneth W. Warren
A. Brian West
Hastings K. Wright
Ralph Wright
Hyman J. Zimmerman

We apologize to anyone whose name was omitted.

many other ways. Dr. Raymond Yesner, who was a close friend and colleague of Gerry's, had been the Chief of Pathology at the West Haven VA Hospital for over 40 years. He helped me to understand some of the subleties of diverse histopathologic controversies. Dr. A. Bryan West, who became Yale's hepatic histopathologist after Gerry's death, filled in gaps by finding in his files beautiful illustrations of hepatic lesions that were first described after Gerry died, or that were otherwise not included. He provided many of the immunoperoxidase-antibody stains presented herein. I will always be grateful to him for his generosity and warm friendship.

I appreciate the careful reading, criticisms, and suggestions of a number of hepatologists, most of whom were Klatskin's ex-fellows, and pathologists who reviewed early versions of chapters or portions of them. These reviewers, whose names appear in the accompanying listing, were helpful in keeping the text integrated and current. I was especially touched by the comment of one of the chapter reviewers, John Craig, who was called upon to complete a similar volume when his senior co-author, Robert Peters, suddenly died. John, who fully understood the issues involved in finishing another's book, commented, "There must be a special place in the Literary Hall of Fame for 'pinch' authors."

Many secretaries spent thousands of hours converting our unintelligible handwritings into legible manuscripts. Without Marie Warner, Camille Paglinco, Josephine Tomei, Irene Cowern, and others, this book would still be a pile of paper.

Many librarians, most prominent among whom are Joan McGuiness, Nancy Baratz-Culkin, Gail LaScola, and Kenny Fry, were instrumental in helping to conduct searches and making available pertinent articles during up-dating of chapters in the later stages of this project.

I am especially grateful for the constant support of my co-worker and companion, my wife, Marilyn Barr Conn. After failing to convince me and the Klatskins that I was too over-committed to accept the invitation to help finish the book, and after the *fait* was *accompli*, she accepted the inevitable and became a full-fledged member of the team. Having served as a

research associate at Yale for many years and as an editorial assistant for *Gastroenterology* and *Hepatology* for almost 15 years, she was well prepared for the task. Marilyn participated in every aspect of completing the book—word processing, editing and critiquing manuscripts, searching for and confirming references, labeling slides and, of course, endless proofreading. When I had completed the final seven chapters, it became painfully clear that the first 20 chapters, which Gerry had written over a period of years, were hopelessly out of date; less than 3% of the references cited had been published after 1980. After seriously considering a number of alternatives, I began a monumental revision. The updating process required literature searches, revision and incorporation of new material into the manuscript, and identification and selection of new histologic images which required the location or preparation of good histologic photomicrographs and/or obtaining permission to include them. The additions, revisions, and responses to the reviewers who critiqued each chapter required more than two years work, about one chapter per month. This was followed by an updating of the revisions. These months were full of stress, and, as my wife put it, "Divorce was not an option, but thoughts of murder? Yes!" The uniformly positive comments of our reviewers sustained us during those difficult days. Penultimately, there was the preparation of the two massive indices. Together they totaled more than 100 manuscript pages. Ultimately, there was the terminal proofreading, which we did during an extended trip abroad. When the galleys were finally finished we could quote large sections of the book verbatim to each other, often out of context. Nevertheless, when the possibility of a second edition was mentioned, I was told that divorce could become an option.

Finally, I thank Jeffrey House, Executive Editor at Oxford University Press, and his colleague, Susan Hannan, Development Editor, for helping us through the hard times.

New Haven, Connecticut   H. O. C.
August 1992

Contents

Histopathology of the Liver

Chapter 1
Techniques

Needle biopsy of the liver

Value

The value of needle biopsy as a diagnostic tool in the investigation of liver disease is well recognized. Not as fully appreciated, however, is the fact that many hepatic lesions are not pathognomonic and that identification of their etiologies often requires consideration of the accompanying clinical and laboratory features. It is evident, therefore, that close collaboration of the clinician and pathologist is essential for the reliable interpretation of liver biopsy material. Serial biopsy studies are useful in following the course of hepatic disease, particularly in assessing the efficacy of therapy, and have shed considerable light on the pathogenesis and natural history of many disorders that affect the liver.

Because of its unique circulation (see schematic drawing, Volume II, p. 2), multiplicity of biochemical activities, and the unusual sensitivity and reactivity of its structural components, the liver is frequently affected in systemic disorders and in a wide variety of diseases that involve other organs primarily. Indeed, such disorders account for a significant fraction of the hepatic lesions encountered in most large biopsy series. Not infrequently such lesions prove to be diagnostic or provide useful collateral evidence to support a diagnosis under consideration for other reasons.

Limitations

Considering the small size of the specimen obtained by needle biopsy, approximately one fifty-thousandth of the liver, the potential for sampling error is great. This is not a serious problem in the case of most diffuse lesions, but, even in these, identification may be difficult if the distinctive morphologic features are irregular in distribution. Focal lesions when small in size or few in number may easily escape detection. However, lesions such as granulomas or metastases are encountered in needle biopsy specimens with surprising frequency. No doubt this reflects the fact that often such lesions are more numerous and widely distributed than is apparent clinically. Our finding of hepatic granulomas in 94% of 247 patients with sarcoidosis, only half of whom had clinical or laboratory evidence of hepatic involvement, illustrates this point. Similarly, a needle biopsy specimen obtained at autopsy revealed malignancy in 48% of those patients who had any evidence of tumor in the liver (1).

Success in sampling focal lesions, particularly tumors, can be enhanced by directing the biopsy needle under peritoneoscopic (2,3), ultrasonic, or computerized tomographic (CT) guidance (4), or by aspirating two cores of tissue through the same puncture site at one sitting, using a different angle of penetration for each (1). Routine examination of serial sections also increases the chances of finding focal lesions. In addition, in the case of diffuse lesions, it often facilitates the detection of sparsely distributed, distinctive, histologic features, such as Mallory bodies, bile thrombi, and degenerating bile ducts, and clarifies the zonal distribution of the lesions that may be of importance diagnostically. In our laboratory, we routinely examined 15 to 20 serial sections on five slides numbered sequentially to permit orientation in three dimensions. When indicated, we prepared additional serial sections for study. These have proved particularly useful in the detection of granulomas and metastatic tumors.

The size and integrity of the biopsy specimen and the quality of its fixation, embedding, sectioning, and staining are of critical importance. Although lesions with distinctive morphologic features, such as metastatic carcinoma and diffuse amyloidosis, can be identified in small fragments, reliable interpretation of needle biopsy material may require an unfragmented core of liver 1 to 2 cm in length. Such intact cores permit assessment of the overall architecture as well as examination of the hepatic parenchyma and of a significant number of portal triads. A well-trained operator using an appropriately selected needle can almost always provide such a specimen. If the first attempt is unsuccessful, reaspiration through the same puncture site, using a different angle of penetration will almost always provide a useful specimen. In the interests of safety, it is probably unwise to puncture the liver more than twice through the same puncture site. If the need for biopsy is urgent and the first two attempts are unsuccessful, we repeat the procedure at another site well removed from the initial point of entry. Failure to obtain tissue may indicate hepatic anatomic anomalies (5).

Advances in ultrasonography and CT imaging have made biopsy of focal lesions more precise and accurate. For neoplasms, fine needle aspiration with cytologic examination has improved diagnostic accuracy (6), and histologic examination may further enhance it (7). Laparoscopic guidance, too, can improve the diagnosis of both focal and generalized lesions such as cirrhosis (8).

Complications

Needle biopsy of the liver is a relatively safe procedure provided it is carried out skillfully and with consideration of a number of precautionary measures and contraindications. However, even under ideal conditions, complications do occur occasionally, and may rarely prove fatal. The mortality rate has been variously estimated to range between 0.009% (9) and

0.194% (10). It varies with the type of needle employed, the status of blood coagulability, and the character of the underlying hepatic lesions. One investigation found no mortality in 20,000 biopsies (11), another no deaths in 1,000 outpatients (12), and six deaths in almost 70,000 biopsies (9).

The most common serious complication of needle biopsy is hemorrhage, usually into the peritoneum, and, less commonly, into the hepatic parenchyma, bile ducts, or the pleural cavity. Other complications include bile peritonitis, bacteremia, pneumothorax, pulmonary bile embolism, arteriovenous fistula, perforation of the gallbladder or colon, suphrenic abscess, intrahepatic hematoma, and nonhemorrhagic shock, presumably of vasomotor origin in most instances, but occasionally due to a reaction to the local anesthetic employed. Most fatalities result from hemorrhage, but occasionally are attributable to bile peritonitis or sepsis. Detailed accounts of needle biopsy complications and references to original reports are available in several comprehensive reviews (9–13). A recent report of more than 9,000 biopsies indicated increased risks of post-biopsy hemorrhage in patients with hepatic neoplasms (14). This article, in turn, stimulated critical comments about complications with different types of needles (15).

Contraindications

Any coagulopathy enhances the potential risk of hemorrhage following needle biopsy. There is general agreement, however, that mild abnormalities of coagulation are not a contraindication to the procedure. The criteria used to define the limits within which deviations from normal are regarded as acceptable in terms of safety vary from one center to another. Our own criteria include a prothrombin time within three seconds of normal, a bleeding time of 10 minutes or less, and a platelet count of at least 50,000 cu mm. If biopsy is urgently needed in a patient with a prolonged prothrombin time that does not respond to vitamin K therapy, the deficit can often be corrected by the infusion of fresh frozen plasma. Infusing two or more units of fresh frozen plasma over the 12 to 18 hours preceding biopsy and again after the procedure almost always permits safe performance of the biopsy. The rate and duration of infusion is based on serial prothrombin time determinations. Plugging the needle track is effective in such patients, but requires some modification of technique (16).

Some of the complications of needle biopsy are not attributable to defects in coagulation, and, in some instances, have been attributed to specific diseases of the liver. These include extrahepatic biliary obstruction, cholangitis, chronic passive congestion of the liver, hepatic neoplasms, amyloidosis, extramedullary hematopoiesis, and ascites. Experience with a few such cases in which other complicating factors may have played a role has led some authors to conclude that these disorders per se are contraindications to biopsy. We have biopsied a number of patients in each of these categories, and, with rare exceptions, have encountered no significant complications (17). With respect to biliary obstruction, our only contraindications to needle biopsy are a suspected hydrops of the gallbladder or overt clinical evidence of suppurative cholangitis. In either case, little is to be gained from needle biopsy. Among the other disorders usually cited as contraindications, only two in our experience have been complicated by significant intraperitoneal hemor-

rhage requiring transfusion. This occurred in one of our 13 patients with hepatic amyloidosis and in two of 26 with extramedullary hematopoiesis. All three survived, but one patient with extramedullary hematopoiesis associated with a malignant histiocytic lymphoma required surgical intervention.

Our only postbiopsy fatality occurred in a patient with moderately severe viral hepatitis whose coagulation parameters were within acceptable limits. Signs of shock appeared within 10 minutes following biopsy, but failed to respond to prompt, massive blood replacement. Death ensued in less than four hours. At autopsy, the peritoneum contained 1.5 liters of clotted blood, far less than the volume transfused, but there was no evidence of a laceration in the liver. The biopsy tract, which measured 1 mm in diameter and 3 cm in depth and contained fresh clot, did not enter, traverse, or lacerate any notable blood vessels judging from a study of serial sections. Accordingly, the explanation for the irreversible shock in this case was not adequately explained.

Needle biopsy is contraindicated in uncooperative patients who cannot or will not suspend respiration in the expiratory phase and lie quietly during the procedure. Infants and young children may be exceptions, since respiratory and other movements can be adequately restrained by an assistant for the brief period required.

Biopsy needles and technique

The selection of a needle for liver biopsy should be based on a consideration of its safety, ease of manipulation, and reliability in providing specimens of good quality and adequate length.

Biopsy needles in current use range in external diameter from 1.0 to 2.0 mm. It is logical to assume that those with the smallest diameters are safest in terms of preventing hemorrhage and other complications. However, the evidence for this is not convincing, since other important factors, such as differences in the biopsy technique employed and the type of patients and the variety of hepatic lesions sampled, make comparisons difficult. The chief objection to the use of needles with diameters of less than 1.2 mm is that they usually provide specimens that are too small and fragmented for reliable histologic interpretation. However, skinny needle biopsy of the liver has been shown to be useful in the cytologic diagnosis of hepatic neoplasms (4,6) and post-transplant rejection reactions (18). In our experience, the thin-walled stainless steel needle with an external diameter of 1.6 mm and internal diameter of 1.3 mm that we have employed for many years has had a good record of safety and has proved reliable in yielding specimens of excellent quality. Both large and fine needles have a place, however (19).

The Menghini needle (Fig. 1) and biopsy techniques have gained wide acceptance since their introduction in 1958 (20). However, the specimens they yield are frequently small and fragmented, particularly in cirrhotic livers. This deficiency appears to be attributable to the blunt, unsharpened cutting tip of the needle, which tends to tear rather than slice through tough collagen, and to the tendency of the specimen to curl and break when it strikes the nail in the hub used to prevent its entrance into the aspirating syringe.

The Klatskin biopsy needle we have used for a number of years with considerable success (No. 1403, Becton, Dickinson and Company, Rutherford, N.J.) is designed to overcome the shortcomings of the Menghini needle by providing it with a sharp point and cutting edge. The cutting edge encircles the entire tip of the needle and is bevelled internally, so that the diameter of the tissue core is 0.32 mm larger than the internal diameter of the needle, a difference determined by the thickness of the needle wall (Figs. 2, 3). This ensures a tight grip on the specimen without crushing, thereby preventing slippage and loss of the core in the needle tract when the needle is withdrawn. With these modifications, the needle provides specimens that are usually longer and less fragmented than those yielded by the original Menghini needle, even when the liver is cirrhotic. The quality of the specimen is further ensured by aspirating it into a 10 ml glass syringe containing 7 ml of saline and using 1.5 to 2.0 ml of suction. This slows the rapidly moving core of tissue as effectively and more gently than the retaining pin of the Menghini needle, and has the additional advantage of allowing the operator to evaluate the quality and size of the specimen immediately. The saline, if drained promptly and replaced by fixative, has no adverse effects on tissue preservation. The saline into which the tissue is aspirated can be examined cytologically in patients in whom tumor is suspected, and additional cases of neoplasia not present in the core of tissue may be detected (21).

Over the years, numerous other biopsy needles have been introduced, almost always designed to increase the reliability of sampling. Of these, only the Vim-Silverman needle, which contains an inner, forked cutting obturator, and the Tru-Cut (Travenol) disposable needle, that depends on an enclosed notched obturator for snaring the specimen, are still in use. Although both are useful occasionally when a specimen of adequate length is unobtainable by the Menghini technique, they are more cumbersome to use, require skill that is not easily mastered, and necessitate manipulation within the liver for two to six seconds, features that may increase the risks of the procedure. The identification of cirrhosis, however, is superior with the Tru-Cut needle than with the Menghini (22). Newly introduced needles include a modification of the Menghini needle with a smaller diameter (0.6 mm) (23) and a biopsy gun (24).

A relatively recent development aimed at permitting needle biopsy in patients with massive ascites or a bleeding tendency is the use of the transvenous (transjugular) biopsy technique (25,26). At first glance, the procedure appears to have great potential, but since it requires the services of an experienced angiographer, often provides specimens that are small and fragmented, and occasionally fails to obtain any tissue at all, it is not likely to be adopted widely. Although not free of complications, experience with this procedure has reduced their frequency and severity (26).

Percutaneous needle biopsy can be carried out transthoracically, subcostally, or in the epigastrium. The transthoracic approach is the method of choice. Infection within the pleura or lower lobe of the right lung and severe respiratory distress are contraindications, and there is the theoretical danger of pneumothorax. However, in our experience, pneumothorax has not been a problem, and small uninfected pleural effusions have not interfered with the procedure. The subcostal approach has the advantage of permitting direct sampling of a palpable nodule or mass, but should not be used without ultrasonic or CT guidance unless the liver edge is palpable at least 6 to 8 cm below the costal margin, and the needle can be directed upward and to the right toward the dome of the right diaphragm. Percutaneous biopsy in the epigastrium may be useful in rare instances when a nodule or mass is palpable close to the costal margin and the left lobe of the liver is significantly enlarged. Unless both these criteria are met, the epigastric approach may be hazardous.

Processing the specimen

Based on our early experience with a wide variety of fixatives recommended for the processing of needle biopsy material, we have routinely used fixation in Carnoy's solution as the method of choice. It ensures rapid and uniform fixation, preserves histologic detail with remarkable clarity, lyses erythrocytes, thereby facilitating visualization of the sinusoids and Kupffer cells, preserves glycogen, and permits more brilliant staining than is possible with other fixatives. The rapidity of fixation, between 30 and 60 minutes, has two advantages. When the specimen has been aligned in a watchglass, and is flooded with Carnoy's solution, it hardens within a minute or two and can then be transferred to a small flat-bottomed specimen jar filled with fixative, without danger of curling. Since the specimen remains rigid and flat throughout the subsequent steps of dehydration, clearing, and embedding, sectioning through the full length of the specimen is assured. The other advantage is that it makes possible a rapid four-hour processing technique.

Biopsy specimens fixed for longer than 60 minutes become excessively hard and are difficult to section. If it is inconvenient to proceed with dehydration within an hour, the specimen must be transferred to 70% alcohol, a solution in which it can be stored indefinitely. Eosinophils are said to stain poorly in Carnoy's-fixed sections. Although we have had no difficulty in identifying eosinophils in such material, we have not established whether or not the number detected is reduced when compared with samples of the same tissue fixed by other methods. Carnoy's-fixed specimens are not suitable for frozen sections to be used for lipid stains, or for some immunofluorescent studies. If these are contemplated, a fragment of the specimen should be fixed in buffered neutral formalin solution. When electron microscopic studies are planned, several 0.5 to 1.0 mm fragments are sliced off the specimen on a glass or paraffin plate with a new, degreased razor blade and immersed in phosphate-buffered 3% glutaraldehyde or other suitable fixative.

Sections cut at 5 microns are suitable for most stains, but we prefer 10 micron sections for demonstrating reticulin.

Stains

No one stain can demonstrate all the morphologic features that may require consideration in the interpretation of hepatic lesions. The routine use of multiple stains has a number of advantages over the common practice of depending on hematoxylin and eosin (H & E) alone, and using additional stains only when they appear to be specially indicated. Routine use of multiple stains not only saves time but also, by providing serial sections and avoiding errors of omission, greatly enhances the reliability of interpretation. The stains we use routinely include Masson, H & E, periodic acid–Schiff following diatase digestion (D-PAS), Gomori Prussian blue stain for hemosiderin, and Laidlaw's reticulin stain. For special purposes we use other stains noted in Volume II.

In our experience, the single most useful stain is the modification of the Masson stain we employ. As illustrated in many of the microphotographs of this book, it visualizes not only the connective tissue but also all the other structural components of the liver in vivid, contrasting colors, thus greatly facilitating assessment of changes in architecture and in the location of lesions within the lobules. The striking differences in the tinctorial properties of hepatocytes and reticuloendothelial cells brought out by the Masson stain are a special advantage, since they simplify identification and localization of small foci of hepatocellular necrosis and dropout, hypertrophy, and hyperplasia of the Kupffer cells and small epithelioid granulomas.

H & E is superior to the Masson stain in demonstrating the character of inflammatory cells, and in identifying bile staining, small bile droplets, lipofuscin and small deposits of hemosiderin in the cytoplasm of both hepatocytes and Kupffer cells, and small bile thrombi within canaliculi. However, dilatation of canaliculi that do not contain bile thrombi usually escapes detection in H & E sections, but often is demonstrable in Masson-stained sections.

The D-PAS stain is useful in detecting and identifying cytoplasmic deposits of lipofuscin, particularly in Kupffer cells, and small bile thrombi in canaliculi, and in demonstrating mucin production in metastatic tumors. In addition, it is invaluable in detecting and identifying the characteristic cytoplasmic globules of α_1-antitrypsin deficiency, which often escape detection by other stains unless relatively large.

The Prussian-blue stain is useful for assessing the degree and distribution of hemosiderin deposition. Although large deposits are readily identified in H & E and Masson-stained sections, small deposits may frequently be overlooked, particularly with the Masson stain.

Although alterations in the lobular architecture are usually readily apparent in Masson-stained sections, they often are more impressive in sections specially stained for reticulin, so that sections provide important confirmatory evidence. Moreover, they facilitate differentiation between zones of recent collapse and fibrosis, clearly visualize the contour and thickness of the hepatocyte plates, and demonstrate any increase in reticulin within the space of Disse, a distinctive feature of some lesions, and the loss, paucity, or absence of reticulin fibers characteristic of others.

Among the many stains available for special purposes, those we employ most frequently and have found most useful include: (a) orcein, Victoria blue, and aldehyde-fuchsin for demonstrating the presence of HBs antigen copper-binding protein, and elastic tissue; (b) PAS for visualizing the content and distribution of glycogen (for confirmation an adjacent section must be stained similarly following diastase digestion); (c) rhodanine for demonstrating copper deposits; (d) alcian blue for the detection of mucin; (e) methyl green pyronine for demonstrating the number and distribution of plasma cells; (f) Kinyoun's acid-fast stain for tubercle bacilli and lipofuscin; (g) Gridely, Grocott, and Gomori stains for fungi; (h) Hall stain for bile; (i) Congo red stain with polarization microscopy and thioflavin-T and toluidine blue with fluorescence microscopy for amyloid; and (j) oil red O and frozen sections for lipid.

Immunohistochemical techniques. Immunohistochemical methods are in increasing use for a variety of purposes. These techniques may be used for the identification of specific cell types, such as Kupffer cells, the antigens of the Hepatitis B virus, or for the demonstration of specific substances such as α_1-antitrypsin, or specific processes such as bile duct regeneration (27). Where there is an antigen there is a way. Examples of such techniques appear in this volume as appropriate.

Surgical wedge biopsy

Because of its larger size and its content of larger bile ducts and blood vessels that may be selectively affected, and because the site of sampling can be selected on the basis of gross appearances, surgical biopsy of the liver is less subject to sampling errors than needle biopsy. An additional advantage is that the procedure rarely gives rise to complications. However, unless a wedge biopsy specimen is of adequate size and has been excised from an appropriate site, it may prove to be misleading and inferior to a needle biopsy specimen. Subcapsular fibrosis is a relatively common finding in sections through the inferior margin of the liver and may be misinterpreted as evidence of cirrhosis if the specimen is too superficial to demonstrate the underlying, normal lobular architecture. To avoid this problem, the wedge of tissue should be excised from the anterior or inferior surface of the liver well away from its lower edge and should measure at least 1 cm in each of its dimensions. An alternative recommended by some authorities is that intraoperative needle biopsy replace wedge biopsy routinely. This is unfortunate, since, with few exceptions, wedge biopsies, if carried out properly, are more informative. The three situations in which intraoperative needle biopsies are preferable and when sampling is indicated in a highly vascular tumor that cannot be resected, when multiple lesions of differing appearance require individual sampling, and when a mass is palpable deep in the liver and is not accessible for direct biopsy. Intraoperative needle biopsies may be obtained from the site of a wedge biopsy just after the wedge has been excised. This method gives good homeostasis and permits examination of a large surgical wedge and a deeper core that may avoid the surgical artifact seen in more superficial specimens. These lesions are characterized by scattered, minute foci of hepatocellular necrosis and infiltrating neutrophils, apparently attributable to anoxia and handling of the liver (28). These are of no diagnostic or prognostic significance but may be misleading if their nature is not recognized. This artifact has also been observed after transjugular venous liver biopsy (29). More complete descriptions and illustrations of these lesions are presented in Chapter 4.

Wedge biopsy specimens should be fixed promptly to avoid artifacts due to autolysis. This can best be ensured by providing the operating room with specimen jars filled with fixative and instructing the staff on the importance of prompt fixation. If the specimen is thicker than 1 cm, it should be sliced into thinner sections to ensure rapid and complete penetration of the fixative. Since Carnoy's solution penetrates liver tissue relatively slowly, it is unsuitable for fixing large surgical specimens. We routinely use neutral buffered formalin for such material. In addition, a 2 mm sliver can be sliced from the edge of the specimen for fixation in Carnoy's solution to permit more rapid processing. We have used this procedure to compare the relative merits of the two fixatives.

Postmorten specimens

In histopathologic studies of autopsy material, due consideration must be given to artifacts produced by postmortem autolysis. As might be anticipated, these vary in severity and character, depending on the time elapsed between death and tissue fixation. However, a more important factor appears to be the antemortem morphologic status of the liver. Thus, when the structure of the liver is relatively normal or only mildly deranged, postmortem artifacts are trivial, even when autopsy has been delayed for 24 hours. The principal changes seen, which are readily recognizable, include dissociation of the hepatocytes within the parenchymal plates accompanied by sharp multiangulation of their contours, widening of the space of Disse with separation of the endothelial and Kupffer cells from the underlying hepatocytes, and loss of cytoplasmic basophilia and glycogen (21). Some of these changes have been attributed to antemortem agonal events (30). However, evidence based on comparisons that we have made between needle biopsy specimens obtained immediately after death and routine autopsy specimens collected at various intervals following death is more consistent with the view that the changes described are due to postmortem autolysis that may appear within an hour.

In contrast to these minor changes, the postmortem artifacts encountered in livers with significant antemortem, parenchymal inflammation and hepatocellular degeneration or necrosis often are striking, and may lead to errors in interpretation unless their nature is recognized. Such artifacts appear early and rapidly increase in severity and distribution when autopsy is delayed. The most notable features include the rapid disappearance of intralobular inflammatory cells, sparing those in the portal triads to some extent (31), and a distinctive type of hepatocellular destruction characterized by karyolysis with shrinkage, loss of staining, and fragmentation of the cytoplasm. These changes are most frequently seen in cases of severe hepatitis, both viral and drug-induced (32,33), particularly when accompanied by bridging necrosis. Changes of this type may be misinterpreted as evidence of massive hepatic necrosis or of ischemic necrosis, a lesion in which the necrotic hepatocytes are similar in appearance, although they tend to be deeply eosinophilic and more consistently centrilobular in distribution.

Polarization microscopy

Polarization microscopy is required for the identification of amyloid, protoporphyrin crystals, starch granules, and other foreign crystalline material. For these purposes a standard microscope fitted with an accessory polarizer and analyzer will suffice, provided an intense light source is available.

Fluorescence microscopy

Fluorescence microscopy is essential for identifying hepatic deposits of porphyrin and vitamin A histologically. It is also useful for immunofluorescence studies of HB surface and core antigens and of α_1-antitrypsin, although immunoperoxidase techniques based on standard light microscopy may be substituted. We have found a standard microscope fitted with a fluorescence attachment adequate for such routine studies.

References

1. Conn HO, Yesner R: A re-evaluation of needle biopsy in the diagnosis of metastatic cancer of the liver. Ann Intern Med 59:53–61, 1963.
2. Brady PG, Goldschmid S, Chappel G. Stone FL, Boyd WP: A comparison of biopsy techniques in suspected focal liver disease. Gastrointest Endosc 33:289–292, 1987.
3. Ash SR, Manfredi F: Directed biopsy using a small endoscope. Thoracoscopy and peritoneoscopy simplified. N Engl J Med 291:1398–1399, 1974.
4. Jacobsen GK, Gammelgaard J, Fuglo M: Coarse needle biopsy versus fine needle aspiration biopsy in the diagnosis of focal lesions of the liver: ultrasonically guided needle biopsy in suspected hepatic malignancy. Acta Cytol 27:152–156, 1983.
5. Dixson AK, Nunez DJ, Bradley JR, Seymour CA: Failure of percutaneous liver biopsy: anatomical variation. Lancet 2:437–439, 1987.
6. Thomas E, Salazar Y: Fine needle aspiration by biopsy in the diagnosis of hepatic malignancy. South Med J 80: 901–902, 1987.
7. Limberg B, Hopker WW, Kommerell B: Histologic differential diagnosis of focal liver lesions by ultrasonically guided fine needle biopsy. Gut 28:237–241, 1987.
8. Pagliaro L, Rinaldi F, Craxi A, DiPiazza S, Filappazzo G, Gatto G, Genova G, Magrin S, Maringhini A, Orsini S, Pallazzo U, Spinello M, Vinci M: Percutaneous blind biopsy versus laparoscopy with guided biopsy in diagnosis of cirrhosis. A prospective, randomized trial. Dig Dis Sci 28:39–43, 1983.
9. Piccinino F, Sagnelli E, Pasquale G, Giusti G: Complications following percutaneous liver biopsy. A multicentre retrospective study on 68,276 biopsies. J Hepatol 2:165–173, 1986.
10. Zamcheck N, Klausenstock O: Liver biopsy. II. The risk of needle biopsy. N Engl J Med 249:1062–1069, 1953.
11. Wildhirt E, Moller E: Experience with nearly 20,000 blind liver punctures. Med Klin 76:254–256, 1981.
12. Perrault J. McGill DB, Ott BJ, Taylor WF: Liver biopsy: complications in 1000 inpatients and outpatients. Gastroenterology 74:103–106, 1978.
13. Millward-Sadler GH, Whorwell PJ. Liver biopsy: Methods, diagnostic value and interpretation. In Liver & Biliary Disease, edited by R. Wright. 2nd Edition. London, Bailliere Tindall, 1985, pp. 495–516.
14. McGill DB, Rakela J, Zinsmeister AR, Ott BJ: A 21-year experience with major hemorrhage after percutaneous liver biopsy. Gastroenterology 99:1396–1400, 1990.
15. Conn HO: Liver biopsy: increased risks in patients with cancer. Hepatology 1991 (in press).
16. Tobin MV, Gilmore IT: Plugged liver biopsy in patients with impaired coagulation. Dig Dis Sci 34:13–15, 1989.
17. Conn HO: Liver biopsy in extrahepatic biliary obstruction and in other "contraindicated" disorders. Gastroenterology 68:817–821, 1975.
18. Hockerstedt K., Lautenschlager I, Ahonen J, Eklund B, Isoniemi H, Korsback C, Makinen J, Makisalo H, Orko R, Petterson E, Salaspuro M, Scheinin B, Scheinin TM, von Willebrand E: Diagnosis of acute rejection in liver transplantation. J Hepatol 6:217–221, 1988.
19. Hall-Craggs MA, Lees WR: Fine needle biopsy: cytology, histology or both? Gut 28:233–236, 1987.
20. Menghini G: One-second needle biopsy of the liver. Gastroenterology 35:190–199, 1958.
21. Atterbury CE, Enriquez RE, dcSuto-Nagy GI, Conn HO: Comparison of the histologic and cytologic diagnosis of liver biopsies in hepatic cancer. Gastroenterology 76:1352–1357, 1979.
22. Colombo M, Del Ninno E, de Franchis R, De Fazio C, Festorazzi S, Ronchi G, Tommasini MA: Ultrasound-assisted percutaneous liver biopsy: superiority of the Tru-Cut over the Menghini needle for diagnosis of cirrhosis. Gastroenterology 95:487–489, 1988.
23. Torp-Pedersen S, Vyberg M, Smith E: Surecut O.6 mm liver biopsy in the diagnosis of cirrhosis. Liver 10:217–220, 1990.
24. Parker SH, Hopper KD, Yakes WF, Gibson MD, Ownbey JL, Carter TE: Image-directed percutaneous biopsies with a biopsy gun. Radiology 171:663–669, 1989.
25. Lebrec D, Goldfarb G, deGott C, Rueff B, Benhamou J-P: Transvenous liver biopsy. An experience based on 1000 hepatic tissue samlings with this procedure. Gastroenterology 83:338–340, 1982.
26. Gamble P, Colapinto RF, Stronell RD, Colman JC, Blendis L: Transjugular liver biopsy: a review of 461 biopsies. Radiology 157:589–593, 1985.
27. Taylor CR: Immunomicroscopy: A diagnostic tool for the surgical pathologist. In Major Problems in Pathology, 19:23–43, 1986, Philadelphia: WB Saunders.

28. Christoffersen P, Poulsen H, Skeie E: Focal liver necrosis accompanied by infiltration of granulocytes arising during operation. Acta Hepato-Splenologica *17*:240–245, 1970.
29. McDonald GSA, Courtney MG: Operation-associated neutrophils in a percutaneous liver biopsy: effect of prior transjugular procedure. Histopathology *10*:217–222, 1986.
30. Popper H: Significance of agonal changes in the human liver. Arch Pathol *46*:132–144, 1948.
31. Gerber MA: Viral hepatitis in the autopsy specimen. Virchow's Arch [A] *354*:285–292, 1971.
32. Roholm K, Iversen P: Changes in the liver in acute epidemic hepatitis (catarrhal jaundice) based on 38 aspiration biopsies. Acta Pathol Microbiol Scan *16*:427–442, 1939.
33. van Beek C, Haex AJCH: The part of postmortal autolysis in the necrosis of the liver in subacute atrophy. Acta Med Scand *114*:557–564, 1943.

Chapter 2
The Normal Liver

The structural components of the liver, which include the hepatocytes, bile ducts, vasculature, and supporting stroma, are so intimately interrelated both anatomically and functionally, that with few exceptions, alterations in one are accompanied by or lead to changes in the others. For that reason, hepatic lesions tend to be complex and require careful study of all components for interpretation.

The liver is made up of histologically ill-defined, contiguous subunits classified as either lobules or acini depending on how the relationship of the hepatic parenchyma to the terminal branches of the vasculature and bile ducts is visualized. The lobule is defined as an unencapsulated, polyhedral mass of parenchyma, approximately 1 mm in diameter, surrounding a terminal branch of the hepatic vein and delimited by planes that pass through adjacent terminal portal tracts. By virtue of this configuration, the lobule receives its blood supply and secretes bile and lymph through multiple sites at its periphery, and has a centripetal circulation of blood that drains centrally. According to the ascinar concept, the acinus, a globular or pear-shaped mass of parenchyma centered about a terminal portal tract and drained by multiple, peripherally located terminal branches of the hepatic vein, has a centrifugual circulation (1). The acini are arranged very much like grapes on a vine, small clusters stemming from preterminal portal tracts, and more complex groups from large portal tracts, each of the stems being encircled by a cuff of parenchyma.

The acinar pattern of hepatic structure is firmly based on the elegant vascular injection studies of Rappaport (1) and accounts for many of the anatomic features of the liver. However, it is difficult to visualize in cross-section, so that most pathologists prefer to use the lobule as a frame of reference in studying or describing sections of the liver.

Reference to the stereogram of the hepatic lobule prepared by Elias (2) on the basis of a serial section reconstruction (Fig. 1) greatly facilitates visualization of the lobule in three dimensions and appreciation of its appearance on cross-section.

Although hepatocytes from different zones of the lobule are similar histologically in most respects, they are extremely heterogeneous functionally (3,4). This heterogeneity may be mediated by structural differences in the endothelial fenestrae in the senusoidal walls (5), alterations that are detectable by electron microscopy but not by light microscopy.

Lobular architecture

Assessment of the overall lobular architecture at relatively low magnification should always be the first step in examining liver biopsy material. Masson- or reticulin-stained sections are essential for this purpose.

A typical normal lobule is characterized by a centrally located, thin-walled vein surrounded by radiating columns of hepatocytes and bordered peripherally by two to five portal tracts (Fig. 4). Since the apparent size and contours of the lobules and the arrangement of their structural components depend on the plane of section, the central veins and portal tracts of contiguous lobules may appear to be randomly distributed, rather than showing the uniform pattern that might be anticipated if all the lobules were identical in shape and orientation, and were sectioned through the same plane. Thus, the lobule illustrated in Figure 4 shows the expected relationship between the central vein and its satellite portal tracts, whereas an adjacent lobule in the same section contains five portal tracts but no central vein (Fig. 5).

The arboreal pattern of the blood vessels and bile ducts is another factor that influences the histologic appearance of the liver. These structures increase in size and show changes in contour and number as their branches join one another en route to the porta hepatis. This seldom poses a problem in needle biopsy specimens, but may make identification of the lobular architecture difficult in large surgical wedge biopsies and postmortem specimens that contain large trabeculae.

Hepatocytes

Organization

The hepatocytes, cells that are polygonal in shape and measure 20 to 30 μm in diameter, are arranged in the form of one-cell-thick plates. These radiate in an irregular pattern from the central vein toward the portal tracts, and merge imperceptibly with the plates of adjacent lobules. By virtue of their numerous anastomoses and fenestrations, the plates create a labyrinth of intercommunicating channels for the sinusoidal circulation (Fig. 1). In microscopic sections, the plates appear as anastomosing columns of hepatocytes of variable length and contour separated from one another by sinusoids (Fig. 6). Most of the columns are one cell thick, but often appear thicker at anastomotic sites and in tangential sections. The hepatocytes in immediate contact with the portal tracts are arranged in the form of a continuous, smooth limiting plate interrupted only by vessels entering or bile ducts leaving the portal tract.

Cytoplasm

In H & E sections, the cytoplasm of the hepatocytes, which is sharply outlined by a well-defined outer cell membrane, ap-

pears mildly eosinophilic and faintly stippled with fine basophilic granules. Staining is more intense and the granularity of
the cytoplasm is more conspicuous in Masson-stained sections,
particularly following fixation in Carnoy's solution (Fig. 7). In
well-prepared sections, the hepatocytes stain uniformly. Delay
in fixation or use of improperly prepared fixative may result in
shrinkage and condensation of the hepatocytes at the margins
of the specimen (Fig. 8), an artifact that is readily recognizable. However, artifacts attributable to uneven fixation and
characterized by alternating groups of pale, swollen cells and
darkly stained, shrunken cells may be misinterpreted as evidence of disease (Fig. 9). Artifacts of this type are encountered
more commonly following fixation in formalin than in Carnoy's
solution.

Often the cytoplasm of the centrilobular hepatocytes contains a variable number of fine, yellow-brown granules of lipofuscin. Usually, these can be identified in lightly stained
H & E sections, but they are more easily and reliably visualized in D-PAS-stained (Fig. 10) and iron-stained sections
(Fig. 11). Since the granules are contained within lysosomes,
they tend to aggregate around canaliculi and, when numerous,
often outline the course of the canaliculi between contiguous
hepatocytes (Fig. 11). When sparse, the lipofuscin granules tend
to be relatively fine (Fig. 10), but when abundant, they often
appear much coarser (Fig. 11) and may be mistaken for hemosiderin granules in H & E sections, although the latter characteristically occur predominantly in periportal hepatocytes.
Deposition of lipofuscin is rare before the age of 15 years, increases between the ages of 15 and 30, but does not continue
to accumulate thereafter (6). Normally, in well-nourished,
nonfasting individuals, the hepatocytes are uniformly filled with
glycogen that presents as closely packed PAS-positive granules
(Fig. 12). Since the glycogen tends to dissolve in aqueous
solutions, a nonaqueous fixative is required for its demonstration histochemically. Carnoy's solution is suitable for this purpose.

Normal hepatocytes occasionally contain a small number of
scattered fat droplets. Although others have reported the occurrence of small amounts of hemosiderin in the cytoplasm of hepatocytes in a high proportion of presumably normal individuals, ranging from 17% (7) to 78% (8), we have encountered
stainable iron only rarely in nonalcoholic patients with no evidence of hematologic or hepatic disease.

Occasional single, eosinophilic, hyalinized, necrotic hepatocytes, called acidophilic bodies, may be seen in the pericentral
regions of normal livers. These cells represent the process of
apoptosis, the normal mechanism by which hepatocytes die (9)
(Fig. 13). These acidophilic bodies, which represent portions
of fragmented cytoplasm extruded from the dying cell, are smaller
and more eosinophilic than the Councilman-like acidophilic
bodies seen in hepatonecrotic liver, which represent condensation necrosis of whole hepatocytes and which often contain a
pyknotic nucleus. It has been suggested that newly formed hepatocytes normally arise in the periportal areas and migrate slowly
toward the terminal hepatic veins where they undergo apoptosis (10).

As hepatocytes age they tend to increase in size, to become
more hematoxophilic, and to contain more lipofuscin (11). Fat
is found in progressively increasing percentages of normal subjects as they age, i.e., 1% of patients less than 20 years of age,
18% of patients from 20 to 40, and 39% of those older than 60
show some fatty infiltration (12). The amount of fat in normal
livers is mild in degree and is not age-related.

Nuclei

The nuclei of normal hepatocytes vary in size, ranging from 6
to 9 μm in diameter. Their location in the cell may be central
or eccentric. Most contain loosely scattered clumps of chromatin and one or two nucleoli enclosed within a prominent,
nuclear membrane (Fig. 7). Binucleate cells are relatively common, one to four being found in most fields at high magnification, but mitotic figures are rarely encountered in normal liver
sections.

Occasionally, the nuclei of apparently normal periportal hepatocytes are enlarged and appear to be empty except for condensed chromatin on the inner surface of their limiting membranes (Fig. 14). Although this appearance is attributable to
glycogen deposition that is readily demonstrable by electron
microscopy, only a minority of these so-called glycogen nuclei
contain PAS-positive material. The latter occasionally fills the
entire nucleus (Fig. 15), but more commonly appears as ill-
defined threads and granules or as a small, centrally located
droplet. Although glycogen nuclei may be encountered in healthy
individuals, they occur more frequently in patients with diabetes mellitus, Wilson's disease, or glycogenosis.

Rarely, the nucleus contains an invagination of cytoplasm,
which, on cross-section, appears as an inclusion (Fig. 16).
Characteristically, the latter is encircled by a prominent limiting membrane identical to that of the nucleus, and contains
finely granular material resembling cytoplasm. Although these
have no clinical significance, they may be mistaken for viral
nuclear inclusions.

As patients' hepatocyte nuclei increase in size, the percentage of binucleate cells increases slightly, as does the degree of
polyploidy.

Bile canaliculi

The canaliculi are fine, intercommunicating channels formed by
the apposition of grooved, specialized segments of the cytoplasm of two or more contiguous hepatocytes, and are sealed
at their outer margins by specialized junction complexes in the
apposing cell membranes. Normally, the canaliculi are too small
to visualize in routine sections, but they can be demonstrated
with special stains (14).

In cross-sections of one-cell-thick hepatic plates, one and,
occasionally, two canaliculi are transected near the center of
the interface between adjacent hepatocytes, whereas in frontal
sections of the plates or sections through groups of hepatocytes
at anastomotic sites, the canaliculi are likely to be sectioned
lengthwise, revealing a polygonal pattern of intercommunicating channels that outline the hepatocytes (Fig. 1).

The microvilli that line the canaliculi and project into their
lumens require electron microscopy for visualization.

Sinusoids and space of Disse

The sinusoids are relatively slender, cylindrical vessels that in-
tercommunicate freely. In sections, they vary in length, diameter, and contour, conforming to the pattern of the hepatic plates

that surround them (Fig. 6). Occasionally, in formalin-fixed material, the sinusoids in some areas may be collapsed, making their identification difficult.

The sinusoids are lined by a discontinuous layer of endothelial and Kupffer cells that rests directly, without an intervening basement membrane, on a network of reticulin fibers in the space of Disse that separates the sinusoids from the hepatocytes. Because of this arrangement and ultrastructural features of the endothelial cells, plasma can pass freely from the lumen of the sinusoids into the space of Disse and come into direct contact with the cell membranes of the hepatocytes.

Randomly distributed groups of erythrocytes and occasional leukocytes are encountered within the sinusoids. Rarely, an isolated megakaryocyte may be found entrapped within a sinusoid. Such cases represent normally circulating megakaryocytes (15) and are not indicative of extramedullary hematopoiesis, a condition in which the megakaryocytes are usually more numerous and are accompanied by other immature cells of bone marrow origin. As shown in Figure 17, entrapped megakaryoctes exhibit the same features as those in the bone marrow, namely, a large, polylobulated nucleus and abundant D-PAS-positive cytoplasm.

Endothelial cells

In routine sections, only the nuclei of the endothelial cells are seen. These appear as flattened oval or spindle-shaped structures closely adherent to the underlying hepatocytes (Fig. 18). However, on electron microscopy, the cytoplasm can be visualized as slender, finely perforated plates that tend to overlap one another rather than form tight junctions.

Kupffer cells

The Kupffer cells, which are stellate in shape, are less numerous than endothelial cells, but are larger, often protruding into the lumen of the sinusoid, and occasionally traversing it. The nuclei are relatively large and vesicular, vary in shape, and often appeared indented or lobulated (Fig. 19). The cytoplasm of the Kupffer cell and its stellate projections into the lumen can often be visualized in Masson-stained sections fixed in Carnoy's solution (Fig. 18), but are more difficult to identify in H & E sections fixed in formalin. By electron microscopy it can be shown that some of the Kupffer cell cytoplasmic processes extend between the endothelial cells into Disse's space (16).

The Kupffer cells are phagocytic, but under normal conditions their cytoplasm shows no evidence of this at the light microscopic level. Faint D-PAS staining, suggestive of lipofuscin deposition, in occasional Kupffer cells may be an exception.

Space of Disse

Normally, the space of Disse that lies between the sinusoidal aspect of the hepatocytes and the lining of the sinusoids is so narrow that it is not visible in routine sections. However, it is readily demonstrable by electron microscopy, and can be shown to extend between contiguous hepatocytes down to the level of the tight junctions that seal off the canaliculi. In addition, the space may be discernible in routine sections when it is widened as a result of postmortem autolysis (17) or disease.

The contents of Disse's space include reticulin fibers, lipocytes (Ito cells), the microvilli of the hepatocytes (demonstrable only by electron microscopy), and plasma that is washed out during fixation.

Reticulin

Following silver impregnation, the reticulin in Disse's space appears as a network of slender, jet-black fibers resting on the hepatic plates and outlining the sinusoids. The number and configuration of the fibers depends on the thickness of the section. In 10 μm sections, the thickest fibers in contact with the hepatocytes are curved or wavy or both, may be duplicated, and often show fine branches that cross the lumens of sinusoids cut tangentially (Fig. 20). In thinner 5 μm sections, the fibers are seldom duplicated and show relatively few branches (Fig. 21).

Reticulin fibers can also be identified in Masson-stained sections, appearing as single, slender blue lines that outline the sinusoidal surfaces of the hepatic plates (Fig. 6).

Lipocytes (Ito cells)

Available evidence indicates that the lipocytes in Disse's space are inactive precursors of fibroblasts (18). They are most numerous in the pericentral area and may be completely absent in the periportal zones (19). These cells normally store vitamin A and other lipids, and may be involved in the deposition of normal reticulin. However, when stimulated by carbon tetrachloride (20) or in chronic active hepatitis (21), the lipocytes proliferate and undergo transformation to active fibroblasts, suggesting that they may play a role in the fibrogenesis that follows some forms of hepatic injury.

The lipocytes, which resemble Kupffer cells in size and shape, but are less numerous, are impossible to identify with confidence in routine sections of normal liver. However, they are readily visualized in 1 μm, Epon-embedded sections stained with toluidine blue (22). In such preparations, they appear as relatively plump cells with abundant cytoplasm containing multiple lipid droplets that often indent their relatively large vesicular nuclei (Fig. 22). Depending on the vitamin A content of their lipid droplets, the lipocytes in frozen sections often exhibit green fluorescence that characteristically fades rapidly (18). On electron microscopy, the lipocytes are seen to lie just beneath the endothelial lining of the sinusoids and to contain numerous lipid droplets and abundant rough endoplasmic reticulum (18,23).

Portal tracts

The portal tracts are composite structures that contain branches of the portal vein, hepatic artery, and bile ducts bound together by connective tissue and encircled by a continuous limiting plate of hepatocytes. Less conspicuous components include lymphatics, nerves, and rare inflammatory cells. Depending on the plane of sectioning, one or more of the major components may not be visualized.

Configuration

Since the portal tracts seen on microscopy represent sections through the vascular-biliary tree, their size and contour depend on the level and plane of sectioning. Portal tracts of variable size that contain bile ducts lined by cuboidal epithelium are often termed portal triads, whereas those that contain larger ducts lined by columnar epithelium are classified as septa or trabeculae. This distinction has no pathophysiologic significance.

Cross-sections of the small, terminal or preterminal portal tracts at the periphery of the lobules appear as roughly oval or triangular structures that contain relatively little connective tissue and single small branches of the portal vein, hepatic artery, and bile ducts (Fig. 23). In the larger portal tracts formed by the fusion of small tracts, the amount of connective tissue relative to the size of their ducts and vessels is significantly greater, and often multiple ducts and vessels may be seen (Fig. 24).

When sectioned lengthwise, the portal tracts present as elongated structures of variable length and width. The most prominent of these contain large ducts lined by columnar epithelium and comparably large arteries and veins (Fig. 25). Portal tracts sectioned through points where they fuse with one another appear as V- or Y-shaped structures (Fig. 26). Such bifurcating and longitudinally sectioned portal tracts are relatively common in large, surgical wedge and postmortem specimens, but are only rarely encountered in needle biopsy sections. Fibrous tissue tends to become denser and to stain more darkly as normal livers age.

Portal veins

The portal veins, usually the largest structural component of the portal tracts, are remarkably thin-walled, even when relatively large (Figs. 22, 23). Characteristically, they present as a channel lined by endothelial cells resting on a basement membrane surrounded by a thin layer of collagen. Connections with the sinusoids through perforations in the limiting plate are relatively frequent. Many of the larger tracts contain two or more portal vein branches (Fig. 23).

Hepatic arteries and arterioles

Small portal tracts contain one or more arterioles that are readily identified by their sharply defined, double-contoured walls containing a few muscle fibers, and by the beaded appearance of their small lumens produced by the nuclei of their intimal lining (Fig. 23). With special stains, a wavy internal elastic lamina can be demonstrated in some of the larger arterioles.

Large portal tracts and trabeculae contain typical arteries with well-defined internal elastic membranes and a muscularis of variable thickness.

Based on histometric studies, it has been reported that the diameter of the arteries and arterioles normally exceeds that of their accompanying bile ducts (24). However, there are many exceptions, particularly in the case of small portal tracts (Fig. 22).

Occasionally, an arteriole extends beyond the limits of a portal tract and is encountered within the parenchyma, encircled by a thin fibrous cuff, but unaccompanied by a bile duct or vein (Fig. 27).

Bile ducts

The bile secreted into the canaliculi drains through a series of intrahepatic ducts of progressively increasing diameter, ultimately emptying into the common hepatic bile duct. The ducts traversed include the ductules, interlobular ducts, and septal ducts.

The ductules, also termed canals of Hering or cholangioles, are slender channels that connect the canaliculi with the interlobular ducts. The junction between the canaliculi and the ductules may occur at the level of the triadal limiting plate or within the lobule [(25); Fig. 1]. Where it joins a canaliculus, the ductule has a barely visible lumen and is lined by interdigitating hepatocytes and low, cuboidal, ductular, epithelial cells resting on a basement membrane (26). More distally, the ductules are lined exclusively by flat, ductular, epithelial cells with oval nuclei (Fig. 28), and enter the interlobular ducts within the portal tracts (Fig. 29). In cross-section, the intralobular ductules resemble interlobular ducts, but are smaller in diameter (Fig. 30). Because of their small size, the ductules may be difficult to identify in routine H & E sections. However, the slender cuff of collagen that often surrounds them facilitates their visualization in Masson-stained sections.

The interlobular ducts, which range in diameter from 15 to 80 μm, have sharply defined, easily visible lumens and are lined by cuboidal epithelial cells resting on a basement membrane surrounded by the collagen of the portal tracts. Both the basement membrane and the luminal surface of the epithelium are D-PAS-positive (Fig. 31). Terminal portal tracts contain only a single duct (Fig. 23), but larger ones often contain two or more (Fig. 24). In some triads, particularly those sectioned tangentially or lengthwise, the apparent duplication is due to multiple sectioning of the same duct, whereas, in others, the multiplicity of ducts is attributable to the junction of two or more portal tracts.

Large septal ducts are rarely encountered in needle or small, surgical wedge biopsy sections, but are relatively common in large wedge and postmortem specimens. Characteristically, these are lined by columnar epithelial cells resting on a basement membrane surrounded by collagen bundles that tend to be arranged concentrically. In the smaller septal ducts, the epithelium is low columnar with centrally located nuclei, whereas in larger ducts, the epithelium is tall columnar with basal nuclei (Fig. 32). Often, in longitudinal sections of large septal ducts, their lumens are tortuous owing to plication of the epithelium and the presence of small diverticuli (Fig. 33). In addition to the basement membrane, both the luminal surface and the apical cytoplasm of the epithelial cells are D-PAS-positive (Fig. 34).

Occasionally, interlobular ducts telescope into one another, presumably because of artifactual shrinkage during fixation (Fig. 35).

Connective tissue

The interstices between the blood vessels and bile ducts of the portal tracts are occupied by randomly oriented, coarse collagen bundles interspersed with fine reticulin and elastic fibers. In the large triads, the collagen bundles may show a concentric arrangement around large bile ducts.

Lymphatics

The lymphatics are slender, endothelium-lined channels that resemble capillaries or branches of the portal vein, but are smaller than the latter and contain no erythrocytes. They are difficult to identify with certainty in small portal tracts, but are readily apparent in larger ones. Undoubtedly, the lymphatics drain lymph from the space of Disse, but no connections between the two can be demonstrated.

Inflammatory cells

Normal portal tracts occasionally contain a few widely scattered and randomly distributed lymphocytes. Histiocytes are even less common, and when present, are usually D-PAS-negative. Aggregates of either of these cells, or the presence of even small numbers of neutrophils, eosinophils, or plasma cells, should be regarded as abnormal findings.

Nerves

The liver is provided with a rich network of unmyelinated nerve fibers that accompany the branches of the hepatic arteries. Some observations suggest that in addition to their role in vasomotor regulation, some fibers terminate on the hepatocytes and may be implicated in their physiologic activities (27).

The nerves in most portal tracts are inconspicuous, and require special stains for their demonstration. However, they can often be identified within the large septa of routinely stained sections of surgical wedge biopsy and postmortem sections.

Central veins and other branches of the hepatic veins

The sinusoids drain directly into the most proximal branches of the hepatic veins, which because of their location within the lobules, are termed central veins. These enter large, sublobular veins almost perpendicularly. The latter converge to form still larger collecting veins that ultimately unite to form the major hepatic veins.

Although the sublobular veins tend to be larger in diameter and to have thicker walls than the central veins, the latter vary so much in diameter and wall thickness that it is difficult to differentiate between the two on the basis of these criteria alone.

For that reason it is common practice to classify all but the largest efferent veins as central veins.

The central veins are lined by endothelial cells surrounded by a cuff of collagen and reticulin fibers that is often interrupted by entering sinusoids (Fig. 36). In many of the central veins, the collagen bundles surrounding them are coarse and oriented in the axis of the vessel, giving its wall a beaded appearance (Fig. 37).

The sublobular and collecting veins are similar in structure, but are rarely perforated by entering sinusoids.

None of these veins contain muscular fibers in their walls.

Glisson's capsule

The liver is completely enclosed within Glisson's capsule, a relatively, thin, connective tissue membrane made up of compact, collagen bundles interspersed with fine reticulin and elastic fibers. Except for a bare area over the posterior diaphragmatic aspects of the liver and the gallbladder bed, Glisson's capsule is covered by peritoneal mesothelial cells. At the porta hepatis, the capsule thickens and extends into the parenchyma merging with the connective tissue that encloses the major blood vessels and ducts.

Only rarely are fragments of Glisson's capsule encountered in needle biopsy specimens. Usually such fragments are small and contain no blood vessels, bile ducts, or inflammatory cells, so they are not likely to be mistaken for segments of abnormal portal triads or fibrous septa.

In surgical wedge and postmortem sections, Glisson's capsule usually appears as a densely collagenized ribbon, 40 to 70 μm in width, that is devoid of blood vessels or ducts (Fig. 38). Fibrous septa of variable thickness and length frequently project from the inner surface of the capsule, often fusing with underlying portal tracts (Fig. 39). When slender, they contain no blood vessels or ducts, but when broad, usually contain both. Some of the capsular septa curve back toward the surface, partially or completely outlining small nodules of parenchyma, a pattern usually classified as subcapsular fibrosis (Fig. 39). This is seen most frequently in specimens excised from the inferior margin of the liver, and may be mistaken for cirrhosis. However, subcapsular fibrosis rarely extends deeper than 2 mm from the surface (28), so that if the wedge is excised to a depth of 1 cm or more, differentiation from cirrhosis is relatively simple.

Occasionally, the capsule is thickened focally and contains blood vessels and bile ducts (Fig. 40). Such focal thickening may or may not be associated with subcapsular fibrosis.

The organization of the parenchyma immediately beneath Glisson's capsule differs in some respects from that found elsewhere in the liver. Often the portal tracts are larger than expected at the periphery of the lobules (Figs. 39, 41), and may appear crowded together (Fig. 42). In addition, the hepatic plates tend to be less regular in their arrangement than in normal lobules.

The normal liver in childhood

Except in early infancy, the microscopic appearance of the liver in children is identical with that in adults.

During the first few weeks of neonatal life, the liver often contains foci of extramedullary hematopoiesis. These foci appear to be clusters of small, dark-staining cells within focally dilated sinusoids (Fig. 43). When the hematopoiesis is extensive, particularly soon after birth, the portal tracts are similarly involved. On electron microscopy, most of the cells, which are located in the space of Disse, prove to be of erythropoietic origin. However, the precise nature of these cells is difficult to identify in routine sections. Megakaryocytes are only rarely found in this type of extramedullary hematopoiesis.

At birth, the hepatic plates are two cells thick, a feature that may persist for several months (Fig. 44). In adults double plates are seen only during regeneration.

Until the age of about 15 years, the hepatocytes contain no lipofuscin.

References

1. Rappaport AM: *In* Diseases of the Liver, edited by L. Schiff. 4th Edition. Philadelphia, J.B. Lippincott Co., 1975. pp. 1–50.
2. Elias MH: Morphology of the Liver. Trans. 11th Conf. on Liver Injury. Josiah Macy, Jr. Foundation, New York, 1952, pp. 111–199.
3. Gumucio JJ: Functional and anatomic heterogeneity in the liver acinus: impact on transport. Am J Physiol *244:* G578–G582, 1983.
4. Haussinger D: Hepatocyte heterogeneity in glutamine and ammonia metabolism and the role of an intercellular glutamine cycle during ureogenesis in perfused rat liver. Eur J Biochem *133:*269–275, 1983.
5. Wisse E, de Zanger RB, Charels K, Van Der Smissen P, McCuskey RS: The liver sieve: considerations concerning the structure and function of endothelial fenestrae, the sinusoidal wall and the space of Disse. Hepatology *5:* 683–692, 1985.
6. Nomura M, Klatskin G: Unpublished data based on a study of 1361 consecutive needle biopsy specimens, including 126 showing a completely normal liver.
7. Edwards CQ, Carroll M, Bray P, Cartwright GE: Hereditary hemochromatosis. Diagnosis in siblings and children. N Engl J Med *297:*7–13, 1977.
8. Weinfeld A, Lundin P, Lundvall O: Significance for the diagnosis of iron overload of histochemical and chemical iron in the liver of conrol subjects. J Clin Pathol *21:*35–40, 1968.
9. Searle J, Kerr JFR, Bishop CJ. Necrosis and apoptosis: distinct modes of cell death with fundamentally different significance. Pathol Annu *17*(Part 2):229–259, 1982.
10. Zajicek G, Oren R, Weinreb M Jr: The streaming liver. Liver *5:*293–300, 1985.
11. Popper H: Aging and the liver. *In* Progress in Liver Disease, edited by H. Popper, F. Schaffner. Vol VIII. New York, Grune & Stratton, 1986, pp. 659–683.
12. Hilden M, Christoffersen P, Juhl E, Dalgaard JB: Liver histology in a 'normal' population: examinations of 503 consecutive fatal traffic casualties. Scand J Gastroenterol *12:* 593–597, 1977.
13. Watanabe T, Tanaka Y: Age-related alterations in the size of human hepatocytes: a study of mononuclear and binucleate cells. Virchows Arch (Cell Pathol) *39:* 9–20, 1982.
14. Luna LG, Ishak KG: A new stain for bile canaliculi. Am J Stain Techn *33:*459–466, 1967.
15. Kaufman RM, Airo R, Pollack S, Crosby WH: Circulating megakaryocytes and platelet release in the lung. Blood *26:*720–731, 1965.
16. Wisse E: Ultrastructure and function of Kupffer cells and other sinusoidal cells in the liver. Med Chir Digest *6:*409–418, 1977.
17. Popper H: Significance of agonal changes in the human liver. Arch Pathol *46:*132–144, 1948.
18. Kent G, Inouye T, Minick OT, Bahu RM: Fat-storing cells (lipocytes) in the liver. Their role in vitamin A storage and fibrogenesis. Med Chir Digest *6:*425–428, 1977.
19. Giampieri MP, Jezequel A-M, Orlandi F: The lipocytes in normal human liver: a quantitative study. Digestion *22:*165–169, 1981.
20. McGee JO, Patrick R: The role of perisinusoidal cells in hepatic fibrogenesis. An electron microscopic study of acute carbon tetrachloride injury. Lab Invest *26:*429–440, 1972.
21. Jezequel A-M, Koch MM, Orlandi F: Hepatic fibrosis. Role of perisinusoidal cells? Ital J Gastroenterol *4:*560–565, 1980.
22. Bronfenmajer S, Schaffner F, Popper H: Fat-storing cells (lipocytes) in human liver. Arch Pathol *82:*447–453, 1966.
23. Tanuma Y, Ito T: Electron microscopic study on the hepatic sinusoidal wall and fat storing cells in the bat. Arch Histol Jpn *41:*1–39, 1978.
24. Nakanuma Y, Ohta G: Histometric and serial section observations of the intra-hepatic bile ducts in primary biliary cirrhosis. Gastroenterology *76:*1326–1332, 1979.
25. Elias H, Sherrick JC: Morphology of the Liver. New York, Academic Press, 1969, pp. 107–108.
26. Steiner JW, Carruthers JS: Studies on the fine structure of the terminal branches of the biliary tree. I. The morphology of normal bile canaliculi, bile pre-ductules (ducts of Hering) and bile ductules. Am J Pathol *38:* 639–661, 1961.
27. Forssmann WG, Ito S: Hepatocyte innervation in primates. J Cell Biol *74:*299–313, 1977.
28. Petrelli M, Scheuer PJ: Variation in subcapsular liver structure and its significance in the interpretation of wedge biopsies. J Clin Pathol *20:*743–748, 1967.

Chapter 3
Abnormalities of the Lobular Architecture

The normal lobular architecture may be distorted or obscured by fibrosis, hepatocellular necrosis, or by a variety of infiltrative lesions. Such alterations in lobular architecture are most easily identified at low magnification of Masson- or reticulin-stained sections.

The changes in lobular architecture are not always uniformly distributed and, occasionally, are limited to focal lesions fortuitously sampled by needle biopsy. Both may lead to errors in interpretation, but, in at least some instances, these may be avoided by studying serial sections.

Fibrosis

Fibrosis limited to the portal or central zones of the lobules does not affect the lobular architecture. The architecture may be significantly altered, however, when the fibrosis is extensive and bridges adjacent portal and/or central zones, dissects the lobules, or replaces them.

Bridging fibrosis

When fibrosis is progressive, or is the sequela of antecedent hepatocellular necrosis that links adjacent portal and/or central zones, portal-portal, portal-central, or central-central bridging fibrosis may ensue. Often these three types of bridging occur in various combinations. In needle biopsy sections, bridging fibrosis may mimic cirrhosis. However, if the specimen is of sufficient length, cirrhosis can usually be excluded by the presence of normal, one-cell-thick hepatic plates, and the absence of nodules or alterations in lobular architecture in other fields. Since some cirrhotic lesions contain areas of bridging fibrosis without nodules, the presence of cirrhosis may escape detection in small biopsy sections.

Portal-portal bridging fibrosis occurs under a variety of conditions, but especially in some forms of chronic hepatitis, prolonged biliary obstruction, early primary biliary cirrhosis, and as a residual of antecedent viral or drug-induced bridging hepatocellular necrosis. Figure 45 illustrates a typical example of portal-portal fibrous bridging in a case of chronic active hepatitis. Although a similar pattern of fibrosis was seen in many other areas, there was no evidence of nodule formation, and, as shown in Figure 46, the lobular architecture was intact in some fields. Moreover, the normal arrangement of the hepatocytes in one-cell-thick radiating plates evident in both illustrations provides further evidence that cirrhosis was not present.

Pure central-central bridging fibrosis is relatively rare, but

does occur occasionally in alcoholic hepatitis (Fig. 47) and chronic passive congestion (Fig. 48).

By far the most common type of bridging fibrosis is a combination of both portal-portal and portal-central fibrosis, as in the case of the noncirrhotic chronic alcoholic hepatitis illustrated in Figure 49.

Cirrhosis

In cirrhosis, the liver is traversed by fibrous septa that encircle nodules of parenchyma and obscure the normal lobular architecture. Depending on their pathogenesis, the septa may be broad or slender, and smooth or irregular in contour. Similarly, the parenchymal nodules may be small or large. Based on the size of the nodules, cirrhotic lesions are often classified as micronodular or macronodular. Although the size of the nodules affords no clue as to their etiology, the distinction merits consideration, since macronodular cirrhosis is more often complicated by hepatocellular carcinoma than micronodular cirrhosis, and usually is more difficult to identify in needle biopsy specimens. Unfortunately, there are no universally accepted criteria for distinguishing between micronodules and macronodules. Since normal lobules measure approximately 1 mm in diameter, it would appear reasonable to limit micronodules to this size. However, many authorities include in this category nodules up to 5 mm in diameter. The committee on standardization of nomenclature sponsored by the World Health Organization recommends that only nodules less than 3 mm in diameter be classified as micronodules (1). To compound further the problem of classifying cirrhosis on the basis of nodule size is the fact that many cirrhotic livers contain both large and small nodules, and must, therefore, be classified as mixed cirrhosis. Finally, the size of nodules in cirrhosis does not remain constant; they tend to decrease in size. In a series of 75 cirrhotic patients who were classified as having micronodular cirrhosis (defined as all nodules less than 1.5 mm in diameter), 90% converted to macronodular cirrhosis during a follow-up period of 10 years (2). The median interval for conversion was just above two years. Abstinence from alcohol and the administration of adrenocorticosteroid therapy tended to accelerate the transformation rate.

It is generally assumed that the parenchymal nodules in cirrhosis represent islands of regenerating hepatocytes derived from intact normal lobules, or fragments thereof, spared during the destructive process that leads to fibrosis. However, not all nodules show evidence of regeneration, and some of the largest often contain what appear to be normal lobules, suggesting that some nodules represent remnants of uninvolved intact parenchyma.

The pattern of fibrosis and the size of the nodules in micronodular cirrhosis tend to be relatively uniform. However, there are exceptions, particularly during the early phases of its development, when an occasional intact lobule or areas of focal or bridging fibrosis can still be found. Nevertheless, micronodular cirrhosis can usually be identified in needle biopsy specimens provided the core is at least a centimeter in length. Shown in Figure 50 is a typical example of micronodular alcoholic cirrhosis. Although the nodules illustrated vary in size, they all are less than 1 mm in diameter. During the active, progressive stage of the lesion, the hepatocytes in such nodules show evidence of regenerative activity, as indicated by their arrangement in the form of thick, irregular plates (Fig. 51). However, when the lesion is quiescent, the plates often revert to a normal one-cell-thick pattern.

Identification of macronodular cirrhosis is relatively simple in surgical wedge or postmortem specimens. The typical appearance is illustrated in Figure 52. This specimen was obtained at laparotomy in a patient with inactive postnecrotic cirrhosis who had bled from esophageal varices. At operation, most of the nodules ranged in size from 3 to 10 mm. However, as can be seen in Figure 53, some were significantly smaller. Moreover, as is often the case in macronodular cirrhosis, many of the largest nodules were partially subdivided by slender fibrous septa (Fig. 54), or contained large areas of parenchyma that appeared normal except for an irregular arrangement of the portal tracts and an absence of central veins (Fig. 55). As shown in Figure 56, the hepatic plates were one-cell-thick and had a normal radial pattern. However, in many cases of macronodular cirrhosis, the hepatic plates, even when one-cell-thick, show a more irregular pattern than is seen in Figures 55 and 56. In general, the contours of the septa in inactive macronodular cirrhosis tend to be smooth, except for fine extensions into the parenchymal nodules. However, when the lesion is active, the septa often show ill-defined, irregular margins due to periseptal, hepatocellular necrosis and inflammation. Usually, the width of the septa varies, being slender in some areas (Figs. 52, 54) and broad in others (Fig. 53). However, in some cases, the septa are uniformly thick or uniformly thin. Occasionally, Glisson's capsule is significantly thickened in macronodular cirrhosis, a feature not seen in the lesion illustrated in Figures 52 and 54.

As might be anticipated, macronodular cirrhosis may be difficult to identify in needle biopsy specimens, not only because the nodules are larger in diameter than the width of the section, but also because relatively normal areas and areas of bridging fibrosis are more common than in micronodular cirrhosis. Obviously, a large nodule sectioned through its center will appear as two widely separated septa crossing the section, whereas one sectioned tangentially will appear as a curved, elongated septum partially outlining a mass of parenchyma, and, thus, will resemble a fibrous bridge. Fortunately, in many cases, nodules sufficiently small to be included in the needle biopsy section accompany the large nodules (Fig. 53). However, if these are not present, identification of macronodules may have to depend on the presence of thick hepatic plates or rosettes and the absence of abnormal distribution of portal tracts and central veins within 1 mm areas of parenchyma corresponding to the size of normal lobules.

The appearance of macronodular cirrhosis in a needle biopsy section is shown in Figure 57. It is evident that the nodules are significantly larger than those in micronodular cirrhosis (Fig. 51), but smaller than those seen in surgical wedge biopsy sections of macronodular cirrhosis (Figs. 52–54). Multiple well-defined nodules, as seen in Figure 57, are relatively infrequent in needle biopsy specimens of macronodular cirrhosis. More common, fibrous septa partially outline nodules of parenchyma (Fig. 58), representing tangential sections through large nodules, or a long segment of apparently normal parenchyma (Fig. 59) bounded by septa, representing a section through the center of a large nodule.

Unfortunately, aspiration needle biopsy of the cirrhotic liver, particularly of the macronodular type, but of the micronodular type as well, often yields fragments of parenchyma and fibrous tissue, but no frank nodules or well-defined septa, making identification of the cirrhosis exceedingly difficult. Such fragmentation is attributable to failure of the biopsy needle to obtain an intact core of liver tissue that contains segments of the fibrous septa it traverses. The softer parenchyma within the nodules is readily aspirated intact. Use of a biopsy needle with a tip that is sharply pointed and provided with a sharp cutting edge around its entire circumference (Figs. 2, 3) will usually avoid this problem. If, nevertheless, the specimen is fragmented, careful examination of serial Masson- or reticulin-stained sections may reveal slender remnants of the septa along the margins of the parenchymal fragments not evident in routine H & E sections. In addition, if the fragments are sufficiently large, cirrhosis may be suggested by the absence of normal central veins and portal tracts, and the presence of thickened hepatic plates.

The reader is referred to Chapter 9 for a more comprehensive discussion of cirrhosis in general, and to Chapters 10 to 13 for details of specific types.

Diffuse fibrosis

Occasionally, the lobular architecture is destroyed by a diffuse fibrotic process. In needle biopsy sections, no nodules of parenchyma are seen in such lesions. However, in most, if not all, cases, nodules are readily demonstrable at laparotomy or autopsy, so that the finding on biopsy of diffuse fibrosis without nodules usually indicates an underlying cirrhosis. This occurs most frequently following the collapse of reticulin and subsequent collagenization of large areas of the liver in the late stages of submassive viral hepatic necrosis. The appearance of such a broad zone of fibrosis is illustrated in Figure 60. This lesion was encountered at autopsy in a patient who died nine months following a biopsy-documented episode of posttransfusion submassive hepatitis. Although more than half the liver was occupied by broad zones of fibrosis, numerous small regenerating nodules were demonstrable in the unaffected areas (Fig. 61).

Another, but rarer form of diffuse fibrosis, sometimes classified as interstitial fibrosis, may be generalized. It is characterized by an irregular pattern of fine, fibrous bands interspersed with disorganized strands of hepatocytes. This may be seen in some forms of congenital syphilis, as a late sequela in some cases of neonatal giant cell hepatitis, and, rarely, in severe alcoholic liver disease. Perisinusoidal fibrosis, also termed capillarization of the sinusoids, which occurs under a wide variety of conditions (Chapter 4), may in its late stages resemble interstitial fibrosis. However, it is seldom universal in distribution, and usually does not obscure the lobular landmarks to the same extent. Similarly, pericellular fibrosis, a relatively common finding in some forms of chronic hepatitis, alcoholic liver disease, and along the septa in many types of cirrhosis, tends to be focal in distribution. Figure 62 illustrates an example of diffuse interstitial fibrosis without nodule formation in a case of severe alcoholic liver disease. As can be seen at higher magnification in Figure 63, the hepatocytes are arranged in the form of short, irregular cords separated by fine strands of collagen.

Congenital hepatic fibrosis

This form of hepatic fibrosis represents a congenital anomaly related to polycystic disease rather than a response to antecedent hepatic injury; it is discussed more fully in Chapter 4. The subject is introduced at this point because the lesion may be mistaken for cirrhosis.

Characteristically, as shown in Figure 64, the liver in congenital hepatic fibrosis is traversed by relatively broad, smooth-contoured, collagenized septa that outline nodules of parenchyma. The septa contain numerous dilated, branching bile ducts lined by cuboidal epithelium, and show few if any portal vein radicules. Occasionally, some of the ducts contain inspissated bile, and, often, there are elongated slender ducts that lie close to the limiting plates (Fig. 65). Usually, there are few or no inflammatory cells. Except for the septa, the remainder of the liver is normal, and usually contains intact lobules in some areas.

Nodular regenerative hyperplasia

Under a variety of conditions the hepatic parenchyma undergoes nodular regenerative hyperplasia. This may be focal in nature or generalized. When generalized, the lesion mimics cirrhosis both grossly and microscopically. However, in contrast to cirrhosis, the development of nodules is not accompanied by fibrosis.

Characteristically, the nodules measure from 5 to 10 mm in diameter, and are outlined by a ring of dilated sinusoids with intervening, atrophic hepatocytes (Fig. 66). Often, the nodules contain centrally located or eccentric portal triads, giving the impression of reversed lobulation. At higher magnification, the hepatocytes are seen to be arranged in the form of thick plates, indicative of regenerative activity (Fig. 67), and, in reticulin-stained sections, the nodules are outlined by bands of collapsed reticulin corresponding to the encircling zone of sinusoidal congestion and hepatocellular atrophy (Fig. 68).

Hepatocellular necrosis

Hepatocellular necrosis, whether focal or confluent, does not alter the normal anatomic relationship between the central veins and portal tracts as long as it is limited to the portal or central zones of the lobules. However, zones of necrosis that bridge adjacent portal tracts or central veins or both, or involve entire lobules distort the normal lobular architecture.

Bridging hepatocellular necrosis

When adjacent zones of periportal hepatocellular necrosis are large, they may merge to produce portal-portal bridging (Fig.

69). In addition, the necrosis extends to involve central zones (Fig. 70), resulting in a combination of portal-portal and portal-central bridging necrosis. Lesions of this type are seen most frequently in severe, acute, viral or drug-induced hepatitis.

Pure central-central bridging necrosis is far less common than portal-portal and portal-central bridging. Although it may be encountered in severe acute viral or drug-induced hepatitis, it is more characteristic of severe ischemic hepatic necrosis (Fig. 71) and, less commonly, of the acute Budd-Chiari syndrome. Occasionally, large zones of centrilobular necrosis extend to adjacent portal tracts producing central-portal rather than central-central bridging (Fig. 72).

Not infrequently in severe acute viral and drug-induced hepatitis, the necrosis is extensive in both the central and periportal zones, resulting in widespread bridging of all types (Fig. 73).

At an early stage, the necrotic bridges may appear as a loose meshwork of fine bundles of reticulin outlining patent sinusoids that contain a variable number of inflammatory cells and swollen Kupffer cells (Fig. 74). More often, however, the reticulin framework is collapsed, obscuring the sinusoids (Fig. 75). Later in its development, as the inflammatory reaction abates, the reticulin fibers appear to fuse, forming relatively thick fibers suggestive of collagen in Masson-stained sections (Fig. 76). However, in silver-impregnated sections, they can be identified as condensed reticulin fibers (Fig. 77).

Identification of bridging necrosis is most reliable in Masson-stained sections. While extensive bridging can be recognized in H & E sections, slender or irregular zones of bridging necrosis may be difficult to identify in such sections, particularly when accompanied by an intense, intralobular, inflammatory reaction.

Massive and panlobular hepatic necrosis

In the fulminant form of acute viral or drug-induced hepatitis, all or most of the hepatocytes may undergo rapid massive necrosis, in which only the portal triads, proliferating ductules, and the reticulin are spared (Fig. 78). Such lesions invariably prove fatal. However, if sufficiently large areas of parenchyma are spared, recovery with residual postnecrotic cirrhosis may ensue (Chapter 6).

Occasionally, bridging hepatic necrosis due to acute viral or drug-induced hepatitis is accompanied by destruction of scattered whole lobules, a lesion termed panlobular necrosis (Fig. 79). Such panlobular necrosis, if not extensive, is not necessarily manifested clinically by features of fulminant hepatic failure, and may heal either completely or with variable degrees of postnecrotic scarring.

Infiltrative lesions

Metastatic tumors

By far the most common infiltrative lesion encountered in needle biopsy specimens is metastatic carcinoma. Occasionally, the tumor occupies the entire specimen, but more commonly, it presents as masses or strands of neoplastic tissue that distort or destroy the normal lobular architecture. Rarely, the entire liver is diffusely infiltrated by strands of metastatic tumor cells and fibrous tissue producing a picture that on gross inspection at autopsy closely mimics cirrhosis. Lesions of this type have been classified as carcinomatous cirrhosis (3).

Although the malignant nature of hepatic metastases is usually obvious, their differentiation from anaplastic hepatocellular carcinoma may be difficult in some cases. Only rarely can their sites of origin be identified.

The reader is referred to Chapter 25 for a more detailed discussion and illustrations of hepatic metastases.

Primary hepatic tumors

Among primary tumors of the liver, hepatocellular carcinoma is the one encountered most frequently in needle biopsy specimens. Except when highly undifferentiated, such lesions are usually readily identified.

Recognition of the malignant nature of a primary hepatic cholangiocarcinoma rarely, if ever, poses a problem. However, its differentiation from a metastatic adenocarcinoma arising in the gallbladder, extrahepatic bile ducts, or other sites is difficult, if not impossible.

Identification of benign primary hepatic tumors in needle biopsy specimens may be exceedingly difficult. Thus, the differentiation between hepatic cell adenoma and hepatocellular regeneration, on one hand, and between focal nodular hyperplasia and cirrhosis, on the other, is often not possible on histologic grounds alone.

A more complete discussion and illustrations of primary tumors of the liver are presented in Chapter 25.

Lymphoma

Lymphomatous infiltration of the liver is encountered far less frequently than carcinomatous metastases. Such lymphomatous infiltrates are often focal and predominantly portal in distribution. Although the affected portal tracts are expanded and often accompanied by extension of the infiltrate into the parenchyma, the overall lobular architecture is usually not affected. However, extensive, lymphomatous infiltrates may distort or destroy the normal lobular architecture, as illustrated in Figure 80.

Extramedullary hematopoiesis

When the liver is the site of extramedullary hematopoiesis, the sinusoids and, to a lesser extent, the portal tracts contain scattered foci of hematopoietic cells. Occasionally, the proliferation of such cells is extensive, leading to expansion of the portal tracts, destruction of periportal parenchyma, and bridging

fibrosis. As illustrated in Figure 81, the portal infiltration and fibrosis may be sufficiently severe to produce portal hypertension and esophageal varices. No doubt the extensive invasion and obstruction of the sinusoids by hematopoietic cells, as shown in Figure 82, are contributory factors in the development of the portal hypertension in such cases.

See Chapter 24 for a further discussion and illustrations of hepatic extramedullary hematopoiesis.

Granulomas

Usually, the granulomas in systemic granulomatous diseases, such as sarcoidosis and brucellosis, are focal in character and randomly distributed, especially in the portal zones. Rarely, such lesions are confluent and distort or destroy the normal lobular architecture. In time, progressive fibrosis may lead to disappearance of the granulomas and the development of cirrhosis. We have documented this sequence of events in several cases of sarcoidosis and brucellosis. Shown in Figures 83 and 84 is an example of extensive granulomatous portal-portal bridging with only minimal fibrosis in a patient with sarcoidosis. Serial biopsies over a period of several years demonstrated progressive fibrosis and the development of cirrhosis with gradual disappearance of the granulomas. The cirrhosis was complicated by portal hypertension and recurrent bleeding from esophageal varices, leading ultimately to hepatic failure and death.

The problem of hepatic granulomas is discussed more fully in Chapter 22.

Amyloidosis

When the liver is involved in amyloidosis, the deposits of amyloid are usually found within the spaces of Disse outlining the sinusoids, and, to a variable degree, in the blood vessel walls and stroma of the portal tracts. As the deposits increase, the hepatocytes atrophy and ultimately disappear, the sinusoids are compressed and obliterated, and the masses of unstructured, intralobular amyloid merge with those in the portal tracts, thereby destroying the normal lobular architecture (Fig. 85).

For a more complete discussion and other illustrations of hepatic amyloidosis, see Chapter 24.

References

1. Anthony PP, Ishak KG, Nayak NC, Poulsen HE, Scheuer PJ, Sobin LH: The morphology of cirrhosis: definition, nomenclature, and classification. Bull WHO 55:521–540, 1977.
2. Fauerholdt L, Schlichting P, Christensen E, Poulsen H, Tygstrup N, Juhl E, and The Copenhagen Study Group for Liver Diseases. Hepatology 3:928–931, 1983.
3. Micolonghi T, Pineda E, Stanley MM: Metastatic carcinomatous cirrhosis of the liver. Report of a case in which death followed hemorrhage from esophageal varices and hepatic coma. Arch Pathol 65:56–62, 1958.

Chapter 4
Abnormalities of the Hepatic Parenchyma

Hepatocellular necrosis

Cell death in normal individuals occurs primarily by the process of apoptosis (1), which appears to take place mainly in pericentral areas (2). It has been suggested that hepatocytes originate in zone 1 and migrate slowly to zone 3 where they die (2). When the acidophilic bodies are seen, the process is recognized, but such bodies are often not seen and the process usually goes unnoticed.

Several types of cell death may be involved in hepatocellular necrosis. In some, the necrotic cells remain *in situ*, whereas in others, they vanish without a trace. Since cytolysis, a presumably rapid process of cell dissolution, cannot be distinguished from the loss of hepatocytes that ultimately follows other forms of hepatocellular necrosis, degeneration, or atrophy, it is common practice, when the nature of cell death is uncertain, to use the less specific term *cell dropout*.

In any given lesion, more than one type of necrosis may be involved, and often its distribution within the lobules varies. Nevertheless, the character of the necrosis and its distribution often prove to be of assistance in identifying the etiology of hepatic lesions.

Cell dropout

Cell dropout is a characteristic feature of viral and drug-induced hepatitis, but may be encountered under a wide variety of other conditions. In acute hepatitis, cell dropout is almost always accompanied by acidophilic bodies (see later), hepatocellular degeneration, a predominantly mononuclear inflammatory reaction, and hypertrophy and proliferation of Kupffer cells. The foci of necrosis tend to be relatively small, involving only a small number of adjacent hepatocytes, but usually are widely scattered throughout the lobules, a distribution termed *spotty necrosis* (Fig. 86). Not infrequently, the loss of contiguous hepatocytes is more conspicuous in the centrilobular zones (Fig. 87). Less commonly, similar larger areas of cell loss occur around the portal tracts (Fig. 88), link adjacent portal tracts and/or central veins *(bridging necrosis)* (Figs. 69, 70, 72–75), or involve entire lobules *(panlobular necrosis)* (Figs. 78, 79). Zones of necrosis involving large numbers of contiguous hepatocytes, irrespective of their distribution and extent, are often classified as confluent (3). Unfortunately, the term *confluent necrosis* is also used in a more limited sense to imply bridging or panlobular necrosis, so that it should always be qualified by the terms *focal, centrilobular, periportal, bridging,* or *panlobular,* to avoid misinterpretation. When bridging necrosis is found, it may be portal-portal, portal-central, or central-central bridging. The nature of the cell death responsible for the cell dropout in acute viral and drug-induced hepatitis is uncertain. Although the formation of acidophilic bodies is undoubtedly an important factor, it is not clear what role other forms of hepatocellular degeneration and cytolysis play.

In the case of *centrilobular ischemic necrosis,* the cell dropout seen in its late phases clearly is the result of antecedent coagulation necrosis. As shown in Figure 89, such zones of centrilobular cell dropout may superficially resemble those of acute viral or drug-induced hepatitis. However, the distinction is not difficult, since, in the late stages of ischemic necrosis, the zones are more sharply circumscribed, may be infiltrated with neutrophils, often show sinusoidal congestion, and are unaccompanied by spotty necrosis elsewhere in the lobules.

Centrilobular cell dropout is also seen in severe alcoholic hepatitis, a condition in which the loss of cells appears to be the result of hepatocellular degeneration. As shown in Figure 90 the cell dropout is always accompanied by ballooned, degenerating hepatocytes, some of which contain Mallory bodies, a neutrophilic exudate, and a variable degree of reticulin collapse. Differentiation from other forms of centrilobular necrosis and cell dropout is relatively simple. In more chronic alcoholic hepatitis, or following its resolution, centrilobular collapse and fibrosis are the prominent features, whereas the balloon cells, Mallory bodies, and neutrophilic infiltrate may be inconspicuous or absent.

Periportal hepatocellular dropout is relatively common in acute drug-induced hepatitis, and in chronic active hepatitis (Fig. 91). It has been suggested that the cell loss in this situation is the result of a cell-mediated immune reaction leading to acidophilic body formation (4). While acidophilic bodies can occasionally be found in the periportal zones, it is not certain that this is the only type of hepatocellular destruction responsible for cell loss.

Focal hepatocellular dropout is a feature of a wide variety of lesions. These include all forms of chronic hepatitis, residuals of antecedent viral hepatitis, and primary biliary cirrhosis, among other, which are discussed more fully in relevant chapters that follow. One type that merits consideration at this point is *nonspecific focal hepatitis,* a lesion characterized by the loss of a few hepatocytes, often accompanied by degeneration of adjacent cells, and a predominantly mononuclear infiltrate (Fig. 92). Often, only a single focus is found in the entire section. When multiple, and especially when associated with an inflammatory reaction in some of the portal tracts, such lesions are often classified as *nonspecific reactive hepatitis.* Both types are relatively common, and are associated with a wide variety of systemic and extrahepatic disorders.

It should be noted that foci of cell dropout, especially when they are small or have been replaced by numerous inflammatory cells and swollen Kupffer cells, may be difficult to identify in H & E sections, but are readily visualized in Masson-stained sections.

Acidophilic bodies

Acidophilic bodies are hepatocytes undergoing a distinctive type of degeneration and necrosis characterized by condensation of the cytoplasm with preservation of the organelles (5) and by pyknosis of the nuclei and subsequent karyolysis. As the cytoplasm shrinks, the acidophilic bodies become spheroid and smaller in size, ultimately fragmenting and undergoing lysis. This form of cell death, termed *apoptosis,* is said to be a normal phenomenon in the steady-state kinetics of cell turnover in many healthy tissues, and in the involution of endocrine-dependent organs after trophic hormone withdrawal (1). In addition, in the case of the liver, it may be provoked by a number of injurious factors, including cell-mediated immune reactions (4). Characteristically, apoptosis affects single cells rather than groups of contiguous cells. However, the number of acidophilic (apoptotic) bodies produced varies, being rare in some hepatic lesions, and widely scattered through the lobules in others (Fig. 13). Apoptosis does not appear to provoke an inflammatory reaction or to lead to fibrosis (1,4). Consistent with this view is the occasional finding of individual acidophilic bodies in the absence of any inflammatory reaction. Although acidophilic bodies are usually associated with inflammation and proliferation of Kupffer cells, the two may represent independent reactions to a common noxious stimulus.

Because acidophilic bodies were first described by Councilman in the hepatic lesions of yellow fever [(6); Fig. 93], they are commonly termed Councilman-like bodies. Since the advent of needle biopsy, it has become apparent that acidophilic bodies occur in a wide variety of hepatic lesions. Although most numerous in acute viral and drug-induced hepatitis, some may be encountered in any form of hepatic injury. Rarely, acidophilic bodies may be found in the centrilobular zone of normal subjects as part of the normal life cycle of hepatocytes (1,2).

The most distinctive feature of an acidophilic body is its intensely eosinophilic, homogeneous cytoplasm that often contains a pyknotic nucleus (Fig. 94). Early in its development, an acidophilic body may be found within an intact hepatic plate (Fig. 95), but, more commonly, it is encountered within the space of Disse (Fig. 94) or in a sinusoid, having previously been extruded from the hepatic plate. Even at an early stage, the affected cell shrinks in size, becomes round or oval in shape, and separates from contiguous hepatocytes (Fig. 95). Ultimately, the acidophilic body loses its nucleus, and is phagocytized by a Kupffer cell (Fig. 96), or undergoes fragmentation (Fig. 97).

Although the cytoplasm of the acidophilic body usually appears homogeneous in H & E sections, fine vacuoles can often be identified in Masson-stained sections (Fig. 96). Rarely, in lesions with marked cholestasis, the acidophilic body may contain small bile droplets.

Councilman bodies in yellow fever, which tend to be located in the midzone, appear to be similar to the acidophilic bodies seen in a variety of other hepatic disorders (7). Acidophilic bodies may contain remnants of whatever normal substances that were present in the cells before they underwent necrosis such as bile droplets, lipid, or iron (7).

Usually, acidophilic bodies are diastase-resistant, PAS-positive (8). They occasionally stain positively with the Shikata orcein stain, a phenomenon that is regarded as falsely positive. Such cells are readily differentiated from HBsAg-positive ground glass cells by their extracellular location in the sinusoids, and by their denser, more homogeneous staining properties.

Coagulation necrosis

This type of necrosis occurs most frequently following ischemic and toxic hepatic injury, but may be seen under other conditions.

Ischemic necrosis, as a result of shock or acute left ventricular heart failure, is characterized by relatively sharply defined, but irregularly contoured zones of centrilobular, hepatocellular, coagulation necrosis that spare the periportal hepatocytes (Fig. 98). When extensive, the zones of necrosis may bridge adjacent central veins and portal tracts. Not infrequently, similar zones of ischemic necrosis are encountered within the nodules of cirrhotic livers following episodes of shock attributable to hemorrhage or sepsis (Fig. 99). In such cases, the lesions are randomly distributed, involving portions or all of some nodules, but sparing others.

Characteristically, the hepatocytes that have undergone ischemic coagulation necrosis retain their location within the hepatic plates, and show intense eosinophilia and condensation of their cytoplasm, and pyknosis, or loss of their nuclei (Fig. 100). Occasionally, the cytoplasm is finely vacuolated or fragmented or both (Fig. 100). Despite extensive hepatocellular necrosis, the reticulin is not affected. When ischemic necrosis is the result of cardiac failure, congestion of the sinusoids and zones of hemorrhage may be additional histologic features.

Early in the ischemic process, there may be no inflammatory reaction (Fig. 98). However, in some cases, some neutrophils may be seen as early as 24 hours following the onset of shock (Fig. 100). In survivors, the necrotic hepatocytes ultimately undergo lysis, producing centrilobular zones of cell dropout. Characteristically, these are relatively sharply circumscribed, contain dilated sinusoids separated by fine bundles of reticulin fibers, and a variable number of lipofuscin-filled pigmented macrophages, mononuclear cells, and neutrophils (Fig. 89). Although we have seen collapse of the reticulin in such lesions, we have never noted postnecrotic residual scarring.

Centrilobular hepatotoxic coagulation necrosis, produced by agents such as carbon tetrachloride and acetaminophen, resembles ischemic necrosis in many respects. However, the neutrophilic inflammatory reaction tends to be more intense, many of the surviving hepatocytes within and around the zones of necrosis show degenerative changes, such as fatty infiltration, ballooning and condensation, and residual fibrosis may ensue. Figure 101 illustrates a lesion of this type produced by repetitive, nonlethal doses of acetaminophen.

A few hepatotoxins, such as yellow phosphorus, produce *periportal coagulation necrosis.* A similar distribution is seen in the hepatic lesions of eclampsia, but the lesions show other distinctive features (Chapter 24).

Focal coagulation necrosis is a relatively common feature of many hepatic lesions. Typical examples are the walls of pyogenic abscesses, the necrotic lesions produced by systemic infections with fungi or viruses, such as herpes simplex and yellow fever, and the necrosis seen in hepatocytes entrapped by infiltrating tumors and granulomas.

A unique form of focal coagulation necrosis is seen exclusively in needle and wedge biopsy specimens obtained during laparotomy. To emphasize its pathogenesis and lack of significance, we prefer to classify such lesions as *surgical artifacts* rather than *focal liver cell necrosis with infiltration of neutrophils,* a term commonly used by others (9). Characteristically, groups of hepatocytes around the central veins and in the subcapsular zones show coagulation necrosis, and are infiltrated with neutrophils (Fig. 102). It has been suggested that such lesions are attributable to anoxia (9). The observation that they occur deep in the liver and only after prolonged operative procedures is consistent with this interpretation. However, more extensive lesions of the same type are occasionally encountered beneath areas of Glisson's capsule that show marked edema and hemorrhage (Fig. 103).

This suggests that mechanical injury to the liver by the prolonged use of retractors may play an equally important role. Of course, one may argue that such retraction compresses the liver and interferes with its circulation, so that the necrosis produced may be the result of local hypoxemia rather than mechanical trauma.

This lesion has also been reported in a specimen obtained from a percutaneous, transjugular liver biopsy (10). Its presence deep in the liver, without general anesthesia or evident hypoxemia, although it was a prolonged procedure, compounds the mystery (11).

Occasionally, small scattered lesions similar to those seen in surgical artifacts are encountered in the needle biopsy specimens of individuals with extrahepatic biliary obstruction, particularly when complicated by bacterial cholangitis, and in patients with sepsis. As a rule, such lesions are either randomly distributed or periportal in location. Rarely, we have encountered a few scattered, necrotic hepatocytes infiltrated with neutrophils in the otherwise normal livers of individuals with no evidence of biliary tract disease, sepsis, or anoxemia.

Significance of bridging and panlobular necrosis

In acute viral hepatitis, bridging necrosis is followed, in a significant number of cases, by the development of chronic hepatitis, cirrhosis, or hepatic failure that results in death (12,13). Although chronic hepatitis may occur in the absence of antecedent bridging necrosis, we have never seen progression to cirrhosis or hepatic failure in such cases. As a rule, bridging necrosis is demonstrable within the first few weeks of illness, but, rarely, its appearance is delayed for several months, often coinciding with a clinical recrudescence or relapse, and may then be followed by progression to cirrhosis. It must be emphasized that bridging, even if accompanied by panlobular necrosis, does not invariably lead to the development of cirrhosis or hepatic failure, and that full recovery without residual fibrosis is possible (12,14), although, in most recovered cases, some degree of scarring occurs.

It has been reported that the bridging necrosis produced by drugs may have less serious consequences than in viral hepatitis (15). Our own experience confirms the impression that progression to cirrhosis is unusual under such conditions (16,17), unless drug administration is continued following the appearance of the hepatitis (17,18). Nevertheless, bridging necrosis is an ominous prognostic sign indicative of the potential for hepatic failure. Our own experience with halothane-induced hepatitis

illustrates this point. Thus, of the 15 patients who exhibited bridging necrosis, 7 died of hepatic failure, while all 7 with unbridged lesions recovered. In most, but not all of our fatal cases, the bridging was accompanied by zones of panlobular necrosis.

Some authorities draw a distinction between portal-portal and portal-central bridging necrosis (19). Indeed, they limit the term to the portal-central type, and classify portal-portal bridging as a form of piecemeal necrosis. Considering its dictionary definition, the term *piecemeal,* as applied to necrosis, implies destruction of hepatic parenchyma bit by bit, a description appropriate for the type of lesion commonly seen in the periportal zones of chronic active hepatitis, but inappropriate for large zones of portal-portal bridging necrosis in which numerous contiguous hepatocytes are destroyed simultaneously. To be sure, as the periportal parenchyma is progressively destroyed by piecemeal necrosis in chronic active hepatitis, adjacent portal tracts and central zones may be linked by bridges containing fibrous tissue, inflammatory cells, degenerating hepatocytes, bile ductules, and blood vessels. Lesions of this type should be classified as *fibrous bridging.* The same term should also be applied to zones of bridging necrosis that have undergone fibrosis.

The question of why bridging necrosis is followed by fibrosis in some cases, but not in others, cannot be answered at this time. Since full restitution of the parenchyma without residual scarring is possible (12,15), it is evident that hepatocellular necrosis, inflammation, and collapse of reticulin, either singly or in combination, cannot account for the collagenization when it occurs. In some as yet unknown way, the fibroblasts, and possibly the Ito cells, are activated, leading to fibrogenesis. It is possible that multiple factors are involved, and that these may differ depending on the etiology of the necrosis.

Death from hepatic failure as a result of acute hepatocellular necrosis occurs when the mass of parenchyma destroyed reaches a critical level, which, on the basis of stereologic studies of biopsy material, has been estimated to be approximately 65% (20). It has been suggested that a defect in the regenerative response, possibly related to advancing age, may be an equally important factor, particularly when the progression to hepatic failure is not fulminant (14). While it is clearly evident that the regenerative response is inadequate to cope with the massive loss of parenchyma, there is no convincing evidence to implicate a primary defect in the regenerative response in the development of hepatic failure. At autopsy, the remaining parenchyma in such cases almost always shows evidence of active regeneration, particularly if the patient survives for a week or longer.

Often, the loss of parenchyma in cases of acute hepatitis with bridging necrosis that prove fatal does not appear massive in antemortem needle biopsy specimens. However, in our own experience, the liver at autopsy in such cases is invariably reduced in weight, ranging from 500 to 1200 g, and, in most instances, exhibits large zones of panlobular necrosis. Thus, the bridging necrosis encountered in needle biopsy specimens may be indicative of more massive necrosis elsewhere in the liver and, hence, may serve as an important prognostic sign of possible impending hepatic failure.

The term *subacute hepatic necrosis,* once used as a synonym for bridging necrosis, needs a word of explanation, since it is often misinterpreted. Long before the term was first used to describe such lesions in needle biopsy specimens (12), pathologists classified massive hepatic necrosis found at autopsy as acute hepatic necrosis, and submassive hepatic necrosis as "subacute hepatic necrosis." Since the latter lesion invariably exhibited not only panlobular but also bridging necrosis, the term subacute hepatic necrosis was adopted to describe bridging necrosis in the lesions found in biopsy specimens (12). Thus, the term subacute hepatic necrosis refers to the distribution and extent of the necrosis, and not to histologic or clinical features that suggest a slow evolution of the lesions, and certainly not to the duration of the disorder.

Piecemeal necrosis

This form of necrosis is characterized by destruction of the hepatocytes in the limiting plates of the portal tracts and of septa that encircle the parenchymal nodules in active forms of cirrhosis. The hepatocellular necrosis is invariably accompanied by an inflammatory exudate that extends out into the surrounding parenchyma. Often the lesion is progressive, and is further characterized by fibrosis that follows in the wake of the advancing zone of hepatocellular destruction, and usually extends into the surviving parenchyma beyond its borders.

Although piecemeal necrosis is a distinctive feature of chronic active hepatitis, it is a nonspecific lesion that may be seen in a wide variety of other disorders, including acute viral and drug-induced hepatitis, the precirrhotic phase of primary biliary cirrhosis, sclerosing cholangitis, the "pericholangitis" associated with ulcerative colitis and Crohn's disease, extrahepatic biliary obstruction, some forms of Wilson's disease, and the active phase of most other forms of cirrhosis.

Depending on the activity and severity of the lesions, the destruction of the limiting plates may be segmental or complete around individual portal tracts or septa, and may vary both in extent and distribution. Often the distribution is patchy, and only rarely are all the portal tracts or septa involved.

As a result of piecemeal necrosis, the portal tracts appear enlarged and irregular in contour, often being stellate in shape (Fig. 104). The enlargement is due primarily to the loss of periportal hepatocytes, and not to expansion of the portal tract by the fibrous tissue and inflammatory cells that are always present, or by the proliferating ductules found in many cases. At an early stage, the original portal tract is surrounded by a mesh of loosely arranged reticulin bundles outlining fine, vascular channels and corresponding to the zone of cell dropout. This is most clearly visualized in Masson-stained sections (Fig. 105). As the reticulin in the zone of cell dropout collapses and undergoes collagenization, the newly formed collagen merges with that of the original portal tract, so that the outlines of the latter may be difficult to identify (Fig. 104). As indicated previously, both the inflammatory cells and fibrous tissue of the expanded portal tract extend into the surrounding parenchyma, usually along the walls of the sinusoids, and often encircle individual hepatocytes or groups arranged in the form of rosettes (Fig. 106).

Hepatocellular degeneration

Following various forms of injury, hepatocytes often exhibit degenerative changes. Although potentially reversible, such changes may lead to cell death. Not infrequently, degenerating hepatocytes are accompanied by frankly necrotic cells. It is not clear, however, whether the loss of hepatocytes that follows degeneration is the result of progression to coagulation necrosis or acidophilic body formation, or is due to other forms of cytolysis.

Ballooning

Ballooning of the hepatocytes occurs under a wide variety of conditions, which is one of the most common forms of hepatocellular degeneration. Characteristically, the affected cells are large and pale owing to swelling of their cytoplasm. Often, their cytoplasmic granules are aggregated in the perinuclear zone, while the remaining peripheral cytoplasm has a finely reticulated appearance (Fig. 107). As a rule, the nuclei are normal.

While ballooned hepatocytes may be seen in any form of hepatic injury, they are encountered most frequently in the centrilobular zones in acute viral hepatitis (Fig. 108), toxic hepatitis (Fig. 107), and alcoholic hepatitis (Fig. 90), in the periportal zones in chronic active hepatitis (Fig. 106), and in the limiting plates of the septa in most forms of active cirrhosis (Fig. 109). Ballooning of the hepatocytes may also be seen in areas of marked cholestasis (Fig. 110), although pseudoxanthomatous degeneration is more common (see later).

At least in the case of alcoholic liver disease, it has been suggested that ballooning may be due to the retention of protein (21) that results from a defect in secretion induced by alcohol (22).

Formalin fixation artifacts (Fig. 9) may be mistaken for ballooning. However, the pale, swollen cells produced by poor fixation differ from ballooned hepatocytes in several respects. In general, the distribution of the artifactually affected cells is random rather than zonal. In addition, they usually alternate with shrunken, deeply stained cells, their cytoplasm is coarsely granular, and they are unaccompanied by other evidence of degeneration, necrosis, or inflammation.

Acidophilic degeneration

Occasionally, degeneration of hepatocytes is manifested by shrinkage and condensation of their cytoplasm and nuclei. The affected cells, which usually occur singly, are relatively small in size, have straight or concave, sharply defined borders that form acute angles where they meet, and contain pyknotic nuclei and intensely eosinophilic, homogeneous, opaque cytoplasm (Figs. 13, 111). Although the appearance of the cytoplasm resembles that in coagulation necrosis (Fig. 100), hepatocytes undergoing acidophilic degeneration are smaller in size, more angulated in shape, and contain intact shrunken nuclei.

Acidophilic degeneration, although less common and usually less extensive than ballooning, may also be found in any type of hepatic injury, and is often associated with other types of hepatocellular degeneration and necrosis. Although it is highly probable that the process is reversible in some cases, it is not known whether it ever progresses to coagulation necrosis.

Surgical wedge biopsy specimens occasionally contain a few cells that appear to be undergoing acidophilic degeneration. Since these may occur in the absence of other evidence of hepatic injury, it is highly probable that such cells are created artifactually by handling the liver during surgery. This interpretation is supported by the observation that scattered, shrunken, acidophilic hepatocytes are relatively common in wedge biopsy specimens of rat liver fixed by immersion in glutaraldehyde, but are almost never encountered when the liver is fixed *in situ* by infusing glutaraldehyde via the portal vein (23).

Fatty degeneration

Accumulation of lipid in the cytoplasm of hepatocytes, chiefly in the form of triglyceride, is by far the most common abnormality encountered in the liver. In most instances, such deposits are indicative of alterations in lipid metabolism or transport unrelated to hepatocellular injury, and are usually classified as *fatty infiltration*. When lipid accumulates as a result of hepatocellular injury, it is commonly termed *fatty degeneration*. The rationale for distinguishing between fatty infiltration and degeneration may be questioned, since in the last analysis, both reflect changes in lipid metabolism or transport. However, the behavior of the hepatocytes in the two conditions appears to differ. Thus, simple *fatty infiltration* is a readily reversible lesion that seldom impairs hepatic function, and rarely results in loss of hepatocytes, whereas *fatty degeneration* may be associated with hepatocellular dysfunction, and may lead to cell death. The distinction between fatty infiltration and degeneration is not possible on the basis of light microscopic features alone.

Fatty degeneration is a relatively frequent finding in alcoholic liver disease. Characteristically, the affected hepatocytes are enlarged, exhibit pale, foamy cytoplasm, shrinkage or loss of nuclei, and, occasionally, disruption of plasma membranes (Fig. 112). Early in the disease, the degenerating lipid-containing cells are seen in the centrilobular zones, but later may be found around enlarged fibrotic portal tracts or along the limiting plates of fibrous septa. Often, adjacent hepatocytes show other degenerative changes, such as ballooning or Mallory bodies. However, as shown in Figure 112, these may be absent. This lesion, termed *alcoholic foamy degeneration* of the liver, has been described in detail (24), and represents microvesicular (small droplet) fat deposition (Fig. 113).

That fatty degeneration alone may be accompanied by marked hepatocellular dysfunction is illustrated by the patient whose biopsy section is shown in Figure 112. This patient presented with the typical features of alcoholic hepatitis, including fever, leukocytosis, hepatomegaly, jaundice, and ascites. However, careful search of a large biopsy section failed to reveal any Mallory bodies or intralobular neutrophils, the only findings of note being fatty degeneration, fatty infiltration and ballooning of the hepatocytes, and mild portal fibrosis and lymphocytosis. Of note is the fact that in the areas of fatty degeneration, there was evidence of focal cell dropout and fibrosis (Fig. 112), suggesting that some of the affected cells had disintegrated or undergone cytolysis. Conceivably, this process accounts, in part at least, for the occurrence in alcoholic patients of hepatic fibrosis in the absence of antecedent alcoholic hepatitis (21).

Microvesicular fat deposition is a relatively common feature of the hepatic lesions produced by a variety of toxins. Of particular interest are those produced by excessive intravenous doses of tetracycline, a lesion encountered most frequently in pregnant women with urinary tract infections (25), and, less often, under other conditions (26), or in males (27). Both the clinical

and morphologic features are remarkably similar to those of the acute fatty liver of pregnancy (see Chapter 24). In the absence of a history of tetracycline administration, the two are indistinguishable. Characteristically, the fat deposition involves the centrilobular hepatocytes, but when severe, may extend into the midzones or even into the periportal zones. The cytoplasm of the affected cells is usually filled with minute, closely packed, lipid droplets, giving it a foamy appearance. However, larger droplets may be seen in some hepatocytes (Fig. 114). In both pregnancy and tetracycline-induced fat deposition, the cytoplasm of the hepatocytes is distended by innumerable, fine, lipid droplets that may mimic pseudoxanthoma or balloon cells (Fig. 115). To avoid errors, it is wise to confirm the lipid nature of the deposits by staining a frozen section with oil red O (Fig. 116). Some hepatocytes are enlarged, while others appear small and shrunken. Usually, the nuclei are preserved, but are often shrunken and displaced to the periphery by the lipid droplets. Disruption of cell membranes with the formation of syncytial multinucleated giant cells has been reported (25), but we have not seen this lesion.

The hepatic lesions of Reye's syndrome, a disorder of young children, are also characterized by hepatocellular fatty degeneration with innumerable fine, cytoplasmic, microvesicular lipid droplets. However, in this condition, the lesions are panlobular rather than centrilobular in distribution. The hepatocytes often appear normal except for the presence of numerous small, sharply defined lipid droplets (Fig. 117), which, in general, tend to be larger in the periportal zones. In some cases, however, the lipid droplets are so small and tightly packed that the strands of cytoplasm between them may be difficult to visualize (Fig. 118). An oil red O–stained frozen section may be required to differentiate such cells from degenerating ballooned hepatocytes.

Pseudoxanthomatous degeneration

As a consequence of cholestasis, both the hepatocytes and the Kupffer cells may undergo a unique type of degeneration characterized by swelling, pallor, and fine vacuolization of their cytoplasm, and contraction or pyknosis of their nuclei. Because of their resemblance to the lipid-containing histiocytes of xanthomas in other tissues, the affected cells are commonly classified as *pseudoxanthoma cells*. The alternative descriptive term, *feathery degeneration,* does not portray the character of the cytoplasmic changes nearly so well.

Circumstantial evidence suggests that the formation of pseudoxanthoma cells is attributable to absorption of some constituent of bile, presumably bile acids. However, this has not been established experimentally.

When few in number, the pseudoxanthomatous hepatocytes and Kupffer cells may be found in their normal locations, within the hepatic plates and sinusoids, respectively (Fig. 119). More commonly, however, they occur in sharply circumscribed groups of variable size in which the plate pattern and sinusoids are obscured, so that the distinction between pseudoxanthoma cells of hepatocyte and Kupffer cell origin is no longer possible (Fig. 120). Not infrequently, such lesions contain strands of atrophic, but otherwise normal hepatocytes. Bile staining and bile droplets may be seen in the pseudoxanthoma cells, but are inconstant findings. Usually, the lesions contain no inflammatory cells. However, in some, the pseudoxanthoma cells undergo further degeneration and necrosis, leading to an inflammatory reaction (Fig. 121).

Occasionally, free bile extravasates into the parenchyma producing a *bile lake* (Fig. 122). Characteristically, the pool of bile is surrounded by a zone of pseudoxanthoma cells, histiocytes, or, less commonly, foreign-body giant cells.

Rarely, the extravasation of bile produces a *bile infarct,* a lesion characterized by a sharply circumscribed zone of hepatocellular coagulation necrosis in which the affected cells are deeply bile stained and surrounded by free bile (Fig. 123). The term *bile infarct* is often used to describe circumscribed clusters of pseudoxanthoma cells or bile lakes, but this appears inappropriate, since such lesions do not exhibit the type of coagulation necrosis common to all other forms of infarction.

The reticulin is well preserved in lesions characterized by clusters of pseudoxanthoma cells, but is destroyed in those that contain bile lakes or bile infarcts.

Pseudoxanthomatous degeneration may be seen in any form of cholestasis. It is generally held that large areas of involvement are indicative of extrahepatic bile duct obstruction. However, as illustrated in Figures 119 through 123, we have frequently encountered large foci of pseudoxanthomatous degeneration, bile lakes, and even bile infarcts in nonobstructive hepatocellular forms of cholestasis. The development of such lesions appears to depend on the severity and duration of the cholestasis, and on the occurrence of cholangiolar or interlobular duct degeneration, necrosis, or rupture rather than on the etiology of the cholestasis.

Collections of pseudoxanthoma cells may be found anywhere in the lobule, and are usually accompanied by bile thrombi in the canaliculi of the adjacent parenchyma. However, small foci may be seen occasionally in the absence of histologic evidence of cholestasis. We have encountered this most frequently in patients with partial obstruction of the extrahepatic bile ducts who exhibit high serum levels of bile acids, but only minimally increased concentrations of serum bilirubin.

With rare exceptions, *bile lakes* and *bile infarcts* are found in the periportal zones of the lobules, and almost always are associated with dilated, degenerating or necrotic cholangioles, and/or interlobular bile ducts.

Hepatic oncocytes

Epithelial cells with intensely eosinophilic, granular cytoplasm found within endocrine and exocrine glands under some conditions have been classified as oncocytes (27). On electron microscopy the cytoplasmic granules of *hepatic oncocytes* have been identified as closely packed mitochondria (28). Characteristically, hepatic oncocytes are enlarged hepatocytes that contain innumerable closely packed, intensely eosinophilic, fine cytoplasmic granules (Fig. 124). Their nuclei are preserved, but often appear shrunken. The mitochondrial nature of the granules can be confirmed by the blue color they exhibit when stained with PTAH (Fig. 125).

Hepatic oncocytes may be encountered in any form of active cirrhosis, but also occur occasionally in noncirrhotic lesions, including alcoholic fatty infiltration, alcoholic hepatitis, and some forms of toxic and drug-induced hepatitis. Usually, they appear in groups adjacent to fibrous septa or portal tracts, but occasionally oncocytes involve an entire cirrhotic nodule, or single cells within a nodule.

Multinucleated giant hepatocytes

In neonatal cholestasis due to a variety of causes some or all of the hepatocytes may undergo transformation to multinucleated giant cells arranged in a disorganized pattern of trabeculae or isolated cells (29). Since this may occur in lesions attributable to or associated with various viral infections, heriditary metabolic disorders, and extrahepatic biliary atresia, giant cell transformation appears to be a nonspecific response of fetal and neonatal hepatocytes to injury. On electron microscopy, well-preserved organelles can be demonstrated in the cytoplasm of the affected cells, but almost always there are associated severe degenerative changes, suggesting that giant cell transformation of neonatal hepatocytes is a degenerative rather than a regenerative response. Histochemical studies indicate that many of the metabolic activities of the affected cells are well preserved, but that their capacity to secrete bile is severely impaired. There is suggestive evidence that the giant cells are derived from regenerating hepatocytes arranged in the form of pseudoglands, and that the loss of intercellular plasma membranes and fusion of adjacent cells account for the development of giant cells. However, remnants of degraded plasma membranes have not been successfully demonstrated by electron microscopy. For a more detailed account of giant cell transformation of neonatal hepatocytes, the reader is referred to a comprehensive review (29).

Characteristically, multinucleated giant hepatocytes are greatly enlarged and irregular in contour and contain numerous nuclei (Fig. 126). Such cells may range in diameter up to 400 μm. Usually, the cytoplasm is pale and vacuolated and often contains bile droplets and hemosiderin. The nuclei, which may number up to 20 in a single cell, appear normal in size and contour, and never show evidence of mitotic activity. They may be aggregated in the center or randomly distributed through the cytoplasm. Occasionally, the cells appear to form a syncytium, and they contain structures resembling canaliculi filled with inspissated bile (Fig. 127), features consistent with the view that the giant cells may be formed by fusion of adjacent hepatocytes following loss of their intercellular plasma membranes.

Occasionally, multinucleated giant hepatocytes are encountered in adults (30). In our experience, they have occurred chiefly in severe, acute, viral toxic or drug-induced hepatitis, usually accompanied by bridging or submassive hepatic necrosis, and in severe chronic active hepatitis. It has been suggested that only young adults are affected. However, we have encountered multinucleated giant hepatocytes in a number of middle-aged individuals. With rare exceptions, cells found in adults are much fewer in number than in infants. In many cases, the affected cells are identical in all respects to those encountered in neonatal cholestasis (Fig. 128). However, often, they are much smaller in size. Although they have not been studied by electron microscopy or histochemically, it is highly probable that at least the large type of multinucleated giant hepatocytes illustrated in Figure 128 have the same significance and and pathogenesis as those in neonates. However, the possibility cannot be excluded that some of the smaller giant cells encountered in various forms of adult hepatitis may represent a regenerative response.

The syndrome of *syncytial giant cell hepatitis* was recently described (31). This disorder was reported in 10 patients who ranged in age from three months to 41 years. They appeared to have acute viral hepatitis, presumably NANB because markers for HAV and HBV were negative. After the acute phase subsided, the patients developed chronic active hepatitis, which progressed rapidly, eventually to require liver transplantation or to death. Liver biopsy in all showed that the liver cords were replaced by syncytial giant cells (Fig. 129). These giant cells had from 3 to 20 centrally located nuclei in a large volume of eosinophilic cytoplasm, which had a ground glass appearance. Brown granules of various size, some of which contained bilirubin, were present in the cytoplasm. Bridging necrosis was prominent. The nonsyncytial hepatocytes showed focal necrosis and ballooning degeneration. Intracellular, canalicular, and ductal cholestasis were present. Moderate lymphocytic infiltration of the portal tracts was characteristic. Cirrhosis developed within a year. Electron microscopy showed large numbers of mitochondria and smooth membranes, which explained the ground glass appearance. Spherical particles and filaments were present, which were thought to be typical of the nucleocapsids of paramyxoviruses. Virologic studies supported the hypothesis that the infectious agent is a paramyxovirus, perhaps the measles virus.

Hepatocellular cytoplasmic inclusions

Mallory bodies

Mallory bodies, distinctive hepatocellular cytoplasmic inclusions, were once regarded as a pathognomonic feature of alcoholic liver disease and, hence, were termed *alcoholic hyalin* deposits. However, it is now recognized that such inclusions may occur not only in alcoholic liver disease but also in a number of other disorders, including primary biliary cirrhosis (32), Wilson's disease (33), Indian childhood cirrhosis (34), nonalcoholic cirrhosis associated with diabetes mellitus and obesity (35), chronic cholestasis of varied etiology (36), the hepatic lesions that appear following jejunoileal bypass for massive obesity (37), hepatocellular carcinoma (38), focal nodular hyperplasia (hamartoma; 39), and the hepatitis and cirrhosis produced by the drugs amiodarone (40) and perhexiline maleate (41). In addition, Mallory bodies can be produced experimentally in mice by prolonged administration of griseofulvin (42) and other oncogenic substances (43).

Three types of Mallory bodies can be identified electron microscopically: Type 1, composed of filaments in parallel arrays; Type 2, the one encountered most commonly, made up of closely packed, randomly oriented filaments; and Type 3, composed of granular or amorphous material devoid of filaments except at their periphery (44). None of the inclusions is membrane-bound. There is suggestive evidence that the three types of Mallory bodies may represent successive stages in their aging. In isolated, purified preparations of Type 2 Mallory bodies, the filaments exhibit a hollow core and measure 175 to 250 nm in length and 14 to 20 nm in diameter (45). In many respects they resemble the intermediate sized filaments of the tonofilament class, but differ in being shorter and thicker and having an outer fimbricated coat. By means of immunofluorescence, using a guinea-pig antibody against purified bovine prekeratin, it has been shown that the filaments of Mallory bodies contain a prekeratin-like protein (45). Since many epithelial cells, including the hepatocytes, contain a prekeratin cytoskeleton, it has been suggested that the formation of Mallory bodies may represent a type of keratinization due to injury. It is still uncertain whether the aggregates of prekeratin in Mallory bodies represent material specifically synthesized by the hepatocytes in response to injury, or are derived from normal constituents of the cells. They appear to form as a result of condensation or collapse of

intermediate sized filaments (46). That prekeratin is not the only constituent of Mallory bodies is clearly evident from histochemical studies indicating that they contain not only protein but also phospholipid (47,48). Moreover, it is apparent from the variability of their staining properties and histochemical reactivity that Mallory bodies are not uniform in composition.

On routine light microscopy, *Mallory bodies* appear as groups of sharply defined globules of variable shape and size, made up of homogeneous material and arranged in the form of beaded chains (Fig. 130). The chains are usually irregular or serpiginous in contour, but may be horseshoe-shaped or circular, partially or completely encircling the nucleus. Occasionally, Mallory bodies present as single or multiple, large, round hyalin globules. These must be differentiated from other types of circumscribed cytoplasmic inclusions. Usually, the true nature of such hyalin globules is suggested by the presence of more typical, beaded, Mallory bodies and transitions between beaded and globular inclusions in adjacent cells, and by their failure to stain with PAS following diastase digestion, a feature shared by all Mallory bodies.

As a rule, Mallory bodies are acidophilic, and stain a brilliant orange-red in Masson sections (Fig. 130), and a less intense, violaceous red in H & E sections (Fig. 131). Variations in the intensity of the staining within the same section are relatively common. Occasionally, some of the Mallory bodies in Masson-stained sections are basophilic, appearing light blue in color, or blue with a bright red central core (Fig. 132). Basophilic Mallory bodies are unusual in H & E sections, except in the case of formalin-fixed postmortem specimens in which they may appear pale and slate-gray in color. In such cases, the inclusions may be overlooked, unless searched for with care under high magnification.

Special stains, such as chromotrope aniline blue (CAB)(49), are often used to confirm the identity or to facilitate the detection of Mallory bodies. In our experience, none of these has proved superior to the Masson stain for these purposes.

The character of the hepatocytes in which Mallory bodies are found varies. Often, the involved cells are ballooned or show other evidence of degeneration, but usually they contain intact nuclei (Fig. 132). However, they may be encountered in enlarged, but otherwise normal hepatocytes with prominent nuclei and nucleoli (Fig. 130). Rarely, inclusions with the typical histologic and electron microscopic features of Mallory bodies may be seen within the epithelial cells of ductules or interlobular bile ducts [(39); Fig. 133].

Hepatocytes that contain Mallory bodies are often surrounded and occasionally invaded by neutrophils, particularly in the case of alcoholic hepatitis (Fig. 131). It has been suggested that the neutrophils are attracted in some unknown way by such cytoplasmic inclusions, and that invariably they can be demonstrated in serial sections (50). While neutrophils are commonly found in areas containing Mallory bodies, it has been our experience that only a minority of the hepatocytes bearing such inclusions are encircled by neutrophils. Indeed, we have occasionally failed to find any neutrophils, even in serial sections, in areas containing innumerable Mallory bodies (Fig. 130).

The number and distribution of Mallory bodies vary, depending on the etiology and severity of the underlying hepatic lesion. In some instances, they occur in only a few scattered hepatocytes, whereas in others, numerous contiguous cells are involved.

Characteristically, in alcoholic hepatitis, Mallory bodies are found in the centrilobular hepatocytes. However, when the lesion is severe, Mallory bodies may be panlobular in distribution, although they never affect all cells. When present in cirrhosis, Mallory bodies occur in periseptal and periportal hepatocytes. In prolonged cholestasis, their distribution may be periportal or centrilobular, depending on the zonal distribution of the cholestasis. However, the involved hepatocytes rarely contain bile droplets and often do not lie in close proximity to bile-filled canaliculi.

The fate of Mallory body–containing hepatocytes is not clear. Certainly, the frequency with which such cells show degenerative changes, and lie adjacent to foci of cell dropout and fibrosis, particularly in alcoholic hepatitis (Fig. 90), suggests that Mallory body formation is an irreversible, degenerative process that leads to disintegration and dissolution of hepatocytes. However, the possibility cannot be excluded that some such cells recover. No Mallory body–containing cell has ever been biopsied more than once.

Although the formation of Mallory bodies is generally regarded as a process limited to the liver, it is of interest that hyalin inclusions with identical ultrastructural and histochemical features have been identified in the pulmonary alveolar cells in cases of asbestosis (51).

Megamitochondria

When the mitochondria are greatly enlarged, they can be visualized at the light microscopic level, and appear as distinctive cytoplasmic inclusions. Such megamitochondria occur most frequently in chronic alcoholic patients, and, therefore, provide a useful diagnostic clue in the identification of alcohol abusers (52). They may be more common in mild than in severe alcoholic hepatitis (53). In one reported series (54), megamitochondria were encountered in 72% of the liver biopsy sections of heavy drinkers, and in only 10% of those with little or no alcohol intake. The incidence in our own series of alcoholic patients has been significantly lower, approximately 5%, a discrepancy possibly reflecting our failure to search diligently for megamitochondria in all cases. Nevertheless, we too regard such cytoplasmic inclusions as presumptive evidence of excessive drinking. However, in our group of 50 patients with megamitochondria, 5 were nonalcoholic. These included 2 with fatty infiltration of the liver related to diabetes mellitus, a child with fatty infiltration of unknown etiology, one with cryptogenic cirrhosis, and a young woman with a normal liver who was a heterozygous carrier of ornithine transcarbamylase deficiency.

Giant cell mitochondria were found in liver biopsies of 13 of 14 patients with systemic scleroderma, none of whom had clinical evidence of liver disease (55).

Megamitochondria present as sharply defined, membrane-bound, cytoplasmic inclusions that contain fine, closely packed eosinophilic granules. They may be found within otherwise normal appearing hepatocytes (Fig. 134), or within cells that are ballooned or infiltrated with fat (Fig. 135). Usually, they are round in shape, although cigar-shaped structures containing elongated, crystalline inclusions, demonstrable by electron microscopy, have been reported (56). Megamitochondria vary in size, ranging from the barely detectable to structures as large as or even larger than the nucleus of the involved cell. Often, several inclusions are present within a single hepatocyte (Fig. 134). Although they have no predilection for any particular area of the lobules or nodules, they are frequently encountered in groups of contiguous hepatocytes (Fig. 134). In alcoholic patients, neither their number nor size bears any relationship to

the character of the hepatic lesions found, occurring with about equal frequency in fatty infiltration, alcoholic hepatitis, and portal cirrhosis; they are rarely found in a completely normal liver. Available evidence suggests that their occurrence correlates with the magnitude and duration of alcohol consumption, and that they may disappear following abstention (54).

Although megamitochondria characteristically are PAS-negative (54), we have occasionally encountered one that appeared to be diastase-resistant, PAS-positive. We have not had the opportunity to document the mitochondrial nature of such inclusions by electron microscopy.

Lysosomal cytoplasmic "ring body" inclusions

A new type of cytoplasmic inclusion body has recently been described in patients with chronic hepatitis, especially post-transfusion, nonA, nonB chronic hepatitis (56A). These bodies are not visible with H & E stain, but are seen with Victoria blue and other stains (Fig. 135A, B, C, D).

HB surface antigen-positive ground glass cells

Chronic infections with the hepatitis B virus (HBV) induce proliferation of the smooth endoplasmic reticulum (SER) in a variable number of hepatocytes, imparting a ground glass appearance to their cytoplasm (57). By electron microscopy, it can be shown that the SER of the affected cells contains tubular and circular structures identical in appearance with those of HBsAg particles (58). Moreover, their identity can be further confirmed by immunofluorescence (57) or immunoperoxidase (59) methods, using an appropriately labeled serum-containing antibody to HBsAg. These methods are applicable to formalin-fixed, paraffin-embedded sections (59), thus obviating the need for frozen sections. Sections fixed in Carnoy's solution serve equally well for this purpose. Although useful in research studies, neither immunofluorescence nor immunoperoxidase compares in simplicity and availability with staining of routine sections with orcein or aldehyde fuchsin (60). This technique is highly specific and is equal in sensitivity to the immunofluorescence and immunoperoxidase methods in the detection of HBsAg. The avidity of HBsAg for orcein and aldehyde fuchsin has been attributed to its content of disulfide bonds.

HBsAg-positive ground glass cells are usually present in variable numbers in the livers of healthy carriers and patients with various forms of chronic hepatitis and cirrhosis accompanied by HBs antigenemia (61), but only rarely in those with acute HBsAg-positive hepatitis (62). Occasionally, orcein-positive ground glass cells are encountered in patients with HBsAg-negative chronic liver disease (63). Rarely, HBsAg can be detected in Kupffer cells by both orcein staining and immunofluorescence (64).

Based on immunofluorescence studies it has been suggested that the distribution and amount of HBsAg in the hepatocytes reflect the immunologic status of the patient and correlate with the histologic features and clinical behavior of the hepatic lesions (65). Thus, it has been proposed that the hepatic lesions in the carrier state, chronic persistent hepatitis, and inactive cirrhosis are characterized by numerous ground glass cells and abundant antigen in the cytoplasm of most hepatocytes, a distribution presumably indicative of an immunologic defect resulting in failure of the host to clear the antigen. According to this view, the hepatocytes containing cytoplasmic antigen are spared destruction in an accompanying cell-mediated immune reaction because their plasma membranes are devoid of antigen. By contrast, in cases of chronic active hepatitis and active cirrhosis, HBsAg is said to be localized in the plasma membranes of the hepatocytes, thus rendering them recognizable as target cells in an immunologic reaction that results in their destruction. Although this is an attractive hypothesis, other investigators have failed to find any correlation between the distribution and amount of HBsAg in the hepatocytes and the character and behavior of the hepatic lesions (62).

The most distinctive histologic feature of a ground glass cell is the presence within its cytoplasm of a sharply circumscribed, non-membrane-bound, pale, eosinophilic, finely granular, homogeneous inclusion. Usually, the inclusion is relatively large, filling the cell and displacing its nucleus and darker staining, more granular cytoplasm to the periphery, and often is encircled by a narrow, clear halo, presumably an artifact of fixation and embedding (Fig. 136). Most inclusions are round or oval, but they may be irregular in shape; in some cells, they occupy only a small portion of the cytoplasm. Occasionally, as shown in Figure 136, some of the inclusions contain fine vacuoles. Most but not all ground glass cells are enlarged. Usually, the inclusions are rich in glycogen and stain a deep red with PAS (Fig. 137), a reaction that is abolished by antecedent diastase digestion.

As a rule, the inclusions are randomly distributed, involving solitary hepatocytes or small groups of cells. Only rarely are they encountered in sheets of contiguous cells, and almost never in an exclusively pericentral or periportal zonal distribution, a pattern relatively common in other types of cytoplasmic inclusions that mimic HBsAg-positive ground glass cells. The number and distribution of ground glass cells encountered in any given case vary greatly.

A distinctive feature of HBsAg-positive ground glass cells that differentiates them from other, similar cytoplasmic inclusions is their avidity for orcein and aldehyde fuchsin. In orcein-stained sections, the cytoplasmic inclusions in HBsAg-positive ground glass cells appear as chocolate-brown bodies against a background of cytoplasm stained light brown or tan (Fig. 138). Unfortunately, orcein varies in its staining properties, so that not all lots are suitable for detecting HBsAg-positive ground glass cells. In addition, orcein occasionally stains sheets of hepatocytes a deep brown at the margins of sections, particularly of formalin-fixed surgical and postmortem specimens. This rarely poses a diagnostic problem, since the stained cells show none of the characteristic histologic features of ground glass cells. Lipofuscin-filled Kupffer cells and portal macrophages also take up orcein, but these are readily differentiated from ground glass cells on the basis of their location and coarse granulation. Coarse, orcein-stained hepatocellular granules may be seen in chronic cholestatic states, especially primary biliary cirrhosis. These are further discussed in the section on hepatocellular cytoplasmic granules and pigments. In this connection, it should be noted that bile thrombi and acidophilic bodies occasionally take up orcein stain.

Aldehyde fuchsin, which has the advantage of being uniform in composition, is just as simple to use as orcein, and is its equal in sensitivity and specificity in the detection of HBsAg-positive ground glass cells. In aldehyde fuchsin–stained sections, the inclusions appear deep purple in color against a background of pink or reddish violet cytoplasm (Fig. 139).

HBsAg-positive ground glass cells must be differentiated from induction cells, Lafora bodies, glycogenosis IV inclusions and

a group of less well defined cytoplasmic inclusions. Although these may mimic HBsAg-positive ground glass cells histologically, they do not stain with orcein or aldehyde fuchsin and they often show a zonal distribution.

HBV core antigen (HBcAg) is found almost exclusively in the nuclei of hepatocytes. When numerous, they may impart a homogeneous, finely sanded, lightly eosinophilic appearance to the nucleus (Fig. 140). Such *sanded nuclei* are rare, even when core particles are readily demonstrable by electron microscopy (66).

HBsAg-negative ground glass cells (induction cells)

Alcohol and a wide variety of drugs induce proliferation of the smooth endoplasmic reticulum of the hepatocytes. When the proliferation is extensive, the affected hepatocytes present as ground glass cells (67). To differentiate them from similar cells that contain HBsAg, they are often classified as *induction cells,* an appropriate and less cumbersome term than HBsAg-negative or orcein-negative ground glass cells. Of the drugs that give rise to the formation of induction cells, those implicated most frequently include barbiturates, diphenylhydantoin, benzodiazepines, such as diazepam (Valium) and chlordiazepoxide (Librium), methotrexate, and cyclophosphamide.

A reliable feature that differentiates induction cells from HBsAg-positive ground glass cells is their resistance to staining with orcein and aldehyde fuchsin. However, other differences between the two are often apparent in routine H & E- and Masson-stained sections. In contrast to HBsAg-positive ground glass cells, induction cells often involve large groups of hepatocytes in a zonal distribution, particularly centrilobular, and occasionally periportal. Although the affected cells are similarly enlarged, and contain finely granular, faintly eosinophilic cytoplasm, the inclusions are less sharply circumscribed, usually fill the entire cell, and only rarely are encircled by a clear halo. Although the nucleus is not always displaced to the periphery, the basophilic and lipofuscin granules of the cytoplasm tend to aggregate along the plasma membranes, particularly in the region of the canaliculi (Fig. 141). Not infrequently, the granules in the inclusions are coarser than those in HBsAg-positive ground glass cells, and, occasionally, they contain fine thread-like structures. However, in some cases, the induction cells are histologically indistinguishable from HBsAg-positive ground glass cells, except for their resistance to orcein and aldehyde fuchsin staining (Fig. 142).

It should be noted that, occasionally, unexplained orcein-negative ground glass cells arc encountered in individuals who are not alcoholic, who have received no inducing drugs, and who exhibit no evidence of Lafora's disease or type IV glycogenosis.

Lafora bodies

Myoclonus epilepsy, or Lafora's disease, is an autosomal recessive hereditary disorder manifested by grand mal seizures that appear during adolescence and are followed by myoclonus and progressive dementia, leading ultimately to death within a few years. The nature of the underlying biochemical defect is not known, but the disease is characterized by the occurrence of distinctive inclusion bodies within the neurons of the central nervous system, the hepatocytes, and, less constantly, in skeletal, smooth muscle and myocardial fibers, and in the cells of other viscera. Since the inclusions occur with regularity in the hepatocytes, liver biopsy has proved to be an invaluable diagnostic tool in the identification of Lafora's disease (68).

In the liver, Lafora bodies are found in numerous periportal hepatocytes and, to a lesser extent in some cases, in midzonal and centrilobular cells. The affected cells are greatly enlarged, and are characterized by the presence of large, round or kidney-shaped, homogeneous or finely granular, faintly eosinophilic inclusions that displace the nuclei to the periphery, and, often, are encircled by a narrow, clear halo (Fig. 143). Although they resemble HBsAg-positive ground glass cells, they differ in that they resist staining with orcein and aldehyde fuchsin, show a striking zonal pattern of distribution, and are diastase-resistant, PAS-positive (Fig. 144). The inclusions lose their property of PAS-binding following digestion with pectinase, and give a strongly positive reaction with the Rinehart-Abul Haj reagent for acid mucopolysaccharide, histochemical features suggesting that they may contain an abnormal form of glycogen or other polysaccharide (68).

On electron microscopy, Lafora bodies appear as non-membrane-bound globular aggregates of randomly distributed, short branching filaments, and scattered deposits of electron dense material suggestive of lipofuscin bodies (68).

Lafora bodies are indistinguishable from the hepatic cytoplasmic inclusions of type IV glycogenosis on the basis of their histologic appearance, ultrastructure, and histochemical reactivity. However, it has been suggested that they may be differentiated on the basis of their staining properties with colloidal iron. Lafora bodies stain homogeneously, while glycogenosis IV inclusions appear craggy or dendritic in shape (68).

Pseudo-Lafora bodies

Inclusion bodies identical in all respects with Lafora bodies have been encountered in chronic alcoholic patients under treatment with disulfiram (Antabuse) (69) or cyanamide (70).

We have found similar pseudo-Lafora bodies in three patients with isoniazid-induced hepatitis. All three exhibited numerous large cytoplasmic inclusions that closely resembled orcein-negative ground glass cells or induction cells (Fig. 145). However, they behaved more like Lafora bodies in that they occurred in large numbers in a periportal zonal distribution, and were strongly PAS-positive following diastase digestion (Fig. 146). Unfortunately, material was not available for electron microscopy, so it was not established that the ultrastructure was identical with that of Lafora bodies, as in the case of the inclusions produced by disulfiram and cyanamide (69,70).

Orcein-negative ground glass cells have also been reported in patients receiving rifampicin (73). Since all of these patients were treated with isoniazid as well, it is conceivable that the inclusions were isoniazid-induced pseudo-Lafora bodies rather than induction cells. Unfortunately, neither the distribution of the inclusions nor their behavior on staining with PAS is described in the reported cases.

Fibrinogen-containing ground glass cells

Fibrinogen-containing ground glass cells indistinguishable from HBsAg ground glass cells have been reported (71, 71a; Figs. 147, 147A, 147B). These inclusions are negative for HBsAg and on PAS staining. They contain fibrinogen by immunohistochemical analysis (Fig. 147C). On electron microscopy the material is amorphous, fluffy or granular within the cisternae of the endoplasmic reticulum. Several histopathologic variants of these inclusion bodies have been observed (71A). Hepatocellular carcinoma cells also may have a variety of cytoplasmic inclusions, some of which resemble HBsAg-positive ground glass cells (see Chapter 25). These may contain fibrinogen (72) or α-1-fetoprotein.

Type IV glycogenosis inclusions

Type IV glycogenosis, also known as Andersen's disease and amylopectinosis, is an autosomal recessive inborn error of metabolism characterized by a deficiency of the glycogen branching enzyme that results in the deposition within the liver of an abnormal glycogen with few branch points and long outer chains that resemble amylopectin. The essential histologic features in the liver are the presence within the hepatocytes of distinctive cytoplasmic inclusions and a progressive portal fibrosis that usually leads to the development of cirrhosis (74)(Chapter 14).

Type IV glycogenosis inclusions closely resemble Lafora bodies histologically, and, characteristically, they are found in numerous enlarged, periportal and periseptal hepatocytes. They appear as large, non-membrane-bound, round or kidney-shaped, pale, homogeneous, or finely granular, faintly eosinophilic inclusions that displace the nuclei to the periphery of the cells and often are encircled by a narrow, clear halo (Fig. 148). In contrast to HBsAg-positive ground glass cells, for which they may be mistaken, glycogenosis IV inclusions do not stain with orcein or aldehyde fuchsin, show a periportal zonal distribution, and are diastase-resistant, PAS-positive (Fig. 149). However, their glycogen content is readily digested by pectinase, thereby abolishing their avidity for PAS (74).

On electron microscopy, the inclusions appear as non-membrane-bound globular masses of randomly arranged, branching filaments intermixed with occasional glycogen rosettes (74).

Cytoplasmic inclusions after bone marrow transplantation

Eosinophilic, cytoplasmic inclusions have been found at autopsy in 3 of 11 patients, 10 to 41 days after bone marrow transplantation (75). These inclusions, which were PAS-negative, did not contain iron, glycogen, lipids, alpha-fetoprotein, or α-1-antitrypsin (Fig. 150). By electron microscopy they contained granular material, but no organelles or virus particles were identified.

Large orcein-negative, PAS-negative cytoplasmic inclusions

On two occasions, we have encountered large cytoplasmic inclusions that resemble ground glass cells or Lafora bodies but differ from both in ultrastructure and in their failure to stain with orcein, aldehyde fuchsin, or PAS. On electron microscopy, the inclusions appear as large, round, sharply circumscribed, non-membrane-bound, punched-out areas filled with a minimally electron-dense, homogeneous material. In some, the contents are separated from the adjacent cytoplasm by an irregular, clear zone. Some of the inclusions contain a few, slender amorphous strands and small, round, electron-dense masses. As a rule, the hepatocytes contain one large inclusion, but, occasionally, multiple smaller inclusions are seen. Making allowances for the poor preservation of the postmortem specimens investigated, we found that the organelles in the unaffected portions of the cytoplasm appeared normal, and there was no evidence of a distinct membrane around the inclusions.

Both cases were encountered postmortem, one in an old man with a fungating carcinoma of the larynx that had been treated unsuccessfully with radiation, bleomycin, and methotrexate; the other was a stillborn infant whose death was unexplained. In neither case did the liver show abnormalities other than the presence of numerous cytoplasmic inclusions.

As shown in Figure 151, the inclusions are large and sharply circumscribed, occur in enlarged hepatocytes located predominantly in the periportal zones, and often displace the nucleus to the periphery of the cell. Usually, they are round, oval or kidney-shaped, and homogeneous in appearance. However, some are finely vacuolated, and, occasionally, two or more are present in a single cell. In H & E sections, they are pale pink, whereas in Masson-stained sections, they are faintly basophilic, appearing pale blue. As previously indicated, the inclusions are not stained by orcein, aldehyde fuchsin, or PAS.

The nature and significance of these inclusions is uncertain. In many respects, they resemble those found in rat livers following partial hepatectomy that have been attributed to the accumulation of serum protein as a result of altered hepatic hemodynamics (76). Similar PAS-negative cytoplasmic inclusions have been reported in human needle biopsy specimens of micronodular cirrhosis and progressive periportal fibrosis of unknown etiology (77). The inclusions in these cases were interpreted as proteinaceous and indicative of a defect in protein synthesis, secretion, or transport. However, they are found within dilated cisternae of rough endoplasmic reticulum, and thus differed from the cytoplasmic inclusions under discussion.

α_1-Antitrypsin, diastase-resistant, PAS-positive cytoplasmic inclusions

α_1-Antitrypsin (A_1AT) deficiency of the homozygous PiZZ or heterozygous PiMZ or SZ phenotypes, an autosomal dominant hereditary disorder, is almost always associated with the presence in the periportal hepatocytes of distinctive, diastase-resistant, PAS-positive, cytoplasmic inclusions. Often, these are accompanied by other changes in the liver, discussed more fully in Chapter 14. On electron microscopy, the inclusions appear as membrane-bound, moderately electron dense, amorphous deposits within dilated cisternae of the endoplasmic reticulum (78) and can be identified as A_1AT by the immunoperoxidase method (79).

In routine sections, A_1AT inclusions appear as lightly stained, homogeneous, acidophilic, cytoplasmic globules in periportal or periseptal hepatocytes (Fig. 152). When small, they may be difficult to identify in H & E sections, but often they are more readily visualized in Masson-stained sections. The globules

usually stain faint pink to red in H & E sections and bright orange-red in Masson sections. However, when minute, they may appear pale blue in Masson-stained sections. Characteristically, the inclusions stain brilliant red with PAS following diastase digestion (Fig. 153).

In noncirrhotic livers, the A_1AT inclusions are found almost exclusively in periportal hepatocytes. However, in cirrhotic lesions, they may be limited to periseptal cells or involve almost all the cells in individual nodules. Often, the involved hepatocytes are enlarged, but usually they appear otherwise normal. However, the inclusions may be encountered in degenerating hepatocytes in the case of active cirrhosis. Under such conditions, A_1AT inclusions occasionally are found lying free or within Kupffer cells, no doubt having been released from necrotic hepatocytes.

A_1AT inclusions vary greatly in size, ranging from 1 to 30 μm in diameter, but small inclusions are more common than large. When small, multiple inclusions frequently fill the entire cell. However, even when large, solitary inclusions are unusual. Often, the larger inclusions are surrounded by a clear halo, undoubtedly due to a fixation or embedding artifact.

A_1AT inclusions may be exceedingly difficult to identify in infants less than 12 weeks old (80), an important point to be considered in trying to establish the role of A_1AT deficiency as an etiologic factor in neonatal cholestasis. However, in one of our cases, the inclusions were demonstrable in D-PAS sections of liver in an infant aged 7 weeks. It has been suggested that the number and size of the inclusions increase with advancing age (81). However, even in adults, the inclusions may escape detection in D-PAS-stained sections, although, in some of these, the presence of A_1AT can be demonstrated by immunofluorescence (82).

Not all PAS-positive, diastase-resistant cytoplasmic inclusions are attributable to the accumulation of A_1AT (83). For that reason, confirmation is always essential, either by documenting a deficiency of A_1AT in the serum, or preferably, by demonstrating the presence in the inclusion of A_1AT by immunofluorescence or by the immunoperoxidase method or by monoclonal antibody (84). Unfortunately, immunofluorescence requires a fresh or formalin-fixed frozen section, which often is not available. However, A_1AT can be detected in formalin-fixed, paraffin-embedded sections by the immunoperoxidase method, and, hence, is readily applicable to routine biopsy material (83,85).

Cytoplasmic bile droplets are frequently diastase-resistant, PAS-positive, so that caution must be exercised in accepting diastase-resistant, PAS-positive cytoplasmic inclusions as evidence of A_1AT deficiency. In the face of overt cholestasis, such deficiency must be documented by measuring the serum level of A_1AT, or by demonstrating A_1AT in the inclusions by immunofluorescence or immunoperoxidase methods. This problem frequently arises in cases of neonatal cholestasis.

Non-α_1-antitrypsin, diastase-resistant, PAS-positive cytoplasmic inclusions

Diastase-resistant, PAS-positive cytoplasmic inclusions are occasionally encountered in individuals with no evidence of A_1AT deficiency (83). It has been reported that such inclusions are found in approximately 10% of routine autopsy specimens, and are almost invariably associated with centrilobular congestion and necrosis (85,86). However, based on our own experience, non-A₁AT diastase-resistant, PAS-positive cytoplasmic inclusions are relatively rare in biopsy material, and appear to be unrelated to centrilobular congestion and necrosis. The few cases we have encountered have occurred predominantly in alcoholic cirrhosis and, less commonly, in other lesions, including nonalcoholic fatty infiltration and portal fibrosis, and in a case of severe extramedullary hematopoiesis secondary to myelofibrosis. As shown in Figure 154, such inclusions are indistinguishable histologically from those due to A₁AT deficiency, and show the same periportal zonal distribution. However, in one of our cases, a nonalcoholic patient with mild portal fibrosis and fatty infiltration and rare Mallory bodies (34), the inclusions were centrilobular in location.

Hepatocellular erythrophagocytosis

In animals, a number of hepatotoxins give rise to both hepatocellular injury and erythrophagocytosis (87). Many years ago, it was reported that similar hepatocellular erythrophagocytosis could be demonstrated at autopsy in patients with either obstructive or hepatocellular cholestasis (88). To our knowledge this observation has not been reported in biopsy material. However, we have seen hepatocellular erythrophagocytosis in liver biopsy sections of five patients. The underlying hepatic lesions included hepatocellular carcinoma in two cases; and one case each of moderately active acute alcoholic hepatitis (Fig. 155), precirrhotic Wilson's disease, and an unusual form of acute, anicteric, HBsAg-negative hepatitis associated with toxemia of pregnancy. Of interest, none of these cases was associated with jaundice or histologic evidence of cholestasis. In all these cases, one or more erythrocytes were encountered within cytoplasmic vacuoles, so that artifactual displacement of the erythrocytes from the sinusoids could be excluded. Only a few of the hepatocytes in each case contained such inclusions.

Hepatocellular cytoplasmic granules and pigments

Hepatocellular lipofuscin

Lipofuscin, a pigment of variable composition found in the lysosomes of the hepatocytes, is an oxidation product of various lipids and lipoproteins. Although its histochemical behavior may vary, lipofuscin usually is diastase-resistant, PAS-positive, often reacts with acid-fast, silver and lipid stains, and may exhibit autofluorescence, appearing bright golden-yellow in unstained sections. A similar, if not identical pigment, classified by some as *ceroid*, may be encountered in Kupffer and other phagocytic cells. Since ceroid cannot be distinguished from lipofuscin histochemically, and since it often appears to be derived from the lipofuscin released by necrotic hepatocytes, there does not appear to be any reason for differentiating between the two.

As previously indicated in Chapter 2, the centrilobular hepatocytes of the normal liver often contain a variable number of fine, yellow-brown lipofuscin granules. Because of their lysosomal location in the cytoplasm, the granules usually appear to be aggregated along the course of the canaliculi (Figs. 10, 11). Although they are rare before the age of 15 and increase

up to the age of 30, they do not increase thereafter (89), so that they cannot be regarded as a "wear and tear" pigment of aging. What factors are responsible for the variations in the number of lipofuscin granules in the normal liver is not known. With a few notable exceptions, hepatocellular injury leads to diminution or loss of such granules (89).

In general, lipofuscin granules, even when numerous, have no diagnostic or prognostic significance when limited to the centrilobular hepatocytes. However, their occurrence in midzonal or periportal hepatocytes is usually indicative of disease.

In Wilson's disease, the periportal hepatocytes often contain coarse, irregularly shaped lipofuscin granules (Fig. 156). Although these may be found at any stage of the disease, they occur most frequently in advanced cirrhotic lesions (90). Usually, the periportal hepatocytes that contain lipofuscin also contain granules that react with rhodanine and rubeanic acid, indicating the presence of copper. However, the number and distribution of the lipofuscin and copper-stained granules in any group of cells often differ, so that it is unlikely that all of the lysosomes visualized always contain both pigments.

Similar, coarse lipofuscin granules ave been encountered in the midzonal and, less commonly, the periportal and centrilobular hepatocytes of individuals who have taken excessive amounts of phenacetin, amidopyrine, or acetylsalicylic acid over a prolonged period (91). Widespread deposition of pigment granules resembling lipofuscin has been observed at autopsy in the hepatocytes, Kupffer cells, dermis, reticuloendothelial system, and in many of the other viscera in young adults who have received large doses of chlorpromazine for several years (92,93).

Periportal cytoplasmic bile droplets may mimic lipofuscin granules. However, as a rule, such droplets are associated with other evidence of cholestasis, such as canalicular bile thrombi, but if the differentiation from lipofuscin is uncertain, especially when both pigments may be present, a special stain for bile may be needed.

Hepatocellular Dubin-Johnson pigment

The Dubin-Johnson syndrome, an autosomal recessive hereditary disorder (94), is characterized by a defect in the hepatic excretion of conjugated bilirubin and the accumulation within the cytoplasm of the hepatocytes of coarse, dark brown, pigment granules (95). The pathogenesis and manifestations of the disease are discussed more fully in Chapter 17.

Characteristically in the Dubin-Johnson syndrome, the cytoplasm of the centrilobular hepatocytes contains numerous large, round or irregularly shaped, dark brown granules (Fig. 157). Rarely, similar granules are found in occasional Kupffer cells, presumably as a result of phagocytosis of pigment released from destroyed hepatocytes. Except for their larger size and deeper brown color and the associated clinical and biochemical features of the disease, the pigment granules of the Dubin-Johnson syndrome closely resemble lipofuscin (95). Both are found within lysosomes (96) and exhibit similar histochemical properties, including inconstant diastase-resistant, PAS-positivity, acid-fastness, and insolubility in a wide variety of polar and nonpolar solvents (95). However, differences in ultrastructure (96) and staining reactions (97) have been reported. These have led to the suggestion that the pigment granules of the Dubin-Johnson syndrome contain melanin. The demonstration of persistent melanuria in a reported case (97) lends some support to this possibility. Also, the pigment isolated from the livers of mutant Corriedale sheep with black liver disease, a disorder similar to the Dubin-Johnson syndrome, exhibits physicochemical properties identical with those of melanin (98). Studies in these animals have suggested that the accumulation of the pigment in the liver may be attributable to a defect in the excretion of epinephrine metabolites (98). In a study of our own (89), pigment isolated from an autopsy specimen of liver in a case of Dubin-Johnson syndrome exhibited identical physicochemical properties, including melting point, solubility, and visible ultraviolet and infrared absorption spectra, with those of DOPA melanin and melanin isolated from a transplantable hamster melanoma. However, using the same techniques, the Dubin-Johnson pigment was indistinguishable from lipofuscin isolated from autopsy specimens of normal liver. Although the apparent identity of the two pigments may account for the overlap of their histochemical properties, it does not follow that lipofuscin and Dubin-Johnson granules are necessarily identical in chemical composition, structure, or origin. In this connection, it should be noted that both types of granule contain not only pigment but also lipid and protein components that have not been characterized. These may be differentiated by electron microscopic examination (99,100).

Cytoplasmic bile droplets may mimic Dubin-Johnson pigment granules. However, they are usually associated with canalicular bile thrombi, a feature not seen in the Dubin-Johnson syndrome. In case of doubt, it is wise to use a special stain for bile to differentiate between the two types of pigment.

Hepatocellular hemosiderin

Normal hepatocytes contain iron as ferritin in the form of micelles of ferric hydroxyphosphate enclosed within a shell of apoferritin protein subunits. On electron microscopy, these can be identified as distinctive particles dispersed through the cytosol and lysosomes (101). Because of their small size and wide dispersion they cannot be visualized in normal hepatocytes by light microscopy or demonstrated by special staining.

Under a variety of conditions that lead to excessive storage of iron, hemosiderin granules may appear in the cytoplasm of the hepatocytes and, in some instances, the Kupffer cells, portal macrophages, and the epithelial cells of bile ducts and ductules. Characteristically, these stain deep blue when treated with acidified potassium ferrocyanide, giving what is generally termed the Prussian blue reaction. On electron microscopy, the hemosiderin granules are found within lysosomes and are made up of aggregated ferritin particles, apparently stripped of their apoprotein coats and occasionally organized in crystalline arrays. In addition, hemosiderin granules contain other forms of ferric iron, possibly bound to polysaccharides that are present, and a variable amount of protein that resembles apoprotein in structure. Often, the granules also contain lipofuscin. Under conditions of iron overload, the cytoplasm of the hepatocytes contains not only lysosomal hemosiderin granules but also numerous ferritin particles dispersed through the cytosol and lysosomes (101).

The occurrence of stainable iron in the liver is usually classified as *hemosiderosis* or *siderosis,* but when associated with progressive portal fibrosis leading to the development of cirrhosis, is categorized as *hemochromatosis.* However, until the cirrhosis has developed, it may be difficult on histologic grounds

alone to distinguish between the two. Since, in the early stages of hemochromatosis, there may be little or no fibrosis, some forms of hemosiderosis are associated with nonprogressive portal fibrosis (102). Recent studies have shown unequivocally that the measurement of hepatic iron concentration when corrected for age can differentiate hemosiderosis in the alcoholic patient from early hemochromatosis, and that there exists a threshold for hepatic iron above which fibrosis is likely to be found (103). Occasionally, hemosiderosis is superimposed on an underlying, unrelated cirrhosis.

The genetic, endogenous and exogenous factors responsible for iron overload, and the types of hepatic lesions they produce are discussed more fully in Chapter 12.

In H & E sections, hemosiderin appears as relatively coarse, greenish-brown granules with sharply defined, refractile edges. Because of their location within lysosomes, they tend to be aggregated along the course of the canaliculi (Fig. 158). The granules vary greatly in size and number, and when small and sparse may be overlooked in routine sections, particularly if the sections are deeply stained. However, even when minute, they are readily visualized as deep blue granules when treated with acidified potassium ferrocyanide in the Prussian blue reaction (Fig. 159). Not infrequently, when the hemosiderosis is extensive, the nongranular portions of the cytoplasm also react, appearing pale blue in color (Fig. 159). This is attributable to the presence of numerous ferritin granules dispersed through the cytosol.

Another but less constant histochemical feature of hemosiderin is its reactivity with PAS following diastase digestion, a property probably attributable to its content of polysaccharide (104) and, in some instances, to the lipofuscin with which it may be associated. Usually, cytoplasmic hemosiderin granules are only weakly D-PAS-positive. However, the granules in adjacent Kupffer cells and in portal macrophages, which tend to be very much larger, almost always stain brilliantly in the D-PAS reaction (Fig. 160).

Characteristically, the deposition of hemosiderin in hepatocytes, irrespective of its etiology, occurs predominantly in the periportal zones. This zonal pattern of distribution persists in both hemosiderosis and hemochromatosis (Fig. 161), although it may be partially obscured in the latter as progressive deposition of hemosiderin tends to involve most, if not all of the hepatocytes.

Often, when the deposition is extensive, particularly in the case of hemochromatosis, exceptionally coarse hemosiderin granules are found in clusters of enlarged Kupffer cells (Fig. 162) and in portal macrophages. This is presumably due to the phagocytosis of pigment released from hepatocytes that have undergone dissolution. However, under some conditions, such as posttransfusional hemosiderosis and certain hemolytic states, the Kupffer cells are the principal primary sites of hemosiderin deposition, although, in time, there is a tendency for some of the pigment to shift to the hepatocytes. Hemosiderin may also be found in the epithelial cells of bile ducts and ductules. This occurs with regularity in all forms of hemochromatosis, but only rarely in other types of extensive hemosiderosis (Chapter 12).

In H & E sections, sparse deposits of small hemosiderin granules may be mistaken for lipofuscin. Although the Prussian blue reaction unequivocally distinguishes between the two, differentiation is almost always possible without special staining. Characteristically, hemosiderin granules are coarse and variable in size, have a pale greenish hue, are refractile on focusing, and are found predominantly in periportal hepatocytes, whereas lipofuscin granules tend to be small and uniform in size, are light brown in color and nonrefractile (Fig. 11), and are usually localized to the centrilobular hepatocytes (Fig. 10).

Hepatocellular copper

Deposits of copper in hepatocytes, even when excessive, are not visualized in routine sections. Under some conditions, however, particularly when the copper is concentrated in lysosomes, it can be demonstrated histochemically. Of the two stains used for this purpose, 5-p-dimethyl-aminobenzylidene rhodanine (rhodanine) is more sensitive and specific than rubeanic acid.

Copper absorbed from the intestinal tract is transported to the tissues bound to serum albumin. Most of the copper is taken up by the liver, where a significant fraction is utilized in the synthesis of ceruloplasmin. Some of the ceruloplasmin is secreted into the plasma, and most of the remainder into bile. Available evidence suggest that this turnover of ceruloplasmin accounts for the zero copper balance in normal individuals (105).

The copper content of the normal liver is less than 100 μg/g of dry weight. Two-thirds of the copper is present in the cytosol bound to two proteins with molecular weights of 10,000 and 40,000, respectively, while the remainder is found in mitochondria, lysosomes, and nuclei. Because of its low concentration and dispersed state, the copper in normal hepatocytes is not demonstrable histochemically (105).

In Wilson's disease and several other types of chronic liver disease, especially primary biliary cirrhosis and other chronic cholestatic states, copper accumulates in the liver and often is detectable histochemically, particularly when concentrated in lysosomes. The retention of copper in the case of Wilson's disease appears to be due to a defect in hepatocellular lysosomes that blocks the normal biliary excretion of copper (105,106). In forms of liver disease characterized by chronic cholestasis, such as primary biliary cirrhosis, the accumulation of copper is also attributable to impairment of its excretion in bile, but, in this instance, the latter is only one expression of a more generalized defect in bile secretion. The pathogenesis of the unusual type of hepatic copper overload seen in Indian childhood cirrhosis is not known, but it does not appear to be dependent on chronic cholestasis (107). There is a close correlation, however, between the amount of bile duct loss and the hepatic copper concentration (108).

It has been suggested that copper may be hepatotoxic when diffusely distributed through the cytoplasm, but not when segregated in lysosomes (105). A number of observations, including the innocuous character of the lysosomal copper deposits in the newborn, and the sequence of events in the development of the hepatic lesions in Wilson's disease, are consistent with this view.

Not infrequently, the accumulation of copper in the liver is accompanied by the deposition of coarse, orcein-positive protein granules. These are discussed in the following section.

In the early presymptomatic phase of Wilson's disease, the copper content of the liver is invariably increased. At this stage, the copper is dispersed predominantly through the cytosol of the hepatocytes, so that often it cannot be detected histochemically. However, as the lesions advance, more and more of the copper tends to concentrate in the lysosomes, so that it can be visualized on staining with rhodanine. Characteristically, the copper-containing lysosomes appear as bright red, coarse granules, almost exclusively localized in periportal hepatocytes (Fig. 163). Not all periportal zones are affected, however, so that granules may escape detection, particularly in needle biopsy specimens. When the lesions have advanced to the stage of cirrhosis, the copper-containing granules tend to aggregate in hepatocytes bordering both fibrous septa and intact portal tracts. However, many of the nodules, particularly those that show evidence of regenerative activity and are presumably made up of younger cells, show no stainable copper (90). Usually, the cytoplasm devoid of copper *granules* fails to take up any of the rhodanine stain, even though it is overloaded with copper. However, in the case of advanced Wilson's disease with overt jaundice of only four weeks' duration illustrated in Figure 163, the cytoplasm of the hepatocytes in some of the nodules was stained light pink, presumably due to its high content of copper. This has not been reported previously in Wilson's disease, but is known to occur in Indian childhood cirrhosis (109). It is noteworthy that as the copper in the hepatocytes shifts from the cytosol into the lysosomes in the late stage of Wilson's disease, a good deal of copper leaves the liver and is deposited in other tissues, particularly the central nervous system, kidneys, and eyes, where it allegedly produces the changes responsible for the extrahepatic manifestations of the disease (105).

For a more complete discussion of the pathogenesis, manifestations, and hepatic lesions of Wilson's disease, the reader is referred to Chapter 13.

In various forms of chronic cholestasis, and particularly primary biliary cirrhosis, copper-containing, rhodanine-positive granules, identical in appearance with those of Wilson's disease, are often demonstrable in the periportal or paraseptal hepatocytes (110). According to some authorities (109), the periportal distribution of the granules is more uniform in primary biliary cirrhosis than in Wilson's disease, but that has not been the case in our experience or that of others (110). However, the subcellular distribution of copper appears to differ in the two conditions, a much higher proportion being found in the supernatant fraction in the case of primary biliary cirrhosis (111).

Rhodanine-stained granules are said to occur in a high proportion of patients with primary biliary cirrhosis and to be of value in differentiating this disorder from other forms of chronic liver disease (110). In our experience, however, such granules are an inconstant feature of primary biliary cirrhosis, tending to occur chiefly in advanced lesions. Moreover, similar granules, although generally fewer in number, are often found in other forms of chronic liver disease, such as chronic active hepatitis, postnecrotic cirrhosis, and alcoholic cirrhosis, particularly when accompanied by chronic cholestasis, so that, on the whole, we have found the presence of rhodanine-positive granules of little or no value in the differential diagnosis of hepatic lesions.

For a more complete discussion of primary biliary cirrhosis, the reader is referred to Chapter 11.

Remarkably high concentrations of hepatic copper are found in Indian childhood cirrhosis, a disorder of unknown etiology that occurs between the ages of one and five years and affects males predominantly. Characteristically, numerous clusters of large and small rhodanine-positive granules are present in the cytoplasm of most hepatocytes and in occasional macrophages (109). In addition, the cytoplasm itself is often stained by the rhodanine because of its high copper content. Some of the large rhodanine-positive granular clusters contain lipofuscin, and, occasionally, the Mallory bodies often found in this disease are surrounded by fine copper granules or are stained by the rhodanine (109,112). The pathogenesis of the copper overload in this condition is poorly understood. Since cholestasis is often absent, or occurs only terminally, it is unlikely that the retention of copper is attributable solely to impairment of bile flow. Two alternative possibilities that have been suggested are that it may be due to an underlying, genetically determined abnormality of copper metabolism that differs from that of Wilson's disease (109), or that it may be attributable to an excessive intake of copper in the form of drinking water, Indian native medicines, or foods cooked in tinned-copper vessels (107). For a more complete discussion of Indian childhood cirrhosis, the reader is referred to Chapter 11.

Hepatocellular orcein-positive copper-protein granules

Under conditions of excessive copper deposition, the cytoplasm of the hepatocytes often contains granules that appear dark brown or black in orcein-stained sections. They also stain with aldehyde fuchsin, but cannot be visualized in routine H & E or Masson sections, and do not take up D-PAS, iron, bile, or melanin stains (113). Based on their histochemical reactions, the granules appear to be copper-protein complexes linked by sulfhydryl and disulfide bonds. In addition, many of the granules contain lipofuscin, as evidenced by their reaction with Schmorl's stain (109). On electron microscopy, the orcein-positive granules are found within large lysosomes or autophagic vacuoles (114).

Orcein-positive cytoplasmic granules are seen most commonly in primary biliary cirrhosis (110), but also occur in Wilson's disease (110), Indian childhood cirrhosis (109,115), and less commonly, in chronic active hepatitis, postnecrotic cirrhosis, and extrahepatic biliary obstruction (116). Although the occurrence of the granules appears to be related, in some unknown way, to cholestasis, they may be found in nonicteric individuals with no histologic evidence of cholestasis.

Following staining with orcein, the granules appear as dark brown or black cytoplasmic deposits of variable shape and size, which often show a perinuclear distribution (Fig. 164). They are usually found in periportal hepatocytes, but in cirrhotic livers they may be limited to the periphery or involve most or all of the hepatocytes in some of the nodules. Although the distribution of orcein-positive granules is similar to that of the rhodanine-stained, copper-containing granules, the two often differ, one or the other type of granule predominating.

As in the case of copper-containing granules, it has been suggested that orcein-positive granules are a useful histologic feature in the differential diagnosis of primary biliary cirrhosis (117). However, in our own experience, such granules are encountered principally in advanced lesions. In early lesions when the differentiation is most difficult, their occurrence is no more frequent than in many other chronic hepatobiliary disorders.

Cytoplasmic bile droplets often stain deep brown with orcein, and may be mistaken for copper-protein granules. However, bile droplets are readily visualized in H & E and Masson-stained sections, and are usually accompanied by canalicular bile thrombi. In cases where both cytoplasmic bile droplets and copper-protein deposits may be present, staining of an adjacent section for bile is required to distinguish between the two.

Large lipofuscin granules in Kupffer cells and portal macrophages also stain dark brown with orcein, but these are not likely to be mistaken for copper-protein complexes, since they are readily visualized in H & E sections.

Hepatocellular bile droplets

Under conditions of moderate to severe cholestasis of either obstructive or hepatocellular origin, the cytoplasm of hepatocytes occasionally contains bile droplets. These appear yellow or brown in H & E sections, and brown or green in Masson-stained sections, and usually are accompanied by other histologic evidence of cholestasis. However, as shown in Figure 165, cytoplasmic bile droplets may be encountered in the absence of bile thrombi in either the canaliculi or Kupffer cells. Under such conditions, particularly when the droplets are centrilobular in location, they may be mistaken for Dubin-Johnson pigment granules. However, they tend to be lighter in color in formalin-fixed sections, often show a greenish hue after Carnoy's fixation, and appear green when stained for bile by Hall's method.

In some cases, cytoplasmic bile droplets are found in periportal hepatocytes. Since they often are PAS-positive after diastase digestion, they may be mistaken for α_1-antitrypsin deposits. Their color, however, in H & E sections is different. The real problem in differentiation arises when α_1-antitrypsin deficiency is suspected in a case of severe neonatal cholestasis. In such cases, the presence of periportal D-PAS-positive deposits should not be interpreted as evidence of α_1-antitrypsin deficiency, unless the latter is confirmed by the finding of a low serum level of the enzyme, or, preferably, by demonstrating the presence of the enzyme within the droplets by the immunofluorescence or immunoperoxidase method.

Cytoplasmic bile droplets often stain dark brown with orcein, and, thus, may mimic the copper-protein deposits seen in chronic cholestasis. However, in contrast to the latter, the former are always readily visualized in routine H & E sections.

Hepatocellular protoporphyrin

Erythropoietic protoporphyria, an autosomal dominant hereditary disorder, is characterized by a deficiency of heme synthetase (ferrochelatase), the enzyme that catalyzes the chelation of ferrous iron to protoporphyrin in the pathway of heme synthesis in the bone marrow and liver. This results in an accumulation of protoporphyrin in marrow normoblasts, circulating reticulocytes, and in Kupffer cells and macrophages in the liver. In the liver, the accumulation of protoporphyrin may lead to hepatocellular degeneration and necrosis, portal fibrosis and inflammation, pigment stone formation, and, less commonly, to bile stasis and the development of a unique type of progressive biliary cirrhosis that almost always proves fatal (118,119). The manifestations of the disease and the histologic features of the hepatic lesions are described more fully in Chapter 18.

When abundant, the protoporphyrin is diffusely distributed throughout the cytoplasm of the hepatocytes, and can be identified in fresh frozen sections by the brilliant red color it emits when examined by fluorescence microscopy, using a Schott B.C. 12 exciter filter (330–500 nm) and a barrier filter that excludes light with wavelengths below 530 nm (Fig. 166). With lesser amounts of protoporphyrin, red fluorescence may be limited to focal pigment deposits. Indeed, such deposits occasionally exhibit red fluorescence in unstained, paraffin-embedded sections. Characteristically, when a mercury vapor lamp is used as the source of ultraviolet light, the red fluorescence of protoporphyrin fades rapidly, usually within 30 to 60 seconds.

This can be obviated by using an iodine-tungsten quartz lamp, which has the virtue of permitting colored microphotography (120). However, by using high speed color film, Ektachrome 400 processed for an ASA rating of 800, and a 15 second exposure, we have had no difficulty in photographing protoporphyrin fluorescence with a mercury vapor light source (Fig. 166).

In routine H & E sections, hepatocellular protoporphyrin appears in the form of coarse, dark brown cytoplasmic granules (Fig. 167). Characteristically, these are birefringent, exhibiting a brilliant gold or red color in polarized light (Fig. 168). This is a pathognomonic feature of protoporphyrin granules and obviates the need for a frozen section (121). Almost always, large and more numerous granules are present in Kupffer cells and portal macrophages and in advanced cases with biliary cirrhosis. These may be globular, and often are found within dilated canaliculi, where they may resemble bile thrombi (Fig. 169). Characteristically, such large, globular Kupffer cell and canalicular deposits appear bright red with a dark central Maltese cross in polarized light (Fig. 170). Although the protoporphyrin deposits are easily visualized and exhibit intense birefringence in H & E or unstained sections, they lose their birefringence in Masson-stained sections. However, the type of fixative employed, such as formalin, Carnoy's, Bouin's, or Zenker's solution, has no effect on the color or birefringence of the pigment (121).

On electron microscopy, the deposits of protoporphyrin in the hepatocytes and canaliculi appear as large, non-membrane-bound arrays of slender, electron-dense, radiating crystals that resemble chrysanthemums, or as masses of randomly distributed bar-like crystals of varying size and shape lying free in the cytoplasm. However, in the Kupffer cells, the crystals, which are long and slender with a hollow core and tapered tips, are found randomly distributed within lysosomes (119,121).

Other hepatocellular cytoplasmic deposits

Fatty infiltration

The liver plays an important role in lipid metabolism. Thus, the hepatocytes take up free fatty acids mobilized from adipose tissue and transported to the liver bound to serum albumin. They incorporate fatty acids split from the triglycerides in chylomicrons of dietary origin, synthesize fatty acids from two-carbon fragments derived from carbohydrate, oxidize some fatty acids to carbon dioxide and water, esterify others to triglyceride, and secrete triglyceride combined with cholesterol and phospholipid in the form of very low density lipoprotein (VLDL). The complex enzymatic reactions involved in this chain of events are under hormonal control and can be modified by dietary factors and extrahepatic metabolic events (122).

The lipid content of the liver is normally less than 5% of its wet weight, and little or no lipid can be visualized histologically in routinely stained, paraffin-embedded sections. However, under a wide variety of conditions leading to the accumulation of lipid, chiefly in the form of triglyceride, droplets of fat of variable size and distribution appear in the cytoplasm of the hepatocytes. Since these are solubilized during the embedding process, they cannot be stained, and present as clear vacuoles. In fresh or formalin-fixed frozen sections, however,

they can be visualized with a number of lipid stains, such as oil red O. Except in rare instances, particularly when minute lipid droplets fill the cytoplasm giving it a foamy appearance that may mimic other conditions (Figs. 115, 116), special stains are not needed for identification.

As indicated previously, fatty infiltration is usually a benign lesion indicative of an alteration in hepatic lipid uptake, metabolism or export, and does not necessarily imply underlying hepatocellular injury. However, under some conditions, the affected hepatocytes not only contain fat droplets but also show cytoplasmic degenerative changes and are associated with evidence of hepatic dysfunction. Such lesions are often classified as fatty degeneration. However, the distinction between fatty infiltration and fatty degeneration is regarded by some as artificial and unnecessary. In this connection, it should be noted that under some conditions, the fat-filled, but otherwise normal hepatocytes are accompanied by other cells that show degenerative changes or necrosis that appear to be unrelated to the deposition of lipid. This is well illustrated in the case of alcoholic hepatitis, a lesion in which the fat-filled cells are usually associated with foci of cell dropout and with hepatocytes that are ballooned and contain Mallory bodies (Fig. 90).

Fatty infiltration is by far the most common abnormality encountered in the liver. Chronic alcoholism, obesity, and diabetes mellitus are the most common causes, but fatty infiltration also occurs under a wide variety of other conditions. These include, among others, protein malnutrition of dietary or of malabsorptive origin, chronic infection, wasting diseases, and a number of hereditary metabolic disorders, such as Wilson's disease, some forms of glycogenosis, galactosemia, and others discussed in Chapters 13, 14, 15, and 16.

The mechanisms responsible for abnormal accumulations of fat include increased delivery of fatty acids to the liver, enhanced hepatic synthesis of fatty acids, impairment of fatty acid oxidation in the liver, and a block in the hepatic synthesis or secretion of VLDL. The pathogenesis of some forms of fatty infiltration has been elucidated, but in most instances remains unknown. However, from what has been learned thus far, it is apparent that multiple mechanisms may be involved (Chapter 15).

The size and distribution of the lipid droplets in fatty infiltration vary considerably, and only rarely afford any clue to the underlying etiology. Large lipid droplets are more common than small. Often, the cytoplasm of the affected hepatocyte is almost completely occupied by a large single vacuole that displaces the nucleus and remaining cytoplasm to the periphery and leads to enlargement of the cell (Fig. 171). The nucleus often appears elongated and flattened. When the lipid droplets in adjacent cells are exceptionally large, they are separated by slender septa made up of cytoplasmic components and the plasma membranes of the two cells. Occasionally, such septa appear to be disrupted (Fig. 171), but almost certainly this is an artifact of processing rather than an early stage of fat cyst formation (see later). When the fatty infiltration is extensive and the hepatocytes are significantly enlarged, the sinusoids are compressed and may be difficult to identify.

In some cases, the cytoplasm of the hepatocytes contains a variable number of small lipid droplets. Even when numerous, these do not often displace the nucleus from its normal location or lead to significant enlargement of the cells (Fig. 172).

Most commonly, fatty infiltration affects the centrilobular hepatocytes predominantly (Fig. 173). However, occasionally, its distribution is exclusively periportal (Fig. 174) or panlobular

(Fig. 175). In addition, the lipid droplets may be randomly distributed, particularly when fatty infiltration is mild.

Large *extracellular* globules of lipid are occasionally encountered in areas of fatty infiltration. Characteristically, these are encircled by histiocytes and lymphocytes (Fig. 176), and less commonly, by a few eosinophils, epithelioid cells, and giant cells. When cut tangentially so that the lipid core is not visualized, such lesions may mimic other types of epithelioid granulomas. Based on observations in choline-deficient rats, it has been suggested that these lesions represent *fat cysts* formed by fusion of large lipid droplets in adjacent hepatocytes, that the surrounding cells are atrophic, altered hepatocytes rather than histiocytes, and that following loss of lipid from the cysts, their walls collapse, leading to the development of the fibrosis seen in choline deficiency (123,124). Considering that the extracellular lipid droplets are no larger in size than those within the adjacent hepatocytes (Fig. 176), and that such structures often disappear without a trace as the fatty infiltration recedes, it is highly improbable that they represent fat cysts or are responsible for the development of fibrosis, at least in the type of fatty infiltration seen in man.

Intralobular extracellular lipid collections surrounded by histiocytes and lymphocytes have also been classified as *lipogranulomas* (125). It has been suggested that these may coalesce and undergo fibrosis, an observation we have not been able to confirm. However, we have frequently encountered another type of lipogranuloma that does show fibrosis, but appears to bear no relationship to fatty infiltration. These occur both in normal livers and in association with a wide variety of apparently unrelated hepatic lesions. Characteristically, this type of lipogranuloma presents as a sharply circumscribed nodule of variable size attached to the wall of a central vein, particularly at bifurcation points, and contains a mixture of lipid droplets, histiocytes, some of which may be finely vacuolated, a few lymphocytes, and strands of collagen (Fig. 177). Of 184 such lesions in our series, only 42% were associated with lipid droplets in the hepatocytes, and then often in only small numbers. Less commonly, similar but less sharply circumscribed lesions are encountered in portal tracts (Fig. 178). Available evidence suggests that both the central and portal lipogranulomas of this type are attributable to the deposition of mineral oil rather than triglyceride, and that the source of this lipid is the mineral oil widely used in commercial baking of bread, the spraying of fruits and vegetables destined for long distance transportation, and the manufacture of wrapping materials used in packaging food (126–129).

In only a few forms of fatty infiltration and degeneration is the pattern of lipid deposition distinctive. In kwashiorkor, a form of protein malnutrition in young children, numerous fine lipid droplets characteristically are found within the periportal hepatocytes initially, but later extend to the midzonal and centrilobular cells as the disease progresses (130,131). Similar, small, lipid droplets are seen in the acute fatty liver of pregnancy and in several forms of toxic hepatitis, such as that induced by excessive intravenous doses of tetracycline, but characteristically these involve the centrilobular and midzonal hepatocytes. In Reye's syndrome, the distinctive feature is the presence of fine lipid droplets in a panlobular distribution.

Fatty infiltration is a reversible process, unless it is accompanied by hepatocellular degeneration and necrosis, as in alcoholic hepatitis. However, the question of whether or not uncomplicated fatty infiltration ever gives rise to fibrosis is still debatable, and is discussed more fully in Chapters 9 and 10.

Cholesterol ester deposits

In some forms of fatty infiltration, the lipid deposits contain not only triglycerides but also cholesterol and cholesterol esters. These can be visualized as birefringent, needle-like crystals on polarization microscopy of fresh or formalin-fixed frozen sections stained with oil red O, and can be identified histochemically by the Schultz modification of the Lieberman-Burchard reaction.

Deposits of cholesterol esters are encountered most frequently in *Wolman's disease* and *cholesterol ester storage disease,* two similar, but distinct hereditary disorders of infants and children, characterized by a severe deficiency of lysosomal acid cholesterol ester hydrolase and acid triglyceride lipase that leads to an accumulation of cholesterol esters and triglycerides in many of the tissues, including the liver (132). Occasionally, similar, but less numerous needle-like birefringent crystals, presumably cholesterol esters, may be encountered in other forms of fatty infiltration. In our experience, these have occurred in several cases of Reye's syndrome, and in a young infant with fatal, familial, neonatal hepatic steatosis (133).

In *Wolman's disease* (134,135) most of the hepatocytes and many of the Kupffer cells and portal macrophages are distended with fine lipid droplets, giving their cytoplasm a foamy appearance (Fig. 179). In frozen sections, the droplets take up lipid stains, such as oil red O and Sudan red, and contain numerous birefringent crystals that can be visualized in polarized light (Fig. 180).

The histologic features of the hepatic lesions in cholesterol ester storage disease (136) are almost identical to those in Wolman's disease, except that the crystals are found predominantly in the hepatocytes.

Glycogen depletion and abnormal storage states

Histologic assessment of the content and distribution of glycogen in the liver is possible in Carnoy's-fixed sections stained with PAS but is only semiquantitative. Aqueous fixatives, such as formalin, solubilize and thus artifactually deplete the liver of its glycogen content. However, when abnormally large amounts are stored, these may still be demonstrable histologically even after prolonged formalin fixation.

As previously indicated, the cytoplasm of the hepatocytes in healthy, well-nourished individuals is normally filled with uniformly distributed glycogen granules (Fig. 12).

Glycogen depletion is a nonspecific response to many types of hepatocellular injury. In the case of acute viral hepatitis, such depletion, which may be accompanied by fasting hypoglycemia, appears to be due to impairment of hepatic glycogen synthesis and gluconeogenesis (137). As shown in Figure 181, the reduction in hepatic glycogen in that disorder is attributable not only to the loss of hepatocytes but also to the depletion of glycogen in otherwise normal-appearing, intact cells. The pathogenesis of the glycogen depletion in other forms of hepatocellular injury is less well understood.

Excessive hepatic *glycogen storage* is a distinctive feature in several types of hereditary glycogenosis, but also occurs as an acquired anomaly, most commonly in diabetes mellitus under treatment with large doses of insulin.

The enzymatic defect and the chemical structure of the glycogen in *Types I and II glycogenosis* differ (see Chapter 14). However, the histologic appearance of the hepatocytes is identical in both. Characteristically, almost all of the hepatocytes are greatly swollen, tightly packed together, and outlined by relatively straight, sharply angulated, prominent, plasma membranes, thereby obscuring the sinusoids and producing a striking mosaic pattern (Fig. 182). Their cytoplasm is unusually pale and contains numerous fine vacuoles separated by slender, beaded strands. Most of the nuclei retain their normal central location, but appear unusually small for the size of the cells. However, the periportal hepatocytes often contain relatively large, vacuolated glycogen nuclei. In PAS-stained sections, the glycogen appears as coarse clumps and strands of smaller granules (Fig. 183) that correspond to the beaded strands outlining the vacuoles seen in H & E and Masson-stained sections (Fig. 182). Portal fibrosis that may progress to cirrhosis is a feature of *Type III glycogenosis,* but is usually absent or only minimal in *Type I glycogenosis.* On electron microscopy, the cytoplasm in both types shows an increase in uniformly distributed glycogen particles that displace the intracellular organelles (138).

In *Type II glycogenosis,* the hepatocytes are only minimally enlarged and do not show the mosaic pattern seen in Types I and III. Characteristically, the cytoplasm contains small vacuoles filled with PAS-positive material, corresponding on electron microscopy to aggregated glycogen particles enclosed within lysosomes (138).

In *Type IV glycogenosis,* the hepatocytes contain deposits of an abnormal glycogen that is diastase-resistant but can be digested by pectinase. These large D-PAS-positive inclusions closely resemble Lafora bodies [(68); Figs. 148, 149].

Acquired glycogenosis is seen most frequently in individuals with moderate to severe diabetes mellitus under treatment with large doses of insulin. However, it is also encountered occasionally in patients with no evidence of diabetes mellitus or hereditary glycogenosis. The appearance of the glycogen-loaded hepatocytes in the *acquired* form of glycogenosis is identical with that in *Types I and II hereditary glycogenosis* (Fig. 184). However, characteristically, only sharply circumscribed groups of hepatocytes are affected (Fig. 185). These foci vary in size and number and may show a random or zonal pattern of distribution. Although the affected hepatocytes are indistinguishable from those of Types I and II glycogenosis, the granular deposits of glycogen seen in PAS-stained sections tend to be smaller and less numerous. Moreover, the deposits rapidly disappear when the insulin dose is sharply reduced or omitted (see Chapter 14).

Mucopolysaccharidosis

A number of autosomal recessive hereditary disorders are characterized by a deficiency of one or another of the enzymes involved in the catabolism of glycosaminoglycans, leading to the accumulation of mucopolysaccharides in the lysosomes of various tissues. In *Hurler's syndrome,* the most common of these, and in several others, hepatosplenomegaly is a prominent feature.

Characteristically, both the hepatocytes and Kupffer cells are swollen, and contain pale, vacuolated cytoplasm (Fig. 186). Since the stored acid mucopolysaccharide is leached out by aqueous fixatives, other methods of fixation, such as Lindsay's dioxane-picrate, are required for its demonstration. In appropriately fixed specimens, the acid mucopolysaccharide is best demonstrated with the colloidal iron stain, and can be digested with hyaluronidase, but not with diastase, usually staining only weakly with PAS after diastase digestion (139).

In routine sections, the hepatocytes resemble those in glycogenosis. However, they can be readily differentiated in 1 μm, plastic-embedded sections fixed in osmium tetroxide. In such sections, the mucopolysaccharide deposits appear as numerous sharply defined vacuoles (140), which on electron microscopy can be identified as lysosomes containing fine, scattered, protein-like precipitates (141).

Hepatocellular uroporphyrin deposits

Porphyria cutanea tarda is a disorder of porphyrin metabolism characterized by a deficiency of hepatic uroporphyrinogen decarboxylase that blocks the conversion of uroporphyrinogen to coproporphyrinogen, thus leading to uroporphyrin accumulation in the liver and excessive excretion in the urine.

Characteristically, the uroporphyrin is distributed uniformly throughout the hepatocellular cytoplasm, and exhibits a distinctive red fluorescence in ultraviolet light that is readily demonstrable in unstained, paraffin-embedded sections (Fig. 187), but is not detectable in routine light microscopy of stained sections. It has been reported that the cytoplasm invariably contains needle-like, birefringent crystals that can be seen in H & E sections examined under polarized light, and that these crystals fluoresce in ultraviolet light, suggesting that they contain uroporphyrin (142). However, we have been unable to confirm these observations in 12 consecutive cases of well-documented porphyria cutanea tarda.

When porphyria cutanea tarda is associated with excessive alcohol consumption, the hepatocytes often contain hemosiderin deposits and show fatty infiltration or other evidence of alcoholic liver disease.

For a more complete discussion of porphyria cutanea tarda the reader is referred to Chapter 18.

Abnormalities of hepatocellular nuclei

Hepatocellular mitoses

Under normal conditions the turnover of hepatocytes is so slow that mitoses are rare. Accordingly, their presence almost always signifies a regenerative response to hepatocellular injury and cell loss. Increased mitotic activity occurs under a wide variety of conditions, but is seen most frequently in all forms of acute hepatitis. Although the extent of the necrosis and other evidence of regeneration, such as pleomorphism, binucleation, and thickening of the hepatic plates, often increase as such lesions advance, the number of mitotic figures tends to decline. The brevity of the mitotic cycle, the persistence of pleomorphism, binucleation, and thickening of the hepatic plates, and a decrease in the rate of cell loss following acute injury probably account for the discrepancy between the number of mitoses and the extent of the necrosis seen in the late stages of acute hepatitis. Undoubtedly, these factors also account for the paucity of mitotic figures found in the regenerating parenchyma in chronic lesions, such as chronic active hepatitis and cirrhosis.

Even at an early stage of acute hepatic injury, the degree of mitotic activity cannot be correlated with the extent of hepatocellular necrosis. Indeed, numerous mitoses may be seen in sections exhibiting only minimal evidence of necrosis or cell loss. We have encountered such lesions most frequently in early mild viral or drug-induced hepatitis, infectious mononucleosis, and leptospirosis. Figure 188 illustrates the numerous mitotic figures seen on the 10th day of illness in a case of mild acute anicteric viral hepatitis. Although the portal tracts are infiltrated with mononuclear cells, only rare acidophilic bodies and foci of cell dropout and Kupffer cell hyperplasia are present in the parenchyma.

Binucleated and multinucleated hepatocytes

Hepatocytes that fail to divide following mitosis present as *binucleate cells*. Since they may persist in that state, they are not necessarily indicative of an abnormal regenerative response. Indeed, normally, up to four such cells may be seen in most high power fields. However, when more numerous, and when accompanied by pleomorphism and cells containing three or more nuclei (Fig. 189), multinucleated cells may be regarded as evidence of increased regenerative activity.

Multinucleated giant hepatocytes occur most frequently in various forms of neonatal cholestasis (Fig. 126, 127) but may be seen occasionally under other conditions in adults [(30,31); Figs. 128, 129]. The relative importance of regeneration and degeneration in their pathogenesis is discussed more fully later.

Glycogen nuclei

Enlarged hepatocellular nuclei containing large, unilocular vacuoles are termed glycogen nuclei because of their glycogen content. They are by far the most common nuclear inclusion encountered in the liver. Although they are seen most frequently in the hepatic lesions of diabetes mellitus, various forms of glycogenosis, and Wilson's disease, they are of little diagnostic significance, since they also occur in association with other hepatic lesions and in normal livers.

As a rule, glycogen nuclei are limited to periportal hepatocytes. However, they may extend to involve midzonal and even centrilobular cells. Characteristically, the affected nuclei are enlarged and appear empty except for condensed chromatin on the inner surface of their limiting membranes (Fig. 14). Although their vacuolization is attributable to glycogen deposition that is readily demonstrable by electron microscopy, only a minority of the vacuolated nuclei are PAS-positive in routine sections appropriately fixed in nonaqueous solutions. In some, the glycogen fills the nucleus (Fig. 15), while in others it appears as PAS-positive granules or threads.

Nuclear cytoplasmic inclusions

Occasionally, the nucleus of a hepatocyte contains an *invagination of cytoplasm,* which, on cross-section, appears as an inclu-

sion. Such nuclei may be seen in both normal and diseased livers, and have no significance except that they may be mistaken for nuclear viral inclusions.

Characteristically, the invaginated cytoplasm is encircled by a prominent limiting membrane identical with that of the nucleus, and contains finely granular material that closely resembles the cytoplasm of the cell (Fig. 16).

Sanded nuclei

The cores of the HB virus replicate in hepatocellular nuclei. Rarely, in immunosuppressed, renal transplant patients with chronic persistent hepatitis and in cases of chronic active hepatitis, excessive accumulation of core particles imparts a sanded or ground glass appearance to the nuclei (66). Such nuclei are relatively rare, even in cases in which core particles are shown by electron microscopy.

Characteristically, as shown in Figure 140, sanded nuclei are devoid of visible nucleoli and chromatin, and are filled with homogeneous, finely granular, eosinophilic material that is both PAS- and orcein-negative.

Cytomegalovirus (CMV) inclusion bodies

The liver is often affected in systemic CMV infections. Both the character of the hepatic lesions and the other manifestation vary, depending on the age and immune status of the host. A distinctive feature of all types of hepatic lesions, but demonstrable in only a minority of cases, is the presence in occasional hepatocytes or bile duct epithelial cells of Cowdry type A nuclear inclusions containing aggregates of virus particles. Generally, the inclusions are found predominantly within hepatocytes in adults, and within bile duct epithelial cells in infants.

As shown in Figure 190, the hepatocytes with CMV nuclear inclusions are usually enlarged, show increased cytoplasmic basophilia, and often lie free in the space of Disse surrounded by histiocytes and/or neutrophils. Characteristically, enclosed within the nucleus is a large, sharply circumscribed, homogeneous, reddish-blue inclusion surrounded by a clear halo.

When bile duct epithelial cells are involved, they too are enlarged and contain similar inclusions that may protrude into the lumen of the duct (Fig. 191).

The diagnosis can be established by specific immunocytochemical staining for CMV antigen (143).

Herpes simplex nuclear inclusions

Disseminated herpes simplex infections, encountered chiefly in neonatal infants and, less commonly, in immunodeficient adults, result in widespread necrosis of the liver, adrenals, and other tissues, and invariably lead to death within a week or two. A distinctive feature of the hepatic lesions is the presence in some hepatocytes of nuclear inclusions containing aggregated viral particles. The inclusions are most easily recognized in the intact hepatocytes bordering the zones of necrosis, but on careful examination, they can almost always be identified within degenerating and necrotic cells as well.

As shown in Figure 192, the affected nucleus is enlarged and exhibits condensation of chromatin in the inner surface of its limiting membrane. It may contain a large, homogeneous or finely ·granular, eosinophilic or amphophilic inclusion surrounded by a clear halo.

The diagnosis can be established by immunocytochemical staining of the viral antigen (144).

Varicella virus nuclear inclusions

Rarely, the varicella virus gives rise to a disseminated infection that often proves fatal. This occurs principally in individuals who are immunologically incompetent or suppressed.

Foci of hepatocellular necrosis are frequently found in such cases, and usually these are accompanied by the presence in some hepatocytes, Kupffer cells, and bile duct epithelial cells of Cowdry type A nuclear inclusions that closely resemble those seen in disseminated herpes simplex infections.

Abnormalities of hepatocellular configuration and organization

Hepatocellular pleomorphism

The hepatocytes and their nuclei are normally relatively uniform in size (Fig. 6). Occasionally, anisocytosis and anisonucleosis are attributable to hepatocellular degeneration, as in early acute viral hepatitis (Fig. 108) and toxic hepatitis (Fig. 107). However, more commonly, such *pleomorphism* is indicative of a regenerative response to antecedent hepatocellular necrosis, and often is accompanied by other evidence of regenerative activity, such as thickening of the hepatic plates, rosette formation, and binucleation of the hepatocytes.

As a rule, *pleomorphism* is encountered during the recovery phase of hepatocellular necrosis. However, in some instances, it occurs in combination with active degeneration and necrosis, as in the case of acute viral hepatitis (Fig. 95). Although hepatocellular anisocytosis and anisonucleosis usually indicate recent cell loss, these changes may persist for a considerable period following recovery from hepatic injury.

Hepatocellular pleomorphism is seen most frequently in the regenerating nodules of cirrhosis, particularly when the lesions are active (Fig. 193), in chronic active hepatitis, and following recovery from acute viral or drug-induced hepatitis. Occasionally, similar anisocytosis and anisonucleosis, often accompanied by rare acidophilic bodies, minimal focal Kupffer cell hyperplasia, and scanty intralobular lymphocytic infiltrates, are encountered in healthy HBsAg-carriers (Fig. 194), and in individuals with mild anicteric viral or drug-induced hepatitis. Lesions of this type are sometimes termed *hepatocellular unrest* (145).

Hepatocellular dysplasia

A form of hepatocellular pleomorphism characterized by enlargement, nuclear pleomorphism, hyperchromasia, and multi-nucleation of the hepatocytes, termed *hepatic cell dysplasia* (Figs. 195, 196), is generally regarded as a precancerous lesion (146,147), although there remains considerable doubt (148,149).

Lesions of this type, which are encountered most frequently in livers bearing hepatocellular carcinoma and in those with cirrhosis, particularly of the macronodular type, are only rarely seen in normal livers (146). In a study of 552 Ugandan Africans, dysplasia was found in 65% of those with cirrhosis complicated by hepatocellular carcinoma, 20% of those with cirrhosis alone, 7% of those with hepatocellular carcinoma without cirrhosis, and 1% of those with normal livers. Moreover, in all groups, the incidence was significantly higher in patients with HB surface antigenemia (146,147). This led to the conclusion that the occurrence of dysplasia can be correlated with both macronodular cirrhosis and HB surface antigenemia, and that patients with dysplasia are at high risk of developing hepatocellular carcinoma. A similar relationship between dysplasia and the occurrence of hepatocellular carcinoma in macronodular cirrhosis has been observed in the United States (150). However, in a study of 50 black South African patients with hepatocellular carcinoma, dysplasia, which occurred in 48% of the groups, could not be correlated with the presence of either cirrhosis or HB surface antigenemia (149).

In our own biopsy series, the incidence of liver cell dysplasia in cirrhosis is significantly lower than that reported from Africa. Moreover, its differentiation from the usual type of pleomorphism, found so frequently in zones of hepatocellular regeneration in both cirrhosis and chronic active hepatitis, has been more difficult than indicated in such reports. This suggests that dysplasia may represent an atypical form of regeneration or hyperplasia, a view held by some experts (151).

As illustrated in Figure 195, dysplasia often affects only small groups of hepatocytes. However, it may involve entire cirrhotic nodules.

Although differentiation between dysplasia and hepatocellular carcinoma seldom poses a problem, it may do so when an entire nodule is involved. Preservation of the reticulin in dysplastic nodules, in contrast to its absence or paucity in carcinoma, is a useful point of differentiation.

Hepatocellular atrophy

Interference with the oxygen and nutrient supply of the hepatocytes, or compression of the hepatic parenchyma by expanding lesions may lead to atrophy and loss of hepatocytes. This is seen most frequently in the type of hepatic congestion produced by right-sided heart failure, constrictive pericarditis, or occlusion of the hepatic veins by fibrosis, thrombi, or tumors, and probably is attributable to both increased sinusoidal hydrostatic pressure and impairment of oxygenation secondary to reduced blood flow (Fig. 197).

Similarly, impairment of blood flow and interference with oxygen and nutrient exchange by deposits of collagen (Fig. 198) or amyloid (Fig. 199) in the spaces of Disse may also result in atrophy and loss of hepatocytes.

As illustrated in Figure 200, compression of the hepatic parenchyma by expanding lesions, such as tumors, cysts, or large, regenerating, hepatocellular nodules, frequently leads to hepatocellular atrophy.

Another but less common cause of such atrophy is occlusion of the intrahepatic portal veins by phlebosclerosis (152) or organized thrombi (153–155), as seen in *"idiopathic"* (noncirrhotic) *portal hypertension.*

With advancing age and under conditions of malnutrition, the liver tends to shrink in size and, at autopsy, often appears unusually brown in color, a condition termed *brown atrophy* (156), which may be associated with impaired drug handling (157).

The hepatocytes in atrophic plates are smaller and flatter than normal, but usually show no other significant changes, except for fine fat droplets in some cases. It has been reported, on the basis of postmortem observations, that atrophic hepatocytes often exhibit increased cytoplasmic basophilia, and that in the brown atrophy of advancing age and undernutrition, the centrilobular hepatocytes contain an excess of lipofuscin (158). However, we have not observed such changes in our own biopsy material.

Thickening and irregularity of the hepatocellular plates

The hepatocytes are normally organized in the form of one-cell-thick plates that radiate from the central veins (Fig. 6), except in early infancy when they characteristically exhibit a twin-cell plate pattern (Fig. 44). As a rule, thickening of the plates is indicative of a regenerative response to a wide variety of hepatic insults. Plates two or more cells in thickness are seen most frequently in cirrhotic nodules (Fig. 51), the late phase of acute viral hepatitis (Fig. 201), prolonged extrahepatic biliary obstruction (Fig. 202), various forms of intrahepatic cholestasis (Fig. 110), and in nodular regenerative hyperplasia (Fig. 67). They may also occur in any other type of lesion characterized by degeneration, necrosis, or loss of hepatocytes.

Often, the thickening of the plates is accompanied by other alterations in their configuration, particularly marked irregularity in their contours (Fig. 51) and rosette formation (Fig. 202).

The hepatocytes in thick plates are usually normal in appearance, but occasionally show changes, such as ballooning or cholestasis (Fig. 110), and fatty infiltration in alcoholic cirrhosis (Fig. 51). Surprisingly, the regenerating cells in thick plates almost never exhibit mitotic activity, and only rarely are they binucleate. Occasionally, foci of active regeneration are encountered within cirrhotic nodules made up of normal, one-cell-thick plates. The cells in such foci are smaller and more basophilic than normal hepatocytes, show a twin-cell arrangement, and usually are binucleated (Fig. 203).

Reversion to a normal plate pattern in areas of regeneration occurs with regularity following recovery from acute viral hepatitis and various forms of cholestasis, but also is often seen within the nodules of advanced cirrhosis (Fig. 56).

Rosettes and pseudoducts (pseudoacini and pseudoglands)

Another feature of regeneration is the formation of rosettes or pseudoacini, a collection of hepatocytes arranged in a circular pattern around a central canaliculus that may be barely visible or dilated. Such rosettes are encountered most frequently in chronic active hepatitis and active forms of cirrhosis, particularly in the periportal and periseptal zones (Fig. 106), but also in acute viral hepatitis (Fig. 204), various forms of cholestasis (Figs. 110, 201), and in other lesions accompanied by hepato-

cellular regeneration. The cells of some rosettes show granular eosinophilia, so-called oncocytes (28).

Not infrequently the lumens of the rosettes contain inspissated bile (Figs. 110, 202). When sectioned longitudinally, the rosettes resemble twin-cell plates (Figs. 203, 204), indicating that they represent cross-sections of tubular structures.

Pseudoducts or *pseudoglands,* a variant of rosettes, are characterized by hepatocytes arranged around a relatively large canalicular lumen, closely resembling interlobular ducts in appearance (Fig. 205). In longitudinal sections, they, too, appear as tubular or glandular structures that occasionally contain inspissated bile (Fig. 206). It has been suggested that the formation of pseudoducts is a genetically determined distinctive feature of galactosemia, fructose intolerance, and tyrosinemia (159). While pseudoducts are found in most such cases, they are also seen in various forms of cirrhosis (Fig. 204) and severe viral hepatitis (Fig. 206), so that a genetic basis for their formation is unlikely.

Abnormalities of the bile canaliculi

Normally, the canaliculi are too slender to visualize at the light microscopic level. However, under conditions of either obstructive or hepatocellular cholestasis, the canaliculi dilate and often contain collections of inspissated bile, termed bile thrombi, that can be readily identified in routine sections.

When sectioned tangentially, the branching, anastomosing pattern of the canaliculi may be outlined by the inspissated bile they contain (Fig. 207). However, more commonly, the bile thrombi are seen in cross-section as round or variably shaped pigment plugs within dilated canaliculi, often surrounded by hepatocytes arranged in the form of rosettes (Fig. 202) or pseudoducts (Fig. 206). It should be noted that in cholestatic lesions many of the dilated canaliculi contain no pigment (Fig. 204). Moreover, in some cases, dilated canaliculi may be seen in the absence of either bile thrombi or hyperbilirubinemia. This phenomenon occurs most frequently in the early stages of primary biliary cirrhosis (Fig. 208), but may be encountered in other cholestatic states. Such observations, supported by a number of electron microscopic studies, indicate that the dilatation is attributable to alterations in the pericanalicular ectoplasm of the hepatocytes rather than to distension of the canaliculi by bile, and that bile thrombi are the result rather than the cause of cholestasis. Experimental evidence suggests that the fundamental defect in cholestasis may be the loss of normal canalicular tone due to disruption of the actin-containing, contractile microfilaments in the pericanalicular ectoplasm of the hepatocytes (160). It appears that this active network is important in the coordinated contractions of bile canaliculi (161,162).

Characteristically, the canalicular changes in most forms of cholestasis are most prominent in the centrilobular zones, but may extend to the mid- and periportal zones of the lobule when the cholestasis is prolonged or severe. In the early stages of primary biliary cirrhosis and in some cases of drug-induced hepatitis, canalicular dilatation and bile thrombi are found in the periportal zones initially, and only later do they extend outward toward the central veins. Similarly, in all forms of advanced cirrhosis accompanied by cholestasis, bile thrombi are most prominent in the periportal and periseptal parenchyma. Whatever the distribution and extent of the cholestatic changes, invariably many of the canaliculi in the involved areas are spared, so that apparently normal and bile-filled, dilated canaliculi are often seen side by side.

Bile thrombi are complex and variable in composition and usually contain not only conjugated bilirubin but also protein, phospholipids, and glycoproteins, apparently derived from hepatocellular membranes and cytoplasmic fragments sloughed into the lumens of the canaliculi. The nonuniform composition of bile thrombi is reflected in their variable staining properties. Usually, in Masson-stained sections, they are light or dark green in color (Fig. 209), whereas in H & E sections, they may appear yellow, brown (Fig. 207), or even black (Fig. 202), depending on the degree of inspissation and amount of bilirubin present. Occasionally, some of the dilated canaliculi contain homogeneous, pink-staining material that appears to be proteinaceous in nature and devoid of pigment.

Most bile thrombi are diastase-resistant, PAS-positive to a variable degree (Fig. 210), a staining reaction that often proves useful in detecting small bile thrombi that may not be evident in routinely stained sections. Special stains for bile, most of which depend on the oxidation of bilirubin to biliverdin, are also useful, particularly in differentiating cytoplasmic bile droplets from other D-PAS-positive inclusions, and in visualizing minute bile droplets in hepatocellular carcinomas.

Most bile thrombi appear homogeneous, but occasionally they exhibit coarse granularity. As previously indicated, the bile thrombi seen in advanced erythropoietic protoporphyria contain both bilirubin and crystalline protoporphyrin. Characteristically, the largest of these are dark brown in color (Fig. 169), and in polarized light exhibit a distinctive red birefringence with a central dark Maltese cross (Fig. 170). Smaller canalicular deposits of protoporphyrin also are birefringent, but appear golden in polarized light, and are finely granular in routine miscroscopy.

It is generally believed that the tight junctions of the hepatocytes sealing the canaliculi are invariably preserved even when the canaliculi are widely dilated. However, as pointed out many years ago (163), rupture of canaliculi and leakage of bile into the spaces of Disse can occasionally be demonstrated histologically in cases of severe cholestasis. This is illustrated in Figure 211, which shows a large, collar button–shaped canalicular bile thrombus projecting into Disse's space encountered postmortem in a patient with advanced primary biliary cirrhosis. Much more frequently, large, sharply circumscribed collections of bile closely resembling canalicular bile thrombi can be demonstrated in the spaces of Disse and within Kupffer cells, as shown in Figure 212, which illustrates this lesion found on needle biopsy in a patient with obstructive jaundice attributable to a metastatic carcinoma of the stomach. That the tight junctions may be permeable even under normal conditions is suggested by experimental evidence indicating that they permit the passage of salt and water via paracellular pathways during normal bile secretion (164).

Abnormalities of the hepatic sinusoids

Centrilobular congestion

Dilatation of the centrilobular sinusoids is a hallmark of right-sided congestive heart failure, constrictive pericarditis, or occlusion of the hepatic veins by fibrosis, thrombi or tumor. Depending on the duration and severity of the congestion, the intervening hepatocytes usually show varying degrees of atrophy [(165) Fig. 197]. The atrophic plates are often interrupted by lost hepatocytes, so that in many areas, truncated columns of cells project into the dilated sinusoids and, in cross-section, appear to be completely surrounded by blood. In long-standing moderate or severe congestion, the sinusoidal dilatation may extend to the midzones, and even to the periportal zones of the lobules. Although the pattern of congestion tends to be uniform, it should be noted that it may vary, and that in mild cases, some lobules may be completely spared.

When the congestion is severe, particularly in constrictive pericarditis and occlusion of the hepatic veins (Budd-Chiari syndrome), striking dilatation of the sinusoids may be accompanied by loss of all the centrilobular hepatocytes, giving the appearance of hemorrhagic necrosis (Fig. 213). However, the outlines of the sinusoids can still be identified in reticulin-stained sections. In some cases, extravasation of blood into the spaces of Disse contributes to the hemorrhagic appearance of the centrilobular zones (Fig. 214). This finding is said to be pathognomonic of the Budd-Chiari syndrome (166). However, we have encountered similar extravasation of blood into the spaces of Disse in other forms of severe hepatic congestion, and in centrilobular ischemic necrosis.

Under conditions of prolonged congestion, loss of centrilobular hepatocytes may be followed by collapse of the sinusoids and fibrosis (Fig. 215). Occasionally, such foci of fibrosis bridge adjacent centrilobular zones (Fig. 48) and, rarely, extend to involve the portal tracts and to outline nodules of parenchyma, thereby giving rise to a lesion usually classified as cardiac or congestive cirrhosis (see Chapter 21).

Another feature of prolonged congestion is the deposition of collagen in the space of Disse surrounding the dilated sinusoids (Fig. 198). This is often accompanied by the development of a continuous basement membrane beneath the endothelium, thereby converting the fenestrated sinusoids into completely enclosed capillaries, a process termed *capillarization,* that may interfere with oxygen and nutrient exchange and thus contribute to the atrophy and loss of hepatocytes (167).

Periportal sinusoidal dilatation

A unique type of sinusoidal dilatation limited to the periportal zones is seen occasionally in women on long-term, oral contraceptive therapy [(168); Fig. 216]. When severe, the dilatation may extend to the midzones, and, occasionally, is accompanied by marked atrophy and loss of the intervening hepatocytes with the formation of relatively large, blood-filled, endothelial-lined cavities suggestive of peliosis hepatis (Fig. 217).

Although the pathogenesis of these lesions is still uncertain, circumstantial evidence suggests that the synthetic estrogens and progesterones in oral contraceptives may exert a toxic effect on the sinusoids, leading to their dilatation. It is noteworthy that similar vascular changes are seen in the benign hepatic cell adenomas encountered in young women on oral contraceptives (Chapter 25), and that synthetic, androgenic anabolic steroids, similar in chemical structure to those used in oral contraceptives, also give rise to peliosis hepatis (see Chapter 21).

Peliosis hepatis

Peliosis of the liver is defined as blood-filled cavities that range in diameter from 1 to 30 mm and are distributed randomly throughout the hepatic parenchyma. These lesions, which appear to be an exaggeration of sinusoidal dilatation, may or may not be lined by sinusoidal cells. They occur under similar circumstances as sinusoidal dilatation, i.e., administration of androgenic or anabolic steroids or diverse pharmaceutical agents, after organ transplantation, probably related to immunosuppression, and in association with various hepatic neoplasms, most notably angiosarcomas in which the peliosis precedes the tumor.

Other forms of sinusoidal dilatation

Focal or randomly distributed zones of sinusoidal dilatation are relatively common in livers bearing metastatic tumors (169). It is highly probable that they are attributable to occlusion or invasion of small branches of the hepatic vein by tumor.

Similar patchy zones of congestion are seen occasionally within cirrhotic nodules. At least in the case of alcoholic cirrhosis, the congestion appears to be the result of the fibrous occlusion of the central veins (170) and the centrilobular perisinusoidal fibrosis that follows antecedent alcoholic hepatitis (171).

Occasionally, centrilobular and, less commonly, midzonal or panlobular sinusoidal dilatation is encountered in the absence of known cases of hepatic congestion. In one study of such cases, the dilatation occurred predominantly in individuals with chronic diseases, and appeared to be correlated with the presence of hypergammaglobulinemia and hypoalbuminemia, leading the authors to suggest that the structural changes in the liver might be related to alterations in hepatic protein synthesis (172). In another study of the problem, sinusoidal ectasia was found to be correlated with the presence of extrahepatic granulomatous disease, including tuberculosis, brucellosis, and Crohn's disease; or extrahepatic malignancy, such as Hodgkin's disease and cancer of the gastrointestinal tract or uterus (173). On the basis of these observations, it was suggested that a humoral factor might be involved, and that the sinusoidal ectasia might represent an early stage of peliosis hepatis. In our biopsies with cryptogenic sinusoidal dilatation, we have found no relationship to the serum levels of albumin or gamma globulin. However, in a few of our cases, the dilatation was associated with extrahepatic granulomatous disease, Hodgkin's disease, or carcinoma. Although needle biopsy failed to demonstrate the specific hepatic lesions of these disorders, the possibility that the liver was involved could not be excluded with certainty. What is needed to resolve the question of whether or not extrahepatic granulomatous disease or malignancy leads to dilatation of the sinusoids is a careful study of postmortem material.

A new hypothesis correlates sinusoidal size inversely with hepatocyte volume (174). Its proponents suggest that in alcoholic liver disease increased hepatocyte volume results in compression of the sinusoids with a reduction in the morphometric area of the sinusoids and an increase in sinusoidal pressure. In nonalcoholic liver disease, in which hepatocytes are not enlarged, the sinusoidal area is not reduced nor is sinusoidal pressure increased. They believe that sinusoidal size is

sufficiently reliable to recommend it as a useful criterion in the differentiation of alcoholic from nonalcoholic liver disease.

Artifactual dilatation of the sinusoids is seen occasionally in aspiration needle biopsy specimens. Characteristically, artifactual dilatation is random in its distribution and is never accompanied by atrophy or loss of the hepatocytes in the intervening hepatic plates, so that its differentiation from congestion and other forms of sinusoidal dilatation is relatively simple.

Cellular distension of sinusoids

In a number of inflammatory, hematopoietic, and infiltrative disorders, cells other than normal erythrocytes may distend the sinusoids and lead to atrophy of the intervening hepatocytes, thus mimicking sinusoidal congestion. The types of cells that can produce these effects include hyperplastic Kupffer cells, aggregated sickled erythrocytes, foci of extramedullary hematopoietic cells, and infiltrating leukemic, neoplastic, or abnormal histiocytic cells. In contrast to passive congestion, the sinusoidal distension produced by such cells tends to be patchy rather than zonal in distribution. Interference with sinusoidal blood flow probably accounts for the atrophy of the intervening hepatocytes, and for the accompanying patchy, sinusoidal congestion often seen in such cases.

Figure 218 illustrates the sinusoidal distension and atrophy of hepatocytes produced by proliferating, swollen Kupffer cells in a case of infectious mononucleosis. A more complete discussion and illustrations of leukemic and histiocytic infiltration of the sinusoids follow.

Sinusoidal fibrin thrombi

In approximately half the fatal cases of eclampsia, sinusoidal fibrin or fibrinogen thrombi (Fig. 219) and foci of hepatocellular necrosis (Fig. 220) are found in the periportal zones. Only rarely are they seen in nonfatal cases. Presumably, thrombus formation is the result of coagulopathy, and is responsible for the development of hepatocellular necrosis. The alternative possibility that the thrombi are secondary to the necrosis appears unlikely, since in preeclampsia, sinusoidal deposits of fibrin have been demonstrated by immunofluorescence in the absence of hepatocellular necrosis (175).

Disseminated intravascular coagulation with sinusoidal fibrin thrombi has been reported in massive hepatic necrosis, and it has been suggested that such thrombi may contribute to progression of the necrosis (176). Although we have found biochemical evidence of disseminated intravascular coagulation in a number of patients with massive hepatic necrosis, in none that have come to autopsy have we found hepatic, sinusoidal, fibrin thrombi.

Alleged fibrinoid necrosis of the sinusoids

Unusual focal lesions characterized by a ring of fibrinoid material encircled by and enclosing endothelial cells, histiocytes, and/or giant cells were first reported in 1965 as a pathognomonic feature of Q fever, and were interpreted as necrotic sinusoids associated with a granulomatous reaction (177). However, in a more recent report, the relationship of these lesions to the sinusoids has been deemphasized, the authors suggesting that they are granulomas undergoing fibrinoid necrosis, and that invariably they contain a large central vacuole, presumably lipid in nature (178). Occasionally, serial sections are required to visualize the central vacuole. In this study, typical ring lesions were demonstrable in 14 of 17 patients with Q fever, but similar lesions were encountered in three patients with Hodgkin's disease.

Our own observations support the view that the ring lesions represent an unusual type of lipogranuloma that may be seen in Q fever and that also occurs under other conditions. Thus, in eight well-documented cases of Q fever, liver biopsy revealed multiple ring lesions in two, in both of which mild or moderate fatty infiltration of the hepatocytes was present (Fig. 221). In addition, identical ring lesions were encountered in six individuals with no clinical or serologic evidence of Q fever. In all instances, the lesions were associated with mild to moderate fatty infiltration, attributable to chronic alcoholism in two, diabetes mellitus in one, and obesity in another. The etiology of the fatty infiltration was uncertain in two, but was associated with streptococcal erythema nodosum in one and giant cell temporal arteritis in the other.

Figure 222 illustrates one of the numerous ring lesions found in the liver biopsy section of a chronic alcoholic patient who had been febrile for two weeks and exhibited moderate fatty infiltration and acute hepatitis of uncertain etiology. Serial serologic and cultural studies over a six-week period failed to reveal evidence of rickettsial, viral, or bacterial infection. Defervescence occurred spontaneously during the fourth week of illness, and was followed two weeks later by clearing of all hepatic functional abnormalities. Follow-up liver biopsy two months later revealed mild portal fibrosis and lymphocytosis, but no evidence of the ring lesions.

The striking resemblance between the ring lesions and the type of intralobular lipogranuloma frequently found in fatty livers (Fig. 176) suggests that they may share a common pathogenesis. However, it is evident that some additional factor, possibly infection, must be involved to account for the deposition of fibrin in the ring lesions.

Abnormalities of the spaces of Disse

Perisinusoidal, intercellular, and pericellular fibrosis

As previously indicated, centrilobular *perisinusoidal fibrosis* due to deposition of collagen in the spaces of Disse is a relatively common feature of chronic passive congestion, and often is accompanied by atrophy of the intervening hepatocellular plates (Fig. 198). When the atrophy and cell loss are extensive, the sinusoids may collapse, giving rise to a centrilobular zone of fibrosis in which the lumens of most sinusoids are obliterated (Fig. 215).

Perisinusoidal fibrosis also occurs under a wide variety of other conditions, in only a few of which there is accompanying sinusoidal congestion. It is seen most frequently in the late phase of alcoholic hepatitis, various forms of cirrhosis, particularly the alcoholic type (179), chronic active hepatitis, and in the residual lesions of severe viral and drug-induced hepatitis. Among less common causes are hypervitaminosis A, radiation hepatitis, myxedema, graft-versus-host disease and chronic hepatotoxicity due to azathioprine, urethane, arsenic, Thorotrast, or vinyl chloride.

As a rule, *perisinusoidal fibrosis* occurs predominantly in the centrilobular zones. However, the distribution is usually periportal in chronic active hepatitis and random in cirrhosis.

Figure 223 illustrates a typical example of noncongestive, centrilobular, perisinusoidal fibrosis in a case of healed alcoholic hepatitis. Occasionally, collagen is deposited not only in the space of Disse but also in the lumens of the sinusoids. A striking example of this is seen in the hepatic lesions of severe hypervitaminosis A illustrated in Figure 224.

In many of the conditions under consideration, the intralobular fibrosis may be *intercellular* and *pericellular,* rather than, or in addition to, perisinusoidal in distribution. When centrilobular, as in the late phase of alcoholic hepatitis, such fibrosis has an arachnoid appearance (Fig. 225), whereas in periportal fibrosis characteristic of chronic active hepatitis, the collagen fibers, often intermixed with inflammatory cells, form an ill-defined mesh in which are embedded groups of hepatocytes. Occasionally, in severe alcoholic liver disease, intercellular and pericellular fibrosis may be diffusely distributed throughout the lobules (Fig. 63), a type of fibrosis often termed interstitial.

Although, in some instances, collapse of collagen-lined sinusoids may account for the appearance of intercellular and pericellular fibrosis, more often, such fibrosis appears to be the result of hepatocellular degeneration and necrosis. It thus resembles the type of intralobular fibrosis that may follow bridging hepatic necrosis (Chapter 3).

There is suggestive evidence that perisinusoidal, intercellular, and pericellular fibrosis may be attributable to activation of the Ito cells (lipocytes) in the spaces of Disse to fibroblastic activity in response to a variety of stimuli (180). Fibrosis of this type is of special interest, since available evidence indicates that it may play an important role in the pathogenesis of some types of portal hypertension (171).

Alterations in reticulin

The reticulin fibers normally present in the spaces of Disse increase in number and often appear thickened in all conditions associated with intralobular fibrosis. In addition, as might be anticipated, they appear condensed in large zones of hepatocellular necrosis that lead to collapse of the sinusoids (Fig. 77).

Destruction of the reticulin is unusual in most forms of hepatocellular necrosis, degeneration, and atrophy, but is seen in the foci of necrosis produced by some viruses, such as herpes simplex, varicella, and yellow fever; certain fungal infections, including candidiasis, cryptococcosis, aspergillosis, and actinomycosis; and in suppurative lesions of bacterial origin. In addition, the reticulin is often destroyed in various types of necrotic granulomas and in areas of tumor infiltration and massive amyloid deposition.

Hemmorhage into the spaces of Disse

As previously indicated, extravasation of blood into Disse's space may be seen in the Budd-Chiari syndrome (Fig. 214), and, less often, in other forms of severe passive congestion, and in centrilobular ischemic necrosis.

Lymphocyte and plasma cell infiltration of Disse's space

In chronic active hepatitis, lymphocytes and plasma cells infiltrate the space of Disse and come into close contact with the hepatocytes in the periportal zones of necrosis and inflammation. Although the intimate relationship between the infiltrating cells and the hepatocytes is suggested by their appearance in routine sections (Fig. 226), it is more convincingly demonstrated by light microscopy in epoxy-resin embedded thin sections, or by electron microscopy. In such preparations, the inflammatory cells are closely adherent to and occasionally invaginate hepatocytes that often show degenerative changes (181).

Cytoplasmic fusion of these cells has been reported, but, on electron microscopy with a goniometer, which permits tilting the specimen, such fusion appears to be an artifact attributable to superimposition of the cells (182).

The intimate relationships between the infiltrating lymphocytes and hepatocytes that show degenerative changes are consistent with the hypothesis that a cell-mediated immune mechanism is involved in the pathogenesis of chronic active hepatitis, a view further supported by the similar relationship occasionally observed in the lesions of hepatic transplant rejection (183).

Perisinusoidal amyloid deposits

The space of Disse is the most common site of amyloid deposition in the liver. In this distribution, amyloid appears as a perisinusoidal band of homogeneous material that stains light pink in H & E and pale blue in Masson-stained sections (Fig. 199). As the deposits increase, the sinusoids are compressed, the intervening hepatocytes undergo atrophy, and ultimately both may be replaced by masses of amyloid (Fig. 82).

Amyloid resembles hyalinized collagen in many respects, so that special methods are required for its identification. Of these, the simplest and most reliable is the demonstration of green birefringence in Congo red–stained sections examined in polarized light (Fig. 227).

The reticulin is unaffected in the early stages of perisinusoidal amyloid deposition but ultimately may be destroyed. Characteristically, following diastase digestion, amyloid stains pink or bright red with PAS.

For a discussion of the pathogenesis and other features of amyloidosis, the reader is referred to Chapter 24.

Kupffer cell hyperplasia and hypertrophy

Kupffer cell hyperplasia

Under a variety of conditions, the cells lining the sinusoids proliferate. Although the endothelial cells may participate in this reaction to a limited extent, most of the cells involved are Kupffer cells, as evidenced by their phagocytic activity. Kupffer cells

can be identified by immunoperoxidase staining using specific antisera (Fig. 228). It has been suggested that the increase in the number of Kupffer cells is attributable to the recruitment and activation of circulating monocytes derived from the bone marrow. However, there is convincing experimental evidence that the Kupffer cells normally present in the sinusoids can proliferate *in situ* when appropriately stimulated (184). Moreover, the frequency with which mitotic figures can be found in aggregates of Kupffer cells in human liver biopsy material is more consistent with a hyperplastic than an infiltrative response.

Kupffer cell hyperplasia, often accompanied by enlargement and pigmentation of the cells, may be focal or diffuse. Focal collections frequently occur at sites of hepatocellular necrosis and cell dropout, presumably in response to the necrosis. Although foci of Kupffer cell hyperplasia are encountered most frequently in viral and drug-induced hepatitis (Fig. 229), they may be seen in any type of lesion accompanied by hepatocellular necrosis and dropout.

Diffuse hyperplasia of the Kupffer cells is relatively common in some forms of disseminated hepatocellular necrosis, such as viral and drug-induced hepatitis, but not in others, as in the case of widespread zonal, ischemic, or toxic necrosis. Moreover, the degree of hyperplasia is often out of proportion to the extent of the necrosis, as is frequently the case in acute necrosis.

Kupffer cell hypertrophy

Proliferating Kupffer cells are almost always enlarged, and often are pigmented because of phagocytosis of lipofuscin released from adjacent necrotic hepatocytes (Fig. 229). Since the hypertrophied, pigmented Kupffer cells often persist following recovery from hepatocellular necrosis (Fig. 230), their presence in an otherwise normal liver usually indicates recent cell loss. However, occasionally, enlarged, pigmented Kupffer cells are encountered long after recovery from hepatic injury. (Fig 231) This is illustrated in Figure 232, which shows the large, pigmented, centrilobular Kupffer cells found one year after complete recovery from severe halothane-induced hepatitis accompanied by extensive bridging necrosis.

Kupffer cell pigments, granules, and crystals

Most of the abnormal pigments, granules, and crystals found in the cytoplasm of Kupffer cells represent phagocytized material. However, it is conceivable that in some instances their accumulation is attributable to alterations in Kupffer cell metabolic activity.

Kupffer cell lipofuscin

By far the most common pigment found in Kupffer cells is lipfuscin, usually deposited as a result of phagocytosis of the normal pigment released from hepatocytes when they are destroyed.

In H & E and Masson-stained sections, the Kupffer cells

containing lipofuscin usually are enlarged and yellow or light brown in color (Fig. 229). Particularly when abundant, the pigment appears finely or coarsely granular, but, occasionally, it stains the cytoplasm diffusely. Characteristically, lipofuscin stains pink or bright red with PAS and resists diastase digestion (Fig. 233).

Frequently, the portal tracts contain lipofuscin-filled macrophages under the same conditions that lead to lipofuscin deposition in Kupffer cells ductules.

Characteristically, the hemosiderin granules in Kupffer cells vary in size and shape, appear light or dark brown in routinely stained sections, and exhibit a pale green hue and sharp, refractile, angulated edges on focusing. Often, the granules are larger than those in the hepatocytes, and fill the cytoplasm (Fig. 162). As in the case of all hemosiderin deposits, the granules stain deep blue in the Prussian blue reaction (Fig. 159), and often are diastase-resistant, PAS-positive owing to their content of lipofuscin and polysaccharides (Fig. 160). In many cases, the D-PAS reaction is more intense in the Kupffer cell deposits than in those of the hepatocytes, probably because of the larger size and greater condensation of their hemosiderin granules (Fig. 234).

Occasionally, scattered, enlarged Kupffer cells are stained diffusely in the Prussian blue reaction (Fig. 235). Such cells are often associated with Kupffer cell lipofuscin deposition. The diffuse character of the iron staining is probably attributable to the uptake of ferritin released from necrotic hepatocytes. Since such ferritin deposits tend to disappear more rappidly than lipofuscin, diffuse iron staining is probably a more reliable sign of recent cell loss.

Kupffer cell bile

Under conditions of either obstructive or hepatocellular cholestasis, the Kupffer cells may be bile-stained or contain droplets of bile. When the cholestasis is severe or prolonged, the pigment retained in the Kupffer cells may be in the form of large, sharply circumscribed structures that closely resemble the bile thrombi seen in adjacent dilated canaliculi (Fig. 236). Moreover, they are often associated with similar structures in Disse's space, which, as previously indicated, supports the view that they probably represent bile thrombi extruded from the canaliculi and phagocytized by the Kupffer cells. For reasons that are not clear, the retention of bile in some cases is more prominent in the Kupffer cells than in the canaliculi.

Kupffer cell pseudoxanthomatous degeneration

As pointed out previously, both the hepatocytes and Kupffer cells may undergo pseudoxanthomatous degeneration under conditions of severe or prolonged cholestasis (Fig. 119). Occasionally, only the Kupffer cells are affected (Fig. 237). Although their foamy, swollen appearance may suggest one of the lipid infiltrates described below, the presence of bile thrombi within adjacent canaliculi and, occasionally, of bile droplets within the cytoplasm of the affected Kupffer cells indicate their pseudoxanthomatous nature.

Kupffer cell protoporphyrin deposits

As pointed out, erythropoietic protoporphyria is characterized by a deficiency of heme synthetase (ferrochelatase) that leads to the accumulation of protoporphyrin in the hepatocytes, Kupffer cells, portal macrophages, and bile canaliculi.

In early lesions, the Kupffer cells contain small, sharply defined, dark brown granules that, characteristically, are birefringent, appearing golden or bright red in polarized light (Figs. 167, 168). Occasionally, the hepatic lesions advance to the stage of cirrhosis and are accompanied by cholestasis. Under such conditions, the largest deposits of protoporphyrin are often found within the Kupffer cells, where they present as large, dark brown globules that resemble bile thrombi (Fig. 169). They often exhibit red fluorescence in ultraviolet light and are birefringent in polarized light, apppearing as bright red, round structures with a central, dark Maltese cross (Fig. 170).

Kupffer cell L-cystine crystals

Cystinosis, an autosomal recessive hereditary disorder, is characterized by the deposition of L-cystine crystals in the eyes and in the lysosomes of the phagocytic reticuloendothelial cells in many other organs, including the liver (Chapter 16). The basic biochemical defect responsible for the accumulation of L-cystine is not known.

Characteristically, the distinctive hexagonal or rectangular crystals of L-cystine are found within enlarged, centrilobular Kupffer cells (Fig. 238) and, less commonly, in portal macrophages, and exhibit striking birefringence in polarized light (Fig. 239). Despite the deposition of crystals, cystinosis has no other adverse effects on the liver.

Since the crystals of L-cystine are water soluble, fresh frozen sections or tissues fixed in alcohol or other nonaqueous solutions are required for their demonstration. Although a nonaqueous type of H & E stain is usually recommended, we have found that the crystals resist solution during routine H & E staining. However, the Masson stain dissolves the crystals, so the affected Kupffer cells appear enlarged and filled with ill-defined granules rather than crystals.

Kupffer cell Thorotrast deposits

Thorotrast, a colloidal solution of thorium dixoide, because of its opacity to x-rays was once widely used for arteriography and hepatosplenography. However, its use as a diagnostic agent was abandoned when its potential hazard as an emitter of alpha, beta, and gamma rays was recognized. Although almost 30 years have elapsed since Thorotrast was last used, hepatic lesions attributable to its prolonged radiation effects continue to appear (see Chapter 25). Normally, Thorotrast injected intravenously or intraarterially is promptly taken up and retained by the reticuloendothelial cells, particularly of the liver and spleen, so that these organs are rendered permanently radiopaque. The adverse radiation effects of Thorotrast in the liver are slowly progressive and become apparent clinically only many years following its deposition. Of the hepatic lesions produced, the most important include progressive portal and intralobular fibrosis, angiosarcoma, hepatocellular carcinoma, cholangiocarcinoma, and malignant lymphoma (185).

Histologically, the deposits of thorium dioxide appear as aggregates of course, irregularly shaped, grayish-brown granules within enlarged Kupffer cells (Fig. 240), portal macrophages, and lying free in the connective tissues of the portal tracts. Although refractile, the granules are not birefringent in polarized light.

Kupffer cell schistosomal pigment

In schistosomal infestations involving the liver, the Kupffer cells and portal macrophages often contain dark brown, small or large, refractile pigment granules (Fig. 241). Characteristically, these do not react with stains for iron or melanin, and are PAS-negative. Available evidence suggests that the pigment is a derivative of host hemoglobin that has been ingested, altered, and regurgitated by the adult schistosomes (186).

Kupffer cell malarial pigment

During the acute phase of malaria, the Kupffer cells are enlarged and contain coarse, dark brown pigment granules. Following recovery, the pigment often shifts to portal macrophages. After repeated attacks of malaria, sufficient malarial pigment may be concentrated in the liver to give it a slate-gray appearance on gross inspection.

The pigment granules derived from host hemoglobin that has been altered within the plasmodia do not react with iron, melanin, or PAS stains, but characteristically exhibit a yellow-orange birefringence in polarized light [(187; Fig. 242].

Kupffer cell anthracotic pigment

Fine, inhaled carbon particles that reach the alveoli of the lungs are phagocytized by macrophages and transported to the lymphatics. Although most of the particles are deposited in the stroma of the lung, the pleura, and hilar lymph nodes, some gain access to the general circulation and may be deposited in the Kupffer cells and portal macrophages of the liver. Such anthracotic pigment presents as coarse, black, nonbirefringent cytoplasmic granules (Fig. 243).

Although Kupffer cell and portal macrophage anthracotic pigment granules are relatively common in individuals with overt pneumonoconiosis, they also occur occasionally in individuals with no history of occupational exposure to carbon-containing dusts.

We have found anthracotic pigment in the Kupffer cells of several patients with pulmonary silicosis. However, in none were the typical birefringent crystals of silica demonstrable in polarized light.

Kupffer cell lipid deposits

In a number of lipid disorders, usually hereditary in nature, metabolites distinctive for each of the disorders are deposited in the reticuloendothelial cells of the liver, spleen, bone marrow, and lymph nodes. In the liver, the Kupffer cells are the principal sites of deposition, but, often, portal macrophages also are involved. Although the composition of the deposits differs, the appearance of the affected cells in the various disorders is remarkably similar, usually being characterized by enlargement of the cells and fine vacuolization of their cytoplasm. Occasionally, the accompanying clinical features and biochemical findings in the serum suggest the nature of the deposits, but, usually, precise identification requires special studies. These may include histochemical studies, fluorescence, polarization or electron microscopy, and enzyme analysis of blood, tissue, or tissue cultures. Unfortunately, not all of these techniques are generally available, and often they require more tissue than can be obtained by needle biopsy, or require specimens that are fresh frozen or specially fixed. For those reasons, the pathologist is often limited to histochemical and electron microscopic studies of paraffin-embedded material, unless a second, appropriately prepared biopsy specimen can be obtained.

For a more complete discussion of lipid disorders, the reader is referred to Chapter 15.

Triglycerides

In disorders accompanied by lipemic serum containing high concentrations of triglycerides, a variable number of Kupffer cells may be enlarged and may contain numerous, small, lipid droplets, giving the cytoplasm a finely vacuolated, foamy appearance. Although the cytoplasm may be pale, it often is tinted tan or light brown owing to the presence of lipofuscin (Fig. 244), which, characteristically, stains with PAS following diastase digestion (Fig. 245).

Foamy Kupffer cells occur in hereditary lipemic states, in types 1, 3, 4, and 5 hyperlipoproteinemia, and in the acquired forms seen in uncontrolled diabetes mellitus, glycogen storage disease, alcoholism, pancreatitis, myxedema, and nephrosis (188).

The pathogenesis of lipemic foam cells has been investigated most thoroughly in the reticuloendothelial cells of type 1 hyperlipoproteinemia (189). Initially, the cells phagocytize chylomicrons, which tend to coalesce and ultimately are enclosed within secondary lysosomes. At this stage, the droplets contain not only triglycerides but also added cholesterol and cholesterol esters, so they exhibit birefringent, needle-like crystals on polarization microscopy. Later, as the lipids are metabolized, the foam cells diminish in size and lose their birefringent crystals, while some of their unsaturated fatty acids undergo oxidation and polymerization to form lipofuscin.

The foam cells in hyperlipemic states closely resemble those in other metabolic disorders. Although precise differentiation usually depends on identification of the underlying enzymatic defect, differences in the character of the autofluorescence and the ultrastructure of the cytoplasmic deposits may be useful in their differentiation (190). Characteristically, the autofluorescence of the lipofuscin granules in hyperlipemic foam cells is yellow-green or golden yellow, whereas the deposits in Tay-Sachs disease and metachromatic leukodystrophy are blue-green, and those in gargoylism light blue. Usually, the deposits in Gaucher's disease, Fabry's disease, and GM_1 gangliosidosis do not exhibit autofluorescence. However, autofluorescence of unspecific character has been reported in some cases of Gaucher's disease (139).

On electron microscopy, the membrane-bound lipofuscin granules in hyperlipemic foam cells contain concentric lamellae of irregular periodicity. The lysosomal deposits in Fabry's disease also contain concentric lamellae, but these exhibit a more regular and well-defined periodicity. In both Gaucher's disease and GM_1 gangliosidosis, the lysosomes of the foam cells contain tubular structures rather than granules, the tubules being longer in Gaucher's disease than in GM_1 gangliosidosis.

The foam cells in hyperlipemia and in Niemann-Pick disease are indistinguishable on the basis of their histochemical reactivity and ultrastructure, so their differentiation usually depends on the associated clinical features, serum lipid findings, and the results of enzyme analysis. Often, in hyperlipemic states, foamy macrophages are found in the portal tracts, and, under some conditions, the hepatocytes are infiltrated with fat (191).

Cholesterol esters

Large, foamy Kupffer cells, characterized by deposits of numerous lipid droplets containing triglycerides and crystals of cholesterol and cholesterol esters, are seen in Wolman's disease, cholesterol ester storage disease, and familial high density lipoprotein deficiency (Tangier disease). In frozen sections, the lipid droplets stain with oil red 0, and react in the Schultz modification of the Lieberman-Burchard reaction for cholesterol. On polarization microscopy of such sections, needle-like, birefringent crystals of cholesterol and cholesterol esters are visualized within the lipid droplets.

Wolman's disease and cholesterol ester storage disease, two closely related autosomal recessive hereditary disorders, are characterized by a deficiency of acid cholesterol ester hydrolase and acid triglyceride lipase that leads to an accumulation of cholesterol, cholesterol esters, and triglycerides in the hepatocytes, Kupffer cells, and portal macrophages (131).

In Tangier disease, a rare inborn error of lipid metabolism transmitted as an autosomal recessive trait, the deposition of cholesterol, cholesterol esters, and triglycerides in the Kupffer cells is attributable to a severe deficiency or absence of high density lipoproteinlipase in the plasma (192).

Although the light microscopic appearance of the foam cells in all three disorders is similar, they differ on electron microscopy in that the lipid deposits in Wolman's disease and cholesterol ester storage disease are found within lysosomes, whereas those in Tangier disease are not membrane-bound (192).

GM₁ gangliosides

The *infantile,* type 1 form of generalized GM_1 gangliosidosis is an autosomal recessive hereditary disorder characterized by a deficiency of all three lysosomal β-galactosidases (A, B, and C) involved in the catabolism of GM_1 ganglioside and keratin-like mucopolysaccharides (193). As a result of this deficiency, both GM_1 ganglioside and mucopolysaccharides accumulate in the lysosomes of Kupffer cells and many other cell types. The affected Kupffer cells are enlarged, and appear foamy owing to the presence in their cytoplasm of numerous fine droplets, which,

because of their GM_1 ganglioside and mucopolysaccharide content, are diastase-resistant, PAS-positive, and react with alcian blue at pH 2.6.

In the *juvenile,* type 2 form of GM_1 gangliosidosis, only two of the three β-galactosidase enzymes (B and C) are deficient. Characteristically, the involved Kupffer cells, which occur in clusters, are enlarged and contain numerous fine fibrils, giving their cytoplasm a wrinkled-paper appearance. The cytoplasm stains with PAS following diastase digestion, and reacts weakly with Sudan black B.

Glycosphingolipids

Fabry's disease, a rare, inborn error of lipid metabolism transmitted as an X-linked recessive trait, is characterized by a deficiency of lysosomal hydrolase, α-galactosidase A, that leads to an accumulation of glycosphingolipids in the lysosomes of reticuloendothelial cells and many other cells types (139).

In the liver, groups of Kupffer cells and some of the portal macrophages are enlarged and finely vacuolated owing to the deposition of glycolipid and cholesterol. The deposits are intensely PAS-positive, resist diastase digestion, and, in frozen section, react in the Schultz modification of the Lieberman-Burchard reaction for cholesterol, and exhibit birefringent crystals on polarization microscopy (139).

Glucocerebroside

Gaucher's disease (195,196), an autosomal recessive hereditary disorder, is characterized by a deficiency of the lysosomal enzyme glucocerebrosidase, involved in the catabolism of glucocerebroside, leading to its accumulation in reticuloendothelial cells. The membranes of senescent leukocytes, platelets, erythrocytes, and, possibly, other tissue cells are the source of the cerebroside phagocytized by the reticuloendothelial cells.

In the liver, the principal site of deposition is in the Kupffer cells, but, occasionally, portal macrophages are also involved.

The affected Kupffer cells, commonly termed Gaucher cells, are greatly enlarged, measuring up to 100 μm in diameter, and contain abundant, pale cytoplasm in relatively small, dark nuclei. Characteristically, as shown in Figure 246, the cytoplasm is filled with numerous thread-like inclusions that give it a crinkled, tissue-paper appearance. The inclusions are diastase-resistant, PAS-positive (Fig. 247), and show intense acid phosphatase activity. Due to an increase in ferritin, some of the Gaucher cells stain diffusely in the Prussian blue reaction. In some, but not all cases, the deposits exhibit autofluorescence.

The distinctive cytoplasmic striations of Gaucher cells may be difficult to identify in H & E sections, but are readily visualized in Masson (Fig. 246) and D-PAS-stained sections (Fig. 247). As illustrated in Figures 246 and 247, large focal collections of Gaucher cells often fill the sinusoids and compress the hepatocytes, leading to their atrophy and ultimate loss.

On electron microscopy, the cytoplasm of Gaucher cells contains numerous membrane-bound, tubular structures made up of aggregated glucocerebroside molecules.

Gaucher cells, identical in all respects to those encountered in Gaucher's disease, are occasionally found in patients with chronic myelogenous leukemia (197). In such cases, the accumulation of glucocerebroside is attributable to overproduction of the cerebroside secondary to increased leukocyte turnover rather than to a hereditary defect in its enzymatic degradation.

Rarely, cells closely resembling Gaucher cells have been found in the bone marrow of patients with multiple myeloma. Although such *pseudo-Gaucher cells* exhibit the typical light microscopic and histochemical features of Gaucher cells, it has been shown by electron microscopy and immunofluorescence that their cytoplasmic inclusions are membrane-bound deposits of crystalline immunoglobulin rather than glucocerebroside (198).

Sulfatide lipids

Metachromatic leukodystrophy, an autosomal hereditary disorder of infants, is characterized by a deficiency of arylsulfatase-A, a lysosomal enzyme that hydrolyzes cerebroside sulfate (galactosyl sulfatide), leading to an accumulation of the latter in the brain, and, to a lesser extent, in the viscera, including the liver (199). Characteristically, the deposits stain metachromatically (200,201).

In paraffin-embedded sections, the liver usually appears normal. However, in frozen sections, metachromatic granules are demonstrable in portal macrophages and, less commonly, in Kupffer cells and periportal hepatocytes. The granules stain red in toluidine blue, mahogany red-brown in cresyl violet, and blue in alcian blue.

On electron microscopy, the granules appear as membrane-bound masses of material arranged in the form of curved, concentric lamellae.

Sphingomyelin

Niemann-Pick disease is an autosomal recessive hereditary disorder characterized by a deficiency of sphingomyelinase, a lysosomal enzyme that normally splits phosphorylcholine from sphingomyelin (202). As a result of this deficiency, sphingomyelin accumulates in the reticuloendothelial cells of many tissues, including the liver, and in the ganglion cells of the central nervous system. Often, the deposits contain other lipids as well, particularly unesterified cholesterol, glucocerebroside, and gangliosides. The accumulated sphingomyelin is derived from plasma membranes released from all cells during their normal turnover.

Two related disorders, the *Nova Scotia variant of Niemann-Pick disease* and *adult non-neuronopathic Niemann-Pick disease,* are also characterized by the deposition of sphingomyelin in the tissues. In neither case is the deposition attributable to a deficiency of sphingomyelinase, the underlying pathogenesis being unknown. Characteristically, in Niemann-Pick disease, the Kupffer cells are greatly enlarged and contain abundant, pale, finely vacuolated, foamy-appearing cytoplasm and small, eccentric, pyknotic nuclei (Fig. 248). Often, the cells contain lipofuscin, so they stain with PAS and resist diastase digestion (Fig. 249). In frozen sections, the lipid deposits stain with oil red O, and give a positive Schultz reaction for cholesterol. On polarization microscopy of such sections, birefringent crystals of cholesterol are demonstrable.

As the disease advances, the number of affected Kupffer cells increase, and similar deposits of sphingomyelin begin to appear in the hepatocytes and portal macrophages.

On electron microscopy, the deposits appear as myelin-like figures composed of concentric, laminated membranes enclosed within large lysosomes.

Ceramide

Farber's lipogranulomatosis is an autosomal recessive hereditary disorder of lipid metabolism characterized by a deficiency of the lysosomal enzyme acid ceramidase, which normally catalyzes the hydrolysis of ceramide (acyl-sphingosine) to sphingosine and fatty acids, a step in the pathway of complex sphingolipid catabolism. As a result of the deficiency, ceramide and mucopolysaccharides accumulate in the lysosomes of neurons, and of phagocytic cells, resulting in the formation of foam cells and granulomas in many tissues (203–205).

In a minority of cases, the Kupffer cells are enlarged and contain finely vacuolated cytoplasm, giving them a foamy appearance. The droplets stain with PAS and are resistant to diastase digestion. In frozen sections, the droplets take up lipid stains, react with phosphomolybdic acid, and exhibit birefringence.

On electron microscopy, the lysosomes of the Kupffer cells contain small tubular structures in an osmiophilic matrix.

Sea blue histiocytes

A number of apparently unrelated disorders are associated with the presence in the bone marrow, spleen, and, less commonly, the liver of large histiocytes containing coarse, cytoplasmic granules that appear deep blue in Giemsa- and Wright-stained sections (see Chapter 15). Such cells have been encountered in chronic myelogenous leukemia, other hematopoietic disorders characterized by rapid turnover of blood or blood precursor cells, Niemann-Pick disease, hyperlipoproteinemia, Tay-Sachs disease, Wolman's disease, chronic granulomatous disease of childhood, familial lecithincholesterol acyltransferase deficiency, and familial lipochrome histiocytosis (206,207).

The *sea blue histiocyte syndrome* has been reported as a specific entity characterized by histiocytic storage of glycosphingolipids and phospholipids. However, on histochemical analysis, the granules have proved to be identical with those in all the other disorders enumerated, so that the existence of a specific storage disease characterized by sea blue histiocytes is in doubt (206–208).

The granules in sea blue histiocytes exhibit all the histochemical properties of lipofuscin (ceroid) (209). These include the uptake of PAS following diastase digestion, acid-fast and Sudan black staining, and golden yellow autofluorescence. On electron microscopy, the granules appear as membrane-bound, electron-dense bodies in a finely granular background, and as whorls of membrane resembling myelin figures (209). These findings are consistent with the currently held view that the inclusions represent phospholipid-containing cell membranes derived from broken down hematopoietic cells and phagocytized circulating lipids.

Sea blue histiocytes are encountered most frequently in the bone marrow and spleen, and only rarely in the liver.

Nonspecific vacuolated Kupffer cells

Occasionally, large, foamy Kupffer cells, often containing lipofuscin, are encountered in individuals with no evidence of
hyperlipemia or any of the storage diseases (Fig. 232). Such
cells are usually few in number and may be found in association with a wide variety of hepatic lesions. Although the vacuolization is probably attributable to lipid deposition, the composition and pathogenesis of the deposits are not known.

Kupffer cell polysaccharide and glycoprotein deposits

For a more complete discussion of polysaccharide and glycoprotein deposits, the reader is referred to Chapter 14.

Amylopectin

As previously indicated, the deposits of amylopectin in *Type IV
glycogenosis* occur primarily in the hepatocytes, producing distinctive cytoplasmic inclusions (Fig. 148). However, occasionally, amylopectin is deposited in the Kupffer cells as well. The
Kupffer cells under such conditions are enlarged and exhibit
finely granular, PAS-positive cytoplasm, but contain no large
inclusions.

Mucopolysaccharides

In *Hurler's syndrome* and a number of other related disorders
characterized by a deficiency of one or another of the enzymes
involved in the catabolism of glycosaminoglycans, mucopolysaccharides accumulate in the lysosomes of both the hepatocytes and Kupffer cells. As a result, the affected cells appear
swollen and contain pale, vacuolated cytoplasm. Because of the
swelling, the sinusoids are often obscured, making the distinction between Kupffer cells and hepatocytes difficult (Fig. 186).
In sections appropriately fixed in a nonaqueous solution, such
as Lindsay's dioxane-picrate, the cytoplasmic acid mucopolysaccharide stains weakly with PAS following diastase digestion, but is deeply stained with colloidal iron.

Fucosides

Fucosidosis, a rare inborn error of lipid metabolism transmitted
as on autosomal recessive trait, is characterized by an absence
of the lysosomal enzyme, α-L-fucosidase, leading to the accumulation in many tissues, including the liver, of fucose-
containing   glycosphingolipids   and   mucopolysaccharides
(210,211).

In the liver, the deposits are found in the Kupffer cells, portal macrophages, hepatocytes, and bile duct epithelium. Characteristically, the affected Kupffer cells are enlarged and contain numerous fine cytoplasmic vacuoles, giving the cells a foamy

appearance (212). The deposits are weakly positive on PAS
staining (210).

On electron microscopy, the cytoplasm of the Kupffer cells
contains numerous large lysosomes, some filled with reticulo-
granular material suggestive of polysaccharide, and others with
groups of lamellae indicative of complex lipids (212).

Mucolipids

A group of autosomal recessive hereditary disorders classified
as *mucolipidoses* are characterized by variable defects in the
metabolism of mucopolysaccharides, lipids, and glycoproteins,
leading to the accumulation of these metabolites in various cell
types, including the Kupffer cells, portal macrophages, and,
occasionally, the hepatocytes (139,213,214). Many lysosomal
hydrolases are deficient in the affected tissues, but high levels
of these enzymes are found in the blood and urine. The primary
defect responsible for this inappropriate distribution of the enzymes is not known.

In *mucolipidosis I,* both the Kupffer cells and portal macrophages are enlarged and contain foamy cytoplasm. On electron
microscopy, the membrane-bound cytoplasmic vacuoles are filled
with reticulorgranular material.

The Kupffer cells and portal macrophages are also foamy in
mucolipidosis II, but the vacuoles contain not only fibrillogran-
ular material but also membranous lamellae and lipid droplets.

In *mucolipidosis III,* the Kupffer cells are vacuolated, and,
on electron microscopy, contain membrane-bound deposits of
unstructured, osmiophilic material.

Kupffer cell erythrophagocytosis and leukophagocytosis

Erythrophagocytosis

Enlarged Kupffer cells containing phagocytized erythrocytes have
been reported in sickle cell disease (215), leptospirosis (216),
P. falciparum malaria (217), and rarely, in severe cholestatic
states. We have encountered such erythrophagocytosis in single
cases of sickle cell disease (Fig. 250), acute Coxsackie virus
hepatitis, hemophilia complicated by peritonitis, and immunoblastic lymphadenopathy.

Kupffer cell hyperplasia with erythrophagocytosis must be
differentiated from infiltrates of the proliferating, abnormal histiocytes seen in histiocytic medullary reticulosis and familial
hemophagocytic reticulosis (see Chapter 24) that also exhibit
erythrophagocytosis (see later).

Leukophagocytosis

Occasionally, a few of the Kupffer cells are enlarged and contain clusters of neutrophils, usually unaccompanied by any significant increase in sinusoidal leukocytes. Although these may
suggest the possibility of biliary tract or systemic infection, they
occur more frequently under other conditions, so that they seldom prove to be diagnostic. Thus, in our own series of 32

patients who exhibited Kupffer cell leukophagocytosis on needle biopsy, only 4 had evidence of biliary tract disease, and only 3 had systemic bacterial infections. Of the remaining 25, 18 had a wide variety of hepatic lesions unassociated with fever or leukocytosis, and 7 who had no clinical evidence of infection had normal livers on biopsy. Figure 251 illustrates the enlargement and leukocytic infiltration of a Kupffer cell encountered in the normal liver of an afebrile patient with unexplained, unilateral, inguinal lymphadenopathy.

Kupffer cell invasion by protozoa and mycotic organisms

Leishmania donovani

In the visceral form of leishmaniasis, *kala-azar, Leishmania donovani* are found in large numbers in swollen, proliferating Kupffer cells (218). The organisms can be identified in H & E sections, but are best visualized with the Giemsa stain. Characteristically, the organisms appear as closely packed, sharply defined, deep blue, round or oval-shaped structures, measuring approximately 1 μm in diameter (Fig. 252). In bone marrow smears, the leishmania appear significantly larger, and can be seen to contain a relatively large nucleus and a short, rod-shaped kinetoplast.

Plasmodium falciparum

In the acute phase of *Plasmodium falciparum* infections, the Kupffer cells enlarge, increase in number, and often contain parasitized erythrocytes (219). These features are not seen in other forms of malaria.

Toxoplasma gondii

The liver is almost always affected in the *acquired* form of *toxoplasmosis,* an infection that often closely resembles infectious mononucleosis both clinically and morphologically (220). In addition to the other features of the hepatic lesions described in Chapter 23, they usually show striking swelling and proliferation of the Kupffer cells. Occasionally, the infecting organisms can be identified in the Kupffer cells, but usually they are few in number and difficult to find. Although best visualized in Giemsa-stained sections, toxoplasma are occasionally demonstrable in routine H & E sections. In such sections, they present as pale, crescentic structures, 2 to 6 μm in diameter, that contain a dark basophilic nucleus at one pole (Fig. 253). The morphology of the organisms is more clearly visualized in Giemsa-stained smears of the peritoneal exudate of mice inoculated intraperitoneally with a fragment of the infected liver (Fig. 254).

Cryptococcus neoformans

Disseminated infections with *Cryptococcus neoformans,* an encapsulated form of yeast, frequently involve the liver, produc-

ing foci of necrosis, granulomas, and proliferation and swelling of the Kupffer cells (221,222). The swollen Kupffer cells in such cases often contain numerous cryptococci. In H & E sections, these appear as small, discrete, circular or oval, eosinophilic bodies encircled by a clear halo (Fig. 255). Since the organisms occasionally stain only faintly in H & E sections, they may be overlooked, particularly if few in number. Grocott's silver methenamine, which stains the capsules of cryptococci, greatly facilitates their demonstration (Fig. 256).

Histoplasma capsulatum

In active forms of *histoplasmosis,* hepatic involvement is relatively common, being manifested by swelling and proliferation of Kupffer cells, and epithelioid granuloma formation (223) (Chapters 22, 23). Occasionally, the affected Kupffer cells contain *H. capsulatum.* In H & E sections, these appear as multiple, small, pale pink dots, each surrounded by a clear halo (Fig. 257). The organisms are more readily identified when their capsules are stained with PAS or Grocott's silver methenamine (Fig. 258).

Hypertrophy and hyperplasia of the lipocytes (Ito cells)

Under normal conditions, the lipocytes in the spaces of Disse store vitamin A and other lipids and serve as inactive precursors of fibroblasts. When appropriately stimulated, the lipocytes proliferate, undergo transformation to active fibroblasts, and probably play a role in the fibrogenesis that follows some forms of hepatic injury (180).

Although lipocytes are readily demonstrable by electron microscopy, and in 1 μm Epon-embedded sections stained with toluidine blue (224), they are difficult to identify by light microscopy in routine sections. However, when the lipocytes contain excessive stores of vitamin A, as in *hypervitaminosis A* (225), they are readily visualized in such sections as large, pale, vacuolated cells with eccentric, indented, pyknotic nuclei projecting into and filling the sinusoidal lumens (Fig. 259). Characteristically, in frozen sections, the affected cells exhibit a distinctive, apple-green autofluorescence that fades rapidly (Fig. 260). Presumably, as a consequence of their activation and transformation to fibroblasts, the proliferating lipocytes are accompanied by deposition of reticulin and collagen in the spaces of Disse (Fig. 224).

Histiocytic and leukemic infiltration of the sinusoids

Histiocytosis X

A group of disorders, including *eosinophilic granuloma of bone, Hand-Schuller-Christian disease,* and *Letterer-Siwe disease,* are regarded by some as variants of a single entity classified as histiocytosis X (226) because of certain overlapping clinical and morphologic features. Although there is general agreement that Hand-Schuller-Christian disease is a multifocal or systemic variant of eosinophilic granuloma of bone, the view that these two disorders are related to Letterer-Siwe disease has been challenged (227).

The systemic form of the disease, usually classified as Letterer-Siwe disease in infants and as histiocytosis X in adults, is a disorder of unknown etiology characterized by proliferation of histiocytes in the liver, spleen, lymph nodes, bone marrow, and skin. Although the histiocytes are well differentiated, their proliferation leads to destructive lesions and a fatal outcome, usually within a few months in infants and after a protracted course in adults.

In the liver, the proliferating histiocytes appear as pale, faintly eosinophilic, finely granular cells with vesicular nuclei (Fig. 261). They tend to form large, randomly distributed aggregates that distend the sinusoids and lead to atrophy and loss of hepatocytes. Occasionally, the histiocytes invade the central veins, filling their lumens (Fig. 262). As a rule, the histiocytic infiltration is most prominent in the portal tracts, which invariably are enlarged and distorted, and often, show destruction or wide separation of their collagen bundles by the infiltrating cells. Occasionally, the infiltrate contains a few eosinophils or giant cells.

Malignant histiocytosis

A neoplastic disease of histiocytes that affects the liver, spleen, bone marrow, and skin has been variously termed *histiocytic medullary reticulosis* (228), *malignant histiocytosis* (229,230), and *aleukemic reticulosis* (231).

The hepatic lesions are characterized by striking proliferation of atypical histiocytes in the sinusoids and portal tracts. The invading cells distend the sinusoids and lead to atrophy and loss of the intervening hepatocytes (Fig. 263). Some of the histiocytes contain relatively large, polylobulated, hyperchromatic nuclei with thick nuclear membranes, irregularly clumped chromatin, and large, irregular nucleoli (Fig. 264). In others, the nuclei are smaller and more vesicular.

In most cases, a few of the histiocytes show evidence of erythrophagocytosis and, less commonly, phagocytosis of leukocytes and platelets. The pancytopenia commonly seen in malignant histiocytosis has been attributed to such phagocytosis (231). A striking feature in many cases is invasion of the central veins by the infiltrating histiocytes (Fig. 265), which is obvious with the Masson stain but may be much less evident with H & E.

Familial hemophagocytic reticulosis (lymphohistiocytosis)

This familial disorder, characterized by widespread infiltration of the liver, spleen, bone marrow, and lymph nodes by large, atypical histiocytes, affects children under two years of age, and is invariably fatal within a few months. Characteristically, the affected histiocytes contain phagocytized erythrocytes and, less commonly, leukocytes and platelets (232–234).

Except for its early age of onset and occurrence in siblings, familial hemophagocytic reticulosis is indistinguishable clinically or morphologically from histiocytic medullary reticulosis (malignant histiocytosis).

Hairy cell leukemia (leukemic reticuloendotheliosis)

This unusual form of leukemia is characterized by the proliferation of a unique type of mononuclear cell that infiltrates many of the tissues, including the liver, but appears in the peripheral blood inconstantly and usually only in small numbers (235–237). Although the precise nature of the cells is uncertain, they resemble monocytes more closely than lymphocytes. Their most distinctive feature histologically is the presence of hair-like, cytoplasmic projections from their surface.

In the liver, the leukemic cells are found in both the sinusoids and portal tracts. The affected sinusoids are usually dilated or even peliotic (235), and contain large cells with prominent nuclei surrounded by radiating strands of pale, eosinophilic cytoplasm (Fig. 266). Because of their large size and stellate shape, they may be mistaken for Kupffer cells. The hairy projections are well visualized in biopsy specimens fixed in Carnoy's solution, but may be difficult to identify in formalin-fixed material. Although difficult to prove at the light microscopic level, there is convincing electron microscopic evidence that the leukemic cells replace the normal endothelial lining cells of the sinusoids (236). Another feature of interest is the increase in sinusoidal reticulin that accompanies the leukemic infiltration (Fig. 267). It is postulated for both peliosis hepatis and hairy cell pseudopeliosis that destruction of reticulin is responsible (235).

The portal lesions of hairy cell leukemia are said to be characterized by numerous fine, vascular channels filled with erythrocytes and lined by hairy cells (236). However, in the only two cases that we have studied, the triads were infiltrated with leukemic cells, but showed no angiomatous features.

Other forms of leukemia

In all forms of leukemia, both the sinusoids and portal tracts may be infiltrated with leukemic cells. Such lesions are encountered at biopsy most frequently in patients with chronic lymphocytic leukemia, but may be seen postmortem in other forms of acute and chronic leukemia. Characteristically, the affected areas show distension of the sinusoids with leukemic cells and atrophy or loss of the intervening hepatocytes (Fig. 268). The portal triads are usually even more heavily infiltrated and show enlargement, erosion of their limiting plates, and separation or destruction of their collagen bundles.

Abnormalities of the central and sublobular veins

Endophlebitis

Under a variety of conditions, the endothelial cells lining the central and sublobular veins proliferate and are often infiltrated with a few inflammatory cells, resulting in significant thickening of the intima (Fig. 269). In some cases, the walls of the affected veins are perforated by strands of proliferating Kupffer cells or histiocytes that project from the subjacent sinusoids into lumens of the veins, and merge with their thickened intima (Fig. 270).

Vascular lesions of this type are encountered most frequently in acute viral hepatitis (Fig. 269), drug-induced hepatitis (Fig. 270), and infectious mononucleosis. However, they may be seen occasionally in other conditions, including, in our own experience, alcoholic hepatitis, extrahepatic biliary obstruction, hepatic metastases, Hodgkin's disease, toxoplasmosis, and bacterial endocarditis.

Veno-occlusive disease

This disorder, which is characterized by subintimal edema, hemorrhage, and inflammation of the central and sublobular hepatic veins that leads ultimately to fibrous occlusion of their lumens and clinical manifestations resembling those of the Budd-Chiari syndrome, was first reported from Jamaica as veno-occlusive disease (239). It is now known that the disease is worldwide in distribution and usually is due to poisoning with one of the pyrrolizidine *(Senecio)* alkaloids (240,241). Similar, if not identical, lesions have been encountered in hepatotoxic reactions to azathioprine (242), 6-thioguanine (243), urethane (244) and excessive vitamin A (225), and in association with myxedema (245), graft-versus-host disease (246), and radiation hepatitis (247).

The *acute* lesions of veno-occlusive disease are characterized by subintimal edema, hemorrhage, and inflammation in the central and sublobular veins, and congestion of the surrounding centrilobular sinusoids. Usually, the affected veins contain no thrombi, and the adjacent hepatocytes show atrophy, but no coagulation necrosis. Figure 271 illustrates these changes in a case of 6-thioguanine hepatotoxicity. In survivors, the affected veins undergo progressive fibrosis with partial or complete occlusion of their lumens, and often are accompanied by extensive centrilobular hepatocellular dropout and fibrosis. *Chronic* lesions of this type may develop insidiously, rather than as a sequela of an antecedent, acute, hepatotoxic reaction. Figure 272 illustrates such a lesion in a case of severe chronic hypervitaminosis A.

Although thrombosis is not a feature of the early vascular lesions in veno-occlusive disease, in the late stages, the occlusions in the veins are indistinguishable histologically from organized thrombi.

Thrombotic occlusions

Fresh clots are rarely encountered in the peripheral branches of the hepatic veins seen in biopsy sections, even when they are present in the proximal, more central branches at autopsy. However, *organized* thrombi, often partially recanalized, are relatively common, being found most frequently in the Budd-Chiari syndrome and in alcoholic liver disease. Rarely, they occur in association with primary and metastatic tumors of the liver, hepatic Hodgkin's disease, and extensive extramedullary hematopoiesis.

In the late stages of alcoholic hepatitis, the lesions are characterized by replacement of centrilobular hepatocytes with fi-

brous tissue, and fibrosis of the central veins. The lumens of the affected veins often contain loosely arranged collagen bundles and fine vascular channels (Fig. 273), features that suggest an organized, recanalized thrombus. However, the possibility cannot be excluded that such vascular lesions are attributable to the same type of endophlebitis and fibrosis seen in veno-occlusive disease. Nevertheless, whatever their pathogenesis, the presence of such fibrotic occluded central and sublobular hepatic veins within the fibrous septa of advanced, inactive cirrhosis may be of diagnostic value in identifying an alcoholic etiology.

Almost always, some of the central veins in the Budd-Chiari syndrome contain organized, partially recanalized thrombi, as illustrated in Figure 215. Since such organized thrombi are encountered so frequently in biopsy specimens, even when fresh clots are found within the major hepatic veins at autopsy, the possibility must be considered that in many cases of the Budd-Chiari syndrome, the thrombotic process begins in the terminal branches of the hepatic venous tree and then extends centrally.

Histiocytic infiltration

As previously indicated, the central veins may be invaded by proliferating histiocytes in both histiocytosis X (Fig. 262) and malignant histiocytosis (Fig. 265).

Granulomatous infiltration

In various granulomatous disorders that affect the liver, and particularly in sarcoidosis and tuberculosis, granulomas are often found closely adherent to central veins (Fig. 274). Occasionally, the granulomas penetrate the walls of the veins and protrude into their lumens (Fig. 275). Such vascular lesions, if numerous, may account for the type of portal hypertension occasionally encountered in patients with sarcoidosis who exhibit high wedged hepatic vein pressure, but no evidence of significant hepatic fibrosis (248).

Prolapse of hepatocytes into the central veins

Transsexual females and impotent males maintained on large doses of methyltestosterone (150 mg daily) for as long as three years frequently exhibit unusual hepatic lesions (249). These are characterized by hepatocellular regeneration, centrilobular and periportal sinusoidal dilatation, and invasion of the central and sublobular veins by proliferating hepatocytes that line and may partially occlude their lumens. The pathogenesis of such lesions, particularly the prolapse of hepatocytes into the hepatic veins, in uncertain, since they may be seen occasionally under conditions other than methyltestosterone therapy. Of the two cases of hepatic vein invasion by hepatocytes that we have encountered, one occurred in a 15-year-old black boy with obstructive jaundice attributable to cholelithiasis and choledocholithiasis unrelated to hemolytic disease, and the other in a 30-year-old man with HBsAg-negative chronic active hepatitis who had been on prednisone-azathioprine immunosuppressive therapy for 14 months following renal transplantation (Fig. 276).

Intralobular inflammatory cells

Under a wide variety of conditions, inflammatory cells infiltrate the parenchyma of the lobules. Often, the portal tracts are similarly involved, and, in some instances, the intralobular exudate appears to represent an extension of inflammatory cells from the portal tracts. The intralobular infiltrates may be focal, zonal, or diffuse in distribution, and may be localized in the sinusoids, foci of necrosis, or, rarely, within hepatocytes or Kupffer cells. Although one or another cell type may predominate, most exudates are of the mixed variety, and often contain proliferating and hypertrophied Kupffer cells.

Intralobular lymphocytes

Lymphocytes are found within the lobules most frequently in various forms of acute and chronic hepatitis, their number and distribution depending on the etiology and the severity of the lesions. In *acute viral hepatitis,* lymphocytes, almost always accompanied by swollen, proliferating Kupffer cells and, in its later stages, by a variable number of plasma cells, are most numerous in the relatively large foci of hepatocellular necrosis usually present in the centrilobular zones (Fig. 230). However, they are also found in the sinusoids and in the small foci of spotty necrosis scattered throughout the lobules (Fig. 86). A similar type of inflammatory reaction is seen in many cases of drug-induced hepatitis (Fig. 270).

The hepatic lesions of *infectious mononucleosis* are characterized by striking Kupffer cell hyperplasia and infiltration of the sinusoids by a variable number of lymphocytes and large mononuclear cells with only minimal or no hepatocellular necrosis (Fig. 218). The striking discrepancy between the intensity of the inflammatory reaction and the extent of the necrosis is a distinctive feature of infectious mononucleosis, but is not pathognomonic. Occasionally, similar lesions are encountered in cases of mild viral and drug-induced hepatitis, and in the mononucleosis syndromes associated with *cytomegalovirus* and *Toxoplasma gondii* infections. Differentiation between these disorders usually depends on the results of serologic studies. Occasionally, however, the finding of cytomegalic inclusions in the hepatocytes (Fig. 190) or bile duct epithelial cells (Fig. 191), or the detection of *Toxoplasma gondii* in Kupffer cells (Fig. 253) makes histologic identification of the etiology possible.

Numerous lymphocytes and plasma cells are found in the advancing edge of periportal hepatocellular necrosis characteristic of *chronic active hepatitis.* The inflammatory cells, usually accompanied by fine strands of collagen, extend out from the portal tracts into the parenchyma, encircling groups of periportal hepatocytes often arranged in the form of rosettes (Fig. 106). In some periportal zones, the lymphocytes and plasma cells infiltrate the sinusoids and spaces of Disse, coming into intimate contact with hepatocytes (Fig. 226), a feature often cited as supporting evidence for the hypothesis that a cell-mediated immune mechanism is involved in the pathogenesis of chronic active hepatitis (181). Although hepatocellular necrosis and inflammation are most prominent in the periportal zones, small foci of cell dropout, Kupffer cell hyperplasia, and lymphocytes frequently are found scattered elsewhere throughout the lobules.

Nonspecific reactive hepatitis and its more localized variant,

nonspecific focal hepatitis, relatively common lesions encountered in a wide variety of systemic and other extrahepatic diseases, are characterized by small foci of hepatocellular degeneration and/or necrosis infiltrated with lymphocytes and macrophages (Fig. 92).

In *tropical splenomegaly,* a disorder thought to be a manifestation of low-grade, chronic, malarial infection, the sinusoids usually are dilated and contain numerous lymphocytes and hypertrophied Kupffer cells (250).

Leukemic infiltrates frequently invade the sinusoids and mimic inflammatory exudates (Fig. 268). The density and uniformity of leukemic infiltrates, their tendency to distend the sinusoids leading to atrophy of intervening hepatocytes, their destructive nature in the portal tracts (Fig. 277) and the occasional presence of immature hematopoietic cells serve to differentiate them from inflammatory exudates.

Intralobular plasma cells

As previously indicated, a variable number of plasma cells are found in the predominantly lymphocytic and histiocytic intralobular inflammatory exudates of *acute viral* and *drug-induced hepatitis,* particularly late in the course of the disease. Usually, however, the plasma cells are more numerous in the portal tracts than in the parenchyma.

The most striking plasma cell infiltrates are seen in *chronic active hepatitis.* Although the portal tracts are invariably involved, plasma cells are most numerous in the advancing edge of periportal hepatocellular necrosis (Fig. 278). This margination of plasma cells is best seen in sections stained with methyl green pyronin, which visualizes the high concentration of ribonucleic acid in the cytoplasm of such cells (Fig. 279). Portal and periportal plasmacytosis of this type is particularly impressive in children with chronic active hepatitis, so that such lesions have been classified by some as plasma cell hepatitis (251).

At autopsy in *multiple myeloma,* the liver often shows diffuse infiltration of the sinusoids and portal tracts by plasma cells, or contains plasma cell tumor nodules. In one large series, such lesions were encountered in 40% of the cases (252). However, they are encountered far less frequently in needle biopsy sections. Thus, of the 13 patients with multiple myeloma whom we have investigated by needle biopsy of the liver, only one exhibited significant portal and intralobular plasmacytosis (Fig. 280).

Intralobular neutrophils

Intralobular exudates contain neutrophils far less frequently than lymphocytes and plasma cells. Neutrophils limited to the sinusoids and unaccompanied by hepatocellular degeneration or necrosis, or by proliferation of Kupffer cells, usually are indicative of *peripheral leukocytosis* and have no significance with respect to the liver.

Neutrophilic infiltration of hepatocytes in centrilobular and subcapsular foci of coagulation necrosis is a relatively common finding in surgical wedge biopsy specimens [(9–11); Figs. 102, 103]. Such lesions, typical of *surgical artifacts,* are attributable to compression of the liver during laparotomy, leading to hepatocellular injury either directly or as a result of interference with the intrahepatic circulation. Although these lesions have no clinical significance, they may be mistaken for microabscesses or other forms of acute hepatocellular necrosis if their nature is not recognized.

Significant numbers of neutrophils are almost always found in the lesions of active *alcoholic hepatitis*. At an early stage, they are encountered principally in the centrilobular zones of degeneration and necrosis that usually contain Mallory bodies. However, once the lesion has advanced to the stage of cirrhosis and remains active, the neutrophils and other features of alcoholic hepatitis are found around the margins of nodules. It is generally held that Mallory bodies exert a chemotactic action that attracts neutrophils, and that in serial sections, neutrophils are invariably demonstrable around hepatocytes that contain Mallory bodies (50). However, this is open to question. Although some hepatocytes containing Mallory bodies may be infiltrated or surrounded by neutrophils (Fig. 131), more commonly, the neutrophils are randomly distributed in areas containing such cells (Fig. 132). Moreover, in some lesions, no neutrophils are found in areas containing numerous Mallory bodies (Fig. 130).

Neutrophils frequently infiltrate the sinusoids and hepatocytes in zones of *ischemic coagulation necrosis* (Fig. 100). As a rule, such infiltrates do not appear until several days after the onset of ischemic injury. A similar neutrophilic reaction is seen occasionally in other forms of coagulation necrosis attributable to hepatotoxins and infection.

Both *suppurative cholangitis* and *pylephlebitis* frequently are associated with periportal foci of hepatocellular coagulation necrosis and cytolysis heavily infiltrated with neutrophils (Fig. 281). Presumably, such lesions are attributable to bacterial infection of the parenchyma. Often, however, no bacteria can be detected in specially stained sections, so that other factors may be involved in some cases. If the infection cannot be brought under control with antibiotics or surgical drainage, the foci of necrosis may expand and undergo liquefaction, giving rise to frank hepatic abscesses (Fig. 282). Such abscess formation entails not only loss of hepatocytes and massive infiltration of neutrophils but also destruction of the supporting reticulin, sinusoids, and portal tracts.

Systemic infections accompanied by *bacteremia* give rise occasionally to small scattered foci of hepatocellular necrosis that contain proliferating, swollen Kupffer cells and a variable number of neutrophils (Fig. 283). However, such lesions are not pathognomonic for systemic bacterial infection, since they are seen occasionally in cases of *extrahepatic biliary obstruction* (Fig. 284), *drug-induced cholestatic hepatitis,* and even in otherwise *normal livers* (Fig. 251) in the absence of infection.

Rarely, similar foci of necrosis containing swollen Kupffer cells and infiltrating neutrophils are attributable to *nonbacterial systemic infections*. Figure 190 illustrates such a lesion in a case of active cytomegalovirus infection.

Intralobular eosinophils

The intralobular exudates in some cases of *drug-induced hepatitis* contain a significant number of eosinophils (Fig. 285), a feature consistent with the view that such lesions are attributable to hypersensitivity reactions. However, intralobular eosinophils are of only limited value as a diagnostic criterion, since they are an inconstant finding in drug-induced hepatitis and may be seen occasionally, although less frequently, in acute viral hepatitis (Fig. 286).

For reasons that are not known, *lipogranulomas* of the type found in livers infiltrated with fat occasionally contain a significant number of eosinophils (Fig. 287). Although such lesions have no diagnostic or clinical significance, they may be misinterpreted as evidence of an underlying hypersensitivity reaction if their nature is not recognized.

The *hypereosinophilic syndrome,* a disorder of unknown and apparently varied etiology that occasionally is a manifestation of eosinophilic leukemia, is characterized by constitutional symptoms, prolonged peripheral eosinophilia, and eosinophilic infiltration of the viscera, central nervous system, and skin. It affects males predominantly and often proves fatal. The liver, one of the organs most frequently affected, usually shows widespread eosinophilic infiltrates in the portal tracts and, less commonly, in the sinusoids and lobular parenchyma (253).

Eosinophilic gastroenteritis, a disorder of uncertain etiology, but probably allergic in nature, is characterized by eosinophilic infiltration of the stomach and small intestine accompanied by peripheral eosinophilia. The clinical manifestations, which tend to be intermittent, include diarrhea, abdominal pain, gastric or intestinal obstruction, or ascites, depending on whether the eosinophilic infiltrate involves the mucosa muscularis, or serosa (254). The liver is enlarged in some cases, but on biopsy, usually shows only sinusoidal eosinophils in numbers consistent with the degree of peripheral eosinophilia. However, in a well-documented case studied here, the portal tracts showed a number of striking changes, described and illustrated in Chapter 5.

The most striking infiltration of the liver by eosinophils is seen in *visceral larva migrans,* a relatively uncommon disorder attributable to the migration of nematode larvae through the tissues that affects young children who swallow soil contaminated with the ova of *Toxocara canis* or *Toxocara cati* (255). Less commonly, the larvae of other nematodes may be implicated (256). Characteristically, the larvae provoke a prolonged and marked peripheral eosinophilia, and give rise to an intense, eosinophilic, inflammatory reaction, granuloma formation, and necrosis in the tissues they invade. The liver, one of the organs most frequently involved, usually contains numerous granulomas made up of loosely arranged epithelioid and giant cells that often show a central zone of necrosis, and invariably are surrounded by a dense band of eosinophils (Figs. 288, 289). In addition, there are large circumscribed zones of liquefaction necrosis that resemble pyogenic abscesses, but are filled with closely packed eosinophils. At the periphery of such zones, remnants of atrophic hepatic plates and widely dilated sinusoids distended with eosinophils can still be identified (Fig. 290). Although the most striking lesions are seen in the parenchyma, the portal tracts also are affected, usually being expanded and heavily infiltrated with eosinophils (Fig. 291). At all sites, the infiltrates are almost exclusively eosinophilic, but, occasionally, they contain a few plasma cells and macrophages. The larvae responsible for provoking the lesions of visceral larva migrans are usually difficult to find in routine sections, but may be detected if multiple serial sections of a large block are examined.

Intralobular macrophages and proliferating Kupffer cells

As previously indicated, proliferating Kupffer cells and other infiltrating macrophages frequently participate in intralobular inflammatory reactions. For a discussion and illustrations of such reactions, the reader is referred to the section on Kupffer cells.

References

1. Searle J, Kerr JFR, Bishop CJ: Necrosis and apoptosis: distinct modes of cell death with fundamentally different significance. Pathol Annu 17 (Part 2): 229–259, 1982.
2. Zajicek G, Oren R, Weinreb M Jr: The streaming liver. Liver 5:293–300, 1985.
3. Bianchi L, DeGroote J, Desmet VJ, Gedick P, Korb G, Popper H, Poulsen H, Scheuer PJ, Schmid M, Thaler H, Wepler W: Morphological criteria in viral hepatitis. Review by an international group. Lancet 1:333–337, 1971.
4. Kerr JFR, Cooksley WGE, Searle J, Halliday JW, Halliday WJ, Holder L, Roberts I, Burnett W, Powell LW: The nature of piecemeal necrosis in chronic active hepatitis. Lancet 2:827–828, 1979.
5. Klion FM, Schaffner F: The ultrastructure of acidophilic "Councilman-like" bodies in the liver. Am J Pathol 48:755–767, 1966.
6. Councilman WT: In Report on the Etiology and Prevention of Yellow Fever, edited by G. M. Sternberg. U.S. Marine Hospital Service, Treasury Dept., Document No. 1328 (Public Health Bulletin 2), Government Printing Office, Washington, D.C., 1890, pp. 141–149.
7. Vieira WT, Gayotto LC, De Lima CP, De Brito T: Histopathology of the human liver in yellow fever with special emphasis on the diagnostic role of the Councilman body. Histopathology 7:195–208, 1983.
8. Child PL, Ruiz A: Acidophilic bodies. Their clinical and physical nature in patients with Bolivian hemorrhagic fever. Arch Pathol 85:45–50, 1968.
9. Christoffersen P, Poulsen H, Skeie E: Focal liver cell necrosis accompanied by infiltration of granulocytes arising during operation. Acta Hepatosplenologica 17:240–245, 1970.
10. McDonald GSA, Courtney MG: Operation-associated neutrophils in a percutaneous liver biopsy: effect of prior transjugular procedure. Histopathology 10:217–222, 1986.
11. Fenster LF: Focal infiltrations of polymorphonuclear leukocytes in liver biopsies: traumatic lesions? Hepatology 7:393–394, 1987.
12. Boyer JL, Klatskin G: Pattern of necrosis in acute viral hepatitis. Prognostic value of bridging necrosis (subacute hepatic necrosis). N Engl J Med 283:1063–1071, 1970.
13. Ware AJ, Eigenbrodt EH, Combes B: Prognostic significance of subacute hepatic necrosis in acute hepatitis. Gastroenterology 68:519–524, 1975.
14. Karvountzis GG, Redeker AG, Peters RL: Long term follow-up studies of patients surviving fulminant viral hepatitis. Gastroenterology 67:870–877, 1974.
15. Spitz RD, Keren DF, Boitnott JK, Maddrey WC: Bridging hepatic necrosis. Etiology and prognosis. Am J Dig Dis 23:1076–1078, 1978.
16. Miller DJ, Dwyer J, Klatskin G: Halothane hepatitis: benign resolution of a severe lesion. Ann Intern Med 89:212–215, 1978.
17. Klatskin G, Kimberg DV: Recurrent hepatitis attributable to halothane sensitization in an anesthetist. N Engl J Med 280:515–522, 1969.
18. Reynolds TB, Peters RL, Yamada S: Chronic active and lupoid hepatitis caused by a laxative, oxyphenisatin. N Engl J Med 285:813–820, 1971.
19. Bianchi L, DeGroote J, Desmet VJ, Gedik P, Korb G. Popper H, Poulsen H, Scheuer PJ, Schmid M, Thaler H, Wepler W: Acute and chronic hepatitis revisited. Review by an international group. Lancet 2:914–949, 1977.
20. Scotto J, Opolon P, Vergoz ED, Thomas M, Caroli J: Liver biopsy and prognosis in acute liver failure. Gut 4:927–933, 1973.
21. Popper H, Lieber CS: Histogenesis of alcoholic fibrosis and cirrhosis in the baboon. Am J Pathol 98:695–715, 1980.
22. Baraona E, Leo MA, Borowsky SA, Lieber CS: Pathogenesis of alcohol-induced accumulation of protein in the liver. J Clin Invest 60:546–554, 1977.
23. Klatskin G: The problem of fixing liver tissue for electron microscopy. (Abst.) J Ultrastruct Res 14:417, 1966.
24. Uchida T, Kao H, Quispe-Sjogren M, Peters RL: Alcoholic foamy degeneration; a pattern of acute alcoholic injury of the liver. Gastroenterology 84:683–692, 1984.
25. Peters RL, Edmondson HA, Mikkelsen WP, Tatter D: Tetracycline-induced fatty liver in nonpregnant patients. A report of six cases. Am J Surg 113:622–632, 1967.
26. Robinson MJ, Rywlin AM: Tetracycline-associated fatty liver in the male. Report of an autopsied case. Am J Dig Dis 15:857–862, 1970.
27. Gerber MA, Thung SN: Hepatic oncocytes. Incidence, staining characteristics and ultrastructural features. Am J Clin Pathol 75:498–503, 1981.
28. Lefkowitch JH, Arborgh BAM, Scheuer PJ: Oxyphilic granular hepatocytes. Mitochondrion-rich liver cells in hepatic disease. Am J Clin Pathol 74:432–441, 1980.
29. Montgomery CK, Ruebner BH: Neonatal hepatocellular giant cell transformation: a review. Perspect Pediatr Pathol 3:85–101, 1976.
30. Thaler H: Post-infantile giant cell hepatitis. Liver 2:393–403, 1982.
31. Phillips MJ, Blendis LM, Poucell S, Patterson J, Petric M, Roberts E, Levy GA, Superina RA, Greig PD, Cameron R, Langer B, Purcell RH: Syncytial giant-cell hepatitis. Sporadic hepatitis with distinctive pathological features, a severe clinical course, and paramyxoviral features. N Engl J Med 324:455–460, 1991.
32. MacSween RNM: Mallory's 'Alcoholic' hyaline in primary biliary cirrhosis. J Clin Pathol 26:340–342, 1973.
33. Levi AJ, Sherlock S, Scheuer PJ, Cumings JN: Presymptomatic Wilson's disease. Lancet 2:575–579, 1967.
34. Nayak NC, Roy S: Morphological types of hepatocellular hyalin in Indian childhood cirrhosis: an ultrastructural study. Gut 17:791–796, 1976.
35. Batman PA, Scheuer PJ: Diabetic hepatitis preceding the onset of glucose intolerance. Histopathology 9:237–243, 1985.
36. Gerber MA, Orr W, Denk H, Schaffner J, Popper H: Hepatocellular hyalin in cholestasis and cirrhosis: its diagnostic significance. Gastroenterology 64:89–98, 1973.
37. Baker AL, Elson CO, Jaspan J, Boyer JL: Liver failure with steatonecrosis after jejunoileal bypass. Recovery with parenteral nutrition and reanastomosis. Arch Intern Med 139: 289–292, 1979.
38. Keeley AF, Iseri OA, Gottlieb LS: Ultrastructure of hyaline cytoplasmic inclusions in a human hepatoma: relationship to Mallory's alcoholic hyalin. Gastroenterology 62:280–293, 1972.
39. Benz EJ, Baggenstoss AH: Focal cirrhosis of the liver: its relation to the so-called hamartoma (adenoma, benign hepatoma). Cancer 6:743–755, 1953.
40. Poucell S, Ireton J, Valencia-Mayoral P, Downar E, Larratt L, Patterson J, Blendis L, Phillips MJ: Amiodarone-associated phospholipidosis and fibrosis of the liver. Gastroenterology 86:926–936, 1984.
41. Pessayer E, Bichara M, Feldmann G, Degott C, Potet F, Benhamou J–P: Perihexiline maleate-induced cirrhosis. Gastroenterology 76:170–177, 1979.
42. Denk H. Gschnait F, Wolff K: Hepatocellular hyalin (Mallory bodies) in long term griseofulvin-treated mice: a new experimental model for the study of hyalin formation. Lab Invest 32:773–776, 1975.
43. Yokoo H, Harwood TR, Racker D, Arak S: Experimental production of Mallory bodies in mice by diet containing 3,5-diethoxycarbonyl-1,4 dihydrocollidine. Gastroenterology 83:109–113, 1982.
44. Yokoo H, Minick OT, Batti F, Kent G: Morphologic variants of alcoholic hyalin. Am J Pathol 69:25–40, 1972.
45. Franke WW, Denk H, Schmid E, Osborn M, Weber K: Ultrastructural biochemical and immunologic characterization of Mallory bodies in livers of griseofulvin-treated mice; fimbricated rods of filaments containing pre-keratin-like polypeptides. Lab Invest 40:207–220, 1979.
46. Oksnour Y, Zohta M, Ou O, Kachi K, Kagawa K, Yuki T, Okuno T, Takino T, French SW: Relationship of Mallory bodies to intermediate filaments in hepatocytes. A scanning electron microscopy study. Lab Invest 53:534–540, 1985.
47. French SW: Present understanding of the development of Mallory body. Arch Pathol Lab Med 107:445–450, 1983.
48. French SW: Mallory bodies in hepatic neoplasms: what does it mean? Hepatology 6:1428–1429, 1986.
49. Roque AL: Chromotrope analine blue method of staining Mallory bodies of Laennec's cirrhosis. Lab Invest 2:15–21, 1953.
50. Christoffersen P: Light microscopical features in liver biopsies with Mallory bodies. Acta Pathol Microbiol Scand 80:705–712, 1972.
51. Kuhn C III, Kuo T-T: Cytoplasmic hyalin in asbestosis. Arch Pathol 95:190–195, 1973.
52. Junge J, Horn T, Christoffersen P: Megamitochondria as a diagnostic marker for alcohol induced centrilobular and periportal fibrosis in the liver. Virchows Arch [A] Pathol Anat Histol 410:553–558, 1987.
53. Chedid A, Mendenhall CL, Tosch T, Chen T, Rabin L, Garcia-Pont P, Goldberg SJ, Kiernan T, Seeff LB, Sorrel M, Tamburro C, Weesner RE, Zetterman R: Significance of megamitochondria in alcoholic liver disease. Gastroenterology 90:1858–1864, 1986.
54. Bruguera M, Bertran A, Bombi JA, Rodes J: Giant mitochondria in

hepatocytes. A diagnostic hint for alcoholic liver disease. Gastroenterology 73:1383–1387, 1977.

55. Feldmann G, Maurice M, Husson JM, Fiessinger JN, Camilieri JP, Benhamou JP, Housset E: Hepatocyte giant mitochondria: an almost constant lesion in systemic scleroderma. Virchows Arch [A] Pathol Anat Histol 374:215–227, 1977.

56. Iseri OA, Gottlieb LS: Alcoholic hyalin and megamitochondria in liver disease associated with alcoholism. Gastroenterology 60:1027–1035, 1971.

56a. Horiuch R, Uchida T, Shikata T: A newly recognized hepatic inclusion body, "ring body"—significance of its occurrence. Acta Hep Japonica 27:945–952, 1986.

57. Hadziyannis A. Gerber MA, Vissoulis C. Popper H: Cytoplasmic hepatitis B antigen in "ground-glass" hepatocytes of carriers. Arch Pathol 96:327–330, 1973.

58. Stein O, Fainaru M, Stein Y: Virus-like particles in the cytoplasm of the livers of Australia antigen carriers. Am J Dis Child 123:313–314, 1972.

59. Huang S-N: Immunohistochemical demonstration of hepatitis B core and surface antigens in paraffin sections. Lab Invest 33:88–95, 1975.

60. Shikata T, Uzawa T, Yoshiwara N, Akatsuka T, Yamazaki S: Staining methods of Australia antigen in paraffin section detection of cytoplasmic inclusion bodies. Jpn J Exp Med 44:25–36, 1974.

61. Deodhar KP, Tapp E, Scheuer PJ: Orcein staining of hepatitis B antigen in paraffin sections of liver biopsies. J Clin Pathol 28:66–70, 1975.

62. Denk H, Radaszkiewicz T, Weirich E: Machweis von Hepatitis-B-Surface (HBs−) Antigen in konventionellem Paraffin eingebetteten Leberbiopsiematerial mittels immunofluoreszens. Wien Klin Wochenschr 89:643–648, 1977.

63. Kostich ND, Ingham CD: Detection of hepatitis B surface antigen by means of orcein staining of liver. Am J Clin Pathol 67:20–30, 1977.

64. Nayak NC, Sachdeva R: Localization of hepatitis B surface antigen in conventional paraffin sections of the liver. Comparison of immunofluorescence, immunoperoxidase, and orcein staining methods with regard to their specificity and reliability as antigen marker. Am J Pathol 81:479–492, 1975.

65. Ray MB, Desmet VJ: Distribution patterns of hepatitis B surface antigen (HBsAg) in the liver biopsies of hepatitis B patients. Acta Gastroenterol Belg 39:307–317, 1976.

66. Bianchi L, Gudat F: Sanded nuclei in hepatitis B. Eosinophilic inclusions in liver cell nuclei due to excess hepatitis B core antigen formation. Lab Invest 35:1–5, 1976.

67. Klinge O, Bannasch P: Zur Vermehrung des glatten endoplasmatischen Retikulum in Hepatocyten menschlicher Leber-punktate. Verh Dtsch Ges Pathol 53:658–573, 1968.

68. Nishimura RN, Ishak KG, Reddick R, Porter R, James S, Barranger JA: Lafora's disease: diagnosis by liver biopsy. Ann Neurol 8:409–415, 1980.

69. Vazquez JJ, Guillen FJ, Zozaya J, Lahoz M: Cyanamide-induced liver injury. A predictable lesion. Liver 3:225–230, 1983.

70. Bruguera M, Lamar C, Bernet M, Rodes J: Hepatic disease associated with ground-glass inclusions in hepatocytes after cyanamide therapy. Arch Pathol Lab Med 110:906–910, 1986.

71. Callea F, De Vos R, Togni R, Taardanico R, Vanstapel MJ, Desmet VJ: Fibrinogen inclusions in liver cells: a new type of ground-glass hepatocyte. Immune light and electron microscopic characterization. Histopathology 10:65–73, 1986.

71a. Callea F. Endoplasmic reticulum storage diseases. Prog Surg Pathol 13: (in press).

72. Stromeyer WF, Ishak KG, Gerber MA: Ground-glass cells in hepatocellular carcinoma. Am J Clin Pathol 74:254–258, 1980.

73. Scheuer PJ, Summerfield JA, Lal S, Sherlock S: Rifampicin hepatitis. A clinical and histological study. Lancet 1:421–425, 1974.

74. Schochet SS Jr, McCormick WF, Zellweger H: Type IV glycogenosis (amylopectinosis). Light and electron microscopic observations. Arch Pathol 90:354–363, 1970.

75. Zubair I, Herrera GA, Pretlow TG, Roper M, Zornes SL: Cytoplasmic inclusions in hepatocytes of bone marrow transplant patients: light and electron microscopic characterization. Am J Clin Pathol 83:65–68, 1985.

76. Doniach I, Weinbren K: The development of inclusion bodies in the cells of the rat's liver after partial hepatectomy. J Exp Pathol 33:499–505, 1953.

77. Pfeifer U, Klinge O: Intracisternal hyalin in hepatocytes of human liver biopsies. Virchows Arch Abt [B] Cell Pathol 16:141–155, 1974.

78. Gordon HW, Dixon J, Rogers JC, Mittman C, Lieberman J: Alpha1-antitrypsin (A1AT) accumulation in livers of emphysematous patients with A1AT deficiency. Hum Pathol 3:361–370, 1972.

79. Feldmann G, Bignon J, Chahinian P, Degott C, Benhamou J-P: Hepatocyte ultrastructural changes in α-1-antitrypsin deficiency. Gastroenterology 67:1214–1224, 1974.

80. Talbot IC, Mowat AP: Liver disease in infancy: histological features and relationship to α-1-antitrypsin phenotype. J Clin Pathol 28:559–563, 1975.

81. Aaganaes O, Matlary A, Elgjo K, Munthe E, Fagerhol M: Neonatal cholestasis in alpha-1-antitrypsin deficient children. Acta Paediatr 61:632–642, 1972.

82. Fisher RL, Taylor L, Sherlock S: α-1-Antitrypsin deficiency in liver disease, the extent of the problem. Gastroenterology 71:646–651, 1976.

83. Callea F, Fevery J, DeGroote J, Desmet VJ: Detection of PiZ phenotype individuals by alpha-1-antitrypsin (A1AT) immunohistochemistry in paraffin-embedded liver tissue specimens. J Hepatol 2:389–401, 1986.

84. Wallmark A, Alm R, Eriksson S: Monoclonal antibody specific for the mutant α-1-antitrypsin and its application in an ELISA procedure for identification of PiZ gene carriers. Proc Natl Acad Sci USA 81:5690–5693, 1984.

85. Palmer PE, DeLellis RA, Wolfe HJ: Immunohistochemistry of liver in alpha1-antitrypsin deficiency. A comparative study. Am J Clin Pathol 62:350–354, 1974.

86. Qizilbash A, Young-Pong O: Alpha1-antitrypsin liver disease. Differential diagnosis of PAS-positive, diastase resistant globules in liver cells. Am J Clin Pathol 79:697–702, 1983.

87. Doljanski L, Rosin A: Studies on the early changes in the liver of rats treated with various toxic agents with special reference to the vascular lesion: the histology of the rat's liver in urethane poisoning. Am J Pathol 20:945–953, 1944.

88. Heinrichsdorff H: Zur Histogenese des Ikterus. Virchows Arch 248:48–94, 1924.

89. Nomura M, Klatskin G: Unpublished data based on a study of 1361 consecutive needle biopsy specimens of liver, including 126 with completely normal morphology.

90. Strohmeyer JW, Ishak KG: Histology of the liver in Wilson's disease. A study of 34 cases. Am J Clin Pathol 73:12–24, 1980.

91. Klinge O: Cytologic and histologic aspects of toxically induced liver reactions. Ergeb Pathol 58:91–116, 1973.

92. Greiner AC, Nicolson GA: Pigment deposition in viscera associated with prolonged chlorpromazine therapy. Can Med Assoc J 91:627–635, 1964.

93. Ishak KG: The liver. In Pathology of Drug-Induced and Toxic Diseases, edited by R. H. Riddell. New York, Churchill Livingstone, 1982, pp. 457–513.

94. Edwards RH: Inheritance of the Dubin-Johnson-Sprinz syndrome. Gastroenterology 68:734–749, 1975.

95. Dubin IN: Chronic idiopathic jaundice. A review of fifty cases. Am J Med 24:268–292, 1958.

96. Baba N, Ruppert RD: The Dubin-Johnson syndrome: electron microscopic observations of hepatic pigment—a case study. Am J Clin Pathol 57:306–310, 1972.

97. Ehrlich JC, Novikoff AB, Platt R, Essner E: Hepatocellular lipofuscin and the pigment of chronic idiopathic jaundice. Bull NY Acad Med 36:488–491, 1960.

98. Arias IM, Bernstein L, Toffler R, Ben-Ezzer J: Black liver disease in Corriedale sheep: metabolism of tritiated epinephrine and incorporation of isotope into the hepatic pigment (Abst). J Clin Invest 44:1026, 1965.

99. Scheuer PJ: In Liver Biopsy Interpretation. London, Bailliere Tindall, 1988, p. 262.

100. Toker C, Trevino N: Hepatic ultrastructure in chronic idiopathic jaundice. Arch Pathol 80:453–460, 1965.

101. Richter GW: The iron-loaded cell: the cytopathology of iron storage. A review. Am J Pathol 91:377–396, 1978.

102. Chapman RW, Morgan MY, Laulicht M: Hepatic iron stores and markers of iron overload in alcoholics and patients with idiopathic hemochromatosis. Dig Dis Sci 27:909–916, 1982.

103. Bassett ML, Halliday JW, Powell LW: Value of hepatic iron measurements in early hemochromatosis and determination of the critical iron level associated with fibrosis. Hepatology 6:24–29, 1986.

104. Kent G: Iron storage diseases and the liver. In Progress in Liver Diseases, Vol. II, edited by H. Popper, F. Schaffner, New York, Grune & Stratton, 1965, pp. 253–271.

105. Scheinberg IH, Sternlieb I: Wilson's Disease. Philadelphia, W.B. Saunders Co., 1984.

106. Sternlieb I, Van den Hamer CJA, Morell AG, Alpert S, Gregoriadis G, Scheinberg H: Lysosomal defect of copper excretion in Wilson's disease (hepatolenticular degeneration). Gastroenterology *64*:99–110, 1973.

107. Tanner MS, Portmann B, Mowat AP, Williams R, Pandit AN, Mills CF, Bremner I: Increased hepatic copper concentration in Indian childhood cirrhosis. Lancet *1*:1203–1208, 1979.

108. Nakanuma Y, Miyamura H, Ohta G, Kobayashi K, Kato Y, Hattori N: Correlation between disappearance of the intrahepatic bile ducts and histologic changes in the liver in primary biliary cirrhosis. Am J Gastroenterol *76*:506–510, 1981.

109. Popper H, Goldfischer S, Sternlieb I, Nayak NC, Madhavan TV: Cytoplasmic copper and its toxic effects. Studies in Indian childhood cirrhosis. Lancet *1*:1205–1208, 1979.

110. Ludwig J, McDonald GSA, Dickson ER, Elveback LR, McCall JT: Copper stains and the syndrome of primary biliary cirrhosis. Evaluation of staining methods and their usefulness for diagnosis and trials of penicillamine treatment. Arch Pathol Lab Med *103*:467–470, 1979.

111. Owen CA Jr, Kickson ER, Goldstein NP, Baggenstoss AH, McCall JT: Hepatic subcellular distribution of copper in primary biliary cirrhosis. Comparison with other hyperhepatocupric states and review of the literature. Mayo Clin Proc *52*:73–80, 1977.

112. Mehrotra R, Randey RK, Nath P: Hepatic copper in Indian childhood cirrhosis. Histopathology *5*:659–665, 1981.

113. Sipponen P: Orcein positive hepatocellular material in long-standing biliary diseases. I. Histochemical characteristics. Scand J Gastroenterol *11*:545–552, 1976.

114. Sipponen P: Orcein positive hepatocellular material in long-standing biliary diseases. II. Ultrastructural studies. Scand J Gastroenterol *11*:553–557, 1976.

115. Portmann B, Tanner MS, Mowat AP, Williams R: Orcein-positive liver deposits in Indian childhood cirrhosis. Lancet *1*:1338–1340, 1978.

116. Salaspuro MP, Sipponen P, Makkonen H: The occurrence of orcein-positive hepatocellular material in various liver diseases. Scand J Gastroenterol *11*:677–681, 1976.

117. Sipponen P, Salapuro MP, Makkonen HM: Orcein positive hepatocellular material in histologic diagnosis of primary biliary cirrhosis. Ann Clin Res *7*:273–277, 1975.

118. Cripps DJ, Scheuer PJ: Hepatobiliary changes in erythropoietic protopophyria. Arch Pathol *80:* 500–508, 1965.

119. Bloomer JR, Phillips MJ, Davidson KL, Klatskin G: Hepatic disease in erythropoietic protoporphyria. Am J Med *58*:869–882, 1975.

120. Cripps DJ, Hawgood RS, Magnus IA: Iodine tungsten fluorescence microscopy for porphyrin fluorescence. A study on erythropoietic protoporphyria. Arch Dermatol *93*:129–134, 1966.

121. Klatskin G, Bloomer JR: Birefringence of hepatic pigment deposits in erythopoietic protoporphyria. Specificity and sensitivity of polarization microscopy in the identification of hepatic protoporphyrin deposits. Gastroenterology *67*:294–302, 1974.

122. Hoyumpa AM Jr, Greene HL, Dunn GD, Schenker S: Fatty liver: biochemical and clinical considerations. Dig Dis *20*:1142–1170, 1975.

123. Hartroft WS: Accumulation of fat in liver cells and in lipodiastaemata preceding experimental dietary cirrhosis. Anat Rec *106*:61–78, 1950.

124. Hartroft WS: Diagnostic significance of fatty cysts in cirrhosis. Arch Pathol *55*:63–69, 1953.

125. Christoffersen P, Braendstrup O, Juhl E, Poulsen H: Lipogranulomas in human liver biopsies with fatty change. A morphological biochemical and clinical investigation. Acta Pathol Microbiol Scand A. *79*:150–158, 1971.

126. Boitnott JK, Margolis S: Saturated hydrocarbons in human tissues. III. Oil droplets in the liver and spleen. Johns Hopkins Med J *127*:65–78, 1970.

127. Dincsoy HP, Weesner RE, MacGee J: Lipogranulomas in non-fatty human livers. A mineral oil induced environmental disease. Am J Clin Pathol *78*:35–41, 1982.

128. Cruickshank B, Thomas MJ: Mineral oil (follicular) lipidosis: II. Histologic studies of spleen, liver, lymph nodes, and bone marrow. Hum Pathol *15*:731–737, 1984.

129. Wanless IR, Geddie WR: Mineral oil lipogranulomata in liver and spleen. Arch Pathol Lab Med *109*:283–286, 1985.

130. Davies JNP: The essential pathology of kwashiorkor. Lancet *1*:317–320, 1948.

131. Webber BL, Freiman I: The liver in kwashiorkor. Arch Pathol *98*:400–408, 1974.

132. Sloan HR, Fredrickson DS: Enzyme deficiency in cholesteryl ester storage disease. J Clin Invest *51*:1923–1926, 1972.

133. Satran L, Sharp HL, Schenken JR, Krivit W: Fatal neonatal hepatic steatosis: a new familial disorder. J Pediatr *75*:39–46, 1969.

134. Lough J, Fawcett J, Wiegensberg B: Wolman's disease. An electron microscopic, histochemical and biochemical study. Arch Pathol *89*:103–110, 1970.

135. Lake BD, Patrick AD: Wolman's disease: deficiency of E600-resistant acid esterase activity with storage of lipids in lysosomes. J Pediatr *76*:262–266, 1970.

136. Schiff L, Schubert WK, McAdams AJ, Spiegel EL, O'Donnell JF: Hepatic cholesterol ester storage disease, a familial disorder. Am J Med *44*:538–546, 1968.

137. Felig P, Brown WV, Levine RA, Klatskin G: Glucose hemeostasis in viral hepatitis. N Engl J Med *283*:1436–1440, 1970.

138. McAdams JA, Hug G. Bove KE: Glycogen storage disease, Types I to X. Criteria for morphologic diagnosis. Hum Pathol *5*:463–487, 1974.

139. Ishak KG, Sharp HL: Metabolic errors and liver disease. In Pathology of the Liver, edited by R.N.M. MacSween, P.P. Anthony, P.J. Scheuer. New York, Churchill Livingstone, 1987, pp. 99–180.

140. Callahan WP, Hackett RL, Loring AE: New observations by light microscopy on liver histology in the Hurler's syndrome. A needle biopsy study of 11 patients utilizing plastic-embedded tissue. Arch Pathol *83*:507–512, 1967.

141. Callahan WP, Loring AE: Hepatic ultrastructure in the Hurler's syndrome. Am J Pathol *48*:277–298, 1966.

142. Waldo ED, Tobias H: Needle-like cytoplasmic inclusions in the liver in porphyria cutanea tarda. Arch Pathol *96*:368–371, 1973.

143. Vanstapel M-J, Desmet VJ: Cytomegalovirus hepatitis: a histological and immunohistochemical study. Appl Pathol *1*:41–49, 1983.

144. Adams RL, Springall DR, Levene MM, Bushell TEC: The immunocytochemical demonstration of Herpes simplex virus in cervical smears: a valuable technique for routine use. J Pathol *143*:241–247, 1984.

145. Berman M, Alter HJ, Ishak KG, Purcell RH, Jones EA: The chronic sequelae of non-A, non-B hepatitis. Ann Intern Med *91*:1–6, 1979.

146. Anthony PB, Vogel CL, Barker LF: Liver cell dysplasia: a premalignant condition. J Clin Pathol *26*:217–223, 1973.

147. Roncalli M, Borzio M, DeBiagi G, Ferrari AR, Macchi R, Tombesi VM, Servida E: Liver cell dysplasia in cirrhosis. Cancer *57*:1515–1521, 1986.

148. Cohen C, Berson SD: Liver cell dysplasia in normal, cirrhotic, and hepatocellular carcinoma patients. Cancer *57*:1535–1538, 1986.

149. Anthony PB: Liver cell dysplasia: what is its significance: Hepatology *7*:394–395, 1987.

150. Kojiro M, Nakashima T: Pathology of hepatocellular carcinoma. *In* Neoplasms of the Liver, edited by K. Okuda, K.G. Ishak. Tokyo, Springer-Verlag, 1987, pp. 81–104.

151. Higginson J, Grobbelaar BG, Walker ARP: Hepatic fibrosis and cirrhosis in man in relation to malnutrition. Am J Pathol *33*:29–53, 1957.

152. Mikkelsen WWP, Edmondson HA, Peters RL, Redeker AG, Reynolds TB: Extra- and intrahepatic portal hypertension without cirrhosis (hepatoportal sclerosis). Ann Surg *162*:602–618, 1965.

153. Nayak NC, Ramalingaswami V: Obliterative portal venopathy of the liver associated with so-called idiopathic portal hypertension or tropical splenomegaly. Arch Pathol *87*:359–369, 1969.

154. Boyer JL, Hales MR, Klatskin G: ''Idiopathic'' portal hypertension due to occlusion of intrahepatic portal veins by organized thrombi. A study based on postmortem vinylite-injection corrosion and dissection of the intrahepatic vasculature in 4 cases. Medicine *53*:77–91, 1974.

155. Okuda K, Kono K, Ohnishi K, Kimura K, Omata M, Kowen H, Nakajima Y, Musha H, Hirashima T, Takashi M, Takayasu K: Clinical study of eighty-six cases of idiopathic portal hypertension and comparison with cirrhosis with splenomegaly. Gastroenterology *86*:600–610, 1984.

156. Popper H, Schaffner F: Liver: Structure and Function. New York, McGraw-Hill, 1957, p. 205.

157. Popper H: Aging and the Liver. *In* Progress in Liver Diseases, Vol. VIII, edited by H. Popper, F. Schaffner. New York, Grune & Stratton, 1986, pp. 659–683.

158. Szanto PB, Popper H: Basophilic cytoplasmic material (pentose nucleic acid). Distribution in normal and abnormal human liver. Arch Pathol *51*:409–422, 1951.

159. Poulsen H, Christofferson P: *Atlas of Liver Biopsies*. Philadelphia, J.B. Lippincott, 1979, p. 72.

160. Phillips MJ, Oda M, Mak E, Fisher MM, Jeejeebhoy KN: Microfilament dysfunction as a possible cause of intrahepatic cholestasis. Gastroenterology *69*:48–58, 1975.

161. Watanabe S, Smith CR, Phillips MJ: Coordination of the contractile activity of bile canaliculi. Evidence from calcium microinjection of triplet hepatocytes. Lab Invest 53:275–279, 1985.
162. Smith CR, Oshio C, Miyairi M, Katz H, Phillips MJ: Coordination of the contractile activity of bile canaliculi. Evidence from spontaneous contractions in vitro. Lab Invest 53:270–274, 1985.
163. Rich AR: The pathogenesis of the forms of jaundice. Bull Johns Hopkins Hosp 47:338–377, 1930.
164. Boyer JL, Elias E, Layden TJ: The paracellular pathway and bile formation. Yale J Biol Med 52:61–67, 1979.
165. Arcidi JM Jr, Moore GW, Hutchins GM: Hepatic morphology in cardiac dysfunction. A clinicopathologic study of 1000 subjects at autopsy. Am J Pathol 104:159–166, 1981.
166. Leopold JG, Parry TE, Storring JK: A change in the sinusoid-trabecular structure of the liver with hepatic venous outflow block. J Pathol 100:87–98, 1970.
167. Schaffner F, Popper H: Capillarization of hepatic sinusoids in man. Gastroenterology 44:239–242, 1963.
168. Winkler K, Poulsen H: Liver disease with periportal sinusoidal dilatation. Scand J Gastroenterol 10:699–704, 1975.
169. Fenster LF, Klatskin G: Manifestations of metastatic tumors of the liver. A study of eighty-one patients subjected to needle biopsy. Am J Med 31:238–248, 1961.
170. Edmondson HA, Peters TB, Reynolds TB, Kuzma OT: Sclerosing hyaline necrosis of the liver in the chronic alcoholic. A recognizable clinical syndrome. Ann Intern Med 59:646–673, 1963.
171. Reynolds TB, Hidemura R, Michel H, Peters R: Portal hypertension without cirrhosis in alcoholic liver disease. Ann Intern Med 70:497–506, 1969.
172. Poulsen H, Winkler K, Christoffersen P: The significance of centrilobular sinusoidal changes in liver biopsies. Scand J Gastroenterol Suppl 7:103–109, 1970.
173. Bruguera M, Aranguibel F, Ros E, Rodes J: Incidence and clinical significance of sinusoidal dilatation in liver biopsies. Gastroenterology 75:474–478, 1978.
174. Vidins EI, Britton RS, Medline A, Blendis LM, Israel Y, Orrego H: Sinusoidal caliber in alcoholic and nonalcoholic liver disease: diagnostic and pathogenic implications. Hepatology 5:408–414, 1985.
175. Arias F, Mancilla-Jiminez R: Hepatic fibrinogen deposits in preeclampsia. Immunofluorescent evidence. N Engl J Med 292:578–582, 1976.
176. Rake MO, Flute PT, Shilkin KB, Lewis ML, Winch J, Williams R: Early and intensive therapy of intravascular coagulation in acute liver failure. Lancet 2:1215–1218, 1971.
177. Bernstein M, Edmondson HA, Barbour BH: The liver lesion in Q fever. Arch Intern Med 116:491–498, 1965.
178. Pellegrin M, Delsol G, Auvergnat JC, Familiades J, Faure H, Guiu M, Voigt JJ: Granulomatous hepatitis in Q fever. Hum Pathol 11:51–57, 1980.
179. Horn T, Junge J, Christoffersen P: Early alcoholic liver injury: changes of the Disse space in acinar zone 3. Liver 5:301–310, 1985.
180. Kent G, Inouye T, Minick OT, Bahu RM: Fat-storing cells (lipocytes) in the liver. Their role in vitamin A storage and fibrogenesis. Med Chir Digest 6:425–428, 1977.
181. Kawanishi H: Morphologic association of lymphocytes with hepatocytes in chronic liver disease. Arch Pathol Lab Med 101:286–290, 1977.
182. Bassewitz V, Roessner A, Nauta R, Themann H: Cytoplasmic fusions between liver parenchyma cells and infiltrating cells in chronic aggressive hepatitis. Virch Arch Abt [A] Pathol Anat 359:309–313, 1973.
183. Starzl TE, Porter KA, Brettschneider L, Penn I, Bell P, Putnam CW, McGuire RL: Clinical and pathological observations after orthotopic transplantation of the human liver. Surg Gynecol Obstet 128:327–339, 1969.
184. Kelly L, Dobson EL: Evidence concerning the origin of liver macrophages. B J Exp Pathol 52:88–99, 1971.
185. Selinger M, Koff RS: Thorotrast and the liver: a reminder. Gastroenterology 68:799–803, 1975.
186. Andrade ZA: Hepatic schistosomiasis. Morphological aspects. In Progress in Liver Diseases, Vol. II, edited by H. Popper, F. Schaffner. New York, Grune & Stratton, 1965, pp. 228–252.
187. Connor DH, Neafie RC, Hockmeyer WT: Malaria. In Pathology of Tropical and Extraordinary Diseases. An Atlas, edited by C.H. Binford, K.H. Connor. Washington, D.C., Armed Forces Institute of Pathology, 1976, pp. 273–283.
188. Roberts WC, Levy RI, Fredrickson KS: Hyperlipoproteinemia. A re-

view of the five types with first report of necropsy findings in type 3. Arch Pathol 90:45–56, 1970.
189. Ferrans VJ, Roberts WC, Levy RI, Fredrickson DS: Chylomicrons and the formation of foam cells in type I hyperlipoproteinemia. A morphologic study. Am J Pathol 70:253–272, 1973.
190. Ferans VJ, Buja LM, Roberts WC, Fredrickson DS: The spleen in type I hyperlipoproteinemia. Histochemical, biochemical, microfluorometric and electron microscopic observations. Am J Pathol 64:67–96, 1971.
191. Bruton OC, Kanter AJ: Idiopathic familial hyperlipemia. Am J Dis Child 82:153–159, 1951.
192. Ferrans VJ, Fredrickson DS: The pathology of Tangier disease. A light and microscopic study. Am J Pathol 78:101–158, 1975.
193. Sandhoff K, Conzelmann E, Neufeld EF, Zaback MM, Suzuki K: The GM2 gangliosidoses. In The Metabolic Basis of Inherited Disease, edited by C.R. Scriver, A.L. Beaudet, W.S. Sly, D. Valle. 6th Edition. New York, McGraw-Hill Inf Svcs Co, 1989, pp. 1807–1859.
194. Desnick RJ, Bishop DF: Fabry disease: alpha-galactosidase deficiency; Schindler disease: alpha-N-acetylgalactosaminidase deficiency. In The Metabolic Basis of Inherited Disease, edited by C.R. Scriver, A.L. Beaudet, W.S. Sly, D. Valle. 6th Edition, New York, McGraw-Hill Inf Svcs Co, 1989, pp. 1751–1796.
195. Peters SP, Lee RE, Glew RH: Gaucher's disease, a review. Medicine 56:425–442, 1977.
196. Barranger JA, Ginns EI: Glucosylceramide lipidoses: Gaucher disease. In The Metabolic Basis of Inherited Disease, edited by C.R. Scriver, A.L. Beaudet, W.S. Sly, D. Valle. 6th Edition. New York, McGraw-Hill Inf Svcs Co, 1989, pp. 1677–1698.
197. Kattlove HE, Williams JC, Gaynor E, Spivack M, Bradley RM, Brady RO: Gaucher cells in chronic myelocytic leukemia: an acquired abnormality. Blood 33:379–390, 1969.
198. Scullin DC Jr, Shelburne JD, Cohen HJ: Pseudo-Gaucher cells in multiple myeloma. Am J Med 67:347–352. 1979.
199. Kolodny EH: Metachromatic leukodystrophy and multiple sulfatase deficiency: sulfatide lipidosis. In The Metabolic Basis of Inherited Disease, edited by C.R. Scriver, A.L. Beaudet, W.S. Sly, D. Valle. 6th Edition. New York, McGraw-Hill Inf Svcs Co, 1989, pp. 1721–1750.
200. Wolfe HJ, Pietra GG: The visceral lesions of metachromatic leukodystrophy. Am J Pathol 44: 921–930, 1964.
201. Resibois A: Electron microscopic studies of metachromatic leucodystrophy. IV. Liver and kidney alterations. Pathol Eur 6:278–298, 1971.
202. Spence MW, Callahan JW: Sphingomyelin-cholesterol lipidoses: the Niemann-Pick group of diseases. In The Metabolic Basis of Inherited Disease, edited by C.R. Scriver, A.L. Beaudet, W.S. Sly, D. Valle. 6th Edition. New York, McGraw-Hill Inf Svcs Co, 1989, pp. 1655–1676.
203. Farber S, Cohen J, Uzman LL: Lipogranulomatosis. A new lipoglycoprotein "storage" disease. J Mt Sinai Hosp 24:816–837, 1957.
204. Moser HW, Moser AB, Chen WE, Schram AW: Ceramidase deficiency: Farber lipogranulomatosis. In The Metabolic Basis of Inherited Disease, edited by C.R. Scriver, A.L. Beaudet, W.S. Sly, D. Valle. 6th Edition. New York, McGraw-Hill Inf Svcs Co, 1989, pp. 1645–1654.
205. Dustin P, Tondeur M, Jonniaux M, Vamos-Hurwitz E, Pele S: La maladie de Farber. Etude anatomo-clinique et ultrastructurale. Bull Acad R Med Belg 128:733–762, 1973.
206. Kattlove HE, Gaynor E, Spivack M, Gottfried EL: Sea-blue indigestion. N Engl J Med 282:630–631, 1970.
207. Rywlin AM, Hernandez JA, Chastain DE, Pardo V: Ceroid histiocytosis of spleen and bone marrow in idiopathic thrombocytopenic purpura (ITP): a contribution to the understanding of the sea-blue histiocyte. Blood 37:587–593, 1971.
208. Silverstein MN, Ellefson RD, Ahern EJ: The syndrome of the sea-blue histiocyte. N Engl J Med 282:1–4, 1970.
209. Rywlin AM, Lopez-Gomez A, Tachmes P, Pardo V: Ceroid histiocytosis of the spleen in hyperlipemia: relation to the syndrome of the sea-blue histiocyte. Am J Clin Pathol 56:572–579, 1971.
210. Durand P, Borrone C, Della Cella G: Fucosidosis. J Pediatr 75:665–674, 1969.
211. Kornfeld M, Snyder RD, Wenger DA: Fucosidosis with angiokeratoma. Electron microscopic changes in the skin. Arch Pathol Lab Med 101:478–485, 1977.
212. Freitag F, Kuchemann K, Blumcke S: Hepatic ultrastructure in fucosidosis. Virchows Arch, Abt B, Zellpathol 7:99–113, 1971.

213. Van Hoof F: Mucopolysaccharidoses and mucolipidoses. J Clin Pathol 27, Suppl 8: 64–93, 1974.
214. Neufeld EF, Muenzer J: The mucopolysaccharidoses. In The Metabolic Basis of Inherited Disease, edited by C.R. Scriver, A.L. Beaudet, W.S. Sly, D. Valle. 6th Edition. New York, McGraw-Hill Inf Svcs Co, 1989, pp. 1565–1587.
215. Green TW, Conley CL, Berthrong M: The liver in sickle cell anemia. Bull Johns Hopkins Hosp 92:99–127, 1953.
216. Dooley JR, Ishak KG: Leptospirosis. In Pathology of Tropical and Extraordinary Diseases, Vol. I, edited by C.H. Binford, D.H. Connor. Washington, Armed Forces Institute of Pathology, 1976,pp. 101–106.
217. Connor KH, Neafie RC: Malaria. In Pathology of Tropical and Extraordinary Diseases, Vol. I, edited by C.H. Binford, D.H. Connor. Washington, Armed Forces Institute of Pathology, 1976, pp. 273–283.
218. Neafie RC, Connor KH: Visceral leishmaniasis. In Pathology of Tropical and Extraordinary Diseases, Vol. I, edited by C.H. Binford, D.H. Connor. Washington, Armed Forces Institute of Pathology, 1976, pp. 265–272.
219. Pounder DJ: Malarial pigment and hepatic anthracosis. Am J Surg Pathol 7:501–502, 1983.
220. Frenkel JK: Toxoplasmosis. In Pathology of Tropical and Extraordinary Diseases, Vol. I, edited by C.H. Binford, D.H. Connor. Washington, Armed Forces Institute of Pathology, 1976, pp. 284–302.
221. Gollan JL, Davidson GP, Anderson K, White TA, Kimber CC: Visceral cryptococcosis without central nervous system or pulmonary involvement: presentation as hepatitis. Med J Aust 1:469–472, 1972.
222. Lefton HB, Farmer RG, Buchwald R, Haselboy R: Cryptococcal hepatitis mimicking primary sclerosing cholangitis. A case report. Gastroenterology 67:511–515, 1974.
223. Silverman FN, Schwarz J, Lahey ME, Carson RP: Histoplasmosis. Am J Med 19:410–459, 1955.
224. Bronfenmajer S, Schaffner F, Popper H: Fat-storing cells (lipocytes) in human liver. Arch Pathol 82:447–453, 1966.
225. Russell RM, Boyer JL, Bagheri SA, Hruban Z: Hepatic injury from chronic hypervitaminosis A resulting in portal hypertension and ascites. N Engl J Med 291:435–440, 1974.
226. Lichtenstein L: Histiocytosis X. Integration of eosinophilic granuloma of bone, Letterer-Siwe disease, and "Hand-Schuller-Christian disease" as related manifestations of a single nosologic entity. Arch Pathol 56:84–102, 1953.
227. Lieberman PH, Jones CR, Dargeon HWK, Begg CR: A reappraisal of eosinophilic granuloma of bone, Hand-Schuller-Christian disease and Letterer-Siwe syndrome. Medicine 48:375–400, 1969.
228. Scott RB, Robb-Smith AHT: Histiocytic medullary reticulosis. Lancet 2:194–198, 1939.
229. Rappaport H: Tumors of the Hematopoietic System. Atlas of Tumor Pathology, Section III-Fascicle 8. Washington DC, Armed Forces Institute of Pathology, 1966, pp. 49–63.
230. Warnke RA, Kim H, Dorfman RF: Malignant histiocytosis (histiocytic medullary reticulosis). I. Clinicopathologic study of 29 cases. Cancer 35:215–230, 1975.
231. Natelson EA, Lynch EC, Hettig RA, Alfrey CP Jr: Histiocytic medullary reticulosis. The role of phagocytosis in pancytopenia. Arch Intern Med 122:223–229, 1968.
232. Farquhar JW, Claireaux AE: Familial haemophagocytic reticulosis. Arch Dis Child 27:519–525, 1952.
233. Bell RJM, Brafield AJE, Barnes ND, France NE: Familial hemophagocytic reticulosis. Arch Dis Child 43:601–606, 1968.
234. Fullerton P, Ekert H, Hosking C, Tauro GP: Haemophagocytic reticulosis. A case report with investigations of immune and white cell function. Cancer 36:441–445, 1975.
235. Zafrani ES, Degos F, Guigui B, Durand-Schneider A-M, Martin N, Flandrin G, Benhamou J-P, Feldmann G: The hepatic sinusoid in hairy cell leukemia: an ultrastructural study of 12 cases. Hum Pathol 18:801–807, 1987.
236. Nanba K, Soban EJ, Bowling MC, Berard CW: Splenic pseudosinuses and hepatic angiomatous lesions. Distinctive features of hairy cell leukemia. Am J Clin Pathol 67:415–426, 1977.
237. Yam LT, Janckila AJ, Chan CH: Hepatic involvement in hairy cell leukemia. Cancer 51:1497–1504, 1983.
238. Grouls V, Stiens R: Hepatic involvement in hairy cell leukaemia: diagnosis by tartrate-resistant acid phosphatase enzyme histochemistry on formalin fixed and paraffin-embedded liver biopsy specimens. Pathol Res Pract 178:332–334, 1984.
239. Stuart KL, Bras G: Veno-occlusive disease of the liver. Q J Med 26:291–315, 1957.
240. Selzer G, Parker RGF: Senecio poisoning exhibiting as Chiari's syndrome. A report of twelve cases. Am J Pathol 27:885–907, 1951.
241. Stillman AE, Huxtable R, Consroe P, Kohnen P, Smith S: Hepatic veno-occlusive disease due to pyrrolizidine (Senecio) poisoning in Arizona. Gastroenterology 73:349–352, 1977.
242. Marubio AT, Danielson B: Hepatic veno-occlusive disease in a renal transplant patient receiving azathioprine. Gastroenterology 69:739–743, 1975.
243. Griner PF, Elbakawi A, Packman CH: Veno-occlusive disease of the liver after chemotherapy of acute leukemia. Report of two cases. Ann Intern Med 85:578–582, 1976.
244. Brodsky I, Johnson, H, Killman S, Cronkite EP: Fibrosis of central and hepatic veins, and perisunusoidal spaces of the liver following prolonged administration of urethane. Am J Med 30:976–980, 1961.
245. Baker A, Kaplan M, Wolfe H: Central congestive fibrosis of the liver in myxedema ascites. Ann Intern Med 77:927–929, 1972.
246. Berk PD, Popper H, Krueger GRF, Decter J, Herzig G, Graw RG Jr: Veno-occlusive disease after allogeneic bone marrow transplantation. Possible association with graft-versus-host disease. Ann Intern Med 90:158–164, 1979.
247. Lewin K, Millis RR: Human radiation hepatitis. A morphologic study with emphasis on the late changes. Arch Pathol 96:21–26, 1973.
248. Maddrey WC, Johns CJ, Boitnott JK, Iber FL: Sarcoidosis and chronic liver disease: a clinical and pathologic study of 20 patients. Medicine 49:375–395, 1970.
249. Paradinas FJ, Bull TB, Westaby D, Murray-Lyon IM: Hyperplasia and prolapse of hepatocytes into hepatic veins during longterm methyltestosterone therapy: possible relationships of these changes to the development of peliosis hepatis and liver tumors. Histopathology 1:225–246, 1977.
250. Pitney WR, Pryor DS, Smith AT: Morphological observations on livers and spleens of patients with tropical splenomegaly in New Guinea. J Pathol Bacteriol 95:417–422, 1963.
251. Page AR, Good RA: Plasma cell hepatitis. Lab Invest 11:351–359, 1962.
252. Thomas FB, Clausen KP, Greenberger NJ: Liver disease in multiple myeloma. Arch Intern Med 132:195–202, 1973.
253. Chusid MJ, Dale DC, West BC, Wolff SM: The hypereosinophilic syndrome. Analysis of fourteen cases with review of the literature. Medicine 54:1–27, 1975.
254. Klein NC, Hargrove RL, Sleisinger MH, Jeffries GH: Eosinophilic gastroenteritis. Medicine 49:299–319, 1970.
255. Beaver PC, Snyder CH, Carrera GM, Dent JH, Lafferty JW: Chronic eosinophilia due to visceral larva migrans. Report of three cases. Pediatrics 9:7–19, 1952.
256. Huntley CC, Costas MC, Lyerly A: Visceral larva migrans: clinical characteristics and immunologic studies in 51 patients. Pediatrics 36:523–536, 1965.

Chapter 5
Abnormalities of the Portal Tracts

Abnormalities of portal tract size and configuration

Enlargement of the portal tracts

Deposition of collagen, infiltration of inflammatory cells, ductular proliferation, and edema, either alone or together, may contribute to enlargement of the portal tracts. However, almost always, loss of periportal hepatocytes is a significant factor in abnormal expansion of the portal tracts. Other less common causes of such expansion include granulomas, foci of extramedullary hematopoiesis, leukemic and lymphomatous infiltrates, benign and malignant histiocytic infiltrates, and amyloid deposits.

Normally, the size of the portal tracts increases as they merge in their course from the periphery of the lobules to the porta hepatitis (Figs. 23–25), i.e. large normal tracts must be differentiated from those that are abnormally expanded. This seldom poses a problem, since large normal portal tracts are smooth in contour, contain relatively large blood vessels and bile ducts and few or no inflammatory cells, and show no evidence of ductular proliferation (Fig. 25).

Portal-portal and portal-central bridging

As the portal tracts enlarge, they may fuse with one another or with adjacent central veins. Such bridging may be attributable to progressive fibrosis (Figs. 45, 49), or to zones of hepatocellular necrosis that present as bands of loosely arranged reticulin fibers devoid of hepatocytes that link adjacent portal triads and/or central veins (Fig. 69). Usually, under both conditions, the portal tracts and bridges contain numerous inflammatory cells.

If bridging fibrosis is extensive, it may ultimately destroy the normal lobular architecture and give rise to cirrhosis.

Portal-portal fibrous bridging must be differentiated from the normal branching pattern of intact portal tracts. The branched portal tracts encountered in biopsy sections of normal liver usually are few in number, exhibit a V- or Y-shaped configuration, and show no evidence of inflammation or fibrosis (Fig. 26). In contrast, abnormal fibrous bridging involves multiple triads in an irregular pattern (Fig. 45), and is usually accompanied by inflammation, ductular proliferation, or erosion of the limiting plates.

Erosion of the limiting plates: piecemeal and acute periportal hepatocellular necrosis

Normally, the portal tracts are encircled by a tightly adherent, single layer of hepatocytes, termed the limiting plate (Figs. 23–

25). Under a variety of conditions, the limiting plates are eroded, either segmentally or circumferentially, but only rarely are all of the portal tracts involved. Such erosion may be the result of the slow progressive loss of hepatocytes, a process often termed piecemeal necrosis, or of acute hepatocellular necrosis characterized by rapid cytolysis of large groups of contiguous periportal hepatocytes. Under both conditions, the loss of hepatocytes involves not only the limiting plates but also many adjacent cells, and is always accompanied by an inflammatory reaction and, less constantly, by collapse of reticulin, fibrosis, ductular proliferation, or edema. Such destruction of periportal parenchyma is the principal factor responsible for enlargement and distortion of the portal tracts.

Piecemeal necrosis

Although the term *piecemeal necrosis* implies a distinctive type of hepatocellular necrosis characterized by slowly progressive, focal destruction of periportal hepatocytes, the term is often defined more broadly to include not only a unique form of necrosis but also the portal and periportal inflammatory and fibrotic reactions that accompany it. Lymphocytes and plasma cells predominate in the portal exudates and, characteristically, migrate into the surrounding parenchyma, often coming to rest in intimate contact with intact or degenerating hepatocytes. Portal fibrosis, another feature of the lesion, also extends out into the parenchyma, chiefly along the walls of the sinusoids, frequently encircling individual hepatocytes, or groups of hepatocytes arranged in the form of rosettes. Often, a small number of acidophilic bodies is found in the advancing edge of the lesion.

Figure 104 illustrates the typical features of piecemeal necrosis in the portal tract of a patient with HBsAg-negative *chronic active hepatitis*. The portal tract is significantly enlarged and fibrotic, shows segmental erosion of its limiting plate, and contains a few proliferating ductules and numerous lymphocytes and plasma cells. As can be seen at higher magnification (Fig. 106), small groups of hepatocytes, arranged in the form of rosettes, are encircled by fine bands of connective tissue and inflammatory cells extending from the portal tract. The intimate contact between the inflammatory cells and the periportal hepatocytes is illustrated in Figure 226, and the presence of occasional acidophilic bodies in the advancing edge of the lesion in Figure 292.

At an early stage in the development of the portal lesion in chronic active hepatitis, it is often possible in Masson-stained sections to identify the original portal tract surrounded by a zone of loosely arranged reticulin fibers interspersed with lymphocytes and histiocytes that correspond to the periportal zone of hepatocellular destruction (Fig. 105). As the lesion advances, the reticulin collapses, undergoes collagenization, and merges with the original portal tract, giving the enlarged portal tract a uniformly fibrotic appearance. In the course of fibrogenesis, solitary or small groups of hepatocytes may be entrapped within the portal tracts. Such entrapped cells, which almost always are indicative of antecedent piecemeal necrosis, may be encountered during periods of remission when the limiting plates are intact or near normal (Fig. 293).

In occasional cases of chronic active hepatitis, some of the periportal zones show relatively large areas of loosely arranged, collapsed reticulin fibers that are interspersed with a few lymphocytes and histiocytes, but are devoid of collagen bundles or hepatocytes (Fig. 294). Such lesions suggest that the loss of periportal hepatocytes in chronic active hepatitis may occasionally be the result of rapid, extensive cytolysis, such as occurs in severe viral hepatitis, rather than of piecemeal necrosis.

Piecemeal necrosis is generally regarded as a key feature in pathogenesis of chronic active hepatitis (1), and has been interpreted as a manifestation of an underlying immune process (2). The presence of acidophilic bodies (3) and the intimate relationship of the infiltrating lymphocytes to the hepatocytes in the margins of the lesion (4) have been emphasized as markers of a cell-mediated, immune response. A growing body of evidence lends support to the hypothesis that an autoimmune process may be involved in the pathogenesis of chronic active hepatitis. However, it is by no means certain that autoimmunity is the only mechanism that provokes piecemeal necrosis. Indeed, similar, if not identical lesions are encountered under a wide variety of conditions, only some of which may have an immunologic basis. The disorders in which piecemeal necrosis may be seen include the active phases of primary biliary cirrhosis and Wilson's disease, extrahepatic biliary obstruction, sclerosing cholangitis, a type of pericholangitis seen in ulcerative colitis and Crohn's disease, and other forms of active cirrhosis in which the periphery of the parenchymal nodules frequently is eroded (5).

In *primary biliary cirrhosis,* as in chronic active hepatitis, many of the portal tracts are enlarged and fibrotic, contain numerous mononuclear inflammatory cells, and often show bridging fibrosis. However, piecemeal necrosis is a less constant feature and, when present, often is limited to segmental erosion of the limiting plates with little or no extension of fibrous tissue and inflammatory cells into the surrounding parenchyma, even when the lesions are florid and contain degenerating interlobular ducts, granulomas, and lymphoid follicles (Fig. 295). Nevertheless, in some cases, piecemeal necrosis is extensive (Fig. 296), so the differentiation of primary biliary cirrhosis from chronic active hepatitis may be difficult. Usually, the distinction is made on the basis of the character of the interlobular ducts, which in primary biliary cirrhosis, show distinctive inflammatory and degenerative changes, and are reduced in number.

Extrahepatic biliary obstruction, particularly when severe or prolonged, often leads to enlargement and fibrosis of the portal tracts and erosion of their limiting plates. Characteristically, periportal hepatocytes are replaced by loose, edematous connective tissue containing proliferating bile ductules and numerous inflammatory cells, many of which are neutrophilic (Fig. 297). In addition, in some cases, the portal tracts appear to be expanded eccentrically by sharply circumscribed zones of large, pale periportal hepatocytes undergoing pseudoxanthomatous degeneration (Fig. 298). Not all of the portal tracts in extrahepatic biliary obstruction show this distinctive pattern of changes.

Thus, some may appear normal, while others contain a mononuclear exudate without neutrophils, ductular proliferation, or erosion of their limiting plates.

The histologic features of the portal tracts in *sclerosing cholangitis* often resemble those of extrahepatic biliary obstruction. However, in some cases, the lesions mimic those of chronic persistent or chronic active hepatitis.

Erosion of the limiting plates due to acute periportal hepatocellular necrosis

Segmental or complete erosion of the limiting plates due to acute loss of periportal hepatocytes that results in enlargement and distortion of the portal tracts is a relatively frequent finding in moderate or severe acute viral or drug-induced hepatitis.

Figure 299 illustrates such a portal lesion in a case of HBsAg-positive *acute viral hepatitis* on the fifth day of illness. As can be seen, the portal tract is enlarged, contains numerous mononuclear inflammatory cells and a few proliferating ductules, and shows extensive erosion of its limiting plate. At higher magnification to visualize the advancing edge of necrosis (Fig. 300), it is evident that many contiguous hepatocytes in the limiting plate and beyond have undergone cytolysis, and have been replaced by swollen, proliferating Kupffer cells, macrophages, lymphocytes, and proliferating ductules. In addition, an occasional acidophilic body can be identified at the edge of the necrotic zone.

Similar enlargement and distortion of the portal tracts due to extensive destruction of periportal hepatocytes may be seen in *acute drug-induced hepatitis.* Figure 88 illustrates such a lesion in a woman with severe isoniazid-induced hepatitis in the eighth week of her illness. Although such lesions superficially resemble those of chronic active hepatitis, they are unaccompanied by fibrosis and show no tendency to progress to cirrhosis.

According to some authorities (1), erosion of the limiting plates is a relatively infrequent feature of acute viral hepatitis, and, when present, may be indicative of "possible transition to chronic hepatitis." Although we have encountered such transitions, in no such case has progression to cirrhosis occurred in the absence of bridging necrosis (6). In a Danish study of 17 patients with acute hepatitis and "possible transition to chronic hepatitis," follow-up biopsies revealed full recovery without residuals in 14, chronic persistent hepatitis in 1, and cirrhosis in 2 (7). However, on reexamination of the biopsy sections in the 2 patients who developed cirrhosis, made possible through the courtesy of one of the authors, Dr. Niels Tygstrup, we found that the early phase lesions exhibited typical portal-portal bridging necrosis in one case, and portal-portal, portal-central, and central-central bridging necrosis in the other. Thus, the results of the Danish study confirm our own observation that the development of cirrhosis that follows acute viral hepatitis correlates with the occurrence of bridging necrosis during the early phase of the disease (6).

Some pathologists regard portal-portal bridging necrosis as a form of piecemeal necrosis (1). However, this view is inconsistent with the fact that bridging necrosis is characterized by rapid cytolysis of numerous contiguous hepatocytes, whereas piecemeal necrosis, by definition, implies slowly progressive, focal destruction of periportal cells. For that reason a distinction should be made between these two types of hepatocellular necrosis.

In cases of acute hepatitis with bridging necrosis that remain active and fail to resolve, the reticulin in the bridges and enlarged portal tracts tends to collapse and undergo collagenization. At this stage, the lesions may be indistinguishable from those of chronic active hepatitis attributable to progressive piecemeal necrosis. However, even in such cases, it is often possible to identify bands of collapsed reticulin connecting portal tracts and central veins. This is illustrated in the lesions encountered in the seventh month of illness of a 42-year-old woman with unresolved acute viral hepatitis who presented with persistent, deep, but fluctuating jaundice, high serum levels of transaminase and globulins, and hypoalbuminemia. Her treatment had been limited to intermittent periods of prolonged bed rest. As illustrated in Figure 301, many of the portal tracts were enlarged and fibrotic, contained numerous mononuclear cells and proliferating ductules, and exhibited erosion of their limiting plates, features consistent with chronic active hepatitis. However, in many areas, the portal tracts and central veins were bridged by bands of collapsed reticulin (Fig. 302). At higher magnification (Fig. 303), it can be seen that the reticulin fibers were thickened and possibly collagenized, but were still separated by collapsed sinusoids, and that the adjacent parenchyma still showed evidence of active hepatitis. A four-month course of adrenocorticosteroid therapy was associated with complete, sustained remission. However, rebiopsy a year later revealed residual inactive postnecrotic cirrhosis.

How often lesions classified as chronic active hepatitis are attributable to acute periportal and bridging necrosis rather than to piecemeal necrosis is uncertain, since, in few published reports is a distinction made between these two types of lesions. However, in at least one study, no less than a third of the 86 cases investigated exhibited panlobular necrosis or submissive collapse (8), features more consistent with diffuse acute hepatocellular necrosis than with piecemeal necrosis.

Since it is still uncertain whether the lesions of chronic active hepatitis that follow acute periportal and bridging necrosis differ from those attributable to piecemeal necrosis, an attempt should be made to distinguish between these two lesions with a view to resolving this question.

Portal inflammatory cells

Normally, the portal tracts contain few if any inflammatory cells. However, under a variety of conditions, the portal tracts may be infiltrated with lymphocytes, plasma cells, neutrophils, eosinophils, or macrophages. As a rule, such exudates are of mixed cellularity, but, often, one or another cell type is relatively conspicuous or predominant. The character of the cellular exudate is seldom diagnostic, but taken together with other histologic features, may provide an important clue to the etiology of the lesion.

Portal lymphocytes

Lymphocytes, the inflammatory cells encountered most frequently in the portal tracts, occur in large numbers and predominate in the portal exudates of many hepatic lesions, but also participate, to some extent, in most other portal inflammatory reactions. In addition, occasional, randomly distributed lymphocytes may be found in the portal tracts of the normal liver.

Dense, predominantly lymphocytic portal infiltrates are characteristic of *acute viral hepatitis* (Figs. 299, 300), *acute drug-induced hepatitis* (Fig. 91), *chronic active hepatitis* (Figs. 104–106), and *primary biliary cirrhosis* (Fig. 295). However, in each of these conditions, other inflammatory cells usually contribute to the exudate (9).

Lymphocytic portal infiltrates of variable extent also occur in a wide variety of other hepatic lesions. In some, such as *chronic persistent hepatitis* and so-called *nonspecific reactive hepatitis,* the lymphocytes usually predominate, but in others, such as alcoholic fatty infiltration, alcoholic hepatitis, and the pericholangitis associated with inflammation or obstruction of the bile ducts, they may be overshadowed by other cell types, particularly neutrophils.

A variable number of lymphocytes are seen in the fibrous septa in most forms of cirrhosis, even when the limiting plates are intact and the lesions are relatively inactive.

Portal lymphoid aggregates and follicles

Under a variety of conditions, some of the portal tracts contain dense, sharply circumscribed aggregates of lymphocytes and occasional plasma cells (Fig. 304). These may contain a germinal center occupied by loosely arranged, large lymphocytes or reticuloendothelial cells with abundant cytoplasm and vesicular nuclei, giving them the appearance of typical lymphoid follicles (Fig. 295). Often, such aggregates lie adjacent to or encircle an interlobular bile duct.

Lymphoid aggregates and follicles are found most frequently in *chronic active hepatitis* (Fig. 304), and in the late stages of *acute viral hepatitis* (Fig. 305), especially HCV (10). Less commonly, they may be seen in *primary biliary cirrhosis* (Fig. 295), *chronic persistent hepatitis, sclerosing cholangitis, prolonged extrahepatic biliary obstruction,* and in various forms of *cirrhosis,* including postnecrotic, alcoholic hemochromatosis, and the type associated with Wilson's disease. In the case of viral hepatitis, follicle formation occurs late in the course of the disease, and, particularly, when bridging necrosis is a feature of the lesions. The earliest we have ever encountered lymphoid aggregates or follicles in acute viral hepatitis is in the sixth week of disease (Fig. 305).

The pathogenesis and prognostic significance of lymphoid aggregates and follicles are uncertain. However, in our experience, the presence of such lesions has not correlated with continued activity or progression of the underlying disease.

At times, it may be difficult to differentiate between lymphoid aggregates and follicles, on the one hand, and chronic lymphocytic, leukemic, or lymphomatous infiltrates, on the other, particularly in those rare instances when the latter contain germinal centers (Fig. 306). However, there are a few distinguishing features that often prove useful in the differentiation. Characteristically, benign lymphoid aggregates and follicles affect only a small minority of the portal tracts, are centrally located, and, rarely, if ever, extend to the limiting plates (Figs. 295, 304, 305). In contrast, lymphocytic leukemic and lymphomatous infiltrates usually involve numerous portal tracts (Fig. 307), often occupying them completely and extending through the limiting plates into the surrounding parenchyma (Fig. 306). Moreover, they tend to be more destructive, so that frequently the affected portal tract appears to be devoid of collagen and blood vessels. Destruction or displacement of portal reticulin and collagen may also occur in benign lymphoid aggregates and follicles, but almost always a significant amount of collagen remains at the periphery, and intact vessels are readily demonstrable. An additional feature of such lesions, particularly those attributable to primary biliary cirrhosis and chronic active hepatitis, is the presence of degenerating interlobular ducts within or adjacent to the lymphoid aggregates (Figs. 295, 308). Such ducts are not seen in portal tracts infiltrated with lymphocytic leukemic or lymphomatous cells, but the frequent absence of ducts in such lesions suggests that often they are destroyed by the infiltrate. Although never a prominent feature, mitotic activity usually is more apparent in such infiltrates than in benign lymphoid aggregates and follicles. Perhaps the most convincing evidence that a portal infiltrate is leukemic or lymphomatous in nature is the presence within the parenchyma remote from the portal tracts of sharply circumscribed, destructive infiltrates of the same type. Figure 309 illustrates such a centrilobular infiltrate replacing hepatocytes and invading the central vein in the patient with lymphocytic lymphoma whose portal lesions are depicted in Figures 300 and 307.

Portal plasma cells

Variable numbers of plasma cells are found in the portal tracts in most chronic inflammatory disorders of the liver and biliary tract, in the lesions of acute viral and drug-induced hepatitis, and, rarely, in multiple myeloma (5). Immunoglobulin-containing plasma cells have been identified in the portal tracts of patients with acute viral hepatitis (11).

Numerous portal plasma cells are a distinctive feature of *chronic active hepatitis,* although not all portal tracts are necessarily equally affected. Characteristically, the plasma cells tend to aggregate in the advancing edge of periportal necrosis and to extend into the adjacent parenchyma (Fig. 278). This margination of the plasma cells is best visualized in sections stained with methyl green pyronine, which demonstrates the high concentration of ribonucleic acid in the cytoplasm of such cells (Fig. 279). In general, the number of plasma cells seen correlates with the activity of the lesions and the degree of hypergammaglobulinemia. Portal plasmacytosis is particularly impressive in children with chronic active hepatitis, so that at one time such lesions were classified as "plasma cell hepatitis" (12).

Almost always, the portal tracts in *primary biliary cirrhosis* contain numerous plasma cells. These are most abundant around degenerating, interlobular ducts (Fig. 310), but also occur in significant numbers elsewhere in the portal tracts.

Variable numbers of plasma cells may be found in the portal tracts in cases of chronic pericholangitis attributable to underlying *biliary tract disease.* Occasionally, they are sufficiently numerous to suggest the possibility of chronic active hepatitis or primary biliary cirrhosis. Figure 311 illustrates such a lesion in an elderly woman with recurrent attacks of cholangitis attributable to a stricture at the distal end of the common bile duct. As can be seen, wedge biopsy of the liver revealed numerous portal lymphocytes and plasma cells, and stratification and lymphocytic infiltration of the epithelium in some of the interlobular ducts, features suggestive of primary biliary cirrhosis. However, repair of the stricture led to full clinical and biochemical

recovery, and serial tests for mitochondrial antibody yielded negative results consistently.

A few plasma cells can be found in the portal exudates in most cases of *acute viral* and *drug-induced hepatitis.* When the illness is prolonged, and particularly when the lesions are accompanied by bridging necrosis, plasma cells may be as numerous as in chronic active hapatitis. The intensity of the portal plasma cell reaction under such conditions is illustrated in Figure 312, which shows the lesion found in the sixth week of severe HBsAg-negative hepatitis, and in Figure 313, which shows similar features in the fifth week of severe methyldopa-induced hepatitis.

In *multiple myeloma,* hepatic plasma cell tumor nodules or plasma cell infiltrates in the sinusoids and portal tracts are said to be relatively common findings at autopsy (13). However, these infiltrates are encountered far less frequently in needle biopsy specimens. In our own series of 13 cases, plasma cell infiltration of the sinusoids and portal tracts was found in only one (Fig. 280).

Portal neutrophils

Neutrophils are found in the portal tracts most frequently in obstructive and inflammatory disorders of the biliary tract, but also occur in some cases of alcoholic, viral, and drug-induced hepatitis. Almost always, the neutrophils are interspersed with a variable number of other types of inflammatory cells. A few scattered neutrophils may be found in many predominantly mononuclear portal exudates, but are never seen in the portal tracts of normal livers.

In *extrahepatic biliary obstruction,* neutrophils characteristically infiltrate the edematous margins of the portal tracts, usually in close association with proliferating bile ducts, some of which may be dilated, filled with bile, or both (Fig. 314). The neutrophilic reaction varies in intensity from one portal tract to another, and often spares some. In severe and prolonged biliary obstruction, neutrophils frequently infiltrate the walls of bile ducts (Fig. 314), and occasionally fill their lumens, even in the absence of complicating bacterial infection (Fig. 315), thereby mimicking the lesions of suppurative cholangitis. Early in the course of biliary obstruction, neutrophils may appear in the portal tracts before the development of ductular proliferation and histologically demonstrable cholestasis.

Obviously, the portal tract lesions produced by obstruction of the major hepatic ducts at their bifurcation within the liver or at the porta hepatis are identical with those seen in extrahepatic biliary obstruction. Moreover, occlusion of smaller intrahepatic ducts produces similar lesions, but these are limited to the areas drained by the affected ducts. This phenomenon occurs most frequently in cases of hepatic metastases.

The portal tract lesions of *acute, pyogenic, bacterial cholangitis* closely resemble those of biliary obstruction. Usually, the bile ducts are heavily infiltrated with neutrophils, and often show evidence of degeneration and necrosis. As a rule, the cholangitis is a complication of underlying biliary obstruction, but, in some cases, is attributable to sepsis secondary to extrahepatic disease. This is illustrated in Figure 316, which shows the suppurative cholangitis found in an elderly woman with *Aerobacter aerogenes* bacteremia secondary to acute pyelonephritis. Laparotomy revealed multiple, small, hepatic abscesses, but on intraoperative cholangiography both the intra- and extrahepatic bile ducts were found to be patent and free of stones.

In some cases of *acute and chronic cholecystitis, acute pancreatitis,* and *sclerosing cholangitis,* the portal lesions may closely resemble those of extrahepatic biliary obstruction or acute bacterial cholangitis. The differentiation of such lesions from those of biliary obstruction and bacterial cholangitis may be impossible on histologic grounds alone, particularly when cholestasis and ductular proliferation are accompanying features. This is illustrated in Figure 317, which shows the ductular proliferation and neutrophilic infiltration found in the portal tracts of a patient with acute and chronic cholecystitis who presented with mild jaundice. Although minimal centrilobular canalicular bile stasis was evident histologically, intraoperative cholangiography revealed patent intra- and extrahepatic bile ducts devoid of stones, and culture of bile aspirated from the common hepatic duct yielded no growth.

The centrilobular, hepatocellular degeneration and necrosis characteristic of *alcoholic hepatitis* are almost always accompanied by a neutrophilic infiltrate of variable extent. In some cases, the portal tracts also contain a significant number of neutrophils (Fig. 318). Usually, this correlates with the severity of the parenchymal lesions, and probably indicates a secondary inflammatory response. However, when the portal neutrophilic reaction is out of proportion to the extent of hepatocellular degeneration and necrosis, and particularly when it is accompanied by ductular proliferation and cholestasis, it often is attributable to complicating alcoholic pancreatitis, or, less commonly, to other inflammatory or obstructive lesions of the biliary tract.

Usually, only a few neutrophils are found in the portal exudates of *acute viral hepatitis.* However, in some cases, they may be numerous, particularly when hepatocellular necrosis is extensive or when cholestasis is a prominent feature. Figure 319 illustrates intense, portal, neutrophilic reaction and ductular proliferation in a case of severe acute viral hepatitis with extensive bridging necrosis. Occasionally, under such conditions, the neutrophils invade the walls and lumens of the bile ducts (Fig. 320). When cholestasis is severe, the ducts may be dilated, contain large bile thrombi or debris, and show atrophy, degeneration, or necrosis of their epithelial lining cells (Fig. 321). Such features may suggest extrahepatic biliary obstruction, but the character of the accompanying intralobular, hepatocellular changes and inflammatory reaction clearly indicates the nature of the lesion.

The hepatic lesions in some forms of *drug-induced hepatic injury,* usually classified as "hepatitic," are indistinguishable from those of viral hepatitis. As in the case of viral hepatitis, when hepatocellular necrosis is extensive, and especially when accompanied by marked cholestasis, the portal tracts may be heavily infiltrated with neutrophils and may contain proliferating, dilated, or degenerating bile ducts (Fig. 322). However, in the type of drug-induced hepatitis usually classified as "cholestatic," the portal tracts may contain numerous neutrophils and proliferating ductules accompanied by canalicular bile stasis in the absence of significant hepatocellular necrosis or intralobular inflammation. Figure 323 illustrates such a lesion in a case of amitryptiline (Elavil)-induced cholestatic hepatitis. Lesions of this type may be difficult to differentiate from those of extrahepatic biliary obstruction on histologic grounds alone. In some cases, the presence of a significant number of eosinophils in the portal tracts may favor a drug-induced hypersensitivity reaction, but, often, identification of the etiology rests on an accurate history of drug ingestion, certain clinical features such as eosinophilia and rash, and on the results of percutaneous, transhepatic or endoscopic, retrograde cholangiography.

Portal eosinophils

The occasional eosinophils commonly found in the portal exudates of a wide variety of hepatic lesions have no diagnostic significance. However, when numerous, portal eosinophils may provide a clue to the etiology of the lesion. As a rule, the eosinophils are interspersed with other inflammatory cells, and only occasionally do they predominate.

The hepatic lesions of *drug-induced hepatitis* usually mimic those of viral hepatitis. However, in some cases, the portal tracts and, occasionally, the parenchyma contain a significant number of eosinophils, a feature consistent with an underlying drug-sensitization reaction. This is illustrated in Figure 324 showing the portal eosinophilia in a case of halothane-induced hepatitis. Unfortunately, portal eosinophilia is not a completely reliable criterion, since it is not found in all cases of drug-induced hepatitis, and may be seen occasionally in acute viral hepatitis [(14); Fig. 325].

The histologic features of *drug-induced cholestasis* often closely resemble those of extrahepatic biliary obstruction. The presence of a significant number of eosinophils in the portal tracts, a feature in some cases (Fig. 326), favors an underlying drug reaction, and lends some support to the view that such lesions are attributable to drug sensitization. Of note in this connection is the fact that synthetic androgenic-anabolic steroids and oral contraceptives that produce cholestasis by a direct action on the bile secretory apparatus do not provoke a similar portal inflammatory reaction. Unfortunately, portal eosinophilia is of only limited value in differentiating between drug-induced cholestasis and biliary obstruction, since it is an inconstant feature in the former and may be seen occasionally in the latter.

Portal eosinophils are commonly seen during *allograft* rejection after liver transplantation (see Chapter 26).

The *biliary tract disorders* in which significant numbers of portal eosinophils may be encountered include acute and chronic cholecystitis, choledocholithiasis, sclerosing cholangitis, and biliary atresia. Although usually associated with histologic evidence of cholestasis under such conditions, portal eosinophilia may be seen occasionally in the absence of cholestatis. This is illustrated in Figure 327, showing the portal eosinophilia in a case of acute and chronic cholecystitis associated with cholelithiasis, but with no evidence of biliary obstruction or infection.

In one reported series, significant numbers of eosinophils were found in the portal tracts in over 20% of patients with *chronic active hepatitis* (15), a feature not encountered in our own cases, probably owing to our routine use of Carnoy's solution for fixation of needle biopsy specimens. As previously pointed out, eosinophils may be difficult to identify in liver biopsy specimens fixed with Carnoy's solution.

The portal tracts in *primary biliary cirrhosis* often contain a small, but significant number of eosinophils. Occasionally, these are numerous and may be accompanied by mild peripheral eosinophilia (Fig. 328).

The most intense portal eosinophilic reactions are seen in

helminthic, larval infestations of the liver and in the *hypereosinophilic syndrome.*

Visceral larva migrans, a disorder attributable to migration of nematode larvae through the tissues, affects young children who swallow soil contaminated with the ova of *Toxocara canis* or *Toxocara cati* (16). Less commonly, the larvae of other nematodes may be implicated (17). Characteristically, the larvae provoke a prolonged and marked peripheral eosinophilia, and give rise to an intense, eosinophilic, inflammatory reaction; necrosis; and granuloma formation in the tissues they invade. In the liver, one of the organs most frequently affected, the parenchyma is the principal site of necrosis and granuloma formation, but almost always both the parenchyma and portal tracts are densely infiltrated with eosinophils [(18); Figs. 288–291]. Only rarely can the larvae be identified in biopsy sections, so usually the diagnosis is presumptive and based on the peripheral eosinophilia and the character of the hepatic lesions. However, a recently developed enzyme-linked immunoabsorbent assay that uses an extract of embryonated *Toxocara canis* ova as antigen is relatively sensitive and specific, so serologic diagnosis of the disease is possible (19).

Significant portal eosinophilia is found in most cases of *acute schistosomiasis* (20). At onset, the eosinophils infiltrate the portal tracts diffusely, but later they tend to aggregate at the periphery of the granulomas that form around ova. In the more common chronic form of schistosomiasis, the portal tracts often contain numerous inflammatory cells, but usually these are predominantly mononuclear rather than eosinophilic in character, although a few eosinophils may be found in the vicinity of granulomas (21).

The *hypereosinophilic syndrome,* a disorder of unknown etiology that affects males predominantly and often proves fatal, is characterized by constitutional symptoms; prolonged, peripheral eosinophilia; and eosinophilic infiltration of the viscera, central nervous system, and skin. The liver, one of the organs most frequently affected, usually shows widespread, intense eosinophilic infiltration of the portal tracts (22,23).

Eosinophilic gastroenteritis, a disorder of uncertain etiology, but probably allergic in nature, is characterized by eosinophilic infiltration of the stomach and small intestine accompanied by peripheral eosinophilia (24). The character of the clinical manifestations, which tend to be intermittent, include diarrhea, abdominal pain, gastric or intestinal obstruction, and ascites, depending on whether the infiltration involves the mucosa, muscularis, or serosa. In some cases, the liver is enlarged, but on biopsy usually shows only sinusoidal eosinophils in numbers consistent with the degree of peripheral eosinophilia. One patient with this syndrome was found to have intense eosinophilic infiltration of the portal tracts (25). In the only well-documented case we have had the opportunity to study, the portal tracts were enlarged and edematous with eroded limiting plates, contained numerous eosinophils and a moderate number of neutrophils, and showed proliferation, inflammation, and degeneration of many of the interlobular bile ducts (Fig. 329). The patient, a young black man, presented with diarrhea and weight loss of two months' duration. In childhood he had had episodic attacks of asthma, and more recently, recurrent urticaria attributed to starchy foods. He was found to have peripheral eosinophilia, hyperglobulinemia, and raised serum levels of alkaline phosphatase and transaminase, but no hyperbilirubinemia or hepatosplenomegaly. Biopsy of the jejunum at laparotomy revealed intense eosinophilic infiltration of the mucosa. On a starch-free diet, the symptoms and eosinophilia

cleared, and follow-up liver biopsy three months later showed a decrease in portal inflammation and disappearance of the edema and duct abnormalities.

Portal histiocytes and macrophages

Histiocytes and macrophages, members of the mononuclear, phagocytic system, are derived from immature mononuclear cells in the bone marrow that are released into the circulation as monocytes, and undergo maturation to histiocytes and macrophages when they are deposited in the tissues. Under appropriate conditions, such cells may undergo further maturation to epithelioid and giant cells (26). At least in the case of the liver, the terms histiocyte and macrophage are used interchangeably, although the former is sometimes defined as a fixed connective tissue cell, and the latter as an infiltrating cell in other tissues (27). Kupffer cells also belong to the mononuclear phagocytic system and show the same reactions as the macrophages in the portal tracts. Indeed, it has been suggested that at least some of the portal macrophages may be derived from wandering Kupffer cells (28).

Because of their phagocytic activity, portal macrophages frequently contain lipofuscin, a feature that greatly facilitates their identification. Under some conditions, portal macrophages, like Kupffer cells, take up hemosiderin, other pigments, and granules or lipids.

As a rule, the macrophages in portal exudates are outnumbered by other inflammatory cells, but occasionally they predominate in small aggregates. When deeply pigmented with lipofuscin or hemosiderin, they are readily identified in H & E- or Masson-stained sections. Small numbers of macrophages may be overlooked in such sections, but usually can be demonstrated in sections stained with PAS following diastase digestion to visualize better their lipofuscin content.

Portal macrophages are significantly larger than lympocytes, and are characterized by pale-staining, vesicular nuclei and abundant cytoplasm with cell borders that may be ill defined (Fig. 330). Frequently, as previously indicated, they contain lipofuscin and appear yellow in H & E-, gray-brown in Masson- (Fig. 331), and bright red in D-PAS-stained sections (Fig. 332).

Lipofuscin-filled, portal macrophages are encountered most frequently in *acute viral* (Fig. 331) and *drug-induced hepatitis* (Fig. 330). Usually, such cells are most numerous late in the disease, and may persist long after apparent full recovery (Fig. 333). In early lesions, pigmented macrophages, in the form of proliferating, hypertrophic Kupffer cells, occur predominantly within the parenchyma (Figs. 229, 230), but even at this stage, a significant number may be found in the portal tracts (Figs. 300, 330).

Although less numerous and less constant a feature, macrophages may be found in the portal exudates of many other hepatic lesions. Of these, *chronic active hepatitis* (Fig. 332), various forms of *active cirrhosis* (Fig. 334), and chronic *inflammatory* and *obstuctive disorders of the biliary tract* (Fig. 335) are the most common. In contrast to chronic active hepatitis, the portal exudates of *chronic persistent hepatitis* rarely contain macrophages.

As a rule, macrophages infiltrate the portal tracts in response to intralobular inflammation and hepatocellular necrosis. However, they may also undergo hyperplasia and hypertrophy as a reaction to the phagocytosis of a variety of pigments and other materials deposited in the portal tracts.

Pigments, granules, and other deposits in portal macrophages

Portal lipofuscin

As previously indicated, lipofuscin is by far the most common pigment encountered in portal macrophages. Usually, such pigment is derived from the lipofuscin normally present in hepatocytes and released when they are destroyed. While some of the lipofuscin-filled macrophages may represent Kupffer cells that have migrated to the portal tracts (28), it is highly probable that many are derived from infiltrating monocytes that have been activated to phagocytize the pigment. The presence of lipofuscin in portal macrophages usually indicates antecedent, hepatocellular destruction. However, since lipofuscin may persist for long periods following recovery from hepatic injury (Fig. 333), the finding of such pigment does not necessarily imply recent cell loss.

Usually, PAS staining following diastase digestion is a reliable method for identifying lipofuscin. However, portal macrophages that contain bile may also take up PAS, so that, in cases of cholestasis, differentiation between deposits of lipofuscin and bile may require special stains.

Portal hemosiderin

Deposits of hemosiderin may be encountered in the portal tracts under any condition of iron overloading, but occur most frequently in hemochromatosis of either the primary (hereditary) (Fig. 336) or secondary type (Fig. 337). Almost always these are accompanied by qualitatively similar deposits in hepatocytes or Kupffer cells, and, less commonly, in the bile ducts (Fig. 336). Most of the hemosiderin in the portal tracts is found within macrophages, but when present in large amounts, it may be extracellular, presumably as a result of macrophage destruction.

Diffuse iron-staining of portal macrophages (Fig. 338) is seen most frequently following acute hepatocellular necrosis, but, in contrast to lipofuscin, tends to clear rapidly following recovery.

Portal deposition of bile

Under conditions of severe cholestasis, due to either biliary obstruction or hepatocellular disease, the portal tracts often contain clusters of large macrophages. Some of these are bile-stained or contain droplets of bile, while others show the type of foamy, pseudoxanthomatous degeneration (Fig. 339) seen more commonly in sharply circumscribed groups of hepatocytes and Kupffer cells in cases of severe cholestasis (Figs. 119–121, 298).

Occasionally, when the ducts undergo necrosis, free bile may be found in the portal tracts (Fig. 339). Such collections may be surrounded by pseudoxanthoma cells, epithelioid cells, or, less commonly, by giant cells.

Portal protoporphyrin deposits

In *erythropoietic protoporphyria,* an autosomal recessive hereditary disorder caused by a deficiency of heme synthetase, the portal tracts almost always contain a variable number of macrophages filled with dark brown, cytoplasmic granules of protoporphyrin [(29); Fig. 340] that characteristically exhibit bright red or golden birefringence on polarization microscopy [(30); Fig. 341]. These are found at an early stage of the disease with regularity, even before there are any other signs of liver disease. In most cases, similar protoporphyrin granules can be found in the hepatocytes and Kupffer cells (Figs. 167–170). Occasionally, the deposits lead to progressive portal fibrosis, cholestasis, and the development of secondary biliary cirrhosis. Under such conditions, protoporphyrin is found in both canalicular and ductular bile thrombi (Figs. 169, 170). When the deposits are large, they often appear globular and characteristically exhibit bright red birefringence with central, dark, Maltese crosses in polarized light (Fig. 170).

Another distinctive feature of the hepatic lesions in erythropoietic protoporphyria is the red fluorescence exhibited by the hepatocytes and pigment deposits when frozen sections are examined in ultraviolet light (Fig. 166).

Both malaria and schistosomal pigments (see below) exhibit birefringence in polarized light. However, they are never deposited in the hepatocytes or canaliculi, do not present as globules, and do not fluoresce in ultraviolet light, so their differentiation from protoporphyrin deposits poses no problem.

Portal malarial pigment

Following attacks of malaria, coarse, dark brown pigment (hemazoin) granules appear in portal macrophages. The pigment is a derivative of host hemoglobin taken up, altered, and released by the parasites. Characteristically, the pigment granules exhibit yellow-orange birefringence in polarized light (Fig. 242), but do not react with PAS or with stains for iron or melanin. The pigment, which resembles carbon, can be differentiated by its solubility in alcoholic picrate (31).

Portal schistosomal pigment

Frequently, dark brown pigment granules of variable size are found in portal macrophages and Kupffer cells in cases of hepatic schistosomiasis (Fig. 241). As in the case of malarial pigment, schistosomal pigment is a derivative of host hemoglobin that has been ingested, altered, and regurgitated by the adult parasite, and exhibits the same type of birefringence in polarized light and the same histochemical properties.

Portal anthracotic pigment

Fine carbon particles that are inhaled and gain access to the pulmonary alveoli are phagocytized by macrophages and transported to the lymphatics. Some of these pigment-laden cells enter the general circulation and migrate to the liver, where the pigment is taken up by Kupffer cells and portal macrophages. Microscopically, these appear as coarse, black granules that are nonreactive histochemically (Fig. 243).

Portal L-cystine crystals

In cystinosis, an autosomal recessive hereditary disorder, birefringent, hexagonal or rectangular crystals of L-cystine are deposited in the centrilobular Kupffer cells (Figs. 238, 239). Occasionally, a few of the portal macrophages contain similar crystals.

Portal Thorotrast deposits

Following its intravenous injection, Thorotrast, a colloidal solution of thorium dioxide, is taken up by the reticuloendothelial cells of the liver and spleen, and, to a lesser extent, by those in the lymph nodes, where it persists for years. In the liver, the deposits are found within Kupffer cells and portal macrophages, or lying free in the connective tissue of the portal tracts. Characteristically, they appear as aggregates of coarse, irregularly shaped, grayish-brown, refractile, but nonbirefringent granules (Fig. 240).

The adverse effects of the deposits with respect to the development of hepatic fibrosis and neoplasia are discussed in Chapters 4 and 25.

Lipid, polysaccharide, and glycoprotein deposits in portal macrophages

In a number of metabolic disorders, mostly hereditary in nature, both the Kupffer cells and portal macrophages contain cytoplasmic deposits of various lipids, polysaccharides, or glycolipids. These are described in Chapter 4, and are discussed more fully in Chapters 14 and 15.

Portal tract granulomas

Portal lipogranulomas

As indicated previously in Chapter 4, intestinal absorption of the mineral oil used in commercial baking, and in spraying fruits and vegetables destined for long-distance transportation, leads to the formation of lipogranulomas in the liver. Usually, these lesions present as sharply circumscribed collections of lipid-containing macrophages interspersed with a few lymphocytes and strands of collagen adherent or close to a central vein (Fig. 177). Less commonly, similar, but less sharply circumscribed lesions are found in the portal tracts (Fig. 178).

Portal epithelioid granulomas

Circumscribed, compact collections of epithelioid and giant cells, classified as granulomas, are encountered under a wide variety of conditions discussed more fully in Chapter 22. Such granulomas may be a feature of lesions that involve the liver primarily, as in primary biliary cirrhosis, but more commonly, they are manifestations of underlying systemic or other extrahepatic disorders such as sarcoidosis, tuberculosis, ulcerative colitis, and Hodgkin's disease.

Granulomas occur not only in the portal tracts but also within the parenchyma of the lobules. With few exceptions, neither the localization nor the histologic features of the granulomas provide a clue to the etiology of the lesions. Usually, identification of the etiology depends on the character of the accompanying hepatic lesions, on a consideration of the clinical and laboratory features, and the results of cultural and serologic studies (32).

In *primary biliary cirrhosis,* the granulomas are found in close proximity to degenerating or inflamed interlobular bile ducts, and are surrounded by dense infiltrates of lymphocytes and plasma cells, occasionally in the form of follicles (Figs. 295, 342). When all of these features are present, there is seldom any difficulty in identifying the nature of the lesion (33). However, similar portal granulomas and degenerating ducts may be found occasionally in cases of *chronic active hepatitis.* In such cases, the erosion of the limiting plates and the extension of fibrous tissue and inflammatory cells into the periportal parenchyma are more impressive than in primary biliary cirrhosis. However, differentiation may be exceedingly difficult, particularly in small, needle biopsy specimens. Occasionally, in cases of primary biliary cirrhosis, sarcoid-like granulomas are found within the parenchyma of the lobules (Fig. 343). These may pose a diagnostic problem in small specimens that do not exhibit the more typical histologic features of the disease.

The portal granulomas in *schistosomiasis* present as sharply circumscribed collections of epithelioid cells surrounding a central giant cell containing an ovum or its chitinous shell (Fig. 344). Often, concentric fibrosis is a prominent feature, which, in late lesions, may obliterate the granuloma except for an occasional giant cell containing an ovum. When cut tangentially, a schistosomal granuloma may resemble a sarcoidal lesion. Impressive concentric fibrosis and the presence of dark brown pigment in adjacent Kupffer cells and portal macrophages (Fig. 241) may suggest the possibility of schistosomiasis, but unequivocal identification requires the demonstration of ova, which almost always can be accomplished by examining serial sections.

Granulomas are found in the portal tracts or hepatic parenchyma in most cases of *sarcoidosis,* particularly if serial sections are examined (32). Characteristically, these present as sharply circumscribed compact collections of epithelioid and giant cells, often surrounded or infiltrated by a few lymphocytes and collagen bundles (Fig. 345). The giant cells, which may not be present in all lesions, usually contain numerous central or eccentric nuclei, and occasionally exhibit cytoplasmic vacuoles. Rarely, the latter contain an asteroid body, a stellate-shaped proteinaceous inclusion. Although more common in sarcoidosis, such inclusions may occur in other granulomas, so that they have no diagnostic significance. Schaumann bodies, laminated cytoplasmic inclusions encrusted with iron and calcium salts, are found occasionally in the giant cells of the lymph node lesions in sarcoidosis. However, we have never encountered one in the liver.

Most of the sarcoidal lesions in the parenchyma of the liver are sharply circumscribed, and contain few inflammatory cells (Fig. 274). However, those in the portal tracts may be ill defined, and heavily infiltrated with lymphocytes (Fig. 346). Although they never show caseation necrosis, sarcoidal granulomas, especially when large, often contain central foci of degeneration and fibrinoid necrosis (Fig. 347). As the lesions advance in age, they tend to undergo central and peripheral fibrosis and hyalinization. However, some disappear without a trace.

Rarely, the portal tracts in sarcoidosis are expanded by numerous granulomas, leading to bridging, progressive fibrosis, destruction of the normal lobular architecture, and the ultimate development of a unique type of granulomatous cirrhosis (Figs. 83, 84).

As might be anticipated, granulomas are found in the liver in most cases of disseminated *tuberculosis*. However, they also occur in other forms of tuberculosis (32). Presumably, such lesions are attributable to hematogenous spread of the infection, but tubercle bacilli are demonstrable by acid-fast staining in only 10% of tuberculous hepatic granulomas, suggesting the possibility that the lesions may represent an immunologic response to extrahepatic infection.

The classic lesions of tuberculosis in most tissues are characterized by a granulomatous reaction accompanied by caseation necrosis. However, such caseation is rare in the liver. In our own series of 70 cases with hepatic tuberculous granulomas, only one lesion exhibited typical caseation necrosis (Fig. 348). Extensive fibrinoid necrosis and diffuse inflammation are more common (Fig. 349), but often the lesions are indistinguishable from those of sarcoidosis (Fig. 350). Accordingly, the differentiation between tuberculous and sarcoidal hepatic granulomas is seldom possible on histologic grounds alone, and usually depends on the demonstration of tubercle bacilli in other tissues or body fluids. Culture of biopsy specimens may be more effective than acid-fast staining in detecting tubercle bacilli in the liver, but, in our own limited experience, this has not proved to be the case. Moreover, the necessity for culture often is not recognized until after the granulomas are discovered following fixation.

At present, atypical tuberculosis caused by *Mycobacteria avium intracellulare* is found much more commonly than true tuberculosis in patients with AIDS (34). The granulomas tend to be less well organized and to contain many more bacteria (see Chapter 27).

Probably the most common type of hepatic granulomas are the lipogranulomas (35). These lesions, which are not associated with any hepatic dysfunction, are found predominantly in the portal or periportal areas.

Noninflammatory cellular infiltrates in the portal tracts

Portal leukemic infiltrates

In many cases of *chronic lymphocytic leukemia,* the portal tracts are heavily infiltrated with lymphocytes. Since the sinusoids may be spared, and the leukemic cells are almost indistinguishable from normal lymphocytes, the infiltrates superficially resemble inflammatory exudates. However, leukemic lymphocytes tend to infiltrate most of the portal tracts, often filling them completely (Fig. 351), show no admixture with other inflammatory cells, and often obscure or destroy the portal collagen and bile ducts (Fig. 352), so their differentiation from inflammatory cells usually poses no problem.

Leukemic infiltration of the portal tracts also occurs in other forms of *acute* and *chronic leukemia,* but usually involves the sinusoids more extensively than in chronic lymphocytic leukemia. Figure 277 illustrates the striking portal and sinusoidal infiltration found in a case of acute monocytic leukemia. As is evident at higher magnification (Fig. 268), the sinusoidal infiltration was so extensive that it led to considerable atrophy and loss of the intervening hepatocytes.

Lymphomatous infiltration of the portal tracts

All forms of lymphoma occasionally infiltrate the portal tracts. In *lymphocytic lymphoma,* the portal infiltrates closely resemble those of chronic lymphocytic leukemias (Figs. 306, 307), although they are more commonly accompanied by intralobular infiltrates (Fig. 309). As a rule, the neoplastic cells show no evidence of mitotic activity and resemble well-differentiated lymphocytes. However, their uniformity and close cohesion, the absence of interspersed inflammatory cells, and their tendency to obscure or destroy the blood vessels, bile ducts, and collagen in the portal tracts, and to replace hepatocytes as they extend into the parenchyma clearly differentiate them from inflammatory lymphocytes. Occasionally, the lymphomatous infiltrates are so extensive that they expand the portal triads, leading to bridging and destruction of the normal lobular architecture (Fig. 80).

The lymphomatous portal infiltrates seen occasionally in *Hodgkin's disease* resemble those found in the lymph nodes. However, they often lack Reed-Sternberg cells and some of the other distinctive features of classic lesions, so an unequivocal diagnosis of Hodgkin's disease may not be possible from liver tissue alone. Differential diagnosis may be aided by immunocytochemical studies (36).

Portal histiocytic infiltrates

Letterer-Siwe disease, a febrile illness of unknown etiology that affects children under the age of three years, is characterized by proliferation of histiocytes in the liver, spleen, lymph nodes, bone marrow, and skin (37) (see Chapter 24). Although the histiocytes are well differentiated and do not appear to be neoplastic, their proliferation leads to destructive lesions and a fatal outcome, usually within a few months. In the liver, the infiltrates are most prominent in the portal tracts (Fig. 353), but may also involve the parenchyma (Fig. 261), and invade the walls and lumens of the central veins (Fig. 262). Characteristically, the infiltrating histiocytes, which are interspersed with lymphocytes and, less commonly, with other inflammatory cells including eosinophils, expand the portal tracts and erode their limiting plates. The histiocytes, which resemble the macrophages found in portal inflammatory exudates, except for an absence of pigment, are relatively large cells with abundant, faintly eosinophilic, finely granular cytoplasm and vesicular nuclei (Fig. 261).

Some authorities regard eosinophilic granuloma of bone, Hand-Schuller-Christian disease, and both the infantile and adult forms of Letterer-Siwe disease as variants of a single entity that they classify as histiocytosis X (38). Although there is general agreement that Hand-Schuller-Christian disease is a multifocal or systemic variant of eosinophilic granuloma of bone, the view that these two disorders are related to Letterer-Siwe disease has been challenged (39).

Malignant histiocytosis, a generalized neoplastic disease of histiocytes, also classified by some as *histiocytic medullary reticulosis,* or *aleukemic reticulosis,* is characterized by proliferation of atypical histiocytes in the liver, spleen, bone marrow, and skin. In the liver, these cells infiltrate and expand the portal tracts, erode their limiting plates as they extend into the parenchyma and destroy or replace their blood vessels, bile ducts, and collagen (Fig. 354). The sinusoids are similarly invaded and distended, resulting in atrophy and loss of the intervening hepatocytes (Fig. 263). In addition, the proliferating histiocytes frequently invade the walls and lumens of central veins (Fig. 265). Characteristically, many of the histiocytes are large and pleomorphic, and contain large polylobulated, hyperchromatic nuclei with thick nuclear membranes, irregularly clumped chromatin, and large, irregular nucleoli (Fig. 264). In most cases, a few of the histiocytes show evidence of erythrophagocytosis, and, occasionally, phagocytosis of leukocytes and platelets.

Familial hemophagocytic reticulosis or *lymphohistiocytosis,* another apparently neoplastic disorder characterized by widespread proliferation of atypical histiocytes that exhibit erythrophagocytosis, affects siblings under the age of two years, and is invariably fatal within a few months. Both the clinical features and character of the lesions, including those in the liver, are indistinguishable from those of histiocytic medullary reticulosis (see Chapter 24).

The *virus-associated hemophagocytic syndrome* (40) (see Chapter 24), a non-neoplastic but often fatal form of histiocytosis, closely mimics malignant histiocytosis clinically and, to some extent, morphologically. The disease is attributable to an acute viral infection, and usually affects immunosuppressed, renal transplant patients. However, it may occur in individuals with no underlying disease, or in patients who are receiving immunosuppressive agents for other reasons. The infectious agents that have been implicated include cytomegalovirus, herpes simplex virus, Epstein-Barr virus, and adenovirus, although, in some reported cases, the diagnosis of viral infection has been presumptive. As in the case of malignant histiocytosis, the disease is manifested by sustained high fever, hepatosplenomegaly, lymphadenopathy, and cytopenia. Characteristically, the liver, spleen, and bone marrow are infiltrated by numerous well-differentiated, proliferating histiocytes that contain many phagocytized erythrocytes. The absence of atypia and the large number of erythrocytes they contain serve to differentiate these cells from the histiocytes of histocytic medullary reticulosis. In the liver, the proliferating cells invade both portal tracts and parenchyma, and often are associated with foci of hepatocelluar necrosis.

The hepatic lesions in one of our cases that presented with a viral-like syndrome, i.e., high fever, chills, leukopenia, elevated SGOT levels, and jaundice, were characterized by extensive infiltration of the sinusoids (Fig. 355) and some of the central veins (Fig. 356) by large, foamy histiocytes containing numerous erythrocytes. Surprisingly, the portal tracts were spared. In many of the centrilobular zones, both the hepato-cytes and invading histiocytes exhibited ischemic necrosis and evidence of cytolysis (Fig. 357). The lesions observed are characteristic of those described in this relatively new syndrome, but, unfortunately, the viral nature of this disorder was not documented serologically or culturally.

Abnormalities of the intrahepatic bile ducts

Proliferation of bile ducts

Biliary obstruction and a wide variety of inflammatory and destructive lesions of the hepatic parenchyma are often accompanied by elongation, tortuosity, reduplication, or extension of the peripheral bile ducts into the parenchyma beyond the boundaries of the portal tracts. Although this process is generally termed ductular proliferation, either or both the ductules and interlobular ducts may be involved.

It is generally agreed that elongation and reduplication of the interlobular ducts are attributable to proliferation of ductal, epithelial cells. However, the origin of proliferating ductules is less certain. According to many authorities, these always arise from ductular or ductal epithelium (41, 42). However, there is suggestive evidence that at least under some conditions, proliferating ductules may stem from hepatocytes (43, 44).

The factors responsible for ductular proliferation have not been clearly identified. Even in the case of biliary obstruction, it is unlikely that increased intraluminal hydrostatic pressure alone plays a major role. Since ductular proliferation also occurs under conditions of hepatocellular cholestasis, it has been suggested that the retention or reflux of bile acids may be involved (45). However, this hypothesis cannot account for the ductular proliferation commonly found in lesions unaccompanied by cholestasis. Of other possibilities that have been considered, the one that appears most plausible is that ductular hyperplasia is attributable to the breakdown products of either periductular inflammatory cells (42) or hepatocytes undergoing necrosis (43).

In most chronic lesions, the ductules that extend into the parenchyma are surrounded by collagen bundles in intimate contact with their basement membranes. This has led to the suggestion that proliferating ductules may play a role in hepatic fibrogenesis (35). However, the possibility cannot be excluded that the two are independent, but attributable to the same stimulus. Also, it has been proposed that at least in the case of severe biliary obstruction, ductular proliferation may be responsible for the edema and neutrophilic infiltrates found at the margins of the portal tracts (46). However, this appears unlikely, since ductular proliferation under other conditions rarely provokes edema and a neutrophilic response.

Characteristically, in *biliary obstruction,* the bile ducts at the margins of the portal tracts are elongated and tortuous, and often extend into the parenchyma beyond the borders of the portal tracts (Figs. 297, 314, 358). The marginal location of the affected ducts has been emphasized as a feature of biliary obstruction (46, 47). However, it cannot be considered diagnostic, since it may be seen in a wide variety of other disorders. Moreover, even in biliary obstruction, the proliferating ducts may not be limited to the periphery of the portal tracts. Nevertheless, the absence of proliferating marginal ducts in any of the portal tracts is a strong point against underlying biliary obstruction. In this connection, it should be noted that, often, some portal tracts are spared, so that marginal ductular proliferation can escape detection in small biopsy sections.

Both the interlobular ducts and ductules are involved in the proliferative response to biliary obstruction. Characteristically, the interlobular ducts are lined by cuboidal epithelial cells, and have a well-defined lumen that may be dilated (Fig. 314). In contrast, the ductules present as slender, branching structures with a fine, often discontinuous lumen outlined by parallel columns of flat epithelial cells (Fig. 358). Stereologic analysis of their configuration has demonstrated that proliferating ductules are flattened cylinders, which accounts for their predominantly elongated appearance in most sections (44). In some cases, the interlobular ducts and, less commonly, the ductules contain inspissated bile, and, under such conditions, may show degenerative changes, especially vacuolization, in the cytoplasm of their epithelial lining cells.

Ductular proliferation is a constant feature in the expanded portal tracts of *severe acute viral and drug-induced hepatitis* (Fig. 88), and often is prominent when periportal necrosis is extensive. Indeed, in cases of bridging, submassive, or massive necrosis, the ductules may extend deep into the lobules, occasionally approaching the central veins (Fig. 78). However, in cases of mild acute hepatitis with little or no periportal hepatocellular necrosis, ductular proliferation is only minimal or absent.

In *chronic active hepatitis,* a variable number of proliferating ductules are always found in the advancing periportal zone of hepatocellular necrosis, inflammation, and fibrosis (Fig. 301). As the lesions progress to cirrhosis, the ductules increase in number, and often are a prominent feature in the fibrous septa that are formed.

As the interlobular ducts are destroyed in *primary biliary cirrhosis,* the portal tracts undergo progressive fibrosis and exhibit ductular proliferation, features that often appear before the development of overt cirrhosis. As shown in Figure 359, most of the proliferating ducts show the typical morphologic features of ductules. However, in some cases, the ductules are accompanied by a small number of proliferating interlobular ducts. These are significantly smaller than the large interlobular ducts that are destroyed in primary biliary cirrhosis, but may lead to the erroneous impression that the number of ducts is not reduced.

Bile duct proliferation can be best demonstrated by immunohistochemical techniques using immunoperoxidase staining with biliary epithelial–specific cytokeratin antibodies (Fig. 360). In Figure 353 extensive bile duct proliferation is shown.

In all forms of *cirrhosis,* the fibrous septa contain a variable number of proliferating ductules. These tend to be most numerous in the postnecrotic cirrhosis that develops as a consequence of chronic active hepatitis or submassive hepatic necrosis, in the late phase of alcoholic cirrhosis, and in a variety of other forms of cirrhosis accompanied by extensive parenchymal destruction. However, the extent of the ductular proliferation does not correlate with the activity of the disease, nor does it give any indication of its etiology.

Dilatation, degeneration, and rupture of portal bile ducts secondary to cholestasis

Under conditions of severe and sustained cholestasis, some of the interlobular ducts may be widely dilated and filled with inspissated bile. Although this may be seen in prolonged, relatively complete *extrahepatic biliary obstruction* (Fig. 361), it is encountered most frequently in severe *hepatocellular cholestasis* attributable to viral hepatitis, particularly when accompanied by bridging necrosis (Fig. 321), drug-induced hepatitis (Figs. 322, 339), and advanced, usually terminal, decompensated cirrhosis (Fig. 362). The epithelial cells lining the involved ducts invariably show atrophy and other degenerative changes, and, occasionally, undergo necrosis leading to extravasation of bile (Figs. 339, 361).

Dilatation of the interlobular ducts with atrophy and degeneration of their epithelium also occurs in the distinctive form of focal or diffuse biliary cirrhosis found in a significant number of patients with *mucoviscidosis* (cystic fibrosis of the pancreas)(48,49). However, the ducts are usually distended with inspissated, eosinophilic mucoid secretions rather than bile (Fig. 363). In advanced lesions, some of the ducts may contain bile as well.

Abnormalities of portal bile duct epithelium not attributable to cholestasis

Although most common in primary biliary cirrhosis, abnormalities of bile duct epithelium may be seen in a number of other disorders, including chronic active hepatitis, acute viral and drug-induced hepatitis, cirrhosis, sclerosing cholangitis, and some forms of granulomatous hepatitis. The pathogenesis of such duct lesions is still uncertain, but there is mounting evidence that an underlying immunologic reaction is responsible (50–53).

In *primary biliary cirrhosis,* randomly distributed ducts, ranging in diameter from 30 to 100 μm, are involved. These include both septal ducts lined by columnar epithelium, and interlobular ducts lined by cuboidal epithelium. Septal duct lesions are encountered most frequently in surgical wedge biopsy specimens (Figs. 364, 365), but may be found occasionally in needle biopsy sections (Fig. 366). Based on studies of serial sections, it has been shown that the lesions involve only short segments of the ducts (54). No doubt this, in part at least, accounts for the relatively small number of affected ducts usually found, even in relatively large sections. However, equally important, is the fact that not all of the ducts are involved at any one time, and that many of those affected are destroyed and disappear as the disease progresses.

The columnar epithelial cells of the affected septal ducts in *primary biliary cirrhosis* show a number of abnormalities. In early lesions, the intercellular and basal cell boundaries are indistinct, some of the cells contain cytoplasmic vacuoles and infiltrating lymphocytes, and the nuclei lose their normal basal polarity and often are reduplicated (Fig. 364). Later in its development, the ductal lesion is characterized by segmental or complete loss of the epithelial basement membrane, and by proliferation and stratification of the epithelial cells, forming papillary projections that deform and compromise the duct lumen (Fig. 365). Often, the ducts show focal areas of epithelial degeneration and necrosis (Fig. 366), and, in some cases, these lead to rupture of the duct (Fig. 367). Although numerous lymphocytes, plasma cells, and macrophages, some of which may show pseudoxanthomatous degeneration, accumulate at the site of rupture, extravasation of bile is never seen. Moreover, the affected ducts never contain bile thrombi. This suggests that they may be occluded proximally, thus interfering with bile flow from the ductules. The observation, based on a study of serial sections, that some of the affected ducts end blindly (54) is consistent with this interpretation. As previously indicated, the duct lesions are segmental, so that, occasionally, the degeneration and necrotic epithelial cells may be found limited to only one sector of the duct circumference (Fig. 367).

Almost always, the abnormal ducts in primary biliary cirrhosis are surrounded by numerous lymphocytes and plasma cells, occasionally aggregated in the form of a follicle (Fig. 295). In addition, the affected duct often lies adjacent to or is surrounded by an epithelioid granuloma (Figs. 295, 365). A few neutrophils may be found in the lumens of the ducts, but, more commonly, they contain exfoliated epithelial cells or cell debris (Figs. 365, 367).

Lesions of the interlobular ducts in primary biliary cirrhosis (Figs. 367, 368) are similar to those of the septal ducts. However, they show less stratification and no papillary hyperplasia of their epithelium. Because their basement membranes may be destroyed, small abnormal interlobular ducts embedded in dense inflammatory infiltrates may be overlooked in H & E sections, but, usually, are readily identified in Masson-stained sections (Fig. 369).

Opinions regarding the specificity of the bile duct lesions in primary biliary cirrhosis vary. Although some authorities consider them pathognomonic (55), most agree that similar lesions may be found in other disorders (56, 57). However, it has been suggested that the bile duct lesions of primary biliary cirrhosis can be differentiated from the others (58), a point of view that has not gained wide acceptance, and is not supported by our own observations.

Abnormalities of bile duct epithelium are encountered in *chronic active hepatitis* far less frequently than in primary biliary cirrhosis, although they may be found in over a third of cases if serial sections are examined routinely (56). The lesions, which affect the interlobular ducts predominantly, are indistinguishable from those in primary biliary cirrhosis. Involvement of the septal ducts is relatively uncommon, but this may be attributable to the infrequency with which surgical wedge biopsy specimens are available for study. The vacuolization, stratification, and lymphocytic infiltration of the ductal epithelium in a case of chronic active hepatitis are illustrated in Figure 370. As can be seen in Figure 371, an adjacent duct in the same section shows focal necrosis and loss of epithelium resulting in disruption of its wall. As in primary biliary cirrhosis, the affected ducts are surrounded by numerous lymphocytes, plasma cells, and macrophages. Although circumscribed portal granulomas are rare in chronic active hepatitis, ill-defined compact collections of macrophages resembling epithelioid cells may be seen occasionally (Fig. 371).

The ductal lesions in chronic active hepatitis, particularly when accompanied by aggregates of epithelioid cells, pose a difficult diagnostic problem. Since they cannot be distinguished from those of primary biliary cirrhosis, differentiation between the two diseases usually depends on a consideration of the accompanying histologic, serologic, and clinical features. Available evidence indicates that the ductal lesions of chronic active hepatitis are encountered frequently in middle-aged women, and can be correlated with the presence of antinuclear antibodies, the absence of antimitochondrial antibody in the serum, increased serum gamma globulin levels, and a propensity for the subsequent development of cirrhosis (58).

Abnormalities of bile duct epithelium, identical with those seen in primary biliary cirrhosis and chronic active hepatitis, are seen occasionally in *acute viral hepatitis*. By examining serial sections, such lesions may be demonstrable in almost 20% of cases (59). With few exceptions, the ductal lesions are encountered in patients with extensive periportal or bridging hepatocellular necrosis, or in those whose hepatic lesions remain active for more than three months. Figure 372 illustrates the degeneration, necrosis, and lymphocytic infiltration of the epithelium of an interlobular duct found in a case of severe acute viral hepatitis with bridging necrosis on the 23rd day of illness. Bile duct lesions of this type never pose a diagnostic problem, since the parenchyma invariably shows the typical features of acute viral hepatitis.

Rarely, the interlobular ducts in acute *drug-induced hepatitis* show the type of epithelial degeneration, necrosis, and inflammation seen in primary biliary cirrhosis. Figure 373 illustrates such a lesion in a case of oxyphenisatin-induced cholestatic hepatitis of one month's duration. Of interest, the etiology of this lesion was not recognized initially, so that oxyphenisatin administration was not interrupted, resulting in the development over the following three years of chronic active hepatitis and postnecrotic cirrhosis, as previously described (60). Other types of interlobular duct lesions are more common in acute drug-induced hepatitis. These include neutrophilic infiltration of the ducts (Fig. 323), and, in cases with severe cholestasis, distension of the ducts with atrophy, degeneration, and necrosis of their lining epithelium (Fig. 339). Loss of interlobular ducts in cases of drug-induced hepatitis has been reported (61,62), but the character of the lesions responsible for their destruction has not been described.

In a study of *"cryptogenic" cirrhosis,* serial sections revealed abnormalities of interlobular bile duct epithelium in 7% of 497 cases (63). Since the ductal lesions were indistinguishable from those of chronic active hepatitis, it was suggested that the cirrhosis in such cases was probably a sequela of antecedent chronic active hepatitis. In our own cases of postnecrotic cirrhosis of insidious onset, only those with accompanying histologic features of chronic active hepatitis have exhibited ductal lesions.

Abnormalities of the interlobular duct epithelium closely resembling those of primary biliary cirrhosis are encountered occasionally in the type of *sclerosing cholangitis* (64–66) seen in patients with ulcerative colitis or Crohn's disease. Figure 374 illustrates such a lesion in a case of sclerosing cholangitis associated with ulcerative colitis. In some cases, the ductal lesions are accompanied by portal granulomas, as shown in Figure 375, which illustrates the lesion found in a woman with active Crohn's disease of 14 years' duration. Differentiation of such lesions from those of primary biliary cirrhosis is not possible on histologic grounds alone, and must depend on the clinical, serologic, and cholangiographic features of the disease. Similar lesions may be seen following antineoplastic chemotherapy (67, 68).

An even more difficult problem in differential diagnosis is posed by cases of *granulomatous hepatitis* accompanied by abnormalities of interlobular duct epithelium. We have encountered such lesions occasionally in sarcoidosis, miliary tuberculosis, and granulomatous hepatitis of unknown etiology. In some, the involved ducts have been in intimate contact with granulomas, whereas in others they have been found in portal tracts free of granulomas. Figure 376 illustrates the proliferation, degeneration, and inflammation of the epithelium in an interlobular duct adjacent to a granuloma found in a case of pulmonary sarcoidosis. A less florid ductal lesion unaccompanied by a granuloma, which was encountered in a patient with sarcoidal hilar and peripheral lymphadenopathy, is shown in Figure 377. Only 2 of our 13 patients with duct lesions associated with granulomatous hepatitis exhibited pruritus or jaundice, and in only 1 was mitochondrial antibody demonstrable. In those with unequivocal clinical and laboratory features of tuberculosis or sarcoidosis, the ductal lesions were attributed to the underlying granulomatous disease. However, in those with granulomas of unknown etiology, the possibility of primary biliary cirrhosis could not be excluded with certainty, since the disease may be asymptomatic and is not always accompanied by the development of mitochondrial antibody (69).

It is well documented that sarcoidosis can destroy the interlobular ducts and give rise to hepatic lesions that mimic primary biliary cirrhosis both clinically and histologically (70). In one such reported case, mitochondrial antibody was detected late in the course of the disease, suggesting the possible coincidence of sarcoidosis and primary biliary cirrhosis (71). We have encountered an almost identical case in which mitochondrial antibody–positive, typical primary biliary cirrhosis appeared 10 years following recovery from biopsy-documented sarcoidosis involving the hilar and cervical lymph nodes. In two other reported cases, serologically and histologically documented primary biliary cirrhosis was followed by the appearance of disseminated, noncaseating granulomas in the lungs and lymph nodes, lesions that were identified at autopsy (72). Since the Kveim reaction in one case was negative, the granulomas were interpreted as manifestations of primary biliary cirrhosis rather than as evidence of complicating or coincidental sarcoidosis.

Bile duct lesions similar to those seen in primary biliary cirrhosis have also been reported in *graft-versus-host disease* following bone-marrow transplantation (73,74) and in liver transplants undergoing *chronic rejection cholangitis* (75) (see Chapter 26).

Although this discussion has drawn attention to the wide variety of conditions under which abnormalities of ductal epithelium may be encountered, it should be emphasized that such ductal lesions, particularly when accompanied by portal granulomas, occur most frequently in primary biliary cirrhosis.

Paucity of interlobular ducts

Under a variety of conditions, the interlobular ducts are reduced in number. Usually, this is attributable to antecedent inflammation and necrosis of the epithelium and destruction of the basement membranes of the ducts, as described in the preceding section. However, in some cases of cirrhosis, it is possible that progressive fibrosis contributes to the obliteration of ducts (76).

In trying to establish whether or not the interlobular ducts are reduced in number, it is important to recognize that even in the normal liver, from 15 to 20% of the portal tracts visualized may be devoid of such ducts (77, 78), presumably due to tangential sectioning. Since under pathologic conditions, ducts may proliferate, only those ducts closely associated with a portal vein and artery should be counted.

As the lesions of *primary biliary cirrhosis* advance, there is progressive destruction of the interlobular ducts, so by the time the stage of fully developed cirrhosis is reached, approximately three-quarters of the portal tracts are devoid of such ducts (77). Often, the original site of the destroyed duct is marked by a circumscribed aggregate of lymphocytes and plasma cells (Fig. 378) or, less commonly, by a granuloma. In addition, the af-

fected portal tracts frequently contain proliferating ductules at their margins (Figs. 359, 379). Usually, these are sectioned lengthwise and are lined by relatively flat epithelial cells, so their differentiation from interlobular ducts is not difficult. However, in some cases, the portal tracts contain cross-sections of proliferating ducts lined by cuboidal epithelium. These are smaller than the interlobular ducts involved in primary biliary cirrhosis, and are not accompanied by branches of the portal vein and hepatic artery.

The *vanishing bile duct syndrome,* which represents acute, irreversible, hepatic allograft rejection, is in effect a temporal telescoping of the loss of bile ducts in primary biliary cirrhosis (79). This uncommon complication of hepatic transplantation runs its fatal course in three to four months (see Chapter 26).

A marked reduction in the interlobular ducts, equal to that seen in primary biliary cirrhosis, may be found occasionally in cases of *drug-induced hepatitis* (62) and the chronic cholestatic lesions produced by *sarcoidosis* (62). Similarly, impressive destruction of the interlobular ducts is a feature of *sclerosing intrahepatic obliterating cholangitis,* a rare disorder that closely resembles sclerosing cholangitis, but affects only the intrahepatic ducts (80). Characteristically, the destroyed ducts are replaced by sharply defined fibrous cords. However, in the two cases we have seen such cords could not be identified in needle biopsy sections.

Idiopathic adult ductopenia is a recently described syndrome in which none of the expected associated factors is present (81).

As a rule, the interlobular ducts in most forms of cirrhosis are not reduced in number (77). However, the type of postnecrotic cirrhosis that follows chronic active hepatitis sometimes appears to be an exception (76).

Discussion of the paucity of interlobular ducts in *neonatal cholestasis* and in *benign recurrent cholestasis* is presented in detail elsewhere (82).

Concentric periductal fibrosis

In the late stage of *primary sclerosing cholangitis* (64–66), the interlobular ducts frequently are encircled by concentric bands of collagen (Fig 380). It has become evident over the past 10 years that the lesion of pericholangitis is identical to the sclerosing cholangitis of ulcerative colitis or Crohn's disease (83). However, this is an inconstant feature, and may be seen in other disorders, including *primary biliary cirrhosis, postnecrotic cirrhosis,* and prolonged *extrahepatic biliary obstruction* (Fig. 381), so that concentric periductal fibrosis has only limited diagnostic significance.

Cytoplasmic deposits and inclusions in bile duct epithelium

Under conditions of severe iron overloading, proliferating ductules and, less commonly, the interlobular ducts may contain deposits of *hemosiderin.* This occurs most frequently in idiopathic hemochromatosis (Fig. 336), but may be seen occasionally in the secondary, posttransfusional type.

In severe alcoholic hepatitis and cirrhosis, typical *Mallory bodies* may be found occasionally in epithelial cells lining proliferating ductules and interlobular ducts [(84); Fig. 133].

Typical *cytomegalovirus inclusions* are encountered in the hepatocytes and bile duct epithelial cells in some cases of active cytomegalovirus infection. Their localization in the bile ducts is said to be more common in infants than in adults, but there are many exceptions. Characteristically, the affected epithelial cell is enlarged and projects into the lumen of the bile duct, shows increased cytoplasmic basophilia, and contains a large nucleus that is almost filled by a sharply circumscribed, homogeneous, reddish-blue inclusion surrounded by a narrow, clear halo (Fig. 191). Biliary obstruction with distal bile duct strictures occur in patients with AIDS and CMV infection (85) often in conjunction with other opportunistic infections (86).

Congenital anomalies of the intrahepatic bile ducts

This group of disorders includes various forms of polycystic disease, choledochal cyst, congenital cystic dilatation of the intrahepatic bile ducts (Caroli syndrome), and von Meyenburg complexes (82). In some cases these occur in combination. With the possible exception of some von Meyenburg complexes and choledochal cysts, most of these disorders appear to be hereditary in nature. Since the ductal lesions usually are accompanied by a variable degree of hepatic fibrosis and may be associated with cystic lesions in other organs, particularly the kidneys, the term "fibropolycystic disease" of the liver has been applied to this group of disorders (87).

For a more complete discussion of the interrelationships, genetics, pathogenesis, and morphologic features of the lesions in these disorders, the reader is referred to Chapter 19.

In *congenital hepatic fibrosis,* the juvenile form of polycystic disease, the hepatic parenchyma is traversed by numerous broad, irregularly shaped but smooth-contoured, densely collagenized septa. Characteristically, these contain numerous dilated, branching bile ducts lined by cuboidal epithelial cells (Fig. 64). Usually, long, slender ducts with relatively flat epithelium and inconspicuous lumens are seen at the margins of the septa in close contact with the limiting plates, and, almost always, some of the ducts contain inspissated bile (Fig. 65). As a rule, few or no portal vein radicles can be identified in the septa.

von Meyenburg complexes, also termed biliary hamartomas (88) or cholangiohamartomas (89), are small, solitary or multiple, sharply circumscribed, wedge-shaped lesions that range in diameter from 2 to 10 mm. Usually, they are found just beneath Glisson's capsule, but may be encountered deeper in the liver when numerous. Although the lesions represent congenital anomalies, and closely resemble a focal form of congenital hepatic fibrosis microscopically, many do not appear to be hereditary in nature. Nevertheless, they frequently are encountered in such hereditary disorders as adult polycystic disease and congenital cystic dilatation of the intrahepatic ducts (Caroli syndrome), which has led to the suggestion that von Meyenburg complexes may represent the first stage in the development of these more complex lesions (89).

Characteristically, von Meyenburg complexes present as sharply circumscribed foci of dense collagen in which are embedded numerous dilated, branching, intercommunicating ducts lined by cuboidal epithelium (Fig. 382). Almost always, a few of the ducts contain inspissated bile. The lesions, which often lie close to or are attached to normal portal tracts, usually contain few or no vascular channels. Although most von Meyenburg complexes are discovered at laparotomy or autopsy, we

and others (76) have encountered them in needle biopsy specimens.

Von Meyenburg complexes must be differentiated from another, probably congenital, but much rarer anomaly of the intrahepatic bile ducts, usually classified as *bile duct adenoma,* benign cholangioma, or cholangioadenoma (90). Such lesions closely resemble von Meyenburg complexes in size, location, and gross appearance, but can be differentiated from them histologically. They too contain many branching ducts, but these are more closely packed, show less dilation, never contain inspissated bile, and are separated by far less fibrous tissue than in von Meyenburg complexes (Fig. 383).

The large macroscopic cysts seen in *adult polycystic disease* of the liver are lined by flat epithelium, and, often, are in direct contact with typical von Meyenburg complexes, a relationship that supports the view that the cysts arise in such complexes. Figure 384 illustrates this combination of lesions in a case of advanced polycystic disease that involved both the liver and kidneys.

In the *Caroli syndrome,* the septal bile ducts are the site of segmental cystic dilatation through their length. Occasionally, one of the affected ducts may be seen in a surgical wedge biopsy section, appearing as a cystic structure lined by low columnar or flattened cuboidal epithelial cells (Fig. 385). More commonly, the portal tracts contain proliferating marginal ductules and dilated, tortuous interlobular ducts, some of which may contain inspissated bile, and an exudate of neutrophils, lymphocytes, plasma cells, and macrophages, features indicative of the cholangitis and biliary obstruction that are frequent complications of the disease. In some cases, congenital cystic dilation of the intrahepatic bile ducts is associated with congenital hepatic fibrosis (82, 91, 92), as illustrated in Figure 386.

Abnormalities of intrahepatic portal veins

Pyelophlebitis

Septic foci in areas drained by the portal vein occasionally give rise to pyelophlebitis. At one time, appendiceal abscess was the most common cause of this complication, but currently other septic foci predominate (93). These include diverticulitis, ulcerative colitis, neonatal omphalitis, pancreatic abscess, splenic abscess, perforated peptic ulcer, erosion of the portal vein by gallstones, infected hemorrhoids, and pelvic abscess.

In pyelophlebitis, septic thrombi form in small veins draining the infected site, and then propagate along the course of the portal vein, or give rise to emboli that lodge in its intrahepatic branches. The thrombi, made up of fibrin and numerous neutrophils, partially or completely occlude some of the veins in the portal tracts. Usually, as shown in Figure 387, there is an accompanying intense, neutrophilic reaction throughout the portal tracts.

Sclerosis, thrombosis, and occlusion of intrahepatic portal veins

Studies based on postmortem vinylite injection corrosion casts, dissection, and histologic examination of the intrahepatic vasculature (94) suggest that most cases of *"idiopathic" portal hypertension* (95) are attributable to thrombotic occlusion of large intrahepatic branches of the portal vein, a lesion termed *obliterative portal venopathy* (96). According to some authorities (97), such occlusions are the result of a primary form of phlebosclerosis, classified as *hepatoportal sclerosis,* that may affect not only the intrahepatic but also the extrahepatic portal veins. However, it is possible that the eccentric, sclerotic, intimal placques that characterize hepatoportal sclerosis represent organized mural thrombi that have been incorporated into the walls of portal vein radicles (95).

In *obliterative portal venopathy,* segments of some of the large septal portal veins contain organized and recanalized thrombi. Although readily demonstrable at autopsy, the thrombi, because of their location deep in the liver, are encountered only occasionally in wedge biopsy sections, and never in needle biopsy specimens. Microscopically, the thrombi present as a loose mesh of collagen bundles perforated by a variable number of thin-walled vascular channels. Characteristically, the thrombi are tightly bound to the walls of the involved veins, partially or completely occluding their lumens (Fig. 388). When localized to one sector of the lumen, organized thrombi resemble the eccentric, intimal, fibrous plaques described in hepatoportal sclerosis. Occasionally, the intima is thickened uniformly around the entire circumference of the portal vein lumen (Fig. 389). It is unclear whether this is indicative of phlebosclerosis of either the primary type, or the secondary type attributable to portal hypertension, or represents thrombotic material that has been incorporated into the intima.

As a consequence of thrombotic occlusion of large septal portal veins, their smaller more distal branches are obliterated and replaced by multiple, fine, venous collaterals. Often, there is accompanying portal fibrosis and an increase in the number and size of hepatic arterioles [(94); Fig. 390]. Changes of this type are demonstrable in most wedge biopsy sections, but only occasionally in needle biopsy specimens. Although such lesions are suggestive of "idiopathic" portal hypertension, they are not pathognomonic. Thus, as illustrated in Figure 391, similar portal fibrosis, replacement of portal veins by fine venous collaterals, and hypertrophy and reduplication of arterioles also occur in *extrahepatic portal obstruction.* Concentric, periportal fibrosis has been emphasized as a feature in the latter disorder (98). However, in our experience, concentric fibrosis is seen only occasionally, and, when present, tends to be periductal or periarterial rather than periportal (Fig. 391).

Granulomatous compression or occlusion of intrahepatic portal veins

In *sarcoidosis* the portal tracts often contain noncaseating, epithelioid and giant cell granulomas. Occasionally, they compress or invade branches of the portal vein, partially or completely occluding their lumens (Fig. 392). Such lesions, if widely disseminated, may account for the type of presinusoidal portal hypertension reported in cases of sarcoidosis unaccompanied by cirrhosis or significant portal fibrosis (99, 100). However, sarcoidal involvement of intrahepatic portal veins is not always associated with portal hypertension. In the eight patients with such lesions that we have investigated, only two exhibited splenomegaly, and none had evidence of esophageal varices.

Neoplastic invasion of intrahepatic portal veins

Hepatocellular carcinomas (101) show a remarkable propensity for invading the portal vein radicles at their periphery and metastatic tumors of the liver do so to a lesser degree (102). As a result, the blood supply of most intrahepatic tumors is largely or exclusively arterial (90). Such tumor thrombi are readily demonstrable in biopsy sections, and, occasionally, are found in the absence of tumor tissue elsewhere in the specimen. This is illustrated in Figure 393, which shows the islet cell tumor thrombus found unexpectedly in a portal vein radicle of a chronic alcoholic patient with prolonged, unexplained cholestasis.

Abnormalities of intrahepatic arteries

Arteriosclerotic and hypertensive arterial lesions

Considering their prevalence in other parts of the body, intrahepatic arterial lesions attributable to arteriosclerosis and hypertensive vascular disease are encountered relatively infrequently in biopsy sections. Arteriosclerotic arterioles are characterized by thickening and fibrosis of their intima and by replacement of medial muscle fibers by collagen (Fig. 394).

In hypertensive vascular disease, particularly when severe, occasional arterioles may appear hyalinized and intensely eosinophilic (Fig. 395), features characteristic of fibrinoid necrosis. The homogeneous, smudged appearance of the arteriolar walls resembles that of "primary" amyloidosis, so that special stains may be required for differentiation.

Amyloidosis of hepatic arteries

In the type of "primary" amyloidosis usually associated with multiple myeloma, some of the hepatic arteries and arterioles may contain amyloid in their walls. Characteristically, the walls of the affected vessels, which appear smudged, contain deposits of hyalinized, homogeneous material that stain deep blue in Masson sections (Fig. 396), and pale pink in H & E sections. Histochemical or electron microscopic confirmation is required for the identification of amyloid. For rapid screening, the most convenient method is the demonstrations of green birefringence in Congo red–stained sections examined in polarized light, as previously illustrated in the case of perisinusoidal amyloidosis (Fig. 227). However, false positive reactions are obtained occasionally (103), so additional histochemical confirmation is recommended. The demonstration of fluorescence in thioflavin-T-stained sections [(104); Fig. 397] or of brilliant red birefringence in toluidine blue–stained sections [(105); Fig. 398] are suitable for this purpose. Although the latter is more reliable and reproducible, it is less sensitive than the former.

Inflammatory lesions of intrahepatic arteries

Some of the intrahepatic arterioles and medium sized arteries are affected in more than half the cases of *periarteritis nodosa*

(106). The lesions, which are segmental, are characterized by fibrinoid necrosis initially (Fig. 399), and, later, by edema, acute inflammation, and destruction of the media and internal elastic lamina (Fig. 400). Usually, the inflammatory cells, chiefly neutrophils with a variable number of lymphocytes, plasma cells, and eosinophils, extend through the adventitia into the connective tissue of the portal tract. In addition, such cells may be found in portal tracts containing intact arteries. Some of the affected arteries may undergo aneurysmal dilatation, resulting in rupture occasionally. Others may be occluded by thrombi leading, in some instances, to foci of hepatic infarction. Healed arterial lesions, characterized by thickening and fibrosis of the intima and media, occasionally accompanied by organized and recanalized thrombi, may be seen during spontaneous or corticosteroid-induced remissions of periarteritis nodosa.

In some cases, infection with the hepatitis B virus has been implicated in the etiology of periarteritis nodosa and mixed cryoglobulinemia (107–109). Available evidence suggests that the deposition of immune complexes containing HBsAg, IgM, and complement is responsible for the development of the arterial lesions (107, 109). Although the arterial lesions have not been reported in liver biopsy sections in HBsAg-associated periarteritis nodosa, they have been demonstrated by arteriography (110). In most instances, the accompanying hepatitis is mild or anicteric. Occasionally, periarteritis nodosa occurs in HBsAg carriers with no evidence of hepatitis (111).

A form of *necrotizing angiitis* involving the small and medium sized arteries of the liver and many other tissues, and indistinguishable from periarteritis nodosa, has been reported in drug abusers (112). Such lesions have been attributed to the use of intravenously injected methamphetamine or other illicit drugs, but the possibility that the hepatitis B virus is implicated has not been adequately explored.

Hypersensitivity angiitis, a generalized vasculitis, usually attributable to drug sensitization, and particularly to sulfonamides, often affects the hepatic vasculature (113). The lesions resemble those of periarteritis nodosa, but affect both portal venous radicles and arterioles, and never become fibrotic.

Giant cell or granulomatous arteritis is a disease of unknown etiology that, in some cases, is associated with syndrome of *polymyalgia rheumatica* (114–116). Although involvement of the temporal arteries is an important feature in many cases, the disease is almost always generalized, involving both large and small arteries in many parts of the body. Characteristically, the walls of the affected vessels are infiltrated with numerous giant cells and other inflammatory cells. Rarely, such arterial lesions are demonstrable in the liver. In the only such case we have seen, in an elderly woman with prolonged fever, weight loss, and hepatomegaly, needle biopsy of the liver revealed a medium sized artery infiltrated with giant cells, neutrophils, and lymphocytes (Fig. 401), a lesion that first suggested the diagnosis of giant cell arteritis. Subsequently, a biopsy of a thickened, tender, temporal artery that had been previously overlooked revealed a similar lesion.

Muscular hyperplasia of intrahepatic arteries and veins

In most cases of *focal nodular hyperplasia,* some of the medium sized vessels in the tumor exhibit striking medial and intimal hyperplasia of smooth muscle and fine elastic fibers, often occluding their lumens [(101, 117); Fig. 402]. Although the affected vessels resemble arteries, it has been suggested that some (101), if not all (117), are veins. Since the vascular lesions resemble those seen in arteriovenous malformations, the possibility has been considered that they represent congenital anomalies, or develop as a result of increased pressure secondary to arterial shunting (117). What role, if any, such vascular lesions play in the pathogenesis of focal nodular hyperplasia is still uncertain.

Although there are no reports of similar vascular lesions in other disorders, we have encountered striking muscular hyperplasia of hepatic arteries in two patients with no evidence of focal nodular hyperplasia. The first, a 69-year-old man with mild, intermittent, systemic hypertension, had had recurrent attacks of cholangitis for 10 years. He was found on biopsy to have secondary biliary cirrhosis and numerous medium sized and large arteries that showed marked hyperplasia of smooth muscle in both the media and intima, often occluding their lumens (Fig. 403). Cholangiography revealed narrowed and bowed intrahepatic bile ducts, but no evidence of stones, strictures, or abnormality of the extrahepatic bile ducts, so that the etiology of the recurrent cholangitis was not established. However, on arteriography, many of the medium sized arteries in the liver, spleen, pancreas, and small intestine were attenuated or occluded, indicating the presence of an unusual type of generalized, occlusive, arterial disease presumably characterized by the same type of muscular hyperplasia found in the hepatic arteries.

The second patient, a 52-year-old man with long-standing acromegaly and systemic hypertension, presented with the typical features of idiopathic portal hypertension. Wedge biopsy of the liver revealed moderate, patchy, portal fibrosis and a number of medium-sized arteries that showed marked muscular hyperplasia in their intima and media. Of particular interest, some of the affected arteries showed extension of smooth muscle fibers into the fibrous tissue of the expanded portal tracts (Fig. 404).

It is highly probable, although not certain, that the arterial lesions in both these cases were coincidental and unrelated to the underlying hepatic lesions.

Abnormalities of the connective tissue in the portal tracts and Glisson's capsule

Portal fibrosis

Under a wide variety of conditions, the amount of collagen deposited in the portal tracts is increased. Usually, the fibrosis is accompanied by an inflammatory reaction and, often, by ductular proliferation. As the fibrosis progresses, the affected portal tracts expand at the expense of periportal hepatocytes that are replaced as a result of either atrophy or necrosis, depending on the nature of the underlying etiology. Neither the cell types nor the stimuli responsible for fibrogenesis have been clearly defined, and may differ under various conditions. Although fibroblasts undoubtedly play an important role in many cases, indirect evidence suggests that other cell types, including lipocytes (Ito cells), myofibroblasts, macrophages, and even hepatocytes, may be involved in some forms of hepatic fibrogenesis (118). Because of their close association with collagen deposition, hepatocellular necrosis, inflammation, and ductular proliferation have been invoked as possible stimuli for the induction of fibrogenesis (119). In addition, the possibility has been considered that certain exogenous factors, such as alcohol, may provoke fibroplasia directly. Thus, it has been reported, on the basis of *in vitro* experiments, that alcohol stimulates collagen production in the liver (120, 121). However, this has not been confirmed in all studies (122, 123). Indeed, it has been shown that in rats maintained on a choline-deficient diet to induce hepatic fibroplasia, the administration of alcohol inhibits collagen synthesis, even though it enhances fibrosis, a paradoxical effect attributed to inhibition of collagen degradation (123). The reversibility of hepatic fibrosis following removal of the etiologic factor responsible for its development, or the administration of certain fibrolytic agents, lends further support to the concept that collagen degradation may play an important role in modulating fibrogenesis (118). Although regulation of collagen degradation often is attributed to variations in collagenase activity, the possibility that other factors are involved has not been excluded.

Portal fibrosis is seen most frequently in various forms of *chronic hepatitis* (Figs. 104, 293), *biliary tract inflammation and obstruction* (Fig. 405), the precirrhotic phase of *primary biliary cirrhosis* (Figs. 295, 296, 378) and hemochromatosis (Figs. 161, 406), *schistosomiasis* (Fig. 407), *"idiopathic" portal hypertension* (Fig. 390), and *extrahepatic portal vein occlusion* (Fig. 405).

As a rule, the fibrosis in *alcoholic hepatitis* is predominantly centrilobular, but, occasionally, it involves the portal tracts as well. In some cases, such portal fibrosis appears to be related to extension of hepatocellular degeneration, necrosis, and fibrosis from the centrilobular to the periportal parenchyma (Figs. 49, 408). However, in others, the fibrotic portal tracts are separated from the affected centrilobular zones by intact parenchyma (Fig. 409). When accompanied by portal neutrophilia, ductular proliferation, and cholestasis, such portal lesions may be attributable to complicating pancreatitis. However, they are often encountered in the absence of pancreatitis, suggesting that they may represent a reaction to the centrilobular lesions, or to the parenchymal fatty infiltration that usually accompanies them.

Some degree of portal fibrosis is relatively common in cases of marked *fatty infiltration*. This association is seen not only in chronic alcoholism (Fig. 410) but also in diabetes mellitus and obesity [(124–126); Fig. 411]. Under such conditions, the fibrosis may involve both the centrilobular and portal zones, or either alone. As in the case of chronic alcoholism, the fatty infiltration and fibrosis attributable to diabetes mellitus or obesity may or may not be associated with centrilobular degeneration, necrosis, inflammation, and Mallory body formation, features indistinguishable from those of alcoholic hepatitis. Moreover, such lesions occasionally lead to the development of cirrhosis.

Prolonged administration of alcohol to baboons leads to progressive centrilobular and portal fibrosis in the absence of any histologic features of alcoholic hepatitis (127). It is still not clear whether the fibrogenesis in this experimental model is attributable to a direct effect of alcohol or its metabolites, or is indicative of a secondary response to alcohol-induced fatty infiltration, ultrastructural alterations in hepatocellular cytoplasm, activation of lipocytes, or accumulation of macrophages. Also uncertain is whether the development of fibrosis is related to or dependent on loss of hepatocytes. Considering the remarkable similarities between the hepatic lesions of diabetes mellitus and obesity and those of chronic alcoholism, direct stimulation of fibrogenesis by alcohol or its metabolites appears unlikely.

As portal fibrosis progresses, it may extend into the lobules and bridge adjacent portal tracts and/or central veins (Fig. 49). Ultimately, if sufficiently widespread, such fibrosis may lead to the development of cirrhosis.

The role of piecemeal acute periportal and bridging necrosis in the pathogenesis of fibrosis and cirrhosis is discussed in Chapters 3, 4, and 9.

Von Meyenburg complexes (Fig. 382) *and congenital hepatic fibrosis* (Fig. 64) are congenital anomalies of the biliary tract that mimic portal fibrosis and cirrhosis, respectively.

Capsular and subcapsular fibrosis

As previously indicated in Chapter 3, focal thickening and fibrosis of Glisson's capsule and subcapsular fibrosis may be seen in otherwise normal livers [(128); Figs. 40, 41]. Characteristically, subcapsular fibrosis is limited to a depth of 1 or 2 mm, so it is readily identified as a normal variant in surgical wedge or postmortem specimens. However, it may be difficult to differentiate from cirrhosis in small, tangential needle biopsy sections.

Degeneration of hepatic collagen

Occasionally, areas of fibrosis in the liver show degenerative changes of an unusual type. These are characterized by disruption and replacement of collagen bundles by deposits of pale-staining, finely fibrillar or granular material, and may be found in zones of fibrosis involving Glisson's capsule and the subcapsular parenchyma (Fig. 412), portal tracts and septa, especially around portal veins (Figs. 413, 414), and the centrilobular parenchyma (Fig. 415). Such changes are best visualized in Masson-stained sections, but can also be identified in H & E sections.

Based on their electron microscopic appearance and their reactions with the Verhoeff-van Gieson, orcein, and reticulin stains, the deposits appear to be made of closely packed, tangled collections of elastic fibers interspersed with reticulin fibers. They stain weakly with D-PAS, and show none of the histochemical reactions of amyloid.

Of the 21 cases of collagen degeneration in our biopsy series, all but 4 were found in surgical wedge biopsy sections. The lesions were located in Glisson's capsule or areas of subcapsular fibrosis in 12, portal tracts or septa in 7, and in zones of centrilobular fibrosis in 2. The underlying fibrosis was attributable to extrahepatic biliary obstruction in 7, various forms of cirrhosis in 4, severe, prolonged drug-induced hepatitis in 2, and miscellaneous hepatic lesions in 8.

Serial biopsy observations over a one-year period in a patient with phenelzine-induced hepatitis with extensive bridging necrosis and fibrosis and collagen degeneration (Figs. 413, 414) suggested that the collagen degeneration was at least partially reversible despite persistence of diffuse fibrosis and nodule formation.

Intrahepatic heterotopic pancreatic tissue

Intrahepatic pancreatic tissue

Intrahepatic, heterotopic pancreatic tissue may be found in large or medium sized portal tracts of patients with normal livers or with a variety of hepatic disorders (129). Such pancreatic tissue, which ranges from 50 to 900 μm in diameter, has been reported in about 4% of autopsies, occurring with equal frequency in subjects with or without hepatic disease [(130); Fig. 416]. The pancreatic cells include acinar cells with eosinophilic, zymogen-like granules, clear cells that resemble centriacinar cells, and ductular structures (Fig. 417). These cells may contain alpha-amylase (Fig. 418) and trypsin. Langerhans islets have not been observed.

The pancreatic tissue appears to communicate with the lumina of bile ducts. It has been suggested that these inclusions arise from the ventral pancreatic bud, are incorporated into anlagen of the hepatobiliary tree, and migrate into large portal tracts during their formation. The secretion of large amounts of pancreatic juice into the bile ducts may induce biliary dilatation of the bile ductules and, perhaps, carcinogenesis (131).

References

1. Bianchi L, De Groote J, Desmet VJ, Gedik P, Korb G, Popper H, Poulsen H, Scheuer PJ, Schmid M, Thaler H, Wepler W: Acute and chronic hepatitis revisited. Review by an international group. Lancet 2:914–919, 1977.
2. Popper H, Paronetto F, Schaffner F: Immune processes in the pathogenesis of liver disease. Ann NY Acad Sci 124:781–799, 1965.
3. Kerr JFR, Cooksley WGE, Searle J, Halliday JW, Halliday WJ, Holder L, Roberts I, Burnett W, Powell LW: The nature of piecemeal necrosis in chronic active hepatitis. Lancet 2:827–828, 1979.
4. Kawanishi H: Morphologic association of lymphocytes with hepatocytes in chronic liver disease. Lab Med 101:286–290, 1977.
5. Baptista A, Bianchi L, DeGroote J, Desmet VJ, Ishak KG, Korb G, Macsween RNM, Popper H, Poulsen H, Scheuer PJ, Schmid M, Thaler H: The diagnostic significance of periportal hepatic necrosis and inflammation. Histopathology 12:569–579, 1988.
6. Boyer JL, Klatskin G: Pattern of necrosis in acute viral hepatitis. Prognostic value of bridging (subacute hepatic necrosis). N Engl J Med 283:1063–1071, 1970.
7. Fauerholdt L, Asnaes S, Ranek L, Schidt T, Tygstrup N: Significance of suspected ''chronic aggressive hepatitis'' in acute hepatitis. Gastroenterology 73:543–548, 1977.
8. Mistilis SP, Blackburn CRB: Active chronic hepatitis. Am J Med 48:484–495, 1970.
9. Alexander GJM, Williams R: Characterization of the mononuclear cell infiltrate in piecemeal necrosis. Lab Invest 50:247–249, 1984.
10. Schmid M, Pirovino M, Altorfer J, Gudat F, Bianchi L: Acute hepatitis non-A, non-B; are there any specific light microscopic features? Liver 2:61–67, 1982.
11. Mietkiewski JM, Scheuer PJ: Immunoglobulin-containing plasma cells in acute hepatitis. Liver 5:84–88, 1985.
12. Page AR, Good RA: Plasma cell hepatitis. Lab Invest 11:351–359, 1962.
13. Thomas FB, Clausen KP, Greenberger NJ: Liver disease in multiple myeloma. Arch Intern Med 132:195–202, 1973.
14. Petersen P, Christoffersen P, Elling P, Juhl E, Dietrichson O, Faber V, Iversen K, Nielsen JO, Poulsen H: Acute viral hepatitis: a survey of 500 patients. Clinical, biochemical, immunological, and morphological features at time of diagnosis. Scand J Gastroenterol 9:607–613, 1974.
15. Christoffersen P, Dietrichson O: Histologic changes in liver biopsies from patients with chronic hepatitis. Acta Pathol Microbiol Scand, Sect A 82:539–546, 1974.
16. Beaver PC, Snyder CH, Carrera GM, Dent JH, Lafferty JW: Chronic eosinophilia due to visceral larva migrans. Report of three cases. Pediatrics 9:7–19, 1952.
17. Huntley CC, Costas MC, Lyerly A: Visceral larva migrans: clinical characteristics and immunologic studies in 51 patients. Pediatrics 36:523–536, 1965.
18. Zuelzer WW, Apt L: Disseminated visceral lesions associated with extreme eosinophilia. Pathologic and clinical observations on a syndrome of young children. Am J Dis Child 78:153–181, 1949.
19. Cypress RH: Visceral larva migrans. Cornell Veterinarian 68:283–296, 1978.
20. Diaz-Rivera RS, Ramos-Morales F, Koppisch E, Garcia-Palmieri MR, Cintron Rivera AA, Marchand EJ, Gonzalez O, Torregrosa MV: Acute Manson's schistosomiasis. Am J Med 21:918–943, 1956.
21. Dimmette RM: Liver biopsy in clinical schistosomiasis. Comparison of wedge and needle types. Gastroenterology 29:219–234, 1955.
22. Chusid MJ, Dale DC, West BC, Wolff SM: The hypereosinophilic syndrome: analysis of fourteen cases with review of the literature. Medicine 54:1–27,1975.
23. Croffy B, Kopelman R, Kaplan M: Hypereosinophilic syndrome. Association with chronic active hepatitis. Dig Dis Sci 33:233–238, 1988.
24. Klein NC, Hargrove RL, Sleisenger MH, Jeffries GH: Eosinophilic gastroenteritis. Medicine 49:299–319, 1970.
25. Robert F, Omura E, Durant JR: Mucosal eosinophilic gastroenteritis with systemic involvement. Am J Med 62:139–143, 1977.
26. Adams DO: The granulomatous inflammatory response. A review. Am J Pathol 84:164–191, 1976.
27. Wilhelm DL: Inflammation and healing. In Pathology, edited by W.A.D. Anderson, J.M. Kissane. 7th Edition. St. Louis, C.V. Mosby Co., 1977, pp. 25–89.
28. Popper H, Schaffner F: Liver: Structure and Function. New York, Blakiston Division, McGraw-Hill Book Co., 1957, p. 241.
29. Bloomer JR, Phillips MJ, Davidson DL, Klatskin G: Hepatic disease in erythropoietic protoporphyria. Am J Med 58:869–882, 1975.
30. Klatskin G, Bloomer JR: Birefringence of hepatic pigment deposits in erythropoietic protoporphyria. Specificity and sensitivity of polarization microscopy in the identification of hepatic protoporphyrin deposits. Gastroenterology 67:294–302, 1974.
31. Pounder DJ: Malarial pigment and hepatic anthracosis. Am J Surg Pathol 7:501–502, 1983.
32. Klatskin G: Hepatic granulomata: problems in interpretation. Mt Sinai J Med 44:798–812, 1979.
33. Hercules HdeC, Bethlem NM: Value of liver biopsy in sarcoidosis. Arch Pathol Lab Med 108:831–834, 1984.
34. Greene JB, Sidhu GS, Lewin S, Levine JF, Masur H, Simberkoff MS, Nicholas P, Good RC, Zolla-Pazner SB, Pollock AA, Tapper ML, Holzman RS: Mycobacterium avium-intracellulare: a cause of disseminated life-threatening infection in homosexuals and drug abusers. Ann Intern Med 97:539–546, 1982.
35. Wanless IR, Geddie WR: Mineral oil lipogranulomata in liver and spleen. Arch Pathol Lab Med 109:283–286, 1985.
36. Verdi CJ, Grogan TM, Protell R, Richter L, Range C: Liver biopsy immunotyping to characterize lymphoid malignancies. Hepatology 6:6–13, 1986.
37. Lahiri K, Dole M, Kamat J, Sane SY, Kandoth P: Letterer-Siwe disease (histiocytosis-X). J Postgrad Med 34:111–113, 1988.
38. Lichtenstein L: Histiocytosis X: integration of eosinophilic granuloma of bone, Letterer-Siwe disease and ''Hand-Schuller-Christian disease'' as related manifestations of a single nosologic entity. Arch Pathol 56:94–102, 1953.
39. Lieberman PH, Jones CR, Dargeon HWK, Begg CF: A reappraisal of eosinophilic granuloma of bone, Hand-Schuller-Christian disease and Letterer-Siwe syndrome. Medicine 48:375–400, 1969.
40. Risdall RJ, McKenna RW, Nesbit ME, Krivit W, Balfour HH Jr, Simmons RL, Brunning RD: Virus-associated hemophagocytic syndrome. A benign histiocytic proliferation distinct from malignant histiocytosis. Cancer 44:993–1002, 1979.
41. Masuko K, Rubin E, Popper H: Proliferation of bile ducts in cirrhosis. Arch Pathol 78:421–431, 1964.
42. Popper H, Schaffner F, Barka T: Has proliferation of bile ductules clinical significance? Acta Hepato-splenologia 9:129–139, 1962.
43. Buyssens N: Ductular proliferation. Gastroenterology 49:702–705, 1965.
44. Jorgensen M: A stereological study of intrahepatic bile ducts. 2. Bile duct proliferation in some pathological conditions. Acta Pathol Microbiol Scand, Sect A 81:663–669, 1973.
45. Desmet VJ: Morphologic and histochemical aspects of cholestasis. In Progress in Liver Diseases, Vol. IV, edited by H. Popper, F. Schaffner. New York, Grune & Stratton, 1972, pp. 97–132.
46. Poulsen H, Christoffersen P: Histologic changes in liver biopsies from

patients with surgical bile duct disorders. Acta Pathol Microbiol, Sect A *78*:571–579, 1970.

47. Christoffersen P, Poulsen H: Histologic changes in human liver biopsies following extrahepatic biliary obstruction. Acta Pathol Microbiol, Suppl *212*:150–157, 1970.

48. di Sant'Agnese PA, Blanc WA: A distinctive type of biliary cirrhosis of the liver associated with cystic fibrosis of the pancreas. Recognition through signs of portal hypertension. Pediatrics *18*:387–409, 1956.

49. Dominick HC: Cystic fibrosis. *In* Liver in Metabolic Diseases, edited by L. Bianchi, W. Gerok, L. Landmann, K. Sickinger, G.A. Stalder. Lancaster, MTP Press, 1983, pp. 283–290.

50. Popper H, Rubin E, Schaffner F: The problem of primary biliary cirrhosis. Am J Med *33*:807–810, 1962.

51. Lindgren S, Laurell A-B, Eriksson S: Complement components and activation in primary biliary cirrhosis. Hepatology *4*:9–14, 1984.

52. Bodenheimer HC, Charland C, Thayer WR, Schaffner F, Staples PJ: Effects of penicillamine in serum immunoglobulins and immune complex-reactive material in primary biliary cirrhosis. Gastroenterology *88*:412–417, 1985.

53. Macsween RNM, Burt AD: The cellular pathology of primary biliary cirrhosis. Mol Aspects Med *8*:269–292, 1985.

54. Williams GED: Pericholangiolithic biliary cirrhosis. J Pathol Bact *89*:23–34, 1965.

55. Portmann B, Macsween RNM: Diseases of the intrahepatic bile ducts. *In* Pathology of the Liver, edited by R.N.M. Macsween, P.P. Anthony, P.J. Scheuer. 2nd Edition. Edinburgh, Churchill Livingstone, 1987, pp. 424–453.

56. Christoffersen P, Dietrichson O, Faber V, Poulsen H: The occurrence and significance of abnormal bile duct epithelium in chronic aggressive hepatitis. A comparative morphological, biochemical, immunological, and prognostic study. Acta Pathol Microbiol Scand, Sect A *80*:294–302, 1972.

57. Scheuer PJ, Texeira MR, Weller IVD: Pathology of acute hepatitis A, B and non-A, non-B. J Pathol *134*:323–332, 1981.

58. Christoffersen P, Poulsen H, Scheuer PJ: Abnormal bile duct epithelium in chronic aggressive hepatitis and primary biliary cirrhosis. Hum Pathol *3*:227–235, 1972.

59. Poulsen H, Christoffersen P: Abnormal bile duct epithelium in liver biopsies with histological signs of viral hepatitis. Acta Pathol Microbiol Scand *76*:383–390, 1969.

60. Reynolds TB, Peters RL, Yamada S: Chronic active hepatitis caused by a laxative, oxyphenisatin, N Engl J Med *285*:813–820, 1971.

61. Zelman S: Liver cell necrosis in chlorpromazine jaundice (allergic cholangiolitis). A serial study of twenty-six needle biopsy specimens in nine patients. *Am J Med* 27:708–729, 1959.

62. Ishak, KG, Irey NS: Hepatic injury associated with the phenothiazines. Clinico-pathologic and follow-up study of 36 patients. Arch Pathol *93*:283–304, 1972.

63. Poulsen H, Christoffersen P, Dietrichson O, Faber V: The occurrence and significance of abnormal bile duct epithelium in cirrhosis. Acta Pathol Microbiol Scand, Sect A *80*:659–664, 1972.

64. Mistilis SP: Pericholangitis and ulcerative colitis. I. Pathology, etiology, and pathogenesis. Ann Intern Med *63*:1–16, 1965.

65. Thorpe MEC, Scheuer PJ, Sherlock S: Primary sclerosing cholangitis, the biliary tree and ulcerative colitis. Gut *8*:435–448, 1967.

66. Barbatis C, Grases P, Shepherd HA, Chapman RW, Trowell J, Jewell DPJ, McGee JO': Histological features of sclerosing cholangitis in patients with chronic ulcerative colitis. J Clin Pathol *38*:778–783, 1985.

67. Herrmann G, Lorenz M, Kirkowa-Reimann M, Hottenrott C, Hubner K: Morphological changes after intra-arterial chemotherapy of the liver. Hepatogastroenterology *34*:5–9, 1987.

68. Kemeny MM, Batifora, H, Blayney DW, Cecci G, Goldberg DA, Leong LA, Margolin KA, Terz JJ: Sclerosing cholangitis after continuous hepatic artery infusion of FUDR. Ann Surg *202*:176–181, 1985.

69. Klatskin G, Kantor FS: Mitochondrial antibody in primary biliary cirrhosis. Ann Intern Med *77*:533–541, 1972.

70. Rudzki C, Ishak KG, Zimmerman HJ: Chronic intrahepatic cholestasis of sarcoidosis. Am J Med *59*:373–387, 1975.

71. Thompson RPH, Williams R: Treatment of chronic intrahepatic cholestasis with phenobarbitone. Lancet *2*:646–648, 1967.

72. Stanley NN, Fox RA, Whimster WF, Sherlock S, James DG: Primary biliary cirrhosis or sarcoidosis—or both. N Engl J Med *287*:1282–1284, 1972.

73. Berman MD, Rabin L, O'Donnell J, Gratwohl AA, Graw RG Jr, Deisseroth AB, Jones EA: The liver in long-term survivors of marrow transplant—chronic graft-versus-host disease. J Clin Gastroenterol *2*:53–63, 1980.

74. Knapp AB, Crawford JM, Rappeport JM, Gollan JL: Cirrhosis as a consequence of graft-versus-host disease. Gastroenterology *92*:513–519, 1987.

75. Demetris AJ, Lasky S, Van Thiel DH, Starzl TE, Dekker A: Pathology of hepatic transplantation: a review of 62 adult allograft recipients immunosuppressed with a cyclosporine/steroid regimen. Am J Pathol *118*:151–161, 1985.

76. Klatskin G: Subacute necrosis and postnecrotic cirrhosis due to anicteric infections with the hepatitis virus. Am J Med *25*:333–358, 1958.

77. Baggenstoss AH, Foulk WT, Butt HR, Bahn RC: The pathology of primary biliary cirrhosis with emphasis on histogenesis. Am J Clin Pathol *42*:259–276, 1964.

78. Nakanuma Y, Ohta G: Histometric and serial section observations of the intrahepatic bile ducts in primary biliary cirrhosis. Gastroenterology *76*:1326–1332, 1979.

79. Ludwig J, Wiesner RH, Batts KP, Pekins JD, Krom RAF: The acute vanishing bile duct syndrome (acute irreversible rejection) after orthotopic liver transplantation. Hepatology *7*:746–783, 1987.

80. Bhatal PS, Powell LW: Primary intrahepatic obliterating cholangitis: a possible variant of 'sclerosing cholangitis.' Gut *10*:886–893, 1969.

81. Ludwig J, Wiesner RH, LaRusso NF: Idiopathic adulthood ductopenia. A cause of chronic cholestatic liver disease and biliary cirrhosis. J Hepatol *7*:193–199, 1988.

82. Alagille D, Odievre M: Liver and Biliary Tract Disease in Children, New York, Wiley-Flammarion, 1979.

83. Wee A, Ludwig J: Pericholangitis in chronic ulcerative colitis: primary sclerosing cholangitis of the small bile ducts? Ann Intern Med *102*:581–587, 1985.

84. Yokoo H, Minick OT, Batti F, Kent G: Morphologic variants of alcoholic hyalin. Am J Pathol *69*:25–40, 1972.

85. Margulis SJ, Honig CL, Soave R: Biliary tract obstruction in the acquired immunodeficiency syndrome. Ann Intern Med *105*:207–210, 1986.

86. Cockerill FR, Hurley DV, Malagelada J-R, LaRusso NF, Edson RS, Katzmann JA, Banks PM, Wiltsie JC, Davis JP, Lack EE, Ishak KG, Van Scoy RE: Polymicrobial cholangitis and Kaposi's sarcoma in blood product transfusion-related acquired immune deficiency syndrome. Am J Med *80*:1237–1241, 1986.

87. Sherlock S: Diseases of the Liver and Biliary System, 8th Edition. London, Blackwell Scientific Publications, 1989, p. 639.

88. Thommsen N: Biliary hamartomas (von Meyenburg complexes) in liver needle biopsies. Acta Pathol Microbiol Scand, Sect A *86*:93–99, 1978.

89. Pollice L, Pagliarulo G: Cholangiohamartomas. Med Chir Digest *5*:19–24, 1976.

90. Ishak KG, Rabin L: Benign tumors of the liver. Med Clin North Am *59*:995–1013, 1975.

91. Hunter FM, Akdamar K, Sparks RD, Reed RJ, Brown CL Jr: Congenital dilatation of the intrahepatic bile ducts. Am J Med *40*:188–194, 1966.

92. Caroli J: Diseases of intrahepatic bile ducts. Israel J Med Sci *4*:21–35, 1968.

93. Klinefelter HF Jr, Grose WE, Crawford HJ: Pyelophlebitis. Bull Johns Hopkins Hosp *106*:65–73, 1960.

94. Boyer JL, Hales MR, Klatskin G: "Idiopathic" portal hypertension due to occlusion of intrahepatic portal veins by organized thrombi. A study based on postmortem vinylite-injection corrosion and dissection of the intrahepatic vasculature. Medicine *53*:71–91, 1974.

95. Nayak NC, Ramalingaswami V: Obliterative portal venopathy of the liver associated with so-called idiopathic portal hypertension or tropical splenomegaly. Arch Pathol *87*:359–369, 1969.

96. Okuda K, Kono K, Ohnishi K, Kimura K, Omata M, Loen II: Clinical study of eight-six cases of idiopathic portal hypertension and comparison with cirrhosis with splenomegaly. Gastroenterology *86*:600–610, 1984.

97. Mikkelson WP, Edmondson HA, Peters RL, Redeker AG, Reynolds TB: Extra and intrahepatic portal hypertension without cirrhosis (hepatoportal sclerosis). Ann Surg *162*:602–618, 1965.

98. Maddrey WC, Sen Gupta KP, Basu Mallik KC, Iber FL, Basu AK: Extrahepatic obstruction of the portal venous system. Surg Gynecol Obstet *127*:989–998, 1968.

99. Kreel L, Williams R: Arteriovenography of the portal system. Br Med J *2*:1500–1503, 1964.

100. Berger I, Katz M: Portal hypertension due to hepatic sarcoidosis. Am J Gastroenterol *59*:147–151, 1973.

101. Edmondson HA: Tumors of the Liver and Intrahepatic Bile Ducts. *In* Atlas of Tumor Pathology, Section VII—Fascicle 25. Washington, Armed Forces Institute of Pathology, 1958.

102. Breedis C, Young G: The blood supply of neoplasms in the liver. Am J Pathol *30*:969–985, 1954.

103. Klatskin G: Nonspecific green birefringence in Congo red-stained tissues. Am J Pathol *56*:1–13, 1969.

104. Saeed SM, Fine, G: Thioflavin-T amyloid detection. Am J Clin Pathol *47*:588–593, 1967.

105. Wolman M: Amyloid, its nature and molecular structure. Comparison of a new toluidine blue polarized light method with traditional procedures. Lab Invest *25*:104–110, 1971.

106. Mowrey FH, Lundberg EA: The clinical manifestations of essential polyangiitis (periarteritis nodosa), with emphasis on the hepatic manifestations. Ann Intern Med *40*:1145–1164, 1954.

107. Gocke DJ, Hsu K, Morgan C, Bombardieri S, Lockshin M, Christian CL: Association between polyarteritis and Australia antigen. Lancet *2*:1149–1153, 1970.

108. Trepo CG, Thivolet J, Prince AM: Australia antigen and polyarteritis nodosa. Am J Dis Child *123*:390–392, 1972.

109. Levo Y, Gorevic PD, Kassab HJ, Tobias H, Franklin EC: Liver involvement in the syndrome of mixed cryoglobulinemia. Ann Intern Med *87*:287–292, 1977.

110. Baker AL, Kaplan MM, Benz WC, Sidel JS, Wolfe HJ: Polyarteritis associated with Australia-antigen hepatitis. Gastroenterology *62*:105–110, 1972.

111. Gerber MA, Brodin A, Steinberg D, Vernace S, Yang C-P, Paranetto F: Periarteritis nodosa, Australia antigen and lymphatic leukemia. N Engl J Med *286*:14–17, 1972.

112. Citron BP, Halpern M, McCarron M, Lundberg GD, McCormick R, Pincus IJ, Tatter D, Haverback BJ: Necrotizing angiitis associated with drug abuse. N Engl J Med *283*:1003–1011, 1970.

113. Zeek PM, Smith CC, Weeter JC: Studies on periarteritis nodosa. III. The differentiation between the vascular lesions of hypersensitivity. Am J Pathol *24*:889–917, 1948.

114. Hamilton CR, Shelley WM, Tumulty PA: Giant cell arteritis: including temporal arteritis and polymyalgia rheumatica. Medicine *50*:1–27, 1971.

115. Litwak KD, Bohan A, Silverman L: Granulomatous liver disease and giant cell arteritis. J Rheumatol *4*:307–312, 1977.

116. Leong AS-Y, Alp MH: Hepatocellular disease in the giant-cell arteritis/polymyalgia rheumatica syndrome. Ann Rheum Dis *40*:92–95, 1981.

117. Fechner RE, Roehm JO Jr: Angiographic and pathologic correlations of hepatic focal nodular hyperplasia. Am J Surg Pathol *1*:217–224, 1977.

118. Rojkind M, Dunn MA: Hepatic fibrosis. Gastroenterology *76*:849–863, 1979.

119. Popper H, Udenfriend S: Hepatic fibrosis. Am J Med *49*:707–721, 1970.

120. Feinman L, Lieber CS: Hepatic collagen metabolism: effect of alcohol consumption in rats and baboons. Science *176*:795, 1972.

121. Chen TSN, Leevy CM: Collagen biosynthesis in liver disease of the alcoholic. J Lab Clin Med *85*:103–112, 1975.

122. Galambos JT, Hollingsworth MA Jr, Falek A, Warren WD: The rate of synthesis of glycosaminoglycans and collagen by fibroblasts cultured from adult human liver biopsies. J Clin Invest *60*:107–114, 1977.

123. Henley KS, Laughrey EG, Appleman HD, Flecker K: Effect of ethanol on collagen formation in dietary cirrhosis in the rat. Gastroenterology *72*:502–506, 1977.

124. Falchuk KR, Fiske SC, Haggitt RC, Federman M, Trey C: Pericentral hepatic fibrosis and intracellular hyalin in diabetes mellitus. Gastroenterology *78*:535–541, 1980.

125. Adler M, Schaffner F: Fatty liver hepatitis and cirrhosis in obese patients. Am J Med *67*:811–816, 1979.

126. Ludwig J, Viggiano TR, McGill DB, Ott BJ: Nonalcoholic steatohepatitis. Mayo Clinic experience with a hitherto unnamed disease. Mayo Clin Proc *55*:434–438, 1980.

127. Popper H, Lieber CS: Histogenesis of alcoholic fibrosis and cirrhosis in the baboon. Am J Pathol *98*:695–716, 1980.

128. Petrelli M, Scheuer PJ: Variation in the subcapsular liver structure and its significance in the interpretation of wedge biopsies. J Clin Pathol *20*:743–748, 1967.

129. Mobini J, Krouse TB, Cooper DR: Intrahepatic pancreatic heteropia: review and report of a case presenting as an abdominal mass. Dig Dis *19*:64–70, 1974.

130. Terada T, Nakanuma Y, Kakita A: Pathologic observations of intrahepatic peribiliary glands in 1000 consecutive autopsy livers: heterotopic pancreas in the liver. Gastroenterology *98*:1333–1337, 1990.

131. Kimura K, Ohto M, Saisho H, Unozawa T, Tsuchiya Y, Morito M, Ebara M, Mafsutani S, Okuda K: Association of gallbladder carcinoma and anomalous pancreaticobiliary union. Gastroenterology *89*:1258–1265, 1985.

Chapter 6
Viral Hepatitis

Viral hepatitis is by far the most common inflammatory disorder that affects the liver. At least five viruses, designated hepatitis A (HAV), hepatitis B (HBV), hepatitis C (HCV), commonly known as non-A, non-B (NANB), delta hepatitis (HDV) and hepatitis E (HEV), an enterically transmitted virus, have been implicated in its etiology. These agents differ not only in their structural and antigenic features but also in their modes of transmission, incubation periods, and potential for producing various types of hepatic lesions. The structure of their genomes, their general properties, and their clinical manifestations have been described (1).

Most hepatitis virus infections that are recognized clinically present with jaundice. However, these are greatly outnumbered by anicteric and inapparent infections. These occult infections are identified either retrospectively by the detection of specific antibodies in the serum, or, during the course of infection, by the demonstration of the virus or its associated antigens in the blood, liver, or excreta, or the appearance of antibodies in the serum, or by the finding of hepatic functional or histologic abnormalities consistent with such infection.

As a rule, viral hepatitis is a self-limited infection, and, characteristically, the associated hepatic lesions heal without significant residuals within a few weeks or months. However, in a small number of HBV and HCV infections, the lesions remain active for months or years, resulting in chronic hepatitis that may progress to cirrhosis. Chronic hepatitis and cirrhosis are especially common consequences of HDV infection. Occasionally, similar chronic hepatitic lesions develop insidiously in healthy carriers who have harbored the HBV or HCV virus for long periods of time without exhibiting any clinical evidence of hepatic disease.

Rarely, viral hepatitis gives rise to massive or submassive hepatic necrosis that often proves fatal within a few days to weeks, but may resolve with or without significant residuals.

In addition to their etiologic roles in hepatitis and cirrhosis, HBV and HCV are important in the pathogenesis of hepatocellular carcinoma. Although such neoplasms may represent a complication of HBV-induced cirrhosis in some instances, there is accumulating evidence that the HB virus may be directly oncogenic.

The cytopathic effects of some viruses that involve the liver, as in the case of yellow fever and disseminated herpes simplex infections, are directly attributable to replication of the virus in hepatocytes. However, in HBV hepatitis, hepatic necrosis and inflammation appear to be the result of an immunologic reaction to the virus rather than to a direct cytopathic effect. Considering the similarity of the hepatic lesions in HAV and HCV infections to those in hepatitis B, it is probable that they too may be attributable to immunologic reactions, although this has not yet been established. On the basis of histologic features, HDV has been suspected of being a cytopathic virus, but since HDV infection requires coinfection with HBV, the mechanism of injury is not clear.

The immunologic reactions in HBV infections occasionally give rise to extrahepatic manifestations that may overshadow the underlying hepatitis.

Features of the hepatitis viruses

Hepatitis A virus

HAV is a 27 nm enterovirus of the family *Picornaviridae* that is transmitted by the fecal-oral route with an incubation period of two to six weeks (1). The genetic material of HAV is a single-stranded RNA that has been introduced into *E. coli* cells and the cloned genome sequenced (2). The infectivity of the virus is destroyed by heating to 100°C for more than one minute (3).

Since the virus is present in the blood only transiently and never gives rise to a chronic carrier state, parenteral transmission occurs only rarely (3). HAV infections involve children and young adults predominantly, but account for almost one-fourth of chronic hepatitis (4). Based on serum studies of anti-HA, it is apparent that a high proportion of such infections are not recognized clinically. Thus, almost half the population of the United States exhibit serologic evidence of antecedent HAV infection, although relatively few can recall an attack of hepatitis in the past (5). The incidence of anti-HA in the population varies geographically, increases with advancing age up to the age of 50, and is highest in low socioeconomic groups.

During the incubation period, the virus probably replicates in the gut. A few days before the onset of symptoms it appears in the blood and is excreted into the feces via the biliary tract for about 15 days after clinical infection appears. Within a week or two, anti-HA appears in the serum, leading to prompt elimination of the virus from the liver, blood, and feces.

The diagnosis of hepatitis A has been made easy by the development of specific antibodies to HAV (3). Anti-HA IgM is invariably elevated at the time clinical signs appear and after three weeks gradually declines (6,7). Anti-HA IgA is also present when symptoms appear, but its titer remains constant. Anti-HA IgG, does not appear until the second or third week of illness, and the titer remains high for months (3).

Using anti-HAV, HAV can be demonstrated in the blood, feces, bile, and sediments of disrupted hepatocytes by means of immune electron microscopy and, in sections of liver, by immunofluorescence (8). Several attenuated or inactivated vaccines are under development (9).

Hepatitis B virus

HBV, a 42 nm, double-shelled, DNA virus of the Hepadnavirus class that characteristically produces hepatitis after a relatively long incubation period of six weeks to six months, is usually transmitted by the parenteral route by transfusion of blood or blood products or the use of blood-contaminated needles by drug addicts and others (1). However, nonparenteral infections are relatively common, although the precise modes of transmission have not been identified. The transmission of HBV between homosexual men (10), the perinatal vertical transmission of HBV from HBV-carrier mothers to their newborn infants (11, 12), and cases of infection that follow close contact with individuals infected with HBV are common (13). There is some evidence that blood-sucking insects, such as mosquitos and bedbugs, may serve as vectors of infection (14), but this route is not an important one. The problem of identifying the precise mode of transmission in many cases is complicated by the fact that the HBV can be found not only in the blood, feces, bile, and liver but also in other body fluids, any of which can, at least theoretically, serve as a source of infection.

Apparently healthy carriers play an important role in transmitting HBV infections. The prevalence of such carriers varies geographically, ranging from approximately 0.1% of the general population in the United States (15) and northern Europe (16) to as high as 10% in other parts of the world (16, 17). Perinatal transmission of HBV from carrier mothers to their newborn infants accounts for many carriers, particularly in areas of high incidence (12). In some instances, the carrier state follows an attack of acute hepatitis, transfusions, or the use of blood-contaminated needles, but, often, neither the source of infection nor its mode of transmission can be identified.

The complete 42 nm hepatitis B virion, usually found in the serum and termed a Dane particle, consists of a 20–25 nm central core that contains a circular, double-stranded DNA and an outer, surrounding coat that differs from the core both biochemically and antigenically (18). These two types of antigen are termed HB core antigen (HBcAg) and HB surface antigen (HBsAg), respectively. In addition to HBcAg and DNA polymerase, the core also contains or is closely associated with a third component, HBe antigen (HBeAg), which may be a degradation product. The surface antigen also contains additional antigenic determinants, but these differ in various strains, so that HBsAg can be subtyped as *adw, adr, ayw,* or *ayr.* Although these subtypes exhibit no differences in behavior, and, hence, have no clinical significance, they provide useful markers for epidemiologic studies, since they retain their specificity when transmitted from one host to another.

The DNA of HBV has a long strand, which contains all of the genomic information (19), and a short strand, which has an incomplete region that is the site of action of the endogenous DNA polymerase. The DNA has been sequenced and found to have four reading frames, which code for surface antigen (S), core antigen (C), probably the polymerase (P), and an unknown (X) antigen (18–20).

Following infection, uncoated HBV cores (HBcAg) penetrate the nuclei of hepatocytes and rapidly replicate. These appear as intranuclear clusters of 20–25 nm spheres on electron microscopy (21), or as punctate nuclear deposits in routine sections by immunohistochemical techniques, using anti-HBc [(22); Fig. 419]. Rarely, numerous HBV cores may impart a sanded appearance to some of the hepatocellular nuclei seen in routinely stained sections [(23); Fig. 140]. Occasionally, a few HBV cores can be demonstrated in the cytoplasm by either electron microscopy or immunofluorescent (21) or immunochemical techniques (24).

Concomitant with the replication of core particles in the nuclei, HBsAg is produced in the cytoplasm of infected hepatocytes. On electron microscopy, HBsAg can be visualized as 20–22 nm rods or spheres within the cisternae of dilated, proliferating endoplasmic reticulum (21). In routine sections treated with labeled, high titer anti-HBs serum and examined by either the immunofluorescence or immunoperoxidase technique (22), cells containing HBsAg exhibit either diffuse cytoplasmic staining (Fig. 420) or a honeycomb pattern of plasma membrane staining. In chronic HBV infections, marked hyperplasia of the endoplasmic reticulum imparts a ground glass appearance to the cytoplasm of affected hepatocytes (Fig. 136) that stains with orcein and aldehyde fuchsin owing to its content of HBsAg [(25); Figs. 138, 139].

HBsAg, which is produced in great excess, appears in the serum during the first or second month of the incubation period, well in advance of the onset of clinically evident hepatitis. The antigen presents in the form of filaments or spheres, 20–22 nm in diameter, that can be identified by electron microscopy of spun serum sediments. During this period of active viral replication, HBsAg, HBeAg, DNA polymerase, and HBV DNA appear in the blood. As the disease becomes clinically evident, the HBV level is at or just past its peak and HBV DNA and DNA polymerase may no longer be found in the serum (26). HBsAg persists in the serum throughout the clinical illness. The significance of its persistence can be determined by the HBeAg level. If HBeAg is absent, viral replication has ceased and the process will subside; if present, HBsAg will persist and the HBV carrier state may ensue (18). HBV DNA is the most sensitive marker of HBV replication (26).

Anti-HBc, both IgM and IgG, are present at the onset of illness. The IgM anti-HBc peaks two to three months after onset and then falls; the IgG titers persist permanently. Anti-HBe develops as the hepatitis subsides. Anti-HBs appears late, after the clinical disorder has subsided, and often after HBsAg has disappeared. As a rule the development of anti-HBs confers immunity to reinfection with HBV, but there are exceptions. Sometimes anti-HBs is not seen at all. Almost all of the soldiers who had developed HBV hepatitis from yellow fever vaccine in 1942 were found to be anti-HBs-positive almost 45 years later (27). There are variations to these patterns, but the changes in titer of anti-HBc IgM provide the most reliable diagnostic information (28).

At about the time or shortly after HBsAg appears in the serum, HBV cores migrate from the nuclei to the cytoplasm where they are coated with HB surface antigen to form complete virions (29, 30). Subsequently, still before the onset of symptoms, these Dane particles are discharged into the serum. Within a week or two, antibody to core antigen (anti-HBc) appears in the serum, followed by a gradual rise in serum transaminase and the occurrence of a mild inflammatory reaction in the liver (31). However, clinically overt signs of hepatitis do not appear until a month or two later. In classic cases, these findings increase in severity over a period of a week or two, and then slowly subside, ultimately to clear completely in a few weeks to months.

In some cases of acute hepatitis B, HBs antigenemia persists. Usually, under such conditions, the hepatic lesions fail to heal. However, even in such cases, clearing of the antigen may ultimately ensue, and may be followed by complete, although delayed recovery. Moreover, the lesions may heal despite persistence of the antigenemia, resulting in an apparently healthy carrier state. Thus, failure to clear the serum of HBsAg is of uncertain prognostic significance. The problem of prognosis is further complicated by the fact that acute hepatitis B may give rise to chronic hepatitis despite rapid clearing of the antigen.

HBe antigenemia correlates with the presence of Dane particles in the blood and a high titer of HBsAg in the serum (32), and is an index of infectivity (33). As a rule, HBsAg-positive blood that contains anti-HBe is less infectious. HBV DNA, however, is the most reliable index of HBV replication and infectivity (34). Active HBV replication bears a close relationship to the development of hepatic lesions, which occurs as replication peaks (35). The presence of HBV in serum parallels active replication, and the detection of HBV DNA by molecular hybridization techniques is a specific, sensitive method to determine the level of HBV replication (36).

Hepatitis delta virus

The delta virus is a defective, hepatotropic RNA virus that is dependent on helper functions provided by HBV (1, 37). HBV surface antigen coats the delta ''core'' and converts it to the complete, spherical HVD, which has a diameter of 36 nm. This relationship is similar to that seen in satellite RNA plant viruses that require a helper virus to replicate (38). The small delta satellite contains a single strand of RNA that has no reverse transcriptase. There is no homology between the HBV DNA and the HDV RNA (39). Because HDV requires HBV for infection, immunity to HBV provides immunity to HDV.

Delta hepatitis, which was first described in 1977 (40), has the propensity to cause severe liver disease. It may occur by simultaneous infection with both viruses, or HDV can superinfect patients who are chronic carriers of HBV. Coinfection by both viruses causes hepatitis of the same severity of HBV infection alone because HDV replication inhibits HBV replication. Occasionally, however, fulminant hepatitis may occur, usually in drug addicts or hemophiliac patients. HDV superinfection of carriers of HBV tends to cause a dramatic acceleration in the course of the underlying hepatitis and often initiates a more aggressive, chronic or fulminant hepatitis. About 20% of HDV-infected carriers develop chronic hepatitis and the remainder run a relatively benign, self-limited course.

The serologic responses to HDV tend to be weak humorally: only two-thirds show any HDV markers (41). In the self-limited type, HD Ag is positive at the onset of illness and anti-HD-IgM appears 10 to 15 days later and anti-HD IgG several weeks thereafter. Antigenemia is short-lived or may not be seen at all. In the aggressive type of delta hepatitis, the antibody response, which is largely anti-HD IgM, is much brisker. It is sometimes found 1 to 2 days after onset, but is almost always present within 5 to 10 days and persists thereafter. Anti-HD IgG appears 6 to 12 weeks later and persists. HD Ag is uncommon in the chronic type.

Delta hepatitis is globally distributed, but tends to be seen in endemic areas. It is uncommon in developed countries, where it is seen almost exclusively in drug addicts or hemophiliacs (42). It can be endemic or epidemic in socially disadvantaged countries (43). Since vertical transmission is rare and infection usually occurs by intimate contact with body fluids, the infection rate is determined by the prevalence of HDV carriers and the degree of promiscuity.

Hepatitis C virus

Non-A, non-B (NANB) viral hepatitis is defined as hepatitis with clear clinical, laboratory, and epidemiologic features of viral hepatitis in the absence of serologic evidence of HAV and HBV infection. Over the past 15 years of working in the dark, i.e., without a serologic marker for HCV infection, epidemiologic studies described the disease as one seen primarily after transfusions and frequently in other high risk groups such as parenteral drug abusers and hemophiliac patients. It also occurs sporadically. It seemed clear that the disease is usually mild clinically or completely asymptomatic, but frequently progresses to cirrhosis, and is often associated with hepatocellular carcinoma. Furthermore, it appears that there are several different NANB viruses (44–46). The recent cloning of the HBC virus (47, 48) has confirmed these observations and permits definitive evaluation of many aspects of the disease.

HCV was cloned by extracting the nucleic acids of highly infective chimpanzee sera and by reverse transcription to complementary DNA. This material was then reacted with antibody presumed to be present in the serum of a patient with chronic NANB hepatitis. Eventually, a recombinant, virus-specific, 363 amino acid, nonstructural protein antigen was synthesized. This antigen is used to test for anti-HCV in serum by ELISA.

HCV is a single-stranded, lipid-coated, RNA virus, which is 50–60 mm in diameter, and contains 10,000 nucleotides (1). It is a flavivirus. Anti-HCV appears in the serum an average of about four months after the acute infection takes place (49). Because of this long latent period the anti-HCV assay is not useful in the diagnosis of acute HCV hepatitis. However, the antibody persists for years. The patients remain infectious during this window period. In the United States about 6% of transfusions are followed by viral hepatitis and in about three-fourths of them anti-HCV can be detected (50). It is also usually positive in intravenous drug abusers (75%) and in hemophiliacs (50–60%). It is present in about one-half of those with sporadic NANB hepatitis. Sexual transmission of HCV hepatitis is uncommon, as determined by the low prevalence of anti-HBC in the sex partners of drug abusers and gay men (51).

The incubation period of HCV hepatitis is 35 to 85 days. Patients are often asymptomatic, and only one-fourth become jaundiced. However, the hepatitis tends to progress rapidly even in the absence of symptoms. In patients who are HIV-positive the disease appears to be more severe and, often, is fulminant (52). Serum transaminases are less elevated than they are in other types of viral hepatitis, showing alanine aminotransferase levels in the hundreds of units rather than in the thousands. Half the patients with acute HCV hepatitis show biochemical evidence of persistence: one year after infection one-half have chronic hepatitis and one-fourth have cirrhosis. Typically, the transaminase values bounce irregularly for months after the acute infection.

The prevalence of anti-HCV is high in cryptogenic cirrhosis, but it varies in different areas (51, 53, 54). It seems to be increased frequently in chronic alcoholic liver disease (55, 56). The ELISA methodology may be overly sensitive, and the recombinant immunoblot assay (RIBA) indicates that false positive tests are frequent. False positives are especially common in autoimmune chronic liver disease (56), which does not appear to be pathogenetically associated with HCV (57). In hepatocellular carcinoma, however, almost two-thirds of patients exhibit HCV antibody (53, 58).

The agent responsible for enterically transmitted NANB hepatitis (NANB-ET) has been tentatively termed *hepatitis E virus* (HEV) (1, 56). This virus has been demonstrated in the stools of patients with focal epidemic hepatitis in Burma, Mexico, Uzbekistan, and elsewhere. The particles are 32–34 nm in diameter. They have spikes and indentations on their surfaces. It has been transmitted to chimpanzees, macaque monkeys, and other experimental animals, using stool suspensions. An immunofluorescent antibody assay for HEV has been developed and the antigen has been demonstrated in the livers of experimental animals. The virus has been cloned and almost completely sequenced. It has a single-stranded, polyadenylated RNA with 8.5 kilobases. It appears to be a calici virus. Increased aminotransferase activity develops 18 to 25 days after experimental inoculation.

The agent that causes parenterally transmitted NANB hepatitis (NANB-PT) has tentatively been termed *hepatitis C virus* (HCV). Although it has not yet been visualized by electron microscopy it has been characterized physiocochemically, and the antigen has been molecularly cloned in recombinant yeast from pooled plasma of chronically infected chimpanzees (57). It is a small (10 kilobase), enveloped RNA virus. It appears to be a flavivirus similar to plant RNA viruses. In experimental infection, elevated aminotransferase levels develop 25 to 35 days after inoculation and peak at 40 to 50 days. An assay for anti-HCV has been developed and is commercially available (58).

HCV is the predominant and, perhaps, the only agent of posttransfusion NANB hepatitis. In the only serologic test currently available (58), the presence of anti-HCV in serum indicates that the interval between infection and the appearance of antibody is often prolonged, sometimes as long as 9 to 12 months. The antibody persists in patients with chronic HCV hepatitis, but disappears with resolution of the infection.

Viral hepatitis variants

Classic acute viral hepatitis

Characteristically, the onset of acute viral hepatitis is abrupt, with anorexia, weakness, and fatigue, often accompanied by nausea, vomiting, abdominal discomfort, and low grade fever, and is followed within a few days to two weeks by overt jaundice. The jaundice tends to deepen rapidly, reaching its peak in a week or two, and then slowly abates over a period of a few weeks to several months, depending on the severity of the hepatic lesions. Usually, recovery is complete, and the lesions heal without significant sequelae. However, in a minority of cases, the hepatitis fails to resolve within six months from onset, and is characterized by lesions variously classified as unresolved or chronic hepatitis (59). Such lesions are encountered most frequently in delta superinfection hepatitis, a little less so in NANB, much less commonly in hepatitis B, and rarely, if ever in hepatitis A infections.

Anicteric acute viral hepatitis

Some acute infections with the hepatitis virus fail to produce jaundice. However, in all other respects, their clinical, biochemical, and histologic features are indistinguishable from those of classic icteric hepatitis. In general, anicteric infections tend to be mild. However, occasionally, even severe lesions accompanied by bridging hepatocellular necrosis may fail to produce jaundice, or do so only after a delay of several months (60, 61).

Anicteric acute viral hepatitis is recognized clinically in a significant number of patients with HBV and NANB infections, largely because such individuals often are screened prospectively following transfusions (59). Considering the frequency of anti-HAV in the general population, it is probable that HAV produces just as many anicteric infections. Since such infections affect children predominantly and tend to be mild, they are more readily overlooked or misinterpreted as other viral infections.

Inapparent viral hepatitis

As previously indicated, surveys in the United States have revealed serologic evidence of antecedent hepatitis A infection in almost half (5), and of antecedent hepatitis B infection in almost 10% of the general population (15). Since only a few of those bearing anti-HA or anti-HB can recall an antecedent attack of hepatitis, it is reasonable to assume that the infections, in most cases, were either asymptomatic or produced only mild symptoms not identified as those of hepatitis. Experience with individuals screened serially for evidence of infection following exposure to any of the hepatitis virus types has clearly demonstrated that many infections are asymptomatic, or produce mild, atypical symptoms that are not suggestive of hepatitis (59).

Cholestatic viral hepatitis

Cholestatic viral hepatitis is usually defined as a clinical variant of acute viral hepatitis, characterized by prolonged jaundice, pruritus, and other features that mimic those of extrahepatic biliary obstruction. In some reports, the syndrome has been ascribed to a specific lesion involving the cholangioles, and has been termed cholangiolitic viral hepatitis (62). However, this has not been confirmed in histologic studies of biopsy material, which usually show the typical lesions of classic viral hepatitis accompanied by cholestasis (63, 64). Rarely, particularly late in the course of the disease, cholestasis and portal inflammation may predominate, making differentiation of the lesions from those of extrahepatic biliary obstruction difficult. Serologic studies suggest that HAV is responsible for most cases of acute cholestatic hepatitis (59).

Both the clinical and morphologic features in cholestatic and classic acute viral hepatitis overlap to a considerable extent. Moreover, there is no evidence that these two variants differ in pathogenesis or prognosis. It is evident, therefore, that cholestatic viral hepatitis is not a well-defined, specific clinical or morphologic entity, but, rather, is a variant in the broad spectrum of manifestations that may be encountered in acute viral hepatitis.

Recrudescent and recurrent viral hepatitis

Occasionally during an apparently uneventful convalescence from acute viral hepatitis, there is an exacerbation of the symptoms and signs of the disease. In some instances, such *recrudesc-*

ences have been attributed to premature resumption of full activity or to excessive alcohol consumption, but, in most, they occur for reasons that cannot be identified.

Most recurrences seen following apparent full clinical recovery from acute viral hepatitis occur within a year of onset. Often, these represent recrudescences of incompletely healed lesions, especially in NANB hepatitis, as evidenced by the finding of persistent or intermittent transaminasemia or histologic evidence of activity during the symptom-free period between attacks. However, rarely, such recurrences, one or more in number, occur following biochemical and biopsy-documented full recovery. Lesions of this type, classified by some as *chronic lobular hepatitis* because of their resemblance to those in classic hepatitis, are said to be limited to NANB infections and to show no tendency to undergo progressive fibrosis. They have been attributed to reactivation of a persistent latent virus (65). However, not all cases of chronic lobular hepatitis are recurrent, and, when accompanied by bridging or panlobular necrosis, may give rise to chronic active hepatitis, progressive fibrosis, and cirrhosis.

Some recurrences of viral hepatitis are attributable to *reinfection*. As a rule, a different virus is responsible for each of the attacks (32). However, reinfection with the hepatitis B virus has been reported following massive transfusions, suggesting that a sufficiently large dose of the virus may overcome naturally acquired immunity to the infection (66). Reinfection with the NANB virus has also been observed (67). In such cases, different strains of the virus may be involved. However, the possibility that the recurrences are attributable to reactivation of the same virus from a state of latency cannot be excluded. Spontaneous recurrences of HBV infection after clinical and serologic resolution have been reported (68).

Unresolved and chronic viral hepatitis

Lesions of acute viral hepatitis that fail to heal within six months of onset may be appropriately termed *unresolved*. However, more commonly, such lesions are classified as *chronic persistent* or *chronic active hepatitis*, depending on whether the limiting plates are intact or eroded. In addition, the term *chronic lobular hepatitis* is applied by some to unhealed lesions that show significant intralobular inflammation and hepatocellular necrosis, resembling those in acute viral hepatitis (69). Allegedly, such lesions invariably heal without significant residuals, although they may relapse. However, in our experience, chronic lobular hepatitis when accompanied by bridging or multilobular hepatocellular necrosis tends to progress to cirrhosis or to fatal hepatic failure.

Since the lesions of unresolved viral hepatitis and chronic lobular hepatitis are indistinguishable, and since those of chronic persistent and chronic active hepatitis often show a variable degree of intralobular inflammation and hepatocellular necrosis, most pathologists limit their classification of such chronic lesions to chronic persistent and chronic active hepatitis, and do not use the terms unresolved hepatitis or chronic lobular hepatitis.

It should be noted that patients with chronic active hepatitis of insidious onset may present with clinical manifestations of short duration suggestive of acute hepatitis. In such cases, the chronicity of the lesions is inferred from the extent of the fibrosis found on biopsy.

The HBV, HCV, HDV, and HEV viruses are capable of producing chronic hepatitis. This occurs in 5 to 10% of HBV infections and in 20 to 40% of the HDV and non-A, non-B infections (37, 70).

Chronic hepatitis may follow an attack of acute hepatitis that fails to resolve. However, in many cases, it develops insidiously as a result of antecedent asymptomatic or unrecognized infection.

The development of chronic hepatitis following HBV infection may be associated with persistence of the virus. Usually, this is shown by the presence of HBsAg in the serum, but, in rare cases, HBsAg or HBcAg can be detected in the liver, but not in the serum (71). However, in such cases, the serum almost always contains anti-HBs, anti-HBc, or both. Persistence of viremia has also been demonstrated by means of chimpanzee transmission in some cases of non-A, non-B chronic hepatitis (50).

Occasionally, acute hepatitis B progresses to chronic active hepatitis despite apparent elimination of the virus (72). It has been suggested that the development of chronicity in such cases is attributable to an antibody-dependent, cell-mediated autoimmune reaction to a liver-specific host antigen in the surface membranes of the hepatocytes.

In addition to its role in the pathogenesis of chronic hepatitis, the HBV has been implicated as an etiologic factor in some cases of cryptogenic cirrhosis (71, 73). Considering the frequency of the NANB viruses in the blood of apparently healthy donors, and the propensity of this agent for producing chronic hepatitis, it is clear that some cases of cryptogenic cirrhosis will result from HEV infection.

Viral hepatitis with bridging necrosis

The clinical features of acute viral hepatitis with bridging necrosis resemble those of classic hepatitis, but, in our experience, differ in several important respects (61). Often, the preicteric phase of the disease is prolonged, the depth and duration of the jaundice tend to be greater, in 25% of the cases there is accompanying ascites, edema, or hepatic encephalopathy, and, in a significant number of cases, the infection gives rise to chronic hepatitis or cirrhosis, or results in fatal hepatic failure. Similar patterns have been reported by others (74). However, in a study of severe acute viral hepatitis in relatively young patients who averaged 27 years of age, were ill for less than a month, and exhibited no evidence of hepatic encephalopathy, ascites, or edema, the incidence of chronicity and the mortality rate were no higher in those with bridging necrosis than in those with classic lesions (75). The apparent discrepancy between these findings and those we reported indicating that bridging necrosis correlates with the development of chronicity, progression to cirrhosis, and death from hepatic failure is probably attributable to important differences between the two patient populations studied. Two-thirds of our bridging necrosis patients were over the age of 40, a significant number had unrelated complicating disease, over one-third had been ill for over a month, and approximately a quarter exhibited ascites, edema, or hepatic encephalopathy, the very clinical features that correlate most closely with severe hepatocellular necrosis. In the Dallas study (75), cases with hepatic encephalopathy were excluded on the assumption that they had massive hepatic necrosis rather than bridging necrosis, an assumption not warranted in the light of the biopsy findings reported in patients with fulminant hepatitis who ultimately recover (76). Thus, those with the most severe lesions were excluded in Ware's study. Taking into consideration the results of both studies, it is reasonable to conclude, at least tentatively, that bridging necrosis in young individuals who have been ill for less than one month may have no prognostic significance, but that when encountered after the fourth week of illness, particularly in older patients, it may be a forerunner of chronic hepatitis, cirrhosis, or fatal hepatic failure.

Although HBV and NANB virus infections account for most cases of acute hepatitis with bridging necrosis, the hepatitis A virus is implicated occasionally, although it rarely gives rise to cirrhosis.

Viral postnecrotic cirrhosis

Infections with either the B or non-A, non-B hepatitis virus may lead to the development of cirrhosis. Such lesions may evolve as the sequelae of antecedent attacks of acute hepatitis with bridging necrosis that fail to resolve, or, more insidiously, as the result of progressive chronic active hepatitis. In addition, chronic hepatitis B infections may give rise to cirrhosis without ever producing antecedent clinical manifestations of either acute or chronic hepatitis. It is highly probable that NANB hepatitis also produces cirrhosis of this type, although the evidence for this is largely indirect, since in only rare instances has the virus been identified serologically, or by chimpanzee transmission.

Viral fulminant hepatitis

Cases of acute viral hepatitis in which hepatic failure with encephalopathy appears early in the course of the disease are usually classified as fulminant. Death occurs in approximately 70% of such cases, the mortality rate increasing with advancing age and the extent of hepatocellular necrosis. Any of the hepatitis viruses may give rise to fulminant hepatitis, but HAV is implicated extremely rarely (77, 78, 78a).

It is uncommon in HCV, especially after transfusion (78a), but appears to occur commonly in intravenous drug abusers (78b). HBV is the most common cause of fulminant viral hepatitis and of fulminant hepatic failure worldwide (78c). HDV is also common, especially in patients with superinfection with HDV and in patients with chronic HBV hepatitis (78d), especially in drug abusers (78e). HEV fulminant hepatic failure is common in the Middle East and India, particularly in patients in the third trimester of pregnancy (78f).

Fulminant hepatic failure has been classified as *hyperacute*, in which the encephalopathy appears within the first week of the onset of hepatitis; *acute*, which appears between the seventh and thirtieth days; and *subacute* or *delayed onset*, which appears from one to six months after the hepatitis. Mortality is lowest in the hyperacute type, highest in the acute type, and intermediate in the subacute type (78g).

The hepatic lesions in fulminant hepatitis may be identical with those in classic viral hepatitis, but usually are more severe, and often are characterized by massive, submassive, or bridging necrosis. Available evidence suggests that survival correlates with the mass of hepatic parenchyma that escapes destruction. Thus, in a stereologic study of liver biopsy material obtained during hepatic coma, it was found that when more than two-thirds of the parenchyma was destroyed, death invariably ensued (79). Neither the depth nor the duration of the coma, nor the severity of any of the other clinical manifestations, correlated with the extent of hepatocellular necrosis. Based on these observations and others, it is evident that the prognosis of fulminant hepatitis is always unpredictable on clinical grounds.

In fatal cases of fulminant hepatitis, the lesions almost always are characterized by massive, submassive, or extensive bridging necrosis. However, in survivors, the lesions are more variable. Thus, in a study of 22 such survivors biopsied early in the course of fulminant hepatitis, the lesions were consistent with mild to moderate classic hepatitis in half the cases, and exhibited bridging necrosis in the remainder (78). All of these patients recovered uneventfully, and none had evidence of residual chronic liver disease, although follow-up biopsy in two cases revealed unresolved hepatitis. It is noteworthy that although almost half the patients in this group exhibited grade IV hepatic coma for 5 to 11 days, none had biopsy evidence of massive or submassive hepatic necrosis, and several had classic lesions. It is conceivable that the discrepancy between the severity of hepatic failure and the extent of hepatocellular necrosis in such cases is attributable to serious impairment of function in the remaining hepatocytes that appear to be intact histologically (80).

In some reports, it is assumed that the occurrence of hepatic encephalopathy during the course of acute viral hepatitis is indicative of underlying massive hepatic necrosis (75). However, it is evident from the data cited above that fulminant hepatitis, as usually defined, and massive hepatic necrosis are not synonymous.

The asymptomatic hepatitis virus carrier state

Apparently healthy individuals may harbor the HBV, HCV, HDV, and HEV viruses and serve as a source of infection to others for many years. The prevalence of HBV carriers in the general population varies geographically, ranging from a low of approximately 0.1% in the United States to rates 10 to 150 times as high elsewhere in the world (17), the highest rates being found in Asia, Africa, southeastern Europe, and South America.

The recent development of a reliable test for anti-HCV has suggested that a carrier rate of about 2% currently exists in the United States (81).

In a minority of cases, the HBV carrier state is the sequela of an antecedent attack of acute viral hepatitis that abates clinically, but is not followed by eradication of the virus. Chronic antigenemia may also result from an inapparent infection acquired during transfusion or the use of blood-contaminated needles. More important than either of these modes of infection in carriers, at least in parts of the world where the carrier rate is high, is neonatal transmission of the HBV virus from infected mothers to their newborn infants. However, in most carriers, no source of infection can be identified.

Although most HBV carriers appear to be healthy, and often show no hepatic functional or histologic abnormalities, except for the presence of orcein-positive ground glass cells, some are found on biopsy to exhibit chronic persistent or chronic active hepatitis, or, rarely, overt cirrhosis (82, 83). Moreover, HBV carriers are uniquely susceptible to the development of hepatocellular carcinoma, even in the absence of cirrhosis (84).

HBsAg-positive healthy carriers whose blood contains HBe antigen can transmit their infection to recipients when they serve as blood donors, whereas those whose blood contains antibody to HBeAg rarely do so (85, 86). Similarly, those with no biochemical or histologic evidence of hepatic disease usually are noninfectious (87).

Failure to eliminate the HBV following infection, and the absence of an appropriate inflammatory reaction and hepatocellular degeneration in most chronic carriers suggest a defect in their immunologic response to the infection. In some cases, this is attributable to underlying diseases often associated with immunoincompetence, such as leukemia, chronic renal failure requiring hemodialysis, Down's syndrome, and lepromatous leprosy, or to the use of immunosuppressive therapeutic agents. Similarly, in carriers whose infection is acquired at birth by perinatal transmission, tolerance to the virus and its persistence may be related to immaturity of the immune system at the onset of infection. However, most healthy carriers exhibit no evidence of impaired immunity, so that their failure to respond to the virus is unexplained.

It has been suggested that susceptibility to infection with the HBV and to the development of the carrier state may be under genetic control (88). Studies of HLA histocompatibility phenotypes lend some support to this hypothesis (89).

Vertically transmitted perinatal HBV infection

Pregnant women who are chronic carriers (90) or who acquire hepatitis B during the last trimester of pregnancy (11) may transmit the infection to their newborn infants. Such perinatal transmission is relatively common when the maternal serum contains HBe antigen (12, 90), but occurs only rarely when it contains antibody to HBeAg (anti-HBe) (91).

The precise mode of viral transmission is uncertain, and may not be the same in all cases. As a rule, neonatal HBs antigenemia does not appear until the second or third month of life, which, considering the usual incubation period of the HB virus, suggests that the infection is acquired at the time of birth. Transmission of the virus by either the oral or percutaneous route as the fetus passes through the birth canal containing maternal blood is a reasonable possibility, particularly since gastric aspirates in such newborns frequently contain HBsAg (92), and abrasions of the scalp, which may serve as a portal of entry, are relatively common.

Infants delivered by cesarean section may also acquire HBV infections (93). Since both HBsAg and Dane particles can be detected in cord blood in some cases (94), transplacental transmission of the virus is possible. This probably accounts for those rare instances in which persistent neonatal HBs antigenemia has its onset within a few days following birth (95). However, the usual delayed appearance of the antigen does not correlate with the cord blood findings. Thus, only a minority of infants who develop delayed antigenemia exhibit HBsAg in their cord blood at birth, whereas many with positive cord blood never become antigenemic (96). Since HBsAg has been detected in amniotic fluid (97), it is conceivable that its aspiration during vaginal delivery or cesarean section may account for the delayed development of neonatal antigenemia.

The breast milk of mothers with HBV infections often contains HBsAg (92), and it has been invoked as a possible source of infection in the newborn (98). However, the infectivity of breast milk has not been established, and there is no evidence that transmission of the virus occurs more frequently in breastfed infants than in those maintained on formula feedings (99).

Considering the relatively uniform incubation period of six weeks to six months, and the fact that infants separated from their mothers immediately following their delivery by cesarean section may also develop neonatal antigenemia (100), it is unlikely that any significant number of such infections are acquired postpartum.

Although neonatal transmission of the HBV has been reported from many parts of the world, it appears to be particularly common in Asia and Africa, where it probably accounts for their unusually high carrier rates. Available evidence suggests that vertical transmission also plays an important role in familial clustering of HBV infections. However, horizontal transmission under such conditions is also possible.

Vertically transmitted neonatal HBV infections usually lead to a chronic carrier state. The duration of such infections and their ultimate effects on the liver are still uncertain. In a few instances, the antigenemia has cleared within six months, and has been followed by the appearance of anti-HBs (100). However, in most cases studied to date, antigenemia has persisted for at least two or three years.

Most infants with vertically transmitted chronic HBV infections appear to remain in good health, although some exhibit hepatomegaly and mild elevations of serum transaminase. Liver biopsy studies in a few such cases have revealed minor changes interpreted as evidence of mild unresolved viral hepatitis (101).

In a minority of cases, vertically transmitted HBV infections result in overt hepatitis that usually appears coincident with the development of antigenemia. Although full recovery with clearing of the antigen and development of anti-HBs may occur (100), the hepatitis often is severe and may prove fatal (102). The lesions encountered in such cases include giant cell hepatitis, chronic active hepatitis, and cirrhosis.

Whether or not the non-A, non-B hepatitis virus can be transmitted vertically by women who are healthy carriers, or who acquire acute infections during pregnancy is unclear.

Childhood viral hepatitis

Hepatitis A is a relatively common infection in children, as evidenced by the fact that approximately 20% exhibit anti-HA in their serum, the incidence rising from approximately 10% in those under the age of five years to 30% in those over nine (103). Most such infections are relatively mild and of short duration, and often are asymptomatic.

Hepatitis B infections are far less common in children than hepatitis A. However, nonparenterally transmitted HBV infections are encountered relatively frequently in the children of low socioeconomic groups living in crowded urban areas (104), and in institutionalized children (105). Also, such infections occur in infants who have received blood transfusions (102).

Although HBV infections in children may present as classic acute hepatitis, more commonly they are associated with chronic hepatitis (106), cirrhosis, or the carrier state (107). Indeed, the incidence of carriers among institutionalized children and those from lower socioeconomic groups is even higher than in adults from the same areas (107).

HBsAg-associated hepatocellular carcinoma

The prevalence of hepatocellular carcinoma (HCC) closely correlates with the HBsAg carrier rate in various parts of the world. In tropical Africa and Asia, where 3 to 15% of the population are carriers, hepatocellular carcinoma is the leading form of cancer in males, and in 40 to 80% of such cases, HBsAg is demonstrable in the serum (108). Although the frequency of HBs antigenemia in patients with HCC is significantly lower in countries with low carrier rates, in at least one study reported from the United States, the incidence was approximately 40% (109). There is suggestive evidence that the risk of developing HCC is greater in carriers infected at birth by their carrier mothers than in those infected later in life (110). This may account, in part at least, for the greater frequency of HCC in the carriers of Africa and Asia than in those elsewhere in the world.

Aflatoxin is another factor that has been invoked in the pathogenesis of HCC, since the incidence of such tumors appears to correlate with the dietary consumption of aflatoxin, an agent known to be carcinogenic in animals (111). However, based on an epidemiologic analysis of the frequency of HCC in carriers of the HBs antigen, it has been estimated that the risk of developing the tumor in male carriers over the age of 50 is approximately 6% per year in New York City, where exposure to aflatoxin is rare, a risk almost identical with that in the carriers of Mozambique, a country where aflatoxin ingestion is common. This risk ratio, which is higher than has been postulated for any other suspected human carcinogen, strongly supports the view that the HBV is oncogenic.

Since HCC is a consequence of many other forms of cirrhosis, it is conceivable that in some cases at least, its occurrence in patients with chronic HBs antigenemia is similarly related to underlying cirrhosis. However, the HBV may be the more important factor in such cases, since in Senegal the incidence of HCC is the same in HBsAg carriers with and without cirrhosis (112). Perhaps the most impressive evidence that the HBV may be directly oncogenic is the demonstration, by means of a hybridization technique using cloned HBV DNA as a probe, that the viral DNA is integrated in the genome of the neoplastic cells in hepatocellular carcinoma (113).

Extrahepatic manifestations of hepatitis B infection

Occasionally, HBV infections give rise to extrahepatic manifestations that may precede, accompany, or overshadow the signs of hepatitis (114). Available evidence suggests that these are attributable to the formation and deposition of immune complexes, particularly in the blood vessels of the affected tissues.

Serum sickness-like syndrome

Skin eruptions, characterized by urticaria, maculopapular rash, or petechiae, and occasionally associated with angioneurotic edema, arthralgia, or arthritis, are seen occasionally early in the course of acute hepatitis B (115, 116).

As a rule, this serum sickness-like syndrome appears a week or two before the onset of jaundice, but jaundice may be delayed for two or three months, or the hepatitis may remain anicteric. Although full recovery usually ensues, the course of the disease is prolonged in some cases. The syndrome appears in about one-third of patients with acute viral hepatitis (117, 118), and HAV, HBV, and NANB virus seem to be involved (114, 119).

Often, circulating immune complexes (120) and low serum levels of complement (115) are demonstrable, features consistent with the widely accepted view that the rash and arthralgia are attributable to immune complex formation.

Glomerulonephritis

Membranous and other forms of glomerulonephritis, some of which present with the nephrotic syndrome, are seen occasionally in cases of HBV infection (121, 122). As a rule, such renal lesions occur in carriers or in patients with chronic active hepatitis or cirrhosis, but may be seen occasionally following acute hepatitis B. Both children and adults may be affected.

By immunofluorescence, deposits of IgG, C3, HBsAg, and HBeAg can be detected in the glomeruli (121, 122). The disease appears to be associated with the consumption of complement (123). Although these findings are consistent with immune complex–induced glomerulonephritis, the possibility cannot be excluded that, at least in some cases, the deposits are attributable to intercurrent infection with the hepatitis B virus in individuals with underlying renal lesions due to other causes.

Periarteritis nodosa

HBs antigenemia is demonstrable in a significant number of patients with periarteritis nodosa (124–126). Often, the manifestations of the vascular disease overshadow those of hepatitis, which usually is mild or anicteric. Occasionally, the periarteritis occurs in carriers who exhibit no histologic evidence of liver disease, or in individuals with chronic active hepatitis. Usually, immune complexes containing HBsAg, immune globulins, and complement can be demonstrated in the vascular lesions, and, less consistently, in the serum.

Infantile papular acrodermatitis (Gianotti's disease)

This disorder, which is characterized by a papular skin eruption, generalized lymphadenopathy, and hepatomegaly, is attributable to infection with the *ayw* subtype of the HB virus (127, 128). Usually, the disease affects children under the age of eight years, but overt hepatitis with jaundice has been encountered in a few adults exposed to their affected children (128). Although limited to Italy initially, the disease has now been reported from other Mediterranean countries and Japan.

The hepatitis associated with the skin lesions is usually mild and anicteric. In many cases, however, HBs antigenemia persists, and the lesions progress to chronic active hepatitis (127). The pathogenesis of this unusual syndrome is still unknown.

Essential mixed cryoglobulinemia

This disorder is characterized biochemically by the presence in the serum of cryoprecipitable, polyclonal IgG and monoclonal or polyclonal IgM with anti-gamma globulin activity, and, clinically, by the occurrence of arthritis, purpura, glomerulonephritis, and generalized vasculitis. The serum complement levels are depressed, and deposits of immunoglobulins and complement may be found in blood vessel walls and in the renal lesions, suggesting that cryoprecipitable immune complexes may play a role in the pathogenesis of the disease. The disorder under discussion must be differentiated from the type of mixed cryoglobulinemia that occurs secondarily in a variety of infectious, neoplastic, and connective tissue diseases.

Based on the observation that a significant number of patients with essential mixed cryoglobulinemia exhibit hepatosplenomegaly, hepatic dysfunction, and a variety of hepatic histologic abnormalities, ranging from nonspecific changes to chronic active hepatitis and postnecrotic cirrhosis, and that HBsAg and anti-HBs can often be detected in their sera and cryoprecipitates (129), it has been suggested that the disease is a manifestation of hepatitis B infection. However, in one study in which patients with essential and secondary mixed cryoglobulinemia were compared, the frequency of detectable HBsAg and anti-HBs in the two groups did not differ, and was low in both (130). Although the results of this study do not exclude the possibility that, rarely, the hepatitis B virus may be implicated in the etiology of essential mixed cryoglobulinemia, they suggest that it is not a major etiologic factor in most cases. Moreover, the possibility cannot be excluded that even when HBsAg is detectable, the occurrence of the hepatitis B virus may be attributable to intercurrent infection in patients who already are chronically ill with essential mixed cryoglobulinemia, and, hence, possibly more susceptible to such infections. Interpretation is complicated when this syndrome is associated with HAV infection (131).

Guillain-Barré syndrome and peripheral neuropathy

The Guillain-Barré syndrome has been reported as a complication of acute icteric HBsAg-positive hepatitis (132, 133). In most cases, the neurologic manifestations have appeared two or three weeks following the onset of jaundice, and, in some instances, coincident with the clearing of HBsAg from the serum. However, the antigen was still detectable in the cerebrospinal fluid at the onset of the syndrome (132). In another, a high titer of smooth muscle antibody appeared in the serum prior to the development of neurologic symptoms, a feature interpreted as possible evidence of an underlying autoimmune reaction (132). The apparent therapeutic effectiveness of ACTH in one reported case is consistent with an immunologic reaction, but its full spontaneous recovery from both the hepatic and neurologic abnormalities has been the rule thus far.

Severe peripheral neuropathy has been reported in patients with both HAV and HBV hepatitis (134). In one patient with mild, anicteric HBV hepatitis (135), the neuropathy improved slowly, but disabling muscular weakness was still present a year later. HBs antigenemia persisted for over a year during which there was progression from a mild lobular hepatitis to chronic active hepatitis and early postnecrotic cirrhosis. Since cryopre-

cipitable immune complexes containing IgM, IgG, and HBsAg were demonstrable in the serum and in the intima of small arteries and veins of skeletal muscle, it appeared likely that the neuropathy was attributable to an immune reaction involving the vasculature of the nerves.

Pathogenesis of the hepatic lesions in viral hepatitis

Most of what is known about the pathogenesis of the hepatic lesions in viral hepatitis is limited to type B infections. Although the mechanisms involved in the evolution of the lesions produced by the A and NANB viruses still remain to be elucidated, the fact that the lesions seen in all types of viral infection are similar suggests that their pathogenesis may be similar.

There is general agreement that the hepatic lesions in hepatitis B are attributable to the immune responses of the host rather than to the cytopathic effects of the virus. This conclusion is based on the failure of the virus to exhibit cytopathic effects in cultures of heptocytes (136) and the fact that healthy carriers, whose sera and hepatocytes usually contain high concentrations of HBsAg, often exhibit no evidence of significant hepatic injury (137), and that, in general, the severity of the hepatic lesions in HBV infections varies inversely with the concentration of viral antigen in the liver (138). Presumably, the A and NANB viruses are similarly noncytopathic, but the evidence for this is till only circumstantial. There is evidence that HDV may be cytopathic (139, 140).

It is widely thought that hepatocytic damage in HBV hepatitis is caused by cellular immune responses to altered hepatocyte membranes. It follows that when a large majority of the liver cells are infected, acute massive necrosis results (141). A recent report demonstrates acute massive necrosis in rats immediately after the intravenous injection of monoclonal antibody against liver cell membranes (142). This finding suggests that antibody-complement-mediated liver cell injury is another possible mechanism in fulminant hepatitis other than T cell–mediated injury (143).

Humoral immunity

As the HB virus emerges from the hepatocytes toward the end of the incubation period, some of its surface antigen is bound by or incorporated within the surface membranes of the hepatocytes. This is evidenced by the honeycomb pattern outlining the hepatocytes exhibited by HBsAg in immunofluorescence studies of the liver during the late incubation period and *early* in the course of acute hepatitis, both in humans (144, 145) and in experimentally infected chimpanzees (146). Later in the disease, when most studies are carried out, little or no antigen can be detected in the liver (147).

HBV on entering the circulation activates B lymphocytes to produce antibody to its surface antigen (anti-HBs). Although the results of conventional assays suggest that the appearance of the antibody in acute hepatitis is delayed at least until HBsAg is cleared from the serum (28), it can be detected early in the course of the disease while HBs antigenemia is still present. Indeed, concurrent HBsAg and anti-HBs is neither rare nor of clinical significance (148). As might be anticipated under such conditions, HBV immune complexes may be demonstrable in both the serum and liver (149).

Such observations are consistent with the view that hepatocytes bearing HBsAg in their surface membranes serve as targets for circulating anti-HBs, and are destroyed as a result of immune complex formation and activation of complement, leading, ultimately, to elimination of the virus and resolution of the lesions. In addition, the antibody may facilitate recovery by binding virus released from necrotic hepatocytes and preventing its reentry into uninfected cells (150) and, perhaps by modulating viral antigen synthesis and expression (151).

The hypothesis that the hepatocellular necrosis in hepatitis B is attributable to the interaction of anti-HBs and HBsAg at the surface of the hepatocytes is supported by a number of observations, including the low serum levels of complement found in some cases of early acute infection (152), the absence of hepatic injury in healthy carriers whose serum contains no immune complexes, the enhanced production of antibody, and the striking prominence of immune complexes in the serum of patients with massive hepatic necrosis (153).

However, a number of other observations are inconsistent with the humoral theory. These include the normal serum levels of complement found in most cases of acute hepatitis (154), the relatively mild character of the hepatic lesions in patients with HBsAg-induced periarteritis nodosa, whose serum and extrahepatic tissues usually contain abundant immune complexes (155), the failure of large infusions of anti-HBs to exacerbate the hepatic lesions in cases of HBsAg-positive chronic active hepatitis (156), and the occurrence of severe acute and chronic hepatitis B in patients with congenital or acquired agammaglobulinemia (157, 158).

From the foregoing, it is evident that the antibody response to HBs antigen alone cannot account for the hepatic lesions in HBV infections. However, there is suggestive evidence that surface antigen may participate in antibody-dependent, cell-mediated immune reactions that lead to hepatocellular necrosis.

Attention has been focused on the possibility that autoimmune humoral response to host antigens may be implicated in the pathogenesis of hepatic injury, particularly in the case of chronic hepatitis (159). Autoantibodies to a liver-specific membrane lipoprotein (anti-LSP) have been detected in the serum of most patients with HBsAg-positive acute hepatitis, HBsAg-positive chronic hepatitis, and HBsAg-negative chronic hepatitis (160). Since anti-LSP occurs only transiently, and since its titer does not correlate with the severity of the lesions in acute hepatitis, it is thought to play no role in their pathogenesis. However, in both HBsAg-positive and HBsAg-negative chronic hepatitis, the titer of anti-LSP closely correlates with the activity of the lesions, suggesting a possible pathogenetic relationship.

The question still to be resolved is: Do these autoimmune antibodies cause liver damage, or merely reflect an immunologic response to host antigens released from disrupted hepatocytes?

T cell immunity

There is convincing evidence that cell-mediated, immune responses are implicated in the pathogenesis of the hepatic lesions in HBV infections. However, still uncertain are the identity of the effector cells involved, how they interact with viral and host antigens and antibodies, and why they induce such a diversity of lesions.

According to one widely held view, circulating HBsAg sensitizes T lymphocytes and induces their proliferation. On reaching the liver, the sensitized lymphocytes interact with hepatocytes bearing HBsAg in their surface membranes, leading to their destruction (161). That the lymphocytes are sensitized has been confirmed in in vitro studies (162,163). Furthermore, T cells predominate over B cells in the hepatic lesions of HBsAg-positive acute and chronic hepatitis, but less in others (164), and that in the absence of surface localization of HBsAg, the hepatocytes of healthy carriers show no evidence of injury (165).

Failure to clear the HB virus in healthy carriers and in those with chronic hepatitis has been attributed to a defect in the T cell–mediated immune response (161). Consistent with this suggestion is the fact that the lymphocytes in such cases are not transformed (161) and macrophage migration is not inhibited when incubated with purified HBsAg in vitro (162). HBsAg does inhibit macrophage migration in HBsAg-positive chronic active hepatitis (163), a lesion allegedly attributable to impaired T cell function.

The susceptibility to chronic infection with the HB virus in individuals with diseases often associated with immunoincompetence, such as leukemia, lymphoma, severe chronic renal failure, Down's syndrome, and lepromatous leprosy, and in those under immunosuppressive therapy emphasizes the importance of the immunologic response in eliminating the virus.

In many cases, the development of chronic persistent or chronic active hepatitis following infection with HBV is associated with persistence of HBs antigenemia, a feature consistent with an underlying defect in humoral or cell-mediated immunity. However, such lesions are encountered occasionally in individuals who have cleared their serum of antigen normally. To account for the development of chronic hepatitis in the absence of replicating HBV, it has been proposed that continued destruction of hepatocytes is attributable to an autoimmune reaction involving antibody-dependent K cell–mediated cytotoxicity.

K cell–mediated antibody-dependent cellular cytotoxicity (ADCC)

Lymphocytes classified as K cells are characterized by surface receptors for the Fc fragment of IgG and by their cytotoxicity for cells coated with IgG antibodies. It has been suggested that if the immune response to hepatitis B fails to eradicate the virus, T cells, continuously activated by viral antigen, stimulate B cells to secrete antibody against the liver specific protein (LSP) normally present on the surface membranes of the hepatocytes, and that K cells then interact with anti-LSP-coated hepatocytes, leading to their destruction (150). In cases of chronic active hepatitis that remain active despite elimination of the virus, and, in those which are etiologically unrelated to HBV, this theory proposes that continued B cell production of anti-LSP is attributable to a defect in suppressor T cell function. Based on the observation that, on histocompatibility typing, a high proportion of individuals with HBsAg-negative chronic active hepatitis carry the HLA-B8 antigen (166,167), and that they exhibit enhanced antibody responses to a wide variety of antigens (166), it has been suggested that the defect in suppressor T cell function and resulting uninhibited antibody production against LSP may be genetically determined (150).

As previously indicated, anti-LSP can be detected in the serum of most patients with HBsAg-positive and HBsAg-negative chronic hepatitis, its titer correlating with the extent of piece-meal necrosis demonstrable histologically (160). Since normal lymphocytes are cytopathic for isolated rabbit hepatocytes pre-treated with the serum of such individuals, a reaction that can be blocked by adding LSP, and since the degree of cytotoxicity also correlates with the extent of hepatocellular necrosis, these observations have been interpreted as evidence of anti-LSP-dependent cell-mediated cytotoxicity (160).

The peripheral blood lymphocytes of patients with either HBsAg-positive or HBsAg-negative chronic active hepatitis are cytopathic for isolated rabbit hepatocytes (168). Since the cy-totoxicity is not shared by T cell fractions of these lympho-cytes, and can be blocked by aggregated IgG, these findings have been cited in support of the theory that a K cell–mediated anti-LSP-dependent autoimmune reaction is involved in the pathogenesis of chronic active hepatitis (168). However, in none of these studies has the presence of Fc receptors on the effector cells and of anti-LSP on the target cells been demonstrated.

Other objections to the interpretation and significance of these *in vitro* studies have been raised (169,170). However, despite its flaws, the theory that a K cell–mediated anti-LSP-dependent reaction is implicated in the pathogenesis of chronic active hep-atitis remains an attractive possibility.

Histopathology of classic acute viral hepatitis

The hepatic lesions of classic acute viral hepatitis are charac-terized by irregular foci of hepatocellular necrosis and degen-eration scattered randomly through all the lobules, a diffuse, predominantly mononuclear inflammatory reaction that in-volves both the parenchyma and the portal tracts, proliferation and swelling of the Kupffer cells, and hepatocellular regenera-tion. The extent of hepatocellular degeneration and necrosis and the intensity of the inflammatory reaction tend to be relatively uniform in the individual lobules in any given case, but vary greatly from case to case, depending not only on the severity of the lesions but also on their stage of development. Although the lesions in the early and late phases of the disease differ, they overlap to such an extent that it is seldom possible to iden-tify the age of the lesions on histologic grounds alone.

Lobular architecture

Irrespective of the extent of hepatocellular degeneration and ne-crosis, the portal tracts and central veins retain their normal anatomic relationships within the lobules. However, the portal tracts are almost always abnormally prominent owing to infil-trating inflammatory cells and, in some cases, their expansion as a result of periportal hepatocellular necrosis. In addition, the loss of hepatocytes, hepatocellular swelling, shrinkage, and re-generation, the infiltration of inflammatory cells, and the pro-liferation and swelling of Kupffer cells distort the normal he-patic plate pattern, a feature aptly termed ''lobular disarray'' (171). As illustrated in Figure 421, the disruption of the hepatic

plates and the diffuse character of the inflammatory reaction are readily apparent even at low magnification.

Hepatocellular necrosis

Most of the hepatocytes that are destroyed undergo rapid cyto-lysis, so relatively few frankly necrotic cells are seen, the loss of cells being evidenced by gaps in the hepatic plates. The cy-tolysis is a result of antecedent hepatocellular degeneration characterized by either ballooning or by shrinkage with the for-mation of acidophilic bodies. However, the relative importance of each of these modes of degeneration in the development of necrosis is uncertain. Since few foci of cell loss contain frankly necrotic hepatocytes, and since their pathogenesis is obscure, they often are designated as foci of hepatocellular ''dropout'' rather than necrosis.

Most of the foci of cell dropout are relatively small, involv-ing only a few hepatocytes, and are scattered through the lob-ules, a type of necrosis usually termed ''spotty.'' The random and wide distribution of such small foci is best seen at low magnification (Fig. 421). As a rule, the sites of cell loss are filled with swollen Kupffer cells and lymphocytes, and, often, contain or are surrounded by a few acidophilic bodies (Fig. 86). The smallest foci of necrosis may be characterized by one or more acidophilic bodies with little or no inflammatory reac-tion or evidence of cell dropout (Fig. 422). As previously in-dicated, acidophilic bodies are hepatocytes that have undergone acidophilic degeneration or necrosis, ultimately to be extruded from hepatic plates into the spaces of Disse where they are engulfed by Kupffer cells (Fig. 423) or undergo apoptosis (172).

In most cases of moderate severity, the loss of hepatocytes is most prominent in the centrilobular zones (Fig. 421). As is evident at higher magnification in Figures 424 and 425, the centrilobular foci of cell dropout involve much larger groups of contiguous hepatocytes than in the intralobular foci of spotty necrosis (Figs. 86, 422). Necrosis of this type is often classified as confluent (173).

Occasionally, centrilobular degeneration and necrosis pre-dominate in the lesions of classic acute viral hepatitis, over-shadowing the spotty necrosis and inflammatory reaction found elsewhere in the lobules (Fig. 87). Such lesions do not correlate with any distinctive clinical or laboratory features, and appear to have no special prognostic significance.

Although the hepatocytes bordering the inflamed portal tracts often are spared, the limiting plates may show foci of cell drop-out and occasional acidophilic bodies (Fig. 426). Less com-monly, as shown in Figure 299, periportal hepatocellular necro-sis is extensive, resulting in complete destruction of the limiting plate and apparent expansion of the portal tract, sometimes being indistinguishable from chronic active hepatitis. As can be seen at higher magnification in Figure 300, the portal tract is sur-rounded by a broad zone in which hepatocytes are replaced by numerous proliferating Kupffer cells, scattered lymphocytes, and occasional acidophilic bodies. According to some authorities (173), erosion of the limiting plates is a relatively rare feature of acute viral hepatitis, and, when present, may be indicative of transition to chronic hepatitis. In a follow-up biopsy study of 17 such lesions, progression to cirrhosis was documented in 2 cases (174). However, review of the initial biopsy sections in these 2 cases revealed bridging necrosis, so that the apparent progression could not be clearly correlated with erosion of the limiting plates. Moreover, in our experience with a large number of patients who exhibited erosion of the limiting plates during the early phase of acute hepatitis, we have never seen progression to cirrhosis in the absence of bridging necrosis (61). Other investigators, however, have reported that a high percentage of patients with piecemeal necrosis, especially those with HBV or NANB hepatitis, develop chronic hepatitis (175).

In occasional cases of acute viral hepatitis, the lesions are characterized by an impressive portal and intralobular inflammatory reaction with only rare small foci of cell dropout and acidophilic bodies. Usually, such lesions are encountered in patients with mild infections that may be either icteric (Fig. 427) or anicteric (Fig. 428).

Hepatocellular degeneration

A variable number of hepatocytes, depending on the severity of the lesions, show ballooning degeneration. The most severely affected cells appear large and pale due to swelling of their cytoplasm, and show marked variations in their size and shape (Figs. 108, 229). Often, their cytoplasmic granules are aggregated in the perinuclear zone, while the remaining peripheral cytoplasm has a finely reticulated appearance. The nuclei in such cells are of variable size, and some show evidence of karyolysis. Occasionally, the intercellular plasma membranes are indistinct, resulting in what appears to be fusion of contiguous hepatocytes (Fig. 229). Less severe ballooning, which is relatively common, is evidenced by enlargement and variations in the size and shape of the hepatocytes with little or no pallor or vacuolization of their cytoplasm (Fig. 95).

Ballooned cells greatly outnumber acidophilic bodies, and usually are most prominent near large centrilobular areas of cell dropout (Figs. 108, 229), suggesting that ballooning may play a more important role in cytolysis than acidophilic degeneration. However, in many of the smaller intralobular foci of spotty necrosis, acidophilic bodies are more numerous than ballooned cells (Fig. 86), so that the relative importance of ballooning and acidophilic degeneration in the pathogenesis of hepatocellular necrosis is uncertain. It has been reported that acidophilic degeneration predominates in cases of mild or anicteric acute viral hepatitis (176). However, this has been an inconstant feature in our experience.

Often, the remaining, apparently intact hepatocytes in acute viral hepatitis are depleted of glycogen (Fig. 181). That this is the result of subtle hepatocellular injury rather than starvation is suggested by the observation that many such patients exhibit a defect in glycogen synthesis and gluconeogenesis (177).

Intralobular inflammation

A diffuse, intralobular, lymphocytic inflammatory reaction is characteristic of acute viral hepatitis. The lymphocytes are most numerous in the large centrilobular zones of necrosis (Figs. 424, 425), but also are found in the small foci of spotty necrosis scattered through the lobules (Fig. 86), and in the sinusoids, even in the absence of cell dropout (Fig. 428).

Plasma cells are relatively infrequent or absent in early lesions, but may be seen from the earliest stages (178), become more numerous at a later stage, particularly when the course of the disease is prolonged. However, when present, plasmacytosis usually is more prominent in the portal tracts than in the parenchyma.

Rarely, eosinophils are encountered in the intralobular exudates of acute viral hepatitis (Fig. 286). Although these have no special significance, they may be misinterpreted as evidence of an underlying drug-sensitization reaction.

Kupffer cell hypertrophy and hyperplasia

The foci of hepatocellular necrosis in acute viral hepatitis almost always contain numerous swollen Kupffer cells that often are pigmented owing to phagocytized lipofuscin (Figs. 86, 108, 229, 300) or iron derived from necrotic hepatocytes (Fig. 235). In addition, focal Kupffer cell proliferation is seen in some of the sinusoids, even in areas where cell dropout is not evident. Occasionally, the sinusoids are filled with swollen, proliferating Kupffer cells out of all proportion to the extent of hepatocellular necrosis (Fig. 230). Not infrequently, some of the hypertrophied Kupffer cells contain phagocytized acidophilic bodies or acidophilic body fragments (Figs. 86, 300, 423).

Hepatocellular regeneration

Signs of hepatocellular regeneration are a constant feature of the lesions throughout the course of acute viral hepatitis. Mitotic figures may be numerous in early lesions, even when hepatocellular necrosis is only minimal (Fig. 188), but, usually, they are relatively infrequent thereafter. As the lesions advance, regeneration is evidenced by the appearance of enlarged intact hepatocytes that contain prominent or reduplicated nuclei (Fig. 429). Late in the disease, particularly when necrosis has been extensive, the regenerated hepatocytes may be arranged in the form of twin-cell-thick plates (Fig. 201) or rosettes (Fig. 204).

It has been suggested that during the course of acute viral hepatitis, most, if not all of the hepatocytes undergo necrosis and are replaced by regenerating cells, and that the spotty character of the necrosis usually found at any given moment is attributable to rapid cell turnover elsewhere in the lobules (179). The complete disappearance of the pigment granules in the Dubin-Johnson syndrome following an attack of acute viral hepatitis (180) has been cited as evidence in support of this hypothesis. However, while this observation is consistent with the complete loss of centrilobular hepatocytes where Dubin-Johnson pigment is localized and where necrosis is usually most extensive, it does not necessarily imply complete cell turnover elsewhere in the lobules.

Cholestasis

In approximately one-third of patients with classic acute viral hepatitis, canalicular bile thrombi are demonstrable in the centrilobular zones (Figs. 206, 430). Injury to the bile duct epithelium is common (181), most frequently in NANB hepatitis. Bile thrombi and bile duct injury may occur as early as the second or third week of illness and often persist for several months, despite clearing of the jaundice (Fig. 206). In general, such cholestasis is encountered in patients with moderate to severe jaundice, but occasionally is found in those with only mild icterus. At times, under such conditions, the canaliculi are dilated but contain no bile thrombi (Fig. 204). As in other forms of cholestasis, the bile thrombi often are encircled by hepatocytes arranged in the form of rosettes (Fig. 430) or pseudoducts (Fig. 206), presumably reflecting a regenerative response.

Central endophlebitis

Occasionally, some of the central veins show proliferation of their endothelial lining cells and a mild lymphocytic infiltrate, resulting in thickening of the intima (Fig. 269). Reactions of this type appear to be related to the generalized reticuloendothelial proliferative response found throughout the lobules. Indeed, in some instances, proliferating Kupffer cells and macrophages extend through the wall of the central vein and merge with its thickened intima (Fig. 269).

Reticulin

Some authorities report that focal disruption of reticulin fibers may occur in large areas of cell dropout (176). However, in our experience, the reticulin is invariably spared, irrespective of the extent of hepatocellular necrosis, although frequently it shows evidence of collapse, particularly in the centrilobular zones (Fig. 431).

Portal tract configuration

As a rule, the portal tracts retain their normal configuration despite their infiltration by inflammatory cells (Figs. 426–428). However, they may appear expanded when periportal hepatocellular necrosis is a prominent feature (Figs. 299, 305).

Portal tract inflammation

Characteristically, most, if not all of the portal tracts are infiltrated by abundant *lymphocytes* that usually greatly outnumber those in the lobules (Figs. 426–428).

Few or no *plasma cells* are found in the portal exudates of early lesions, but often appear in variable numbers late in the disease (Fig. 331), and are especially numerous following bridging necrosis (Fig. 312).

As a rule, the portal infiltrates in acute viral hepatitis contain few, if any *neutrophils*. However, occasionally, when the lesions are characterized by extensive hepatocellular necrosis or marked cholestasis, portal neutrophils may be a prominent feature (Figs. 320, 432).

Mild portal *eosinophilia* has been reported in over a third of patients with acute viral hepatitis (182). However, in our experience, this has been encountered only rarely (Fig. 325), possibly owing to our routine use of Carnoy's solution for fixation, a procedure that appears to obscure eosinophils.

Macrophages appear in the portal tracts in increasing numbers during the course of acute viral hepatitis. Usually, these are pigmented (Fig. 331) owing to the presence of abundant D-PAS-positive lipofuscin (Fig. 234), and, often, they persist following full recovery (Fig. 333).

Portal tract bile ducts

Usually, the interlobular ducts and ductules appear normal. However, mild to moderate *ductular proliferation* may be seen when the limiting plates are destroyed by periportal or bridging hepatocellular necrosis, or when cholestasis is a prominent feature (Figs. 299, 300, 320).

Abnormal interlobular bile duct epithelium of the type seen more commonly in primary biliary cirrhosis has been reported in 20% of patients with acute viral hepatitis (183). In our biopsy material, such lesions have been encountered far less frequently, and only in cases of severe hepatitis with extensive periportal or bridging necrosis (Fig. 372), or an unusually prolonged cholestatic course (Fig. 433).

Portal limiting plates

As previously indicated, most of the limiting plates around the portal tracts appear to be normal, but, on close inspection, they frequently show focal loss of individual hepatocytes and occasional acidophilic bodies (Fig. 426). Moreover, even in cases of moderate severity, some of the limiting plates may be completely eroded (Fig. 299). Such lesions have no prognostic significance.

Late phase lesions

Early in the course of acute viral hepatitis, the regenerative response is overshadowed by hepatocellular degeneration and necrosis. However, once degeneration and necrosis begin to abate, regeneration becomes an increasingly prominent feature of the lesions, leading to gradual replacement of destroyed hepatocytes, and ultimate restoration of normal hepatic volume. Thus, as foci of cell dropout and acidophilic bodies diminish in number, pleomorphic and multinucleated hepatocytes (Fig. 429) and twin-cell-thick hepatic plates (Fig. 201) become increasingly prominent. Although intralobular inflammation tends to diminish as hepatocellular necrosis abates, swollen Kupffer cells filled with either lipofuscin or iron (Fig. 235), and portal exudates (Fig. 234) often persist.

Residuals following recovery

As a rule, the lesions of acute viral hepatitis heal without significant residual abnormalities. However, in some cases, minor abnormalities can still be found a year or more following full clinical and biochemical recovery. These include minimal portal fibrosis and lymphocytosis (Fig. 434), a slight increase in the number of binucleate cells and mild pleomorphism (Fig.

434), and occasional small foci of prominent Kupffer cells and occasional lymphocytes (Fig. 435). Fatty infiltration is said to be a residual feature in some cases (179). However, we have encountered this only rarely since the therapeutic practice of force-feeding carbohydrate was abandoned many years ago.

Unresolved classic acute viral hepatitis

The duration of acute viral hepatitis is highly variable, ranging from a few weeks to several months. The term "unresolved" has never been clearly defined, being used both to indicate incomplete healing of the lesions at any stage of the disease, or only when they remain active for a long, but usually unspecified time. To avoid this confusion, most authorities classify lesions of viral hepatitis that fail to heal within six months as "chronic."

In a comparison of the clinical features and prognosis in our own patients with acute HBsAg-positive hepatitis that failed to resolve within six months, and in those with HBsAg-positive chronic active hepatitis of insidious onset and unknown duration, we could find no significant differences (184). For that reason, the term "chronic" would appear to be more appropriate and less likely to cause confusion than "unresolved" in classifying the lesions of acute viral hepatitis that fail to heal within six months.

The histologic differentiation of acute HAV, HBV, HDV, and NANB viral hepatitis

In general the histologic abnormalities of acute hepatitis caused by HAV, HBV, HCV, HDV, and HEV are indistinguishable and all conform to the histologic patterns described for HBV hepatitis over the past 40 years (171,173,176,185–187). The similarities are far more numerous than the differences (188–191). However, some authors describe certain patterns that suggest that histopathologic differences may identify specific types of viral hepatitis.

HAV

The typical pattern of perivenular ballooning of hepatocytes, spotty necrosis, and multinucleation is usually seen, and HAAg can be demonstrated immunocytochemically in the cytoplasm of hepatocytes and Kupffer cells in the early stages of the disease (192). Several characteristic subpatterns have been described, including periportal necrosis with dense portal infiltrates rich in plasma cells. This periportal lesion may be difficult to differentiate from the piecemeal necrosis of chronic active hepatitis, but the absence of fibrosis may help differentiate. In a second pattern, pericentral cholestasis is the predominant lesion and hepatocellular damage and portal inflammation are minimal (188,189,193,194).

HBV

Most pathologists detect no specific differences between HAV and HBV hepatitis in the absence of the immunocytochemical demonstration of HBsAg and HBcAg in hepatocytes. However, some have found patterns characterized by extensive parenchymal abnormalities and inflammation, but with relatively little portal inflammation (189,190,193). These investigators find piecemeal necrosis and bridging necrosis to be more common in HBV than in HAV hepatitis. Despite more confluent necrosis, several have found these lesions not usually predictive of chronic liver disease (195,196). We have found bridging hepatic necrosis to be a frequent precursor of chronicity and others have found piecemeal necrosis to be a similar ominous marker (175,197). Other investigators have emphasized peripolesis and emperipolesis, the presence of lymphocytes surrounding or within injured hepatocytes, respectively, to be typical of HBV hepatitis (193). The presence of sanded nuclei in HBV infection [(23,198); Fig. 140], but not in HAV infection, can be used to differentiate the two types of hepatitis histologically.

Concomitant infections with HAV and HBV are not uncommon in areas where both infections are endemic (199). The clinical and histologic features in these patients in whom acute HAV hepatitis was superimposed on HBV infection are similar to acute HAV hepatitis alone.

HDV

Acute HDV hepatitis is usually described as having no distinctive histopathologic features (200–202), although HDAg can be demonstrated in the liver, predominantly in nuclei. Sanded nuclei, which have been described in HBV [(23,203); Fig. 140], and which have eosinophiloc nuclear inclusions, have been reported in HDV infection (Figs. 436, 437). Immunohistochemically these sanded nuclei are strongly positive for HDAg but are negative for HBc antigen. HBV core particles are not demonstrable by electron microscopy in these nuclei as they are in HBV sanded nuclei. In concurrent HBV and HDV infection, microvesicular fatty infiltration, sparse lymphocytic infiltration, and increased aggregation of macrophages have been observed (204–206). Microvesicular fatty deposition, however, may occasionally be seen in each of the other types of acute hepatitis. Chronic HDV infection, defined as the presence of HDAg, anti-HD, or HDV RNA in serum and HDAg in the liver, is characterized by cellular inflammation, hepatocyte degeneration, and eosinophilia of the cytoplasm with frequent acidophilic necrosis. Severe piecemeal necrosis is typical.

Studies from Italy have shown an inverse correlation between the histologic activity index (207) and prognosis (208). There was, however, a positive correlation between the degree of portal lymphocytic infiltration and the amount of intracellular HDAg. This led the investigators to speculate that increased expression of HDAg might amplify the inflammatory reaction, thus enhancing elimination of the virus. This hypothesis receives support from the observation of emperipolesis of HDAg-containing hepatocytes (209). Others have not confirmed this association, however (210).

Focal epidemics of chronic fulminant HDV liver disease have been reported in Indians in Venezuela and Colombia (139,211).

In these patients acute hepatitis was characterized by microvesicular fatty infiltration as the earliest abnormality and by focal necrosis that progressed to confluent piecemeal or bridging necrosis. The cytoplasm of the hepatocytes showed eosinophilic granulation, and acidophilic degeneration was common. Portal lymphocytic infiltration varied widely in degree. Cholestasis was mild or absent. HDAg was usually present in the nuclei of hepatocytes (211). This finding is interpreted to be a cytopathic pattern induced by the HDV. The disease tends to progress rapidly to chronic active hepatitis and cirrhosis and is often fatal.

In patients with both HDV infection and hepatocellular carcinoma, HDVAg can be demonstrated in the nuclei of non-neoplastic hepatocytes (Figs. 438, 439), and HBsAg can be found in the cytoplasm of non-neoplastic hepatocytes (Fig. 440). Neither antigen is seen in the neoplastic cells (199).

The report of a single, well-studied case of HDV hepatitis (140) provides insight into these differing histologic observations. This patient, who was from the United States, exhibited a cytopathic type of acute hepatitis characterized, as in the Venezuelan Indians (139,212), by microvesicular steatosis with few parenchymal inflammatory cells. This pattern, which has also been seen in HBV carrier chimpanzees infected with HDV (213), suggests that HDV is a cytopathic, rather than a lymphocytotoxic virus. There may, of course, be different responses in different patients, and, perhaps, there may be more than one strain of HDV.

The intranuclear distribution of HDV RNA as a marker of viral replication, was studied by in situ hybridization in patients with chronic HBV infection who were superinfected with HDV (214). Intranuclear HDV RNA and HDV antigen were often seen in the same cells (Fig. 441). In some patients, HDV RNA in the absence of HDV antigen was found, usually in patients in whom the HDV infection had occurred more than one year before biopsy. Eosinophilic degeneration of hepatocytes, which is characteristic of HDV hepatitis, usually occurs in cells in which neither HDAg or HDV RNA is present. These findings suggest that there is no association between this cytopathologic abnormality and viral replication.

HCV, HEV (NANB)

Acute NANB hepatitis is generally thought to be indistinguishable from type A and B hepatitis, although microvesicular fat may appear early in its course. Several subpatterns have been described. In one, cytopathic changes, including eosinophilia of the cytoplasm, acidophilic degeneration, and multinucleated hepatocytes, have been observed (199,215). In the other, apparently associated with short incubation hepatitis, there is little hepatocellular necrosis, many lymphocytes in the sinusoids, and lymphoid follicles in the portal areas, with some bile duct damage. Both lesions may be seen in the same liver (53).

Cholestasis with severe bile duct damage has also been reported to be more common in NANB hepatitis than in the other types (216,217). This cholestasis is associated with predominantly portal-periportal hepatitis with many lymphocytes and plasma cells, lymph follicles with germinal centers, and bile duct lesions (207). Lymphocytic infiltration of the sinusoids has also been considered characteristic of NANB, but peripolesis is less common in NANB than in HBV hepatitis.

In one controlled comparison, acute HAV, HBV, and NANB hepatitis from Leuven and from Rome were compared (216,217). Type A and B were similar in patients from the two cities, but NANB hepatitis differed. In Leuven, eosinophilia of the cytoplasm, acidophilic bodies, and Mallory bodies were seen. In Rome, lymphocytic and histiocytic infiltrations predominated. Such "geographic" differences may reflect different responses to the same virus or different virus strains in the two cities.

It is not clear that these overlapping histologic patterns in acute viral hepatitis are mutually exclusive. Indeed, many experts do not believe that the different types of viral hepatitis can be differentiated on histologic grounds alone. Certainly, many exceptions occur, even in the interpretations by the proponents of "characteristic" patterns. Some of these variations may be due to differences in the route of transmission, the stage of the disease, or the severity of the disorder, or may be determined by differences in host status, such as the nutritional state or immunologic responsiveness, or in the method of selection of patients for study.

True differences between the various types of viral hepatitis can only be established by objective studies of comparative histopathology in large consecutive series with serologically unequivocal diagnoses from different geographic areas, examined at the same stage of the disease by multiple, experienced pathologists, using the same histologic criteria. The development of a reliable serologic test for HCV (58) will permit such investigations to be performed for the first time.

Histopathology of acute viral hepatitis variants

Anicteric viral hepatitis

The histologic features of the lesions in anicteric viral hepatitis are identical with those in icteric cases, except that, in general, they tend to be milder (Figs. 423, 428). Occasionally, however, they exhibit extensive lesions with bridging necrosis that may progress to chronic active hepatitis and postnecrotic cirrhosis (60). Figure 442 illustrates such a lesion in a 42-year-old woman who presented with nausea, vomiting, anorexia, weight loss, ascites, edema, and right upper quadrant abdominal pain for four months' duration. Although her urine had been dark intermittently, she never exhibited jaundice or hepatomegaly. She underwent laparotomy to exclude an intraabdominal malignancy or biliary tract disease. The only finding of note was a small, soft liver that had a finely wrinkled capsule. Liver biopsy revealed the typical features of severe acute viral hepatitis with extensive bridging necrosis (Fig. 442). Despite supportive therapy, signs of hepatic failure increased, and, in the eighth month of illness, there was biopsy evidence of chronic active hepatitis and postnecrotic cirrhosis. Death ensued two months later.

Cholestatic viral hepatitis

Only a minority of patients with acute viral hepatitis who exhibit histologic evidence of cholestasis present with the combination of jaundice, acholic stools, pruritus, and high serum levels of alkaline phosphatase and cholesterol that characterize the syndrome of cholestatic hepatitis, as it is usually defined (59). Moreover, there is considerable overlap in the histologic features of classic and cholestatic cases, so that, as previously indicated, cholestatic viral hepatitis is not a specific clinical or morphologic entity, but probably represents an ill-defined variant in the broad spectrum of manifestations that may be encountered in acute viral hepatitis.

The early lesions of acute cholestatic viral hepatitis are indistinguishable from those of classic viral hepatitis, although bile stasis is a more constant feature, and tends to be more prominent. However, when the cholestasis persists for four to eight weeks, which often is the case, the distinctive histologic features of acute viral hepatitis may no longer be present. Thus, at this stage, the parenchyma often shows few or no balloon cells, acidophilic bodies, foci of cell dropout, or intralobular inflammatory cells. Instead, the lesions are characterized by the presence of numerous bile thrombi in dilated canaliculi and swollen Kupffer cells, evidence of hepatocellular regeneration with the formation of thick plates and numerous rosettes and pseudoducts, and a variable increase in the number and size of the Kupffer cells (Fig. 443). As a rule, the portal tracts contain a moderate number of lymphocytes and macrophages, and show no significant ductular proliferation. However, in occasional cases, some of the portal tracts are enlarged and edematous, and contain numerous neutrophils and proliferating ductules (Fig. 444), features that mimic those of extrahepatic biliary obstruction. Moreover, when cholestasis is both severe and prolonged, some of the interlobular ducts may be widely dilated and show degeneration of their epithelium (Fig. 321), and circumscribed foci of pseudoxanthomatous degeneration ("bile infarcts") may appear in the periportal parenchyma (Fig. 121).

The evolution of the lesions in cholestatic acute viral hepatitis is well illustrated in the case of the patient whose biopsy section is shown in Figure 443. In this case, jaundice, pruritus, and acholic stools appeared abruptly two months following multiple transfusions for an anemia due to myelofibrosis. Biopsy on the ninth day of illness, at which time the serum bilirubin concentration was 35 mg/dl and the SGOT level 1620 I.U., revealed the features of moderately severe, classic, acute viral hepatitis with bile-staining of the centrilobular hepatocytes, but no canalicular or Kupffer cell bile thrombi. Jaundice, pruritus, and acholic stools, later accompanied by marked steatorrhea and a 30-pound weight loss, despite a drop in serum bilirubin to 20 mg/dl and SGOT to 22 I.U., persisted until the seventh week of disease. Repeat biopsy at this time revealed the features of cholestatic hepatitis illustrated in Figure 443. Over the next six months, the jaundice abated and the patient made an uneventful recovery, except for his underlying chronic anemia.

It has recently been pointed out that acute HAV hepatitis may sometimes be characterized by a cholestatic syndrome (218–220). Of 13 consecutive patients who had been admitted to the hospital and who had undergone liver biopsy, 10 showed total serum bilirubin levels greater than 10 mg/dl. Histologically intracellular and intracanalicular bile plugs were common, and the latter were often surrounded by an acinar arrangement of hepatocytes termed "cholestatic liver cell rosettes." In addition, peculiar, metaplastic bile ductules with irregular epithelium of variable shape and height with vacuolization of cytoplasm, pyknotic nuclei and infiltration with neutrophils were found. Four of the patients developed this syndrome and three

of them died. This atypical series may reflect selection bias in that patients with classic viral hepatitis are rarely hospitalized or biopsied. On the other hand, this report indicates that acute HAV hepatitis does not always conform to its benign clinical and histologic reputation. Others have also reported cholestatic type A viral hepatitis but without these dramatic histologic findings (219–222).

Acute viral hepatitis with bridging necrosis

In the form of acute viral hepatitis characterized by zones of confluent hepatocellular necrosis that bridge adjacent central veins and portal tracts, the unbridged parenchyma shows the usual type of spotty necrosis, diffuse inflammation, and Kupffer cell proliferation seen in classic cases. At one time, such lesions were classified as "subacute hepatic necrosis" (60,61), a term that was ultimately abandoned because it was so often misinterpreted. This lesion is now widely referred to as bridging hepatic necrosis.

The distribution of bridging necrosis may be portal-portal, portal-central, central-central, or any combination of these. Although the extent of bridging varies from case to case, it usually can be identified in most low-magnification microscopic fields, and often involves numerous contiguous lobules. In occasional cases, the bridging is accompanied by confluent, panlobular necrosis that completely destroys one or more lobules.

Periportal necrosis may be mistaken for bridging necrosis if adjacent portal tracts are sectioned close to their branch points. Fortunately, such branch points occur only occasionally in normal liver biopsy sections. Such errors can be obviated if a minimum of three portal-portal bridges is required for identification.

Some authorities (223) draw a distinction between portal-portal and portal-central bridging necrosis. In their view, the term bridging should be limited to portal-central necrosis, since they consider portal-portal bridging as nothing more than a form of piecemeal necrosis. This distinction is both unwarranted and misleading. Considering its dictionary definition, the term "piecemeal" when applied to necrosis implies destruction of hepatic parenchyma bit by bit, a description appropriate for the type of periportal necrosis commonly seen in chronic active hepatitis, but inappropriate for the large zones of confluent, acute necrosis seen in acute viral hepatitis. Moreover, in our own experience, we have found no differences between portal-portal, portal-central, and central-central bridging necrosis in terms of clinical features or prognostic significance.

Both the distribution and histologic features of bridging necrosis are best visualized in Masson-stained sections. When intralobular inflammation is intense, zones of bridging necrosis may be difficult to identify in H&E-stained sections, and, often, the sinusoids and reticulin fibers in the involved areas are obscured.

By far the most frequent pattern of necrosis in cases of bridging is the combination of portal-portal, portal-central, and central-central bridging. Figures 73 and 75 illustrate such a lesion in a patient with severe acute HBsAg-positive hepatitis that proved fatal on the 11th day of illness. A similar pattern is seen in the lesion of a patient with acute HBsAg-positive hepatitis on the 11th day of illness who recovered (Figs. 445, 446).

Less commonly, the bridging is exclusively portal-portal, except for rare extensions of the periportal necrosis to central veins, as can be seen in the lesions found on the ninth day of illness in a case of acute non-A, non-B posttransfusion hepatitis (Figs. 69, 70).

Predominantly centrilobular necrosis with central-portal bridging occurs only rarely (Fig. 72). We have not encountered any examples of exclusively central-central bridging necrosis in cases of acute viral hepatitis.

Occasionally, bridging necrosis is accompanied by complete destruction of a few randomly distributed lobules. The example illustrated in Figure 79 was encountered in the patient with diffuse bridging necrosis whose lesions are shown in Figures 445 and 446. Despite the resemblance of the lesions in some areas to those of submassive hepatic necrosis, the patient exhibited no evidence of hepatic encephalopathy, ascites, or edema, and, during the course of prednisone therapy, cleared her serum of HBsAg in three weeks, and showed complete healing of her lesions without residuals in seven weeks (Fig. 447), a recovery that was sustained following withdrawal of prednisone.

Dissolution of the hepatic plates in the zones of bridging necrosis leads to collapse and coalescence of the reticulin fibers on either side of the affected plates, producing a mesh in which are enclosed sinusoids and a variable number of inflammatory cells and swollen Kupffer cells (Fig. 74). At a later stage, the sinusoids collapse, making them difficult to identify, and resulting in further condensation of the reticulin. Although the condensed reticulin may resemble collagen bundles (Figs. 302, 303), its constituent collapsed fine fibers are readily apparent in silver-impregnated sections (Fig. 448).

As previously indicated, outside the zones of bridging necrosis, the remaining parenchyma and portal tracts show the usual histologic features of classic acute viral hepatitis, including foci of spotty hepatocellular necrosis, scattered acidophilic bodies, diffusely distributed intralobular and portal inflammatory cells, proliferating, swollen Kupffer cells, and evidence of hepatocellular regeneration. However, often, the hepatocellular regenerative response is more prominent and is associated with bile duct proliferation and, occasionally, with the formation of multinucleated giant hepatocytes (Fig. 128). Moreover, erosion of the limiting plates and ductular proliferation are more prominent (Fig. 319), and, frequently, when hepatocellular necrosis occurs, the portal tracts may contain numerous neutrophils (Fig. 319). In acute hepatitis, bridging hepatic necrosis is devoid of elastic fibers, but elastic tissue is characteristic of mature septa (224).

Lesions characterized by bridging necrosis, even when accompanied by foci of panlobular necrosis, may heal without significant residuals (Fig. 447). However, in a number of cases, the lesions either heal with significant residual fibrosis, or remain active, giving rise to chronic active hepatitis with or without complicating postnecrotic cirrhosis. Figure 449 illustrates the inactive postnecrotic cirrhosis found three years following a corticosteroid-induced remission of biopsy-documented, acute viral hepatitis with extensive bridging necrosis. At the time of this biopsy, the patient had been off corticosteroids for 18 months, exhibited normal hepatic function, and was well clinically, but still had an enlarged, firm liver. When last seen four years later, the liver was significantly smaller, and, on biopsy, showed only patchy portal fibrosis with occasional portal-portal fibrous bridges, but no nodule formation or thickening of the hepatic plates.

Shown in Figure 450 are the chronic active hepatitis and postnecrotic cirrhosis found at autopsy in a young HBsAg-positive heroin addict who nine years previously had suffered an attack of acute viral hepatitis with bridging necrosis. Prednisone therapy, begun in the seventh month of illness because the hepatitis failed to resolve, suppressed the activity of the lesions, but failed to prevent their progression to chronic active hepatitis and cirrhosis that led ultimately to hepatic failure and death. As evidence of his chronic HBV infection, occasional clusters of aldehyde-fuchsin-positive ground glass cells were found in some of the parenchymal nodules (Fig. 139).

Massive and submassive hepatic necrosis

The lesions of viral *massive hepatic necrosis* are characterized by almost complete destruction of the hepatocytes in adjacent lobules, a diffuse intralobular and portal mononuclear inflammatory reaction, occasionally accompanied by neutrophils, and marked Kupffer cell swelling and proliferation (Fig. 78). Usually, the portal tracts are spared, but may show mild inflammation or marked proliferation of ductules that often extend deeply into the lobules, occasionally approaching the central veins, so-called ductular hepatocytes. The portal areas are often surrounded by small islands of degenerating hepatocytes. Although the reticulin may be collapsed, it shows no evidence of destruction (Fig. 451).

Postmortem specimens in cases of massive hepatic necrosis tend to undergo unusually rapid autolysis, so that, often, no intralobular inflammatory cells or proliferating Kupffer cells are found at autopsy, and the surviving hepatocytes appear as shrunken cytoplasmic remnants, devoid of nuclei. Usually, the portal tracts and proliferating ductules are unaffected by the autolysis.

Invariably, *massive hepatic necrosis* presents clinically as fulminant hepatitis, and results in death within a few days to weeks.

In *submassive hepatic necrosis,* large areas of parenchyma undergo complete necrosis, as in massive hepatic necrosis, but others are less extensively involved, usually showing the features of acute hepatitis with bridging necrosis. The outcome of such lesions depends on the extent of necrosis and on the regenerative response of the surviving hepatocytes. Patients with the most extensive lesions usually present clinically with the features of fulminant hepatitis and die within a few days or weeks. More commonly, however, hepatocellular regeneration permits survival for months or years. Characteristically, the livers in survivors are cirrhotic, small in size, and contain large or small nodules or regenerating parenchyma separated by slender or broad zones of collapsed reticulin and fibrosis. Figures 60 and 61 illustrate such lesions in an elderly patient who died of hepatic failure nine months following the onset of posttransfusional, viral, submassive hepatic necrosis. At autopsy, his liver weighed 1000 g, and contained broad zones of collapsed reticulin and fibrosis in which were embedded both small and large nodules of regenerating parenchyma. As can be seen in Figure 60, the large zones of collapse contained numerous crowded portal tracts surrounded by collapsed reticulin undergoing collagenization, numerous proliferating ductules, and infiltrating inflammatory cells. In the surviving parenchyma, the hepatocytes showed evidence of active regeneration, and were arranged in the form of either large or small nodules surrounded by slender fibrous septa (Fig. 61).

Histopathology of viral-induced chronic liver disease

The HBV, HDV, HCV, and HEV viruses are capable of producing chronic persistent hepatitis, chronic active hepatitis, and postnecrotic cirrhosis. Although each of these lesions has distinctive morphologic features, they overlap to some extent, so that sharp distinctions between chronic persistent and chronic active hepatitis, on the one hand, and between chronic active hepatitis and postnecrotic cirrhosis, on the other, are not always possible. Moreover, the intensity of the inflammatory reaction, the extent of hepatocellular necrosis and the degree of fibrosis in each of these lesions may vary, depending on the activity and duration of the disease. Furthermore, sampling error can make differentiation difficult for each of these entities.

Some viral-induced chronic hepatitic lesions are the sequelae of antecedent attacks of acute hepatitis, whereas others occur insidiously following unrecognized infections, as in the case of apparently healthy carriers. Those of insidious onset may remain asymptomatic and go unrecognized, unless hepatomegaly, hepatic functional abnormalities, or serologic evidence of active viral infection are discovered during the course of a routine examination. More often, however, the lesions ultimately give rise to clinical manifestations of liver disease. Moreover, once the lesions become clinically evident, their activity may undergo spontaneous exacerbations and remissions, or may be suppressed by corticosteroid therapy.

The clinical features and prognosis of viral-induced chronic liver disease are dependent on the character, extent, and activity of the lesions. Most chronic lesions attributable to HBV infections occur in individuals with persistent HBs antigenemia. Rarely, however, identical lesions may develop following elimination of the virus (72). Although the lesions in HBs antigen-positive and antigen-negative cases are similar, only the former contain orcein-positive ground glass cells, and there is suggestive evidence that such HBsAg-positive lesions may be less responsive to corticosteroid therapy (225).

Chronic persistent hepatitis

The lesions of chronic persistent hepatitis are characterized by a mononuclear inflammatory reaction that involves a variable number of portal tracts. As a rule, the limiting plates are intact, and the parenchyma contains only a few small, scattered foci of inflammation and hepatocellular necrosis. However, during exacerbations of the disease, and in cases of severe acute viral hepatitis that fail to resolve within six months, intralobular inflammation and necrosis often are prominent features, and, occasionally, the portal tracts show segmental erosion of their limiting plates. Lesions of this type, classified by some as chronic lobular hepatitis (69), closely resemble those of acute viral hepatitis.

In minimally active lesions, some of the portal tracts are infiltrated by lymphocytes and plasma cells, which, occasionally, are aggregated in the form of follicles (Fig. 452). A few of the portal tracts may be slightly enlarged and fibrotic, but they show no erosion of their limiting plates or tendency to undergo bridging (Fig. 453), so that the overall lobular architecture is not affected. Ductular proliferation and portal macrophages are relatively uncommon in inactive lesions. However, invariably under such conditions, occasional acidophilic bodies, often accompanied by a few swollen Kupffer cells, lymphocytes, or plasma cells, are found scattered through the lobules (Fig. 454). Less commonly, somewhat larger circumscribed clusters of Kupffer cells, lymphocytes, and plasma cells may replace groups of hepatocytes, especially in the centrilobular zones (Fig. 455). As a rule, the remaining hepatocytes are normal in appearance and show a normal plate pattern (Figs. 452–455). Occasionally, however, some of the hepatocytes exhibit mild anisocytosis and anisonucleosis. Moreover, in cases with chronic HBs-antigenemia, a variable number often contain orcein-positive ground glass inclusions (Figs. 136, 138).

As illustrated in Figure 456, the lesions encountered during acute exacerbations of chronic persistent hepatitis, or those attributable to active unresolved acute hepatitis, may be characterized by a diffuse inflammatory reaction that involves not only the portal tracts but also the parenchyma, accompanied by widely distributed foci of hepatocellular necrosis. Usually, the portal tracts are more uniformly infiltrated with lymphocytes and plasma cells, and show greater expansion than those in relatively inactive lesions. Moreover, they occasionally exhibit segmental erosion of their limiting plates, and may contain a variable number of proliferating ductules and pigmented macrophages (Fig. 457). The predominant features of the intralobular lesions, which vary in severity depending on the activity and duration of the exacerbation, usually include multiple foci of cell dropout that interrupt and distort the normal hepatic plate pattern, a variable number of scattered acidophilic bodies, ballooning hepatocytes, widespread proliferation of swollen Kupffer cells, and diffusely distributed lymphocytes and plasma cells (Fig. 458). Evidence of hepatocellular regeneration in the form of thick plates and binucleate hepatocytes is relatively common, and, occasionally, a few rosettes and pseudoducts may be seen. In some cases, bile thrombi are found within the canaliculi or the Kupffer cells. As a rule, the foci of hepatocellular necrosis are small and spotty in distribution, but, as in the case of classic acute viral hepatitis, may be significantly larger in the centrilobular zones.

When the limiting plates are segmentally eroded in chronic persistent hepatitis, differentiation from chronic active hepatitis may be difficult. The features that favor chronic persistent over chronic active hepatitis include the segmental character of the limiting plate erosion, the minimal extension of fibrous tissue from the portal tracts into the lobules, the paucity of periportal rosettes and proliferating ductules, and the absence of bridging fibrosis or necrosis. However, in some cases, differentiation is not possible on the basis of a single biopsy specimen, so that serial biopsy studies may be required to establish the nature and prognosis of the lesions. Moreover, since the distinctive features of the lesions in both forms of chronic hepatitis are not uniformly distributed, relatively large needle biopsy sections, at least 1 cm in length, are needed to avoid errors in interpretation due to inadequate sampling.

Distinguishing between the lesions of classic acute viral hepatitis and those of chronic persistent hepatitis during recrudescences may pose an equally difficult problem. The presence of orcein-positive ground glass cells in cases with HBs antigenemia clearly establishes the chronicity of the lesions. In the absence of these markers, other histologic features that point to chronicity include prominence of plasma cells in the portal and intralobular exudates, and the presence of significant portal fibrosis. However, these criteria are not always reliable; differentiation must often depend on a consideration of the clinical features.

As a rule, the lesions of chronic persistent hepatitis show no tendency to progress to chronic active hepatitis or cirrhosis, even when they remain active or undergo repeated relapses over a period of years, and, occasionally they regress spontaneously. However, progression to chronic active hepatitis has been reported in a number of cases (226,227), particularly in patients with chronic persistent hepatitis of insidious onset accompanied by persistent HBs antigenemia (226). More recently pathologists have reported that chronic persistent hepatitis may frequently progress to chronic active hepatitis and vice versa.

Chronic active hepatitis

The lesions of chronic active hepatitis are characterized by mononuclear cell infiltration, fibrosis, and expansion of the portal tracts with destruction of periportal hepatocytes and extension of portal inflammatory cells and fibrous tissue into the lobules. As a rule, the portal tracts are larger and more fibrotic, contain more numerous inflammatory cells, and show more complete erosion of their limiting plates than in active chronic persistent hepatitis. However, when relatively inactive, especially during periods of remission, the lesions of chronic active hepatitis may be indistinguishable from those of chronic persistent hepatitis.

As in the case of chronic persistent hepatitis, the lobules in chronic active hepatitis usually contain foci of inflammation and hepatocellular necrosis that vary in number, size, and distribution, depending on the activity of the disease and its mode of onset. In minimally active lesions that develop insidiously, as in the case of some healthy carriers with HBs antigenemia, the intralobular changes tend to be trivial. However, they may be extensive during exacerbations of the disease, and in cases that are attributable to antecedent acute viral hepatitis with bridging hepatocellular necrosis.

Piecemeal necrosis, usually defined as progressive, unicellular destruction of hepatocytes in the limiting plates of the portal tracts accompanied by a predominantly lymphocytic or plasma cell infiltrate, has been regarded as a key feature in the pathogenesis of chronic active hepatitis by some pathologists (223), but not by others (175). It has been interpreted as evidence of an underlying immune process (228). The presence of acidophilic bodies (229) and the intimate relationship of the infiltrating lymphocytes to the hepatocytes in the margins of the lesion (230) have been emphasized as markers of a cell-mediated immune response. Although other evidence, previously cited, also supports this view, it should be recognized that piecemeal necrosis and the formation of acidophilic bodies are not always attributable to an immunologic reaction. Moreover, while the type of slowly progressive, unicellular loss of hepatocytes characteristic of piecemeal necrosis may account for the destruction of periportal parenchyma in many cases of chronic active hepatitis, some lesions contain zones of confluent bridging or panlobular necrosis that appear to evolve by rapid cytolysis of contiguous hepatocytes. Usually, necrosis of this type is attributable to antecedent acute viral hepatitis that fails to resolve. However, rarely, bridging or panlobular necrosis may be a late development during a relapse or recrudescence of chronic active

hepatitis (231). Early in the course of chronic active hepatitis, zones of bridging or panlobular necrosis may be indistinguishable from those of acute viral hepatitis. However, as the lesions mature, the reticulin fibers and sinusoids tend to collapse, forming septa made up of loosely arranged, thick bundles of fibers that often contain only a modest number of inflammatory cells. Ultimately, the septa may undergo collagenization, but there is suggestive evidence that some may disappear, or become less conspicuous, if the disease becomes inactive.

By far the most important feature of the lesions in chronic active hepatitis is their tendency, in some cases, to progress to cirrhosis. Progressive fibrosis leading to distortion of the lobular architecture and the development of cirrhosis may be the result of slowly advancing piecemeal necrosis, or acute bridging necrosis. Judging from the findings in cases studied serially from the onset of disease, bridging appears to be more important than piecemeal necrosis in the pathogenesis of such cirrhosis (61,231). However, in many cases studied only late in the course of the disease, the lesions are characterized by piecemeal necrosis and bands of connective tissue that link adjacent portal tracts. In such cases, it is generally assumed that the fibrosis is attributable to the accompanying piecemeal necrosis. In the absence of biopsy documentation of the early lesions, however, the possibility of antecedent bridging necrosis can never be excluded.

The view that bridging may be more important than piecemeal necrosis in the pathogenesis of cirrhosis in cases of chronic active hepatitis is not shared by all authorities (223). Their concept that portal-portal bridging necrosis is a form of piecemeal necrosis is open to question, since the pathogenesis and prognostic significance of these two lesions appear to differ. Thus, bridging necrosis is characterized by relatively rapid cytolysis of numerous contiguous hepatocytes, which, when healing is delayed, frequently gives rise to cirrhosis, whereas the principal feature of piecemeal necrosis, implied in its definition, is gradual destruction of hepatocytes one or two at a time that leads to cirrhosis only occasionally.

Figure 459 illustrates the typical features of the early lesions in chronic active hepatitis of insidious onset and mild activity. Characteristically, the portal tracts are enlarged and fibrotic, and contain numerous lymphocytes and plasma cells, occasionally aggregated in the form of follicles, but show no evidence of portal-portal, fibrotic bridging or necrosis, so that the overall lobular architecture is not distorted. As can be seen at higher magnification in Figure 460, the portal tracts invariably show significant periportal piecemeal necrosis, as evidenced by erosion of their limiting plates with extension of inflammatory cells and fine strands of collagen into the surrounding parenchyma. Often, the infiltrating lymphocytes and plasma cells in the advancing edge of the piecemeal necrosis lie in intimate contact with the hepatocytes (Fig. 226). At this early stage, ductular proliferation is only minimal or absent. As a rule, a few small foci of lymphocytes, plasma cells, and swollen Kupffer cells are found scattered through the lobules. Occasionally, these are accompanied by rare acidophilic bodies, but, more commonly, the latter are encountered in the advancing edge of piecemeal periportal necrosis (Fig. 292). In early lesions of this type, the remaining hepatocytes appear normal, but their plate pattern may be slightly thickened and irregular in the periportal zones, and, in cases with chronic HBs antigenemia, some may contain orcein-positive ground glass inclusions (Fig. 292).

The more advanced lesions of chronic active hepatitis exhibit the same features as those found at an early stage, but both portal and intralobular fibrosis are more extensive and, invariably, are accompanied by some degree of bridging fibrosis. In addition, evidence of piecemeal necrosis, ductular proliferation, and hepatocellular regeneration usually are more impressive. Such lesions may develop insidiously, or may present as the sequelae of unresolved acute viral hepatitis with bridging necrosis.

Figure 461 illustrates an example of advanced chronic active hepatitis in a patient who 15 months previously had had a biopsy-documented attack of acute HBsAg-positive viral hepatitis with bridging necrosis. Although corticosteroids had completely suppressed all his symptoms, HBs antigenemia and a modest increase in the serum transaminase levels persisted. The diffuse, intralobular, portal and bridging fibrosis with distortion of the lobular architecture are clearly evident, and, at higher magnification (Fig. 106), it can be seen that most of the hepatocytes are arranged in the form of rosettes encircled by bands of collagen and infiltrating lymphocytes and plasma cells, indicative of active piecemeal necrosis. Although not striking in this case, ductular proliferation (Fig. 462), twin-cell hepatic plates indicative of regenerative activity (Fig. 463), foci of pleomorphic and ballooned hepatocytes (Fig. 464), canalicular bile thrombi, and scattered acidophilic bodies, inflammatory cells, and swollen Kupffer cells may be seen in the active phase of advanced chronic active hepatitis. Rarely, some of the interlobular ducts in such cases exhibit vacuolization, stratification, focal necrosis, and lymphocytic infiltration of their epithelial lining cells (Fig. 465). However, ductal changes of this type may be encountered in the nonviral form of chronic active hepatitis (232). Another feature of the late lesions seen occasionally is the presence within the portal tracts of small isolated groups of hepatocytes that often show degenerative changes (Fig. 466). These undoubtedly represent cells that have escaped destruction during active piecemeal necrosis, and may persist as the only evidence of antecedent periportal necrosis when the lesions are no longer active and the limiting plates appear to be intact.

It is noteworthy that the fibrosis found in the late lesion illustrated in Figure 461 was significantly more extensive than the zones of periportal and bridging necrosis observed in the initial biopsy section obtained early in the course of the disease. This change demonstrates the progressive nature of the lesion, and suggests that piecemeal necrosis may have played a more important role in the pathogenesis of the fibrosis than bridging necrosis.

However, in some cases of advanced chronic active hepatitis attributable to antecedent unresolved acute viral hepatitis, zones of bridging necrosis can still be identified late in the course of the disease, and appear to be the major factor in the pathogenesis of the lesions. Shown in Figure 302 are the extensive portal-portal and portal-central zones of cell dropout and collapse found in the lesions of a patient who was still deeply jaundiced and chronically ill seven months after the abrupt onset of typical, acute viral hepatitis. At higher magnification (Fig. 303), it can be seen that the zones of bridging are made up of collapsed reticulin fibers in which are enmeshed, compressed sinusoids, a few lymphocytes, and occasional degenerating hepatocytes. The adjacent surviving parenchyma shows a diffuse inflammatory reaction, swelling and proliferation of Kupffer cells, occasional acidophilic bodies, and an irregular, thickened, and interrupted plate pattern. However, elsewhere in the same section (Fig. 301), some of the unbridged portal tracts were enlarged and fibrotic, contained numerous lymphocytes, plasma cells, and proliferating ductules, and showed erosion of their

limiting plates with extension of inflammatory cells and fibrous tissue into the periportal parenchyma, suggesting that piecemeal necrosis had played a contributory role in the pathogenesis of the fibrosis in this case.

In many cases of chronic active hepatitis seen for the first time only late in the course of the disease, the lesions show both piecemeal necrosis and portal-portal bridging fibrosis. When the onset has been insidious, it is impossible to judge whether the fibrous bridges are attributable to progressive piecemeal necrosis or to antecedent bridging necrosis. However, when such lesions are found following an attack of acute viral hepatitis that has not been biopsy documented, the clinical features of the attack may suggest that it was associated with bridging necrosis. Figure 467 illustrates a lesion of this type in a heroin addict who six months months previously had suffered a severe attack of HBsAg-positive acute hepatitis with deep jaundice that failed to abate for three months. Although the patient was asymptomatic thereafter, HBs antigenemia and raised serum levels of transaminase persisted. As can be seen, despite the absence of symptoms, the lesions were still active, and were characterized by both piecemeal necrosis and portal-portal bridging fibrosis. The history of deep, prolonged jaundice at the onset suggested that bridging necrosis may have been present initially, and may have accounted for the development of bridging fibrosis. However, in the absence of biopsy documentation of the early lesions, the alternative possibility cannot be excluded that the acute illness represented an exacerbation of previously unrecognized, chronic active hepatitis, a type of presentation that is not rare.

Aggregates of oncocytic (oxyphilic) hepatocytes known as oncocytes, which are usually located adjacent to fibrotic portal tracts or septa, are a relatively common finding in the lesions of HBsAg-positive chronic active hepatitis and cirrhosis (233). However, they are not pathognomonic, and may be seen in other forms of active cirrhosis, and, less commonly, in other hepatic lesions. Characteristically, the cytoplasm of oncocytic hepatocytes is distended with innumerable mitochondria that present as fine, closely packed, acidophilic cytoplasmic granules that appear bright red in H&E-stained (Fig. 124) and deep blue in PTAH-stained sections (Fig. 125).

Viral postnecrotic cirrhosis

HBV, HDV, and the NANB hepatitis viruses are important etiologic factors in the pathogenesis of cirrhosis. The evolution of such lesions is characterized by progressive hepatocellular necrosis and advancing fibrosis that ultimately lead to destruction of the normal lobular architecture. Normal lobules are replaced by nodules of regenerating parenchyma separated by bands of fibrous tissue, a process that may follow an attack of acute hepatitis with bridging or submassive necrosis or that may be attributable to more slowly progressive chronic active hepatitis of insidious onset. However, it should be noted that such lesions do not invariably lead to the development of cirrhosis, and that, in the case of chronic active hepatitis of insidious onset, such progression is rare in the absence of portal-portal bridging fibrosis or necrosis.

Although patients with chronic active hepatitis of insidious onset usually exhibit clinical manifestations of liver disease before the development of cirrhosis, some remain asymptomatic until the cirrhosis gives rise to overt signs of hepatic decom-pensation, or results in hemorrhage from esophageal varices, while others never develop symptoms.

Cirrhosis may be demonstrable histologically within a few months following an attack of acute hepatitis with bridging or submassive necrosis, but usually develops much more slowly in cases of chronic active hepatitis of insidious onset.

Of the two descriptive terms most commonly used in classi-fying such lesions, we prefer "viral postnecrotic cirrhosis," although it has the disadvantage that it once was applied exclu-sively to the type of cirrhosis that follows submassive hepatic necrosis and is characterized by broad zones of fibrosis and huge nodules of regenerating parenchyma (234). The alterna-tive designation, "posthepatitic cirrhosis," appears less appro-priate, since usually it implies the type of cirrhosis that follows an attack of acute hepatitis, and, hence, does not include le-sions that develop insidiously. Moreover, the same term has been applied to macronodular cirrhosis with slender fibrous septa, irrespective of its etiology or mode of onset (234).

The activity of the lesions in viral postnecrotic cirrhosis, judging from the extent of hepatocellular degeneration and ne-crosis, and the intensity of the intraparenchymal inflammatory reaction, usually correlates with the severity of the clinical and biochemical manifestations of hepatic dysfunction, and with the potential for progression of the disease. Although the intensity of the inflammatory reaction in the fibrous septa and portal tracts usually parallels that in the parenchyma, portal and septal in-flammation in the absence of hepatocellular degeneration and necrosis has no significance with respect to disease activity. The activity of viral postnecrotic cirrhosis may be graded as mild, moderate, severe, or inactive, but, more commonly, ac-tive lesions are classified as cirrhosis with chronic active hepa-titis, or chronic active hepatitis with cirrhosis, depending on which of the two features of the disease is predominant.

Most of the parenchymal nodules in viral postnecrotic cirrho-sis are larger than normal lobules, so that the lesions usually are classified as macronodular or mixed micro- and macro-nodular. However, if 3 mm is taken as the minimum diameter of a macronodule, as recommended by some authorities (235), many of the lesions, particularly those encountered in needle biopsy sections, would have to be classified as micronodular.

Figure 450 illustrates the macronodular character of the le-sions in a postmortem section of liver in a case of HBsAg-positive active cirrhosis that proved fatal nine years following a biopsy-documented attack of acute hepatitis with bridging ne-crosis. Almost all of the nodules seen at autopsy exceeded 3 mm in diameter, but none was as large as those often found following submassive hepatic necrosis. The nodules in cases of the latter type may measure up to 5 cm in diameter. They often appear lobulated due to indentations of fibrous septa, may con-tain numerous central veins and portal tracts, which suggest multilobular origin, and are separated by broad zones of col-lapsed reticulin and collagen. Figure 468 illustrates the edge of such a large nodule bordered by a large zone of fibrosis in a case of viral postnecrotic cirrhosis three months following the acute onset of submassive hepatic necrosis. At autopsy, the liver was small and grossly distorted by dense, depressed scars that ranged in width from a few millimeters to 6 cm, and separated coarse nodules of regenerating parenchyma that varied from 0.5 to 5 cm in diameter.

Considering that the width of needle biopsy sections rarely exceeds 1.8 mm, it is not surprising that even the largest nod-ules completely encircled by fibrous tissue found in such sec-tions barely qualify as macronodules, even if a diameter ex-ceeding the width of a normal lobule (1 mm) is used as the criterion for their identification. However, if 3 mm is used to define the lower limits of macronodule diameter, none of the nodules would qualify as macronodules. This is illustrated in Figure 57, which shows a group of nodules ranging from 0.8 to 1.8 mm in their largest diameter in a case of mildly active HBsAg-positive postnecrotic cirrhosis. However, midline or tangential sections through nodules often provide more con-vincing evidence of their macronodular character. Thus, as can be seen in Figure 59, a section through the center of a macron-odule may present as a long ribbon of apparently normal paren-chyma, bordered at either end by a fibrous band, or, as in this case, by the nodules seen in Figure 57. Although such tissue may appear to be made up of normal lobules, it is apparent on closer inspection, even at the low magnification of Figure 59, that many of the hepatic plates are more than one cell thick, and that the central veins are more numerous and show an ab-normal relationship to the single portal tract visualized, features more consistent with the interior of a large regenerating nodule than a group of intact lobules.

Tangential sections are more common than midline sections through macronodules in needle biopsy specimens. In these, the nodules present as large hemispherical or semilunar-shaped islands of regenerating hepatocytes partially outlined by long curvilinear or scalloped fibrous septa (Fig. 58).

Although cirrhotic nodules are generally thought to be masses of regenerating hepatocytes, some may represent islands of pa-renchyma that have escaped destruction. Certainly, groups of intact lobules may be encountered in the early stages of all forms of cirrhosis. However, the absence of an irregular, thick-ened hepatic plate pattern in a nodule does not necessarily im-ply that it is a remnant of intact parenchyma, since, late in the course of cirrhosis, particularly when it is inactive, the hepatic plate pattern in large nodules often reverts to normal (Fig. 56).

The histologic features indicative of activity in viral postne-crotic cirrhosis are identical with those in precirrhotic chronic active hepatitis. Characteristically, the margins of the paren-chymal nodules at their junction with fibrous septa show a varying degree of piecemeal necrosis, as evidenced by erosion of their limiting plates with extension of mononuclear inflammatory cells and fibrous tissue into the parenchyma. In mildly active le-sions, the piecemeal necrosis may be only segmental in distri-bution (Fig. 57), but in those that are highly active, it usually involves the margins of most nodules, and extends more deeply into the parenchyma (Fig. 450). As illustrated in the case of chronic active hepatitis, the hepatocytes in highly active cirrho-sis are often arranged in the form of rosettes encircled by fine, fibrous bands and closely adherent mononuclear cells, espe-cially at the periphery of the nodules (Figs. 106, 226), and may be accompanied by occasional acidophilic bodies (Fig. 292). Deeper in the nodules, the hepatic plates usually are thickened and irregular in contour, and may show foci of cell dropout, infiltration with mononuclear cells and proliferating Kupffer cells (Fig. 458), or ballooning and pleomorphism of the hepatocytes (Fig. 464).

In inactive cirrhotic lesions, the contours of the nodules are smooth, and the parenchyma shows no evidence of necrosis, degeneration, or inflammation, although its plate pattern usu-ally is irregular and thickened. This is illustrated in Figure 449, which shows the inactive cirrhosis found three years following a biopsy-documented attack of acute viral hepatitis with bridging necrosis that progressed to chronic active hepatitis, but was brought into a complete and sustained remission by nine months of corticosteroid therapy.

As in chronic active hepatitis, orcein-positive and aldehyde-fuchsin–positive ground glass cells in variable numbers are found frequently in cases with chronic HBs antigenemia (Figs. 138, 139).

Hepatic cell dysplasia, characterized by enlargement, nuclear pleomorphism, hyperchromasia, and multinucleation of contiguous hepatocytes may be encountered in any type of cirrhosis (Figs. 195, 196), but is most common in those with chronic HBs antigenemia (236). Since it occurs most frequently in cirrhotic lesions complicated by hepatocellular carcinoma, such dysplasia has been interpreted as evidence of a precancerous state (236).

The fibrous septa in viral postcirrhosis vary greatly in width, ranging from slender (Fig. 449) to relatively thick (Fig. 57) or broad (Fig. 468). Although they tend to widen with advancing age and activity of the lesions, the broadest septa are seen in the type of cirrhosis that follows healing of submassive hepatic necrosis, irrespective of its age or activity. In the late, inactive phase of postnecrotic cirrhosis, the septa are densely collagenized, contain only a few inflammatory cells and proliferating ductules, and are smooth-contoured, except for occasional slender, fibrous spurs that project into the parenchyma (Figs. 52–54, 449).

In advanced active lesions, the septa are more irregular in contour and less sharply defined, owing to the accompanying piecemeal necrosis, and often appear less densely collagenized, owing to separation of the collagen bundles by numerous infiltrating lymphocytes and plasma cells (Fig. 450). Occasionally, ductular proliferation is a prominent feature in such lesions (Fig. 462), although these tend to disappear with advancing fibrosis.

As in the active phase of chronic active hepatitis, an occasional interlobular duct may show vacuolization, stratification, focal necrosis, or lymphocytic infiltration of its lining epithelial cells (Fig. 465), and, often, the septal lymphocytes and plasma cells are aggregated in the form of lymphoid follicles (Fig. 304).

Not infrequently, some of the large regenerating nodules in postnecrotic cirrhosis contain a number of apparently normal portal tracts and central veins (Fig. 55). Although these may suggest a collection of intact lobules, the abnormal number and organization of these structures, and the presence of thickened, irregular hepatic plates serve to identify them as components of a regenerating nodule. However, such differentiation may be difficult, if not impossible in small needle biopsy specimens.

HBsAg-associated hepatocellular carcinoma

As previously indicated, the hepatitis B virus plays an important role in the pathogenesis of hepatocellular carcinoma, both as a relatively common cause of cirrhosis and as an oncogenic agent (84).

Most cases of hepatocellular carcinoma present as a complication of underlying cirrhosis that may vary in etiology, but usually is of the nacronodular type (237). The reported incidence of cirrhosis in such cases ranges from 40 to 90% (238).

The frequency with which hepatocellular carcinoma develops in different forms of cirrhosis varies, depending, in part at least, on the etiology of the underlying cirrhosis, being relatively low in those of alcoholic origin (2–5%) and highest in those attributable to hepatitis B infection (up to 50%).

In most studies of hepatocellular carcinoma reported from Africa (112) and other areas with high HBsAg-carrier rates, antigenemia has been detectable in approximately 60 to 70% of cases. Although a similarly high incidence of HB viral infection was found in Los Angeles (238), significantly lower rates have usually been reported from this country and others where carrier rates are low.

The frequency with which HBsAg-positive hepatocellular carcinoma occurs in the absence of cirrhosis varies greatly, ranging from approximately 5% of cases in Los Angeles (238) to 63% in Senegal, Africa (112). The explanation for this striking difference is not clear. However, the unusually high incidence of noncirrhotic hepatocellular carcinoma in Senegal may be related to the fact that carrier infections in that country occur primarily during the first few years of life (239), and that the carcinoma usually develops one or two decades earlier than in the United States (109,238).

The cirrhosis associated with HBsAg-positive hepatocellular carcinoma almost always is macronodular or mixed micro- and macronodular in type, and often is relatively inactive (Fig. 469). As a rule, the lesion has no distinctive features, except for the frequent presence of a variable number of orcein- and aldehyde-fuchsin-positive ground glass cells, and the occasional occurrence of hepatic cell dysplasia. In some cases, tumor thrombi may be found in portal vein radicles, but only rarely are the sinusoids similarly invaded, even in areas close to large tumor masses. Histologic evidence of cholestasis is relatively common late in the course of the disease when the liver contains numerous satellite tumor nodules, but may be seen early in the case of large centrally located tumors that impinge on the major hepatic ducts at their bifurcation near the porta hepatitis.

The histologic features of HBsAg-positive hepatocellular carcinoma, whether or not associated with cirrhosis, are identical with those in other forms of the neoplasm. Usually, the neoplastic cells resemble hepatocytes, but tend to be larger and slightly more basophilic, show significant pleomorphism, hyperchromasia, increased nuclear size, prominence of nucleoli, and a variable degree of mitotic activity, and are arranged in an irregular trabecular pattern (Fig. 470). Well-differentiated tumor masses may be difficult to distinguish from nodules of regenerating parenchyma, but usually the sparsity of reticulin fibers and absence of a well-defined sinusoidal pattern and of Kupffer cells in the former serve to differentiate between the two. In the case of highly undifferentiated hepatocellular carcinomas, the absence of a desmoplastic reaction and the occasional presence of bile thrombi or Mallory bodies often prove useful in their differentiation from metastatic, anaplastic neoplasms (see Chapter 25).

Usually, no HBs antigen-bearing, orcein-positive ground glass cells are demonstrable in the neoplastic cells of HBsAg-positive hepatocellular carcinoma, even when they are numerous in adjacent, intact hepatocytes. however, in some cases, antigen-bearing neoplastic cells have been identified by means of immunofluorescence, immunoperoxidase, and orcein-staining (240). Moreover, several human hepatoma cell lines derived from patients with HBs antigenemia have been shown to produce the antigen *in vitro* (241).

Effects of therapy on the lesions of viral hepatitis

Classic acute hepatitis

Corticosteroid therapy is capable of inducing a prompt remission in classic acute viral hepatitis, but, since this disease usually resolves spontaneously, such therapy is seldom employed. It may be used to advantage when the activity of acute viral hepatitis fails to abate over a period of several weeks. Under such conditions, corticosteroids in modest doses, e.g., 20 mg/day tapered over a period of weeks, usually induces resolution of the lesions with few if any minor residuals. However, it has been suggested that corticosteroid therapy may lead to persistence of HBs antigenemia and the development of chronic hepatitis, and, that withdrawal of the drug may result in a transient relapse (161). However, in two well-controlled studies of severe HBsAg-positive acute hepatitis, large dose corticosteroid therapy failed to retard clearing of the antigen from the serum or to potentiate the development of chronic hepatitis (75,242).

Acute hepatitis with bridging necrosis

Both our own experience and that reported from the Mayo Clinic (231) attest to the effectiveness of prednisone therapy in suppressing the activity of the lesions in acute viral hepatitis with bridging necrosis that fail to heal spontaneously. Although such lesions were uniformly classified as chronic in the Mayo Clinic series, they are relevant to this discussion, since some of them were still acute by conventional standards, ranging in duration from 10 to 25 weeks.

Following prednisone therapy, in almost half the cases of acute viral bridging necrosis, the lesions resolve either completely or with only minimal residual portal scarring or relatively inactive chronic persistent hepatitis. In the remaining cases, the activity of the lesions is suppressed to a variable degree, but they progress to chronic active hepatitis or cirrhosis. Such progression is less common than in untreated cases.

As previously reported in a group of young individuals ill for less than a month with predominantly HBsAg-positive acute hepatitis and bridging necrosis, but unaccompanied by ascites, edema, or hepatic encephalopathy, large doses of prednisolone, as compared to a placebo, had no effect on the rate of resolution or progression of the lesions (75). Moreover, it was found that spontaneous healing of such lesions in the placebo-treated controls of this study occurred more frequently than had been observed previously (61).

Chronic active hepatitis and cirrhosis

Despite differences and certain deficiencies in their design (243), all controlled trials of corticosteroids in the treatment of chronic active hepatitis with or without cirrhosis have led to the conclusion that such therapy tends to suppress the activity of the disease, retards or prevents progression of the lesions to cirrhosis, and reduces the mortality rate (244–246). In one of these studies (246), however, the HBsAg-positive patients appeared to be less responsive than those who were HBsAg-negative (225). Azathioprine, perhaps by reducing the dose of corticosteroids required for control of the disease, may be a useful adjuvant in therapy (246), but is ineffective when used alone (245,246).

In evaluating the effects of corticosteroids on the lesions of chronic active hepatitis, due consideration must be given to their histologic features at the onset of therapy, and their natural history in untreated cases. Such data are available only in one controlled trial in which serial liver biopsy was carried out routinely (231,246). Corticosteroid therapy led to a reduction in the activity of the lesions in most cases, although the improvement was not always complete. Similar regression of the lesions was observed in some untreated controls. However, the differences between the behavior of the lesions in the two groups, although not double-blind, were most impressive in the case of lesions characterized by bridging or multilobular necrosis. Thus, in 11 patients with such lesions who received no corticosteroids, there was progression to cirrhosis in 7 (63%), regression to chronic active hepatitis without bridging or multilobular necrosis in 2 or to chronic persistent hepatitis in 1, and no change in the character of the lesions in 1. In contrast, in 17 corticosteroid-treated cases of chronic active hepatitis with bridging or multilobular necrosis, the lesions progressed to cirrhosis in only 4 (24%) (p<0.01), regressed to chronic active hepatitis without bridging or multilobular necrosis in 3 or to chronic persistent hepatitis in 8, and showed no change in their character in 2. The behavior of the lesions in chronic active hepatitis unaccompanied by bridging or multilobular necrosis, however, was similar in the two groups.

Based on our experience and that of others (231,246,247), it is clear that corticosteroids can suppress the activity of the lesions in some cases of cirrhosis accompanied by chronic active hepatitis, some of which are of viral etiology. However, there is no convincing evidence that such therapy increases longevity or prevents cirrhosis. In one study of patients with cirrhosis (247), the survival rate in nonalcoholic women treated with corticosteroids prior to the appearance of ascites was significantly higher than that in controls.

The studies demonstrating the efficacy of corticosteroids in the treatment of chronic active hepatitis were carried out in patients, who, for the most part, had highly active lesions that were symptomatic. Although neither the effects of nor the necessity for such therapy in the case of less severe and asymptomatic lesions has been demonstrated, corticosteroids often are used routinely in all cases of chronic active hepatitis, a practice that cannot be condoned (248).

Chronic active HBV hepatitis

α-Interferon therapy has been used to treat chronic active HBV hepatitis in numerous randomized clinical trials with mixed results (249–255) (see Chapter 8). It appears that more than one-half of the treated patients lose serum HBV DNA and HBeAg, many develop anti-HBe, and about one-fourth become HBSAg-negative, findings that occur significantly less frequently in randomly selected, untreated, control patients (255). Improvement tends to follow a period of clinical and laboratory exacerbation (255). Both biosynthetic and recombinant interferon seem equally efficacious. It appears that women with high serum alanine aminotransferase activity are especially responsive. Asian patients are less responsive. Furthermore, gay men and intravenous drug abusers, presumably immunocompromised patients, tend not to respond. The histologic severity of the hepatic lesions does not predict responsiveness.

These serologic benefits are accompanied by histologic improvement that consists primarily of decreased inflammation and necrosis, findings that are also noted during spontaneous clearance of HBeAg (256–258) and HBsAg (259). These observations support the concept that hepatic damage develops when HBV replicates as mature virions rather than when the HBV DNA is integrated into the host genome (260,261).

Adenine arabinoside 5'-monophosphate has been used in the treatment of chronic active hepatitis B with mixed results in four randomized clinical trials (262–265). About one-half of patients so treated responded with the loss of HBV DNA compared with none of the untreated control patients (265). These changes, which appear inconstant, incomplete, and temporary, are not accompanied by histologic improvement (265). Female patients and patients with high serum alanine aminotransferase levels (ALT) and low serum HBV DNA seem to be more responsive to this therapy than men with low ALT activity and active HBV replication. These characteristics are similar to those that predict responsiveness to alpha-interferon therapy.

Chronic active HDV hepatitis

Recombinant α-interferon suppresses viral replication in chronic active HDV hepatitis as shown by the disappearance of HDV RNA and improved blood tests in a substantial portion of patients so treated (266). So far most such patients have relapsed on cessation of therapy.

Chronic NANB hepatitis

The use of *recombinant* α-interferon in medium to large doses (5–10 million units/day) for periods of three to four months results in improvement in clinical features, in serologic abnormalities, and in hepatic blood tests in more than 90% of patients (267). The improvement, which is usually transient, follows a brief three- to four-day exacerbation of the disease, i.e., a worsening in symptoms and an increase in serum ALT activity. The responses appear to be better in patients with mild or moderate disease by histologic criteria than in those with severe CAH. CAH of short duration is more responsive. Relapses during treatment are common and recurrences when therapy is discontinued are characteristic.

Adrenocorticoids are ineffective in chronic active NANB hepatitis although they are effective in autoimmune chronic hepatitis (268). The existence of an antibody test for HBC CAH will permit for the first time unequivocal differentiation of autoimmune from NANB CAH.

Fulminant viral hepatitis and massive hepatic necrosis

Available evidence, based on the results of three randomized, controlled trials (269–271), suggest that corticosteroids do not increase the survival rate in cases of fulminant hepatitis.

Fulminant hepatitis is a clinical rather than a morphologic entity, usually being defined as an acute hepatitis of less than four to six weeks' duration that is accompanied by hepatic encephalopathy and a prolonged prothrombin time (76,77,269–272). Although it is often assumed that the syndrome is always attributable to underlying massive hepatic necrosis (269), the lesions in such cases are highly variable. In fatal cases, postmortem examination invariably reveals submassive or massive hepatocellular necrosis or extensive bridging necrosis. However, the lesions appear to be less severe in those that survive. Thus, in a biopsy study of 22 patients with fulminant hepatitis who ultimately recovered without significant sequelae, the liver showed mild to moderate centrilobular necrosis in all but one case, and varying degrees of accompanying bridging necrosis in 11 (76). However, in none of the cases was there evidence of massive or submassive hepatic necrosis, even though 13 of the 22 patients had been in stage III or IV hepatic coma for periods of 3 to 10 days. This absence attests to the tremendous regenerative capacity of the liver.

Since the extent of hepatic necrosis undoubtedly is a major factor in determining the outcome of fulminant hepatitis (79), variations in the severity of the lesions, which cannot be identified on the basis of their clinical or biochemical manifestations (76,79), almost certainly account for the wide range of survival rates, which range from as high as 64% to as low as 25% (77).

It is evident, therefore, that valid assessment of the effects of therapy on survival in fulminant hepatitis is not possible, even in the most carefully controlled randomized trials, unless the character of the lesions prior to therapy is documented by biopsy, or a sufficiently large number of patients are investigated to ensure a comparable distribution of the variable lesions in the treatment and control groups. Thus, the negative findings can not be regarded as definitive.

Considering that most of the hepatocytes are destroyed in massive hepatic necrosis, it is highly improbable that any form of therapy can facilitate recovery. However, since immunosuppressive therapy tends to suppress other types of lesions in acute viral hepatitis, it is conceivable that immunosuppressive therapy may facilitate the healing of those lesions in fulminant hepatitis that are characterized by centrilobular, bridging, or multilobular necrosis, and, thus, may permit recovery in occasional cases.

Histologic differential diagnosis of viral hepatitis

Acute viral hepatitis

As a rule, the lesions in the hepatitic form of *drug-induced* hepatitis and in posttransplant rejection may be indistinguishable from those of acute viral hepatitis. The presence of numerous infiltrating eosinophils or occasional granulomas favors a drug-induced lesion, but neither of these findings is a constant feature. Other histologic findings that have been suggested as possible criteria for identifying such lesions include fatty infiltration, early periportal cholestasis, bile-duct damage, and, at least in the type of hepatitis produced by halothane, sharply circumscribed centrilobular zones of confluent necrosis (273,274). However, in our experience, none of these criteria has proved reliable in differentiating between viral and drug-induced hepatitis.

The hepatic lesions of *infectious mononucleosis* (Chapter 23) often resemble those of acute viral hepatitis, but may show other features suggestive of the diagnosis. Of these, the most distinctive is a marked discrepancy between the extent of hepatocellular necrosis and the intensity of the accompanying intralobular and portal inflammatory reaction. Characteristically, the necrosis involves only occasional scattered hepatocytes, whereas the parenchyma and portal tracts are heavily infiltrated by large and small lymphocytes, accompanied by numerous swollen, proliferating Kupffer cells, and, less frequently, by small granulomas. Despite the minimal extent of the necrosis, the hepatocytes often show significantly increased mitotic activity. Unfortunately, these features are not pathognomonic, and may be seen occasionally in cases of mild, acute, viral or drug-induced hepatitis, in liver rejection syndromes, and, less commonly, in the mononucleosis syndrome attributable to infections with the *cytomegalovirus* or *Toxoplasma gondii* (Chapter 23).

In *leptospirosis* (Chapter 23), the hepatic lesions may mimic those of classic acute viral hepatitis, but, more commonly, they resemble those of viral or drug-induced cholestatic hepatitis. Usually, cholestasis is a prominent feature, whereas hepatocellular necrosis, lobular disarray, and intralobular and portal inflammation tend to be mild. Often, hepatocellular regeneration, as evidenced by prominent mitotic activity, binucleation, and pleomorphism is increased out of proportion to the extent of necrosis.

Cholestatic hepatitis

In the early phases of acute viral hepatitis with cholestasis, the prominence of hepatocellular degeneration and necrosis, the lobular disarray, and the diffuse character of the inflammatory reaction serve to differentiate the lesions from those of *extrahepatic biliary obstruction* (Chapter 20). However, when the course of the disease is prolonged, the distinctive intralobular changes tend to disappear, so the lesions may then be characterized exclusively by cholestasis and portal inflammation. Under such conditions, differentiation of the lesions from those of extrahepatic biliary obstruction may be difficult. Although portal neutrophils and marginal ductular proliferation tend to be less conspicuous in prolonged cholestatic hepatitis than in extrahepatic biliary obstruction, the prominence of these features in the two types of lesions overlap to such an extent that they cannot be regarded as reliable criteria for their differentiation.

A number of other less common forms of cholestasis, discussed more fully in Chapter 19, are also characterized by lesions that may be indistinguishable from those in the late stage of unresolved viral cholestatic hepatitis. Included among them are the types of cholestasis that follow the administration of *oral contraceptives* or *synthetic anabolic and androgenic steroids,* and those associated with prolonged *parenteral hyperalimentation,* the *postoperative* state, extrahepatic *Hodgkin's disease, pregnancy,* and the syndrome of *benign recurrent intrahepatic cholestasis.* Histologic differentiation of such lesions from those of viral cholestatic hepatitis, as in the case of extrahepatic biliary obstruction, is not difficult when the cholestasis is of relatively brief duration, but may not be possible when it

is prolonged. Under such conditions, differentiation almost always depends on the accompanying clinical features.

Massive and submassive hepatic necrosis

Any of the hepatitis viruses and a number of drugs (Chapter 7) are responsible for most cases of massive or submassive hepatic necrosis. As a rule, histologic differentiation between the lesions of viral and drug or toxin-induced hepatitis is not possible, unless the latter contain numerous eosinophils, granulomas, or both.

Although usually confined to the centrilobular zones, *ischemic necrosis* due to shock, hypovolemia, or left ventricular heart failure, when severe may be panlobular in distribution, at least in some areas. The acidophilic, coagulative character of the hepatocellular necrosis, the absence of inflammatory cells in the portal tracts initially and their neutrophilic nature later, and the frequency of accompanying sinusoidal congestion and intralobular hemorrhage serve to differentiate such lesions from those of viral or drug-induced submassive hepatic necrosis. However, in autopsy specimens of viral and drug-induced hepatic necrosis, postmortem autolysis may lead to artifactual cytoplasmic coagulation and loss of nuclei in the hepatocytes of surviving parenchyma, and to dissolution of the accompanying inflammatory exudate, so the lesions may superficially resemble those of ischemic necrosis.

A number of other viral agents have been implicated in the pathogenesis of extensive and often fatal hepatic necrosis. *Yellow fever,* disseminated *Herpes simplex,* the arenavirus of *Lassa fever,* and the *Marburg virus* produce such lesions regularly, whereas the *Coxsackie* and *adenoviruses* do so only rarely. Each of these lesions has distinctive features that are described in Chapter 23.

Chronic active hepatitis

At least three etiologic factors have been implicated in the pathogenesis of chronic active hepatitis: (1) infection with the HBV, HCV, or HDV virus, (2) reactions to certain drugs (Chapter 7), and (3) autoimmunity (Chapter 8). Except for the presence of orcein-positive ground glass cells in many cases attributable to hepatitis B infection, these etiologically diverse lesions are histologically indistinguishable from one another.

The problem of differentiating between chronic active hepatitis, *chronic persistent hepatitis,* and *unresolved acute hepatitis* has been discussed previously.

The lesions of *primary biliary cirrhosis* (Chapter 11) resemble those of chronic active hepatitis, but have a number of distinctive features, so that differentiation between the two usually poses no problem. However, in a minority of cases, the histologic features in the two disorders overlap to such an extent that a clear distinction between them is difficult, if not impossible. Indeed, it has been suggested that mixed forms of chronic active hepatitis and primary biliary cirrhosis occur, and that these can be identified by the presence in the serum of a unique type of mitochondrial antibody. The principal features of the lesions in classic primary biliary cirrhosis that serve to distinguish them from those of chronic active hepatitis include the following: (1) piecemeal necrosis is an inconstant finding, and, when present, tends to be segmental, and rarely involves more than an occasional portal tract; (2) degeneration, necrosis, and inflammation of the epithelial lining cells, and disruption of the basement membranes of medium sized interlobular and septal bile ducts are found more frequently and tend to be more severe; (3) epithelioid granulomas in the portal tracts, especially adjacent to degenerating ducts, and, occasionally, in the parenchyma are relatively common; (4) often, the periportal hepatocytes are ballooned, and, occasionally, contain Mallory bodies; and (5) bile thrombi may be found in periportal canaliculi before they appear in the centrilobular zones.

As a rule, the hepatic lesions of *primary sclerosing cholangitis* (Chapters 19 and 24) are characterized by expansion, fibrosis, and inflammation of the portal tracts, and often exhibit segmental erosion of their limiting plates, so that they may be mistaken for those of chronic active hepatitis. However, the portal exudates usually contain more neutrophils and eosinophils, and fewer lymphocytes and plasma cells than in chronic active hepatitis, and periportal hepatocellular necrosis and extension of fibrous tissue and inflammatory cells into the lobules tend to be more limited in extent. Periductal concentric lamellar fibrosis and fibrotic obliteration of septal bile ducts, features generally regarded as distinctive of primary sclerosing cholangitis, are rarely encountered in needle biopsy specimens, and are demonstrable in only a third of cases in surgical wedge biopsy sections.

In some cases of *Wilson's disease* the hepatic lesions may closely resemble those of chronic active hepatitis. As a rule, such lesions have advanced to the stage of cirrhosis by the time that they are recognized. Although not always demonstrable, the features found in routine sections that may suggest the diagnosis of Wilson's disease include the presence of Mallory bodies, numerous glycogen nuclei, fatty infiltration, or coarse cytoplasmic lipofuscin granules in periportal hepatocytes. The detection of numerous copper-containing cytoplasmic granules in rhodanine- and orcein-stained sections tends to support the diagnosis, and may be found in the absence of the other features just described (Chapter 13).

Chronic persistent hepatitis

The lesions of *unresolved acute viral hepatitis* that fail to heal within six months, if unaccompanied by significant piecemeal necrosis, are usually classified as chronic persistent hepatitis. Except for the presence of orcein-positive ground glass cells in those with persistent HBs antigenemia, the lesions are indistinguishable from those of nonviral etiology.

As previously indicated, significant piecemeal necrosis is the critical feature that distinguishes between *chronic active hepatitis* and *chronic persistent hepatitis.*

Minor histologic abnormalities, classified by some as *nonspecific reactive hepatitis,* may be encountered in a wide variety of extrahepatic systemic and infectious disorders. Such lesions are characterized by variable combinations of portal fibrosis and inflammation, ductular proliferation, focal hepatocellular necrosis or degeneration, hepatocellular regeneration, fatty infiltration, and focal collections of swollen Kupffer cells. In cases with predominantly portal abnormalities, the lesions may be indistinguishable from those of chronic persistent hepatitis. Included in this group by some are the lesions classified by others

as *triaditis* or *pericholangitis* that may be associated with chronic inflammatory disease in the biliary tract or pancreas (Chapters 19 and 20) or with inflammatory bowel disease (Chapter 24).

Cirrhosis

In its late inactive phase, viral postnecrotic cirrhosis usually is indistinguishable from other forms of macronodular cirrhosis (Chapter 9), except for the presence of orcein-positive ground glass cells in cases with persistent HBs antigenemia.

Late in its course, particularly following prolonged abstention from alcohol, *alcoholic cirrhosis* frequently is macronodular in type (Chapter 10). When inactive, the lesions may show no distinctive features. However, in some cases, they may exhibit features suggestive of antecedent alcoholic hepatitis, such as extensive fibrous capillarization of the sinusoids or the presence within the septa of central veins that are occluded by fibrous tissue, and often are partially recanalized. In lesions that are more active, hepatocellular ballooning, Mallory bodies, neutrophils, or fatty infiltration may be seen.

In cases of advanced *Wilson's disease* that present with predominantly neurologic manifestations, the hepatic lesions almost always are characterized by an inactive form of macronodular cirrhosis. These invariably contain numerous irregularly distributed, copper-containing cytoplasmic granules, and may, in addition, exhibit other features suggestive of Wilson's disease, such as numerous glycogen nuclei, fatty infiltration, and coarse, periportal cytoplasmic lipofuscin granules (Chapter 13).

Cryptogenic cirrhosis, an appropriate designation for any type of cirrhosis of unknown etiology, includes some lesions that are indistinguishable from those of macronodular, inactive, viral postnecrotic cirrhosis (Chapter 9).

References

1. McIntyre N, Benhamou J-P, Bircher J, Rizzetto M, Rodes J. Viral hepatitis. *In* Oxford Textbook of Clinical Hepatology. Oxford, Oxford University Press, 1991. p. 529–626.
2. Ticehurst JR, Racaniello VR, Baroudy BM. Molecular cloning and characterization of hepatitis A virus cDNA. Proc Natl Acad Sci USA *80:*5885–5889, 1983.
3. Mijch AM, Gust ID: Clinical, serologic and epidemiologic aspects of Hepatitis A virus infection. Semin Liver Dis *6:*42–45, 1986.
4. Lemon SM: Type A viral hepatitis: new developments in an old disease. N Engl J Med *313:*1059–1067, 1985.
5. Szmuness W, Dienstag JL, Purcell RH, Harley EJ, Stevens CE, Wong DC: Distribution of antibody to hepatitis A antigen in urban adult populations. N Engl J Med *295:*755–759, 1976.
6. Kao HW, Ashcavai M, Redeker AG: The persistence of hepatitis A IgM antibody after acute clinical hepatitis A. Hepatology *4:*933–936, 1984.
7. Slusarczyk J, Hansson BG, Nordenfelt K: Etiopathogenic aspects of hepatitis A: specific and non-specific humoral immune response during the course of infection. J Med Virol *14:*269–277, 1984.
8. Mathiesen LR, Feinstone SM, Purcell RH, Wagner JA: Detection of hepatitis A antigen by immunofluorescence. Infect Immun *18:*524–530, 1977.
9. Provost PJ, Hughes JV, Miller WJ: An inactivated hepatitis A viral vaccine of cell culture origin. J Med Virol *19:*23–31, 1986.
10. Heathcote J, Sherlock S: Spread of acute type-B hepatitis in London. Lancet *1:*1468–1473, 1973.
11. Centers for Disease Control: Update on hepatitis B prevention. Ann Intern Med *107:*353–360, 1987.
12. Chang M-H, Hsu H-C, Lee C-Y, Wang T-R, Kao C-L: Neonatal hepatitis: a follow-up study. J Pediatr Gastroenterol Nutr *6:*203–207, 1987.
13. Szmuness W, Much MI, Prince AM, Hoofnagle JH, Cherubin CE,

Harley EJ, Block GH: On the role of sexual behavior in the spread of Hepatitis B infection. Ann Intern Med 83:489–495, 1975.

14. Newkirk MM, Downe AER, Simon JB: Fate of ingested Hepatitis B antigen in blood-sucking insects. Gastroenterology 69:982–987, 1975.

15. Szmuness W, Prince AM, Brotman AM, Hiroch RL: Hepatitis B antigen and antibody in blood donors: an epidemiologic study. J. Infect Dis 127:17–25, 1973.

16. Sherlock, S: Viral hepatitis. In Diseases of the Liver and Biliary System, edited by S. Sherlock. 8th Edition. London, Blackwell Scientific Publications, 1989, p. 338.

17. Botha JF, Ritchie MJJ, Dusheiko GM: Hepatitis B virus carrier state in black children in Ovamboland: role of perinatal and horizontal infection. Lancet 1:1210–121, 1984.

18. Hoffnagle JH, Schafer DF: Serologic markers of Hepatitis B virus infection. Semin Liver Dis 6:1–10, 1986.

19. Summers J, O'Connell A, Millman I: Genome of hepatitis B virus: restriction enzyme cleavage and structure of DNA extracted from Dane particles. Proc Natl Acad Sci USA 72:4597–4601, 1975.

20. Meyer zum Buschenfelde K-H, Gerken G, Hess G. The significance of the pre-S region of the hepatitis B virus. J Hepatol 3:273–279, 1986.

21. Gudat F, Bianchi L, Sonnabend W, Thiel G, Aenishaenslin W, Stalder GA: Pattern of core and surface expression in liver tissue reflects state of specific immune response in hepatitis B. Lab Invest 32:1–9, 1975.

22. Lamothe F, Laurencin-Piche J, Cote J, Guevin R, Viallet A, Richer G: Detection of surface and core antigens of hepatitis B virus in the liver of 164 human subjects. A study of immunoperoxidase and orcein staining. Gastroenterology 71:102–108, 1976.

23. Bianchi L, Gudat F: Sanded nuclei in hepatitis B. Eosinophilic inclusions in liver cell nuclei due to excess hepatitis B core antigen formation. Lab Invest 35:1–5, 1976.

24. Gowans EJ, Burrell CJ: Widespread presence of cytoplasmic HBcAg in hepatitis B infected liver detected by improved immunochemical methods. J Clin Pathol 38:393–398, 1985.

25. Shikata T, Uzawa T, Yoshiwara N, Akatsuka T, Yamazaki S: Staining methods of Australia antigen in paraffin section: detection of cytoplasmic inclusion bodies. Jpn J Exp Med 44:25–36, 1974.

26. Krogsgaard JM, Kryger P, Aldersvile J: Hepatitis B virus DNA in serum from patients with acute hepatitis B. Hepatology 5:10–13, 1985.

27. Seeff LB, Beebe GW, Hoofnagle JH, Norman JE, Buskell-Bales Z, Waggoner JG, Kaplowitz N, Koff RS, Petrini JL, Schiff ER, Shorey J, Stanley MM: A serologic follow-up of the 1942 epidemic of post-vaccination hepatitis in the United States Army. N Engl J Med 315:965–970, 1987.

28. Hoofnagle JH: Serodiagnosis of acute viral hepatitis. Hepatology 3:267–268, 1983.

29. Taylor PE, Zuckerman AJ, Bird RG: Electron microscopy of hepatitis associated antigens. Vox Sang 19:246–253, 1970.

30. Zuckerman AJ (ed.): Viral Hepatitis and Liver Disease, New York, Alan R. Liss, 1988, p. 1158.

31. Krugman S, Hoofnagle JH, Gerety RJ, Kaplan PM, Gerin JL: Viral hepatitis, type B. DNA polymerase activity and antibody to hepatitis B core antigen. N Engl J Med 290:1331–1335, 1974.

32. Koretz RL: The serology of viral hepatitis. Making sense out of alphabet soup. In Modern Concepts of Acute and Chronic Hepatitis, edited by G. Gitnick. New York, Plenum Medical Book Company, 1989, p. 51–66.

33. Alter HJ, Seeff LB, Kaplan PM, McAuliffe VJ, Wright EC, Gerin JL, Purcell RH, Holland PV, Zimmerman HJ: Type B hepatitis: the infectivity of blood positive for e antigen and DNA polymerase after accidental needlestick exposure. N Engl J Med 295:909–913, 1976.

34. Tassopoulos NC, Papaevangelou GJ, Roumeliotou-Karayannis A, Ticehurst JR, Feinstone SM, Purcell RH: Detection of hepatitis B virus DNA in asymptomatic hepatitis B surface antigen carriers: relation to sexual transmission. Am J Epidemiol 126:587–591, 1987.

35. Seeff LB, Koff RS: Evolving concepts of the clinical and serologic consequences of hepatitis B virus infection. Semin Liver Dis 6:11–22, 1986.

36. Weller IVD, Fowler MJF, Monjardino J: The detection of HBV DNA in serum by molecular hybridization: a more sensitive method for detection of complete HBV particles J Med Virol 9:273–280, 1982.

37. Bonino F, Rizzetto M: Hepatitis delta virus in acute and chronic liver disease. In Modern Concepts of Acute and Chronic Hepatitis, edited by G. Gitnick. New York, Plenum Medical Book Company, New York, 1989, pp. 113–126.

38. Rizzetto M, Canese MG, Bonino F, Ponzetto A, Smedile A: The hepatitis delta virus (HDV): a common origin with plant viruses? Ital J Gastroenterol 19:235–238, 1987.

39. Bonino, F, Smedile A: Delta agent (Type D) hepatitis. Semin Liver Dis 6:28–32, 1986.

40. Rizzetto M, Canese MG, Arico S: Immunofluorescence detection of a new antigen-antibody system (delta/anti-delta) associated to the hepatitis B virus in the liver and in the serum of HBsAg carriers. Gut 18:997–1003, 1977.

41. Aragona M, Caredda F, Lavarini C, Farci P, Macagno S, Crivelli O, Maran E, Purcell RH, Rizzetto M: Serological response to the hepatitis Delta virus in hepatitis D. Lancet 1:478–481, 1987.

42. Jackson, IM, Dienstag JL, Werner BG, Brettler DB, Levine PH, Mushahwar IK: Epidemiology and clinical impact of hepatitis D virus (delta) infection. Hepatology 5:188–191, 1985.

43. Purcell, RH, Gerin JL: Epidemiology of the delta agent: an introduction. Prog Clin Biol Res 143:113–119, 1983.

44. Bradley DW, Maynard JE, Popper H: Posttransfusion non-A, non-B hepatitis: physicochemical properties of two distinct agents. J Infect Dis 148:254–265, 1983.

45. Hollinger FB, Mosley JW, Szmuness W: Transfusion-transmitted viruses study: experimental evidence for two non-A, non-B agents. J Infect Dis 142:400–407, 1980.

46. Tabor E: The three viruses of non-A, non-B hepatitis. Lancet 1:743–745, 1985.

47. Choo Q-L, Kuo G, Weiner AJ, Overby LR, Bradley DW, Houghton M: Isolation of a cDNA clone derived froma blood-borne non-A, non-B viral hepatitis genome. Science 244:359–362, 1989.

48. Kuo G, Choo Q-L, Alter HJ, Gitnick GL, Redeker AG, Purcell RH, Miyamura T, Dienstag JL, Alter MJ, Stevens CE, Tegtmeier GE, Bonino F, Colombo M, Lee W-S, Kuo C, Berger K, Shuster JR, Overby LR, Bradley DW, Houghton M: An assay for circulating antibodies to a major etiologic virus of human non-A, non-B hepatitis. Science 244:361–364, 1989.

49. Alter HJ, Purcell RH, Shih JW: Detection of antibody to hepatitis C virus in prospectively followed transfusion recipients with acute and chronic non-A, non-B hepatitis. N Engl J Med 321:1494–1500, 1989.

50. Weiner AJ, Kuo G, Bradley DW: Detection of hepatitis C viral sequences in non-A, non-B hepatitis. Lancet 335:1–3, 1990.

51. Esteban JI, Esteban R, Viladomiu L: Hepatitis C virus antibodies among risk groups in Spain. Lancet 2:294–297, 1989.

52. Martin P, Di Bisceglie AM, Kassianides C: Rapidly progressive non-A, non-B hepatitis in patients with human immunodeficiency virus infection. Gastroenterology 97:1550–1555, 1989.

53. Colombo M, Choo Q-L, Ninno ED: Prevalence of antibodies to hepatitis C virus in Italian patients with hepatocellular carcinoma. Lancet 2:1006–1008, 1989.

54. Sanchez-Tapias JM, Barrera JM, Costa J, Ercilla MG, Gares A, Comalrrena L, Soley F, Bruix J, Calvet X, Gil MP, Mas A, Bruguera M, Castillo R, Rodes J: Hepatitis C virus infection in patients with nonalcoholic chronic liver disease. Ann Intern Med 112:921–924, 1990.

55. Pares A, Barrera JM, Caballeria J, Ercilla G, Bruguera M, Caballeria L, Castillo R, Rodes J: Hepatitis C virus antibodies in chronic alcoholic patients: association with severity of liver injury. Hepatology 12:1295–1299, 1990.

56. McFarlane IG, Smith HM, Johnson PJ, Bray GP, Vergani D, Williams R: Hepatitis C virus antibodies in chronic active hepatitis: pathogenetic factor or false-positive result? Lancet 335:754–757, 1990.

57. Mitchel LS, Jeffers LJ, Moreda R, Reddy KR, de Medina M, Hill M, Altman R, Manns MP, Schiff ER: The prevalence of hepatitis C virus antibody (anti-HCV) among patients with autoimmune chronic active hepatitis (AI-CAH), supplemented by RIBA. Hepatology (Abstract) 12:904, 1990.

58. Bruix J, Calvet X, Costa J: Prevalence of antibodies to hepatitis C virus in Spanish patients with heaptocellular carcinoma and hepatic cirrhosis. Lancet 2:1004–1006, 1989.

59. Koff RS: The clinical features of acute viral hepatitis. In Modern Concepts of Acute and Chronic Hepatitis, edited by G. Gitnick. New York, Plenum Medical Book Company, 1989, pp. 11–18.

60. Klatskin G: Subacute hepatic necrosis and postnecrotic cirrhosis due to anicteric infections with the hepatitis virus. Am J Med 25:333–358, 1958.

61. Boyer JL, Klatskin G: Pattern of necrosis in acute viral hepatitis. Prognostic value of bridging (subacute necrosis). N Engl J Med 283:1063–1071, 1970.

62. Eliakim M, Rachmilewitz M: Cholangiolitic manifestations in virus hepatitis. Gastroenterology 31:369–383, 1956.

63. Dubin IN, Sullivan BH, Le Golvan PC, Murphy LC: The cholestatic form of viral hepatitis. Experiences with viral hepatitis at Brooke Army Hospital during the years 1951 to 1953. Am J Med 29:55–72, 1960.

64. Gordon SC, Reddy KR, Schiff L: Prolonged intrahepatic cholestasis secondary to acute hepatitis A. Ann Intern Med 101:635–637, 1984.

65. Wilkinson SP, Portmann B, Cochrane AMG, Tee DEH, Williams R: Clinical course of chronic lobular hepatitis. Report of five cases. Q J Med 47:421–429, 1978.

66. Holland PV, Walsh JH, Morrow AG, Purcell RH: Failure of Australia antibody to prevent post-transfusion hepatitis. Lancet 2:553–555, 1969.

67. Norkrans G, Frosner G, Hermodsson S, Iwarson S: Multiple hepatitis attacks in drug addicts. JAMA 243:1056–1058, 1980.

68. Davis GL, Hoofnagle JH: Reactivation of chronic type B hepatitis presenting as acute viral hepatitis. Ann Intern Med 102:762–765, 1985.

69. Popper H, Schaffner F: The vocabulary of chronic hepatitis. N Engl J Med 284:1154–1156, 1971.

70. Rakela J. Redeker AG: Chronic liver disease after acute non-A, non-B viral hepatitis. Gastroenterology 72:1200–1202, 1979.

71. Omata M, Afroudakis A, Liew C-T, Ashcavai M, Peters RL: Comparison of serum hepatitis B surface antigen (HBsAg) and serum anticore with tissue HBsAg and hepatitis B core antigen (HBcAg). Gastroenterology 75:1003–1009, 1978.

72. Nielsen JO, Dietrichson O, Elling P, Christoffersen P: Incidence and meaning of persistence of Australia antigen in patients with acute viral hepatitis: development of chronic hepatitis. N Engl J Med 285:1157–1160, 1971.

73. Faber V, Christoffersen P, Nielsen PE, Nielsen JO, Poulsen H: Au antigen in liver cirrhosis. Lancet 2:825–826, 1970.

74. Ware AJ, Eigenbrodt EH, Combes B: Prognostic significance of subacute hepatic necrosis in acute hepatitis. Gastroenterology 68:519–524, 1975.

75. Ware AJ, Cuthbert JA, Shorey J, Gurian LE, Eigenbrodt EH, Combes B: A prospective trial of steroid therapy in severe viral hepatitis. The prognostic significance of bridging necrosis. Gastroenterology 80:219–224, 1980.

76. Karvountzis GG, Redeker AG, Peters RL: Long term follow-up studies of patients surviving fulminant viral hepatitis. Gastroenterology 67:870–877, 1974.

77. Mathiesen LR, Skinoj P, Nielsen JO, Purcell RH, Wong D, Ranek L: Hepatitis Type A, B, and non-A, non-B in fulminant hepatitis. Gut 21:72–77, 1980.

78. Bismuth H, Samuel D, Gugenheim J, Castaing D, Bernuau J, Rueff B, Benhamou J-P: Emergency liver transplantation for fulminant hepatitis. Ann Intern Med 107:337–341, 1987.

78a. Dienstag JL. Non-A, non-B hepatitis. I. Recognition, epidemiology, and clinical features. Gastroenterology 85:439–462, 1983.

78b. Bernuau J, Marcellin P, Loriot MA, Courouce AM, Martinot-Peignoux M, Erlinger S, Benhamou JP. Prevalence of anti-HCV antibody in patients with fulminant hepatitis. Hepatology 12:875, 1990 (abstract).

78c. Sarraco G, Macagno S, Rosina F, Caredda F, Antinori S, Rizzetto M. Serologic markers with fulminant hepatitis in persons positive for hepatitis B surface antigen. A worldwide epidemiology and clinical review. Ann Intern Med 108:380–383, 1988.

78d. Govindarajan S, Chin KP, Redeker AG, Peters RL. Fulminant B viral hepatitis: role of delta agent. Gastroenterology 86:1417–1420, 1988.

78e. Lettau LA, McCarthy JG, Smith MH, Hadler SC, Morse LJ, Ukena T, Bessette R, Gurwitz A, Irvine WG, Fields HA, Grady GF, Maynard JE. Outbreak of severe hepatitis due to delta and hepatitis B viruses in parenteral drug abusers and their contacts. N Engl J Med 317:1256–1262, 1987.

78f. Ramalingaswami V, Purcell RH. Waterborne non-A, non-B hepatitis. Lancet 1:571–573, 1988.

78g. Williams R, Gimson AE. Intensive liver care and management of acute hepatic failure. Dig Dis Sci 36:820–826, 1991.

79. Scotto J, Opolon P, Eteve J, Vergoz D, Thomas M, Caroli J: Liver biopsy and prognosis in acute liver failure. Gut 14:927–933, 1973.

80. Horney JT, Galambos JT: The liver during and after fulminant hepatitis. Gastroenterology 73:639–645, 1977.

81. Alter H: Epidemiologic studies of hepatitis non-A, non-B using a new test. In Frontiers in Molecular Biology, Virology and Immunology of Hepatitis Non-A, Non-B. Eur Assoc Study Liver, Aug 30, 1989.

82. Bolin TD, Davis AE, Liddelow AG: Liver disease and cell-mediated immunity in hepatitis-associated antigen (HAA) carriers. Gut 14:365–368, 1973.

83. Singleton JW, Fitch RA, Merrill DA, Kohler PF, Rettberg, WAH: Liver disease in Australia-antigen-positive blood donors. Lancet 2:785–787, 1971.

84. Beasley RP, Hwang L-Y: Hepatocellular carcinoma and hepatitis B virus. Semin Liver Dis 4:113–121, 1984.

85. Alter HJ, Seeff LB, Kaplan PM: Type B hepatitis: the infectivity of blood positive for e antigen and DNA polymerase after accidental needlestick exposure. N Engl J Med 295:909–913, 1976.

86. Weiner BG, Gradey GF: Accidental hepatitis-B-surface-antigen-positive inoculations. Ann Intern Med 97:367–369, 1982.

87. Reinicke V, Dybkjaer E, Poulsen H, Banke O, Lylloff K, Nordenfelt E: A study of Australia-antigen-positive blood donors and their recipients, with special reference to liver histology. N Engl J Med 286:867–870, 1972.

88. Blumberg BS, Friedlaender JS, Woodside A, Sutnick I, London WT: Hepatitis and Australia antigen: autosomal recessive inheritance of susceptibility to infections in humans. Proc Natl Acad Sci 62:1108–1115, 1969.

89. Hillis WD, Hills A, Bias WB, Walker WG: Associations of hepatitis B surface antigenemia with HLA locus B specificities. N Engl J Med 296:1310–1314, 1977.

90. Okada K, Kamiyama I, Inomata M, Imai M, Miyakawa Y, Mayumi M: e Antigen and anti-e in the serum of asymptomatic mothers as indicators of positive and negative transmission of hepatitis B virus to their infants. N Engl J Med 294:746–749, 1976.

91. Skinhoj P, Cohn J, Bradburne AF: Transmission of hepatitis type B from healthy HBsAg-positive mothers. Br Med J 1:10–11, 1976.

92. Lee AKY, Ip HMH, Wong VCW: Mechanism of maternal-fetal transmission of hepatitis B virus. J Infect Dis 138:668–671, 1978.

93. Buckholz HM, Frosner GG, Ziegler GB: HBsAg carrier state in an infant delivered by caesarean section. Lancet 2:343, 1974.

94. Boxall EIJ, Davies H: Dane particles in cord blood. Lancet 2:1513, 1974.

95. Okada K, Yamada T, Miyakawa Y, Mayumi M: Hepatitis B surface antigen in the serum of infants after delivery from asymptomatic carrier mothers. J Pediatr 87:360–363, 1975.

96. Gerety RJ, Schweitzer IL: Viral hepatitis type B during pregnancy, the neonatal period and infancy. J Pediatr 90:368–374, 1977.

97. Matsuda S, Tada K, Shirachi R, Ishida N: Australia antigen in amniotic fluid. Lancet 1:1117, 1972.

98. Krugman S: Vertical transmission of hepatitis B and breast feeding. Lancet 2:916, 1975.

99. Beasley RP, Stevens CE, Shiao I-S, Meng H-C: Evidence against breast feeding as a mechanism of vertical transmission of hepatitis B. Lancet 2:740–741, 1975.

100. Giraud P, Drouet J, Dupuy JM: Hepatitis-B virus infection of children born to mothers with severe hepatitis. Lancet 2:1088–1089, 1975.

101. Dunn AEG, Peters RL, Schweitzer IL, Spears RL: Virus-like particles in livers of infants with vertically transmitted hepatitis. Arch Pathol 94:258–264, 1972.

102. Dupuy JM, Frommel D, Alagille D: Severe viral hepatitis type B in infancy. Lancet 1:191–194, 1975.

103. Stevens CE, Cherubin CE, Dienstag JL, Purcell RH, Szmuness W: Antibody to hepatitis A antigen in children. J Pediatr 91:436–438, 1977.

104. Cherubin CE, Szmuness W, Harley EJ, Much MI, Roldman E: Evidence of hepatitis B infection in hospitalized children in New York. J Pediatr 88:893–894, 1976.

105. Krugman S, Giles JP: Viral hepatitis. New light on an old disease. JAMA 212:1019–1029, 1970.

106. Brzosko WJ, Mikulska BE, Biedrzycka R, Roszkowska K, Rudkowski Z, Rabenda C, Oziemska-Lozinska H, Debski R: Hepatitis B in children. Lancet 2:259, 1973.

107. Gerety RJ, Hoofnagle JH, Markenson JA, Barker LF: Exposure to hepatitis B virus and development of the chronic HBsAg carrier state in children. J Pediatr 84:661–665, 1974.

108. Ohta Y: Viral hepatitis and hepatocellular carcinoma. In Hepatocellular Carcinoma, edited by K. Okuda, R.L. Peters. New York, John Wiley & Sons, 1976, pp. 73–81.

109. Tabor E, Gerety RJ, Vogel CL, Bayley AC, Anthony PP, Chan CH, Barker LF: Hepatitis B virus infection and primary hepatocellular carcinoma. J Natl Cancer Inst 53:1197–1200, 1977.

110. Larouze B, London WT, Saimot G, Werner BG, Lustbader ED, Payet M, Blumberg BS: Host responses to hepatitis B infection in patients

with primary hepatic carcinoma and their families. A case/control study in Senegal, West Africa. Lancet 2:534–538, 1976.

111. Wogan GN: Aflatoxins and their relationship to hepatocellular carcinoma. In Hepatocellular Carcinoma, edited by K. Okuda, R.L. Peters. New York, John Wiley & Sons, 1976, pp. 25–41.

112. Prince AM, Szmuness W, Michon J, Demaille J, Diebolt G, Linhard J, Quenum C, Sankale M: A case/control study of the association between primary liver cancer and hepatitis B infection in Senegal. Int J Cancer 16:376–383, 1975.

113. Shafritz DA, Kew MC: Identification of integrated hepatitis B virus DNA sequences in human hepatocellular carcinomas. Hepatology 1:1–8, 1981.

114. Bartels J, Gocke DJ: Viral hepatitis. Extrahepatic manifestations. In Modern Concepts of Acute and Chronic Hepatitis, edited by G. Gitnick. New York, Plenum Medical Book Company, 1989, pp. 35–50.

115. Alpert E, Isselbacher KJ, Schur PH: The pathogenesis of arthritis associated with viral hepatitis. Complement-component studies. N Engl J Med 285:185–189, 1971.

116. Duffy J, Lidsky MD, Sharp JT, Davis JS, Person DA, Hollinger FB, Mink K-W: Polyarthritis, polyarteritis and hepatitis B. Medicine 55:19–37, 1976.

117. Niermeijer P, Gips CH: Natural history of acute hepatitis B in previously healthy patients. A prospective study. Acta Hepatogastroenterol 24:317–325, 1977.

118. Stewart JS, Farrow LJ, Clifford RE: A three-year survey of viral hepatitis in West London. Q J Med 47:365–384, 1978.

119. Routenberg JA, Dienstag JL, Harrison WO: Foodborne outbreak of hepatitis A: clinical and laboratory features of acute and protracted illness. Am J Med Sci 278:123–137, 1979.

120. Wands JR, Mann E, Alpert E, Isselbacher KJ: The pathogenesis of arthritis associated with acute hepatitis B surface antigen-positive hepatitis. Complement activation and characterization of circulating immune complexes. J Clin Invest 55:930–936, 1975.

121. Combes B, Stastny P, Shorey J, Eigenbrodt EE, Barrere A, Hull AR, Carter NW: Glomerulonephritis with deposition of Australia antigen-antibody complexes in glomerular basement membrane. Lancet 2:234–237, 1971.

122. Kniescr MR, Jcnis EII, Lowenthal DT, Bancroft WH, Barns W, Shalhoub R: Pathogenesis of renal disease associated with viral hepatitis. Arch Pathol 97:193–200, 1974.

123. Thomas HC, Potter BJ, Elias E, Sherlock S: Metabolism of the third component of complement in acute type B hepatitis, HBs antigen-positive glomerulonephritis, polyarteritis nodosum and HBs antigen positive and negative chronic liver disease. Gastroenterology 76:673–679, 1979.

124. Gocke DJ, Hsu K, Morgan C, Bombardieri S, Lockshin M, Christian CL: Association between polyarteritis and Australia antigen. Lancet 2:1149–1153, 1970.

125. Trepo CG, Zuckerman AJ, Bird RC, Prince AM: The role of circulating hepatitis B antigen/antibody immune complexes in the pathogenesis of polyarteritis nodosa. J Clin Pathol 27:863–868, 1974.

126. Michalak T: Immune complexes of hepatitis B surface antigen in the pathogenesis of periarteritis nodosa. A study of seven necropsy cases. Am J Pathol 90:619–628, 1978.

127. Columbo M, Gerber MA, Vernace SJ, Gianotti F, Paronetto F: Immune response to hepatitis B virus in children with papular acrodermatitis. Gastroenterology 73:1103–1106, 1977.

128. Toda G, Ishimaru Y, Mayumi M, Oda T: Infantile papular acrodermatitis (Gianotti's disease) and intrafamilial occurrence of acute hepatitis B with jaundice: age dependency of clinical manifestations of hepatitis B infection. J Infect Dis 138:211–216, 1978.

129. Levo Y, Gorevic PD, Kassab HJ, Zucker-Franklin D, Franklin EC: Association between hepatitis B virus and essential mixed cryoglobulinemia. N Engl J Med 196:1501–1504, 1977.

130. Popp JW, Dienstag JL, Wands JR: Essential mixed cryoglobulinemia without evidence for hepatitis B virus infection. Ann Intern Med 92:379–386, 1980.

131. Inman RD, Hodge M, Johnston MEA, Wright J, Heathcote J: Arthritis, vasculitis and cryoglobulinemia associated with relapsing hepatitis A virus infection. Ann Intern Med 105:700–703, 1986.

132. Niermeijer P, Gips CH: Guillain-Barre syndrome in acute HBsAg-positive hepatitis. Br Med J 4:732–733, 1975.

133. Penner E, Maida E, Mamoli B, Gange A: Serum and cerebrospinal fluid immune complexes containing hepatitis B surface antigen in Guillain-Barre syndrome. Gastroenterology 82:576–580, 1982.

134. Pelletier G, Elghozi D, Trepo C: Mononeuritis in acute viral hepatitis. Digestion 32:53–56, 1985.

135. Ferivar M, Wands JR, Benson GD, Dienstag JL, Isselbacher KJ: Cryoprotein complexes and peripheral neuropathy in a patient with chronic active hepatitis. Gastroenterology 71:490–493, 1976.

136. Zuckerman AJ: Laboratory investigation in the aetiology of human viral hepatitis. Br Med Bull 28:134–137, 1972.

137. Dudley FJ, Fox RA, Sherlock S: Relationship of hepatitis-associated antigen (H.A.A.) to acute and chronic liver injury. Lancet 2:1–3, 1971.

138. Krawczynski K, Nazarewicz T, Brzosko WT, Nowoslawski A: Cellular localization of hepatitis-associated antigen in livers of patients with different forms of hepatitis. J Infect Dis 126:372–377, 1972.

139. Popper H, Tjing SN, Gerber MA: Histologic studies of severe Delta agent infection in Venezuelan Indians. Hepatology 3:906–912, 1983.

140. Lefkowitch JH, Goldstein H, Yatto R, Gerber MA: Cytopathic liver injury in acute delta virus hepatitis. Gastroenterology 92:1262–1266, 1987.

141. Dudley FJ, Fox FA, Sherlock S: Cellular immunity and hepatitis-associated Australia-antigen liver disease. Lancet 1:723–726, 1972.

142. Kurebayashi Y, Stao K, Ikeda T, Katami K, Ogawa H, Osada Y: Acute hepatic injury induced by an intravenous injection of monoclonal antibody to rat liver cell membrane in rats. Igakunoayumi (Tokyo) 146:179–180, 1988.

143. Okuda K: Acute massive necrosis of the liver induced by antibody/complement, not by T-cells. Hepatology 9:118–119, 1989.

144. Edgington TS, Ritt DJ: Intrahepatic expression of serum hepatitis virus-associated antigens. J Exp Med 134:871–885, 1971.

145. Alberti A, Realdi G, Tremolada F, Cadrobbi P: HBAg in liver-cell surface in viral hepatitis. Lancet 1:346, 1975.

146. Barker LF, Chisari FV, McGrath PP, Dalgard DW, Kirchstein RL, Almeida JD, Edgington TS, Sharp DG, Peterson MR: Transmission of type B viral hepatitis to chimpanzees. J Infect Dis 127:648–662, 1973.

147. Ray MB, Desmet VJ, Bradburne AF, Desmyter J, Fevery J, De Groote J: Hepatitis B core antigen immune complexes in the liver of hepatitis B patients. Clin Exp Immunol 37:15–24, 1979.

148. Tsang T-K, Blei AT, O'Reilly DJ, Decker R: Clinical significance of concurrent hepatitis B surface antigen and antibody positivity. Dig Dis Sci 31:620–624, 1986.

149. Kater L, Schmitz du Moulin F, Borst-Eilers E: Acute viral hepatitis B: an immune complex disease? Lancet 1:364, 1974.

150. Eddleston ALWF, Williams R: Inadequate antibody response to HBAg or suppressor T-cell defect in the development of active chronic hepatitis. Lancet 2:1543–1545, 1974.

151. Edgington T, Chisari PW: Immunological aspects of hepatitis B virus infection. Am J Med Sci 270:213–227, 1975.

152. Kosmidis JC, Leader-Williams LK: Complement levels in acute infectious hepatitis and serum hepatitis. Clin Exp Immunol 11:31–35, 1972.

153. Woolf IL, El Sheik N, Cullens H, Lee WM, Eddleston ALWF, Williams R, Zuckerman AJ: Enhanced HBsAb production in the pathogenesis of fulminant viral hepatitis. Br Med J 2:669–671, 1976.

154. Fox RA, Dudley FJ, Sherlock S: The serum concentration of the third component of complement B1c/B1a in liver disease. Gut 12:574–578, 1971.

155. Gocke DJ, Hsu K, Morgan C, Bombardieri S, Lockshin M, Christian CL: Association between polyarteritis and Australia antigen. Lancet 2:1149–1153, 1970.

156. Reed WD, Eddleston ALWF, Cullens H, Williams R, Zuckerman AJ, Peters KD, Williams KG, Maycock WDIA: Infusion of hepatitis B antibody in antigen-positive chronic hepatitis. Lancet 2:1347–1351, 1973.

157. Good RA, Page AR: Fatal complications of virus hepatitis in two patients with agammaglobulinemia. Am J Med 29:804–810, 1960.

158. Tong MJ, Nies KM, Redeker AG: Rapid progression of chronic active type B hepatitis in a patient with hypogammaglobulinemia. Gastroenterology 73:1418–1421, 1977.

159. Meyer zum Buschenfelde K-H, Hutteroth TH, Arnold W, Hopf U: Immunologic liver injury: the role of hepatitis B viral antigens and liver membrane antigens as targets. In Progress in Liver Diseases, Vol. VI, edited by H. Popper, F. Schaffner. New York, Grune & Stratton, 1979, pp. 407–424.

160. Jensen DM, McFarlane IG, Portmann BS, Eddleston ALWF, Williams R: Detection of antibodies against a liver-specific membrane lipoprotein in patients with acute and chronic active hepatitis. N Engl J Med 299:1–7, 1978.

161. Dudley FJ, Fox RA, Sherlock S: Cellular immunity and hepatitis-associated Australia antigen liver disease. Lancet *1*:723–726, 1972.

162. Howlett SA, McGuigan JE: Inhibition of macrophage migration in response to hepatitis Bs antigen. Gastroenterology *69*:960–964, 1975.

163. Tong, MJ, Wallace, AM, Peters, RL, Reynolds, TB: Lymphocyte stimulation in hepatitis B infections. N Engl J Med *293*:318–322, 1975.

164. Miller DJ, Dwyer JM, Klatskin G: Identification of lymphocytes in percutaneous liver biopsy cores. Different T:B ratio in HBsAg-positive and -negative hepatitis. Gastroenterology *72*:1199–1203, 1977.

165. Ray MB, Desmet VJ, Bradburne AF, Desmyter J, Fevery J, De Groote J: Differential distribution of hepatitis B surface antigen and hepatitis B core antigen in the liver of hepatitis B patients. Gastroenterology *71*:462–467, 1976.

166. Galbraith RM, Eddleston ALWF, Williams R, Webster ADB, Pattison J, Doniach D, Kennedy LA, Batchelor JR: Enhanced antibody responses in active chronic hepatitis: relation to HLA-B8 and HLA-B12 and portosystemic shunting. Lancet *1*:930–934, 1976.

167. Mackay I, Tait BD: HLA association with autoimmune type chronic active hepatitis: identification of B8-BRW3 haplotype by family studies. Gastroenterology *79*:95–98, 1980.

168. Cochrane AMG, Moussouros A, Thomson AD, Eddleston ALWF, Williams R: Antibody-dependent cell-mediated (K cell) cytotoxicity against isolated hepatocytes in chronic active hepatitis. Lancet *1*:441–444, 1976.

169. Dienstag JL, Isselbacker KJ: Liver-specific protein: more questions than answers. Gastroenterology *299*:40–42, 1978.

170. Behrens UJ, Vernace S, Paronetto F: Studies on "liver-specific" antigens. II. Detection of serum antibodies to liver and kidney cell membrane antigens in patients with chronic liver disease. Gastroenterology *77*:1053–1061, 1979.

171. Mallory TB: The pathology of epidemic hepatitis. JAMA *134*:655–662, 1947.

172. Searle J, Kerr JFR, Bishop CJ: Necrosis and apoptosis: distinct modes of cell death with fundamentally different significance. Pathol Annu *17* (Part 2):229–259, 1982.

173. Bianchi L: Liver biopsy interpretation in hepatitis. Pathol Res Pract *178*:2–19, and *178*:180–213, 1983.

174. Fauerholdt L, Asnaes S, Ranek L, Schodt T, Tygstrup N: Significance of suspected "chronic aggressive hepatitis" in acute hepatitis. Gastroenterology *73*:543–548, 1977.

175. Vanstapel MJ, Van Steenbergen W, DeWolf-Peeters C, Desmyter J, Fevery J, De Groote J, Desmet VJ: Prognostic significance of piecemeal necrosis in acute viral hepatitis. Liver *3*:46–57, 1983.

176. Ishak KG: Light microscopic morphology of viral hepatitis. Am J Clin Pathol *65*:787–827, 1976.

177. Felig P, Brown WV, Levine RA, Klatskin G: Glucose homeostasis in viral hepatitis. N Engl J Med *283*:1436–1440, 1970.

178. Mietkiewski JM, Scheuer PJ: Immunoglobulin-containing plasma cells in acute hepatitis. Liver *5*:84–88, 1985.

179. Bianchi L, Zimmerli-Ning M, Gudat F: Viral hepatitis. *In* Pathology of the Liver, edited by R.N.M. MacSween, P.P. Anthony, P.J. Scheuer. New York, Churchill Livingstone, 1979, pp. 164–191.

180. Ware AJ, Eigenbrodt EH, Shorey J, Combes B: Viral hepatitis complicating the Dubin-Johnson syndrome. Gastroenterology *63*:331–339, 1972.

181. Bardadin KA, Scheuer PJ: Endothelial cell changes in acute hepatitis. A light and electron microscopic study. J Pathol *144*:213–220, 1984.

182. Petersen P, Christoffersen P, Elling P, Juhl E, Dietrichson O, Faber M, Iversen K, Nielsen JO, Poulsen H: Acute viral hepatitis: a survey of 500 patients. Clinical, biochemical, immunological, and morphological features at time of diagnosis. Scand J Gastroenterol *9*:607–613, 1974.

183. Poulsen H, Christoffersen P: Abnormal bile duct epithelium in liver biopsies with histologic signs of viral hepatitis. Acta Pathol Microbiol Scand *76*:383–390, 1969.

184. Klatskin G: Persistent HB antigenemia: associated clinical manifestations and hepatic lesions. Am J Med Sci *270*:33–40, 1975.

185. Peters RL: Viral hepatitis: a pathologic spectrum. Am J Med Sci *270*:17–31, 1975.

186. Phillips MJ, Pottcell S: Modern aspects of the morphology of viral hepatitis. Hum Pathol *12*:1060–1084, 1981.

187. Desmet VJ: Acute viral hepatitis. *In* Modern Concepts of Acute and Chronic Hepatitis, edited by G. Gitnick. New York, Plenum Medical Book Company, 1989, pp. 87–111.

188. Okuno T, Sano A, Deguchi T, Katsuna Y, Ogasawara T, Okanoue T, Takino T: Pathology of acute hepatitis A in humans; comparison with acute hepatitis B. Am J Clin Pathol *81*:162–169, 1984.

189. Tanaka K, Mori W, Suwa S: Victoria blue-nuclear fast red stain for HBs antigen detection in paraffin sections. Acta Pathol Jpn *31*:93–98, 1981.

190. Teixeira MR Jr, Weller IVD, Murray A, Bamber M, Thomas HC, Sherlock S, Scheuer PJ: The pathology of hepatitis A in man. Liver *2*:53–60, 1982.

191. Scheuer PJ: Viral hepatitis. *In* Pathology of the Liver, edited by R.N.M MacSween, P.P. Anthony, P.J. Scheuer. 2nd Edition Edinburgh, Churchill Livinstone, 1987, pp. 202–223.

192. Shimizu YK, Shikata T, Beninger PR, Sata M, Setoyama H, Abe H: Detection of hepatitis A antigen in human liver. Infect Immun *36*:320–324, 1982.

193. Abe H, Beninger PR, Ikejiri N, Setoyama H, Sata M, Tanikawa K: Light microscopic findings of liver biopsy specimens from patients with hepatitis type A and comparison with type B. Gastroenterology *82*:938–947, 1982.

194. Sciot R, Van Damme B, Desmet VJ: Cholestatic features in hepatitis A. J Hepatol *3*:172–181, 1986.

195. Houthoff HJ, Niermeijer P, Gips CH, Arends A, Hofstee N, van Guldener M: Hepatic morphologic findings and viral antigens in acute hepatitis B: a longitudinal study. Virchow's Arch Pathol Anat *389*:153–166, 1980.

196. Bianchi L, Spichtin HP, Gudat F: Chronic hepatitis. In *Pathology of the Liver*, Second Ed. edited by R.N.M. MacSween, P.P. Anthony, P.J. Scheuer. New York, Churchill Livingstone, 1987, pp. 310–341.

197. Vanstapel MJ, Van Steenbergen W, DeWolf-Peeters C, Desmyter J, Fevery J, De Groote J, Desmet VJ: Prognostic significance of piecemeal necrosis in acute viral hepatitis. Liver *3*:46–57, 1983.

198. Yasui H, Fujitani Y, Sugimura H: An autopsy case of delta agent-positive hepatocellular carcinoma with liver cirrhosis. Acta Hepatol Jpn *28*:466–471, 1987.

199. Tassopoulos N, Papaevangelou G, Roumeliotou-Karayannis A, Kalafatas P, Engle R, Gerin J, Purcell RH: Double infections with hepatitis A and B viruses. Liver *5*:348–353, 1985.

200. Verme G, Amoroso P, Lettieri G, Pierri P, David E, Sessa F, Rizzi R, Bonino F, Recchia S, Rizzetto M: A histological study of hepatitis delta virus liver disease. Hepatology *6*:1303–1307, 1986.

201. Kanel GC, Govindarajan S, Peters RL: Chronic delta infection and liver biopsy changes in chronic active hepatitis B. Ann Intern Med *101*:51–54, 1984.

202. Thung SN, Gerber MA: Immunohistochemical study of delta antigen in an American metropolitan population. Liver *3*:392–397, 1983.

203. Moreno A, Ramon y Cajal S, Marazuela M, Carreno V, Milicua JM, Cerezo E, Cuesta C, Oliva H: Sanded nuclei in delta patients. Liver *9*:367–371, 1989.

204. Popper H, Thung SN, Gerber MA, Hadler SC, de Monzon M, Ponzetto A, Anzola E, Rivera D, Mondolfi A, Bracho A, Francis DP, Gerin JL, Maynard JE, Purcell RH: Histologic studies of severe delta agent infection in Venezuelan Indians. Hepatology *3*:906–912, 1983.

205. Rizzetto M, Verme G, Gerin JL, Purcell RH: Hepatitis delta virus disease. *In* Progress in Liver Diseases, Vol. VIII, edited by H. Popper, F. Schaffner. New York, Grune & Stratton, 1986, pp. 417–431.

206. Smedile A, Verme G, Cargnel A: Influence of delta infection on severity of hepatitis B. Lancet *2*:945–947, 1982.

207. Knodell RG, Ishak DG, Black WC: Formulation and application of a numerical scoring system of assessing histological activity in asymptomatic chronic active hepatitis. Hepatology *1*:431–435, 1981.

208. Negro F, Baldi M, Bonino F, Rocca G, Demartini A, Passarino G, Maran E, Lavarini C, Rizzetto M, Verme G: Chronic HDV (hepatitis delta virus) hepatitis. Intrahepatic expression of delta antigen, histologic activity and outcome of liver disease. J Hepatol *6*:8–14, 1988.

209. Kojima T, Callea F, Desmyter J, Sasaki H, Desmet VJ: Hepatitis Delta antigen (HDAg) in hepatocytes and lymphocyte reaction: immune light and electron microscopic studies. Hepatology *6*:793, 1986 (abstract).

210. De Cock KM, Govindarajan S, Redeker AG: Natural course of Delta superinfection in chronic hepatitis B virus infected patients. Histopathologic study. *In* The Hepatitis Delta Virus (HDV) and Its Infection, edited by H. Rizzetto, J.L. Gerin, R.H. Purcell. New York, Alan R. Liss, 1987, pp. 167–180.

211. Buitrago B, Popper H, Hadler SC, Thung SN, Gerber MA, Purcell RH, Maynard JE: Specific histologic features of Santa Marta Hepatitis: a severe form of Hepatitis Delta Virus infection in Northern South America. Hepatology *6*:1285–1291, 1986.

212. Hadler SC, DeMonzon M, Ponzetto A: Delta virus infection and se-

vere hepatitis. An epidemic in the Yucpa Indians of Venezuela. Ann Intern Med *10:*339–344, 1984.

213. Govindarajan S, De Cock KM, Redeker AG: Natural course of Delta superinfection in chronic Hepatitis B Virus-infected patients: histopathologic study with multiple liver biopsies. Hepatology *6:*640–644, 1986.

214. Negro F, Bonino F, Di Bisceglie A, Hoofnagle JH, Gerin JL: Intrahepatic markers of hepatitis delta virus infection: a study by *in situ* hybridization. Hepatology *10:*916–921, 1989.

215. Spichtin HP, Gudat F, Schmid M, Pirovino M, Altorfer J, Bianchi L: Microtubular aggregates in human chronic non-A, non-B hepatitis with bridging necrosis and multinucleated hepatocytic giant cells. Liver *2:*355–360, 1982.

216. Kryger P, Christoffersen P: Liver histopathology of the hepatitis A virus infection: a comparison with hepatitis type B and non-A, non-B. J Clin Pathol *36:*650–654, 1983.

217. Schmid M, Pirovino M, Altorfer J, Gudat F, Bianchi L: Acute hepatitis non-A, non-B; are there any specific light microscopic features? Liver *2:*61–67, 1982.

218. Poulsen H, Christoffersen P: Abnormal bile duct epithelium in liver biopsies with histologic signs of viral hepatitis. Acta Pathol Microbiol Scand *76:*383–390, 1969.

219. Rugge M, Vanstapel MJ, Ninfo V, Realdi G, Tremolada F, Montanari PG, van Damme B, Fevery J, De Groote J, Desmet V: Comparative histology of acute hepatitis B and non-A, non-B in Leuven and Padova. Virchows Arch Pathol Anat *401:*275–288, 1983.

220. Sciot R, Van Damme B, Desmet VJ: Cholestatic features in hepatitis A. J Hepatol *3:*172–181, 1986.

221. Gordon SC, Reddy KR, Schiff L: Prolonged intrahepatic cholestasis secondary to acute hepatitis A. Ann Intern Med *101:*635–637, 1984.

222. Huang GT, Chen DS, Lai MY: Cholestatic viral hepatitis. Clin Gastroenterol *1:*186–191, 1984.

223. Bianchi L, De Groote J, Desmet VJ, Gedigk P, Korb G, Popper H, Poulsen H, Scheuer PJ, Schmid M, Thaler H, Wepler W: Acute and chronic hepatitis revisited. Review by an international group. Lancet *2:*914–919, 1977.

224. Thung SN, Gerber MA: The formation of elastic fibers in livers with massive hepatic necrosis. Arch Pathol Lab Med *106:*468–469, 1982.

225. Schalm SW, Summerskill WHJ, Gitnick GL, Elveback LR: Contrasting features of severe chronic liver disease with and without hepatitis Bs antigen. Gut *17:*781–786, 1976.

226. Chadwick RG, Galizzi Jr J, Heathcote J, Lyssiotis T, Cohen BJ, Scheuer PJ, Sherlock S: Chronic persistent hepatitis: hepatitis B virus markers and histological follow-up. Gut *20:*372–377, 1979.

227. Seeff LB, Kiernan T, Zimmerman HJ, Leevy CM, Wright EC, Tamburro CH, Schiff ER, Ishak KG: Hepatic disease in asymptomatic parenteral narcotic drug abusers: a Veterans Administration collaborative study. Am J Med Sci *270:*41–47, 1975.

228. Popper H, Paronetto F, Schaffner F: Immune processes in the pathogenesis of liver disease. Ann NY Acad Sci *124:*781–799, 1965.

229. Kerr JFR, Cooksley WGE, Searle J, Halliday JW, Halliday WJ, Holder L, Roberts I, Burnett W, Powell LW: The nature of piecemeal necrosis in chronic active hepatitis. Lancet *2:*827–828, 1979.

230. Kawanishi H: Morphologic association of lymphocytes with hepatocytes in chronic liver disease. Lab Med *10:*286–290, 1977.

231. Baggenstoss AH, Soloway RD, Summerskill WHJ, Elveback LR, Schoenfield LJ: Chronic active liver disease. The range of histologic lesions, their response to treatment, and evolution. Hum Pathol *3:*183–198, 1972.

232. Christoffersen P, Dietrichson O, Faber V, Poulsen H: The occurrence and significance of abnormal bile duct epithelium in chronic aggressive hepatitis. A comparative morphological, biochemical, immunological, and prognostic study. Acta Pathol Microbiol Scand, Sect A *80:*294–302, 1972.

233. Lefkowitch JH, Arborgh BAM, Scheuer PJ: Oxyphilic granular hepatocytes. Mitochondrion-rich liver cells in hepatic disease. Am J Clin Pathol *74:*432–441, 1980.

234. Gall BA: Posthepatitic, postnecrotic, and nutritional cirrhosis. A pathologic analysis. Am J Pathol *36:*241–271, 1960.

235. Anthony PP, Ishak KG, Nayak NC, Poulsen HE, Scheuer PJ, Sobin LH: The morphology of cirrhosis: definition, nomenclature, and classification. Bull WHO *59:*521–540, 1977.

236. Anthony PP, Vogel CL, Barker LF: Liver cell dysplasia: a premalignant condition. J Clin Pathol *26:*217–223, 1973.

237. Shikata T: Primary liver carcinoma and liver cirrhosis. *In* Hepatocel-

lular Carcinoma, edited by K. Okuda, R.L. Peters. New York, John Wiley & Sons, 1976, pp. 53–71.

238. Peters RL: Pathology of hepatocellular carcinoma. *In* Hepatocellular Carcinoma, edited by K. Okuda, R.L. Peters. New York, John Wiley & Sons, 1976, pp. 107–168.

239. Szmuness W, Prince AM, Diebolt G, Leblanc L, Baylet R, Massayeff R, Linhard J: The epidemiology of hepatitis B infections in Africa: the results of a pilot study in the Republic of Senegal. Am J Epidemiol *98:*104–110, 1973.

240. Nayak NC, Sachdeva R: Localization of hepatitis B surface antigen in conventional paraffin sections of the liver. Comparison on immunofluorescence, immunoperoxidase, and orcein staining methods with regard to their specificity and reliability as antigen marker. Am J Pathol *81:*479–492, 1975.

241. MacNab GM, Alexander JJ, Lacatsas G, Bey EM, Urbanowicz JM: Hepatitis B surface antigen produced by a human hepatoma cell line. Br J Cancer *34:*509–515, 1976.

242. Greenberg HB, Robinson WS, Knauer CM, Gregory PB: Hepatitis B viral markers in severe viral hepatitis: influence of steroid therapy. Hepatology *1:*54–57, 1981.

243. Wright EC, Seeff LR, Berk PD, Jones A, Plotz PH: Treatment of chronic active hepatitis. An analysis of three controlled trials. Gastroenterology *73:*1422–1430, 1977.

244. Cook GC, Mulligan R, Sherlock S: Controlled prospective trial of corticosteroid therapy in active chronic hepatitis. Q J Med *40:*159–185, 1971.

245. Murray-Lyon IM, Stern RB, Williams R: Controlled trial of prednisone and azathioprine in active chronic hepatitis. Lancet *1:*735–737, 1973.

246. Soloway RD, Summerskill WHJ, Baggenstoss AH, Geall MG, Gitnick GL, Elveback LR, Schoenfield LJ: Clinical, biochemical, and histological remission of severe chronic active liver disease: a controlled study of treatments and early prognosis. Gastroenterology *63:*820–833, 1972.

247. Copenhagen Group for Liver Diseases: Effect of prednisone on the survival of patients with cirrhosis of the liver. Lancet *1:*119–121, 1969.

248. Berk PD, Jones EA, Plotz PH, Seeff LB, Wright EC: Corticosteroid therapy for chronic active hepatitis. Ann Intern Med *85:*523–525, 1976.

249. Alexander GJM, Fagan EA, Guarner P: A controlled trial of 6 months thrice weekly lymphoblastoid interferon versus no therapy in chronic hepatitis B virus infection. J Hepatol *3:* (Suppl 2):183–188, 1986.

250. Thomas HC, Scully LJ, McDonald JA: Lymphoblastoid and recombinant alpha-A interferon therapy of chronic hepatitis B virus infection. The Royal Free Hospital experience. J Hepatol 3 (Suppl 2):193–197, 1986.

251. Dusheiko GM, Paterson AC, Pitcher L: Recombinant leucocyte interferon treatment of chronic hepatitis B. An analysis of two therapeutic trials. J Hepatol 3 (Suppl 2):199–207, 1986.

252. Lok ASF, Lai C-L, Wu PC: Interferon therapy of chronic hepatitis B virus infection in Chinese. J Hepatol 3 (Suppl 2):209–215, 1986.

253. Anderson MG, Harrison TJ, Alexander GJM: Randomized controlled trial of lymphoblastoid interferon for chronic active hepatitis B. J Hepatol 3 (Suppl 2):225–227, 1986.

254. Barbara L, Mazzella G, Baraldini M: A randomized controlled trial with human lymphoblastoid interferon versus no treatment in chronic hepatitis B virus infection. Preliminary results. J Hepatol 3 (Suppl 2):235–238, 1986.

255. Saracco G, Mazzella G, Rosina F, Cancellieri C, Lattore V, Raise E, Rocca G, Giorda L, Verme G, Gasbarrini G, Barbara L, Bonino F, Rizzetto M, Roda E: A controlled trial of human lymphoblastoid interferon in chronic hepatitis B in Italy. Hepatology *10:*336–341, 1989.

256. Hoofnagle JH, Dusheiko GM, Seeff LB: Seroconversion from hepatitis B e entigen to antibody in chronic type B hepatitis. Ann Intern Med *94:*744–748, 1981.

257. Realdi G, Alberti A, Rugge M: Seroconversion from hepatitis B e antigen to anti-HBe antigen seroconversion in chronic hepatitis B virus infection. Gastroenterology *79:*195–199, 1980.

258. Liaw YF, Chu CM, Su IJ: Clinical and histological events preceding hepatitis B antigen seroconversion in chronic type B hepatitis. Gastroenterology *84:*216–219, 1983.

259. Sampliner RE, Hamilton RA, Iseri OA: The liver histology and frequency of clearance of the hepatitis B surface antigen (HBsAg) in chronic carriers. Am J Med Sci *277:*17–22, 1979.

260. Hoofnagle JH, Alter HJ: Chronic viral hepatitis. *In* Viral Hepatitis

and Liver Disease, edited by G.H. Vyas, J.L. Dienstag, J.H. Hoofnagle. New York, Grune & Stratton, 1984, pp. 97–113.

261. Thomas HC, Montano L, Goodall A: Immunological mechanisms in chronic HBV infection. Hepatology 2:116 S–121 S, 1982.

262. Weller IVD, Lok ASF, Mindel A: Randomized controlled trial of adenine arabinoside 5′-monophosphate (ARA-AMP) in chronic hepatitis B virus infection. Gut 26:745–751, 1985.

263. Hoofnagle JH, Hanson RG, Minuk GY: Randomized controlled trial of adenine arabinoside monophosphate for chronic type B hepatitis. Gastroenterology 86:150–157, 1984.

264. Garcia G, Smith CI, Weissberg JI: Adenine arabinoside monophosphate (vidarabine phosphate) in combination with human leucocyte interferon in the treatment of chronic hepatitis B. Ann Intern Med 107:278–285, 1987.

265. Marcellin P, Ouzan D, Degos F, Brechot C, Metman E-H, Degott C, Chevalier M, Berthelot P, Trepo C, Benhamou J-P: Randomized controlled trial of adenine arabinoside 5′-monophosphate in chronic active hepatitis B: comparison of the efficacy in heterosexual and homosexual patients. Hepatology 10:328–331, 1989.

266. Rosina F, Pintus C, Meschievitz C, Rizzetto M. A randomized controlled trial of a 12-month course of recombinant human interferon-a in chronic delta (type D) hepatitis: a multicenter Italian study. Hepatology 13:1052–1056, 1991.

267. Di Bisceglie AM, Rustgi VK, Kassianides C, Lisker-Melman M, Park Y, Waggonner JG, Hoofnagle JH: A randomized, double-blind, placebo-controlled trial of interferon alfa therapy for chronic non A, non B hepatitis. Hepatology 11:266–270, 1990.

268. Hoofnagle JH: Antiviral treatment of chronic type B hepatitis. Ann Intern Med 107:413–415, 1987.

269. Ware AJ, Jones RE, Shorey JW, Combes B: A controlled trial of steroid therapy in massive hepatic necrosis. Am J Gastroenterol 62:130–133, 1974.

270. Redeker AG, Schwertzer IL, Yamahiro HS: Randomization of corticosteroid therapy in fulminant hepatitis. N Engl J Med 294:728–729, 1976.

271. EASL Study Group: Randomised trial of steroid therapy in acute liver failure. Gut 20:620–624, 1979.

272. Redeker AG, Yamahiro HS: Controlled trial of exchange-transfusion in fulminant hepatitis. Lancet 1:3–6, 1973.

273. Bianchi L, De Groote J, Desmet V, Gedigk P, Korb G, Popper H, Poulsen H, Scheuer PJ, Schmid M, Thaler H, Wepler W: Guidelines for diagnosis of therapeutic drug-induced liver injury in liver biopsies. Review of an International Group. Lancet 1:854–857, 1974.

274. Zimmerman HJ: Hepatotoxicity. New York, Appleton-Century-Crofts, 1978, p. 597.

Chapter 7
Toxic and Drug-Induced Hepatic Injury

Hepatotoxins, a heterogeneous group of natural and synthetic chemical agents, are capable of producing a variety of acute and chronic hepatic lesions, usually classified as manifestations of *toxic hepatic injury.* Although such lesions may differ in morphology and pathogenesis, they share a number of features. Characteristically, (1) all exposed individuals are susceptible to such injury; (2) signs of hepatic injury following acute intoxication appear promptly within 12 to 48 hours; (3) the severity of the lesions is dose-related; (4) the lesions exhibit a histologic pattern distinctive for each agent; and (5) most important, identical lesions to those seen in humans can be induced in experimental animals. As a rule, the lesions of acute hepatotoxicity are characterized by zonal hepatocellular degeneration and necrosis, often accompanied by fatty infiltration, but with little or no inflammatory reaction. Some hepatotoxins, particularly after prolonged administration, give rise to cholestasis or various forms of intrahepatic vascular injury. Some agents may give rise to a mixed type with features of both hepatocellular and cholestatic injury. Chronic hepatic injury may lead to the development of hepatic fibrosis, cirrhosis, or neoplasia.

Many drugs are capable of producing hepatic injury, but few in current use are true hepatotoxins. This paradox is not surprising since all new drugs are tested in animals; if the drugs are found to be hepatotoxic, they are not released for clinical use, unless the ratio of the toxic to the therapeutic dose is very low, or unless they possess unique therapeutic properties.

In most forms of *drug-induced hepatic injury,* the lesions exhibit a number of distinctive features that distinguish them from those produced by hepatotoxins: (1) only a small minority of exposed individuals, ranging from 1 in 50 to 1 in 10,000, are susceptible to this type of injury; (2) the signs of acute hepatic injury appear one week to several months following the initiation of drug therapy, but may occur within a few hours or days when the drug is readministered at a later date; (3) neither the occurrence nor the severity of such lesions is dose-related; (4) the acute lesions are characterized by widely disseminated foci of hepatocellular necrosis and a diffuse inflammatory reaction that mimic the lesions of acute viral hepatitis, and/or by cholestasis and portal inflammation that resemble the histologic features of extrahepatic biliary obstruction; and (5) most important, the lesions cannot be reproduced in experimental animals.

Idiosyncratic drug-induced hepatic injury can be distinguished from the lesions produced by true hepatotoxins by the fact that the former affect only a small minority of exposed individuals, are not dose-related, and fail to produce similar lesions in experimental animals. Circumstantial evidence strongly suggests that in many cases such lesions are attributable to hypersensitivity reactions, and the agents that produce them are often referred to as *sensitizing drugs.*

Although differentiation between hepatotoxic and sensitizing drugs seldom poses a problem, classification is complicated for those that behave as hepatotoxins under some conditions and as sensitizing agents under others. Thus, a number of drugs, such as *α-methyldopa,* exhibit mild hepatotoxicity in 5 to 20% of recipients, as shown by elevated levels of the serum transaminase activity and scattered small foci of hepatic necrosis that regress following withdrawal of the drug. These same agents in rare instances may give rise to hypersensitivity reactions with overt acute hepatitis apparently unrelated to antecedent hepatotoxic injury. Although the hepatotoxic effects of such drugs usually are mild and independent of the dose, there are exceptions, as in the case of *arsphenamine,* an organic arsenical preparation once widely used in the treatment of syphilis. Massive doses of arsphenamine invariably produce moderate or severe toxic hepatitis in both humans and in animals, while small, intermittently administered doses may give rise to typical hypersensitivity reactions, characterized by fever, exfoliative dermatitis, and cholestatic hepatitis in humans, but not in animals.

Pathogenesis of hepatotoxin-induced hepatic injury

Hepatotoxins are of diverse origin. Many are synthetic, organic, or inorganic chemical agents that pose occupational risk for workers in industry and agriculture, or an environmental hazard when such hepatotoxins are allowed to pollute the environment. A number of drugs contain agents of this type, and may lead to hepatic injury if used injudiciously or with suicidal intent. Other hepatotoxins that are used medicinally, and occasionally occur as food contaminants, are of plant or fungal origin. Finally, endotoxins and some exotoxins produced endogenously by bacteria are capable of injuring the liver.

The adverse effects of most hepatotoxins are attributable to metabolites produced during their biotransformation by the liver. Such metabolites, in contrast to the agents from which they are derived, are highly reactive substances that bind and alter structural and biochemical components of hepatocytes essential for their maintenance. As might be anticipated, agents that induce the microsomal enzymes responsible for the biotransformation of hepatotoxins, such as alcohol and phenobarbital, may enhance the toxicity of such hepatotoxins by accelerating the rate at which the toxic metabolites are produced. Furthermore, the inherited deficiency of one of these enzymes, as has been demonstrated for phenytoin (epoxide hydrolase), renders some patients predictably susceptible to the development of hepatic injury (1,2).

Considering the diversity of the chemical structure of hepatotoxins and the variable character of the lesions they produce, it is obvious that multiple mechanisms must be involved in the pathogenesis of hepatotoxic injury. Some of these have been identified, but many remain obscure. Moreover, the biochemical and ultrastructural changes observed during the evolution of hepatotoxic lesions are complex and vary not only with the chemical nature of the agent involved but also with its concentration and duration of action, so understanding their interrelationships and the chain of events that lead to cell injury and death is difficult.

Some hepatotoxins attack hepatocellular membranes directly, resulting in alterations of their structure and function, whereas others block essential metabolic processes in the hepatocytes by interacting with specific biochemical components of metabolic pathways, leading secondarily to similar changes in membrane structure and function. These two classes of agents are classified as *direct* and *indirect hepatotoxins,* respectively. However, the actions of both are biochemical in nature, and sooner or later lead to membrane injury and impairment of metabolic activities, so that fundamentally the effects of direct and indirect hepatotoxins are similar, at least in the final pathway that leads to cell death. The ultimate causes of hepatocellular necrosis are still only poorly understood, but involve membrane injury, inhibition of protein synthesis and energy production, activation or release of lysosomal hydrolytic enzymes, and alterations in pH or in cytoplasmic electrolyte concentrations.

Direct effects of hepatotoxins on cell membranes

Under the influence of microsomal mixed function oxidase activity, *carbon tetrachloride* undergoes homolytic cleavage in the liver to form a highly reactive free radical, CCl_3 (3). This metabolite promptly interacts with the endoplasmic reticulum leading to peroxidative denaturation of its structural lipids and impairment of protein synthesis (4). Inhibition of lipoprotein synthesis, and possibly other factors, blocks the transport of lipids out of the hepatocytes, resulting in the rapid accumulation of triglycerides, a characteristic feature of the lesions produced by carbon tetrachloride (5). Subsequently, striking changes in the mitochondria occur. These include an increase in permeability, loss of DPN, a decline in the activity of the DPN-dependent dehydrogenases of the Krebs' cycle, a decrease in ATP, and uncoupling of oxidative phosphorylation (6), effects that appear to be due primarily to impaired synthesis of proteins essential to the maintenance of mitochondrial structure and function (7). However, there is suggestive evidence that increased intracellular concentrations of calcium, secondary to leakage from hepatocellular organelles, may play a contributory role (8). It has been unequivocally established that the plasma membranes are injured by CCl_3 derived from CCl_4 (9).

A number of other halogenated hydrocarbons, including *chloroform* and *chlorinated naphthalenes* and *diphenyls,* also damage the membranes of the hepatocytes, leading to fatty deposition and necrosis, as in the case of carbon tetrachloride.

In *yellow phosphorus* poisoning, alterations in the membranes of the endoplasmic reticulum, mitochondria, and lysosomes appear early (10), and are followed by inhibition of protein synthesis (11) and impaired transport of lipid out of the liver (12). Although these features are similar to those in CCl_4-induced hepatic injury, the role of lipoperoxidation in phosphorus poisoning is still controversial (10,12), and there is no conclusive evidence that a reactive metabolite is involved (12).

Phalloidin and *amanitine,* the cyclic polypeptides responsible for the hepatotoxic effects of the poisonous mushroom *Amanita phalloides,* are other agents that injure the plasma membranes of the hepatocytes, leading initially to an increase in permeability and later to their disruption (13,14). This is followed by an increase in mitochondrial permeability and uncoupling of oxidative phosphorylation (13). Disruption of lysosomes with the release of hydrolytic enzymes appears to play an important role in the hepatocellular necrosis that ensues. However, available evidence suggests that lysosomal damage is a secondary phenomenon attributable to changes in cytoplasmic electrolytic concentration and pH rather than to a direct effect of phalloidin (13). Destruction of endothelial cells lining the sinusoids with the formation of blood-filled, peliotic cavities is a feature of the hepatic lesions produced by phalloidin in the rat (14), but not in humans.

Metabolic effects of hepatotoxins that lead to hepatic injury

A number of naturally occurring and synthetic chemical agents, only a few of which are of clinical significance, produce fatty deposition, degeneration, or necrosis of hepatocytes by selective interference with various metabolic activities essential for the maintenance of their structural and functional integrity. The net effects of these biochemical reactions, which usually are complex for any given agent, are inhibition of protein synthesis, lipid transport, and key enzyme activities. The molecular basis of such reactions is diverse, and includes, among others, covalent binding, alkylation and arylation of proteins, inhibition of the synthesis of sources of energy, and depletion of ATP, UTP, and other essential cofactors (12,15,15a).

Agents of clinical significance that fall into the category of indirect hepatotoxins that interfere with the metabolic activities of the liver include *tetracycline, puromycin, L-asparaginase, azaserine,* and *azacytidine,* which produce fatty infiltration, and *urethane, 6-mercaptopurine, 5-fluoro-2'deoxyuridine* (FUDR), and *mithramycin,* which produce hepatocellular necrosis.

Inorganic compounds of *arsenic, beryllium, copper,* and *iron* known to damage the liver are usually classified as indirect hepatotoxins, since, in some cases at least, they interact with essential enzymes and other proteins. However, they may also damage plasma membranes and organelles, so the validity of this classification is open to question.

Observations that, under experimental conditions, diets deficient in sulfur-containing amino acids (16), and poisoning with agents that bind cysteine, such as bromobenzene (17), lead to hepatic necrosis were once interpreted as evidence that the action of some hepatotoxins might be directly attributable to depletion of sulfhydryl groups in the liver. However, more recent studies indicate that the toxic metabolites of agents, such as bromobenzene and acetaminophen, are detoxified in the liver by enzymatic conjugation with sulfhydryl-containing glutathione, and that when the dose of toxin is sufficiently large to deplete glutathione stores, their toxic metabolites bind hepatic proteins covalently, leading to necrosis (18,19). Moreover, if administered sufficiently early following acetaminophen intoxication, sulfhydryl-containing compounds like methionine (20), cysteamine (21), or N-acetylcysteine (22) may prevent the progression of hepatocellular necrosis.

Hepatotoxic cholestasis (15,23)

A number of drugs, particularly the synthetic C-17 alkylated *androgenic, anabolic,* and estrogenic steroids, impair canalicular bile secretion without provoking hepatocellular degeneration or necrosis. Since this is reproducible and dose-dependent in animals, such agents qualify as hepatotoxins. However, overt cholestasis occurs only sporadically in humans, so that, in this respect, such reactions appear to be idiosyncratic. At least in the case of oral contraceptives that contain mixtures of C-17 alkylated estrogenic and progestational steroids, sporadic susceptibility to cholestasis appears to be a genetically determined exaggerated responsiveness to estrogens that becomes evident not only following the use of oral contraceptives but also during the gravid state in the form of recurrent cholestasis of pregnancy (24,25).

However, the C-17 alkylated steroids give rise, in some cases, to vascular damage, peliosis hepatis, or neoplasia.

Lithocholic acid (26), a metabolite of chenodeoxycholic acid produced in the gut by bacterial action, and *endotoxin* (27), produced by gram-negative bacteria, behave as cholestatic hepatotoxins under experimental conditions, and may be of clinical significance, although this has not yet been established.

Total parenteral nutrition may also induce cholestasis (28–30) that sometimes mimics large bile duct obstruction (29,30). Although the pathogenesis of this lesion is not known, lipid and calorie overload have been blamed (29,31).

Although *phalloidin* and *amanitine* produce hepatocellular necrosis and fatty infiltration in humans, they also give rise to cholestasis under experimental conditions (32).

Other naturally occurring cholestatic hepatotoxins, some of which are of importance in veterinary medicine but have no clinical significance in humans, have proved to be useful tools in investigating the pathogenesis of cholestasis. These include *icterogenin*, a plant alkaloid that produces jaundice and leads to photosensitization in sheep that feed on *Lippia rhemanni* (33), *sporidesmin*, a fungal toxin (34), and *cytochalasin B,* a fungal alkaloid (35).

Many drugs that impair bile flow, as, for example, *chlorpromazine* and *erythromycin estolate,* appear to be sensitizing rather than hepatotoxic agents, since the cholestasis they produce occurs only sporadically, is not dose-dependent, and often is accompanied by clinical and histologic features indicative of a hypersensitivity reaction. However, some of these drugs exhibit a dose-dependent cholestatic effect in experimental models, suggesting that they are both sensitizing and hepatotoxic agents. Although there can be little doubt that the cholestasis in humans produced by these drugs is due to hypersensitivity reactions, the possibility that hepatotoxicity plays a contributory role in its pathogenesis cannot be excluded.

What little is known about the pathogenesis of cholestasis is based largely on studies of the effects of *chlorpromazine, phalloidin, estrogens,* and *cytochalasin B* in experimental animals. Although no unified concept has emerged from such studies, a number of functional, biochemical, and ultrastructural changes have been identified as possible factors responsible for the impairment of canalicular bile flow produced by these agents. Of these, the two most important appear to be (1) a decrease in NaK-ATPase activity in the canalicular and plasma membranes, resulting in impairment of the sodium pump involved in bile salt–independent, canalicular bile secretion (36), and (2) distortion or disruption of the actin-containing microfilaments

of the pericanalicular ectoplasm and microvilli that appear to be responsible for canalicular tone and contractility (35,37). There is suggestive evidence, at least in the case of *chlorpromazine* and *ethinyl estradiol,* that the decrease in NaK-ATPase activity is related to an increase in the viscosity of the membranes, attributable to an alteration in their constituent lipids induced by these cholestatic agents (36).

It has been suggested that patients with phenotypically defective hepatic sulfoxidation but who are good hydroxylators are especially susceptible to develop chlorpromazine jaundice (38). Thus, as has been proposed for halothane, a double metabolic defect may predispose to hepatotoxicity (see below).

Vascular effects of hepatotoxins

It has been suggested that CCl$_4$, by stimulating the central autonomic nervous system, may produce intrahepatic vasoconstriction that ultimately leads to centrilobular ischemia and necrosis (39). However, direct measurements have failed to demonstrate impairment of hepatic blood flow (40), and it has been suggested that cordotomy reduces the hepatotoxicity of CCl$_4$ by inducing hypothermia rather than by preventing vasoconstriction (41). Moreover, it is now clear that the lobular, zonal localization of hepatocellular necrosis produced by many hepatotoxins may be determined by the zonal distribution of the enzymes rather than by circulatory factors.

Oral contraceptives containing synthetic C-17 alkylated steroids occasionally produce striking *periportal sinusoidal dilatation* with atrophy of the intervening hepatic plates (42). The pathogenesis of this lesion is obscure.

Peliosis hepatis, another vascular lesion associated with the prolonged use of synthetic *C-17 alkylated steroids* and, probably, oral contraceptives (42) with androgenic and anabolic activities (43), is a disorder characterized by the presence in the hepatic parenchyma of blood-filled cystic cavities devoid of lining by endothelial or Kupffer cells. Other drugs have also been associated with this lesion (44), although the fact that such cavities may be surrounded by and communicate with dilated sinusoids is consistent with the widely held view that the lesions evolve as a result of injury to sinusoidal walls. The loss of hepatocytes and reticulin in the center of these cavities suggests the possibility that necrosis of these structures may be the primary event.

In some cases, prolonged administration of *methyltestosterone* leads to hyperplasia and *prolapse of hepatocytes into the central veins,* a lesion that may be accompanied by sinusoidal ectasia or peliosis hepatis (45). Occasionally, the invading hepatocytes disrupt the walls of the affected veins and partially occlude their lumens. It has been suggested that such lesions are attributable to hepatocellular regeneration induced by the anabolic actions of methyltestosterone, and that occlusion of the central veins may account for the development of sinusoidal ectasia and peliosis hepatis.

Veno-occlusive disease is a disorder characterized by subintimal edema, hemorrhage, and inflammation of the central and sublobular hepatic veins that ultimately leads to fibrous occlusion of their lumens. Its clinical manifestations sometimes resemble those of the Budd-Chiari syndrome. It usually is attributable to hepatotoxic injury, but may occur under other conditions, including myxedema (46), graft-versus-host disease (47), alcoholic liver disease, and radiation hepatitis (48).

Poisoning with the *pyrrolizidine* (senecio) *alkaloids* of plant origin, as a result of food contamination or the use of herbal teas as medicinal agents, accounts for most cases of veno-occlusive disease (49,50). However, a number of drugs, including *azathioprine* (51), *6-thioguanine* (52), *urethane* (53), and other oncotherapeutic combinations, particularly after bone marrow transplantation (54), can also induce this disorder. Excessive doses of *vitamin A* may also produce such lesions. Patients in whom this disease develops appear to have an underlying myeloproliferative disorder that increases susceptibility to veno-occlusive disease (55). Azathioprine can cause similar lesions (56).

Centrilobular necrosis and hemorrhage are early features of the lesions produced by the pyrrolizidines, and have been attributed to impairment of hepatic blood flow secondary to occlusion of the central veins (50). However, signs of hepatocellular injury appear before there is any evidence of venous occlusion, so that it is highly probable that the lesions of veno-occlusive disease are the result of toxic injury to hepatocytes or blood vessels.

Rarely, prolonged use of *oral contraceptives* leads to *thrombotic occlusion of the major hepatic veins*, resulting in an outflow block and the development of congestive hepatomegaly, ascites, and portal hypertension, features characteristic of the *Budd-Chiari* syndrome (57). Although the propensity of these agents to produce thromboembolic disease (58) and to induce intimal thickening in blood vessels (59) is well known, the precise mechanism responsible for thrombotic occlusion of the hepatic veins is still uncertain.

Hepatic fibrosis and cirrhosis

Most acute hepatotoxic lesions are readily reversible, and heal without significant residuals. However, hepatic fibrosis and cirrhosis may ensue if: (1) exposure to a hepatotoxin is intermittent or prolonged, as in the case of *carbon tetrachloride* (60) or *methotrexate* (61) or FUDR intoxication (62); (2) vascular injury leads to sustained impairment of hepatic blood flow, as in veno-occlusive disease (49), and the Budd-Chiari syndrome (57); or (3) hepatic necrosis is massive or submassive instead of zonal, a rare type of lesion produced by only a few hepatotoxins, including *chlorinated naphthalenes* and *diphenyls* (63), *tetrachlorethane* (64), *trinitrotoluene*, and *alcohol*. Under all of these conditions, fibrosis appears to be the result of progressive hepatocellular degeneration and necrosis, but the precise stimulus responsible for fibrogenesis is still uncertain.

Hepatic fibrosis may develop insidiously following prolonged exposure to a number of hepatotoxins, including *potassium arsenite* (Fowler's solution) used medicinally (65), other *inorganic arsenicals* (66), and *copper sulfate* and other compounds contained in insecticide sprays employed by vineyard workers (67), *thorium dioxide* (Thorotrast), a radioactive agent previously used as a contrast medium in radiography (68), *vinyl chloride*, an industrial hepatotoxin (69), and excessive doses of *vitamin A* (54). Thus, there is suggestive evidence that excessive doses of vitamin A may stimulate fibrogenesis directly by activating Ito cells. It is conceivable that the radioactivity of Thorotrast may have similar effects.

Hepatic neoplasia

A wide variety of natural and synthetic chemical agents induce hepatic tumors in experimental animals (70,71). Of these, only a few have been implicated as hepatocarcinogens in humans.

Thorotrast, a colloidal solution of radioactive thorium dioxide once widely used as a contrast medium in arteriography, is one of the well-recognized etiologic factors in the pathogenesis of hepatic angiosarcoma (72,73) accounting for approximately 15% of reported cases. In addition, it has been implicated etiologically in some cases of hepatocellular carcinoma (72,74), cholangiocarcinoma (72,74), and, rarely, Hodgkin's disease. In one of our own cases of Hodgkin's disease, the liver was massively invaded by lymphomatous tissue in which numerous Thorotrast-filled macrophages were present, but there was evidence of widespread similar lymphomatous infiltration and Thorotrast deposits throughout the reticuloendothelial system in other tissues, so the primary site could not be established.

Neoplasms attributable to Thorotrast, which are not necessarily limited to the liver, usually appear 20 to 30 years following its administration (75). Since the colloid is an alpha ray emitter and is permanently retained in tissues rich in reticuloendothelium, it is reasonable to assume that neoplasia is the direct result of radiation. In this connection, it is noteworthy that there are rare reports of hepatic angiosarcoma attributed to *radium* implantation in adjacent tissues (76), and hepatocellular carcinoma following exposure to *x-irradiation* (77), or prolonged administration of *radioactive phosphorus* (78).

Vinyl chloride is also an important etiologic factor in the pathogenesis of hepatic angiosarcoma, accounting for 10 to 20% of reported cases (73,79). Characteristically, the tumor occurs in industrial workers who have been heavily exposed to vinyl chloride for long periods of time, ranging from 4 to 28 years (80).

Studies in the rat, a species in which vinyl chloride induces hepatic angiosarcoma, suggest that the carcinogenicity of the agent is dependent on one of its highly reactive metabolites that binds hepatocellular macromolecules (81).

In experimental animals, chronic administration of inorganic *arsenicals* induces tumors in the skin and lungs (82), but not in the liver (15). Nevertheless, there is convincing clinical and epidemiologic evidence that arsenicals are hepatocarcinogenic in humans. Thus, hepatic angiosarcomas have been reported in a significant number of vineyard workers exposed for 15 to 30 years to insecticide sprays and dusts containing high concentrations of arsenic trioxide (82,83), and in occasional patients medicated with potassium arsenite (Fowler's solution) for similarly long periods (84). Based on published reports, it has been estimated that arsenicals account for 2 to 3% of hepatic angiosarcomas (73,79). However, chronic arsenical intoxication rarely leads to the development of hepatocellular carcinoma or cholangiocarcinoma.

Both benign and malignant hepatic tumors are encountered in a small, but significant number of young women on long-term therapy with *oral contraceptive agents* that contain synthetic estrogenic and progestational steroids (85,86). Hepatic cell adenomas are by far the most common lesions found in this group.

Only a small number of hepatocellular carcinomas and single cases of combined hepatocellular-cholangiocarcinoma and mixed hepatoblastoma have been reported in women taking oral contraceptives (85,86).

Considering the rapid rise in the reported incidence of hepatic cell adenoma in young women since the introduction of oral contraceptives, and the regression of such tumors that follows withdrawal of these agents (85,86), it is highly probable that they are oncogenic. The prevalence of such tumors is three times greater in patients on oral contraceptive agents than in the general population (86).

Although too few hepatocellular carcinomas have been reported in women on oral contraceptives to provide firm epidemiologic evidence of a relationship between the two, the occurrence of such tumors in noncirrhotic young women and the remarkably benign clinical course in some cases following withdrawal of the steroids strongly suggest that the steroids may be hepatocarcinogenic. The short duration of exposure reported (86) is in striking contrast to the uniformly long latent period of 15 to 30 years exhibited by most known hepatocarcinogens, such as vinyl chloride, Thorotrast, and arsenic.

As in the case of oral contraceptives, prolonged administration of synthetic C-17 alkylated *androgenic-anabolic steroids,* usually used in the treatment of Fanconi's symdrome or aplastic anemia, may be associated with the development of hepatic neoplasia. However, such tumors are predominantly malignant, affect males more frequently than females, and often occur in children. Of the first 30 cases reported up to 1979, 20 were classified as hepatocellular carcinoma (85,87), 5 as hepatic cell adenoma (85), 1 as cholangiocarcinoma (88), and 4 as angiosarcoma (89).

Considering the rarity of hepatocellular carcinoma in children under other conditions, the reported regression of such tumors following withdrawal of the steroids (90), and experimental evidence in animals that androgens may enhance the hepatocarcinogenicity of other agents (91), it is highly probable that androgenic-anabolic steroids are hepatocarcinogenic in humans. However, the evidence supporting this view must be regarded as circumstantial rather than conclusive. Moreover, it has been pointed out that hepatocellular carcinomas may arise spontaneously in Fanconi's syndrome (92), and that, in some reported cases, the histologic features and behavior of the tumor have not been those of hepatocellular carcinoma (93).

Aflatoxins, metabolites of *Aspergillus flavus,* a ubiquitous fungus frequently found in moldy food, is a potent hepatocarcinogen in experimental animals (94). In areas of the world with a warm, humid climate and inadequate facilities for storage and refrigeration of food, moldy food is often consumed, and seems to be associated with a high incidence of hepatocellular carcinoma. Indeed, a number of surveys have demonstrated a remarkably close correlation between the estimated daily intake of aflatoxin and the prevalence of such neoplasms in various population groups in Africa and Southeast Asia (94). However, there is compelling evidence that chronic infection with the hepatitis B virus is the principal factor responsible for the high prevalence of hepatocellular carcinoma in areas of high aflatoxin intake. Although the possibility that aflatoxins serve as cocarcinogens cannot be excluded, this appears unlikely, since it has been shown that the risk of developing hepatocellular carcinoma in chronic HBsAg-carriers is as high in New York City, where aflatoxin intake is negligible, as in Mozambique, where it is inordinately high (95). Nevertheless, it has been suggested that aflatoxins may play an indirect role in the pathogenesis of hepatocellular carcinoma by enhancing the susceptibility to infection with the HBV, a theory based on observations indicating that, under some conditions, aflatoxins may inhibit cell-mediated immunity (96). However, there is no good evidence that aflatoxins play a role in the development of the chronic carrier state.

There is a single case report of hepatocellular carcinoma that appeared seven years following acute *carbon tetrachloride* poisoning (97), but the role of carbon tetrachloride as a carcinogen in this case is in doubt. One case of angiosarcoma has been reported in a vintner who had been exposed for 35 years to insecticide sprays and dusts containing *copper sulfate* (67). Since both the liver and tumor contained inordinately high concentrations of copper, it is highly probable that copper was the etiologic agent involved. Moreover, other vintners similarly exposed often exhibit hepatic fibrosis or cirrhosis (67), so that, in many respects, the actions of copper in the liver resemble those of vinyl chloride and inorganic arsenicals.

Nodular regenerative hyperplasia

Transformation of the hepatic parenchyma into regenerating nodules, outlined and separated by slender bands of atrophic hepatocytes and collapsed reticulin, a lesion usually classified as nodular regenerative hyperplasia may be associated with a variety of disorders, including *rheumatoid arthritis, Felty's syndrome,* the *CRST syndrome* (calcinosis, Raynaud's phenomenon, sclerodactyly, and telangiectasia), and *myeloproliferative disorders* (98,99). In many cases, including those with the disorders just cited, the lesions appear following the prolonged use of *oral contraceptives, androgenic-anabolic steroids, corticosteroids,* or *antineoplastic agents* (98). Nodular regenerative hyperplasia has also been observed after the toxic oil syndrome (100).

The pathogenesis of nodular regenerative hyperplasia is still unknown, but considering the wide variety of conditions under which it may occur, it is likely to be multifactorial. It has been suggested, on the basis of morphometric studies of the hepatic vasculature, that the hepatocellular regeneration and atrophy characteristic of the lesions are attributable to obliteration of intrahepatic venous radicles secondary to their embolization by platelet aggregates arising in the portal system or spleen (90) or secondary to vascular lesions induced by the unknown toxic contaminants in the toxic oil syndrome (100). While this may account for some cases, vascular lesions of this type are rarely demonstrable (98). Alternatively, it has been proposed that the regeneration may be a response to the drugs frequently employed in this group (98). In support of this view, it has been pointed out that the lesions closely resemble the precancerous hyperplastic nodules produced by carcinogens in experimental animals, and that nodular regenerative hyperplasia may also be a precancerous lesion, since, rarely, it has been associated with the development of hepatic cell adenoma or hepatocellular carcinoma (98).

Hepatic granulomas

Beryllium and copper compounds are unique among hepatotoxins in that they may induce granulomatous reactions in both the lung and liver.

Inhalation of *beryllium,* particularly as its oxide, may provoke either an acute pneumonitis or a delayed, chronic granulomatous pneumonitis. The chronic pulmonary lesions closely resemble those of sarcoidosis, and may be accompanied by similar granulomas in the liver. A number of features suggest that the granulomatous lesions are manifestations of a sensitization reaction to beryllium. These clues include their sporadic occurrence in exposed individuals, the long period of latency between exposure to beryllium and the appearance of such lesions, the granulomatous dermal reaction provoked by beryllium salts in affected individuals, and the *in vitro* transformation of their lymphocytes on exposure to beryllium (23).

In vineyard workers, prolonged exposure to insecticide sprays and dusts that contain *copper sulfate* and other compounds of copper may lead to the development of granulomatous pulmonary lesions (101). In approximately a third of individuals so affected, the liver contains either histiocytic or noncaseating, epithelioid granulomas in which stainable copper-containing granules can be demonstrated (67). Experimental animals exposed to copper-containing sprays also exhibit pulmonary granulomas, but these are unaccompanied by similar lesions in the liver.

The mechanism responsible for granuloma formation on exposure to copper is obscure. Although its presence in the lesions suggests a direct etiologic role for copper, the possible involvement of other constituents of Bordeaux mixture, the spray commonly used in vineyards, cannot be excluded, since similar granulomas have not been encountered under other conditions of excessive copper storage.

Pathogenesis of idiosyncratic drug-induced hepatic injury

There are few problems in medicine as controversial as the pathogenesis of idiosyncratic, drug-induced, hepatic injury. At least three mechanisms have been proposed to account for such reactions: (1) hypersensitization; (2) initiation of injury by a toxic metabolite followed by sensitization; and (3) the formation of aberrant hepatotoxic drug metabolites. Since the lesions encountered in idiosyncratic drug reactions are not uniform, being characterized by cholestasis predominantly in some cases, and by a diffuse hepatitis in others, and since some drugs appear to behave as hepatotoxins under some conditions and as sensitizing agents under others, formulation of a unified concept of the pathogenesis that is generally applicable to all idiosyncratic drug reactions is not possible at the present time. Indeed, none of the available evidence marshalled in support of any of the proposed mechanisms can be regarded as conclusive, so resolution of this problem must await the results of further studies.

Drug hypersensitivity

A number of clinical features in many forms of idiosyncratic drug-induced hepatic injury strongly suggest an underlying hypersensitivity reaction (23). These include: (1) a period of latency between the initiation of drug administration and the appearance of hepatic injury that ranges from one to four weeks, but that often is reduced to a few hours or days when the agent is subsequently readministered; (2) the prompt recurrence of hepatic injury if the agent is readministered following recovery; (3) the frequent concurrent appearance of fever, rash, lymph-

adenopathy, or eosinophilia; (4) the independence of either the appearance or severity of hepatic injury on the dose of drug employed; and (5) the increased susceptibility to such reactions of individuals with a history of antecedent, allergic disease or reactions to other drugs. Similarly, the occurrence of numerous eosinophils and granulomas in many of the hepatic lesions induced by drugs is consistent with a hypersensitivity reaction. However, it must be emphasized that even in the case of an unequivocal sensitization reaction, many or all of these clinical and histologic features may be lacking, so that their absence does not necessarily exclude an allergic basis for the lesion. The importance of this point is illustrated in the case of the controversial issue of the pathogenesis of *isoniazid-induced hepatitis*. On the basis of a retrospective study of 114 cases (102), the authors concluded that the lesions are attributable to the toxic metabolites of isoniazid in most instances, but in a few that are accompanied by fever, rash, or eosinophilia, they may be manifestations of a hypersensitivity reaction. The length of the latent period before the appearance of hepatitis in this study was cited as evidence against an immunologic basis for the lesions. In another study in which the patients were followed closely (102), the appearance of jaundice almost always was preceded by a prodromal period of constitutional symptoms.

Phenelzine (Nardil), a substituted hydrazine, is metabolized by the same biochemical pathways, and may cause a clinically and histologically similar type of liver injury (104). It has been postulated that liver injury in exposed patients may be related to their ability to acetylate hydrazines rapidly.

A unique hepatic lesion produced by phenelzine has been described (104). After two months of therapy, liver biopsy showed a parenchymal-cholestatic hepatitis with portal-portal bridging, diffuse parenchymal and portal injury and inflammation, and the presence of a unique extracellular material thought to be premature collagen (Figs. 471, 472). As the hepatitis subsided under corticosteroid-azathioprine therapy, the collagenous material diminished in amount. Micronodular cirrhosis developed promptly.

Drug-induced sensitization reactions occur more frequently in women than in men, and seldom affect children. Although no explanation can be offered for these differences in susceptibility, they do not appear to be related to the relative frequency of exposure to drugs, and serve to emphasize further the difference between sensitization and hepatotoxic reactions.

In experimental animals, simple chemical compounds can serve as antigens provided that they are covalently bound to protein (23). Under such conditions, sensitization is of the *humoral* type, and is characterized by the appearance of circulating specific antibody and skin sensitivity. Attempts to demonstrate such evidence of humoral sensitization in patients with idiosyncratic drug-induced hepatitis are only rarely successful. The occasional finding of so-called markers of autoimmunity, such as LE cells, antinuclear factor, antimitochondrial antibody, rheumatoid factor, and a positive Coombs' test, suggests an altered immunologic response, but does not necessarily imply that humoral drug-sensitization has occurred, or that such a reaction is responsible for the accompanying hepatic lesions. Such lesions have been attributed to immune complexes, i.e., the Schwartzman reaction (23).

The possibility that the cholestatic and hepatic forms of drug-induced hepatic injury are manifestations of *cell-mediated* immune reactions is suggested by the observation that many of the drugs involved stimulate lymphocyte transformation or inhibit macrophage migration in *in vitro* cultures of the lymphocytes from affected individuals. Such evidence of a cell-mediated immune response has been reported in reactions to *halothane, sulfonamides, nitrofurantoin, gold compounds, chlorpropamide, indomethacin,* and *disulfiram* among others (23). However, the results of such tests have been inconsistent in the case of some drugs, and uniformly negative in others. The reasons for this are not clear. One possibility is that the metabolites of the offending drugs are sufficiently reactive to bind protein covalently and to serve as antigens, but the parent drugs usually employed in *in vitro* studies of cell-mediated immunity may not react with lymphocytes or macrophages sensitized by their metabolites. Another is that a *K cell–mediated antibody-dependent cellular cytopathic* mechanism may be involved. There is suggestive evidence that this may be the case in *halothane-*induced hepatitis. *In vitro* tests of cell-mediated immunity using halothane as the antigen have yielded inconclusive or contradictory results, while homogenates of liver obtained from rabbits previously anesthetized with halothane inhibit the migration of leukocytes of most patients with severe halothane-induced hepatitis during the acute phase of their disease (105). Moreover, an antibody to the surface membranes of halothane-pretreated rabbit hepatocytes has been demonstrated in the serum of most patients with fulminant halothane-induced hepatitis, and it has been shown that normal lymphocytes are cytotoxic for such antibody-coated hepatocytes (106). Although the validity and interpretation of these observations have been questioned (107), they appear to be consistent with the hypothesis that halothane or its metabolites interact with the surface membranes of the hepatocytes to form a neoantigen that incites an antibody-dependent, cell-mediated, cytopathic immune reaction. Scanning electron microscopic evidence that exposure to halothane produces significant alterations in the plasma membranes of isolated rat hepatocytes lends further support to this view (108).

Many of the clinical features of *halothane-induced hepatitis* also are more consistent with a sensitization than with a hepatotoxic reaction. These include: (1) the abrupt onset with high fever, often accompanied by chills; (2) the higher incidence of hepatitis following multiple than single exposures; (3) the shorter latent period to the onset of hepatitis following multiple exposures than after single exposures: (4) the occurrence of eosinophilia in approximately 50% of cases; (5) the predominance of women among those affected; and (6) the lesser susceptibility of children (109). Moreover, it was shown that in an anesthetist who had experienced recurrent attacks of hepatitis following occupational exposure to halothane, the administration of a nonanesthetic dose of halothane for five minutes provoked high fever and severe myalgia within 4 hours, and biopsy-documented evidence of recurrent acute hepatitis within 24 hours (110). On cessation of exposure to halothane, the lesions healed and remained inactive, as documented by biopsy, over the following seven years. Nevertheless, a number of investigators attribute the hepatic lesions produced by halothane to their hepatotoxic metabolites, a conclusion based on the results of animal experiments that will be discussed later. The possibility that susceptibility to halothane-induced hepatitis, whatever its pathogenesis, may be genetically determined is suggested by the report of such reactions in three pairs of closely related women of Mexican extraction—a mother and daughter, two sisters, and two first cousins (111).

Other evidence of genetically determined susceptibility to halothane-associated hepatic injury has appeared. Investigations using phenytoin-exposed lymphocytes as a nonspecific precipi-

tant of lymphocyte-mediated sensitization have shown that patients who had halothane-induced hepatic injury and their close relatives gave positive responses in the experimental test system employed, but that controls did not (112–114). These observations suggest that the combination of a genetic abnormality of halothane metabolism and sensitization may be required to cause halothane-induced hepatic injury (112–114). The use of such tests may permit recognition of those patients who are at increased risk of developing halothane-induced hepatic injury.

Disulfiram-induced hepatic injury fulfills all criteria for drug hypersensitivity. Indeed, of 12 reported cases, 7 have been challenged by the readministration of the drug with prompt recurrence of the disease (115). Disulfiram is an especially interesting hepatotoxic drug in that in addition to inducing acute hypersensitivity hepatitis, it and cyanamide can cause a chronic hepatic lesion that is characterized by the presence of distinctive cytoplasmic inclusions that resemble Lafora's disease and the ground glass cells of HBV infection (116).

Occasionally, agents such as *azathioprine* (117) and *captopril* (118) appear to induce idiosyncratic mixed cholestatic-hepatocellular injury.

In weighing the evidence on which to establish whether drugs or their metabolites are hepatotoxic or sensitizing agents, due consideration must be given to the nature of the hepatic lesions they produce. Characteristically, in the hepatotoxic form of idiosyncratic drug-induced injury, the lesions are characterized by diffuse, spotty, or bridging hepatic necrosis, a diffuse mononuclear inflammatory reaction, and proliferation of Kupffer cells, features that are readily distinguishable from the zonal necrosis, fatty infiltration, and sparse inflammatory reaction that characterize hepatotoxic lesions.

Aberrant drug metabolism

As an alternative to the hypersensitivity hypothesis, it has been proposed that some idiosyncratic drug reactions are attributable to aberrations in drug metabolism, resulting in the production of hepatotoxic metabolites that, in some individuals, are abnormal in either chemical structure or concentration. Clinical features that are said to differentiate idiosyncratic reactions due to toxic metabolites from these attributable to hypersensitivity include: (1) absence of fever, rash, or eosinophilia; (2) a more variable and often more prolonged period of latency, ranging between one week to 12 months or longer, between the institution of drug administration and the appearance of hepatitis; and (3) a delay in the response to rechallenge with the drug following recovery (102).

Normally, the metabolic pathway of *isoniazid* in the liver involves its acetylation to acetylisoniazid and subsequent hydrolysis to acetylhydrazine, two metabolites that, under special conditions, are hepatotoxic in experimental animals (119,120). In rats, even massive doses of *isoniazid* or *acetylisoniazid* have no adverse effects on the liver, but when administered following pretreatment with phenobarbital, which induces microsomal enzymes involved in their metabolism and, thus, accelerates the rate at which their metabolites are generated, these agents produce acute centrilobular and midzonal hepatocellular necrosis (119). With the aid of radiolabeled acetylisoniazid, it has been demonstrated that its metabolites bind covalently with macromolecules in the liver, particularly in the zones of necrosis, which supports the view that such metabolites play a critical role in the pathogenesis of the lesions produced in the rat (119). The idiosyncratic type of isoniazid-induced hepatitis seen in humans has been said to occur predominantly in subjects with genetically determined fast acetylation, but this hypothesis has not been confirmed (120).

On the basis of experimental evidence similar to that obtained in the study of isoniazid, it has been proposed that the hepatic lesions produced by *iproniazid* (Marsilid) also are attributable to aberrant hepatotoxic metabolities (119). However, the interpretation of the evidence is open to the same criticisms as in the isoniazid experiments.

As previously indicated, both the clinical and histologic features of halothane-induced hepatitis are more consistent with a hypersensitivity than a hepatotoxic reaction (109). Nevertheless, several groups of investigators contend that such lesions are attributable to toxic metabolites, a conclusion based on their observations in animal experiments (121–123). Halothane alone has only minimal or no adverse effects on the liver of animals (124,125). However, when administered to rats pretreated with phenobarbital (124), particularly in an atmosphere relatively low in oxygen content (14%), conditions that induce microsomal drug-metabolizing enzymes, halothane produces extensive centrilobular or multifocal hepatocellular necrosis (123,124).

Although there is evidence that both oxidative and reductive metabolites are generated during the biotransformation of halothane in the liver, it has been suggested that reductive metabolites may play the key role in the pathogenesis of the hepatic necrosis produced by halothane in *animals* (125). These observations have been interpreted as indicating that such lesions in humans may also reflect aberrations in halothane metabolism that are dependent on concomitant exposure to enzyme inducers, resulting in enhanced generation of normally produced hepatotoxic metabolites, or on genetically determined, alternative, biochemical pathways that lead to the formation of unique, toxic metabolites.

Although the results of these experiments are consistent with the hepatotoxic metabolite theory in the case of the rat, their relevance to the pathogenesis of halothane-induced hepatitis in humans is doubtful for a number of reasons: (1) the lesions produced in the rat are characterized by centrilobular or multifocal coagulation necrosis with little or no intralobular or portal inflammation, features that bear no resemblance to the diffuse, viral-like hepatitis in humans; (2) in the rat, the lesions appear within 24 hours, while those in humans are delayed for about six days following an initial exposure to halothane; (3) the abrupt onset of high fever, often accompanied by chills, the frequent occurrence of peripheral eosinophilia, the greater susceptibility of women and its rare occurrence in young children, and (4) the shorter latent period following multiple exposures to halothane are all features of the hepatitis in humans that are inconsistent with a hepatotoxic reaction (109).

The results of the metabolic studies of isoniazid and iproniazid have encouraged speculation that many other idiosyncratic drug-induced reactions, previously considered allergic in nature, may be attributable to aberrant hepatotoxic drug metabolites. However, the biotransformation of such agents in the liver has not been adequately investigated, so no potentially hepatotoxic metabolites have been identified. Moreover, in many instances, what evidence is available is more consistent with a hypersensitivity than a hepatotoxic reaction, as, for example, in the case of *cinchophen*-induced hepatitis (23), a lesion often classified as hepatotoxic (15). Nevertheless, a number of drugs

that give rise to idiosyncratic hepatic reactions that are not reproducible in animals and exhibit no clinical or histologic features of hypersensitization may well prove to be attributable to hepatotoxic metabolites. *Sodium valproate,* an anticonvulsant that rarely produces microvesicular fatty infiltration and may produce extensive hepatocellular necrosis, may be an example of such an agent (126).

Combined hepatotoxicity and hypersensitivity

Experimental evidence indicates that chemical agents that bind protein covalently may serve as antigens (23). Since only the metabolites of drugs are sufficiently reactive to bind protein covalently, it is highly probable that in the case of sensitizing drugs, such metabolites provoke a cell-mediated immune response either directly by forming conjugates with protein, or indirectly by injuring hepatocellular membranes leading to the formation of neoantigens.

That the metabolites of drugs can bind covalently to the membranes of hepatocytes has been convincingly demonstrated in the case of such presumed sensitizing agents as *isoniazid* (119), *iproniazid* (119), and *halothane* (121). Additional evidence usually cited in support of the hypothesis that the development of hypersensitivity reactions in the liver is dependent on antecedent hepatocellular injury is the frequency with which minor hepatic functional and histologic abnormalities are found in patients receiving drugs known to induce sensitization reactions in only a few, uniquely susceptible individuals. Such agents include *isoniazid* (119), *halothane* (127), *α-methyldopa* 8,129), *chlorpromazine* (130), *diphenylhydantoin* (131), and phenytoin.

Hepatic injury following α-methyldopa administration may present as two different syndromes (129). Patients who develop hepatic injury within the first six months of therapy tend to develop acute hepatocellular necrosis that is often severe with malaise, abdominal discomfort, and jaundice. Bilirubin levels and transaminase and alkaline phosphatase activity may be elevated 10-fold. Histologically, these patients usually show acute hepatitis with mild to moderate necrosis. The more common, delayed onset disorder occurs after one to five years of therapy. Clinically, this late syndrome is benign. Laboratory tests show minimal abnormalities, and liver biopsy is characterized by moderate or severe fatty infiltration. Most show minimal evidence of active hepatitis. Chronic persistent or chronic active hepatitis may be present.

Chronic active hepatitis

A number of drugs have been implicated in the pathogenesis of *chronic active hepatitis.* These include *oxyphenisatin,* the most common offender that is no longer in use (132–134), *α-methyldopa* (Aldomet) (135,136), *nitrofurantoin* (137), *chlorpromazine* (138), *isoniazid* (103), *sulfonamides* (139), *propylthiouracil* (140), *dantrolene* (141), papavarine (142), and clometazine (143). Two alleged cases of *halothane*-induced chronic active hepatitis have been reported (144,145). The diagnosis in the first case was based on the biopsy findings at three months from the onset of acute hepatitis, but there were no follow-up observations, so the chronicity of the lesion was not truly established.

The second case, a 60-year-old woman with carcinoma of

the cervix, had had halothane three years before and then twice more four weeks apart. She had had enflurane in between the second and third administrations of halothane (143). One day after the third halothane anesthetic, the patient developed fever and jaundice. Liver biopsy 10 days later showed bridging and piecemeal hepatic necrosis with advanced collagenization of the septa, which showed well-developed nodules. She developed ascites but recovered completely within one month. Ten months later liver biopsy showed cirrhosis with chronic active hepatitis. Although there was no other obvious cause of cirrhosis, it seems clear that well-advanced chronic liver disease was present at the time the first biopsy had been performed within 10 days of the onset of the liver disease. It is unlikely that cirrhosis could have developed so rapidly. In this case, it seems likely that chronic liver disease actually preceded the halothane injury.

In all of our own cases of severe, acute halothane-induced hepatitis with extensive bridging necrosis that resolved slowly, the lesions ultimately healed with only minimal residual fibrosis and fatty infiltration (146), suggesting that progressive chronic active hepatitis is unlikely to evolve following an episode of acute halothane-induced hepatitis. However, chronic occupational exposure to halothane may occasionally give rise to such lesions. In one of our own patients, an anesthetist who had experienced repeated episodes of acute hepatitis apparently provoked by intermittent exposure to halothane, the lesions ultimately were indistinguishable from those of classic chronic active hepatitis. During a biopsy-documented remission, challenge with a brief nonanesthetic exposure to halothane provoked a prompt exacerbation that was demonstrated histologically (110). When exposure to halothane was discontinued, the hepatic lesions healed and remained inactive without treatment. Biopsy at that time revealed no evidence of acute or chronic hepatitis and only minimal fibrosis.

Five additional cases of chronic hepatitis with cirrhosis attributed to halothane have been reported (147), but no individual data about these patients were presented and it is difficult to assess these cases.

Available evidence suggests that most, if not all of the drugs that induce chronic active hepatitis are sensitizing agents. In many cases, the onset is abrupt with an acute hepatitis, often accompanied by bridging necrosis that fails to resolve, but, in others, the development of chronic hepatitis is insidious. As a rule, the lesions remain active and progress because of continued drug administration, and characteristically, tend to heal when the drug is withdrawn and to recur when it is readministered following recovery. However, occasionally, withdrawal of the drug is not followed by healing. Under such conditions, the etiologic relationship of the drug to the hepatic lesions may be questioned. However, it has been suggested, at least in some cases, that perpetuation of the lesions may be attributable to an autoimmune reaction triggered by the drug, and possibly dependent on a defect in suppressor T cell function that is genetically determined, as evidenced by the increased frequency of HLA-B8 antigen in such individuals (143,147).

Chronic drug-induced cholestatic injury

Chronic cholestatic injury that occasionally progresses to secondary biliary cirrhosis, accompanied by xanthomatosis in some cases, has been reported as a rare consequence of acute drug-induced reactions to *chlorpromazine* (148,149), *prochlorpera-*

zine (Compazine) (150), *organic arsenicals* (arsphenamine) (151), *tolbutamide* (Orinase) (152), *haloperidol* (153), and *ajmaline* (154). Available evidence suggests that all these drugs are sensitizing agents. However, the factors responsible for perpetuation and progression of the lesions are not known. In some cases, continued administration of the drug may be the cause, but, usually, cholestasis, portal inflammation, and fibrosis persist long after the drug has been withdrawn (155). Although inflammation, necrosis, and, ultimately, fibrous obliteration of interlobular bile ducts are seen in some cases (149), they are inconstant features and may be the result, rather than the cause of protracted cholestasis. Although no convincing supporting evidence is available at present, it is conceivable that an autoimmune reaction triggered by drugs is responsible for the perpetuation of such lesions.

A significant percentage of patients who receive continuous, hepatic arterial infusions of FUDR for the treatment of hepatic metastases develop sclerosing cholangitis (156). The lesions are clinically, radiologically, and pathologically indistinguishable from the usual, idiopathic form of the disease. The pathogenesis of this disorder is unknown.

Drug-induced hepatic granulomas

As previously indicated, the occurrence of granulomas in the liver in many forms of idiosyncratic drug-induced hepatitis lends support to the hypothesis that such lesions are manifestations of hypersensitivity reactions.

Hepatic granulomas have been encountered in reactions to *halothane* (155,157), *α-methyldopa* (155,158), *hydralazine* (Apresoline) (155,159), *quinidine* (155,160), *chlorpromazine* (155), *diazepam* (Valium) (155), *amitryptiline* (Elavil) (155), *imiprimine* (Tofranil) (155), *diphenylhydantoin* (Dilantin) (155), *carbamazepine* (Tegretol) (161), *oxyphenisatin* (155), *phenylbutazone* (155,162), *allopurinol* (163), *sulfonamides* (164), *nitrofurantoin* (Furadantin) (165), *penicillin* (166), *tolbutamide* (Orinase) (167), *procainamide* (Pronestyl) (168), and others (169).

Histopathology of hepatotoxin-induced hepatic injury

Most *acute* hepatotoxic lesions are characterized by hepatocellular degeneration, necrosis, or fatty infiltration, either alone or in various combinations, depending on the nature of the hepatotoxin, the severity of the lesions, and their age (170). As a rule, the lesions are zonal in distribution, most commonly centrilobular, and are accompanied by little intralobular or portal inflammation. Extensive necrosis may result in bridging, but massive or submassive necrosis is relatively rare, even in fatal cases.

In the case of some *acute* hepatotoxic lesions, the intrahepatic blood vessels or bile ducts are the principal sites of injury.

Chronic exposure to some hepatotoxins may give rise to cholestasis, hepatic fibrosis, cirrhosis, vascular lesions, or hepatic neoplasia, either alone or in combination. In some instances, these features represent the sequelae of antecedent acute hepatocellular injury, but more often they develop insidiously.

Hepatotoxin-induced zonal necrosis

Zonal hepatocellular necrosis. The *acute* lesions produced by many hepatotoxins are characterized by *centrilobular necrosis* accompanied by a variable degree of hepatocellular degeneration and fatty infiltration. Figures 473 and 474 illustrate such a lesion in a patient with severe *carbon tetrachloride*–induced hepatic injury on the eighth day of an illness manifested by increasing jaundice, oliguria, and azotemia that first appeared 24 hours following exposure for several hours to a high concentration of carbon tetrachloride fumes. As is evident at low magnification in Figure 473, there has been extensive centrilobular hepatocellular dropout, resulting in collapse of reticulin and central-central bridging. At higher magnification (Fig. 474), it can be seen that the zones of necrosis contain a few ballooned, degenerating hepatocytes and rare inflammatory cells, and are surrounded by scattered hepatocytes filled with large fat droplets. Of particular note are the intact portal tracts and periportal hepatocytes. In less severe lesions of this type, the zones of necrosis are smaller, and show no tendency to link adjacent centrilobular zones. Occasionally, in mild cases, the lesions are characterized by centrilobular hepaotcellular degeneration and fatty infiltration with little or no necrosis.

Other hepatotoxins that induce centrilobular necrosis and fatty infiltration include a number of other halogenated hydrocarbons, such as *chloroform, naphthalenes* and *trichlorethylene, halothane, pyrrolizidine alkaloids, phalloidin, amanitine,* and *cocaine* (171).

Acetaminophen is unique among the hepatotoxins in this group in that it produces centrilobular necrosis but no fatty infiltration. In fatal cases, the necrosis often is hemorrhagic, owing to disruption of sinusoidal walls, and may be massive, resulting in the destruction of most hepatocytes, except for some in the periportal zones that are arranged in the form of pseudoducts (ductular hepatocytes). Under such conditions, ductular proliferation, bile stasis, and infiltration of the collapsed reticulin by lymphocytes and histiocytes may be prominent features. Figure 475 illustrates a lesion of this type in a patient who died on the 32nd day of an acute hepatitis that followed the self-administration of massive doses of acetaminophen for the relief of intractable pain associated with advanced carcinoma of the neck. At autopsy, the liver was small and shrunken, weighing only 1025 g. Of note in this photomicrograph are the large centrilobular zone of necrosis, hemorrhage and congestion, the loss of most hepatocytes, except for the few at the periphery of the lobule, which are arranged in the form of pseudoducts, many of which contain inspissated bile. Note also the numerous histiocytes and lymphocytes in the reticulin mesh at the margins of the hemorrhagic zone, and a minimal inflammatory reaction in the portal tracts.

In nonfatal cases of *acetaminophen*-induced hepatitis, necrosis is less extensive, and usually presents as centrilobular zones of cell dropout that encircle and often bridge adjacent central veins. As a rule, the surviving loose reticulin mesh contains only a few macrophages and lymphocytes. Figure 476 illustrates a lesion of this type in a patient who had taken acetaminophen, 4 g daily, over a period of one year for the relief of arthritis. On admission, he exhibited hepatomegaly and moderately raised levels of SGOT and SGPT, but had no other signs or symptoms of liver disease. Of note in this section are the sharply circumscribed zones of cell dropout and collapsed reticulin surrounding and bridging two adjacent central veins, and the normal appearance of the portal tracts and periportal paren-

chyma. Ceroid-containing macrophages in the centrilobular regions are typical of acetaminophen-induced hepatotoxicity.

Susceptibility to acetaminophen-induced hepatotoxicity is enhanced in alcoholic patients and by alcohol (172).

Early in the course of *acetaminophen* hepatotoxicity, particularly in cases of mild intoxication, the centrilobular hepatocytes may show evidence of coagulation necrosis (Fig. 477), ballooning (Fig. 107), or acidophilic degeneration (Fig. 111) rather than cytolysis. Occasionally, the hepatocytes undergoing coagulation necrosis in such lesions are infiltrated with neutrophils (Fig. 101), and there may be an accompanying inflammatory reaction in the portal tracts (Fig. 478).

Cocaine, a narcotic substance that can be taken by inhalation, by absorption through the nasal membrane, or intravenously, has been shown to cause hepatic injury (171). Although uncommonly reported in the past, a recent publication describes a relatively consistent syndrome in patients shown to have a specific metabolite of cocaine in their urine. Within a few hours of ingestion a sharp increase in transaminase activity develops, falling rapidly within a few days. Although serum bilirubin levels were only moderately elevated, increased CPK activity, myoglobinuria, and disseminated intravascular coagulopathy were common. Histologically, there was severe centrilobular necrosis with cholestasis and steatosis but only a minimal inflammatory reaction (Figs. 479–481). Since cocaine usage is common and this syndrome is uncommon, an individual susceptibility factor appears to be operative.

In rats, *beryllium compounds* produce *midzonal hepatic necrosis* when administered intravenously, but are innocuous when inhaled (23). It is not surprising, therefore, that midzonal hepatic necrosis is not a feature of either acute or chronic beryllium intoxication in humans, which invariably is acquired through the respiratory route. The more common finding in acute pulmonary berylliosis is centrilobular hepatic necrosis, which may be attributable to respiratory failure and anoxia rather than beryllium intoxication. Characteristically, in chronic beryllium intoxication, both the lungs and the liver contain noncaseating, epithelioid granulomas that resemble those of sarcoidosis.

A number of other hepatotoxins produce midzonal hepatic necrosis in animals, but none of these is of clinical significance in humans.

Periportal hepatic necrosis, often accompanied by some degree of fatty infiltration, characterizes the lesions produced by a number of hepatotoxins, of which only yellow phosphorus and ferrous sulfate are of clinical significance in humans.

The hepatic lesions of *yellow phosphorus* poisoning are variable in character. Although periportal hepatocellular degeneration, necrosis, and fatty infiltration are the features usually emphasized in most reports (173), the periportal distribution of the lesions and the prominence of fatty infiltration are not seen in all cases. The only case we have studied was found by biopsy in a man with deep jaundice and hepatic encephalopathy that followed the suicidal ingestion of one ounce of rat poison containing 1 to 4% of yellow phosphorus 15 days previously. The outstanding histologic features included marked ballooning of the hepatocytes, widespread formation of hepatocellular rosettes of the ''hepatitis'' type (174), and marked cytoplasmic and canalicular bile stasis throughout the lobules, involving the centrilobular (Fig. 482) and periportal zones (Fig. 483) equally, accompanied by striking expansion of the portal tracts by edema, fibrous tissue, proliferating ductules, and a mixed exudate of neutrophils and lymphocytes (Fig. 484). Although fat-stained frozen sections were not available, no lipid droplets could be identified in routine sections. The lesions illustrated ultimately healed, but residual patchy portal and portal-portal bridging fibrosis were still evident five months afterward.

Poisoning with *ferrous sulfate,* which often proves fatal, usually occurs as a result of its accidental ingestion by young children. The hepatic lesions produced are characterized by extensive coagulation necrosis of periportal hepatocytes that usually contain fine lipid droplets and hemosiderin deposits (175).

Hepatotoxin-induced massive and submassive hepatic necrosis

Although bridging necrosis is seen occasionally in cases of severe hepatotoxin-induced hepatitis, massive or submassive necrosis is rare, even when the lesions are sufficiently extensive to result in hepatic failure and death. This is in striking contrast to the frequency with which such lesions are encountered in fatal cases of idiosyncratic drug-induced hepatic injury.

As previously indicated, *acetaminophen* occasionally produces massive or submassive hepatic necrosis (Fig. 475). Other agents that produce such lesions more frequently include *tetrachlorethylene* (176), *trinitrotoluene* (177,178) and *chlorinated naphthalenes* and *diphenyls* (64).

Figure 485 illustrates a typical example of submassive hepatic necrosis produced by *chlorinated naphthalene.* This lesion was found postmortem in a man with jaundice of six months' duration that had appeared following a five-month occupational exposure to molten Halowax, a mixture of chlorinated naphthalenes used to coat electrical wire for purposes of insulation. Because of the jaundice and increasing malaise, he had stopped work for three months, leading to some improvement of his symptoms, although the jaundice persisted. Following this period of convalescence, he returned to work and again was exposed to Halowax, resulting in deepening of the jaundice, the appearance of ascites and edema, and, ultimately, progressive hepatic failure that led to his death six months from the onset of jaundice. At autopsy, the liver was small, weighing only 1027 g, and showed broad, deep, red, depressed zones of recent multilobular necrosis and collapse that alternated with areas containing large nodules of regenerating parenchyma separated by relatively thick collagenized septa, typical of postnecrotic cirrhosis. One of the zones of recent multilobular necrosis is illustrated in Figure 485. As can be seen, there has been loss of all hepatocytes and collapse of reticulin in a large group of contiguous lobules that are outlined by numerous proliferating ductules interspersed with many infiltrating plasma cells and lymphocytes. In an adjacent section (Fig. 486) are seen the typical features of an advanced, but inactive macronodular cirrhosis. The absence of any inflammatory reaction, ductular proliferation, or evidence of hepatocellular degeneration or necrosis is in striking contrast to the activity of the lesions in the zones of more recent multilobular necrosis (Fig. 485).

Hepatotoxic fatty infiltration

As previously indicated, fatty infiltration often accompanies the zonal hepatic necrosis produced by many hepatotoxins (Fig. 474). Occasionally, in cases of mild intoxication, the lesions exhibit fatty infiltration and hepatocellular degeneration with little or no necrosis. A lesion of this type in a case of mild *carbon tetrachloride*–induced hepatitis, manifested by slight hyperbilirubinemia and moderately raised levels of SGOT that appeared 12 days previously following the ingestion of a small volume of carbon tetrachloride in an unsuccessful suicide attempt, is illustrated in Figures 487 and 488. The centrilobular pattern of fatty infiltration and absence of necrosis are evident in Figure 487, and, at higher magnification in Figure 488, it can be seen that most of the affected hepatocytes are filled with small fat droplets, and that some show ballooning, karyolysis, and acidophilic degeneration.

A few hepatotoxins, including tetracycline, aflatoxin, and hypoglycin A, can produce severe, and even fatal hepatic injury that is characterized by extensive centrilobular or panlobular microvesicular steatosis with no evidence of hepatocellular necrosis.

The intravenous administration of large doses of *tetracycline* frequently results in severe hepatic injury that often proves fatal. Such reactions are encountered most frequently in pregnant women with urinary tract infections (179), but may occur in men and under other conditions (180,181). Characteristically, the hepatocytes in the centrilobular zones or in a panlobular distribution are distended by numerous small and large lipid droplets, and show evidence of degeneration, but little or no necrosis. Often, in severe cases, the fatty deposition is accompanied by cholestasis, an inflammatory reaction in the portal tracts, and ductular proliferation. Figure 489 illustrates the panlobular micro- and macrovesicular fatty deposition found in a case of severe but nonfatal tetracycline-induced hepatitis that had begun 16 days previously following the intravenous administration of 10 g of tetracycline over a period of four days. The ballooning and distension of the hepatocytes by both small and large lipid droplets, the apparent disruption of the plasma membranes in some cells, resulting in their coalescence, a feature emphasized by some observers (180), and the pyknosis of some nuclei and the dissolution of others are clearly evident at higher magnification in Figure 114. Many of the midzonal canaliculi were dilated and contained inspissated bile (Fig. 490), and most of the portal tracts were enlarged and edematous, showed segmental erosion of their limiting plates, and contained proliferating ductules, occasional small pools of free bile, and numerous macrophages, neutrophils, and lymphocytes (Fig. 491).

The microscopic features of the hepatic lesions produced by tetracycline are indistinguishable from those of acture fatty liver of pregnancy and Reye's syndrome. Although the liver tends to be enlarged in the former and reduced in size in the latter, this is not a reliable criterion for differentiating between these two disorders.

Based on epidemiologic, toxicologic, and experimental evidence, it has been proposed that *aflatoxin,* the toxic metabolite of the fungus *Aspergillus flavus,* commonly found in moldy food, may be the etiologic agent responsible for some cases of Reye's syndrome (182,183). As in the case of tetracycline-induced hepatic injury, the lesions in this disorder also are characterized by panlobular microvescular fatty infiltration and degeneration of the hepatocytes, usually unaccompanied by necrosis.

The akee fruit of the *Blighia sapida* tree in Jamaica contains a potent hypoglycemic and hepatotoxic agent, *hypoglycin A.* Ingestion of the raw fruit, particularly by children, leads to severe vomiting and profound hypoglycemia, an illness known as Jamaica vomiting sickness that often proves fatal. As in the case of Reye's syndrome, the associated hepatic lesions are characterized by panlobular microvesicular hepatocellular fatty infiltration and degeneration without accompanying necrosis (184).

Reye's syndrome, which presents almost the same clinical and histologic picture, is inextricably intertwined with aspirin toxicity. It seems likely that aspirin plays a major role in the pathogenesis in some cases of this disorder (185).

Hepatotoxin-induced cholestasis

Histologic evidence of cholestasis is a relatively common feature of the lesions in acute hepatotoxic injury. When present, bile thrombi usually are found in the dilated canaliculi of surviving parenchyma in the centrilobular or midzones of the lobules, as in the case of mild *carbon tetrachloride*–induced toxic hepatitis illustrated in Figure 492. However, when necrosis is extensive, as in the lesions of severe *acetaminophen*-induced hepatitis shown in Figure 475, the bile thrombi may be located in periportal canaliculi and ductules. Moreover, in instances in which the cholestasis of severe toxic hepatitis resolves slowly, the parenchyma occasionally contains sharply circumscribed foci of foamy pseudoxanthoma cells that often encircle a central collection of free bile, forming so-called bile infarcts (Fig. 122), while the portal tracts are expanded, and may contain widely dilated, degenerating, and necrotic interlobular ducts filled with bile that may extravasate into the surrounding connective tissue. In such instances the bile is usually surrounded by pseudoxanthoma cells and a variable number of lymphocytes, neutrophils, and histiocytes (Fig. 339). The lesions illustrated in Figures 122 and 339 were found on biopsy during the fifth week of severe *tetracycline-induced* hepatitis that began abruptly immediately following the intravenous adminstration of 8 g of tetracycline over a period of four days.

Prolonged administration of *oral contraceptives* and synthetic C-17 alkylated *analbolic-androgenic steroids* may lead to a type of cholestasis that is unique in two respects. First, although a cholestatic effect is producible in animals, thus qualifying these agents as hepatotoxins, jaundice is produced in humans only sporadically. This feature, at least in the case of oral contraceptives, appears to be related to a genetically determined enhanced susceptiblity to the effects of estrogens (24,25). Second, in contrast to most other hepatotoxins, anabolic-androgenic steroids produce cholestasis with little or no accompanying hepatocellular degeneration or necrosis and little portal inflammation. In addition to cholestasis, these steroids may give rise to hepatic vascular lesions and neoplasia, which are described in sections that follow.

As a rule, the principal feature of the lesions in steroid-induced cholestasis is the presence of numerous bile thrombi in dilated centrilobular canaliculi, occasionally accompanied by bile-staining or accumulation of fine bile droplets in the cytoplasm of adjacent hepatocytes and Kupffer cells. A lesion of this type found on the sixth day of jaundice in a patient who had been receiving *norethandrolone* (Nilevar) for six months is illustrated in Figure 493. Although hepatocellular degeneration and necrosis, and intralobular or portal inflammation are never prominent features in steroid-induced cholestasis, rare acidophilic bodies (Fig. 494), occasional focal collections of swollen Kupffer cells, lymphocytes, and neutrophils (Fig. 495), and mild to moderate infiltration of the portal tracts by lymphocytes and neutrophils (Fig. 496) may be seen in early lesions, particularly when the cholestasis is severe. In the patient with *norethandrolone*-induced cholestasis whose lesions are illustrated in Figures 493–496, the serum bilirubin reached a peak level of 25 mg/dl on the 13th day of jaundice, and took five months to return to normal.

Late in the course of severe prolonged steroid-induced cholestasis, the lesions may show extension of bile stasis to the periportal zones, ballooning of centrilobular hepatocytes, swelling and pseudoxanthomatous degeneration of Kupffer calls, more extensive portal inflammation, ductular proliferation, and, occasionally, distension of interlobular ducts with retention of inspissated bile and atophy of their walls. Severe duct abnormalities of this type in a case of *oxymethalone* (Adroyd)-induced cholestasis of six weeks' duration are illustrated in Figure 497. In this same case, a number of centrilobular and periportal hepatocytes contained typical Mallory bodies (Fig. 498). Since these parenchymal and portal abnormalities tend to increase with persistence of the cholestasis following withdrawal of the drug, it is highly probable that they are attributable to the cholestasis rather than to the direct effects of the steroids.

Hepatotoxic injury to bile ducts

A small number of chemical agents that induce cholestasis in animals under experimental conditions injure the intrahepatic bile ducts. Of these, only *methylenedianiline* (4, 4′-diaminodiphenyl methane), a hardening agent used in the production of epoxy resins, is of clinical significance in humans, having been implicated as an etiologic factor in the pathogenesis of cholestatic jaundice in industrial workers exposed to the agent (186) and in a large group of individuals with an illness known as *Epping jaundice* that developed following the ingestion of bread made of flour accidentally contaminated with *methylenedianiline* (187).

In addition to histologic evidence of centrilobular cholestasis, the lesions in Epping jaundice exhibited expansion and infiltration of the portal tracts by inflammatory cells, including numerous eosinophils, inflammation and necrosis of interlobular ducts, ductular proliferation, small foci of hepatocellular necrosis, and increased mitotic activity in the hepatocytes (187). Except for the cholangitis, the lesions resembled those in idiosyncratic drug-induced cholestatic hepatitis. Moreover, some of the patients with Epping jaundice exhibited fever, rash, and eosinophilia, features suggestive of a hypersensitivity reaction. Although no explanation can be offered to account for these manifestations, there can be no doubt that *methylenedianiline* is a hepatotoxin, since the lesions it produces in humans are readily reproducible in animals, and since a high proportion of exposed individuals appear to be susceptible to its adverse effects. Obviously, the unusual clinical and histologic manifestations of Epping jaundice have led to speculation that a similar unique type of hepatotoxic reaction may be involved in the pathogenesis of idiosyncratic forms of cholestatic hepatitis induced by drugs thought to be sensitizing agents (15). Certainly, this is an interesting possibility that merits further investigation. Despite the severity of the lesions produced by *methylenedianiline* in some cases, the lesions usually heal without significant residuals (186,188).

Some drug-induced lesions, such as those produced by *paraquat*, may be biphasic, causing hepatocellular damage early in the course and cholangiocellular lesions later (189).

Hepatotoxin-induced vascular lesions

Prolonged use of *oral contraceptives* can lead to striking *periportal sinusoidal dilatation* with atrophy of the intervening hepatic plates (Figs. 216, 217), a lesion often manifested clinically by hepatomegaly and minor hepatic functional abnormalities that regress when contraceptive therapy is discontinued (42).

Another hepatic vascular lesion that may appear following prolonged use of C-17 alkylated *anabolic-androgenic steroids* or *oral contraceptives* (43,44) is *peliosis hepatis,* a disorder characterized by the presence in the hepatic parenchyma of multiple blood-filled cystic cavities unlined by either endothelial or Kupffer cells. A typical example of such a lesion in a child with Fanconi's anemia under prolonged treatment with *oxymethalone* is illustrated in Figure 499. Another example was induced by testosterone enanthate (Fig. 500). Peliotic cavities vary in size and number, and, often, are asymptomatic, being discovered unexpectedly in biopsy sections or at autopsy. Occasionally, however, they are massive and may rupture into the peritoneal cavity, or lead to hepatic failure that results in death (44).

Occasionally, peliotic cavities are surrounded by and communicate with widely dilated sinusoids, a type of peliosis that has been termed "phlebectatic" (190). A lesion of this type, attributable to prolonged *oral contraceptive* therapy, is illustrated in Figure 217. However, in most cases of peliosis, the cavities do not show an intimate relationship to dilated sinusoids, although such sinusoids may be present elsewhere in the section. An example of this type of peliosis, usually classified as "parenchymal," (184) is illustrated in Figure 499, which shows the lesion in a child with Fanconi's anemia on prolonged *oxymethalone* therapy.

There is general agreement that the "parenchymal" form of peliosis probably is attributable to antecedent focal necrosis that leads to destruction of the sinusoids, reticulin, and hepatocytes. Indeed, in some cases, transitions between such zones of focal necrosis and peliotic cavities can be demonstrated. Figure 500 illustrates such a sharply circumscribed zone of hepatocellular necrosis in which there is partial destruction of the reticulin in a patient with peliosis hepatis due to the prolonged administration of *testosterone enanthate.*

The pathogenesis of the phlebectatic type of peliosis is still controversial. It has been suggested that since the cavities are in continuity with dilated sinusoids and allegedly are lined by endothelium, they represent ectatic sinusoids (190). However, in none of the phlebectatic lesions that we have examined have the cavities been lined by endothelium, nor have they been encircled by condensed reticulin, as might be expected if they developed as a result of progressive dilatation of the sinusoids and atrophy of the intervening hepatocytes. Accordingly, it appears more likely that both the phlebectatic and parenchymal forms of peliosis are attributable to a type of focal necrosis that destroys the sinusoidal walls, reticulin, and hepatocytes.

In addition to *oral contraceptives* and *anabolic-androgenic steroids,* other etiologic factors that have been implicated in the pathogenesis of peliosis hepatis include advanced *tuberculosis* (191), *carcinomatosis* (185), hypervitaminosis A (192), and other wasting diseases.

One of the most serious but fortunately rare complications of *oral contraceptive* therapy is *hepatic vein thrombosis* and its sequela, the *Budd-Chiari syndrome,* a disorder manifested by hepatomegaly, often accompanied by abdominal pain and tenderness, signs of portal hypertension, including ascites, splenomegaly, and esophageal varices, and, ultimately, hepatic failure or hemorrhage from varices, which often proves fatal.

In addition to oral contraceptives, other etiologic factors that have been implicated in the pathogenesis of the Budd-Chiari syndrome include *polythemia vera, paroxysmal nocturnal hemoglobinuria, ulcerative colitis, pregnancy, abdominal trauma, aspergillosis,* primary and metastatic *hepatic neoplasms,* and *congenital anomalies* of the hepatic veins or inferior vena cava. Although some of these disorders have distinctive clinical features, the hepatic lesions they produce are indistinguishable.

The early lesions of the Budd-Chiari syndrome are characterized by severe centrilobular sinusoidal congestion with atrophy and loss of the intervening hepatocytes, features resembling those produced by right-sided heart failure or constrictive pericarditis. However, some of the sublobular and central veins contain distinctive, organized thrombi. Hemorrhage into the spaces of Disse is said to be another diagnostic feature of the Budd-Chiari syndrome (193), but, in our own experience, this is a nonspecific histologic criterion, since it may be seen in centrilobular ischemic necrosis (Fig. 89), hemorrhagic necrosis produced by hepatotoxins (Fig. 475), and in severe passive congestion due to heart failure or constrictive pericarditis (Fig. 214).

The typical histologic features of the early lesions in the Budd-Chiari syndrome are illustrated in the case of a young woman with inactive ulcerative colitis who presented with intractable ascites of 10 months' duration. The diagnosis of hepatic vein thrombosis was established by needle biopsy of the liver and subsequently was confirmed by hepatic venography. As can be seen in Figure 501, there was extensive centrilobular sinusoidal dilatation and loss of hepatocytes, resulting in central-central bridging. The reticulin was intact and the portal tracts and periportal parenchyma were unaffected. Scattered through the section were occasional central veins that contained organized, partially recanalized thrombi, as shown in Figure 502. Although progression to cirrhosis occurred in this case, the ascites ultimately abated and the patient remained in relatively good health for over eight years.

As the hepatic lesions in the Budd-Chiari syndrome progress, the centrilobular zones of congestion and cell loss extend to the portal tracts, the reticulin in these zones collapses and undergoes collagenization, and there is accompanying expansion and fibrosis of the portal tracts. As a result, the normal lobular architecture is destroyed and replaced by a homogeneous form of cirrhosis, usually termed "congestive," that, except for the presence of thrombosed hepatic veins, is identical with the type of "cardiac" cirrhosis encountered occasionally in cases of severe, long-standing, recurrent, right-sided heart failure or constrictive pericarditis. A reversal of the lobular pattern, characterized by nodules that contain a centrally located, intact portal tract, and are encircled by central veins joined by dilated sinusoids and bands of collagen, has been emphasized as a distinctive feature of congestive cirrhosis due to either hepatic vein thrombosis or cardiac disease. However, nodules of this type are relatively uncommon. More often the portal tracts are enlarged and fibrotic, and merge with the fibrous septa that radiate from the central zones, so that the nodules formed are devoid of portal tracts, and are surrounded by both central veins and portal tracts. Characteristically, the prominence of congestion, fibrosis, and nodule formation varies from one area to another in any given section, and even intact lobules may be present in some. The combination of these features plus the presence of organized thrombi in central or sublobular veins provide firm histologic criteria for identifying the Budd-Chiari syndrome. This is illustrated in the case of a young woman who presented with ascites of six weeks' duration that appeared following eight years of oral contraceptive therapy. As illustrated in Figure 503, needle biopsy revealed numerous small, irregular, parenchymal nodules separated by relatively coarse, irregularly contoured, fibrous septa that occupied most of the section. Note that none of the nodules contained portal tracts, the sinusoids were only minimally dilated, and no central veins could be identified in the fibrous septa, but some septa contained proliferating ductules, venous channels, and an occasional arteriole, suggesting that they arose from portal tracts. However, some fields were noncirrhotic, and showed extensive centrilobular congestion with atrophy and loss of hepatocytes (Fig. 504) and occasional central veins that contained organized, recanalized thrombi (Fig. 215). Although reversal of the lobular pattern was not evident anywhere in this needle biopsy specimen, it was found in a few areas at autopsy two months later. One such area is illustrated in Figure 505, which shows a parenchymal nodule with a centrally located intact portal tract that is surrounded at its periphery by central veins linked by dilated sinusoids and fine bands of collagen. Also seen in this nodule are the irregular, two-cell-thick hepatic plates, indicative of regeneration, a feature of congestive cirrhosis that is relatively uncommon, as compared with most other forms of cirrhosis. In this case, the diagnosis of the Budd-Chiari syndrome was established by needle biopsy and subsequently confirmed by hepatic venography and autopsy.

The unusual features in this case were the advanced degree of fibrosis found at seven weeks, and the rapid progression to hepatic failure that led to death within four months from the onset of symptoms. These findings are in striking contrast to the absence of significant fibrosis at 10 months and to the subsequent clinical remission despite progression to cirrhosis in a patient with the Budd-Chiari syndrome associated with ulcerative colitis whose biopsy sections are illustrated in Figures 501 and 502. Although it is generally assumed that the thrombosis in the Budd-Chiari syndrome starts in the major hepatic veins and then extends in retrograde fashion to involve the more peripheral branches, it is conceivable that, in some cases at least, the thrombosis starts peripherally and then extends along the direction of blood flow to involve the larger hepatic veins. Under such conditions, hepatic congestion and fibrosis tends to progress slowly and may lead to the development of advanced cirrhosis, even before the appearance of overt clinical signs of the Budd-Chiari syndrome.

The *pyrrolizidine alkaloids,* the most frequent cause of *veno-occlusive disease,* produce lesions that may be acute, subacute, or chronic (49,50). Those that occur following the administration of *6-thioguanine* usually are acute (52), whereas those attributable to *hypervitaminosis A* (54), and *azathioprine* (51) tend to be chronic. In the case of *radiation* (48,194) and *urethane-* induced hepatic injury (53,195), the lesions may be either acute or chronic.

The *acute* lesions of *veno-occlusive disease* are characterized by edema, hemorrhage, and inflammation in the intima of central and sublobular veins, and by severe centrilobular congestion, hemorrhage into the spaces of Disse, and hepatocellular lysis. As a rule, the affected veins contain no thrombi, and the hepatocytes show no evidence of coagulation necrosis. The typical lesions of acute veno-occlusive disease of about two weeks' duration are illustrated in Figures 271 and 506. These were encountered in a boy with acute myelogenous leukemia who

had been under treatment with *6-thioguanine* for two months. As shown in Figure 271, the intima in all of the central veins was edematous and infiltrated by numerous erythrocytes and occasional lymphocytes, but did not occlude their lumens. In addition, all the centrilobular zones showed striking congestion of the sinusoids, hemorrhage into the spaces of Disse, and loss of hepatocytes (Fig. 506). Death from hepatic failure ensued three weeks from the onset of symptoms, At autopsy, the liver was massively enlarged, severely congested, and showed the same vascular and parenchymal lesions found in the biopsy specimen illustrated in Figures 271 and 506. A careful search revealed no evidence of hepatic vein thrombosis.

In the *chronic* form of *veno-occlusive disease,* the central and sublobular veins undergo progressive fibrosis, leading to partial or complete occlusion of their lumens. Characteristically, these vascular changes are accompanied by a variable degree of centrilobular congestion and atophy or loss of hepatocytes. Under some conditions, the sinusoids are lined or partially occluded by collagen bundles, whereas in others, there is collapse and collagenization of the reticulin in the congested areas, leading, in some cases, to the development of congestive cirrhosis, as in the Budd-Chiari syndrome. Chronic lesions may be encountered during the recovery phase of acute veno-occlusive disease, as in the case of individuals who survive an attack of acute Senecio poisoning, or may develop insidiously, as in patients with hypervitaminosis A. Shown in Figure 272 are the lesions of chronic veno-occlusive disease found at autopsy in a patient with severe hypervitaminosis A who died of progressive hepatic failure. For several years this individual had taken massive doses of vitamin A for the treatment of a pharyngeal carcinoma. The two central veins illustrated in Figure 272 show fibrous thickening of the intima, resulting in partial occlusion of the lumen. In the surrounding centrilobular parenchyma are seen a broad zone of severe sinusoidal congestion, complete loss of hepatocytes, and, in some areas, condensation and early collagenization of the reticulin. A less advanced lesion of chronic veno-occlusive disease in another case of hypervitaminosis A is illustrated in Figure 224. Of particular note in this centrilobular field are the numerous collagen bundles within the lumens of dilated sinusoids and the spaces of Disse, and the atrophy and loss of hepatocytes. Throughout the section, but especially in the centrilobular zones, many of the sinusoids contained large, pale, vacuolated Ito cells (Fig. 259) that, in frozen sections, exhibited the typical, transient, apple-green autofluorescence of vitamin A (Fig. 260), findings consistent with the view that the sinusoidal deposition of collagen in hypervitaminosis A is attributable to activation and transformation of Ito cells to functioning fibroblasts (54).

Full recovery without significant residuals is possible in veno-occlusive disease, but occurs in only a minority of cases (49,50).

Hepatotoxin-induced hepatic fibrosis and cirrhosis

Acute zonal necrosis produced by hepatotoxins like *carbon tetrachloride, phosphorus,* and *acetaminophen* usually heal without significant residuals following cessation of exposure, even when the zones of necrosis bridge adjacent central veins or portal tracts. Occasionally, however, some degree of zonal or bridging fibrosis may be found following recovery, but it tends to regress with time, and does not progress. This is illustrated in the case of *phosphorus*-induced toxic hepatitis shown in Figures 482–484. Thus, two months following apparent recovery, liver biopsy revealed significant portal-portal bridging fibrosis with occasional nodule formation (Fig. 507). However, four months later, only minimal portal fibrosis with no evidence of bridging or nodule formation was demonstrable. Similarly, in the case of acute *carbon tetrachloride*–induced toxic hepatitis illustrated in Figures 473 and 474, biopsy following recovery demonstrated significant central-central bridging fibrosis. Although the patient's refusal to permit rebiopsy made it impossible to document whether it had regressed or remained stable, no clinical or biochemical evidence of liver disease could be demonstrated during a prolonged follow-up period.

Massive hepatic necrosis due to such agents as *chlorinated naphthalenes* and *diphenyls* (63), *tetrachlorethane* (64), and *trinitrotoluene* (177) usually proves fatal. However, if the necrosis is *submassive* and the patient survives sufficiently long, progression to macronodular postnecrotic cirrhosis usually ensues. Figure 486 illustrates a lesion of this type in a patient who died six months following the acute onset of *chlorinated naphthalene*–induced submassive hepatic necrosis.

Hepatic fibrosis and cirrhosis may develop insidiously, in the absence of antecedent *acute* hepatocellular necrosis, following *prolonged* or *intermittent exposure* to a number of hepatotoxins. These include *carbon tetrachloride* (60), *methotrexate* (61), *inorganic arsenicals* (66), *copper sulfate* (67), *thorium dioxide* (68), and *vinyl chloride* (69).

Long-term exposure to *carbon tetrachloride* fumes is a rare cause of cirrhosis. In the only well-documented case that we have seen, the patient, who was teetotal, presented with jaundice, ascites, and edema that appeared following occupational exposure to high concentrations of carbon tetrachloride fumes for over 10 years. At autopsy, the liver was small, and on microscopic examination, showed an inactive, mixed micronodular and macronodular cirrhosis with no distinctive features indicative of its etiology (Fig. 508).

Hepatic fibrosis and cirrhosis were recognized as complications of prolonged *methotrexate* administration soon after it was first used in the treatment of acute leukemia (190,196). Although the indications for such therapy soon were extended to include other neoplastic and chronic inflammatory disorders, it was not until its use in severe psoriasis became widespread that the risk of chronic methotrexate hepatotoxicity became a matter of serious concern and the subject of intensive investigation. Based on studies in patients with psoriasis, it seems that such hepatotoxicity is dose-dependent. The incidence of hepatic fibrosis and cirrhosis increases progressively as the duration of administration lengthens (197) and the cumulative dose exceeds 2 to 4 g (198). Moreover, small frequent doses appear to be more hepatotoxic than large intermittent doses (197), and that advanced age, obesity, and, particularly, alcohol abuse may potentiate the adverse effects of the drug (198,199). The problem of monitoring patients under prolonged methotrexate therapy for evidence of hepatotoxicity is complicated by the fact that routine tests of hepatic function often fail to detect the development of hepatic fibrosis and cirrhosis (197,198), and that almost half the patients with psoriasis exhibit hepatic lesions before such therapy is instituted (200). Fatty infiltration is by far the most common abnormality found, but nonspecific focal hepatitis, varying degrees of portal fibrosis, and nonspecific granulomas are not rare. No doubt obesity, diabetes mellitus, and alcohol abuse account for the lesions in some cases, but, in others, no etiologic factors can be identified. It is conceivable that some of the hepatic lesions in psoriasis are attrib-

utable to associated skin infection, or to absorption of the tars and salicylates frequently applied topically. Since the development of hepatic fibrosis may escape detection by routine tests of hepatic function, and since structural abnormalities of the liver are relatively common in untreated psoriatic patients, it is common practice to biopsy the liver prior to the institution of methotrexate therapy, and at annual or biennial intervals thereafter for as long as the treatment is continued.

The reported incidence of hepatic fibrosis and cirrhosis in psoriatic patients undergoing prolonged methotrexate therapy ranges from as low as 12% (199) to as high as 46% (197). In early lesions, the fibrosis is limited to the portal tracts, and appears to be the result of the degeneration and necrosis of periportal hepatocytes accompanied by a mononuclear inflammatory reaction, features resembling the type of piecemeal necrosis seen in chronic active hepatitis (201). With progression, the fibrosis extends to bridge adjacent portal tracts and central veins, ultimately resulting in destruction of the normal lobular architecture and the development of cirrhosis that may be either micronodular or mixed micro- and macronodular in type (197–199). There is suggestive evidence that activation of Ito cells may play a role in the fibrogenesis provoked by methotrexate (202). At all stages in their development, the lesions may be accompanied by fatty infiltration, small scattered foci of inflammation and necrosis in the parenchyma, and occasional acidophilic bodies.

Figure 509 illustrates the enlarged and fibrotic portal tracts and the fatty infiltration found in a patient with psoriasis following intermittent methotrexate administration for eight years. At higher magnification, it can be seen that the portal tracts are infiltrated with numerous lymphocytes and show segmental erosion of their limiting plates with extension of the lymphocytes into the periportal parenchyma (Fig. 510), and that the latter may contain an occasional acidophilic body (Fig. 511). That this lesion may be attributed to the methotrexate is supported by the fact that liver biopsy four years previously had revealed only mild fatty infiltration, and that no other etiologic factors could be identified.

An example of advanced inactive methotrexate-induced cirrhosis is shown in Figure 512. This lesion was encountered in an elderly woman with Wegener's granulomatosis that had been completely suppressed for six years by almost continuous methotrexate administration. She presented with asymptomatic, slowly progressive splenomegaly that had first appeared one year previously. Particularly noteworthy is the fact that despite the presence of advanced cirrhosis, the results of all tests of hepatic function were within normal limits.

Some investigators have questioned the association of methotrexate and cirrhosis (203,204). They suggest that other known causes of cirrhosis, such as alcohol, are usually present and that methotrexate may act as a cofactor in potentiating such toxicity.

The occurrence of hepatic granulomas in psoriasis is of particular interest, since these lesions may be mistaken for evidence of sarcoidosis or tuberculosis if their relationship to psoriasis is not recognized. Obviously, such lesions, which are common in psoriasis, cannot be attributed to methotrexate when they are encountered before the drug is used. In our own series of 49 psoriatic patients subjected to liver biopsy before the institution of methotrexate therapy, 11 (22%) exhibited hepatic granulomas. The results of Kveim tests in this group were uniformly negative, except in one patient with concomitant sarcoidosis, and in none of the cases was there evidence of tuberculosis or other granulomatous disorders. The resemblance of such granulomas to those of sarcoidosis and tuberculosis is clearly evident in Figure 513. The possibility that the granulomas in psoriasis may be indicative of a response to tars or salicylates absorbed from the skin is suggested by the fact that all of our psoriatic patients with hepatic granulomas had previously been treated for long periods with ultraviolet light and ointments containing mixtures of tars and salicylates, and that, often, their serum levels of salicylate during such therapy had been significantly elevated. Perhaps granulomas may occasionally occur in untreated psoriasis.

Chronic ingestion of *inorganic arsenicals,* as, for example, in the form of Fowler's solution used medicinally (205), lengthy industrial exposure to *vinyl chloride* (206), or the prolonged inhalation and ingestion of *copper sulfate and other compounds* found in insecticide sprays used by vineyard workers (67) may lead to the development of portal fibrosis and severe presinusoidal portal hypertension with hemorrhage from esophageal varices. Unless the exposure to these agents is known and their significance as etiologic factors is recognized, these clinical and morphologic features may be misinterpreted as manifestations of idiopathic portal hypertension. An example of *vinyl chloride*–induced hepatoportal sclerosis associated with severe portal hypertension that led to hemorrhage from esophageal varices is illustrated in Figure 514. As can be seen, even in the area most severely affected, the portal tracts were only moderately enlarged and fibrotic, contained few inflammatory cells or ductules, and showed no erosion of the limiting plates. Although there was minimal portal-portal fibrous bridging, the lobular architecture was well preserved, and there was no evidence of nodule formation to suggest cirrhosis. Usually, histologic identification of the etiology in such lesions is not possible. However, in those lesions attributable to copper compounds, the fibrosis may be accompanied by granulomas containing granules that take up copper stains (67).

In some cases of chronic *arsenical, vinyl chloride,* and *copper* intoxication, fibrosis is more extensive, leading to the development of cirrhosis.

Hepatotoxin-induced hepatic neoplasia

A number of hepatotoxins are known to produce a variety of benign and malignant hepatic neoplasms. These are also discussed and illustrated in Chapter 25.

Hepatotoxin-induced hepatic granulomas

The hepatic granulomas produced by *copper* sulfate and other compounds in the insecticide sprays used in vineyards (100), and by *beryllium* compounds to which machinists, metallurgists, and manufacturers of ceramics, radio tubes, fluorescent bulbs, and neon signs are exposed (207) invariably are secondary manifestations of chronic granulomatous pneumonitis induced by prolonged inhalation of these agents.

The hepatic granulomas associated with *copper*-induced vineyard sprayer's lung disease are of two types: (1) well-defined nodules made up of histiocytes, and (2) sharply circumscribed aggregates of epithelioid cells that resemble the lesions of sarcoidosis. Often, the granulomas are infiltrated by a few lymphocytes, and may show varying degrees of fibrosis, but contain no giant cells. Characteristically, yellow-brown granules that exhibit the histochemical properties of copper compounds are found in the epithelioid cells and in scattered foci of proliferating Kupffer cells (100).

The hepatic granulomas found in *berylliosis,* which occur exclusively in association with the delayed form of chronic pneumonitis seen in that disease, are indistinguishable from those of sarcoidosis. The lesions may be found in the parenchyma or portal tracts, and present as masses of epithelioid and giant cells interspersed or surrounded by a variable number of lymphocytes. In general, those in the parenchyma are more sharply circumscribed and more compact than those in the portal tracts. The granulomas show no evidence of necrosis or tendency to undergo fibrosis. Differentiation from sarcoidosis is not possible histologically, and usually depends on a history of occupational exposure to beryllium and a positive patch test with one of the soluble beryllium salts. Application of such solutions to the skin provokes an inflammatory reaction that appears in 48 hours and then persists for at least three to five weeks, at which time it is found to be granulomatous in nature on biopsy (208). A typical example of a hepatic granuloma in berylliosis is illustrated in Figure 515. The patient involved, a young woman who had been exposed to beryllium phosphors in the manufacture of fluorescent bulbs for over a year, presented with dyspnea, fatigue, and weight loss, and showed a fine, diffuse interstitial infiltrate throughout both lungs on X-ray, and a positive beryllium nitrate patch test.

Histologic differential diagnosis of hepatotoxic lesions

Hepatotoxic zonal necrosis. Lesions of toxic hepatitis characterized by *centrilobular* degeneration, necrosis, and fatty infiltration, as in the case of carbon tetrachloride intoxication (Fig. 474) may resemble those of *alcoholic hepatitis* (Fig. 130). However, in the latter, the necrotic zones tend to be less sharply circumscribed, fatty infiltration usually is more widely distributed, the degenerating hepatocytes often contain Mallory bodies (Fig. 130), neutrophilic infiltrates are relatively common (Fig. 131), fibrous bands often line the centrilobular sinusoids (Fig. 223) and encircle individual hepatocytes (Fig. 225), and some of the intact hepatocytes within the lobules may contain megamitochondria (Fig. 134).

Late in the course of *hepatotoxic centrilobular necrosis,* cytolysis of damaged hepatocytes may lead to the appearance of sharply circumscribed zones of cell dropout and collapsed reticulin that encircle the central veins, as in the case of acetaminophen-induced hepatitis illustrated in Figure 476. Similar lesions may be seen during the recovery phase of *centrilobular ischemic necrosis,* but, usually, the reticulin is not collapsed, and presents as a fine mesh in which are enclosed numerous dilated sinusoids (Fig. 89).

Hepatic fatty deposition. When *centrilobular fatty deposition* is the predominant feature in toxic hepatitis, as in the lesion produced by carbon tetrachloride shown in Figures 487 and 488, differentiation from the more common types of fatty infiltration due to *alcoholism* (Fig. 173), *diabetes mellitus,* or *obesity* may be difficult, if not impossible. Although microvesicular fatty infiltration, hepatocellular ballooning, and acidophilic degeneration favor a hepatotoxic etiology (Fig. 488), these features are not diagnostic, since they may be seen in other forms of centrilobular fatty infiltration, as illustrated by the microvesicular character of the lipid droplets in a case of alcoholic liver disease (Fig. 172).

Panlobular microvesicular fatty deposition, while characteristic of tetracycline intoxication (Figs. 114, 489), also occurs in the *acute fatty liver of pregnancy* (Figs. 115, 116), in *Reye's syndrome* (Fig. 117), and in alcoholic liver disease, so-called *alcoholic foamy degeneration* [(209); Fig. 113], so differentiation between these lesions depends on the history and clinical features.

Hepatotoxic cholestasis. As illustrated in the case of phosphorus poisoning, hepatotoxic lesions characterized by *zonal hepatic necrosis,* if sufficiently severe, often show centrilobular bile stasis (Fig. 482), expansion and edema of the portal tracts, ductular proliferation, and a portal neutrophilic exudate (Fig. 484), features that may suggest *extrahepatic biliary obstruction.* Usually, however, the toxic nature of such lesions is apparent from the prominence of the accompanying hepatocellular degenerative changes (Fig. 482), the evidence of active hepatocellular regeneration in the form of thick plates and rosettes (Fig. 483), and the presence of periportal bile thrombi (Fig. 483). Although bile thrombi may be encountered in the periportal zones in severe and prolonged extrahepatic biliary obstruction, they occur more frequently and at an earlier stage in all forms of hepatocellular cholestasis. "Hepatocellular cholestasis," however, is currently used to describe an entity in which hepatocellular necrosis is minimal or absent.

Centrilobular cholestasis, portal inflammation, and ductular proliferation also occur in cases of toxic *panlobular microvesicular fatty infiltration,* as, for example, in tetracycline intoxication (Figs. 490, 491). Such lesions are not likely to be mistaken for those of extrahapatic biliary obstruction because of the prominence of the microvesicular lipid droplets. However, when the cholestasis is prolonged, the lipid droplets tend to disappear, whereas the evidence of bile stasis and the portal changes may become more prominent, suggesting extrahepatic biliary obstruction.

The cholestatic lesions produced by *synthetic estrogenic* and *anabolic-androgenic* steroids also resemble those of extrahepatic biliary obstruction, as is evident in Figures 493 and 496, which show a lesion of this type induced by norethandrolone. Since such lesions have no distinctive features, identification of their steroidal etiology is impossible on histologic grounds alone, so the diagnosis invariably depends on the history of drug administration and the exclusion of concomitant biliary obstruction by cholangiography.

Pseudoxanthomatous degeneration of Kupffer cells and hepatocytes, and the formation of *bile "infarcts,"* although often considered pathognomonic of extrahepatic biliary obstruction, may be seen occasionally in severe and prolonged hepatocellular cholestasis. An example of such a lesion in a case of tetracycline-induced severe cholestasis is illustrated in Figure 122. Changes in the portal tracts are minimal or absent.

Another lesion associated with severe hepatocellular cholestasis that may be misleading is marked *dilatation, atrophy, and necrosis* of the *interlobular bile ducts,* often accompanied by stasis or extravasation of bile. In our experience, such duct changes are encountered more commonly in hepatocellular disease than in biliary obstruction. Examples of such duct lesions in cases of tetracycline and oxymethalone intoxication are illustrated in Figures 339 and 497, respectively.

Hepatotoxic vascular lesions. The *late* lesions of *chronic veno-occlusive disease* are characterized by centrilobular sinusoidal dilatation, atrophy or loss of the intervening hepatocytes, and perisinusoidal fibrosis (Fig. 224), features that resemble those of *chronic passive congestion* due to long-standing right-sided heart failure or constrictive pericarditis (Fig. 198). However, the presence of central veins that show intimal fibrosis and occlusion of their lumens (Fig. 272) serves to identify the lesions of chronic veno-occlusive disease. In the case of hypervitaminosis A, an additional diagnostic feature is the occurrence in the sinusoids of large, pale, vacuolated Ito cells (Fig. 259) that, characteristically, in frozen sections, exhibit the transient, apple-green autofluorescence of vitamin A (Fig. 260).

In the *early* stages of the *Budd-Chiari syndrome* induced by oral contraceptives (Fig. 501), the lesions closely resemble those of *chronic passive congestion* (Figs. 197, 198), and, in the *late* stages (Fig. 505) those of *congestive (cardiac) cirrhosis* (Fig. 516). However, both in the early and the late lesions of the Budd-Chiari syndrome, some of the central veins invariably contain organized, recanalized thrombi (Figs. 215, 502). Similar occlusions of the central veins may be encountered in the late stages of *alcoholic hepatitis* and *alcoholic cirrhosis* (Fig. 273), but neither of these lesions shows the areas of impressive congestion seen in veno-occlusive disease or the Budd-Chiari syndrome (Figs. 504, 505).

Histopathology of idiosyncratic drug-induced acute cholestatic hepatitis

The hepatic lesions encountered in *acute* idiosyncratic drug reactions are of three major types: (1) *cholestatic,* characterized by features that closely resemble those of biliary obstruction; (2) *hepatitic,* with features that mimic those of acute viral hepatitis; and (3) *mixed.* Although the type of lesion is distinctive in the case of some drugs, often it is variable. Thus, the lesions produced by *chlorpromazine* and *erythromycin estolate* are characteristically cholestatic, whereas those produced by *halothane* and *isoniazid* are invariably hepatitic. However, reactions to α-*methyldopa, phenylbutazone, sulfonurea derivatives, propylthiouracil,* and others may give rise to either cholestatic or hepatitic lesions, although one or the other tends to predominate. To complicate further the problem of classification, the lesions in many idiosyncratic drug reactions exhibit both cholestatic and hepatitic features, the so-called *mixed hepatocellular* type (15). Although this is an appropriate histologic descriptive term, it may be misleading, since it is often applied to hepatic lesions associated with high serum levels of alkaline phosphatase, but no histologic evidence of cholestasis (15).

A wide variety of drugs have been implicated as etiologic factors in drug-induced cholestatic hepatitis. The incidence of such reactions is relatively low, ranging from 0.01 to 1.0% of exposed individuals. Those encountered most frequently are attributable to *chlorpromazine,* other *phenothiazine derivatives,* and *erythromycin estolate* and other esters of erythromycin. Drugs less commonly involved include *chlordiazepoxide* (Librium), *diazepam* (Valium), *meprobamate* (Equanil), *carbamazepine* (Tegretol), *tolbutamide* (Orinase), *chlorpropamide* (Diabinase), *methimazole* (Tapazole), *demecolcine* (Colcemid), *chlorothiazide, chlorthalidone* (Hygroton), *quinethazone, nitrofurantoin,* and *thiobendazole.* In addition, drugs that may produce either cholestatic or hepatitic lesions include among others, *phenylbutazone indomethacin, diphenylhydantoin, carbamazepine, thiouracil, metahexamide, prochlorperazine* (Compazine), and *imipramine* (Tofranil).

Bile stasis

Characteristically, the centrilobular zones contain a variable number of bile thrombi within dilated canaliculi (Fig. 517). Often, adjacent Kupffer cells show focal hyperplasia and hypertrophy, and may be bile-stained or contain droplets of bile (Fig. 518). Under conditions of severe or prolonged cholestasis, bile thrombi may be found in periportal canaliculi (Fig. 519), or, less commonly, in ductules or interlobular ducts.

Hepatocellular degeneration and necrosis

Although hepatocellular degeneration and necrosis seldom are prominent features in the lesions of drug-induced cholestasis, occasional, randomly distributed acidophilic bodies are relatively common (Fig. 520). In addition, particularly when the cholestasis is severe, some of the hepatocytes in the vicinity of bile thrombi may show ballooning (Fig. 521) or pseudoxanthomatous degeneration (Fig. 522), while others may undergo cytolysis, resulting in focal disruption of the hepatic plates (Fig. 518). Under similar conditions, the limiting plates of some portal tracts may show segmental erosion due to the loss of periportal hepatocytes (Fig. 519).

Hepatocellular regeneration

Often, drug-induced cholestasis provokes a hepatocellular regenerative response. Most frequently this is evidenced by pleomorphism, binucleation, and trinucleation of hepatocytes (Fig. 520), and, less commonly, by increased mitotic activity or the formation of thick hepatic plates (Fig. 519), pseudoducts, or rosettes (Fig. 517, 518).

Kupffer cells

Focal *swelling* and *proliferation* of Kupffer cells, and staining or infiltration of their cytoplasm by *bile* are relatively common, particularly in the zones of most marked cholestasis (Fig. 518). In addition, some may show foamy *pseudoxanthomatous degeneration* of their cytoplasm (Fig. 522).

Intralobular inflammation

As a rule, relatively few inflammatory cells are found within the lobules. However, in some cases, the sinusoids may contain occasional lymphocytes (Figs. 518, 520) and eosinophils.

Portal tracts

Almost always, some of the portal tracts show an inflammatory reaction. Usually, lymphocytes predominate, but, in some cases, a variable number of eosinophils and neutrophils may be present (Fig. 523). When cholestasis is severe or prolonged, the portal tracts often contain macrophages, some of which may show pseudoxanthomatous degeneration of their cytoplasm. Although the lesions of drug-induced cholestatic hepatitis are classified as "pericholangitic" by some authorities (15), the inflammatory cells in small and medium sized portal tracts usually show a random distribution (Fig. 523), but may be localized around the large ducts found in septa (Fig. 524).

As a rule, the portal tracts are not enlarged or fibrotic, and are enclosed within intact limiting plates (Fig. 523). However, under conditions of prolonged or severe cholestasis, the portal tracts may be *expanded,* and show *fibrosis* and *erosion* of their *limiting plates* (Fig. 519, 525).

Ductular proliferation is another inconstant feature of drug-induced cholestatic hepatitis.

Hepatic granulomas are rare in the cholestatic lesions induced by drugs, but we have encountered them in reactions to *chlorpromazine* in two cases (158) and to *diazepam* (Valium) and *amitryptiline* (Elavil) in one case each. Characteristically, the granulomas are sharply circumscribed, consist of a compact mass of epithelioid and occasional giant cells, and are found in small numbers in either the parenchyma or the portal tracts (Fig. 526). Since they closely resemble the lesions of sarcoidosis and many other systemic granulomatous diseases, the possibility that the granulomas are attributable to such disorders must always be excluded before they are accepted as manifestations of a drug reaction.

Histopathology of idiosyncratic drug-induced chronic cholestatic hepatitis and biliary cirrhosis

Rarely, *chlorpromazine* (148,149), *prochlorperazine* (149), *organic arsenicals* (151), and *tolbutamide* (152) produce a type of chronic cholestatic hepatitis that fails to resolve following withdrawal of the drug. In some cases, the lesions are characterized by cholestasis and portal fibrosis, but show no tendency to progress, and may even heal (152). However, in others, the fibrosis is progressive, leading ultimately to the development of cirrhosis (148–150,152).

Figure 525 illustrates an example of apparently nonprogressive, chronic, cholestatic hepatitis in a young black man who presented with jaundice, severe pruritus, and generalized xanthomatosis. His illness had begun abruptly with jaundice seven months previously following a four-week course of chlorpromazine therapy. Although drug administration was discontinued promptly, signs of cholestasis persisted. Almost all the portal tracts were enlarged and fibrotic, contained a moderate number of lymphocytes and neutrophils and a few eosinophils, and showed ductular proliferation. Although the limiting plates were eroded, there was no evidence of bridging fibrosis, and the overall lobular architecture was normal. Many of the canaliculi and some of the ductules contained bile thrombi. The epithelial cells lining the ducts that contained inspissated bile were vacuolated, but showed no evidence of inflammation or necrosis. The fate of this lesion is not known, since the patient was not seen again following biopsy.

A more advanced lesion in a case of chlorpromazine-induced chronic cholestatic hepatitis is illustrated in Figure 526. The patient, a middle-aged schizophrenic woman, presented with mild icterus, severe pruritus, hepatomegaly, and xanthomata of four years' duration. These had appeared following the administration of chlorpromazine, but since the relationship of the cholestasis to the drug was not recognized, chlorpromazine administration had been continued throughout her illness. As can be seen in Figure 527, all portal tracts were enlarged and fibrotic, showed segmental erosion of their limiting plates, and contained numerous lymphocytes and histiocytes and occasional neutrophils. In many areas, adjacent portal tracts showed fibrous bridging that partially or completely outlined nodules of parenchyma. There was evidence of ductular proliferation, but the interlobular ducts were normal in number and structure. Only a few bile thrombi were found within canaliculi. Withdrawal of chlorpromazine led to a significant fall in the serum bilirubin, alkaline phosphatase, and SGOT levels, but mild pruritus persisted.

Figure 528 illustrates a case of advanced chlorpromazine-induced biliary cirrhosis in a young woman who presented with jaundice, severe pruritus, xanthomatosis, and hepatosplenomegaly. Jaundice had appeared abruptly five years previously following a one-week course of chlorpromazine, which was continued for another four weeks. Despite withdrawal of the drug at that point, the jaundice failed to abate, and signs of slowly progressive biliary cirrhosis appeared. As can be seen in Figure 528, a needle biopsy section revealed advanced micronodular cirrhosis with marked canalicular bile stasis and moderate ductular proliferation. The interlobular ducts were normal in number and showed no evidence of degeneration, necrosis, or inflammation, and there were no portal lymph follicles or granulomas to suggest primary biliary cirrhosis. Two years following this biopsy, the patient bled massively from esophageal varices and died of progressive hepatic failure.

In two of these three cases of chlorpromazine-induced chronic cholestatic hepatitis, the lesions appeared to be self-perpetuating in that they showed progression following withdrawal of the drug. In the third case, their progression may have been due to continued drug administration.

Histopathology of idiosyncratic drug-induced acute hepatitic lesions

Idiosyncratic reactions to a wide variety of drugs give rise to lesions, usually classified as *hepatic,* that closely resemble those of acute viral hepatitis. The incidence of such reactions is relatively low, ranging from 0.01 to 1.0% of exposed individuals. The drugs most frequently implicated include *halothane, alpha-methyldopa,* and *isoniazid.* Among others may be cited *methoxyflurane* (Penthrane), *allopurinol, cinchophen* and its derivatives, *gold salts, trimethadione, ethionamide, sulfonamides, propylthiouracil, carbutamide, iproniazid, isocarboxazide* (Marplan), *phenelzine* (Nardil), pheniprazine (Catron), and *trimethobenzamide* (Tigan). In addition, a number of drugs may produce either cholestatic or hepatitic lesions. Among these, the most common include *indomethacin, phenylbutazone,*

diphenylhydantoin, thiouracil, metahexamide, prochlorperazine (Compazine), and *imipramine* (Tofranil).

Although the hepatitic lesions in drug-induced reactions resemble those of acute viral hepatitis, they are characterized more frequently by cholestasis, eosinophilic infiltrates, granulomas, and bridging hepatic necrosis. Unfortunately, these features are neither constant nor pathognomonic, so they are of only limited value in differential diagnosis.

Many of the lesions are readily reversible following withdrawal of the offending drug. However, progression to *chronic active hepatitis* and *cirrhosis* may ensue. As indicated in Chapters 8 and 9, such progression may be attributable to continued drug administration, but, rarely, it may be self-perpetuating. Although chronic lesions often are the sequelae of unresolved antecedent acute hepatitis, they may develop insidiously. Acute lesions characterized by bridging necrosis are less likely to progress to chronic active hepatitis and cirrhosis in drug reactions than in viral hepatitis (210) provided drug administration is promptly discontinued. This is well illustrated in the case of severe halothane-induced bridging necrosis, which heals without significant residuals in individuals who survive the first few weeks of their acute hepatic disease and are not reexposed to halothane (146). However, intermittent or continuous exposure to the offending drug once bridging necrosis has appeared often leads to chronic active hepatitis and cirrhosis (103,110,135).

Hepatocellular necrosis

As illustrated in the lesion produced by *halothane* (Fig. 529), all of the lobules in drug-induced hepatitis show foci of necrosis (cell dropout) that tend to be relatively large and *confluent* in the *centrilobular* zones and *spotty* elsewhere in the parenchyma. The pattern of necrosis is often indistinguishable from CCl_4-induced hepatic injury. The spectrum of halothane-induced hepatic necrosis varies widely in lobular distribution and degree. The severity of the necrosis appears to be more closely related to the frequency with which the patients received halothane than to any other factor (142). Occasionally, *periportal necrosis* also occurs, so that the portal tracts appear expanded and show erosion of their limiting plates (Fig. 530). The prominence of centrilobular confluent necrosis in many cases of halothane-induced hepatic injury often is cited as evidence that the lesions are manifestations of hepatotoxicity rather than hypersensitivity. However, as illustrated in Figure 531, periportal necrosis may predominate in some cases.

Bridging necrosis is a relatively common feature of the hepatic lesions produced by *halothane, isoniazid, cinchophen* and its derivatives, *indomethacin, phenylbutazone, diphenylhydantoin, thiouracil, metahexamide, tolbutamide, iproniazid, phenelzine, pheniprazine, imipramine,* and any other drugs capable of causing severe necrosis. As illustrated in the case of *halothane*-induced hepatitis (Fig. 532), the distribution of the bridging necrosis may be central-central, central-portal, or portal-portal, or, more commonly, a combination of these. Although the bridging usually is found in all fields, some lobules may be spared. Lesions of this type may result in hepatic failure and death, or give rise to chronic active hepatitis, but may also heal without significant residuals, as in the case of *halothane*-induced bridging necrosis illustrated in Figure 532.

Drugs that produce bridging necrosis occasionally give rise to *massive* or *submassive hepatic necrosis*. Almost always such lesions prove fatal within a few weeks. At autopsy in such cases, the liver is greatly reduced in weight and shows large areas of necrosis in which most of the hepatocytes have been destroyed. Characteristically, the portal tracts are spared, and, often, are encircled by proliferating ductules or small groups of hepatocytes. A lesion of this type in a case of *halothane*-induced massive hepatic necrosis is illustrated in Figure 533. The patient, an elderly woman who had had two previous exposures to halothane, experienced shaking chills and fever 11 days following her third exposure, and soon thereafter showed signs of progressive hepatic failure that promptly proved fatal.

Hepatocellular degeneration

Many of the surviving hepatocytes in drug-induced hepatitis show *ballooning*, as is evident at higher magnification (Fig. 534) in one of the centrilobular zones of the *halothane*-induced lesion shown in Figure 529. In addition, a variable number of *acidophilic bodies* are found scattered through the lobules, both in the centrilobular (Fig. 534) and periportal zones (Fig. 530). As shown in Figure 535, some of the hepatocytes may be both swollen and finely *vacuolated*.

Hepatocellular regeneration

When hepatocellular necrosis is moderate to severe, the surviving hepatocytes often show evidence of increased regenerative activity. Usually the hepatocytes are arranged in the form of two-cell-thick plates, and *rosettes or pseudoacini* that enclose bile thrombi, as illustrated in the case of halothane-induced hepatitis shown in Figure 535. In severe lesions, marked *pleomorphism* and *multinucleated giant hepatocytes* may be seen, as illustrated in the lesion of *ibuprofen* (Motrin)-induced hepatitis shown in Figure 270.

Cholestasis

Histologic evidence of cholestasis is a relatively common feature of the hepatitic lesions produced by drugs, and, often, is even more impressive than in drug-induced cholestasis. Most frequently, *bile thrombi* are found within dilated canaliculi and swollen Kupffer cells in the centrilobular zones, as illustrated in the case of *paraminosalicylic acid*–induced hepatitis shown in Figure 209. However, when the cholestasis is severe or prolonged, midzonal and periportal bile thrombi are relatively common (Fig. 535).

Typical *bile "infarcts,"* often erroneously regarded as a pathognomonic feature of extrahepatic biliary obstruction, may be seen in severe drug-induced hepatitic lesions accompanied by marked cholestasis. Such infarcts characteristically appear as sharply circumscribed foci of foamy hepatocytes and Kupffer cells that are undergoing pseudoxanthomatous degeneration. Often, they contain extravasated bile, and usually are located in the periportal parenchyma, although they may be found in

other zones in severe cholestasis. In some cases, the infarcts lie close to distended, necrotic, or degenerating interlobular bile ducts filled with inspissated bile. A typical lesion of this type is illustrated in Figure 536, in a fatal case of *propylthiouracil*-induced hepatitis with bridging necrosis.

Intralobular inflammation

Characteristically, the parenchyma is infiltrated by a variable number of inflammatory cells that usually are most numerous in the foci of necrosis. As can be seen in Figure 534, lymphocytes and proliferating Kupffer cells predominate. However, in some cases, a variable number of eosinophils may be seen, as is evident in the lesion of *halothane*-induced hepatitis illustrated in Figure 285. Occasionally, plasma cells and neutrophils are seen.

Kupffer cells

Almost always, the Kupffer cells are swollen and greatly increased in number. Usually, they are most prominent in the foci of necrosis, but often appear to fill the sinusoids in some areas (Figs. 531, 534). Many of the Kupffer cells are pigmented, and are stained by PAS following diastase degeneration, indicating their increased content of ceroid pigments (lipofuscin).

As previously indicated, foci of Kupffer cells may show pseudoxanthomatous degeneration when cholestasis is prominent. Often, such cells are found in bile infarcts (Fig. 536), but smaller groups may be encountered within the sinusoids.

Hepatic granulomas

Available evidence suggests that most, but not necessarily all granulomatous lesions are attributable to delayed hypersensitivity reactions (211). Accordingly, the occurrence of granulomas in some of the hepatic lesions induced by idiosyncratic drug reactions lends support to the view that such reactions are manifestations of hypersensitivity. Whatever their pathogenesis, it is not clear why hepatic granulomas appear in only a minority of cases, or why they are encountered more frequently in hepatitic than in cholestatic lesions. As previously indicated, hepatic granulomas have been seen in hepatitic reactions to *halothane, methyldopa, hydralazine, quinidine, imipramine, diphenylhydantoin, oxyphenisatin, phenylbutazone, allopurinol, sulfonamides, nitrofurantoin,* and *penicillin*.

Although some reports suggest that granulomas may be the only feature of the hepatic lesions induced by idiosyncratic drug reactions, in our biopsy material, they have invariably been accompanied by histologic evidence of diffuse hepatitis or cholestasis. For that reason, we prefer to classify such lesions as hepatitic or cholestatic drug-induced hepatitis with granulomas, rather than as granulomatous hepatitis.

Usually, only a few granulomas are found within the parenchyma or portal tracts. Characteristically, they are made up of epithelioid giant cells interspersed with a few lymphocytes. Those in the parenchyma tend to be more compact and sharply circumscribed than those in the portal tracts. Figure 537 illustrates such a large, ill-defined epithelioid giant cell granuloma in a portal tract in a case of *halothane*-induced hepatitis.

In some cases, the granulomas appeared to be circumscribed masses of proliferating, swollen Kupffer cells that are beginning to undergo transformation to epithelioid and giant cells. A granuloma of this type in another case of *halothane*-induced hepatitis is illustrated in Figure 231.

In one unique case, *allopurinol* induced a typical hypersensitivity syndrome involving liver, skin, and muscles in a patient after four weeks of therapy (212). The biopsy showed focal hepatocellular necrosis, a mixed inflammatory reaction, and intralobular, noncaseating, epithelioid *fibrin-ring granulomas*. Each granuloma consisted of an empty, fat vacuole surrounded by a concentric ring of fibrinoid material that stained positive with Masson trichrome stain. These ''doughnut'' granulomas are similar to those seen in Q fever. There were no organisms visible and no exposure to nor serologic evidence of Q fever.

In a restrospective review of 95 cases of ''granulomatous hepatitis'' the authors concluded that 15% were probably drug-related (169). The diagnosis was based largely on the temporal relationship between the drug administration and the onset of the adverse effect and the exclusion of other common causes of granulomatous disease. In the absence of such diseases the cases were considered *probably* drug-related; when these other diseases could not be excluded definitively, they were classified as *possibly* related to drug administration. Among the toxic drugs most frequently responsible were sulfonamide, alphamethyldopa, penicillin, and isoniazid. Unfortunately, it is rarely possible to exclude definitively all of the large number of granuloma-stimulating diseases.

Central vein endophlebitis

A feature of the lesions in some cases of idiosyncratic drug-induced hepatitis is an endophlebitis that involves the central veins. Characterisitically, the intima of the affected veins is thickened, and shows proliferation of its endothelial lining cells and a mononuclear exudate. The intimal reaction appears to be related to the Kupffer cell proliferation and inflammatory reaction in the adjacent sinusoids, since frequently these cells invade and disrupt the walls of the involved central veins and fuse with the intima. A lesion of this type in a case of *ibuprofen*-induced hepatitis is illustrated in Figure 270.

Since a similar type of central vein endophlebitis occurs in acute viral hepatitis, a disorder in which the hepatic lesions are clearly attributable to an immunologic reaction, the finding of such vascular lesions in idiosyncratic drug-induced hepatitis is more consistent with an underlying hypersensitivity reaction than with hepatotoxic injury.

Portal tracts

Invariably, most, if not all of the portal tracts in drug-induced hepatitis are *expanded*, owing primarily to *destruction* of their *limiting plates* and *loss of periportal hepatocytes* (Figs. 530,

531). Portal *fibrosis* is unusual, except late in the course of severe unresolved drug-induced hepatitis.

Characteristically, the portal tracts are infiltrated by inflammatory cells. Usually, *lymphocytes* predominate, and, often, are accompanied by a variable number of *macrophages,* as can be seen in the case of *sulfasalazine* (Azulfidine)-induced hepatitis illustrated in Figure 330.

Frequently, a few *plasma cells* are found in the portal tracts, but, in some cases, particularly those accompanied by extensive bridging necrosis, they may be numerous, as in the case of *α-methyldopa*-induced hepatitis illustrated in Figure 313.

Usually, only a few *neutrophils* are found in the portal triads, but occasionally they are present in large numbers. They are most frequently found in cases with extensive necrosis or marked cholestasis, but may be seen in lesions of only moderate severity, as illustrated in the case of *α-methyldopa*-induced hepatitis shown in Figure 538.

Portal *eosinophilia* is generally regarded as a hallmark of idiosyncratic, presumably allergic hepatitis. However, in our experience, only a minority of cases show a large number of eosinophils, as seen in the case of halothane-induced hepatitis shown in Figure 324. More commonly, the portal tracts contain no eosinophils or only a few.

Ductular proliferation of mild degree is a relatively common finding in drug-induced hepatitis (Fig. 538), but often is extensive when necrosis is massive or submassive in character (Fig. 533).

Under conditions of extensive hepatocellular necrosis and severe cholestasis, the *interlobular ducts* may show *dilatation, bile stasis, degeneration,* and *necrosis.* Such ductular lesions may be associated with *extravasation of bile* and the formation of *bile infarcts.* A lesion of this type in a fatal case of *propylthiouracil*-induced hepatitis is illustrated in Figure 536. Less commonly, some of the interlobular ducts in cases of only moderate severity show inflammation, degeneration, and necrosis in the absence of ductal bile stasis, duct lesions that resemble those in primary biliary cirrhosis. A typical example in a case of acute *oxyphenisatin*-induced hepatitis is illustrated in Figure 373.

Histopathology of idiosyncratic drug-induced chronic hepatitis and cirrhosis

The onset of chronic drug-induced lesions is often abrupt with an acute hepatitis that fails to resolve and may progress to cirrhosis in patients with continued exposure to the drug. Withdrawal of the drug usually is followed by a remission, but varying degrees of residual fibrosis may persist. This is illustrated in one of our cases of *oxyphenisatin*-induced hepatitis. The patient, an elderly woman who had used oxyphenisatin (Dialose Plus) regularly for one year, presented with the typical clinical and laboratory features of an acute hepatitis. Because the serum alkaline phosphatase level was high and jaundice failed to abate, exploratory laparotomy was carried out to exclude extrahepatic biliary obstruction. The extrahepatic ducts were found to be patent, and wedge biopsy of the liver revealed an acute hepatitis. In addition to moderate cholestasis, the parenchymal lesions were characterized by lobular disarray, spotty hepatocellular necrosis, and a diffuse intralobular mononuclear inflammatory reaction (Fig. 539). All of the portal tracts were expanded and infiltrated with numerous mononuclear cells, showed erosion of the limiting plates, and contained occasional interlobular ducts that showed degeneration, necrosis, and inflammation (Fig. 373). Unfortunately, the role of oxyphenisation as an etiologic factor in acute hepatitis had not yet been reported, so that the patient was allowed to continue taking the drug. Over the next two and a half years, despite a course of prednisone therapy, the jaundice failed to abate and was followed by the appearance of ascites. This led to a second exploratory laparotomy, which demonstrated the presence of advanced, macronodular, postnecrotic cirrhosis that was confirmed histologically (Fig. 540). In addition, biopsy revealed evidence of chronic active hepatitis (Fig. 541). Tests for HBsAg, and antimitochondrial, smooth-muscle, and antinulcear antibodies yielded uniformly negative results. By this time, the etiologic role of oxyphenisation was recognized for the first time (132), and its use was discontinued, as was the prednisone therapy. This was followed promptly by improvement, and ultimately by disappearance of the jaundice and ascites, and apparent complete clinical recovery.

In some cases of drug-induced chronic active hepatitis, the signs of liver disease appear insidiously. This is illustrated in the case of one of our patients with an α-methyldopa-induced lesion. The patient was a middle-aged woman who was begun on methyldopa therapy for hypertension. Four months later she noted the insidious onset of ascites and edema, and, on presentation a month later, exhibited ascites, edema, and hepatosplenomegaly, but no jaundice, although her serum bilirubin concentration was increased to 3.6 mg/dl. Tests for HBsAg and anti-smooth-muscle and antimitochondrial antibodies were negative, but antinulcear antibodies were present in a titer of 1:16. Liver biopsy revealed the typical features of chronic active hepatitis with extensive bridging and, in some areas, panlobular hepatocellular necrosis (Fig. 542). Withdrawal of α-methyldopa was followed promptly by a decrease in serum bilirubin, alkaline phosphatase, and transaminase, and a rise in the serum albumin level, and more gradually by loss of ascites and edema. However, the serum transaminase level remained modestly elevated, suggesting that the lesion was still active, so that small doses of prednisone and azathioprine were administered. Within two months, the transaminase level had returned to normal and remained so thereafter, so that prednisone-azathioprine therapy was discontinued. Although the patient remained well and showed no biochemical evidence of hepatic dysfunction, follow-up biopsy 18 months later revealed an inactive postnecrotic cirrhosis (Fig. 543), a lesion that has shown no clinical or biochemical evidence of renewed activity over the past few years.

Usually, withdrawal of the drug responsible for chronic active hepatitis results in remission of the disease, but when the lesions are extensive, they may fail to heal completely. Under such conditions, the lesions appear to be self-perpetuating. However, the alternative possibility that the suspected drug is not the etiologic factor involved must always be excluded. Although lesions attributable to hepatitis B infections can be ruled out readily, those due to non-A, non-B viral infection and those considered to be "autoimmune" or "lupoid," cannot be excluded with certainty, although they present a characteristic clinical picture. Challenge with the suspected drug to demonstrate that it is capable of provoking a reaction can be useful in confirming the diagnosis of drug-induced chronic active hepatitis. However, it entails some risk, so it is best avoided, unless the drug involved is urgently needed for therapy, and no suitable substitute is available.

Histopathology of minor hepatotoxic lesions produced by drugs capable of provoking idiosyncratic reactions

As previously indicated, a number of drugs that rarely induce overt cholestatic or hepatitic lesions in uniquely susceptible individuals often produce minor hepatic functional abnormalities in a relatively high proportion (5–30%) of recipients. Included in this group are *isoniazid* (119), *halothane* (127), *methyldopa* (128), *chlorpromazine* (130), *diphenylhydantoin* (131), and many others.

Considering their frequency and the fact that they may be reproducible in animals, such reactions appear to be manifestations of minor hepatotoxicity. However, their behavior is atypical in that they often subside spontaneously in the face of continued drug administration and are not dose-related. As previously indicated, there is no convincing evidence that such reactions are the forerunners of overt hepatitis.

Unfortunately, the character of the lesions in these relatively common transient episodes of drug-induced hepatic dysfunction has not been adequately investigated. In the only three biopsy-documented reactions of this type that we have seen, two attributable to *isoniazid*, and the other to α-*methyldopa*, the lesions were characterized by a mild nonspecific focal hepatitis, as evidenced by the presence of rare acidophilic bodies, a few small, scattered foci of lymphocytes and proliferating Kupffer cells, and a mild portal lymphocytic reaction. In all three cases, the serum levels of alkaline phosphatase and transaminase were modestly elevated and returned to normal despite continued drug administration.

Histopathology of unique lesions encountered in some idiosyncratic drug reactions

Perhexiline maleate, a drug widely used abroad for the relief of angina pectoris, may give rise rarely to hepatic lesions that closely resemble those of alcoholic hepatitis and cirrhosis. They are characterized by different degrees of fatty infiltration, hepatocellular ballooning, Mallory body formation, neutrophilic infiltration, and fibrosis (213–215). Following withdrawal of the drug, the lesions tend to regress, but in some cases, they lead to progressive hepatic failure and death (213–215).

Since lesions of this type occur only after one to three years of perhexiline administration and are unaccompanied by any features suggestive of a hypersensitivity reaction, it is reasonable to assume that they represent hepatotoxicity. However, they occur only sporadically, are not dose-related, and are not reproducible in animals. This suggests that an aberrant toxic metabolite may be involved in their pathogenesis.

The elimination from the body of perhexiline is dependent on hepatic oxidation of the drug (216). The hepatic oxidation of some drugs is under single gene control, and genetic polymorphism can be shown (217). Oxidation of debrisoquine appears to be regulated by two alleles, one a rapid oxidation phenotype and the other a slow oxidation phenotype. In Britain about 9% of the population are slow oxidizers (217). Since it is not possible to measure the oxidation of perhexiline easily in humans, the oxidation of debrisoquine was studied in four patients who had had perhexiline hepatotoxicity (218). All four patients showed decreased oxidation of debrisoquine and, presumably, therefore, of perhexiline, compared with only 6 of 70 patients (9%) with a variety of chronic liver disorders. Three of the four were considered to have a genetically determined deficiency in oxidation capacity. This highly significant difference ($p < 0.005$) indicates that patients who develop perhexiline hepatotoxicity are probably poor hydroxylators of drugs. In turn, these observations suggest that the susceptibility to develop liver injury while taking perhexiline is genetically determined to a large extent.

A similar syndrome that mimics alcoholic liver disease has been reported after the long-term administration of *amiodarone* (219–222). Amiodarone is an iodinated, amphophilic drug that has many actions and reactions (223), and which is extremely efficacious in the management of arrythmias that are intractable to other antiarrythmic agents. It has many side effects that involve the skin, lungs, thyroid, cornea, muscle, peripheral nervous system, and the liver, and which have been attributed to diffuse lysosomal injury. Its hepatotoxic effects are uncommon, occurring in only about 1% of patients, but may give rise to transaminase elevations in 15 to 20% of patients receiving the drug (224).

Amiodarone hepatotoxicity causes few symptoms referable to the liver, and it is recognized because of abnormal aminotransferase activity or hepatomegaly. It may develop in as many as half the patients so treated (225). It has been reported within 24 hours of the parenteral administration of amiodarone (226). Occasionally, amiodarone may induce cholestatic injury (227). In advanced cases, cirrhosis may develop, and any of the symptoms and signs of advanced chronic liver disease may be present in such cases. It rarely appears before at least 12 months of administration of the drug. The abnormalities progress with the duration of therapy. Serum alkaline phosphatase activity is usually increased, but bilirubin, prothrombin, and albumin levels usually remain normal (228). Corneal deposits of phospholipids are almost invariably present. The syndrome is reversible and the hepatomegaly and functional abnormalities gradually disappear after the agent is discontinued.

The syndrome can be distinguished from alcoholic liver disease by (1) its appearance in patients who do not consume alcohol; (2) by the absence of acute hepatic injury as shown by normal bilirubin levels and prothrombin times; (3) the high SGPT:SGOT ratio; (4) the presence of many portal polymorphonuclear neutrophils; (5) the absence of extensive hepatocellular necrosis; and (6) the ultimate disappearance of the syndrome after stopping the offending agent.

Histologically, the liver shows fibrosis, which may have progressed to cirrhosis, large droplet fatty infiltration, and polymorphonuclear infiltration in the portal and periportal areas. Often there are small foci of necrosis and a few Mallory bodies. The cytoplasm in the earliest stages shows granularity of hepatocytes, which, on electron microscopy is caused by cytoplasmic inclusions with membranous, lamellar structures (229,230) indistinguishable from those observed in phospholipidoses like Tay-Sachs disease (231). These lesions are PAS-positive, diastase resistant, and contain iodine. Some of the hepatocytes may

contain ground glass cytoplasmic inclusions typical of induction cells (229,230). On electron microscopy phospholipids appear as concentric, lamellar, lysosomal myelin bodies in hepatocytes, bile duct epithelium, endothelial cells, and Kupffer cells, identical to those seen in perhexiline-induced hepatic injury (229,232,233). This type of reaction is characteristic of the drug-induced phospholipidosis induced by chloroquine, 4,4′-diethylaminoethoxybestrol, and perhexilene maleate, which are, like amiodarone, amphophilic, cationic agents (234). Whether the phospholipid deposits cause cell injury or represent merely a morphologic expression of a biochemical effect is not clear. Similar lamellar bodies have been seen in the cytoplasm of cells of the zona glomerulosa of the adrenal glands of *all* patients who are receiving spironolactone. These bodies known as "spironolactone bodies" are interpreted to be histologic evidence of the metabolic inhibition of aldosterone synthesis at a specific biochemical site, in the biosynthetic pathway of aldosterone and at a specific anatomic site in the adrenal glands (235).

Amiodarone and its major metabolite desethylamiodarone disappear from the plasma promptly after cessation of the agent, but persist for months in liver tissue. Iodine can be detected exclusively in lysosomes, the site of the phospholipidotic lesion (230).

The similarity of hepatic lesions of perhexilene maleate and amiodarone indicates that their mechanisms of inducing hepatic injury are similar. Although no genetic pattern has been reported for amiodarone, as has been suggested for perhexilene, it is reasonable to assume that the infrequency of the lesion indicates that the oxidation of amiodarone, like that of perhexilene, is under genetic control. Presumably, pretreatment testing should be able to identify patients with a high propensity for drug-induced hepatotoxicity.

In halothane-induced hepatic injury, too, a genetically determined susceptibility has been postulated and demonstrated (112), and, presumably, application of such tests before therapy may be able to exclude from treatment patients who are highly likely to develop drug-related injury.

Sodium valproate (Depakene), an anticonvulsant effective in the treatment of all forms of epilepsy, occasionally induces an unusual type of hepatic injury that often leads to fulminant hepatic failure and death (236–238). At least 57 such fatalities had been reported by 1982 (236,237).

One type of valproate-induced hepatic lesion is characterized by centrilobular hepatocellular degeneration and necrosis (Fig. 544). In the other type, which resembles Reye's syndrome, microvesicular fatty infiltration predominates [(238); Fig. 545]. Although the clinical and some of the morphologic features of valproate reactions, especially the microvesicular fatty infiltration and striking alterations in the mitrochondria of the hepatocytes (236–238), mimic those of Reye's syndrome, the presence of extensive hepatocellular necrosis in the former clearly differentiates it from the latter. The simultaneous administration of other drugs often complicates interpretation of the hepatic lesions.

Most of the fatal reactions to valproate have been encountered in infants and young children, but some have occurred in adults. The patient whose postmortem liver sections are illustrated in Figures 544 and 545 was a 21-year-old black man. As a rule, the signs of hepatic injury appear 2 to 12 weeks following the institution of valproate therapy, but may occur as early as three days.

Since the distinctive lesions produced by valproate occur only rarely, are not dose-dependent, and are not reproducible in animals, there is reason to suspect that an aberrant toxic metabolite of the drug may be implicated in their pathogenesis.

Hepatocellular adaptive changes induced by hepatotoxins and drugs

Induced cells

Prolonged administration of alcohol and a number of drugs that are metabolized in the liver induce proliferation of the smooth endoplasmic reticulum of the hepatocytes, resulting in the formation of induced or "turned on" cells, also termed orcein-negative ground glass hepatocytes (239). These closely resemble the orcein-positive and aldehyde fuchsin–positive ground glass cells that contain HBsAg in cases of chronic hepatitis B infection (Figs. 136, 138, 139). The drugs most frequently implicated in the formation of induction cells include *phenobarbital, diphenylhydantoin, diazepam* (Valium), *chlordiazepoxide* (Librium), *methotrexate,* and *cyclophosphamide*. Instances of induction cells in patients taking rifampicin (240) and chlorpromazine (241) have been reported.

Characteristically, the affected hepatocytes are enlarged and contain a single, large, faintly eosinophilic, finely granular cytoplasmic inclusion body that often fills much of the cell, displacing the nucleus and the normal cytoplasmic basophilic and lipofuscin granules to the periphery. A group of such cells in a patient with chronic alcoholism, but no other evidence of liver disease is illustrated in Figure 141. Although absence of staining with orcein and aldehyde fuchsin, and the failure to bind antibody to HBsAg in immunofluorescence or immunoperoxidase reactions are the only completely reliable ways of differentiating induction cells from HBsAg-containing ground glass cells, these two types of cells often show other differences in routinely stained sections. Thus, in contrast to HBsAg-positive ground glass cells, induction cells often involve large groups of hepatocytes in a predominantly centrilobular location, the inclusions are less sharply circumscribed, contain coarser granules and thready material, and only rarely are encircled by a clear halo.

Lafora bodies

In *myoclonus epilepsy* (LaFora's disease), an autosomal recessive hereditary disorder manifested by grand mal seizures initially and by myoclonus and progressive dementia later, the periportal hepatocytes characteristically contain large cytoplasmic inclusions termed *Lafora bodies* (Fig. 143) that exhibit PAS-staining that resists digestion by diastase, but not by pectinase [(242); Fig. 144]. On electron microscopy, the inclusions are non-membrane-bound and contain aggregates of randomly distributed, short, branching filaments, and scattered deposits of electron dense material resembling lipofuscin bodies that are predominantly periportal.

Pseudo-Lafora bodies, identical in all respects to the periportal cytoplasmic inclusions of myoclonus epilespy, are encountered rarely in alcoholic patients under treatment with *disulfiram* (Antabuse) (243), or *cyanamide* (Dipsan) (244,245). As a rule, these are unaccompanied by alterations in hepatic function or structure, although hepatomegaly has been observed in some cases (243). At least in one reported case, withdrawal of cyanamide led to disappearance of the inclusions over a period of three years (243). Whether the inclusions are indicative of an adaptive response or are attributable to a unique type of hepatotoxicity is not known.

Cytoplasmic ground glass cells similar to those seen in alcoholic patients treated with cyanamide can be regularly produced in rats given cyanamide (246). The ground glass inclusions in which glycogen is deposited as beta-granules, in both humans and rats, are preceded by the appearance of homogeneous areas of cytoplasm that contain alpha-glycogen granules and smooth endoplasmic reticulum. Glycogen deposition and proliferation of the smooth endoplasmic reticulum are well-recognized morphologic findings in drug toxicity (247).

Similar *pseudo-Lafora bodies* were encountered in three of our cases of *isoniazid*-induced acute hepatitis, all of which were relatively mild. As shown in Figure 145, many of the periportal hepatocytes contained large, pale inclusions that stained with PAS following diastase digestion (Fig. 146). Unfortunately, material was not available for electron microscopic study, so it was not possible to establish whether the ultrastructure of the inclusions is identical to that in the Lafora bodies of myoclonus epilepsy or the pseudo-Lafora bodies induced by disulfiram and cyanamide.

Fibrinogen bodies, which are morphologically indistinguishable from ground glass cells and which are orcein-negative and PAS-negative, have been reported in patients with chronic active hepatitis (248) and in acute non-A, non-B hepatitis (249). These deposits are more homogeneous than the granular bodies seen in LaFora's disease. They are probably the same as the homogeneous inclusions seen in fibrolamellar carcinoma of the liver (250), which have been shown to contain fibrinogen (251). Electron microscopically these inclusions are well demarcated, non-membrane-bound, electron-dense, and amorphous or slightly fibrillar. They are postulated to arise from a secretory block due to an intrinsic defect in the fibrinogen molecule.

These fibrinogen bodies and other inclusions may be differentiated from globular deposits of amyloid [(252); Fig. 147] by their failure to stain with Congo red or to show dichroism.

Type IV glycogenosis (amylopectinosis), another autosomal recessive hereditary disorder, which bears no relationship to myoclonus epilepsy, also exhibits periportal, hepatocellular, cytoplasmic inclusions that are indistinguishable from Lafora bodies [(253); Figs. 148, 149]. Curiously, despite the similarity of the inclusions in these two disorders, the hepatic lesions in glycogenosis IV are characterized by progressive hepatic fibrosis that leads to cirrhosis, whereas those in myoclonus epilepsy show only minimal or no fibrosis.

Histologic differential diagnosis of the hepatic lesions in idiosyncratic drug reactions

Acute idiosyncratic drug-induced cholestasis

Differentiation between the lesions of drug-induced cholestasis and *extrahepatic biliary obstruction* on histologic grounds alone may be exceedingly difficult. Although a number of morphologic features may favor an underlying drug reaction, they are not seen in all cases and are never pathognomonic. In general, portal edema, neutrophilic infiltration, and ductular proliferation are less prominent, whereas eosinophilic infiltrates are more common and more impressive in drug-induced cholestasis, particularly in its early stages. Although bile infarcts occur more frequently in extrahepatic biliary obstruction, they may be encountered in cases of prolonged and severe drug-induced cholestasis. Often, drug reactions, even when predominantly cholestatic, produce mild, but significant intralobular changes out of proportion to the degree of cholestasis. These include occasional acidophilic bodies, small foci of cell dropout, and scattered aggregates of swollen, proliferating Kupffer cells. When cholestasis is prolonged and severe, differentiation of the lesions from those of extrahepatic biliary obstruction usually is impossible. In such cases, even more important than the histologic findings are (1) an accurate history of the drugs the patient has received; (2) the interval between the institution of therapy and the appearance of jaundice; and (3) the presence or absence of fever, eosinophilia, or rash at or prior to its onset. However, even when there is a reliable history of drug use, failure of the jaundice to abate following withdrawal of the suspected drug often necessitates transhepatic or endoscopic retrograde cholangiography when imaging techniques are inconclusive to establish whether or not the biliary tract is patent.

Usually, the lesions in the early phase of *acute cholestatic viral hepatitis* are readily differentiated from those of drug-induced cholestasis, since invariably they show evidence of spotty necrosis, Kupffer cell proliferation, and a diffuse mononuclear inflammatory reaction. However, late in the course of such viral infections, the lesions are characterized by prominent cholestasis and show little evidence of parenchymal inflammation or necrosis, so they may be indistinguishable from those of drug-induced cholestasis. Usually, in such cases, differentiation depends on a history of exposure to drugs or the hepatitis virus, the character of the initial symptoms, and the results of serologic tests for evidence of infection with the hepatitis A, B, or C virus, cytomegalovirus, infectious mononucleosis, or toxoplasmosis.

Chronic idiosyncratic drug-induced cholestasis

The rare chronic cholestatic lesions produced by drugs like *chlorpromazine, prochlorperazine, organic arsenicals,* and *tolbutamide* usually are manifested by chronic jaundice, pruritus, hyperpgimentation, xanthomatosis, and hepatosplenomegaly, clinical features identical with those in *primary biliary cirrhosis.* However, such lesions are readily differentiated from those of primary biliary cirrhosis, because they do not show the paucity of interlobular ducts, the ductal degenerative and inflammatory changes, the follicle formation, and the granulomas characteristic of the latter. Moreover, the abrupt onset of overt jaundice early in the course of the disease and the absence of antimitochondrial antibodies are inconsistent with the diagnosis of primary biliary cirrhosis.

Histologic differentiation between the lesions of chronic drug-induced cholestasis and those of *extrahepatic biliary obstruction,* however, is impossible. As a rule, the diagnosis depends on the absence of symptoms suggestive of antecedent biliary tract disease and a history of drug ingestion followed shortly by the abrupt onset of jaundice. If the history is uncertain, im-

aging techniques are required to establish patency of the biliary tree.

Acute idiosyncratic drug-induced hepatitic lesions

As a rule, the histologic features of acute drug-induced hepatitis are indistinguishable from those of acute viral hepatitis. However, in some cases, the prominence of eosinophils in the intralobular or portal exudates, and the presence of granulomas point to an underlying drug reaction. Since patients on drug therapy may acquire infections with any of the hepatitis viruses, this possibility must always be excluded by appropriate serologic studies. Challenge with the suspected drug may confirm the diagnosis of drug-induced hepatitis. However, failure to induce a relapse does not necessarily exclude the diagnosis. Moreover, induced relapses may be severe, so challenge is not recommended unless the suspected drug is urgently needed for therapy, and no suitable substitute is available.

Drug-induced chronic active hepatitis

The lesions of chronic active hepatitis induced by *oxyphenisatin* (132,133), *α-methyldopa* (136), *nitrofurantoin* (137), *chlorpromazine* (138), *isoniazid* (103), *sulfonamides* (139), *propylthiouracil* (140), and *dantrolene* (141) usually are indistinguishable from those induced by infections with the B or non-A, non-B hepatitis viruses, or those of unknown etiology, usually classified as ''autoimmune'' or ''lupoid.'' The one exception is the presence of orcein-positive ground glass cells, which are diagnostic of chronic hepatitis B infection. Identification of drug-induced lesions usually depends on their regression when the offending drug is withdrawn. As in the case of acute drug-induced lesions, the results of a drug challenge may lend further support to the diagnosis, but is not recommended for the reasons previously given.

Essential features of the hepatic lesions produced by individual hepatotoxins and drugs

Itemization of the histologic features of the hepatic lesions produced by individual hepatotoxins and drugs is beyond the scope of this volume. For detailed descriptions of such lesions and the drugs that cause them the reader is referred to several comprehensive reviews of this topic (15,254,255). The latter two references, published in 1979 and 1983, respectively, are tabulations of drugs reported to induce liver disease. In addition, we have appended selected references of hepatotoxic drugs reported since the 1983 tabulation or apparently omitted by these authors and not specifically mentioned elsewhere in this chapter.

References

1. Farrell GC: Hepatic drug reactions: how unpredictable are they? J Gastroenterol Hepatol *1*:267–271, 1986.
2. Spielberg, SP, Gordon GB, Blake DA, Goldstein DA, Herlong HF:

Predisposition to phenytoin toxicity assessed *in vitro*. N Engl J Med *305*:722–727, 1981.

3. Recknagel RO, Glende EA Jr: Carbon tetrachloride hepatotoxicity: an example of lethal cleavage. Crit Rev Toxicol *2*:263–297, 1973.

4. Smuckler EA, Iseri OA, Benditt EP: Studies on carbon tetrachloride intoxication. I. The effect of carbon tetrachloride on incorporation of labelled amino acids into plasma proteins. Biochem Biophys Res Commun *5*:270–275, 1961.

5. Recknagel RO, Lombardi B, Schotz MC: A new insight into pathogenesis of carbon tetrachloride fat infiltration. Proc Soc Exp Biol Med *104*:608–610, 1960.

6. Calvert DN, Brody TM: Biochemical alterations of liver function by the halogenated hydrocarbons. I. *In vitro* and *in vivo* changes and their modification by ethylene-diamine tetraacetate. J Pharmacol Exp Ther *124*:273–281, 1958.

7. Smuckler EA, Iseri OA, Benditt EP: Studies on carbon tetrachloride intoxication. II. Depressed amino acid incorporation into mitochondrial protein and cytochrome C. Lab Invest *13*:531–538, 1964.

8. Thiers RE, Reynolds ES, Vallee BL: The effect of carbon tetrachloride poisoning on subcellular metal distribution in rat liver. J Biol Chem *235*:2130–2133, 1960.

9. Le Page RN, Dorling PR: Plasma membranes in acute liver injury. Biochemical changes induced by carbon tetrachloride. Aust J Exp Biol Med Sci *49*:345–350, 1971.

10. Ghoshal AK, Porta EA, Hartroft WS: The role of lipoperoxidation in the pathogenesis of fatty livers induced by phosphorus poisoning in rats. Am J Pathol *54*:275–291, 1969.

11. Barker EA, Smuckler EA, Benditt EP: Effects of thioacetamide and yellow phosphorus poisoning on protein synthesis *in vivo*. Lab Invest *12*:955–960, 1963.

12. Dianzani MU: Toxic liver injury by protein synthesis inhibitors. *In* Progress in Liver Diseases, Vol. V, edited by H. Popper, F. Schaffner. New York, Grune & Stratton, 1976, pp. 232–245.

13. Frimmer M: Toxic cyclopeptides of the toadstool Amanita phalloides and related species. Naunyn-Schmiedebergs Arch Pharmacol *269*:152–163, 1971.

14. Tuchweber B, Kovacs K, Khandekar JD, Garg BD: Peliosis-like changes induced by phalloidin in the rat liver. A light and microscopic study. J Med *4*:327–345, 1973.

15. Zimmerman HJ: Hepatotoxicity: The Adverse Effects of Drugs and Other Chemicals on the Liver. New York, Appleton-Century-Croft, 2nd Edition, 1989.

15a. Pessayre D, Larrey D. Drug-induced liver injury. *In* Oxford Textbook of Clinical Hepatology, Edited by N McIntyre, J-P Benhamou, J Bircher, M Rizzetto, and J Rodes. Oxford, Oxford University Press, 1991, p. 875–902.

16. Glynn LE, Himsworth HP, Neuberger A: Pathological states due to deficiency of the sulphur-containing amino-acids. Br J Exp Pathol *26*:326–337, 1945.

17. Koch-Weser D, De La Huerga J, Popper H: Hepatic necrosis due to bromobenzene and its dependence upon available sulfur amino acids. Proc Soc Exp Biol Med *79*:196–198, 1952.

18. Mitchell JR, Jollows DJ: Metabolic activation of drugs to toxic substances. Gastroenterology *68*:392–410, 1975.

19. Seeff LB, Cuccherini BA, Zimmerman HJ, Adler E, Benjamin SB: Acetaminophen hepatotoxicity in alcoholics. Ann Intern Med *104*:399–404, 1986.

20. Crome P, Vale JA, Volans GN, Widdop B, Goulding R: Oral methionine in the treatment of severe paracetamol (acetaminophen) overdose. Lancet *2*:829–830, 1976.

21. Hughes RD, Gazzard BG, Hanid MA, Trewby PN, Murray-Lyon IM, Davis M, Williams R, Bennett JR: Controlled trial of cysteamine and dimercaprol after paracetamol overdose. Br Med J *4*:1395, 1977.

22. Prescott LF, Park J, Ballentyne A, Adriaenssens P, Proudfoot AT: Treatment of paracetamol (acetaminophen) poisoning with N-acetylcysteine. Lancet *2*:432–434, 1977.

23. Klatskin G: Toxic and drug-induced hepatitis. *In* Diseases of the Liver, edited by L. Schiff. 4th Edition. Philadelphia, J.B. Lippincott Co., 1975, pp. 604–710.

24. Kreek MJ, Weser E, Sleisenger MH, Jeffries GH: Idiopathic cholestasis of pregnancy. The response to challenge with the synthetic estrogen, ethinyl estradiol. N Engl J Med *277*:1391–1395, 1967.

25. De Pagter AGF, van Berge Henegouwen GP, Ten Bokkel Huinink JA: Familial benign recurrent intrahepatic cholestasis. Interrelation with intrahepatic cholestasis of pregnancy and from oral contraceptives? Gastroenterology *71*:202–207, 1976.

26. Fisher MM, Magnusson R, Miyai K: Bile acid metabolism in mammals. I. Bile acid induced intrahepatic cholestasis. Lab Invest *21*:88–91, 1971.

27. Utili R, Abernathy CO, Zimmerman HJ: Cholestatic effects of *Escherichia coli* endotoxin on the isolated perfused rat liver. Gastroenterology *70*:248–253, 1976.

28. Benjamin DR: Hepatobiliary dysfunction in infants and children associated with long-term total parenteral nutrition. A clinicopathologic study. Am J Clin Pathol *76*:276–283, 1981.

29. Body JJ, Bleiberg H, Bron D, Maurage H, Bigirimana V, Heimann R: Total parenteral nutrition-induced cholestasis mimicking large bile duct obstruction. Histopathology *6*:787–792, 1982.

30. Dahms BB, Halpin TC: Serial liver biopsies in parenteral nutrition-associated cholestasis of early infancy. Gastroenterology *81*:136–144, 1981.

31. Lowry SF, Brennan MF: Abnormal liver function during parenteral nutrition: relation to infusion excess. J Surg Res *26*:300–307, 1979.

32. Dubin M, Michele M, Feldmann G, Erlinger S: Phalloidin-induced cholestasis in the rat: relation to changes in microfilaments. Gastroenterology *75*:450–455, 1978.

33. Rimington C, Quin JI, Roets GCS: Studies upon the photosensitization of animals in South Africa. I. The icterogenic factor in geeldikkop. I. Isolation of acitve principles from Lippia rhemanni pears. Onderstepoort J Vet Sci *9*:225–255, 1937.

34. Slater TF, Griffiths DB: Effects of sporidesmin on bile flow rate and composition in the rat (Abst). Biochem J *88*:60P–61P, 1963.

35. Phillips MJ, Oda M, Mak E, Fisher MM, Jeejeebhoy KN: Microfilament dysfunction as a possible cause of intrahepatic cholestasis. Gastroenterology *69*:48–58, 1975.

36. Keefe EB, Blankenship NM, Scharschmidt BF: Alteration of rat liver plasma membrane fluidity and ATPase activity by chlorpromazine hydrochloride and its metabolites. Gastroenterology *79*:222–231, 1980.

37. Phillips MJ, Oshio C, Miyairi M: Microfilament dysfunction as a mechanism in intrahepatic cholestasis: evidence from time-lapse cinemicrophotography (Abst). Gastroenterology *79*:1120, 1980.

38. Watson RGP, Olomu A, Clements D, Waring RH, Mitchell S, Elias E: A proposed mechanism for chlorpromazine jaundice-defective hepatic sulphoxidation combined with rapid hydroxylation. J Hepatol *7*:72–78, 1988.

39. Glynn LE, Himsworth HP: The intralobular circulation in acute liver injury by carbon tetrachloride. Clin Sci *6*:235–245, 1948.

40. Calvert DN, Brody TM: Role of the sympathetic nervous system in CCl$_4$ hepatotoxicity. Am J Physiol *198*:669–676, 1960.

41. Stoner HB: The effect of anesthesia and laparotomy on the blood flow through the necrotic liver. Br J Surg *45*:81–82, 1957.

42. Winkler K, Poulsen H: Liver disease with periportal sinusoidal dilatation. A possible complication to contraceptive steroids. Scand J Gastroenterol *10*:699–704, 1975.

43. Pliskin M: Peliosis hepatis. Radiology *114*:29–30, 1975.

44. Nadell J, Kosek J: Peliosis hepatis. Twelve cases associated with androgen therapy. Arch Pathol Lab Med *101*:405–410, 1977.

45. Paradinas FJ, Bull TB, Westaby D, Murray-Lyon IM: Hyperplasia and prolapse of hepatocytes into hepatic veins during longterm methyltestosterone therapy: possible relationships of these changes to the development of peliosis hepatis and liver tumours. Histopathology *1*:225–246, 1977.

46. Baker A, Kaplan M, Wolfe H: Central congestive fibrosis of the liver in myxedema ascites. Ann Intern Med *77*:927–929, 1972.

47. Berk PD, Popper H, Krueger GRF, Decter J, Herzig G, Graw RG Jr: Veno-occlusive disease after allogenic bone marrow transplantation. Possible association with graft-versus-host disease. Ann Intern Med *90*:158–164, 1979.

48. Lewin K, Millis RR: Human radiation hepatitis. A morphologic study with emphasis on the late changes. Arch Pathol *96*:21–26, 1973.

49. Kumana CR, Ng M, Lin HJ, Ko W, Wu P-C, Todd D: Herbal tea induced hepatic veno-occlusive disease: quantification of toxic alkaloid exposure in adults. Gut *26*:101–104, 1985.

50. Hu SY: An enumeration of Chinese materia medica. Hong Kong, Chinese University Press, 1980.

51. Marubio AT, Danielson B: Hepatic veno-occlusive disease in a renal transplant patient receiving azathioprine. Gastroenterology *69*:739–743, 1975.

52. Griner PF, Elbadawi A, Packman CH: Veno-occlusive disease of the liver after chemotherapy of acute leukemia. Report of two cases. Ann Intern Med *85*:578–582, 1976.

53. Brodsky I, Johnson H, Killman S, Cronkite EP: Fibrosis of central and hepatic veins, and perisinusoidal spaces of the liver following prolonged administration of urethane. Am J Med *30*:976–989, 1961.

54. Ceci G, Bella M, Melissari M, Gabrielli M, Bocchi P, Cocconi G: Fatal hepatic vascular toxicity of DTIC. Is it really a rare event? Cancer *61:*1988–1991, 1988.

55. McLean E: The toxic actions of pyrrolizidine (Senecio) alkaloids. Pharmacol Rev *22:*429–483, 1970.

56. Gerlag PGG, Lobatto S, Driessen WMM, Deckers PFL, Van Hooff JP, Schroder E, Assmann KM, Van Haelst UJG: Hepatic sinusoidal dilatation with portal hypertension during azathioprine treatment after kidney transplantation. J Hepatol *1:*339–348, 1985.

57. Wu S-M, Spurny OM, Klotz AP: Budd-Chiari syndrome after taking oral contraceptives. A case report and review of 14 reported cases. Am J Dig Dis *22:*623–628, 1977.

58. Subcommittee of the Medical Research Council: Risk of thromboembolic disease in women taking oral contraceptives. A preliminary communication to the Medical Research Council by a subcommittee. Br Med J *2:*355–359, 1967.

59. Irey NS, Norris HJ: Intimal vascular lesions associated with female reproductive steroids. Arch Pathol *96:*227–234, 1973.

60. Cameron GR, Karunaratne WAE: Carbon tetrachloride cirrhosis in relation to liver regeneration. J Pathol Bact *42:*1–21, 1936.

61. Coe RO, Bull FE: Cirrhosis associated with methotrexate treatment of psoriasis. JAMA *206:*1515–1520, 1968.

62. Doria Jr. MI, Shepard KV, Levin B, Riddell RH: Liver pathology following hepatic arterial infusion chemotherapy. Hepatic toxicity with FUDR. Cancer *58:*855–861, 1986.

63. Strauss N: Hepato-toxic effects following occupational exposure to Halowax (chlorinated hydrocarbons). Rev Gastroenterol *11:*381–396, 1944.

64. Wilcox WW: Toxic jaundice. Lancet *2:*57–63, 1931.

65. Franklin M, Bean WB, Hardin RC: Fowler's solution as an etiologic agent in cirrhosis. Am J Med Sci *219:*589–596, 1950.

66. Luchtrath H: Cirrhosis of the liver in chronic arsenical poisoning of vintners. Germ Med *2:*127–128, 1972.

67. Pimental JC, Menezes AP: Liver disease in vineyard sprayers. Gastroenterology *72:*275–283, 1977.

68. Sellinger M, Koff RS: Thorotrast and the liver. A reminder. Gastroenterology *68:*799–803, 1975.

69. Gedigk P, Muller R, Bechtelsheimer H: Morphology of liver damage among polyvinyl chloride production workers. A report on 51 cases. Ann NY Acad Sci *246:*278–285, 1975.

70. Miller EC, Miller JA: Hepatocarcinogenesis by chemicals. *In* Progress in Liver Diseases, Vol. V, edited by H. Popper, F. Schaffner. New York, Grune & Stratton, 1976, pp. 699–711.

71. Farber E: On the pathogenesis of experimental hepatocellular carcinoma. *In* Hepatocellular Carcinoma, edited by K. Okuda, R.L. Peters. New York, John Wiley & Sons, 1976, pp. 3–22.

72. Rubel LR, Ishak KG: Thorotrast-associated cholangiocarcinoma. An epidemiologic and clinicopathologic study. Cancer *50:*1408–1415, 1982.

73. Locker GY, Doroshow JH, Zwelling LA, Chabner BA: The clinical features of hepatic angiosarcoma: a report of four cases and a review of the English literature. Medicine *58:*48–64, 1979.

74. Smoron GL, Battifora HA: Thorotrast-induced hepatoma. Cancer *30:*1252–1259, 1972.

75. Wegener K, Leipolz-Angermuller S: Double tumours of the liver following intravenous Thorotrast injection. Virchows Arch A Pathol Anat Histol *382:*63–71, 1979.

76. Ross JM: A case illustrating the effects of prolonged action of radium. J Pathol Bacteriol *15:*899–912, 1932.

77. Moore TA, Ferrante WA, Crowson TD: Hepatoma occurring two decades after hepatic irradiation. Gastroenterology *71:*128–132, 1976.

78. Chudecki B: Primary cancer of the liver following treatment of polycythemia vera with radioactive phosphorus. Br J Radiol *45:*770–774, 1972.

79. Popper H, Thomas LB, Telles NC, Falk H, Selikoff IJ: Development of hepatic angiosarcoma in man induced by vinyl chloride, thorotrast, and arsenic. Comparison with cases of unknown etiology. Am J Pathol *92:*349–376, 1978.

80. Makk L, Delorme F, Creech JL Jr, Ogden LL II, Fadell EH, Songster CL, Clanton J, Johnson MN, Christopherson WM: Clinical and morphologic features of hepatic angiosarcoma in vinyl chloride workers. Cancer *37:*149–163, 1976.

81. Berk PD, Martin JF, Young RS, Creech J, Selikoff IJ, Falk H, Watanabe P, Popper H, Thomas L: Vinyl chloride-associated liver disease. Ann Intern Med *84:*717–731, 1976.

82. Roth F: Uber die chronischer Arsenvergiftung der Moselwinzer unter besonderer Berücksichtingung des Arsenkrebses. Ztschr Krebsforsch *61:*287–319, 1956.

83. Roth F: Zur Pathologie der chronischen Arsenvergiftung. Zentralblatt Allg Pathol *100:*529–530, 1959.

84. Lander JJ, Stanley RJ, Sumner HW, Boswell DC, Aach RD: Angiosarcoma of the liver associated with Fowler's solution (potassium arsenite). Gastroenterology *68:*1582–1586, 1975.

85. Klatskin G: Hepatic tumors: possible relationship to use of oral contraceptives. Gastroenterology *73:*386–394, 1977.

86. Ishak KG: Hepatic neoplasms associated with contraceptive and anabolic steroids. *In* Recent Results in Cancer Research, Vol 66, edited by C.H. Lingeman. New York, Springer-Verlag, 1979, pp. 73–128.

87. Shapiro P, Ikeda RM, Ruebner BH, Connors MH, Halsted CC, Abildgaard CF: Multiple hepatic tumors and peliosis hepatis in Fanconi's anemia treated with androgens. Am J Dis Child *131:*1104–1106, 1977.

88. Stromeyer FW, Smith DW, Ishak KG: Anabolic steroid therapy and intrahepatic cholangiocarcinoma. Cancer *43:*440–443, 1979.

89. Falk H, Thomas LB, Popper H, Ishak KG: Hepatic angiosarcoma associated with androgenic-anabolic steroids. Lancet *2:*1120–1122, 1979.

90. Farrell GC, Joshua DE, Uren RF, Baird PJ, Perkins KW, Kronenberg H: Androgen induced hepatoma. Lancet *1:*430–431, 1975.

91. Johnson FL: Androgenic-anabolic steroids and hepatocellular carcinoma. *In* Hepatocellular Carcinoma, edited by K. Okuda, R.L. Peters. New York, John Wiley & Sons, 1976, pp. 95–103.

92. Cattan D, Vesin P, Wautier J, Kalifat R, Mergnan S: Liver tumours and steroid hormones. Lancet *1:*878, 1974.

93. Anthony PP: Hepatoma associated with androgenic steroids. Lancet *1:*685–686, 1975.

94. Wogan GN: Aflatoxins and their relationship to hepatocellular carcinoma. *In* Hepatocellular Carcinoma, edited by K. Okuda, R.L. Peters. New York, John Wiley & Sons, 1976, pp. 25–41.

95. Prince AM: Evidence suggesting that hepatitis B virus is a tumor-inducing virus in man: an estimate of the risk of development of hepatocellular carcinoma in chronic HBsAg carriers and controls. *In* The Role of Viruses in Human Cancer, Vol. 1, edited by G. Giraldo, E. Beth. New York, Elsevier North Holland, 1980, pp. 141–155.

96. Lutwack LI: Relation between aflatoxin, hepatitis B virus, and hepatocellular carcinoma. Lancet *1:*755–757, 1979.

97. Tracey JP, Sherlock P: Hepatoma following carbon tetrachloride poisoning. NY State J Med *68:*2202–2204, 1968.

98. Stromeyer FW, Ishak KG: Nodular transformation (nodular regenerative hyperplasia) of the liver. A clinicopathologic study of 30 cases. Hum Pathol *12:*60–71, 1981.

99. Wanless IR, Godwin TA, Allen F, Feder A: Nodular regenerative hyperplasia of the liver in hematologic disorders: a possible response to obliterative portal venopathy. A morphometric study of nine cases with an hypothesis on the pathogenesis. Medicine *59:*367–379, 1980.

100. Solis-Herruzo JA, Vidal JV, Colina F, Santalla F, Castellano G: Nodular regenerative hyperplasia of the liver associated with the toxic oil syndrome: report of five cases. Hepatology *6:*687–693, 1986.

101. Pimental JC, Menezes AP: Liver granulomas containing copper in vineyard sprayer's lung. A new etiology of hepatic granulomatosis. Am Rev Respir Dis *111:*189–195, 1975.

102. Black M, Mitchell JR, Zimmerman HJ, Ishak KG, Epler GR: Isoniazid-induced hepatitis in 114 patients. Gastroenterology *69:*289–301, 1975.

103. Maddrey WC, Bortnott JK: Isoniazid hepatitis. Ann Intern Med *79:*1–12, 1973.

104. Bonkovsky HL, Blanchette PL, Schned AR: Severe liver injury due to phenelzine with unique hepatic deposition of extracellular material. Am J Med *80:*689–692, 1986.

105. Vergani D, Tsantoulas D, Eddleston ALWF, Davis M, Williams R: Sensitization to halothane-altered liver components in severe hepatic necrosis after halothane anaesthesia. Lancet *2:*801–803, 1978.

106. Vergani D, Mieli-Vergani G, Alberti A, Neuberger J, Eddleston ALWF, Davis M, Williams R: Antibodies to the surface of halothane-altered rabbit hepatocytes in patients with severe halothane-associated hepatitis. N Engl J Med *303:*66–71, 1980.

107. Dienstag JL: Halothane hepatitis. Allergy or idiosyncrasy? N Engl J Med *303:*102–104, 1980.

108. Dujovne CA: Alterations of liver-cell membranes after exposure to halothane. N Engl J Med *303:*1367, 1980.

109. Klatskin G: Halothane-induced hepatitis. *In* Drugs and the Liver, ed-

ited by W. Gerok, K. Sickinger. New York, FK Schattauer Verlag, 1975, pp. 289–296.

110. Klatskin G, Kimberg DV: Recurrent hepatitis attributable to halothane sensitization in an anesthetist. N Engl J Med 280:515–522, 1969.

111. Hoff RH, Bunker JP, Goodman HI, Gregory PB: Halothane hepatitis in three pairs of closely related women. N Engl J Med 304:1023–1024, 1981.

112. Farrell G, Prendergast D, Murray M: Halothane hepatitis. Detection of a constitutional susceptibility factor. N Engl J Med 313:1310–1314, 1985.

113. Ranek L: Halothane hepatitis: a double defect?: Hepatology 6:538–539, 1986.

114. Frost L, Prendergast D, Farrell G: Halothane hepatitis: damage to peripheral blood mononuclear cells produced by electrophilic drug metabolites is CA 2+-depdenent. J Gastroneterol Hepatol 4:1–9, 1989.

115. Bartle WR, Fisher MM, Kerenyi N: Disulfiram-induced hepatitis. Report of two cases and review of the literature. Dig Dis Sci 30:834–837, 1985.

116. Vasquez JJ: Hepatic lesions induced by alcohol sensitizing drugs: two lesions for the price of one. Hepatology 6:748–749, 1986.

117. DePinho RA, Goldberg CS, Lefkowitch JH: Azathioprine and the liver. Gastroenterology 86:162–165, 1984.

118. Rahmat J, Gelfand RL, Gelfand MC, Winchester JF, Schreiner GE, Zimmerman HJ: Captopril-associated cholestatic jaundice. Ann Intern Med 102:56–58, 1985.

119. Mitchell JR, Jallows DJ: Metabolic activation of drugs to toxic substances. Gastroenterology 68:392–410, 1975.

120. Bernstein RE: Isoniazid hepatotoxicity and acetylation during tuberculosis chemoprophylaxis. Am Rev Respir Dis 121:429–430, 1980.

121. Sipes IG, Brown BR Jr: An animal model of hepatotoxicity associated with halothane anesthesia. Anesthesiology 45:622–628, 1976.

122. Cousins MJ, Sharp JH, Gourlay GK, Adams JF, Haynes WD, Whitehead R: Hepatotoxicity and halothane metabolism in an animal model with application for human toxicity. Anaesth Intensive Care 7:9–24, 1979.

123. Cousins MJ: Halothane and the liver: "firm ground" at last? Anaesth Intensive Care 7:5–8, 1979.

124. Norris FH Jr, Geisler PH, Pritchard WL, Hall KD: Lack of necrosis in dog liver after anesthesia with halothane. Arch Int Pharmacodyn Ther 145:405–412, 1963.

125. Ross WT Jr, Cardell RR Jr: Effects of halothane on the ultrastructure of rat liver cells. Am J Anat 135:5–22, 1972.

126. Suchy FJ, Balistreri WF, Buchino JJ, Sondheimer JM, Bates SR, Kearns GL, Stull JD, Bove KE: Acute hepatic failure associated with the use of sodium valproate. Report of two fatal cases. N Engl J Med 300:962–966, 1979.

127. Dawson B, Adson MA, Dockerty MB, Fleisher GA, Jones RR, Hartridge VB, Schnelle N, McGuckin WF, Summerskill WHF: Hepatic function tests: postoperative changes with halothane or diethyl ether anesthesia. Mayo Clin Proc 41:599–607, 1966.

128. Leonard JW, Gifford RW Jr, Humphrey DC: Treatment of hypertension with methyldopa alone or in combination with diuretics and/or guanethidine. Am Heart J 69:610–618, 1965.

129. Arranto AJ, Sotaniemi EA: Morphologic alterations in patients with alpha-methyldopa-induced liver damage after short- and long-term exposure. Scand J Gastroenterol 16:853–863, 1981.

130. Dickes R, Schenker V, Deutsch L: Serial liver-function and blood studies in patients receiving chlorpromazine. N Engl J Med 256:1–7, 1957.

131. Andreason PB, Lyngbye J, Trolle E: Abnormalities in liver function tests during long-term diphenylhydantoin therapy in epileptic outpatients. Acta Med Scand 194:261–264, 1973.

132. Reynolds TB, Peters RL, Yamada S: Chronic active and lupoid hepatitis caused by laxative, oxyphenisatin. N Engl J Med 285:813–820, 1971.

133. Dietrichson O, Juhl E, Nielsen JO, Oxlund JJ, Christoffersen P: The incidence of oxyphenisatin-induced liver damage in chronic nonalcoholic liver disease. Scand J Gastroenterol 9:473–478, 1974.

134. Dietrichson O: Chronic active hepatitis. Aetiological considerations based on clinical and serological studies. Scand J Gastroenterol 10:617–624, 1975.

135. Goldstein G, Lam KC, Mistilis SP: Drug-induced active chornic hepatitis. Am J Dig Dis 18:177–184, 1973.

136. Maddrey WC, Boitnott JK: Severe hepatitis from methyldopa. Gastroenterology 68:351–360, 1975.

137. Black M, Rabin L, Schatz N: Nitrofurantoin-induced chronic active hepatitis. Ann Intern Med 92:62–64, 1980.

138. Russell RI, Allan JG, Patrick R: Active chronic hepatitis after chlorpromazine ingestion. Br Med J 1:655–656, 1973.

139. Tonder M, Nordoy A, Elgio K: Sulfonamide-induced chronic liver disease. Scand J Gastroenterol 9:93–96, 1974.

140. Fedotin MS: Liver disease caused by propylthiouracil. Arch Intern Med 135:319–321, 1975.

141. Utili R, Boitnott JK, Zimmerman HJ: Dantrolene-associated hepatic injury: incidence and character. Gastroenterology 72:510–516, 1977.

142. Poupon RY, Poupon RE, Erlinger S, Darnis F: Hepatite chronique associee a la prise prolongee de papaverine. Gastroenterol Clin Biol 2:305–312, 1978.

143. Pessayre D, Degos F, Feldmann G, Degott C, Bernuau J, Benhamou J-P: Chronic active hepatitis and multinulceated hepatocytes in adults treated with clometacin. Digestion 22:66–72, 1981.

144. Thomas FB: Chronic aggressive hepatitis induced by halothane. Ann Intern Med 81:487–489, 1974.

145. Kronborg IJ, Evans DTP, Mackay IR, Bhathal PS: Chronic hepatitis after successive halothane anesthetics. Digestion 27:123–128, 1983.

146. Miller DJ, Dwyer J, Klatskin G: Halothane hepatitis: benign resolution of a severe lesion. Ann Intern Med 89:212–215, 1978.

147. Eddleston ALWF, Williams R: Inadequate antibody response to HBAg or suppressor T-cell defect in development of active chronic hepatitis. Lancet 2:1543–1545, 1974.

148. Dossing M, Andreasen PB: Drug-induced liver disease in Denmark. An analysis of 572 cases of hepataotoxicity reported to the Danish Board of Adverse Reactions to Drugs. Scand J Gastroenterol 17:205–211, 1982.

149. Walker CO, Combes B: Biliary cirrhosis induced by chlorpromazine. Gastroenterology 51:631–640, 1966.

150. Ishak KG, Irey NS: Hepatic injury associated with phenothiazines. Clinico-pathologic and follow-up study of 36 patients. Arch Pathol 93:283–304, 1972.

151. Stolzer BL, Miller C, White WA, Zuckerbrod M: Postarsenical obstructive jaundice complicated by xanthomatosis and diabetes mellitus. Am J Med 9:124–132, 1950.

152. Gregory DA, Zaki GF, Sarcosi GA, Carey JB Jr: Chronic cholestasis following prolonged tolbutamide administration associated with destructive cholangiolitis. Arch Pathol 84:194–201, 1967.

153. Dincsoy HP, Saelinger DA: Haloperidol-induced chronic cholestatic liver disease. Gastroenterology 83:694–700, 1982.

154. Larrey D, Pessayre D, Duhamel G, Casier A, Degott C, Feldman G, Erlinger S, Benhamou J-P: Prolonged cholestasis after aimaline-induced acute hepatitis. J Hepatol 2:81–87, 1982.

155. Klatskin G, Conn HO: Personal observations.

156. Kemeny MM, Battifora H, Blayney DW, Cecchi G, Goldberg DA, Leong LA, Margolin KA, Terz JJ: Sclerosing cholangitis after continuous hepatic artery infusion of FUDR. Ann Surg 202:176–181, 1985.

157. Dordal E, Glagov S, Orlando RA, Platz C: Fatal halothane hepatitis with transient granulomas. N Engl J Med 283:357–359, 1970.

158. Miller AG, Reed W: Methyldopa-induced granulomatous hepatitis. JAMA 235:2001–2002, 1976.

159. Jori GP, Peschle C: Hydralazine disease associated with transient granulomas in the liver. A case report. Gastroenterology 64: 1163–1167, 1973.

160. Chajek T, Lehrer B, Geltner D, Levy IS: Quinidine-induced granulomatous hepatitis. Ann Intern Med 81:774–776, 1974.

161. Levander HG: Granulomatous hepatitis in a patient receiving carbamazepine. Acta Med Scand 208:333–335, 1980.

162. Ishak KG, Kirchner JP, Dhar JK: Granulomas and cholestatic-hepatocellular injury associated with phenylbutazone. Report of two cases. Am J Dig Dis 22:611–617, 1977.

163. Espirutu CE, Alulu J, Glueckauf LG, Lubin J: Allopurinol-induced granulomatous hepatitis. Am J Dig Dis 21:804–806, 1976.

164. Espiritu CR, Kim TS, Levine RA: Granulomatous hepatitis associated with sulfadimethoxine hypersensitivity. JAMA 202:985–988, 1967.

165. Strohscheer H, Wegener HH: Nitrofurantoin-induzierte granulomatose Hepatitis. Munch Med Wchschr 119:1535–1536, 1977.

166. Waugh D: Myocarditis, arteritis, and focal hepatic, splenic and renal granulomas apparently due to penicillin sensitivity. Am J Pathol 28:437–447, 1952.

167. Bloodworth JMB Jr: Morphologic changes associated with sulfonurea therapy. Metabolism 12:287–301, 1963.

168. Rotmensch HH, Yust I, Siegman-Ingra Y, Liron M, Ilie B, Var-

dinon N: Granulomatous hepatitis: a hypersensitivity response to procainamide. Ann Intern Med 89:646–647, 1978.
169. McMaster KR III, Hennigar GR: Drug-induced granulomatous hepatitis. Lab Invest 44:61–73, 1981.
170. Stricker BH Ch, Spoelstra P: Drug-induced hepatic injury: a comprehensive survey of the literature on adverse drug reactions up to January 1985. Amsterdam, 1985, p. 314.
171. Wanless IR, Dore S, Gopinath N, Tan J, Cameron R, Heathcote EJ, Blendis LM, Levy G: Histopathology of cocaine hepatotoxicity: report of four patients. Gastroenterology 98:497–501, 1990.
172. Seeff LB, Cuccherini BA, Zimmerman HJ: Acetaminophen hepatotoxicity in alcoholics: a therapeutic misadventure. Ann Intern Med 104:399–404, 1986.
173. Greenberger NJ, Robinson WL, Isselbacher KJ: Toxic hepatitis after the ingestion of phosphorus with subsequent recovery. Gastroenterology 47:179–183, 1964.
174. Nagore N, Howe S, Boxer L, Scheuer PJ: Liver cell rosettes: structural differences in cholestasis and hepatitis. Liver 9:43–51, 1989.
175. Luongo MA, Bjornson SS: The liver in ferrous sulfate poisoning. A report of three fatal cases in children and an experimental study. N Engl J Med 251:995–999, 1954.
176. Spilsbury BH: Toxic jaundice in munitions workers and troops. Br Med J 1:156, 1917.
177. Stewart MJ: Toxic jaundice in munition workers and troops. Br Med J 1:153–155, 1917.
178. Himsworth HP, Glynn LE: Toxipathic and trophopathic hepatitis. Lancet 1:457–461, 1944.
179. Schultz JC, Adamson JS Jr, Workman WW, Norman TD: Fatal liver disease after intravenous administration of tetracycline in high dosage. N Engl J Med 269:999–1004, 1963.
180. Peters RL, Edmondson HA, Middelsen WP, Tatter D: Tetracycline-induced fatty liver in nonpregnant patients. A report of six cases. Am J Surg 113:622–632, 1967.
181. Robinson MJ, Rywlin AM: Tetracycline-associated fatty liver in the male. Report of an autopsied case. Am J Dig Dis 15:857–862, 1970.
182. Bourgeois CH, Shank RC, Grossman RA, Johnsen DO, Wooding WL, Chandavimol P: Acute aflatoxin B1 toxicity in the macaque and its similarities to Reye's syndrome. Lab Invest 24:206–216, 1971.
183. Hogan GR, Ryan NJ, Hayes AW: Aflatoxin B1 and Reye's syndrome. Lancet 1:561–563, 1978.
184. Bourgeois C, Olson L, Comer D, Evans H, Keschamras N, Cotton R, Grossman R, Smith T: Encephalopathy and fatty degeneration of the viscera: a clinicopathologic analysis of 40 cases. Am J Clin Pathol 56:558–571, 1971.
185. Starko KM, Mullick FG: Hepatic and cerebral pathology findings in children with fatal salicylate intoxication: further evidence for a causal relation between salicylate and Reye's syndrome. Lancet 1:326–330, 1983.
186. McGill DB, Motto JD: An industrial outbreak of toxic hepatitis due to methylene-dianiline. N Engl J Med 291:278–282, 1974.
187. Kopelman H, Scheuer PJ, Williams R: The liver lesion of the Epping jaundice. Q J Med 35:553–564, 1966.
188. Kopelman H: The Epping jaundice after two years. Postgrad Med J 44:78–81, 1968.
189. Mullick FG, Ishak KG, Mahabir R, Stromeyer FW: Hepatic injury associated with paraquat toxicity in humans. Liver 1: 209–221, 1981.
190. Yanoff M, Rawson AJ: Peliosis hepatis. An anatomic study with demonstration of two varieties. Arch Pathol 77:159–165, 1964.
191. Zak FG: Peliosis hepatis. Am J Pathol 26:1–15, 1950.
192. Zafrani ES, Bernuau D, Feldmann G: Peliosis-like ultrastructural changes of the hepatic sinusoids in human chronic hypervitaminosis A: report of three cases. Hum Pathol 15:1166–1170, 1984.
193. Leopold JG, Parry TE, Storring FK: A change in the sinusoid-trabecular structure with hepatic venous outflow block. J Pathol 100:87–98, 1979.
194. Ingold JA, Reed GB, Kaplan HS, Bagshaw MA: Radiation hepatitis. Am J Roentgenol 93:200–208, 1965.
195. Hazlett BE, Taylor HE, Whitelaw DM: Fulminating hepatic necrosis in a patient with multiple myeloma treated with urethane. Report of a case. Blood 10:76–80, 1955.
196. Colsky J, Greenspan EM, Warren TN: Hepatic fibrosis in children with acute leukemia after therapy with folic acid antagonists. Arch Pathol 59:198–206, 1955.
197. Dahl MGC, Gregory MM, Scheuer PJ: Liver damage due to methotrexate in patients with psoriasis. Br Med J 1:625–630, 1971.
198. Nyfors A: Liver biopsies from psoriatics related to methotrexate therapy. 3. Findings in postmethotrexate liver biopsies from 160 psoriatics. Acta Pathol Microbiol Scand Sect A 85:511–518, 1977.
199. Nyfors A, Poulsen H: Liver biopsies from psoriatics related to methotrexate therapy. 2. Findings before and after methotrexate therapy in 88 patients. A blind study. Acta Pathol Microbiol Scand Sect A 84:262–270, 1976.
200. Nyfors A, Poulsen H: Liver biopsies from psoriatics related to methotrexate therapy. 1. Findings in 123 consecutive non-methotrexate treated patients. Acta Pathol Microbiol Scand Sect A 84:253–261, 1976.
201. Nyfors A, Poulsen H: Morphogenesis of fibrosis and cirrhosis in methotrexate treated patients with psoriasis. Am J Surg Pathol 1:235–243, 1977.
202. Nyfors A, Hopwood D: Light microscopic and ultrastructural findings in liver biopsies from 8 psoriatics before and after methotrexate therapy. A preliminary report of a prospective study. Acta Dermatovener 56:465–471, 1976.
203. Zachariae H, Sogaard H: Methotrexate-induced liver cirrhosis: a follow-up. Dermatologica 175:178–182, 1987.
204. Kaplan MM: Methotrexate treatment of chronic cholestatic liver diseases: friend or foe? Q J Med 268:757–761, 1989.
205. Huet PM, Guillaume E, Cote J, Legare A, Lavoie P, Viallet A: Noncirrhotic presinusoidal portal hypertension associated with chronic arsenical intoxication. Gastroenterology 68:1270–1277, 1975.
206. Villeneuve JP, Huet PM, Joly JG, Marleau D, Legare A, Lafortune M, Lavoie P, Viallet A: Idiopathic portal hypertension. Am J Med 61:459–464, 1976.
207. Van Orstrand HS: Current concepts of beryllium poisoning. Ann Intern Med 35:1203–1217, 1951.
208. Sneddon IB: Beryllium disease. Postgrad Med J 34:262–267, 1958.
209. Uchida T, Kao H, Quispe-Sjogren M, Peters RL. Alcoholic foamy degeneration: a pattern of acute alcoholic injury of the liver. Gastroenterology 84:683–692, 1983.
210. Spitz RD, Keren DF, Boitnott JK, Maddrey WC: Bridging hepatic necrosis. Etiology and prognosis. Am J Dig Dis 23:1076–1078, 1978.
211. Adams DO: The granulomatous inflammatory response. A review. Am J Pathol 84:164–191, 1976.
212. Vanderstigel M, Zafrani ES, Lejonc JL, Schaeffer A, Portos JL: Allopurinol hypersensitivity syndrome as a cause of hepatic fibrin-ring granulomas. Gastroenterology 90:188–190, 1986.
213. Beaugrande M, Chousterman M, Callard P, Camilleri J-P, Petite J-P, Ferrier J-P: Hepatites au maleate de perhexiline (Pexid) evoluant vers la cirrhose malgre l'arret due traitement (2 cas). Gastroenterol Clin Med 1:745–750, 1977.
214. Lewis D, Wainwright HC, Kew MC, Zwi S, Isaacson C: Liver damage associated with perhexiline maleate. Gut 20:186–189, 1979.
215. Pessayre D, Bichara M, Feldmann G, Degott C, Potet F, Benhamou J-P: Perhexiline maleate-induced cirrhosis. Gastroenterology 76:170–177, 1979.
216. Wright GJ, Leeson GA, Zeiger AV, Lang JW: The absorption, excretion and metabolism of perhexiline maleate by the human. Postgrad Med J 49:Suppl 3:8–15, 1973.
217. Sloan TP, Mahgoub A, Lancaster R, Idle JR, Smith RL: Polymorphism of carbon oxidation of drugs and clinical implications. Br Med J 2:655–657, 1978.
218. Morgan MY, Reshef R, Shah RR, Oates NS, Smith RL, Sherlock S: Impaired oxidation of debrisoquine in patients with perhexiline liver injury. Gut 25:1057–1064, 1984.
219. Lim PK, Trewby PN, Storey GCA: Neuropathy and fatal hepatitis in a patient receiving amiodarone. Br Med J 288:1638–1639, 1984.
220. Poucell S, Ireton J, Valencia-Mayoral P: Amiodarone-associated phospholipidosis and fibrosis of the liver. Light, immunohistochemical, and electron microscopic studies. Gastroenterology 86:926–936, 1984.
221. Simon JB, Manley PN, Brien JF: Amiodarone hepatotoxicity simulating alcoholic liver disease. N Engl J Med 311:167–172, 1984.
222. Babany G, Mallat A, Zafrani ES, Girardin M-F S-M, Carcone B, Dhumaux D: Chronic liver disease after low daily doses of amiodarone. J Hepatol 3:228–232, 1986.
223. Mason JE: Amiodarone. N Engl J Med 316:455–466, 1987.
224. Rigas B, Rosenfeld LE, Barwick KW, Enriquez R, Helzberg J, Batsford WP, Josephson ME, Riely CA: Amiodarone hepatotoxicity. A clinicopathologic study of five patients. Ann Intern Med 104:348–351, 1986.

225. Fogoros RN, Anderson KP, Winkle RA, Swerdlow CD, Mason JW: Amiodarone: clinical efficacy and toxicity in 96 patients with recurrent, drug-refractory arrhythmias. Circulation 68:88–94, 1983.
226. Pye M, Northcote RJ, Cobbe SM: Acute hepatitis after parenteral amiodarone administration. Br Heart J 59:690–691, 1988.
227. Morse RM, Valenzuela GA, Greenwald TP, Eulie PJ, Wesley RC, McCallum RW: Amiodarone-induced liver toxicity. Ann Intern Med 109: 838–840, 1988.
228. Lewis JH, Ranard RC, Caruso A, Jackson LK, Mullick F, Ishak KG, Seeff LB, Zimmerman HJ: Amiodarone hepatotoxicity: prevalence and clinicopathologic correlations among 104 patients. Hepatology 9:679–685, 1989.
229. Poucell S, Ireton J, Valencia-Mayoral P, Downar E, Larratt L, Patterson J, Blendis L, Phillips MJ: Amiodarone-associated phospholipidosis and fibrosis of the liver. Gastroenterology 86:926–936, 1984.
230. Shepherd NA, Dawson AM, Crocker PR, Levison DA: Granular cells as a marker of early amiodarone hepatotoxicity: a pathological and analytical study. J Clin Pathol 40:418–423, 1987.
231. Ishak KG: The liver. In Pathology of Drug-Induced and Toxic Diseases, edited by R.H. Ridell. New York: Churchill Livingston, 1982, pp. 472–473.
232. Guigui B, Perrot S, Berry JP, Fleury-Feith J, Martin N, Metreau JM, Chumeaux D, Zafrani ES: Amiodarone-induced hepatic phospholipidosis: a morphological alteration independent of pseudoalcoholic liver disease. Hepatology 8:1063–1068, 1988.
233. Pessayre D, Bichara M, Feldmann G, Degott D, Potet F, Benhamou J-P: Perhexiline maleate-induced cirrhosis. Gastroenterology 76:170–177, 1979.
234. Lullmann H, Lullmann-Rauch R, Wassermann O: Lipidosis induced by amphilphilic cationic drugs. Biochem Pharmacol 27:1103–1108, 1978.
235. Conn JW, Hinerman DL: Spironolactone-induced inhibition of aldosterone biosynthesis in primary aldosteronism: morphological and functional studies. Metabolism 26:1293–1307, 1977.
236. Zimmerman HJ, Ishak KG: Valproate-induced hepatic injury: analysis of 23 fatal cases. Hepatology 2:648–649, 1982.
237. Zafrani ES, Berthelot P: Sodium valproate in the induction of unusual hepatotoxicity. Hepatology 2:591–597, 1982.
238. Powell-Jackson PR, Tredger JM, Williams R: Hepatotoxicity to sodium valproate: a review. Gut 25:673–681, 1984.
239. Klinge O, Bannasch P: Zur Vermehrung des glatten endoplasmatischen Retikulum in Hepatocyten menschlicher Leberpunktate. Verhandl dtsch Ges Pathol 53:568–573, 1968.
240. Scheuer PJ, Summerfield JA, Lal S, Sherlock S: Rifampicin hepatitis. A clinical and histological study. Lancet 1:421–425, 1974.
241. Popper H: Drug induced liver injury. In The Liver, edited by E.A. Gall, F.K. Mostofi. Baltimore: Williams & Wilkins, 1973, p. 1822.
242. Nishimura RN, Ishak KG, Reddick R, Porter R, James S, Barranger JA: Lafora's disease: diagnosis by liver biopsy. Ann Neurol 8:409–415, 1980.
243. Vazquez JJ, Pardo-Mindan J: Liver cell injury (bodies similar to Lafora's) in alcoholics treated with disulfiram (Antabuse). Histopathology 3:377–384, 1979.
244. Vazquez JJ, Guillen FJ, Zozaya J, Lahoz M: Cyanamide-induced liver injury. A predictable lesion. Liver 3:225–230, 1983.
245. Thomsen P, Reinicke V: Ground glass inclusions in liver cells in an alcoholic treated with cyanamide (Dipsan). Liver 1:67–73, 1981.
246. Guillen FJ, Vazquez JJ: Cyanamide-induced liver cell injury: experimental study in the rat. Lab Invest 50:385–393, 1984.
247. MacKay IR: Induction by drugs of hepatitis and autoantibodies to cell organelles: significance and interpretation. Hepatology 5:904–906, 1985.
248. Callea F, DeVos R, Togni R, Tardanico R, Vanstapel MJ, Desmet VJ: Fibrinogen inclusions in liver cells: a new type of ground-glass hepatocyte. Immune light and electron microscopic characterization. Histopathology 10:65–73, 1986.
249. Desmet VJ, DeVos R: Ultrastructural findings in non-A, non-B viral hepatitis. In Hepatology: A Festschrift for Hans Popper, edited by H. Brunner, H. Thaler. New York, Raven Press, 1985, 159–175.
250. Strohmeyer FW, Ishak KG, Gerber MA, Mathew T: Ground-glass cells in hepatocellular carcinoma. Am J Clin Pathol 74:254–258, 1980.
251. Goodman ZD, Ishak KG, Langlos JM, Sesterhenn IA, Rabin L:

Combined hepatocellular-cholangiocarcinoma. A histologic and immunohistochemical study. Cancer 55:124–135, 1985.
252. Livni N, Behar AJ, Lafair JS: Unusual amyloid bodies in human liver. Ultrastructural and freeze-etching studies. Israel J Med Sci 13:1163–1170, 1977.
253. Schochet SS Jr, McCormick WF, Zellweger H: Type IV glycogenosis (amylopectinosis). Light and electron microscopic observations. Arch Pathol 90:354–363, 1970.
254. Ludwig J, Axelsen R: Drug effects on the liver. An updated tabular compilation of drugs and drug-related hepatic diseases. Dig Dis Sci 28:651–666, 1983.
255. Ludwig: Drug effects on the liver: a tabular compilation of drugs and drug-related hepatic diseases. Dig Dis Sci 24:785–796, 1979.

Additional reported hepatotoxic drugs

256. Miller MA: Reversible hepatotoxicity related to amphotericin B. Can Med Assoc J 131:1245–1247, 1984.
257. Goudie BM, Birnie GF, Watkinson G, MacSween RNM, Kissen H, Cunningham NE: Jaundice associated with the use of benoxaprofen. Lancet 1:959, 1982.
258. Parker WA: Captopril-induced cholestatic jaundice. Drug Intell Clin Pharm 18:234–235, 1984.
259. Williams SJ, Ruppin DC, Grierson JM, Farrell GC: Carbamazepine hepatitis: the clincopathological spectrum. J Gastroenterol Hepatol 1:159–168, 1986.
260. Lunzer M, Huang S-N, Ginsberg J, Ahmed M, Sherlock S: Jaundice due to carbimazole. Gut 16:913–917, 1975.
261. Gjone E, Orning OM: Jaundice due to chloramphenicol. Acta Hepato-Spleno 13:288–292, 1966.
262. Elmore M, Rissing JP, Rink L, Brooks GF: Clindamycin-associated hepatotoxicity. Am J Med 57:627–630, 1974.
263. Perino LE, Warren GH, Levine JS: Cocaine-induced hepatotoxicity in humans. Gastroenterology 93:176–180, 1987.
264. Aubrey DA: Massive hepatic necrosis after cyclophosphamide. Br Med J 3:588, 1970.
265. Pearson K, Zimmerman HJ: Danazol and liver damage. Lancet 1:645–646, 1980.
266. Stone SP, Goodwin RM: Dapsone-induced jaundice. Arch Dermatol 114:947, 1978.
267. Velasco HA, Sokal JE: Cholestatic jaundice in association with desacetyl-methylcolchicine. N Engl J Med 260:1280–1281, 1959.
268. Stricker BHCh, Blok APR, Bronkhorst FB, Van Parys GE, Desmet VJ: Ketoconazole-associated hepatic injury: a clinicopathological study of 55 cases. J Hepatol 3:399–406, 1986.
269. Loiudice TA, Buhac I, Peng SK, Dillard P: Hepataic dysfunction following methylprylon intoxication. Am J Dig Dis 23:33–37, 1978.
270. Reshev R, Lok ASF, Sherlock S: Cholestatic jaundice in fascioliasis treated with niclofolan. Br Med J 285:1243–1244, 1982.
271. Winter SL, Boyer JL: Hepatic toxicity from large doses of vitamin B3 (nicotinamide). N Engl J Med 289:1180–1182, 1973.
272. Vaz FG, Singh R, Nurussaman M: Hepatitis induced by nomifensine. Br Med J 289:1268, 1984.
273. Den Boer W, Loehger EA: Phenprocouman-induced jaundice. Lancet 1:912, 1976.
274. Hartman H, Fischer G, Janning G: Prolonged cholestatic jaundice and leucopenia associated with piroxicam. Zeitschrift Gastroenterologie 22:343–345, 1984.
275. Munoz SJ, Jariello R, Maddrey WC: Submassive hepatic necrosis associated with the use of progabide: a GABA receptor agonist. Dig Dis Sci 33:375–380, 1988.
276. Lauristen K, Havelund T, Rask-Madsen J, Fenger C: Ranitidine and hepatotoxicity. Lancet 2:1471, 1984.
277. Gulley RM, Mirza A, Kelly CE: Hepatotoxicity of salcylazosulfapyridine. A case report and review of the literature. Am J Gastroenterol 72:561–564, 1979.
278. Millikan LE, Harrell ER: Drug reactions to sulfones. Arch Dermatol 102:220–224, 1970.
279. Blackburn AM, Amierl SA, Millis RR, Rubens RD: Tamoxifen and liver damage. Br Med J 2:288, 1984.
280. Jalota R, Freston JW: Severe intrahepatic cholestasis due to thiobendazole. Am J Trop Med 23:676–678, 1974.

Chapter 8
Chronic Hepatitis

Definition

A wide variety of disorders that affect the liver are characterized by clinical, biochemical, and histologic features indicative of chronic hepatic inflammation, degeneration, and necrosis, which often are accompanied by a variable degree of fibrosis. However, by convention, use of the term *chronic hepatitis* is limited to a small group of disorders of varied etiology that share a number of distinctive clinical and morphologic features. The remaining chronic inflammatory, degenerative, necrotic, and fibrotic lesions that affect the liver are classified under other rubrics, including: alcoholic hepatitis and cirrhosis (Chapter 10), primary biliary cirrhosis (Chapter 11), hemochromatosis (Chapter 12), Wilson's disease (Chapter 13), chronic biliary tract disease (Chapter 20), hepatic lesions associated with chronic inflammatory bowel disease (Chapter 24), and a number of infections and hereditary metabolic disorders that affect the liver in infancy. With few exceptions, the histologic features of chronic hepatitis are readily differentiated from those in other forms of chronic liver disease. However, in individual cases, identification of the etiology almost always depends on a synthesis of clinical, biochemical, serologic, and histologic evidence.

Chronic persistent and *chronic active hepatitis,* the two major variants of chronic hepatitis, differ clinically and histologically. The former usually runs a benign course, produces no clinical manifestations or only mild ones, and shows virtually no tendency to progress (1). The latter is usually accompanied by overt clinical signs of hepatic disease and progressive hepatocellular destruction and fibrosis that may ultimately result in the development of cirrhosis or hepatic failure. Occasionally, chronic persistent hepatitis can progress to chronic active hepatitis (1,2) and vice versa, either spontaneously or during immunosuppressive therapy.

Chronic persistent or chronic active hepatitis may develop as a consequence of antecedent overt acute hepatitis, or may evolve silently. By convention, acute hepatitis that fails to resolve within six months is classified as chronic hepatitis. However, such lesions are often classified as *unresolved acute hepatitis.* No significant differences between unresolved acute hepatitis and chronic hepatitis of insidious onset have been identified (3). Except in investigative studies, differentiation between the two appears to serve no useful purpose, and may be misleading if no distinction is made between lesions of less than and more than six months' duration. To avoid such confusion, the term unresolved acute hepatitis should be limited to lesions of less than six months' duration.

Often, the age of the histologic lesions of chronic hepatitis of insidious onset cannot be determined from the clinical or laboratory features. This is particularly true in asymptomatic cases and in those that present abruptly with clinical and laboratory features that suggest an acute hepatitis. Recognition of the chronic nature of the lesions in such cases depends on their histologic features, particularly the presence of portal fibrosis, the prominence of piecemeal necrosis, the paucity of intralobular inflammatory cells and necrotic hepatocytes, and, in the case of HBV infections, the presence of orcein-positive ground glass cells. The demonstration of elastic fibers in septa may help to estimate the age of the lesion. Elastic tissue is not present in acute hepatitis, but increases as the process matures (4).

In some cases of chronic hepatitis, particularly those that evolve when acute hepatitis fails to resolve, or recurs repeatedly, intralobular inflammation and necrosis may be prominent features. Lesions of this type are classified by some as *chronic lobular hepatitis* (5,6). It has been suggested that such lesions occur almost exclusively in men with non-A, non-B hepatitis virus infections, show no tendency to undergo progressive fibrosis, and may be due to fluctuations in the activity of the underlying viral infection (6). However, in our experience such lesions are not limited to men, sometimes occur in hepatitis B infections, and when accompanied by bridging necrosis, may progress to cirrhosis. Moreover, intralobular inflammation and hepatocellular necrosis of variable degree are relatively common findings in chronic persistent and chronic active hepatitis, particularly in those that are the sequelae of antecedent unresolved acute hepatitis, so that differentiation between chronic lobular and other forms of chronic hepatitis usually is based on ill-defined and arbitrary criteria. Since there is no convincing evidence that the clinical features or prognosis in these two types of chronic hepatitis differ, there appears to be little reason to include chronic lobular hepatitis as a separate entity in the classification of liver disease. The changes of chronic lobular hepatitis have been reported to occur frequently in HBV carriers in the Far East (7).

Histologic variants of chronic hepatitis include *chronic persistent, chronic active,* and *chronic cholestatic hepatitis.* Although the clinical and laboratory features in each type differ to some extent, there is general agreement that classification of such lesions should be based on their morphologic features. Classification of chronic hepatitis on the basis of clinical and laboratory criteria, however, often results in diagnostic errors, and may lead to confusing or inconclusive results in clinical investigations. Such ambivalence is illustrated in the case of a frequently cited controlled trial of corticosteroid therapy in what was termed *chronic active liver disease* (8,9). Although liver biopsy material was available in all cases, the criteria used in selecting patients for study were clinical, namely, an illness of at least 10 weeks' duration that showed no evidence of improvement, and biochemical findings indicative of severe hepatic injury. Of note, only 34 of the 63 patients investigated exhibited lesions that met the histologic criteria for chronic persistent hepatitis, chronic active hepatitis, or cirrhosis, while 29 exhibited severe acute hepatitis with bridging or multilobular necrosis. Moreover, of the 44 patients with noncirrhotic lesions, only 4 treated cases and 3 control subjects had histologic evidence of either chronic persistent or chronic active hepatitis. Thus, the results of this study appear to demonstrate the effects of corticosteroid therapy in a group of patients, many of whom had severe acute hepatitis and who are generally regarded to have had autoimmune chronic active hepatitis of less than six months' duration (10), but provide only equivocal evidence of its effects in other types of *chronic active hepatitis*. The inclusion of patients with hepatic disease of viral, drug, and cryptogenic origin in that study renders interpretation of the results inconclusive. Some such uncertainties can be avoided in clinical investigations by the use of a standardized, semiquantitative assessment of histologic activity (11,12).

Often, chronic active hepatitis is accompanied by *progressive portal fibrosis,* which may destroy the normal lobular architecture and may lead to the development of *cirrhosis.* In the early stages of such cirrhosis, nodule formation tends to be patchy in distribution, so cirrhosis may escape detection in small needle biopsy sections. However, in such cases, *portal-portal bridging fibrosis* is often demonstrable. As an indication of how far the fibrosis has progressed, and as a sign of possible early cirrhosis, the presence or absence of bridging fibrosis should always be noted in the histologic diagnosis of chronic active hepatitis.

Since the clinical features and prognosis in chronic active hepatitis are greatly influenced by the existence of cirrhosis, its presence or absence should always be considered in the diagnosis of such lesions. Depending on whether the clinical and histologic features are predominantly hepatitic or cirrhotic, such complex lesions are classified as *chronic active hepatitis with postnecrotic cirrhosis,* or *postnecrotic cirrhosis with chronic active hepatitis,* respectively.

Bridging hepatocellular necrosis is another feature that greatly worsens the prognosis in chronic active hepatitis, so it, too, should be included in the classification of such lesions (13–15). Some authorities distinguish between *bridging* and *multilobular hepatocellular necrosis* (9). In our experience, the prognosis and clinical features in these two types of lesions are similar. Moreover, based on observations of surgical wedge and postmorten specimens, we have found that bridging necrosis is often accompanied by multilobular necrosis that may have escaped detection in needle biopsy specimens. For these reasons, we draw no distinctions between these two types of necrosis.

Etiology

Although the causes of chronic active hepatitis may be changing (16), at least five etiologic factors have been implicated in the pathogenesis of chronic hepatitis: *hepatitis B virus* (HBV), *hepatitis D virus* (HDV), *non-A, non-B* (NANB or HCV) *hepatitis virus, idiosyncratic drug-induced reactions,* and *autoimmune chronic active hepatitis.* The last category, *autoimmune hepatitis,* has also been termed *lupoid hepatitis* (17), *HBsAg-negative hepatitis, plasma cell hepatitis* (18), *active juvenile cirrhosis* (19), and *chronic liver disease of young women* (20). Each of these terms is open to criticism. The assumption that

such lesions are manifestations of an autoimmune reaction is based on circumstantial rather than conclusive evidence, although support for an autoimmune pathogenesis is accumulating (21–27). Moreover, there is accumulating evidence that autoimmunity may also play a role in the pathogenesis of HBV-induced and drug-related chronic hepatitis (28–30). Only a small minority of patients in this group exhibit LE cells in their blood or have clinical features suggestive of disseminated lupus erythematosus, so the term ''lupoid'' often is inappropriate (31,32). Unfortunately, the absence of HBsAg in the serum does not always exclude an underlying HBV infection, since HBsAg or HBcAg are sometimes undetectable in the liver (33). Undue emphasis on the prominence of plasma cell infiltrates, as implied in the term ''plasma cell hepatitis,'' is unwarranted, since the number of plasma cells does not clearly distinguish between chronic hepatitis of known and unknown etiology. The terms ''active juvenile cirrhosis'' and ''chronic liver disease of young women'' have even less merit, since chronic hepatitis may occur at any age and in either sex, and is not always accompanied by cirrhosis. The most appropriate term and the one used hereafter is *autoimmune chronic active hepatitis.* The availability of an accurate serologic test for HCV and, presumably, for HEV will allow identification of the etiology of cases of ''cryptogenic'' chronic active hepatitis, and will help define more precisely the autoimmune types (34–36).

Hepatitis B virus

Based on prospective liver biopsy studies, it has been estimated that in 5 to 10% of cases, *acute HBV hepatitis* fails to resolve within six months, and gives rise to either chronic persistent or chronic active hepatitis. In patients who fail to clear their serum of HBsAg within four months, the incidence of chronicity approaches 100% (33,37,38). Extremes of age (39) and bridging hepatocellular necrosis (40) are two other features that predispose to chronicity in acute B hepatitis.

Often, chronic hepatitis has an insidious onset. There may be a history of possible exposure to HBV from blood transfusions, from sharing needles, from intimate contacts with HBsAg carriers, or from exposure to blood or blood products in health care professionals. In addition, vertical transmission of HBV and other viruses accounts for some chronic infections, particularly in parts of the world where carrier rates are high. Moreover, in many cases, the source of infection cannot be identified. α-fetoprotein is frequently elevated in chronic HBV hepatitis (41) and must be differentiated from hepatocellular carcinoma. These elevations are sometimes, but not always, preneoplastic abnormalities (42).

Many patients with HBsAg-positive chronic hepatitis of insidious onset present with signs or symptoms of liver disease (43,44). However, in some, the lesions are asymptomatic, although, usually, they are accompanied by increased transaminase activity or other biochemical evidence of hepatic dysfunction. The reported incidence of biopsy-documented chronic hepatitis in presumably healthy carriers of HBsAg is highly variable, ranging from 0% (45) to 84% (46). In a combined series of 250 healthy carriers reported in the literature, liver biopsy revealed chronic active hepatitis in 6%, chronic persistent hepatitis in 28%, nonspecific reactive hepatitis in 46%, normal liver in 10%, and other lesions in 10% (45–53).

In general, the frequency of HBs antigenemia in cases of

chronic hepatitis varies with the prevalence of HBV infections in any given area, ranging from as low as 4% in countries where the carrier rate is negligible (54), to as high as 90% in Taiwan where the carrier rate is 13% (55). However, other factors must be involved, since in some countries with low carrier rates, such as Denmark, the incidence of HB surface antigenemia in chronic hepatitis may be as high as 65% (56). Similarly, in New Haven, where the carrier rate is less than 0.1%, HBsAg was detected in 26% of patients with chronic active hepatitis (3). In this group, no single epidemiologic factor could be identified to account for this relatively high rate of chronic HBV infection.

Identification of the hepatitis B virus as the etiologic factor in chronic hepatitis depends on the detection of HBsAg, HBcAg, or HBV DNA in the serum or liver (33) or the finding of orcein-positive ground glass cells in liver biopsy sections. The polymerase chain reaction for HBV DNA is the most sensitive test, being able to detect as few as three HBV DNA genomes in a serum sample (57). Since antibody to HBsAg is a relatively common finding in the general population, it has little diagnostic significance. However, a high titer of anti-HBc usually indicates virus replication, and, thus, provides convincing evidence that the lesion is attributable to infection with HBV (58). When both HBsAg and anti-HBc are absent, the diagnosis of HBV-induced chronic hepatitis is warranted only when transient HBs antigenemia had been documented at the onset of illness. Quiescent, chronic HBV hepatitis with anti-HBs and anti-HBe in serum may undergo spontaneous severe reactivation (59,60).

Hepatitis D virus

The acute lesions of HDV infection are indistinguishable from those of HBV hepatitis, but tend to be more abrupt in onset and more severe, and are much more likely to progress to chronic active hepatitis (61). When HDV causes superinfection in a patient who is a chronic HBV carrier, it occasionally causes severe acute even fulminant hepatitis (62,63). HBV replication is suppressed (64), and the episode is self-limited, even though it may end fatally. More frequently, HDV superinfection induces an acute episode of hepatitis, which is followed by an aggressive form of chronic active hepatitis in which HDV may persist for years (65). In patients with coinfection with HBV and HDV simultaneous infection with HIV inhibits the inhibition of HBV replication (64,66).

In patients in whom low grade chronic hepatitis, either chronic persistent or chronic active, had been present, superinfection with HDV rapidly accelerates the histologic abnormalities to severe chronic active hepatitis (61,67,68). Frequently the process progresses rapidly to cirrhosis (61,62,69,70). The diagnosis of HDV chronic hepatitis can be established by the demonstration of anti-HDAg or HDV RNA in the serum and HDAg in the nuclei of hepatocytes.

Non-A, Non-B hepatitis viruses

In many respects, the *acute* lesions produced by HCV and HEV resemble those of acute hepatitis B. However, they tend to be milder, and to run a prolonged course that is characterized by periodic, transient elevations of serum transaminase activity usually accompanied by the recurrence of symptoms. They frequently give rise to chronic persistent or chronic active hepatitis (71). Indeed, the incidence of such chronic lesions has been found to be as high as 40% in some studies (72). The recent description of late onset hepatic failure, which as many features of fulminant hepatic failure, has a high prevalence of residual chronic active hepatitis in the survivors (73). The type of NANB virus in delayed-onset fulminant hepatic failure has not yet been identified.

Identification of NANB viral infections has depended on clinical and laboratory features consistent with viral hepatitis in the absence of serologic evidence of HAV or HBV infection. Although these diagnostic criteria are reasonably reliable in cases of *acute hepatitis,* they are not as dependable in the case of *chronic hepatitis* or in *carriers* of the NANB viruses. Under such conditions, identification requires not only the exclusion of HAV, HBV, and other viral infections and drug-induced hepatitis but also the demonstration of HCV infection (34–36). A number of studies indicate that chronic NANB hepatitis and chronic HCV hepatitis are often responsive to therapy with interferon, at least transiently (74–76). Histologic patterns typical of NANB acute viral hepatitis have been described (77), and some of these abnormalities may persist with chronic hepatitis, including lymphoid aggregates and follicles in the portal zones.

Chronic active hepatitis secondary to NANB hepatitis has been associated in a few cases with abnormal bile duct epithelium that appears to represent the development of microdiverticula of the small bile ducts (78).

Idiosyncratic drug-induced reactions

Drugs have been implicated as possible etiologic factors in 28 to 67% of cases of *chronic active hepatitis* (79–82). This probably represents an overestimate, since in only a minority of cases has the etiologic role of the suspected drug been established by documentation of a remission following withdrawal of the drug or an exacerbation on rechallenge. Nevertheless, drugs probably play a more important role in the pathogenesis of chronic active hepatitis than is generally appreciated, and certainly should always be considered as a possible etiologic factor.

Well-documented cases of *chronic active hepatitis* have been encountered following reactions to *oxyphenisatin* (79–83) and, less commonly, to *α-methyldopa* (Aldomet) (81,84), *nitrofurantoin* (85), *chlorpromazine* (86), *isoniazid* (87), *sulfonamides* (88), *propylthiouracil* (89), *phenylbutazone* (83,90), *dantrolene* (91), and *acetaminophen* (92).

In many cases of *drug-induced chronic active hepatitis,* the onset is abrupt with an acute hepatitis, often accompanied by bridging hepatocellular necrosis that fails to resolve. In others, the development of chronic hepatitis is insidious. As a rule, the lesions remain active and progress if administration of the drug is continued. They tend to heal when the drug is withdrawn (93) and to recur when the agent is readministered. However, occasionally, withdrawal of the drug is not followed by recovery. Under such conditions, the etiologic relationship of the drug to the hepatic lesions is not established. In some cases, at least perpetuation of the lesions may be attributable to an autoimmune reaction triggered by the drug, and possibly dependent on a defect in suppressor T cell function that is genetically determined, as suggested by the high frequency of the HLA-B8 phenotype in affected individuals (21,83).

Chronic cholestatic hepatitis is a rare sequela of acute drug-induced cholestasis. Such lesions, characterized by persistent cholestasis and progressive portal inflammation and fibrosis that may ultimately give rise to an unusual type of *biliary cirrhosis,* occasionally accompanied by xanthomatosis, have been encountered in reactions to *chlorpromazine* (94,95), *prochlorperazine* (Compazine) (96), *arsphenamine* (97), and *tolbutamide* (Orinase) (98).

The factors responsible for perpetuation and progression of the lesions in chronic cholestatic hepatitis are not known. In some cases (98) continued administration of the drug may be the cause, but, usually, cholestasis, portal inflammation and fibrosis persist and progress long after the drug is withdrawn. Inflammation, necrosis, and ultimate fibrous obliteration of the interlobular bile ducts are seen in some cases (96,98), but these are inconstant features, and may be the result rather than the cause of the protracted cholestasis. Although there is no conclusive supporting evidence at present, it is conceivable that an autoimmune reaction triggered by the offending drug is responsible for the perpetuation and progression of such lesions, as has been proposed in the case of drug-induced chronic active hepatitis.

Whether this disorder represents a discrete syndrome or the concurrence of both chronic hepatitis and primary biliary cirrhosis is not known. These cases may show antimitochondrial antibodies, but these antibodies are heterogeneous and differ from the primary biliary cirrhosis–specific antibody (anti-M$_2$) (81) or antibody to the E2 subunits (99–101).

Autoimmune chronic active hepatitis

Although the morphology and behavior of the lesions in autoimmune chronic active hepatitis are relatively uniform, their clinical, biochemical, and serologic features are more variable, suggesting that the disease may include a heterogeneous group of disorders that differ in etiology and pathogenesis (102). Characteristic, distinctive features differentiate *lupoid hepatitis,* the variant that has attracted the greatest attention, from other forms of chronic active hepatitis. These include: a propensity for attacking both young (103,104) and elderly women (104), a predisposition for HLA hapolotypes B8 and DR3 (105,105A), often the presence of LE cells in the blood (103,104), high serum levels of gamma globulin (103,104), high serum antibody titers against smooth muscle (actin)(106), organ-specific antigens (107,108), microsomes (109) and double-stranded DNA (110), the absence of antimitochondrial antibodies (111), an association with other presumably autoimmune disorders, such as ulcerative colitis (112), or hypereosinophilic syndromes (113), and clinical manifestations resembling those in systemic lupus erythematosus, such as rash, pericarditis, pleurisy, glomerulonephritis, and polyarthritis (103,104,112). An increased frequency of hyperglobulinemia and serologic markers of autoimmunity in relatives is often present (114,115). However, in our experience and that reported by others (116), neither the clinical manifestation nor the laboratory findings differ in patients with or without LE cells in the blood. Moreover, we have encountered LE cells, smooth muscle and nuclear antibodies, and hypergammaglobulinemia in cases of HBsAg-positive and drug-induced chronic active hepatitis, so it is doubtful that lupoid hepatitis represents a distinct etiologic or clinical entity. Moreover, it is highly probably that more than one etiologic factor is involved in the pathogenesis of HBsAg-negative chronic active hepatitis. In addition to lupoid hepatitis, NANB viral hepatitis, unrecognized drugs, or environmental hepatotoxins may play a role.

Cryptogenic chronic active hepatitis

Cryptogenic chronic active hepatitis is defined as chronic active hepatitis that has none of the markers that identify autoimmune chronic active hepatitis, such as HLA haplotype B8 or DR3, LE cells, or antibodies to smooth muscle or nuclear membranes. This disorder, however, cannot otherwise be differentiated from autoimmune chronic active hepatitis by clinical, biochemical, or histologic features, although gamma-globulin levels appear to be lower in cryptogenic chronic active hepatitis. The response to corticosteroid therapy is equally good in both groups and the prognosis is similar (117). It is probable that some of these cases will be shown to be HCV chronic active hepatitis (118), but other etiologic agents may also be involved in some cases.

Hepatitis A virus

Rare cases of chronic hepatitis caused by HAV have been reported (119–123). The disease does not appear to differ from the patterns seen in HBV chronic hepatitis. It may appear without signs or symptoms (121) or as chronic active hepatitis with piecemeal necrosis (119,120,124). It is characterized by the persistence of IgM antibodies. It is a transient type of chronic hepatitis (124), the longest reported case having lasted only three years. It does not differ histologically from chronic hepatitis of other etiologies.

Pathogenesis

A number of observations suggest that the progressive destruction of hepatocytes in chronic active hepatitis may be attributable to a K cell–mediated, antibody-dependent, or cytotoxic T cell immune reaction directed at an antigenic determinant in the surface membranes of hepatocytes (125–127). In some cases, a defect in suppressor T cell activity is responsible for the perpetuation of this process (128–131). It has been proposed that failure to eliminate the hepatitis B virus in cases of *HBsAg-positive chronic active hepatitis* is attributable to a defect in anti-HBs production, and that persistence of the virus activates helper T cells continuously, resulting in stimulation of B cells to produce antibody directed against a liver-specific protein or liver membrane antigen normally present in hepatocellular surface membranes. Secondarily, such antibody coating of hepatocytes leads to their destruction by circulating K cells. In contrast, perpetuation of the lesions in *HBsAg-negative chronic active hepatitis* of viral origin is ascribed to a defect in suppressor T cell activity that permits unrestricted anti-liver–specific protein production by B cells that subtly react in hepatocellular surface membranes that have been altered by antecedent viral injury. A similar mechanism has been invoked to account for the development of *drug-induced chronic active hepatitis*. The demonstration of anti-liver–specific protein (128) and *in vitro* evidence of reduced suppressor T cell activity (127–131) in most cases of chronic active hepatitis, both HBsAg-positive and negative, are consistent with the hypothesis that a K cell–mediated, anti-liver–specific protein-dependent autoimmune reaction is involved in the pathogenesis of the disease (132).

Even if the role of autoimmunity as a major factor in the pathogenesis of chronic active hepatitis can be established unequivocally, an important question still to be resolved is the nature of the agent that triggers the autoimmune mechanism in *HBsAg-negative chronic active hepatitis of unknown etiology*. In some cases, such as those in which HBsAg is detectable in the liver but not in the serum (21), and in those that exhibit *in vitro* evidence of cell-mediated immunity to purified HBsAg in the absence of antigenemia (133), it is highly probable that the hepatitis B virus is responsible for initiating the injury that leads to an autoimmune reaction. In others, the NANB hepatitis virus may be implicated, a possibility suggested by the occurrence of chronic active hepatitis in cases of well-documented infections with this agent. However, assessment of the relative importance of the NANB hepatitis virus as an etiologic factor must await further development of reliable serologic diagnostic methods.

Recent investigations in patients with chronic HBV hepatitis have shown greater than normal interleukin-1 (IL-1) levels in cultured mononuclear cells (134). This evidence of the presence of activated monocytes was not accompanied by increased activity of interleukin-2 (IL-2). This elevation is not simply an effect of active hepatic inflammation, since IL-1 is not increased in patients with primary biliary cirrhosis (134). Among the patients studied, IL-1 activity was higher in patients with chronic active hepatitis than in those with chronic persistent hepatitis and was highest in those with cirrhosis. There is a positive correlation between the presence of fibrosis and the degree of IL-1 activity. These observations are of great interest, since one of the biologic properties of IL-1 is its stimulation of fibroblasts to produce collagen (135,136). These findings are in accord with the clinicopathologic observations that chronic persistent hepatitis is a benign disease while chronic active hepatitis is a more severe disorder that often progresses to cirrhosis.

The possibility that the proposed defect in immunoregulation in autoimmune chronic active hepatitis is genetically determined is suggested by the relatively high frequency of the HLA-B8, DR3 (137), and B12 (138) histocompatibility phenotypes reported in affected individuals (137–139). However, the relationship between reduced suppressor T cell activity and HLA-B8 and HLA-B12 antigens has not been confirmed in some studies (131,140). It has also been suggested that a genetically determined defect in suppressor T cell synthesis of specific hepatocyte protein antigens unrelated to HLA antigens may play a role in the pathogenesis of autoimmune chronic hepatitis (141,142). Objections have been raised to the interpretation and significance of the evidence cited in support of the autoimmune theory (132). Nevertheless, despite its flaws, the theory remains an attractive possibility that merits further investigation (143). Circulating antibodies have been noted in autoimmune chronic active hepatitis, but their role in the pathogenesis of chronic active hepatitis is not clear (144).

The immunology of chronic active hepatitis has been thoughtfully and concisely reviewed (145).

Relationship of chronic active hepatitis to other hepatic disorders

Primary biliary cirrhosis

As previously indicated, acute drug-induced cholestasis occasionally fails to resolve, and gives rise to a type of *chronic cholestatic hepatitis* that may progress to a cirrhotic picture that mimics primary biliary cirrhosis (95–98). However, in such cases, the clinical manifestations, characterized by an abrupt onset of jaundice, often accompanied by features of a hypersensitivity reaction that appear following exposure to a drug known to produce cholestasis, the absence of antimitochondrial antibodies, and the histologic character of the lesions differ from those of primary biliary cirrhosis.

Occasionally, cholestasis is a conspicuous feature, both clinically and histologically, in cases of *chronic active hepatitis* of unknown etiology, or in those associated with HBs antigenemia (146–149). Differentiation from primary biliary cirrhosis may be difficult, since in some cases the serum contains antimitochondrial antibodies that may differ from those of primary biliary cirrhosis (99,146,147,149), and the lesions show some of the features of primary biliary cirrhosis, particularly hyperplasia, degeneration, and inflammation of bile duct epithelium (148), and a reduction in the number of interlobular ducts (146,149). As in the case of primary biliary cirrhosis, lesions of this type usually are refractory to prednisone therapy (149) and to have a worse prognosis than those in classic chronic active hepatitis (147).

It has been suggested that chronic active hepatitis and primary biliary cirrhosis may be manifestations of a single autoimmune process that affects either the hepatocytes or the intrahepatic bile ducts predominantly, resulting in the development of either chronic active hepatitis or primary biliary cirrhosis, respectively, but occasionally affects both, thereby producing mixed lesions (150). Although overlapping lesions of this type and the occurrence of antimitochondrial antibodies in some cases of chronic active hepatitis appear to support the hypothesis that chronic active hepatitis and primary biliary cirrhosis share a common pathogenesis, the striking difference between their responses to corticosteroid therapy (149), the frequency with which chronic active hepatitis can be related to hepatitis B infection, and the observation that the antimitochondrial antibodies in the two diseases differ in antigenic specificity (151) are more consistent with the view that they are distinct etiologic entities. Both may be autoimmune disorders.

Recent investigations confirm the overlap in histologic and laboratory features in the two disorders, but point out that histologic examination can differentiate them in more than 90% of cases and that antimitochondrial antibody titers (>1:160), immunoglobulin M levels (>6 mg/ml), serum alkaline phosphatase activity (>fourfold the upper limit of normal), and cholesterol (>300 mg/dl) can differentiate more than 80% of patients (152,153). Chronic active hepatitis with low levels of antimitochondrial antibody seems to respond to steroid therapy.

Cryptogenic cirrhosis

Obviously, by definition, cryptogenic cirrhosis is neither an etiologic nor a morphologic entity. The occurrence of smooth muscle and antinuclear antibodies in some cases has led to the suggestion that cryptogenic cirrhosis is a manifestation of an autoimmune disease closely related pathogenetically to chronic active hepatitis and primary biliary cirrhosis (150). The possibility that the lesions, at least in some cases, may be the sequelae of antecedent unrecognized chronic active hepatitis is supported not only by the presence of serologic markers of autoimmunity but also by the occasional detection of HBsAg in the serum of such cases (154,155), and by the close resemblance of the lesions to those of inactive postnecrotic cirrhosis that may appear following spontaneous or induced remission in chronic active hepatitis. However, lesions classified as cryptogenic cirrhosis, which exhibit a macronodular pattern, show little or no evidence of activity, and usually present with signs of portal hypertension and little clinical evidence of hepatocellular failure (156,157), undoubtedly include disorders of other etiologies that either cannot be identified or have been overlooked. The most common of these include: (1) the late inactive phase of alcoholic cirrhosis; (2) the late inactive form of cirrhosis in Wilson's disease when neurologic signs and Kaiser-Fleischer rings are absent or overlooked, the serum levels of ceruloplasmin and copper have not been investigated, and the sections have not been stained for copper; and (3) the macronodular cirrhosis associated with α_1-antitrypsin deficiency in the adult, when the characteristic α_1-antitrypsin cytoplasmic inclusions are not evident in routine H & E sections, and no attempt is made to visualize them in D-PAS-stained sections or by the use of specific antibodies or immunologic-staining techniques.

The frequency with which cirrhotic lesions are classified as cryptogenic in most large series of cases is remarkably variable, ranging from as low as 14% to as high as 62% (157). However, the criteria used to identify the etiology in such cases are so poorly defined that the classification is open to question in some instances. Moreover, published reports rarely give any indication of the extent to which the search for known causes of cirrhosis was carried out, so the incidence of truly cryptogenic cases is uncertain. Obviously, the more precise the histologic criteria used in identifying the nature of the lesions, and the more exhaustive the search for etiologic factors, the fewer the number of cases categorized as cryptogenic chronic active hepatitis.

Histopathology of chronic hepatitis

Three major types of lesions are encountered in chronic hepatitis: *chronic persistent hepatitis, chronic active hepatitis,* and *postnecrotic cirrhosis.* Although each of these lesions has distinctive morphologic features, they overlap to some extent, so sharp distinctions between chronic persistent and chronic active hepatitis, on the one hand, and chronic active hepatitis and postnecrotic cirrhosis, on the other, are not always possible (12). Under such conditions, classification often depends on the result of serial biopsy studies. Moreover, during the course of the disease, transitions from one type of lesion to another may occur, the sequence depending on whether the disease is progressing, or is undergoing spontaneous or treatment-induced remission. In each of the lesions, the intensity of the inflammatory reaction, the extent of hepatocellular necrosis, and the degree of fibrosis may vary with the activity and duration of the disease. A semiquantitative method of assessing these histologic features has been proposed and validated (158).

Occasionally, cholestasis is a prominent feature in chronic hepatitis. Since the clinical and histologic manifestations of such lesions may differ to some extent from those in classic lesions, they often are classified separately as *chronic cholestatic hepatitis.* However, some degree of cholestasis is common in chronic active hepatitis and postnecrotic cirrhosis, so distinctions between cholestatic and noncholestatic lesions cannot be sharply defined.

As previously indicated, all forms of chronic hepatitis may be induced by infections with HBV, HDV, or the NANB hepatitis viruses, by idiosyncratic drug reactions, or by presumed autoimmune mechanisms triggered by unknown etiologic factors. Except for the occurrence of orcein-positive ground glass cells in many cases with persistent HBs antigenemia, the lesions of varied etiology are indistinguishable histologically. When acute viral hepatitis of the classic type fails to resolve within six months, the resulting lesion is almost always chronic persistent hepatitis. In contrast, acute viral hepatitis with bridging necrosis that fails to heal usually gives rise to chronic active hepatitis.

Chronic persistent hepatitis

As a rule, the lesions of chronic persistent hepatitis are characterized by a portal inflammatory reaction with only minimal intralobular inflammation and necrosis. However, during exacerbations of the disease and in cases of *severe* acute hepatitis that fail to resolve, the intralobular changes may be more prominent, giving rise to a lesion that resembles acute viral hepatitis, often classified as *chronic lobular hepatitis* (2,3).

Characteristically, many of the portal tracts are infiltrated with numerous lymphocytes, plasma cells, and macrophages, but only a few are expanded and fibrotic, or show evidence of ductular proliferation, and, invariably, their limiting plates are intact (Figs. 452, 453). Occasionally, as shown in Figure 452, the portal lymphocytes and plasma cells are aggregated in the form of follicles. Almost always, acidophilic bodies, often accompanied by small clusters of swollen Kupffer cells, lymphocytes, or plasma cells, are found scattered through the lobules (Fig. 454). Less commonly, larger foci of proliferating Kupffer cells and infiltrating lymphocytes and plasma cells are encountered in centrilobular zones of hepatocellular dropout (Fig. 455). Usually, the remaining hepatocytes are normal in appearance and arrangement (Figs. 452–455), but in some cases they exhibit mild anisocytosis and anisonucleosis. Moreover, in cases with chronic HBs antigenemia, a variable number of hepatocytes contain orcein-positive ground glass cytoplasmic inclusions (Figs. 136, 138).

During the *active phase* of *chronic persistent hepatitis,* the lesions are characterized by a diffuse inflammatory reaction that involves not only the portal tracts but also the parenchyma, and is accompanied by widely distributed foci of spotty hepatocellular necrosis (Fig. 456). Usually, the portal tracts are more uniformly infiltrated with lymphocytes and plasma cells, often are expanded and fibrotic, contain proliferating ductules and pigmented macrophages, and may show segmental erosion of their limiting plates (Fig. 457). The predominant features of the intralobular lesions, which vary in severity depending on their activity and age, usually include multiple small foci of cell dropout that interrupt and distort the hepatic plate pattern, scattered acidophilic bodies, ballooning of hepatocytes, widespread proliferation and swelling of Kupffer cells, and diffusely distributed lymphocytes and plasma cells (Fig. 458). Hepatocellular regeneration, as evidenced by the presence of thickened hepatic plates, an increased number of binucleate and trinucleate cells, and hepatocellular pleomorphism, is a relatively common feature, and, occasionally, a few rosettes and pseudoducts may be seen. In some cases, bile thrombi are found within canaliculi or Kupffer cells. As a rule, the foci of hepatocellular necrosis are small and randomly distributed. However, as in the case of acute viral hepatitis, they may be significantly larger in the centrilobular zones.

When the limiting plates are eroded in chronic persistent hepatitis, differentiation from chronic active hepatitis may be difficult (159). The features that favor chronic persistent hepatitis include the segmental character of the limiting plate erosion, the minimal extension of fibrous tissue from the portal tracts into the lobules, the paucity of periportal rosettes and proliferating ductules, and the absence of bridging fibrosis or necrosis. However, in some cases, differentiation is not possible on the basis of a single biopsy specimen, so serial biopsy studies may be required to establish the character and prognosis of the lesions. Moreover, because the distinctive features of the lesions in both forms of chronic hepatitis often are not uniformly distributed, relatively large needle biopsies are needed to avoid errors in interpretation due to inadequate sampling. They should be at least 1 cm in length, and 2 to 3 cm are ideal.

Some authorities believe that in chronic persistent hepatitis there is no necrosis of periportal hepatocytes, by definition (160), and that the presence of any "piecemeal" necrosis indicates that the lesion is chronic active hepatitis (161).

Distinguishing between the lesions of classic acute viral hepatitis and those of chronic persistent hepatitis during exacerbations may pose an equally difficult problem. The presence of orcein-positive ground glass cells clearly establishes the chronicity of the lesions. In the absence of this marker, other histologic features that point to chronicity include prominence of plasma cells in the portal exudates, and the presence of significant portal fibrosis. However, these findings are variable, and, therefore, these criteria are not always reliable. Often, differentiation must depend on the clinical history to determine the duration of the disease.

As a rule, the lesions of chronic persistent hepatitis show little tendency to progress to chronic active hepatitis or cirrhosis, even when they remain active or undergo repeated relapses over a period of years. Moreover, they are often asymptomatic, and, occasionally, regress spontaneously. However, progression to chronic active hepatitis has been reported (2,162), a sequence said to occur most frequently in lesions of insidious onset that are accompanied by persistent HBs antigenemia. Conversion from chronic persistent to chronic active hepatitis and vice versa may occur (161), but the nonspecificity of the lesions and sampling error make differentiation difficult.

Chronic active hepatitis

By far the most distinctive feature of the lesions in chronic active hepatitis, in contrast to those in chronic persistent hepatitis, is its tendency to progress, leading to the development of cirrhosis or hepatic failure. This is particularly true of patients with delta superinfection or patients with chronic HBV hepatitis (163). Although usually accompanied by clinical manifestations of acute or chronic liver disease, some lesions are asymptomatic and show no tendency to progress.

The lesions of chronic active hepatitis are characterized by lymphocytic and plasma cell infiltration, expansion, and fibrosis of the portal tracts with destruction of periportal hepatocytes and extension of portal inflammatory cells and fibrous tissue into the lobules. As a rule, the portal tracts are larger and more fibrotic, contain more numerous inflammatory cells and proliferating ductules, and show more complete erosion of their limiting plates than in the active phase of chronic persistent hepatitis. During periods of remission, the lesions of chronic active hepatitis may be indistinguishable from those of chronic persistent hepatitis. The lobular architecture may be distorted by portal-portal bridging fibrosis or zones of bridging necrosis, features never seen in chronic persistent hepatitis. The cirrhosis that develops from chronic active hepatitis may be micronodular or macronodular. The nodules that are created by the necrotic process may increase in size by regenerative activity. The regenerative nodules may sometimes simulate pseudotumors of the liver by various imaging techniques (164).

Almost always, the lobules in chronic active hepatitis contain foci of hepatocellular necrosis and inflammatory cells that vary in size, number, and distribution depending on the activity of the disease and its mode of onset. In minimally active lesions, as in the case of some healthy HBsAg carriers, the intralobular changes may be trivial. However, during exacerbations of the disease and, in cases attributable to antecedent acute hepatitis with bridging necrosis, intralobular inflammation and necrosis often are prominent features.

Piecemeal necrosis is usually defined as the entrapment or destruction of hepatocytes of the limiting plates of the portal tracts within the expanding portal inflammation and fibrosis. It is accompanied by a predominantly lymphocytic and plasma cell infiltrate that is generally regarded as the key feature in the pathogenesis of chronic active hepatitis (165), and has been interpreted as evidence of an underlying immune process (166). It is generally agreed that the presence of periportal piecemeal necrosis in acute hepatitis accurately predicts the progress of the lesion to chronic hepatitis (167). Furthermore, its persistence thereafter is considered a reliable sign that it will be responsive to immunosuppressive therapy (168,169). The presence of acidophilic bodies (170) and the intimate relationship of the infiltrating lymphocytes to the hepatocytes along the margins of necrosis (171) have been emphasized as markers of a cell-mediated immune response. Moreover, while slowly progressive unicellular loss of hepatocytes characteristic of piecemeal necrosis may account for the destruction of the periportal parenchyma in many cases of chronic active hepatitis, some lesions exhibit zones of bridging or multilobular necrosis that appear to evolve by rapid cytolysis of contiguous hepatocytes. Usually, necrosis of this type is attributable to antecedent acute hepatitis that fails to resolve. However, rarely, bridging or multilobular necrosis may be a late development in exacerbations of chronic active hepatitis (9). Early in the course of chronic active hepatitis, zones of bridging or multilobular necrosis may be indistinguishable from those in acute hepatitis. However, as the lesions mature, the reticulin fibers and sinusoids tend to collapse, forming septa made up of loosely arranged bundles of thick fibers that often contain only a modest number of inflammatory cells. Ultimately, the septa may undergo collagenization, but there is suggestive evidence that some may disappear, or become less conspicuous if the disease becomes inactive.

Progressive fibrosis leading to distortion of the lobular architecture and the development of *cirrhosis* may be the sequela of slowly advancing piecemeal necrosis or acute bridging necrosis. Judging from the findings in cases studied serially from the onset of disease, bridging appears to be more important than piecemeal necrosis, both prognostically and pathogenetically, in the development of cirrhosis (9,40). However, in many cases studied for the first time late in the course of the disease, the lesions are characterized by piecemeal necrosis and portal-portal bridging fibrosis. In such cases, it is generally assumed that the bridging fibrosis is the sequela of piecemeal necrosis (158). However, in the absence of biopsy documentation of the early lesions, the possibility of antecedent bridging necrosis can never be excluded.

The view that bridging necrosis may be more important than piecemeal necrosis in the pathogenesis of cirrhosis in chronic active hepatitis is not shared by all authorities (165). However, since these pathologists classify portal-portal bridging necrosis as a form of piecemeal necrosis, their contention that piecemeal necrosis is the key factor in the pathogenesis of cirrhosis is not necessarily contradictory. Nevertheless, their concept that portal-portal bridging necrosis is a form of piecemeal necrosis is open to question, since the pathogenesis and prognostic significance of these two types of necrosis differ. Thus, bridging necrosis is characterized by the rapid, simultaneous cytolysis of numerous contiguous hepatocytes, which when healing is delayed, may lead to the development of cirrhosis. In contrast, the principal feature of piecemeal necrosis, implied in its definition, is the gradual, unicellular destruction of periportal hepatocytes, which, in our experience and that of others (5), seldom progresses to cirrhosis unless it is accompanied by bridging necrosis. Chronic active hepatitis without cirrhosis or bridging hepatic necrosis is a relatively benign disease, but in the presence of bridging necrosis, especially central-portal bridging, it has a much worse prognosis (172-173).

Portal hypertension, as documented by an increased occluded hepatic venous pressure gradient, often appears before histologically detectable cirrhosis has developed (174). The hypertension seems primarily related to an increase in hepatocyte size that is often associated with increased collagen deposition in the space of Disse. These phenomena, which are accompanied by other histologic indices of hepatic injury, also are seen in chronic alcohol-induced liver injury (175).

The histologic pattern of *HBV chronic active hepatitis* evolves as the disease runs its course. Then HBeAg is present in the serum, the histologic pattern tends to that of chronic persistent hepatitis or of mild chronic active hepatitis. As anti-HBe appears, lobular necrosis abruptly increases (176). When viral replication decreases, an event often associated with the loss of HBsAg from the serum, the inflammation and periportal necrosis subside and the picture may resemble that of chronic persistent hepatitis (177).

Illustrated in Figure 459 are the typical features of *early chronic active hepatitis*. In such lesions, the portal tracts are enlarged and fibrotic, contain numerous lymphocytes and plasma cells, occasionally aggregated in the form of follicles, and show erosion of their limiting plates. However, there is no evidence of bridging fibrosis or necrosis, so the overall lobular architecture is not distorted. As can be seen at higher magnification in Figure 460, this portal tract shows significant periportal piecemeal necrosis, as evidenced by the erosion of its limiting plate and the extension of inflammatory cells and fine fibrous strands into the surrounding parenchyma. Often, as shown in Figure 226, the infiltrating lymphocytes and plasma cells in the advancing edge of piecemeal necrosis lie in intimate contact with hepatocytes. At this early stage, ductular proliferation is only minimal or absent. Almost always, the parenchyma contains small scattered collections of lymphocytes, plasma cells and swollen Kupffer cells, and minute foci of cell dropout that occasionally are accompanied by a few acidophilic bodies, particularly in the periportal zones (Fig. 292). As a rule, the remaining hepatocytes appear normal, but often show a thickened plate pattern and some degree of pleomorphism. In cases with persistent HBs antigenemia, some of the hepatocytes contain orcein-positive cytoplasmic inclusions or ground glass cytoplasmic inclusions (Fig. 292).

In the absence of bridging fibrosis or necrosis, the lesions of early chronic active hepatitis rarely progress to cirrhosis or hepatic failure. Similar lesions may be seen in alcoholic liver injury (178). Furthermore, fatty infiltration may be a manifestation of chronic active hepatitis (179).

The lesions of more *advanced chronic active hepatitis* exhibit the same features as those just described, but portal and intralobular fibrosis, piecemeal necrosis, ductular proliferation, and hepatocellular regeneration are more extensive, and are almost always accompanied by bridging fibrosis. Such lesions may develop insidiously, or may present as the sequelae of antecedent acute hepatitis with bridging necrosis.

Figure 461 illustrates an example of *advanced chronic active hepatitis* encountered in a patient 15 months following an attack of HBsAg-positive acute hepatitis with bridging necrosis that failed to resolve. The diffuse intralobular portal and bridging fibrosis with distortion of the lobular architecture are clearly evident at this low magnification. At higher magnification (Fig. 106), it can be seen that the periportal hepatocytes are arranged in the form of rosettes encircled by fine bands of collagen and infiltrating lymphocytes and plasma cells, indicative of active piecemeal necrosis. Although not prominent in this case, ductular proliferation (Fig. 462), two-cell-thick hepatic plates indicative of regeneration (Fig. 463), foci of pleomorphic and ballooned hepatocytes (Fig. 464), canalicular bile thrombi, and scattered acidophilic bodies, inflammatory cells, and swollen Kupffer cells are relatively common features in chronic active hepatitis. Occasionally, a few of the interlobular ducts in such cases exhibit vacuolization, stratification, focal necrosis, and lymphocytic infiltration of their epithelial lining cells (Fig. 465). Although the bile ductal lesion illustrated in Figure 465 was encountered in a patient with HBs antigenemia, such lesions are said to occur more commonly in NANB or nonviral forms of chronic active hepatitis (180). Another feature seen occasionally in chronic active hepatitis is the presence within the portal tracts of entrapped hepatocytes that often show degenerative changes (Fig. 466). They undoubtedly represent cells that have escaped destruction during antecedent active piecemeal necrosis, and may persist as the only evidence of such necrosis when the lesions no longer are active, and the limiting plates appear to be intact.

It is noteworthy that the fibrosis found in the late lesion illustrated in Figure 461 was significantly more extensive than the zones of bridging necrosis found in the initial biopsy section obtained early in the course of the disease, clearly demonstrating the progressive nature of the lesion, and suggesting that continuing piecemeal necrosis probably played a more important role than bridging necrosis in the pathogenesis of the progressive fibrosis in this particular case. Sampling error could have contributed to this discrepancy.

However, in many cases of severe chronic active hepatitis

attributable to unresolved antecedent acute hepatitis, zones of bridging necrosis can still be identified late in the course of the disease, and appear to be the principal factor responsible for progressive fibrosis. An example of such *chronic active hepatitis with bridging necrosis* is illustrated in Figure 302. As can be seen, this lesion, encountered in a patient who was still deeply jaundiced and chronically ill seven months following the abrupt onset of typical acute viral hepatitis, shows extensive portal-portal and portal-central zones of cell dropout and collapse. At higher magnification (Fig. 303), it is evident that the bridged zones contain collapsed reticulin fibers in which are enmeshed and compressed sinusoids, a few lymphocytes, and occasional degenerating hepatocytes. The adjacent surviving parenchyma shows a diffuse inflammatory reaction, swelling and proliferation of Kupffer cells, occasional acidophilic bodies, and an irregular, thickened, and interrupted hepatic plate pattern. However, elsewhere in the same section (Fig. 301), some of the portal tracts are enlarged and fibrotic, but unbridged, and contained numerous lymphocytes, plasma cells, and proliferating ductules, and show erosion of their limiting plates with extension of inflammatory cells and fibrous tissue into the periportal parenchyma. These findings suggest that piecemeal necrosis may have played a contributory role in the pathogenesis of the fibrosis in this case.

As previously indicated, in many cases of advanced chronic active hepatitis seen for the first time late in the course of the disease, the lesions show both piecemeal necrosis and portal-portal bridging fibrosis. In cases with an insidious onset, it is impossible to determine whether the fibrous bridges are attributable to progressive piecemeal necrosis or to antecedent bridging necrosis. However, antecedent bridging necrosis may be suspected in patients whose illness starts abruptly and is severe. An example of advanced *chronic active hepatitis with piecemeal necrosis and portal-portal bridging fibrosis* is illustrated in Figure 467. Although not documented, antecedent bridging necrosis was suspected, since the lesion was encountered in a heroin addict who had had an abrupt onset of acute severe HBsAg-positive hepatitis six months previously that had failed to resolve.

Chronic active hepatitis with postnecrotic cirrhosis

All etiologic types of chronic active hepatitis may give rise to postnecrotic cirrhosis. The evolution of such lesions is characterized by progressive hepatocellular necrosis and advancing fibrosis that ultimately lead to the destruction of the normal lobular architecture, and its replacement by nodules of regenerating parenchyma separated by bands of connective tissue. Such cases of cirrhosis may be the consequence of acute hepatitis with bridging or submassive hepatic necrosis that fails to resolve, but more frequently is attributable to slowly progressive chronic active hepatitis of insidious onset. However, progression to cirrhosis is not an invariable outcome of such lesions, and, in cases of chronic active hepatitis without bridging necrosis, the development of cirrhosis is relatively rare. The propensity to develop cirrhosis is related to the severity of bridging necrosis and microinflammatory lobular changes (181).

Although patients with chronic active hepatitis of insidious onset usually exhibit clinical manifestations of liver disease before the development of cirrhosis, some remain asymptomatic until the cirrhosis gives rise to overt signs of hepatic decompensation or results in hemorrhage from esophageal varices. Others may never develop symptons.

The severity of the clinical and biochemical manifestations of hepatic dysfunction, and the potential for progression in chronic active hepatitis correlate with the activity of the necroinflammatory lesions, as judged from the extent of hepatocellular degeneration and necrosis, and the intensity of the intraparenchymal inflammatory reaction. Although the intensity of the inflammatory reaction in the fibrous septa and portal tracts usually parallels the activity of the lesions, portal and septal inflammation in the absence of parenchymal necrosis and inflammation have no clinical or prognostic significance.

Most of the parenchymal nodules in postnecrotic cirrhosis are larger than normal lobules (1 mm), so usually the lesions are classified as macronodular or mixed micro/macronodular. However, if 3 mm is taken as the minimum diameter of a macronodule (182), many of the lesions, particularly those in needle biopsy sections, would qualify as micronodular. By contrast, the nodules in alcoholic cirrhosis are usually less than 1 mm in diameter, although the size of the nodules tends to increase with the duration of the disease (183).

Figure 450 illustrates the macronodular character of the cirrhosis in a patient with HBsAg-positive chronic active hepatitis who died of hepatic failure nine years following the onset of acute hepatitis with bridging necrosis that was refractory to corticosteroid therapy. At autopsy, almost all of the nodules exceeded 3 mm in diameter, but none was as large as those often found following submassive hepatic necrosis. The nodules in cases of the latter type may measure up to 5 cm in diameter, often appear lobulated owing to indentations of fibrous septa that penetrate the parenchyma to a variable depth, may contain numerous central veins and portal tracts that suggest a multilobular origin, and are separated by broad zones of collapsed reticulin and collagen. Figure 468 illustrates the edge of such a large nodule bordered by a zone of fibrosis in a patient with chronic active hepatitis and postnecrotic cirrhosis three months after the acute onset of submassive hepatic necrosis. At autopsy, the liver was small and grossly distorted by dense, depressed scars, ranging in width from a few millimeters to 6 cm, which separated coarse, regenerating nodules of parenchyma that varied from 0.5 to 5 cm in diameter.

Considering that the width of needle biopsy sections rarely exceeds 1.6 mm, it is not surprising that the largest nodules completely encircled by fibrous tissue found in such sections barely qualify as macronodules, even if 1 mm, the diameter of a normal lobule, is used as the criterion for distinguishing between micronodules and macronodules. However, if 3 mm is used, as recommended (182), none of the nodules seen can qualify as macronodules. This is illustrated in Figure 57, which shows a group of nodules ranging from 0.8 to 1.6 mm in diameter, in a case of HBsAg-positive chronic active hepatitis and macronodular cirrhosis. However, midline or tangential sections through nodules often provide more convincing evidence of their macronodular character. Thus, as shown in Figure 59, a section through the center of a macronodule may present as a long ribbon of apparently normal parenchyma, bordered at each end by a fibrous band, or, as in this case, by the nodules illustrated in Figure 57. Although such tissue may appear to be made up of multiple normal lobules, it is apparent on closer inspection, even at the low magnification of Figure 59, that many of the hepatic plates are more than one-cell thick, and that the central veins are more numerous than normal and show an abnormal relationship to the single portal tract in the field, features more consistent with a large, regenerating nodule than a group of intact lobules.

Tangential sections are more common than midline sections through macronodules in needle biopsy sections. In such sections the nodules present as large, hemispheric or semilunar islands of regenerating hepatocytes partially outlined by long, curvilinear or scalloped fibrous septa (Fig. 58).

Although cirrhotic nodules are generally regarded as masses of regenerating hepatocytes, some may represent islands of parenchyma that have escaped destruction. Certainly, groups of intact lobules may be found in the early stages of any type of cirrhosis. However, the absence of a thickened hepatic plate pattern in a nodule does not necessarily imply that it is a remnant of intact parenchyma, since late in the course of inactive cirrhosis, the hepatic plate pattern in regenerated nodules may revert to normal.

The *fibrous septa* in chronic active hepatitis with postnecrotic cirrhosis vary greatly in width, ranging from slender (Fig. 449) to relatively thick (Fig. 57) or broad (Fig. 468). Although they tend to broaden with advancing age and activity of the lesions, the broadest septa are seen in the type of cirrhosis that follows healing of submassive hepatic necrosis, irrespective of its age or activity. In the late inactive cirrhotic phase, the septa are densely collagenized, contain only a few inflammatory cells and proliferating bile ductules, and are smooth-contoured, except for spurs that project into parenchyma (Figs. 52–54, 449). In active lesions, the septa are irregular in contour and less sharply defined, owing to erosion of their limiting plates and infiltration of inflammatory cells, and often appear less densely collagenized because of separation of their collagen bundles by infiltrating lymphocytes and plasma cells (Fig. 450). Occasionally, bile ductular proliferation is a prominent feature in such lesions (Fig. 462), but tends to regress as the fibrosis advances.

As in chronic active hepatitis, occasional degenerating interlobular ducts (Fig. 465) and lymph follicles (Fig. 304) may be found in the septa of active postnecrotic cirrhosis.

Hepatic cell dysplasia may be encountered in cases of posthepatitic cirrhosis. Such lesions, which are characterized by enlargement of the hepatocytes, nuclear pleomorphism, hyperchromatism, and multinucleation of contiguous hepatocytes (Figs. 195, 196), occur frequently in HBsAg-positive cases. Since their presence may correlate with the development of hepatocellular carcinoma, they are regarded by some as precancerous lesions (184). More recent analysis both confirm and deny the association of hepatic cell dysplasia and hepatocellular carcinoma (185–187). Recent studies indicate that hepatocellular dysplasia occurs with NANB chronic active hepatitis as well as with HBV chronic active hepatitis (188), both of which may be associated with hepatocellular carcinoma.

Aggregates of *oncocytic (oxyphilic) hepatocytes,* usually located adjacent to portal tracts or fibrous septa, are a relatively common finding in chronic active hepatitis and postnecrotic cirrhosis, particularly in HBsAg-positive cases (189). However, they may also occur in almost any other type of chronic liver disease. Characteristically, the cytoplasm of these oncocytes is distended with innumerable mitochondria that present as fine, closely packed, cytoplasmic granules that appear reddish in routine H & E sections (Fig. 124) and deep blue in PTAH-stained sections (Fig. 125).

The histologic criteria used in assessing the *activity* of the lesions in postnecrotic cirrhosis are identical with those in precirrhotic chronic active hepatitis. In *active postnecrotic cirrhosis,* the margins of the parenchymal nodules, are irregular where they come in contact with portal tracts and septa owing to erosion of the limiting plates with extension of portal inflammatory cells and fibrous tissue into the parenchyma. In mildly active lesions, such piecemeal necrosis may be segmental in distribution (Fig. 57), whereas in those that are highly active it usually involves the periphery of all nodules and extends more deeply into the parenchyma (Fig. 450). Often in active lesions, the hepatocytes at the periphery of the nodules are arranged in the form of rosettes encircled by fine bands of collagen and infiltrating lymphocytes (Figs. 106, 226), and, occasionally, acidophilic bodies are found in the margins of piecemeal necrosis (Fig. 292). Deeper in the nodules, the hepatic plates usually are thickened and irregular in contour, and may show small foci of cell dropout, clusters of lymphocytes, plasma cells, and proliferating swollen Kupffer cells (Fig. 458), or ballooning and pleomorphism of hepatocytes (Fig. 464). Proliferation of bile ductules may be a prominent feature in some cases.

In *inactive postnecrotic cirrhosis,* the contours of the nodules are smooth, and the parenchyma shows no evidence of necrosis, degeneration, or inflammation (Fig. 449). Usually, the septa contain few inflammatory cells or proliferating ductules. However, in some cases, the septa contain numerous lymphocytes, plasma cells, and occasional lymph follicles despite the absence of parenchymal inflammation and necrosis. Although the hepatic plate pattern may be thickened and irregular, it may appear perfectly normal, except for the absence of a normal complement of central veins and portal triads (Fig. 52).

Cholestatic chronic active hepatitis

Drug-induced reactions occasionally give rise to *chronic cholestatic hepatitis.* Initially, the lesions are characterized by cholestasis, expansion and fibrosis of the portal tracts, infiltration of the portal tracts by a variable number of lymphocytes, neutrophils, and eosinophils, ductular proliferation, and erosion of the limiting plates. Although they may remain active following prompt withdrawal of the drug, such lesions do not always progress, as in the case of chlorpromazine-induced chronic cholestasis illustrated in Figure 525. Withdrawal of the offending drug soon after the onset of symptoms in this case was followed by a decrease in jaundice, but pruritus persisted, and the lesions remained active, although they showed no tendency to progress over a period of seven months, despite the development of generalized xanthomatosis.

If administration of the drug involved is not discontinued, the lesions of drug-induced, chronic, cholestatic hepatitis may progress, leading to portal-portal fibrous bridging (Fig. 527), and, ultimately, to a form of portal or biliary cirrhosis (Fig. 528) that often results in hemorrhage from esophageal varices or hepatic failure. The *early,* patchy *cirrhotic lesion* illustrated in Figure 527 was encountered in a patient who presented with mild icterus, severe pruritus, and xanthomas of four years' duration that had appeared following a brief course of chlorpromazine. Because the relationship of the cholestasis to the drug was not recognized, chlorpromazine administration had been continued throughout her illness. The *advanced cirrhosis* with marked cholestasis illustrated in Figure 528 was found in a woman who presented with jaundice, pruritus, and xanthomatosis of five years' duration, which had appeared following a one-week course of chlorpromazine that had been continued for an additional four weeks. Despite withdrawal of the drug at this point, the jaundice failed to abate and signs of slowly progressive biliary cirrhosis appeared. Two years following this biopsy, the patient had a massive hemorrhage from esophageal varices, and shortly thereafter died of hepatic failure.

As a rule, corticosteroid therapy is ineffective in cases of drug-induced chronic cholestatic hepatitis, although, occasionally, it may induce a partial remission.

In occasional cases, the clinical manifestations of chronic active hepatitis include prolonged jaundice, persistent pruritus, high serum levels of alkaline phosphatase and cholesterol, and, less commonly, xanthomatosis (146–149), features that mimic those of primary biliary cirrhosis. However, the two disorders differ both clinically and histologically. In a group of 11 patients with *cholestatic chronic active hepatitis* that we have had the opportunity to investigate, the disease had an abrupt onset with overt jaundice more frequently (5 of 11 cases), and affected males more often (4 of 11 cases) than occurs in typical, primary biliary cirrhosis (unpublished observations). Moreover, in none of the cases was antimitochondrial antibody demonstrable in the serum. However, in other respects, the clinical manifestations resembled those of primary biliary cirrhosis in that pruritus was a prominent feature in 8 of the 11 cases, generalized xanthomatosis occurred in 2, the course was prolonged and progressive in all, and, in none of the 5 treated with corticosteroids was a sustained remission induced. Despite these clinical similarities, the lesions in cholestatic chronic active hepatitis did not resemble those of primary biliary cirrhosis. Except for a paucity of interlobular bile ducts in 3 and prominent cholestasis in all 11 cases, the lesions were indistinguishable from those of classic chronic active hepatitis complicated by postnecrotic cirrhosis. Of particular note is the fact that in none of the cases was degenerating interlobular ducts or portal granulomas found in the lesions. However, others have reported finding such duct lesions in cases of cholestatic chronic active hepatitis (148).

A pseudodiverticular lesion of small bile ducts has been reported in chronic NANB hepatitis (78).

Effects of immunosuppressive therapy on the lesions of chronic hepatitis

Controlled therapeutic trials in patients with *relatively severe* autoimmune chronic active hepatitis have demonstrated that corticosteroids suppress the activity of the lesions, prevent or retard their progression to cirrhosis, and reduce the mortality of the disease (8,9,190,191).

In only one of the reported therapeutic trials of corticosteroids in chronic active hepatitis were serial liver biopsies carried out routinely (8,9). From this study, it is evident that the prognosis and response to therapy are greatly influenced by the histologic character of the lesions, so assessment of the therapeutic efficacy of corticosteroids must depend on a comparison of treated and untreated patients with identical lesions. Thus, in this study, it was found that although corticosteroids reduced the activity and progression of the lesions in most cases, the effects appeared to be most impressive in those with bridging or multilobular necrosis, and that lesions of this type were the most aggressive and least likely to show evidence of spontaneous regression. Thus, in 11 patients with bridging or multilobular necrosis who received no corticosteroids, the lesions progressed to cirrhosis in 7, and showed evidence of spontaneous regression in only 3 (to chronic active hepatitis without bridging necrosis in 2 and to chronic persistent hepatitis in 1). In contrast, similar lesions in 17 corticosteroid-treated patients progressed to cirrhosis in only 4, and regressed in 11 (to chronic active hepatitis without bridging or multilobular necrosis in 3 and to chronic persistent hepatitis in 8). The observed differences between the behavior of treated and untreated lesions unaccompanied by bridging or multilobular necrosis were less impressive, possibly owing to the small number of cases investigated.

It should be kept in mind that these numbers are small and that these trends do not achieve statistical significance. Furthermore, as mentioned earlier, these were nonhomogeneous cases; they were termed "chronic active *liver disease,*" and included patients with viral, drug-induced, and idiopathic origin. In retrospect, it was realized that some patients with primary biliary cirrhosis had been inadvertently included (149). The beneficial effects of corticosteroid therapy were not observed in the patients with primary biliary cirrhosis or in those patients with persistent HBs antigenemia (192) and those who had developed cirrhosis by the time therapy started (193). By exclusion it has been concluded that autoimmune chronic active hepatitis in the precirrhotic stage is responsive to adrenocorticosteroid therapy (10).

Based on our experience and that reported by others (8,9,172,173), lesions of chronic active hepatitis characterized by portal fibrosis and piecemeal necrosis that are unaccompanied by bridging fibrosis or necrosis rarely progress to cirrhosis or lead to hepatic failure. Moreover, such lesions may be asymptomatic, particularly in the case of presumably healthy HBsAg carriers.

In some studies (192–195) but not in others (196), the lesions of *HBsAg-positive chronic active hepatitis* have appeared to be less responsive to corticosteroids than those in HBsAg-negative cases (192). A "histological activities index" that employs semiquantitative grading of (1) piecemeal necrosis, (2) lobular necrosis, (3) portal inflammation, and (4) portal fibrosis has been reported to be useful in predicting responsiveness to steroid therapy (63). Those patients with multilobular necrosis, which correlates closely with persistent hyperbilirubinemia, appear to have the worst prognosis (197).

Azathioprine, perhaps by reducing the dose of corticosteroids required for the control of autoimmune chronic active hepatitis, may be a useful adjuvant in therapy (8), but is ineffective when used alone (8,191,192). Cyclosporine has been shown to be beneficial in autoimmune chronic active hepatitis in one study (198).

Combination therapy with corticosteroid and other immunosuppressive or antiviral agents, including azathiaprine (199), adenosine arabinoside, acyclovir (200), interferon, and interleukins has been tried on patients with chronic HBV hepatitis. Among the most promising are those in which long-term interferon therapy had been administered after steroid withdrawal (201) had induced enhanced cellular immune responses (202). Impressive clinical improvement which has been documented by the loss of HBV DNA, HBeAg, and HBsAg, and improvement in laboratory tests and in "hepatic histology" has been reported." In one such study, portal zone lesions, lobular inflammation, and the progression to cirrhosis decreased (P.J. Scheuer, unpublished observations).

α-Interferon has now been shown to be effective in chronic viral hepatitis (203). Randomized clinical trials in patients with chronic HBV hepatitis have shown that 3 million units three times per week induces remission in 15 to 25% of patients (204–206), characterized by normalization of transaminase activity, and reduction of portal and lobular inflammation and necrosis. A smaller percentage lose their HBsAg, HBeAg, HBV DNA, and later become anti-HBs-positive. Those who lose HBV DNA and HBeAg from their serum no longer show evidence of active HBV replication (207). The most responsive patients are those with greatly elevated transaminase activity and low levels of HBV DNA, especially women. Cirrhotic patients (208) and those who acquired the infection in infancy (209) appear to be less responsive.

In chronic HDV hepatitis treatment has been less impressive (210), although in one study larger doses of interferon (5–10 million units three times per week) have induced clinical and laboratory improvement (211).

In chronic HCV hepatitis, interferon has caused biochemical and histologic remission (Figs. 546–551) in about half the patients treated with smaller doses (1–2 million units three times per week) (212,213).

Thymosin (fraction 5), which is considered a modifier of immune responses, has been shown to be effective in a small randomized trial in chronic HBV hepatitis (214). Its use has been followed by reduction in transaminase levels, cleared HBsAg and HBV DNA from the serum, and reduction in portal inflammation (Figs. 552–555).

Prolonged immunosuppressive therapy after transplantation (215) or for autoimmune disorders (216) has been associated with the development of neoplasia (217). Conceivably, the hepatic dysplasia and hepatocellular carcinoma reported in some instances of chronic liver disease (187) may be associated with immunosuppressive therapy as well as with the underlying liver disease.

Histologic differential diagnosis of chronic hepatitis

Chronic persistent hepatitis

The histologic features of the lesions of chronic persistent hepatitis that differentiate them from those of chronic active hepatitis include the absence of piecemeal necrosis and of bridging fibrosis or necrosis.

Nonspecific reactive hepatitis, an ill-defined lesion characterized by variable combinations of portal fibrosis and inflammation, ductular proliferation, focal hepatocellular necrosis, hepatocellular regeneration, and focal collections of swollen Kupffer cells, may be encountered in a wide variety of extrahepatic systemic and infectious disorders (218) or in association with chronic inflammatory disease in the biliary tract, pancreas, or bowel (219). When portal tract changes are prominent, such lesions are indistinguishable from those of chronic persistent hepatitis.

Chronic active hepatitis

During the more active phases of chronic active hepatitis, when intralobular inflammation and necrosis are prominent features, the lesions may be difficult to differentiate from those of *acute hepatitis*. However, as a rule, such lesions show more impressive portal fibrosis, erosion of the limiting plates, and plasma cell infiltration, and may contain lymph follicles, occasional degenerating interlobular ducts, and, in HBsAg-positive cases, orcein-positive ground glass cells.

The concurrence of chronic alcoholism and HBV infection may complicate the diagnosis of either disorder, and results in more severe liver disease and earlier development of cirrhosis than with either disease alone (220).

The lesions of *primary biliary cirrhosis* (Chapter 11) may closely resemble those of chronic active hepatitis (Fig. 296). However, usually, they exhibit a number of distinctive features that make differentiation possible: (1) piecemeal necrosis is an inconstant finding, and, when present, tends to be segmental, and only occasionally involves multiple portal tracts (Fig. 295); (2) degeneration, necrosis, and inflammation of the epithelial lining cells, and disruption of the basement membranes of medium sized interlobular and septal ducts are found more frequently and tend to be more severe than in chronic active hepatitis (Fig. 364–368); (3) the number of bile ducts is reduced; (4) epithelioid granulomas in the portal tracts, especially adjacent to degenerating bile ducts (Figs. 295, 342), are relatively common; occasionally, similar granulomas are found within the lobules (Fig. 343); (5) often, in more advanced lesions, the periportal hepatocytes are ballooned (Fig. 109) and may contain Mallory bodies (Fig. 556); (6) bile thrombi may be found in periportal canaliculi before they appear in the centrilobular zones (Fig. 557); and (7) when present, bile ductular proliferation is very extensive. Despite these differential clues, experienced pathologists reading such sections blindly are not always able to differentiate chronic active hepatitis from primary biliary cirrhosis as shown by the erroneous inclusion of 6 patients with primary biliary cirrhosis among the 64 studied in the Mayo Clinic randomized clinical trial of chronic active hepatitis (8,9,192).

Occasionally, the hepatic lesions of *primary sclerosing cholangitis* (Chapter 24) resemble those of chronic active hepatitis (221–223). Figure 558 illustrates a lesion of this type in a young woman who presented with malaise, mild jaundice and pruritus, hepatosplenomegaly, and elevated levels of serum alkaline phosphatase, transaminase, gamma globulin, and cholesterol. Test for HBsAg and for antimitochondrial and smooth muscle antibodies yielded negative results. Although the histologic findings appeared to be typical of chronic active hepatitis, endoscopic retrograde cholangiography, carried out because corticosteroids failed to suppress the activity of the disease, revealed the classic features of primary sclerosing cholangitis. In more typical cases of primary sclerosing cholangitis, the hepatic lesions usually are characterized by features suggestive of extrahepatic biliary obstruction, such as cholestasis (Fig. 559), and portal fibrosis, ductular proliferation, and neutrophilic infiltration (Fig. 560), plus what are generally considered to be the more distinctive features of primary sclerosing cholangitis, namely, concentric periductal fibrosis (Fig. 380) and deposition of copper-containing granules in the cytoplasm of periportal hepatocytes (Fig. 561). Unfortunately, periductal fibrosis and copper deposits are not found in all cases, and are not pathognomonic, so that in the last analysis, identification of primary sclerosing cholangitis depends on the cholangiographic findings.

As illustrated in Figure 562, the *active* hepatic lesions of *Wilson's disease,* usually encountered in children and adolescent patients, may closely resemble those of chronic active hepatitis. However, such lesions usually exhibit a variable number of distinctive features, including periportal, hepatocellular, copper-containing granules (Fig. 163), orcein-positive copper/protein granules (Fig. 164), coarse D-PAS-positive lipofuscin granules (Fig. 156), numerous glycogen nuclei (Fig. 156), and Mallory bodies (Fig. 563) and foci of hepatocellular fatty infiltration (Fig. 564). Although these features are characteristic of Wilson's disease, they are not pathognomonic; the diagnosis must be confirmed by the demonstration of low serum levels of ceruloplasmin and high concentrations of copper in the urine and liver (Chapter 13).

References

1. Scheuer PJ: Changing views on chronic hepatitis. Histopathology *10:*1–4, 1986.
2. Aldershvile J, Dietrichson O, Skinhoj P, Kryger P, Mathiesen LR, Christoffersen P, Nielsen JO, and the Copenhagen Hepatitis Acuta Programme. Chronic persistent hepatitis: serological classification and meaning of the hepatitis B e system. Hepatology *2:*243–246, 1982.
3. Klatskin G: Persistent HB antigenemia: associated clinical manifestations and hepatic lesions. Am J Med Sci *270:*33–40, 1975.
4. Scheuer PJ, Maggi G: Hepatic fibrosis and collapse: histological distinction by orcein staining. Histopathology *4:*487–490, 1980.
5. Popper H, Schaffner F: The vocabulary of chronic hepatitis. N Engl J Med *284:*1154–1156, 1971.
6. Wilkinson SP, Portmann B, Cochrane AMG, Tee DEH, Williams R: Clinical course of chronic lobular hepatitis. Report of five cases. Q J Med *47:*421–429, 1978.
7. Liaw Y-F, Chu C-M, Chen T-J, Lin D-Y, Chang-Chien C-S, Wu C-S: Chronic lobular hepatitis: a clinicopathological and prognostic study. Hepatology *2:*258–262, 1982.
8. Soloway RD, Summerskill WHJ, Baggenstoss AH, Geall MG, Gitnick GL, Elveback LR, Schoenfield LJ: Clinical, biochemical, and histological remission of severe chronic active liver disease: a controlled study of treatments and early prognosis. Gastroenterology *63:*820–833, 1972.
9. Baggenstoss AH, Soloway RD, Summerskill WHJ, Elveback LR, Schoenfield LJ: Chronic active liver disease. The range of histologic lesions, their response to treatment, and evolution. Hum Pathol *3:*183–198, 1972.
10. Kirk AP, Jain S, Pocock S: Late results of Royal Free Hospital controlled trial of prednisolone therapy in hepatitis B surface antigen-negative chronic active hepatitis. Gut *21:*78–93, 1980.
11. Knodell RG, Ishak KG, Black WC, Chen TS, Craig R, Kaplowitz N, Kiernan TW, Wollman J: Formulation and application of a numerical scoring system for assessing histological activity in asymptomatic chronic active hepatitis. Hepatology *1:*431–435, 1981.
12. Scheuer PJ: Changing views on chronic hepatitis. Histopathology *10:*1–6, 1986.
13. Cooksley WGE, Bradbear RA, Robinson W, Harrison M, Halliday JW, Powell LW, Han-Seung Ng, Chen-Siang S, Okuda K, Scheuer PJ, Sherlock S: The prognosis of chronic active hepatitis without cirrhosis in relation to bridging necrosis. Hepatology *6:*345–348, 1986.
14. Combes, B: The initial morphologic lesion in chronic hepatitis, important or unimportant? Hepatology *6:*518–522, 1986.
15. Soloway RD, Baggenstoss AH, Schoenfield LJ, Summerskill WHJ: Observer error and sampling variability tested in evaluation of hepatitis and cirrhosis by liver biopsy. Am J Dig Dis *16:*1082–1086, 1971.
16. Bradbear RA, Robinson WN, Cooksley WGE, Halliday JW, Harris OD, Powell LW: Are the causes and presentation of chronic hepatitis changing? An analysis of 104 cases over 15 years. Q J Med *53:*279–288, 1984.
17. Mackay IR, Taft LI, Cowling DC: Lupoid hepatitis. Lancet *2:*1323–1326, 1956.
18. Page AR, Good RA: Plasma cell hepatitis. Lab Invest *11:*351–359, 1962.
19. Read AE, Sherlock S, Harrison CV: Active 'juvenile' cirrhosis considered part of a systemic disease and the effect of corticosteroid therapy. Gut *4:*378–393, 1963.
20. Bearn AG, Kunkel HG, Slater RJ: The problem of chronic liver disease in young women. Am J Med *21:*3–15, 1956.
21. Kilby AE, Albertini RJ, Krawitt EL: HLA typing and autoantibodies in hepatitis B surface antigen-negative chronic hepatitis. Tissue Antigens *28:*214–221, 1986.
22. Vergani D, Wells L, Larcher VF: Genetically determined low C4: a predisposing factor to autoimmune chronic active hepatitis. Lancet *2:*294–297, 1985.
23. Manns M, Gerken G, Kyriatsoulis A: Characterization of a new subgroup of autoimmune chronic active hepatitis by autoantibodies against a soluble liver antigen. Lancet *1:*292–294, 1987.
24. Buffet C, Homberg J-C, Pelletier G: Chronic active hepatitis associated with liver-kidney microsomal antibody of an autoimmune type: two familial cases. Dig Dis Sci *31:*1273–1276, 1986.
25. Penner E: Nature of immune complexes in autoimmune chronic active hepatitis B: is a little too much? Gastroenterology *92:*304–308, 1987.
26. Maddrey WC: Subdivisions of idiopathic autoimmune chronic active hepatitis. Hepatology *7:*1372–1374, 1987.
27. Robertson DAF, Zhang SL, Guy EG: Persistent measles virus genome in autoimmune chronic active hepatitis Lancet *2:*9–11, 1987.
28. Mondelli M, Vergani GM, Alberti A, Vergani D, Postmann B, Eddleston ALWF, Williams R: Specificity of T lymphocyte cytotoxicity to autologous hepatocytes in chronic hepatitis B virus infection: evidence that T cells are directed against HBV core antigen expressed on hepatocytes. J Immunol *129:*2773–2778, 1982.
29. Meyer zum Buschenfelde KH, Hutteroth TH, Manns M, Moller B: The role of liver membrane antigens as targets in autoimmune type liver disease. Springer Semin Immunopathol *3:*297–316, 1980.
30. Mieli-Vergani G, Vergani D, Portmann B, White Y, Murray-Lyon I, Marigold JH: Lymphocyte cytotoxicity to autologous hepatocytes in HBsAg positive chronic liver disease. Gut *23:*1029–1036, 1982.
31. Gurian LE, Rogoff TM, Ware AJ: The immunologic diagnosis of chronic active 'auto-immune' hepatitis: distinction from systemic lupus erythematosus. Hepatology *5:*397–402, 1985.
32. Hall S, Czaja AJ, Kaufman DK: How lupoid is lupoid hepatitis? J Rheumatol *13:*95–96, 1986.
33. Omata M, Afroudakis A, Liew CT, Ashcavai M, Peters RL: Comparison of serum hepatitis B surface antigen (HBsAg) and serum anticore with tissue HBsAg and hepatitis B core antigen (HBcAg). Gastroenterology *75:*1003–1009, 1978.
34. Choo Q-L, Kuo G, Weinder AJ, Overby LR, Bradley DW, Houghton M: Isolation of a cDNA clone derived from a blood-borne non-A, non-B viral hepatitis genome. Science *244:*359–362, 1989.
35. Kuo G, Choo Q-L, Alter HJ, Gitnick GL, Redeker AG, Purcell RH, Miyamura T, Dienstag JL, Alter MJ, Stevens CE, Tegtmeier GE, Bonino F, Colombo M, Lee W-S, Kuo C, Berker K, Shuster JR, Overby LR, Bradley DW, Houghton M: An assay for circulating antibodies to a major etiologic virus of human non-A, non-B hepatitis. Science *244:*361–364, 1989.
36. Alter HJ, Purcell RH, Shih JW, Melpolder JC, Houghton M, Cho Q-L, Kuo G: Detection of antibody to hepatitis C virus in prospectively followed transfusion recipients with acute and chronic non-A, non-B hepatitis. N Engl J Med *321:*1494–1500, 1989.
37. Nielsen JO, Dietrichson O, Elling P, Christoffersen P: Incidence and meaning of persistence of Australia antigen in patients with acute viral hepatitis: development of chronic hepatitis. N Engl J Med *285:*1157–1160, 1971.
38. Kamada T, Akeyama T, Koyama T, Abe H: Relation of protraction of acute viral hepatitis to Australia antigen. Acta Hepato-Gastroenterol *21:*358–363, 1974.
39. Lesnicar J, Ferluga D, Lesnicar G: Sequelae of acute viral hepatitis type B. Acta Hepato-Gastroenterol *24:*241–249, 1977.
40. Boyer JL, Klatskin G: Pattern of necrosis in acute viral hepatitis. Prognostic value of bridging (subacute hepatic necrosis). N Engl J Med *283:*1063–1071, 1970.
41. Czaja AJ, Beaver SJ, Wood JR, Klee GG, Go VLW: Frequency and significance of serum *α*-fetoprotein elevation in severe hepatitis B surface antigen-negative chronic active hepatitis. Gastroenterology *93:*687–692, 1987.
42. Lok ASF, Lai C-L: Alpha-fetoprotein monitoring in Chinese patients with chronic hepatitis B virus infection: role in the early detection of hepatocellular carcinoma. Hepatology *9:*110–115, 1989.
43. Bonino F, Rosina F, Rizzetto M, Chiaberge E, Tardanico R, Callea F, Verme G: Chronic hepatitis in HBsAg carriers with serum HBV-DNA and anti-HBe. Gastroenterology *90:*1268–1273, 1986.
44. Hoofnagle JH, Shafritz DA, Popper H: Chronic type B hepatitis and the 'healthy' HBsAg carrier state. Hepatology *7:*758–762, 1987.
45. Vittal SBV, Dourdourekas D, Shobassy N, Gerber M, Telischi M, Szanto PB, Steigmann F, Clowdus BF: Asymptomatic hepatic disease in blood donors with hepatitis B antigenemia. Am J Clin Pathol *62:*649–654, 1974.

46. Villeneuve JP, Richer G, Cote J, Guevin R, Marleau D, Joly JG, Viallet A: Chronic carriers of hepatitis B antigen (HBsAg). Histological, biochemical, and immunological findings in 31 voluntary blood donors. Am J Dig Dis *21*:18–25, 1976.

47. Anderson KE, Sun S-C, Berg HS, Chang N-K: Liver function and histology in asymptomatic Chinese military personnel with hepatitis B antigenemia. Am J Dig Dis *19*:693–703, 1974.

48. Bolin TD, Davis AE, Liddlelow AG: Liver disease and cell-mediated immunity in hepatitis-associated antigen (HAA) carriers. Gut *14*:365–368, 1973.

49. Papadopoulos NM, Traianos GP, Thomakos AP, Tiniakos G: Biochemical findings compared with histologic observations in carriers of hepatitis B carriers. Proc Soc Exp Biol Med *143*:323–325, 1973.

50. Piccinino F, Manzillo G, Sagnelli E, Balestrieri GG, Maio G, Pasquale G, Felaco FM: The significance of the Australia antigen (HBsAg) persistent healthy carrier ''status'': a long-term follow-up study of 34 cases. Acta Hepato-Gastroenterol *25*:171–178, 1978.

51. Reinicke V, Dybkjaer E, Poulsen H, Banke O, Lylloff K, Nordenfelt E: A study of Australia-antigen-positive blood donors and their recipients with special reference to liver histology. N Engl J Med *286*:867–870, 1972.

52. Sampliner R: Chronic active hepatitis in hepatitis B surface antigen (HBsAg) carriers. The need for liver biopsy. JAMA *237*:50–51, 1977.

53. Simon JB, Patel SK: Liver disease in asymptomatic carriers of hepatitis B antigen. Gastroenterology *60*:1020–1028, 1974.

54. Cooksley WGE, Powell LW, Mistilis SP, Mackay IR, Barker LF: Hepatitis B antigen and antibody in active chronic hepatitis and other liver diseases in Australia. A multicenter collaborative study. Am J Dig Dis *20*:110–114, 1975.

55. Chen D-S, Sung J-L: Hepatitis B virus infection on Taiwan. Lancet *2*:668–669, 1977.

56. Skinho JP, Nielsen JO, Dietrichson O: Serologic evidence of hepatitis B infection in patients with chronic liver diseases: radioimmunoassay of HBsAg and anti-HBs. Scand J Gastroenterol *12*:615–619, 1977.

57. Kaneko S, Miller RH, Feinstone SM, Unoura M, Kobayashi K, Hattori N, Purcell RH: Detection of serum hepatitis B virus DNA in patients with chronic hepatitis using the polymerase chain reaction assay. Proc Natl Acad Sci USA *86*:312–316, 1989.

58. Hoofnagle JH, Gerety RJ, Ni LY, Barker LF: Antibody to hepatitis B core antigen. A sensitive indicator of hepatitis B replication. N Engl J Med *290*:1336–1340, 1974.

59. Davis GL, Hoofnagle JH, Waggoner JG: Spontaneous reactivation of chronic hepatitis B virus infection. Gastroenterology *86*:203–207, 1984.

60. Levy P, Marcellin P, Martinot-Peignoux M, Degott C, Nataf J, Benhamou J-P: Clinical course of spontaneous reactivation of hepatitis B virus infection in patients with chronic hepatitis B. Hepatology *12*:570–574, 1990.

61. Rizzetto M, Gerin JL, Purcell RH (eds): The hepatitis delta virus and its infection. *In* Progress in Clinical and Biological Research, Vol. 234, New York, Alan R. Liss, 1987.

62. Hadziyannis SJ: Delta antigen positive chronic liver disease in Greece: clinical aspects and natural course. *In* Viral Hepatitis and Delta Infection, edited by G. Verme, F. Bonino, M. Rizzeto. New York, Alan R. Liss, 1983, pp. 209–218.

63. Moestrup T, Hansson BG, Widell A, Nordenfelt E: Clinical aspects of delta infection. Br Med J *286*:87–90, 1983.

64. Frommel D, Allain JP, Courouce AM, Derose S, Trepo C, Crivelli O, Rizzetto M: Long-lasting abatement of HBsAg synthesis induced by acute delta infection. Lancet *1*:656–657, 1983.

65. Stocklin E, Gudat F, Krey G, Durmuller U, Gasser M, Schmid M: Antigen in hepatitis B: immunohistology of frozen and paraffin-embedded liver biopsies and relation to HBV infection. Hepatology *1*:238–242, 1981.

66. Govindarajan S: Inhibition of HBV replication during co-infection with HBV and HDV: inhibition of the inhibition by co-infection with HIV. Hepatology *11*:703–704, 1990.

67. Colombo M, Cambieri R, Rumi MG, Ronchi G, Del Ninno E, DeFranchis R: Long-term delta superinfection in hepatitis B surface antigen carriers and its relationship to the course of chronic hepatitis. Gastroenterology *85*:235–239, 1983.

68. Sagnelli E, Felaco FM, Filippini P, Pasquale G, Peinetti P, Buonaguiro E, Aprea L, Pulella C, Piccinino F, Giusti G: Influence of HDV infection on clinical, biochemical and histological presentation of HBsAg positive chronic hepatitis. Liver *9*:229–234, 1989.

69. Govindarajan S, De Cock KM, Redeker AG: Natural course of delta superinfection in chronic hepatitis B virus-infected patients: histopathologic study with multiple liver biopsies. Hepatology *6*:640–644, 1986.

70. Raimondo G, Longo G, Squadrito G: Exacerbation of chronic liver disease due to hepatitis B surface antigen after delta infection. Br Med J *286*:845–846, 1983.

71. Berman M, Alter HJ, Ishak KG, Purcell RH, Jones EA: The chronic sequelae of non-A, non-B hepatitis. Ann Intern Med *91*:1–6, 1979.

72. Rakela J, Redeker AG: Chronic liver disease after acute non-A, non-B viral hepatitis. Gastroenterology *72*:1200–1202, 1979.

73. Gimson AES, O'Grady J, Ede RJ, Portmann B, Williams R: Late onset hepatic failure: clinical, serological and histological features. Hepatology 6:288–294, 1986.

74. Thomson BJ, Doran M, Lever AML: α interferon therapy for non-A, non-B hepatitis transmitted by gamma globulin replacement therapy. Lancet *1*:539–541, 1987.

75. Jacyna MR, Brooks MG, Loke RHT, Main J, Murray-Lyon IM, Thomas HC: Randomised controlled trial of interferon alfa (lymphoblastoid interferon) in chronic non-A, non-B hepatitis. Br Med J *298*:80–82, 1989.

76. DiBisceglie AM, Martin P, Kassianides C, Lisker-Melman M, Murray L, Waggoner J, Goodman Z, Banks SM, Hoofnagle JH: Recombinant interferon α therapy for chronic hepatitis C: a randomized, double-blind, placebo-controlled trial. N Engl J Med *321*:1506–1510, 1989.

77. Lefkowitch JH, Apfelbaum TF: Non-A, non-B hepatitis: characterization of liver biopsy pathology. J Clin Gastroenterol *11*:225–232, 1989.

78. Vyberg M: Diverticular bile duct lesion in chronic active hepatitis. Hepatology *10*:774–780, 1989.

79. Cooksley WGE, Cowen AE, Powell LW: The incidence of oxyphenisatin ingestion in active chronic hepatitis: a prospective controlled study of 29 patients. Aust N Z J Med *3*:124–128, 1973.

80. Dietrichson O: Chronic active hepatitis. Aetiological considerations based on clinical and serological studies. Scand J Gastroenterol *10*:617–624, 1975.

81. Goldstein GB, Lam KC, Mistilis SP: Drug-induced chronic hepatitis. Am J Dig Dis *18*:177–184, 1973.

82. Reynolds TB, Peters RL, Yamada S: Chronic active and lupoid hepatitis caused by a laxative, oxyphenisatin. N Engl J Med *285*:813–820, 1971.

83. Lindberg J, Linholm A, Lundin P, Iwarson S: Trigger factors and HL-A antigens in chronic active hepatitis. Br Med J *4*:77–79, 1975.

84. Maddrey WC, Boitnott JK: Severe hepatitis from methyldopa. Gastroenterology *68*:351–360, 1975.

85. Black M, Rabin L, Schatz N: Nitrofurantoin-induced chronic active hepatitis. Ann Intern Med *92*:62–64, 1980.

86. Russell RI, Allan JG, Patrick R: Active chronic hepatitis after chlorpromazine ingestion. Br Med J *1*:655–656, 1973.

87. Maddrey WC, Boitnott JK: Isoniazid hepatitis. Ann Intern Med *79*:1–12, 1973.

88. Tonder M, Norday A, Elgio K: Sulfonamide-induced chronic liver disease. Scand J Gastroenterol *9*:93–96, 1974.

89. Fedotin MS: Liver disease caused by propylthiouracil. Arch Intern Med *135*:319–321, 1975.

90. Benjamin SB, Ishak KG, Zimmerman HJ, Grushka A: Phenylbutazone liver injury: a clinical-pathologic survey of 23 cases and review of the literature. Hepatology *1*:255–263, 1981.

91. Utili R, Boitnott JK, Zimmerman HJ: Dantrolene-associated hepatic injury: incidence and character. Gastroenterology *72*:510–516, 1977.

92. Bonkowsky H, Mudge GH, McMurty RJ: Chronic hepatic inflammation and fibrosis due to low doses of paracetanol. Lancet *1*:1016–1018, 1978.

93. Wright R: Drug-induced chronic hepatitis. Springer Semin Immunopathol *3*:331–338, 1980.

94. Myers JD, Olson RE, Lewis JH, Moran TJ: Xanthomatous biliary cirrhosis following chlorpromazine, with observations indicating overproduction of cholesterol, hyper-prothrombinemia, and the development of portal hypertension. Trans Assoc Am Physicians *70*:243–260, 1957.

95. Walker CO, Combes B: Biliary cirrhosis induced by chlorpromazine. Gastroenterology *51*:631–640, 1966.

96. Ishak KG, Irey NS: Hepatic injury associated with phenothiazines. Clinico-pathologic and follow-up study of 36 patients. Arch Pathol *93*:283–304, 1972.

97. Stolzer BC, Miller C, White WA, Zuckerbrod M: Postarsenical obstructive jaundice complicated by xanthomatosis and diabetes mellitus. Am J Med *9*:124–132, 1950.

98. Gregory DA, Zaki GF, Sarcosi GA, Carey JB Jr: Chronic cholestasis following prolonged tolbutamide administration associated with destructive cholangitis. Arch Pathol *84:*194–201, 1967.

99. Baum H, Berg PA: The complex nature of mitochondrial antibodies and their relation to primary biliary cirrhosis. Semin Liver Dis *1:*309–321, 1981.

100. Gershwin ME, Coppel RL, Mackay IR: Primary biliary cirrhosis and mitochondrial autoantigens: insights from molecular biology. Hepatology *8:*147–151, 1988.

101. Berg PA, Klein R, Lindenborn-Fotinos J: Anti-mitochrondrial antibodies in primary biliary cirrhosis. J Hepatol *2:*123–131, 1986.

102. Maddrey WC: Subdivisions of idiopathic autoimmune chronic active hepatitis. Hepatology *7:*1372–1374, 1987.

103. Mackay IR, Wood IJ: Lupoid hepatitis: a comparison of 22 cases with other types of chronic liver disease. Q J Med *31:*485–507, 1962.

104. Reynolds TB, Edmondson HA, Peters RL, Redeker A: Lupoid hepatitis. Ann Intern Med *61:*650–666, 1964.

105. Krawitt EL, Kilby AE, Albertini RJ, Schanfield MS, Chasteney BF, Harpe PC, Mickey RM, McAuliffe TL: Immunogenetic studies of autoimmune chronic active hepatitis: HLA, immunoglobulin allotypes and autoantibodies. Hepatology *7:*1305–1310, 1987.

105a. Czaja AJ, Rakela J, Hay JE, Moore SB: Clinical and prognostic implications of HLA B8 in corticosteroid-treated severe autoimmune chronic active hepatitis. Gastroenterology *98:*1587–1593, 1990.

106. Doniach D, Roitt IM, Walker JG, Sherlock S: Tissue antibodies in primary biliary cirrhosis, active chronic (lupoid) hepatitis, cryptogenic cirrhosis and other liver diseases and their clinical implications. Clin Exp Immunol *1:*237–262, 1966.

107. Manns M, Gerken G, Kyriatsoulis A: Characterization of a new subgroup of autoimmune chronic active hepatitis by autoantibodies against a soluble liver antigen. Lancet *1:*292–295, 1987.

108. Homberg J-C, Abuaf N, Bernard O, Islam S, Alvarez F, Khalil SH, Poupon R, Darnis F, Levy V-G, Grippon P, Opolon P, Bernuau J, Benhamou J-P, Alagille D: Chronic active hepatitis associated with antiliver-kidney microsome antibody type 1: a second type of "autoimmune" hepatitis. Hepatology *7:*1333–1338, 1987.

109. DeLemos-Chiarandini C, Alvarez F, Bernard O, Homberg JC, Kreibich G: Anti-liver kidney microsome antibody is a marker for the rat hepatocyte endoplasmic reticulum. Hepatology *7:*468–473, 1987.

110. Wood JR, Czaja AJ, Beaver SJ: Frequency and significance of antibody to double-stranded DNA in chronic active hepatitis. Hepatology *6:*976–981, 1986.

111. Berg PA, Baum H: Serology of primary biliary cirrhosis. Springer Semin Immunopathol *3:*355–373, 1980.

112. Gray N, Mackay IR, Taft LI, Weiden S, Wood IJ: Hepatitis, colitis, and lupus manifestations. Am J Dig Dis *3:*481–491, 1958.

113. Croffy B, Kopelman R, Kaplan M: Hypereosinophilic syndrome. Association with chronic active hepatitis. Dig Dis Sci *33:*233–239, 1988.

114. Cowell B, Leonhardt T: Hereditary hyperglobulinemia and lupoid hepatitis. Acta Med Scand *177:*751–759, 1965.

115. Galbraith RM, Smith RM, Mackenzie RM, Tee DE, Doniach D, Williams R: High prevalence of seroimmunologic abnormalities in relatives of patients with active chronic active hepatitis or primary biliary cirrhosis. N Engl J Med *290:*63–69, 1974.

116. Soloway RD, Summerskill WHJ, Baggenstoss AH, Schoenfield LJ: "Lupoid" hepatitis, a nonentity in the spectrum of chronic active liver disease. Gastroenterology *63:*458–465, 1972.

117. Czaja AJ, Hay E, Rakela J: Clinical features and prognostic implications of severe corticosteroid-treated cryptogenic chronic active hepatitis. May. Clin Proc *65:*23–30, 1990.

118. Weiner AJ, Kuo G, Bradley DW, Bonino F, Saracco G, Lee C, Rosenblatt J, Choo Q-L, Houghton M: Detection of hepatitis C viral sequences in non-A, non-B hepatitis. Lancet *335:*1–3, 1990.

119. Routenberg JA, Dienstag JL, Harrison WO: Foodborne outbreak of hepatitis A: clinical and laboratory features of acute and protracted illness. Am J Med Sci *278:*123–137, 1979.

120. Cornu C, Lamy ME, Geubel A, Galanti L: Persistence of immunoglobulin M antibody to hepatitis A virus and relapse of hepatitis A infection. Eur J Clin Microbiol *3:*45–46, 1984.

121. Kao HW, Ashcavai M, Redeker AG: The persistence of hepatitis A IgM antibody after acute clinical hepatitis A. Hepatology *4:*933–936, 1984.

122. Teixeira MR, Weller IVD, Murray A, Bamber M, Thomas HC, Sherlock S, Scheuer PJ: The pathology of hepatitis A in man. Liver *2:*53–60, 1982.

123. McDonald GSA, Courtney MG, Shattock AG, Weir DG: Prolonged

124. Meier E, Richte K, Fruhmorgen P: Vorubergehend-chronische Hepatitis nach akuter Virushepatitis A. Dtsch Med Wochenschr *107:*46–50, 1982.

125. Cochrane AMG, Moussouros A, Thomson AD, Eddleston ALWF, Williams R: Antibody-dependent cell-mediated (K cell) cytotoxicity against isolated hepatocytes in chronic active hepatitis. Lancet *1:*441–444, 1976.

126. Montano L, Aranguibel F, Boffill M, Goodall AH, Janossy G, Thomas HC: An analysis of the composition of the inflammatory infiltrate in autoimmune and hepatitis B virus-induced chronic liver disease. Hepatology *3:*292–296, 1983.

127. Kawaniski H, MacDermott RP: K-cell mediated antibody-dependent cellular cytotoxicity in chronic active liver disease. Gastroenterology *76:*151–158, 1979.

128. Hopf U, Meyer zum Buschenfelde KH, Arnold W: Detection of a liver-membrane autoantibody in HBsAg-negative chronic active hepatitis. N Engl J Med *294:*578–582, 1976.

129. Hodgson HJF, Wands JR, Isselbacher KJ: Alteration in suppressor cell activity in chronic active hepatitis. Proc Natl Acad Sci USA *75:*1549–1553, 1978.

130. Kakumu S, Yata K, Kashio T: Immunoregulatory T-cell function in acute and chronic liver disease. Gastroenterology *79:*613–619, 1980.

131. Wiedmann KH, Bartholemew TC, Brown DJC, Thomas HC: Liver membrane antibodies detected by immunoradiometric assay in acute and chronic virus-induced and autoimmune liver disease. Hepatology *4:*199–204, 1984.

132. Dienstag JL: Immunologic mechanisms in chronic viral hepatitis. *In* Viral Hepatitis and Liver Disease, edited by G.N. Vyas, J.L. Dienstag, J.H. Hoofnagle. New York, Grune & Stratton, 1984, pp. 135–166.

133. Trevisan A, Realdi G, Alberti A: Core antigen specific immunoglobulin G bound to the liver cell membrane in chronic hepatitis B. Gastroenterology *82:*218–222, 1982.

134. Anastassakos Ch, Alexander GJM, Wolstencroft RA, Avery JA, Portmann BC, Panayi GS, Dumonde DC, Eddleston ALWF, Williams R: Interleukin-1 and interleukin-2 activity in chronic hepatitis B virus infection. Gastroenterology *94:*999–1005, 1989.

135. Dinarello CA: Interleukin-1. Rev Infect Dis *6:*51–95, 1984.

136. Postelthwaite AE, Smith GN, Mainardi CL, Seyer JM, Kang AH: Lymphocyte modulation of fibroblast function in vitro: stimulation and inhibition of collagen production by different effector molecules. J Immunol *132:*2470–2479, 1984.

137. Mackay IR: Genetic aspects of immunologically mediated liver disease. Semin Liver Dis *4:*13–24, 1984.

138. Galbraith RM, Eddleston ALWF, Williams R, Webster ADB, Pattison J, Doniach D, Kennedy LA, Batchelor JR: Enhanced antibody responses in active chronic hepatitis: relation to HLA-B8 and HLA-B12 and porto-systemic shunting. Lancet *1:*930–934, 1976.

139. Lindberg J, Lindholm A, Iwarson S: Genetic factors in the development of chronic active hepatitis. Lancet *1:*67–68, 1977.

140. Scott BB, Rajah SM, Losowsky MS: Histocompatibility antigens in chronic liver disease. Gastroenterology *72:*122–125, 1977.

141. Wiedmann KH, Bartholomew DJC, Brown DJC: Liver membrane antibodies detected by immunoradiometric assay in acute and chronic virus-induced and autoimmune liver disease. Hepatology *4:*199–206, 1984.

142. O'Brien CJ, Vento S, Donaldson PT, McSorley CG, McFarlane IG, Williams R, Eddleston ALWF: Cell-mediated immunity and suppressor-T-cell defects to liver-derived antigens in families of patients with autoimmune chronic active hepatitis. Lancet *1:*350–353, 1986.

143. Robertson DAF Zhang SL, Guy EG: Persistent measles virus genome in autoimmune chronic active hepatitis. Lancet *2:*9–14, 1987.

144. Black FL: Persistent measles virus genome in autoimmune chronic active hepatitis: cause of coincidence: Hepatology *8:*186–187, 1988.

145. Eddleston ALWF: Immunology of chronic active hepatitis. Q J Med *55:*191–198, 1985.

146. Cooksley WG, Powell LW, Kerr JF, Bhathal PS: Cholestasis in active chronic hepatitis. Am J Dig Dis *17:*495–504, 1972.

147. Shouval D, Levij IS, Eliakim M: Chronic active hepatitis with cholestatic features. I. A clinical and immunological study. Am J Gastroenterol *72:*542–550, 1979.

148. Shouval D, Eliakim M, Levij IS: Chronic active hepatitis with cho-

lestatic features. II. A histopathological study. Am J Gastroenterol 72:551–555, 1979.

149. Geubel AP, Baggenstoss AH, Summerskill WHJ: Responses to treatment can differentiate chronic active liver disease with cholangitic features from the primary biliary cirrhosis syndrome. Gastroenterology 71:444–449, 1976.

150. Doniach D, Walker JG: A unified concept of autoimmune hepatitis. Lancet 1:813–815, 1969.

151. Kloppel G, Seifert G, Lindner H, Dammermann R, Sack HJ, Berg PA: Histopathologic features in mixed types of chronic active hepatitis and primary biliary cirrhosis. Correlations of liver histology with mitochondrial antibodies of different specificity. Virch Arch A 373:143–160, 1977.

152. Kenny RP, Czaja AJ, Ludwig J, Dickson ER: Frequency and significance of antimitochondrial antibodies in severe chronic active hepatitis. Dig Dis Sci 31:705–711, 1986.

153. Williamson JMS, Chalmers DM, Clayden AD, Dixon MF, Ruddell WSJ, Losowsky MS: Primary biliary cirrhosis and chronic active hepatitis: an examination of clinical, biochemical, and histopathological features in differential diagnosis. J Clin Pathol 38:1007–1012, 1985.

154. Sadikali F, Doniach D: Autoimmune factors in African cirrhosis. Correlations with hepatitis B surface antigen and antibody. Am J Gastroenterol 64:484–489, 1975.

155. Faber V, Christoffersen P, Nielsen PE, Nielsen JO, Poulsen H: Au antigen in liver cirrhosis. Lancet 2:825–826, 1970.

156. Summerskill WHJ, Davidson CS, Dible JH, Mallory GK, Sherlock S, Turner MD, Wolfe SJ: Cirrhosis of the liver. A study of alcoholic and nonalcoholic patients in Boston and London. N Engl J Med 262:1–9, 1960.

157. MacSween RNM, Scott AR: Hepatic cirrhosis: a clinico-pathological review of 520 cases. J Clin Pathol 26:936–942, 1973.

158. Lindh G, Weiland O, Glaumann H: The application of a numerical scoring system for evaluating the histological outcome in patients with chronic hepatitis B followed in long term. Hepatology 8:98–103, 1988.

159. Popper H, Schaffner F: The vocabulary of chronic hepatitis. N Engl J Med 284:1154–1156, 1971.

160. MacSween RNM, Anthony PP, Scheuer PJ (eds): Pathology of the Liver, 2nd Edition, Churchill Livingstone, London, 1987.

161. Bianchi L, Spichtin HP, Gudat F: Chronic hepatitis. In Pathology of the Liver, edited by R.N.M. MacSween, P.P. Anthony, P.J. Scheuer. 2nd Edition. London, Churchill Livingstone, 1987; pp. 310–341.

162. Seeff LB, Kiernan T, Zimmerman HJ, Leevy CM, Wright EC, Tamburro CH, Schiff ER, Ishak KG: Hepatic disease in asymptomatic parenteral narcotic drug abusers: a Veterans Administration Collaborative Study. Am J Med Sci 270:41–47, 1975.

163. Govindarajan S, DeCock KM, Redeker AG: Natural course of delta superinfection in chronic hepatitis B virus-infected patients: histopathologic study with multiple liver biopsies. Hepatology 6:640–644, 1986.

164. Kong K, Kelly JK, Lee SS: Pseudotumor appearance in chronic hepatitis. J Clin Gastroenterol 12:437–440, 1990.

165. Bianchi L, De Groote J, Desmet VJ, Gedigk P, Korb G, Popper H, Poulsen H, Scheuer PJ, Schmid M, Thaler H, Wepler W: Acute and chronic hepatitis revisited. Review by an international group. Lancet 2:914–919, 1977.

166. Popper H, Paronetto F, Schaffner F: Immune process in the pathogenesis of liver disease. Ann NY Acad Sci 124:781–799, 1965.

167. Vonstapel MJ, vanSteenbergen W, de Wolf-Peeters C: Prognostic significance of piecemeal necrosis in acute viral hepatitis. Liver 3:46–57, 1983.

168. Schalm SW: Treatment of chronic active hepatitis. Liver 2:69–76, 1982.

169. Schlichting P, Fauerholdt L, Christense E: Prednisone treatment of chronic liver disease. I. Chronic aggressive hepatitis as a therapeutic marker. Liver 2:271–273, 1974.

170. Kerr JFR, Cooksley WGE, Searle TJ, Halliday JW, Halliday WJ, Holder L, Roberts I, Burnett W, Powell LW: The nature of piecemeal necrosis in chronic active hepatitis. Lancet 2:827–828, 1979.

171. Kawanishi H: Morphologic association of lymphocytes with hepatocytes in chronic liver disease. Lab Med 10:286–290, 1977.

172. Okuno T, Okanoue T, Takino T, Mori K: Prognostic significance of bridging necrosis in chronic active hepatitis. Gastroenterol Jpn 18:577–584, 1983.

173. Cooksley WGE, Bradbear RA, Robinson W, Harrison M, Halliday JW, Powell LW, N HS, Seah CS, Okuda K, Scheuer PJ, Sherlock

S: The prognosis of chronic active hepatitis without cirrhosis in relation to bridging necrosis. Hepatology 6:345–348, 1986.

174. van Leeuwen DJ, Howe SC, Scheuer PJ, Sherlock S: Portal hypertension in chronic hepatitis: relationship to morphological changes. Gut 31:339–343, 1990.

175. Poynard T, Degott C, Munoz C, Lebrec D: Relationship between degree of portal hypertension and liver histologic lesions in patients with alcoholic cirrhosis. Dig Dis Sci 32:337–343, 1987.

176. Liaw Y-F, Yang S-S, Chen T-J, Chu C-M: Acute exacerbation in hepatitis B e antigen positive chronic type hepatitis. J Hepatol 1:227–233, 1985.

177. Chu C-M, Karayiannis P, Fowler MJF, Monjardino J, Liaw Y-F, Thomas HC: Natural history of chronic hepatitis B virus infection in Taiwan: studies of hepatitis B virus DNA in serum. Hepatology 5:431–434, 1985.

178. Crapper RM, Bhathal PS, Mackay IR: Chronic active hepatitis in alcoholic patients. Liver 3:327–337, 1983.

179. Bruguera M, Zambon D, Ros E, Sanchez-Tapias JM, Rodes J: Chronic hepatitis: a possible etiology of fatty liver. Liver 5:111–116, 1985.

180. Christoffersen P, Dietrichson O, Faber V, Poulsen H: The occurrence and significance of abnormal bile duct epithelium in chronic aggressive hepatitis. A comparative morphological, biochemical, immunological, and prognostic study. Acta Pathol Microbiol Scand Section A: 80:294–302, 1972.

181. Liaw Y-F, Tai D-I, Chu C-M, Chen T-J: The development of cirrhosis in patients with chronic type B hepatitis: a prospective study. Hepatology 8:493–496, 1988.

182. Anthony PP, Ishak KG, Nayak NC, Poulsen H, Scheuer PJ, Sobin LH: The morphology of cirrhosis: definition, nomenclature, and classification. Bull WHO 59:521–540, 1977.

183. Fauerholdt L, Schlichting P, Christensen E, Poulsen H, Tygstrup N, Juhl E: The Copenhagen Study Group for Liver Diseases. Conversion of micronodular cirrhosis into macronodular cirrhosis. Hepatology 3:928–931, 1983.

184. Anthony PP, Vogel CL, Barker LF: Liver cell dysplasia: a premalignant condition. J Clin Pathol 26:217–223, 1973.

185. Roncalli M, Borzio M, DeBiagi G, Ferrari AR, Macchi R, Tombesi VM, Servida E: Liver cell dysplasia in cirrhosis. Cancer 57:1515–1521, 1986.

186. Cohen C, Berson SD: Liver cell dysplasia in normal, cirrhotic, and hepatocellular carcinoma patients. Cancer 57:1535–1538, 1986.

187. Anthony PP: Liver cell dysplasia. What is its significance? Hepatology 7:394–395, 1987.

188. Lefkowitch JH, Apfelbaum TF: Liver cell dysplasia and hepatocellular carcinoma in non-A, non-B hepatitis. Arch Pathol Lab Med 111:170–173, 1987.

189. Lefkowitch JJ, Arborgh BAM, Scheuer PJ: Oxyphilic granular hepatocytes, mitochondrian-rich liver cells in hepatic disease. Am J Clin Pathol 74:432–441, 1980.

190. Cook GC, Mulligan R, Sherlock S: Controlled prospective trial of corticosteroid therapy in active hepatitis. Q J Med 40:159–185, 1971.

191. Murray-Lyon IM, Stern RB, Williams R: Controlled trial of prednisone and azathioprine in active chronic hepatitis. Lancet 1:735–737, 1973.

192. Schalm SW, Summerskill WHJ, Gitnick GL, Elveback LR: Contrasting features and responses to treatment of severe chronic active liver disease with and without hepatitis Bs antigen. Gut 17:781–786, 1976.

193. Summerskill WHJ: Chronic active liver disease evaluation and treatment. Viewpoints Dig Dis 5:9–12, 1973.

194. Wu PC, Lai CL, Lam KC: Prednisolone in HBsAg-positive chronic active hepatitis. Histologic evaluation in a controlled prospective study. Hepatology 2:777–783, 1982.

195. European Association for the Study of the Liver: A multicenter randomized clinical trial of low-dose steroid treatment in chronic active HBsAg positive liver disease. Gastroenterology 86:1317, 1984 (abstract).

196. Dudley FJ, Scheuer PJ, Sherlock S: Natural history of hepatitis-associated antigen positive chronic liver disease. Lancet 2:1388–1393, 1972.

197. Czaja AJ, Rakela J, Ludwig J: Features reflective of early prognosis in corticosteroid-treated severe autoimmune chronic active hepatitis. Gastroenterology 95:448–453, 1988.

198. Hyams JS, Ballow M, Leichtner AM: Cyclosporine treatment of autoimmune chronic active hepatitis. Gastroenterology 93:890–893, 1987.

199. Stellon AJ, Keating JJ, Johnson PJ, McFarlane IG, Williams R: Maintenance of remission in autoimmune chronic active hepatitis with

azathioprine after corticosteroid withdrawal. Hepatology 8:781–784, 1988.

200. Guarascio P, DeFelici AP, Migliorini D, Alexander GJM, Fagan EA, Visco G: Treatment of chronic HBeAg-positive hepatitis with acyclovir. A controlled trial. J Hepatol 3:S143–S147, 1986.

201. Perrillo RP, Regenstein FG, Peters MG, DeSchryver-Kecskemeti K, Bodicky CJ, Campbell CR, Kuhns MC: Prednisone withdrawal followed by recombinant α interferon in the treatment of chronic type B hepatitis. Ann Intern Med 109:95–100, 1988.

202. Hanson RG, Peters MG, Hoofnagle JH: Effects of immunosuppressive therapy with prednisone on B and T lymphocyte function in patients with chronic type B hepatitis. Hepatology 6:173–179, 1986.

203. Hoofnagle JH, Di Bisceglie AM: Antiviral therapy of viral hepatitis. In Antiviral Agents and Viral Diseases of Man, edited by G.J. Galasso, R.J. Whitley, T.C. Merigan. 3rd Edition. New York, Raven Press, 1989, pp. 415–460.

204. Perrillo RP, Schiff ER, Davis GL, Bodenheimer HC, Lindsay K, Payne J, Dienstag JL, O'Brien C, Tamburro C, Jacobson IM, Sampliner R, Feit D, Lefkowitch J, Kuhns M, Meschievitz C, Sanghvi B, Albrecht J, Gibas A: A randomized, controlled trial of interferon α-2b along and after prednisone withdrawal for the treatment of chronic hepatitis B. N Engl J Med 323:295–301, 1990.

205. Hoofnagle JH, Peters MG, Mullen KD: Randomized controlled trial of a four-month course of recombinant human α interferon in chronic type B hepatitis. Gastroenterology 95:1318–1325, 1988.

206. Brook MG, McDonald JA, Karayiannis P: Randomised controlled trial of interferon α 2a (rbe) (Roferon-A) for the treatment of chronic hepatitis B virus (HBV) infection: factors that influence response. Gut 30:1116–1122, 1989.

207. Lok ASF, Ma OCK, Lau JYN: Interferon α therapy in patients with chronic hepatitis B virus infection. Effects on hepatitis B virus DNA in the liver. Gastroenterology 100:756–761, 1991.

208. Kassianides C, Di Bisceglie AM, Hoofnagle JH: α interferon therapy in patients with decompensated chronic type B hepatitis. In Viral Hepatitis and Liver Disease, edited by A.J. Zuckerman. New York, Alan R Liss, 1988, pp. 840–843.

209. Lok ASF, Lai CL, Wu PC, Leung EKY: Long-term follow-up in a randomised controlled trial of recombinant α-2 interferon in Chinese patients with chronic hepatitis B infection. Lancet 2:298–302, 1988.

210. Rosina F, Rizzetto M: Treatment of chronic type D (delta) hepatitis with α interferon. Semin Liver Dis 9:264–266, 1989.

211. Farci P, Mandas A, Lai ME: Randomized controlled trial of high and low doses of interferon α-2a (Roferon-A) in chronic HDV hepatitis. In Viral Hepatitis and Liver Disease, edited by F.B. Hollinger. Baltimore, Williams & Wilkinson, 1991.

212. Di Bisceglie AM, Kassianides C, Lisker-Melman M: Randomized, double-blind, placebo-controlled trial of α interferon therapy for chronic non-A, non-B hepatitis. N Engl J Med 321:1506–1510, 1989.

213. Davis GL, Balart L, Schiff E: Multicenter randomized controlled trial of α interferon treatment for chronic non-A, non-B hepatitis. N Engl J Med 321:1311–1316, 1989.

214. Mutchnick MG, Appelman HD, Chung HT, Aragona E, Lee HH, Gupta TP, Cummings GD, Waggoner JG, Hoofnagle JH, Shafritz DA: Thymosin treatment of hepatitis B virus chronic active hepatitis: a randomized, double-blind, controlled pilot trial. Hepatology 14:409–415, 1991.

215. Penn I: Tumor incidence in allograft recipients. Transplant Proc 11:1047–1051, 1979.

216. Kinlen LJ: Incidence of cancer in rheumatoid arthritis and other disorders after immunosuppressive treatment. Am J Med 78: (Suppl. 1A) 44–49, 1985.

217. Wang KK, Czaja AJ, Beaver SJ, Go VLW: Extrahepatic malignancy following long-term immunosuppressive therapy of severe hepatitis B suface antigen-negative chronic active hepatitis. Hepatology 10:39–43, 1989.

218. Schaffner F, Popper H: Nonspecific reactive hepatitis in aged and infirm people. Am J Dig Dis 4:388–399, 1959.

219. Popper H, Schaffner F: Liver: Structure and Function. New York, McGraw-Hill Book Company, 1957, pp. 404–407.

220. Chung H-T, Lai C-L, Wu P-C, Lok ASF: Synergism of chronic alcoholism and hepatitis B infection in liver disease. J Gastroenterol Hepatol 4:11–16, 1989.

221. La Brecque DR, Klatskin G: The various histopathologic presentations of sclerosing cholangitis (Abst). Gastroenterology 78:1310, 1980.

222. Wiesner RH, La Russo NF: Clinicopathologic features of the syndrome of primary sclerosing cholangitis. Gastroenterology 79:200–206, 1980.

223. Chapman RWG, Marborgh BA, Rhodes JM, Summerfield JA, Dick R, Scheuer PJ, Sherlock S: Primary sclerosing cholangitis: a review of its clinical features, cholangiography, and hepatic histology. Gut 21:870–877, 1980.

Chapter 9
Cirrhosis

Definition

The hepatic lesions in all forms of cirrhosis, irrespective of their varied etiology and pathogenesis, are characterized by a diffuse fibrosis that destroys the normal lobular architecture and replaces the normal lobules with nodules of parenchyma encased in fibrous tissue (1). Although the fibrosis affects the entire liver, its distribution is not necessarily uniform, so occasionally, intact lobules escape destruction.

Most of the nodules cirrhosis represent masses of regenerating hepatocytes that are arranged in the form of irregular, thickened hepatic plates separated by sinusoids, but unaccompanied by central veins or portal tracts. However, as the regenerating nodules enlarge with advancing age of the lesions, the hepatocytes may revert to a normal, one-cell-thick, radiating plate pattern, and newly formed central veins and portal tracts may appear (2), a sequence of events also seen in normal regenerating liver tissue following partial hepatectomy. Although nodules of this type resemble islands of intact lobules that have escaped destruction, the number and orientation of the central veins and portal tracts seldom conform to the pattern found in normal lobules.

Also classified as cirrhosis are hepatic lesions characterized by a diffuse, uniformly distributed, perisinusoidal and pericellular fibrosis that destroys the normal lobular architecture, but does not provoke a nodular regenerative response. Lesions of this type, classified as *diffuse interstitial* (3) or *florid cirrhosis* (4), are relatively rare, but may be encountered in *alcoholic liver disease* (3–5), *congenital syphilis* (6), drug-induced phospholipidosis (7), and the late phase of progressive *neonatal giant cell hepatitis* (6).

Hepatocellular degeneration and necrosis play an important role in the pathogenesis of cirrhosis, and, usually, are readily demonstrable in active progressive lesions. However, the hepatocytes may appear normal in the late inactive phase of the disease, so histologic evidence of hepatocellular damage is not an essential criterion in the definition of cirrhosis.

Hepatic fibrosis or nodule formation are not necessarily indicative of cirrhosis. *Noncirrhotic fibrosis* with nodules may be seen in subcapsular hepatic fibrosis, congenital hepatic fibrosis, and focal nodular hyperplasia.

Subcapsular hepatic fibrosis, a relatively common finding in both normal and abnormal livers, presents as fibrous bands that project into the liver from a normal, thickened Glisson's capsule, outlining small nodules of parenchyma (Figs. 39,40). Such lesions are readily differentiated from those of cirrhosis, since they never extend to a depth greater than 2 mm below Glisson's capsule (8). However, they may be misinterpreted as evidence of cirrhosis in small, superficial or tangential biopsy sections.

In *congenital hepatic fibrosis,* an autosomal recessive hered-itary anomaly related to juvenile polycystic disease (9,10), the liver is traversed by numerous relatively broad, smoothly contoured, densely collagenized septa that contain numerous dilated, branching bile ducts lined by cuboidal epithelium, but few or no portal veins or inflammatory cells [(11,12); Figs. 63, 64]. Although the septa may enclose a variable number of parenchymal nodules, they show no evidence of regenerative activity, and the lobular architecture in the remaining liver is well preserved.

The lesions of *nodular regenerative hyperplasia* are characterized by nodules of regenerating hepatocytes outlined by narrow bands of congested sinusoids, atrophic hepatic plates, and collapsed reticulin (Figs. 65–67). In contrast to cirrhosis, the hepatocellular regeneration is unaccompanied by fibrosis. The etiology and pathogenesis of such lesions are obscure. However, they are known to occur in association with a wide variety of disorders, including rheumatoid arthritis, Felty's syndrome, the CRST syndrome (calcinosis, Raynaud's phenomenon, sclerodactyly, and telangectasia) and myeloproliferative diseases (13,14), early primary biliary cirrhosis (15), and following the prolonged use of oral contraceptives, androgenic-anabolic steroids, corticosteroids, and antineoplastic agents (13). It has been proposed that obliteration of small intrahepatic portal veins is the critical lesion in the pathogenesis of nodular regenerative hyperplasia. Such obliteration can result from a variety of mechanisms, including aggregated platelets arising in the spleen or elsewhere in the portal venous system (16,17). Alternatively, it has been suggested that nodular regenerative hyperplasia represents a regenerative-vascular response to drugs that results in the formation of nodules analogous to the precancerous, hyperplastic nodules produced by carcinogens in experimental animals (13).

Focal nodular hyperplasia, a benign hepatic tumor, mimics cirrhosis histologically [(18); Fig. 565]. However, even when multiple, the lesions are focal in character, and are separated by large areas of normal hepatic parenchyma, so their differentiation from cirrhosis seldom poses a problem. The only exception is in the case of needle biopsy sections of large tumors that are not recognized as focal lesions.

For reasons that are not clear, the lesions of hepar lobatum and hepatic hereditary telangiectasia are not classified as cirrhosis. In *hepar lobatum,* a manifestation of late, untreated, acquired syphilis, chronic inflammation and healing of gummas lead to the development of numerous widespread, contracted scars that deform the liver, giving it an irregular, coarsely lobulated appearance (19). On microscopic examination, the lesions are characterized by large, irregular nodules of parenchyma separated by broad fibrous septa (Fig. 566), many of which are heavily infiltrated with lymphocytes and plasma cells, and contain granulomas (Fig. 567). Often, the granulomas show varying degrees of fibrosis, fibrinoid necrosis, and giant cells.

Except for the presence of granulomas, the histologic appearance of the lesions closely resembles that seen in postnecrotic cirrhosis after recovery from submassive hepatic necrosis (Fig. 468).

In some cases of *hereditary hemorrhagic telangiectasia* (Osler-Weber-Rendu syndrome), the liver shows lesions that are usually classified as *pseudocirrhosis* (20) or *telangiectatic hepatic fibrosis* (21). When advanced, the fibrosis may be diffuse with accompanying nodule formation (Fig. 568), as in other forms of cirrhosis. The only distinctive feature is the presence of numerous dilated, thin-walled, blood-filled vascular channels within the septa (Fig. 569).

Etiology

A wide variety of etiologic factors have been invoked to account for the development of cirrhosis. Some of these have been clearly identified, whereas others are still only speculative. Moreover, in many cases, the etiology remains obscure.

Listed in Table 9–1 are the recognized forms of cirrhosis, classified on the basis of their established, presumed, or unknown etiology. With the exceptions of alcoholic, posthepatitic, and cryptogenic cirrhosis, which occur commonly, and

hemochromatosis and primary biliary cirrhosis, which occur only occasionally, the other forms of cirrhosis cited are rare.

Schistosomiasis in its late "pipestem" stage is a cirrhotic process (22), but may require coinfection with hepatitis B virus (23).

Classification

Etiologic

Whenever possible, cirrhotic lesions should be classified on the basis of their etiology. In many cases, however, the etiology is unknown, so descriptive terms based on morphologic, clinical, or laboratory features are often employed. Cirrhosis secondary to autoimmune chronic active hepatitis and primary biliary cirrhosis are examples of such lesions.

Although the histologic features in some forms of cirrhosis are sufficiently distinctive to permit recognition of the underlying etiology, identification depends on a consideration of both the character of the lesions and the accompanying clinical and laboratory manifestations. Even in the case of cirrhotic lesions with distinctive features, collateral evidence may be needed, as in the differentiation of alcoholic and nonalcoholic portal cirrhosis, or between hereditary and acquired hemochromatosis.

Table 9–1. Etiology of cirrhosis

A. *Established Etiology*
  1. Toxic
    a. Alcohol
    b. Hepatotoxins
    c. Drugs
  2. Infections
    a. Hepatitis B, D, and C (non-A, non-B) viruses
    b. Brucellosis
    c. Syphilis
  3. Biliary obstruction
  4. Hepatic circulatory disorders (outflow obstruction)
    a. Congestive "cardiac" cirrhosis
    b. Budd-Chiari syndrome
    c. Veno-occlusive disease
  5. Hereditary metabolic disorders
    a. Metals
      (1) Hemochromatosis
      (2) Wilson's disease
    b. Carbohydrates
      (1) Type IV glycogenosis
      (2) Galactosemia
      (3) Hereditary fructose intolerance
    c. Glycoproteins
      (1) Alpha$_1$-antitrypsin deficiency
      (2) Mucopolysaccharidosis
    d. Lipids
      (1) Abetalipoproteinemia
      (2) Wolman's disease
      (3) Cholesterol ester storage disease
    e. Amino acids
      (1) Tyrosinemia
    f. Porphyrins
      (1) Erythropoietic protoporphyria

Established Etiology—Continued
  6. Other hereditary disorders
    a. Mucoviscidosis
    b. Progressive neonatal cholestasis (Byler's disease)
    c. Familial intrahepatic duct hypoplasia with defective bile acid metabolism
    d. Familial cirrhosis of unknown etiology
    e. Hereditary hemorrhagic telangiectasia

B. *Presumed Etiology*
  1. Autoimmunity
    a. Autoimmune ("lupoid") chronic active hepatitis
    b. Primary biliary cirrhosis
    c. Primary sclerosing cholangitis
    d. Scleroderma
  2. Metabolic
    a. Diabetes mellitus
    b. Obesity
    c. Malnutrition (kwashiorkor)

C. *Unknown Etiology*
  1. Neonatal cirrhosis
  2. Biliary atresia
  3. Indian childhood cirrhosis
  4. Cirrhosis following ileojejunal bypass
  5. Cryptogenic cirrhosis

Morphologic

Often, cirrhotic lesions are classified as *micronodular, macronodular,* or *mixed* on the basis of their parenchymal nodule size. Unfortunately, there are no universally accepted criteria for distinguishing between micronodules and macronodules; consequently this classification lacks precision and uniformity. The diameter of a normal hepatic lobule, approximately 1 mm, is a logical basis for defining the upper limits of a micronodule. However, two international committees on standardization of nomenclature have recommended 3 mm (24) and 10 mm (25), respectively. The problem of definition is further complicated by the fact that in some forms of cirrhosis the nodules tend to enlarge with advancing age of the lesions, so that, often, micronodules are converted to macronodules (26). Although nodule size is variably defined and does not correlate with the underlying etiology, its retention as a qualifying term in the classification of cirrhosis has been recommended, since hepatocellular carcinoma, which usually arises in cirrhotic livers, occurs predominantly in macronodular lesions (24). However, there is evidence that the prevalence of such neoplasms not only is related to the size of the nodules but also to the width of the fibrous septa. Hepatocellular carcinoma occurs only rarely in cirrhosis with septa more than 1 mm in width, irrespective of nodule size (27).

State of development and activity of cirrhotic lesions

The classification of cirrhotic lesions should include an assessment of their stage of development and their activity. The criteria used in defining early, moderately advanced, and advanced cirrhosis, and in distinguishing between mildly, moderately, and severely active lesions are discussed below.

Cirrhosis of ill-defined or unknown etiology

Most descriptive terms used to classify cirrhosis are based on generally accepted etiologic, morphologic, or pathogenetic criteria. Some of the terms that cause confusion, which are cited in the next few paragraphs, serve to illustrate how they may complicate the classification of cirrhosis (28). Use of the recently revised nomenclature of the International Association of the Study of the Liver (25), which parallels the World Health Organization classification (24), should minimize the confusion.

Postnecrotic cirrhosis at one time was limited to the healed phase of viral or drug-induced submassive hepatic necrosis, and implied a small, misshapen liver traversed by broad scars, containing remnants of multiple, collapsed lobules interspersed with large, multilobular nodules of regenerating parenchyma. More recently, some authorities use the term to define any type of cirrhosis that contains broad fibrous septa, regardless of the underlying etiology or the size of the accompanying regenerating nodules (29,30). Others, however, classify all forms of macronodular cirrhosis as postnecrotic, whether or not the fibrous

septa are broad or narrow and contain remnants of collapsed lobules or not.

As a rule, the term *posthepatitic cirrhosis* implies a form of cirrhosis attributable to antecedent viral- or drug-induced acute hepatitis (31). However, the same term has been used to define a type of macronodular cirrhosis characterized by uniform nodules ranging in diameter from 0.5 to 1.5 cm separated by relatively slender fibrous septa that do not exceed 0.3 cm in width. Others have classified identical lesions in chronic alcoholic patients as *coarsely nodular cirrhosis* (32).

Nutritional or *Laennec's cirrhosis* was originally introduced as a synonym of alcoholic cirrhosis at a time when such lesions were regarded as the sequelae of malnutrition alone or in conjunction with the alcohol. Since abandonment of this view, the term nutritional or portal cirrhosis has been applied to any form of uniformly micronodular cirrhosis accompanied by fatty infiltration without regard to the underlying etiology (29), but these terms are no longer in wide use.

The frequency with which *cryptogenic cirrhosis* is reported varies geographically, ranging from as low as 20% in some areas (33) to as high as 60% in others (34), depending, in part at least, on the prevalence of chronic alcoholism and infection with the B and non-A, non-B hepatitis viruses, two major causes of cirrhosis. As more sensitive and reliable techniques for their detection have become available, HBV and the NANB viruses are proving to be of increasing importance as etiologic factors in types of chronic hepatitis and cirrhosis previously classified as cryptogenic (35,36).

Although patients with cryptogenic cirrhosis undoubtedly comprise an etiologically heterogeneous group, they usually exhibit inactive, macronodular lesions, and often are asymptomatic or present with complications of portal hypertension such as hemorrhage from esophageal varices or ascites rather than signs of hepatocellular failure. The demonstration of inherited differences in the metabolism of drugs, as shown for halothane (37,38), debrisoquine (39), and perhexiline (40), suggests that drug-induced liver injury should occur statistically more frequently in family members than in unrelated individuals.

Most examples of *familial cirrhosis* are attributed to hereditary metabolic disorders, such as Wilson's disease or hereditary hemochromatosis (see Table 9–1), or, perhaps, to hereditary abnormalities of immune regulation that render individuals susceptible to presumed autoimmune disorders, such as primary biliary cirrhosis and nonviral chronic active hepatitis. Less frequently shared exposure to environmental factors, such as alcohol and hepatitis B or C viruses (41), HBV and schistosomiasis (21,22), vitamins (42) alone or in combination with alcohol (43), or occupational hepatotoxic substances may be involved. The role of heredity and other factors in the various forms of familial cirrhosis are discussed individually for each type of cirrhosis.

A number of cases of familial cirrhosis have been reported in which all known hereditary and environmental etiologic factors have been excluded (40). In most instances, only siblings have been affected, so it has been proposed that the disease or the susceptibility to it is probably inherited as an autosomal recessive trait. However, many of these cases were investigated before methods were available for excluding the possibility of underlying infection with the hepatitis B or C viruses. Nevertheless, in the few cases we observed there was no serologic evidence of such infection.

Pathogenesis

Available evidence suggests that in most, if not all forms of cirrhosis, fibrosis and hepatocellular regeneration are the result of hepatocellular degeneration and necrosis.

Hepatic fibrogenesis

Surprisingly little is known about the factors that induce fibrogenesis following hepatocellular degeneration and necrosis. Loss of hepatocytes and collapse of reticulin alone cannot account for the diffuse fibrosis seen in cirrhosis. This is illustrated in the case of viral- and drug-induced acute bridging and multilobular necrosis, lesions characterized by extensive loss of hepatocytes and collapse of reticulin, resulting in the formation of what have been termed "passive septa" (44). Although such septa undergo collagenization and lead to the development of cirrhosis in some cases (44,45), they may also heal without significant residual fibrosis (46,47). It is apparent, therefore, that other factors must be responsible for triggering fibrogenesis, and transforming growth factors (TGF) such as TGF β-1, a cytokine, have been identified (48). Of these, infiltrating inflammatory cells that usually accompany hepatocellular degeneration and necrosis are promising candidates (45). However, progressive fibrosis can occur in the absence of significant inflammation, as seen in cardiac cirrhosis. Ductular proliferation is another factor that has been invoked as a possible stimulus for fibrogenesis (49). Although the intimate relationship between proliferating ductules and encircling collagen bundles appears consistent with this interpretation, ductular proliferation is not a feature in all cirrhotic lesions.

The possibility has been considered that some of the exogenous factors responsible for the hepatocellular degeneration and necrosis in cirrhosis may also stimulate fibrogenesis directly. Attempts to demonstrate this in the case of alcohol have led to conflicting results (50–53), More recent studies have shown that acetaldehyde, the primary metabolite of ethanol, stimulates procollagen synthesis in human fibroblasts (54, 55) and lipocytes and may be directly fibrogenic in man. Evidence implicating excessive doses of vitamin A as a direct stimulant of fibrogenesis, by inducing the proliferation and activation of lipocytes (Ito cells) to fibroblastic activity (56), is more suggestive, but still only circumstantial. The experimental synergism of alcohol and vitamin A suggest that such mechanisms may be of clinical significance (43). Whether or not other etiologic factors involved in the pathogenesis of cirrhosis can induce collagen synthesis directly has not been adequately investigated. Such factors may prove to be important in the types of hepatic fibrosis and cirrhosis that develop insidiously in the apparent absence of overt hepatocellular degeneration and necrosis, as, for example, in chronic vinyl chloride intoxication (57,58), or even in alcoholic cirrhosis in baboons (59) and humans (60).

Although fibroblasts undoubtedly play an important role in the fibrogenesis of cirrhosis, a number of other cell types, including perisinusoidal lipocytes (Ito cells), myofibroblasts, monocytes (61), and even hepatocytes, are capable of synthesizing collagen (62). The relative importance of these different cell types in the fibrogenesis of cirrhosis is not known.

Collagen is the most abundant protein in the extracellular matrix. In the normal liver, types I, III, IV, and V, make up 90% of the collagen. Type I, which is an interstitial collagen found in large fibrils primarily in portal tracts, makes up one-third of hepatic collagen. Type III, which is an interstitial collagen found in fine fibrils largely in reticulin, constitutes another third. Types IV and V, each of which make up 10%, are basement membrane collagens found in the space of Disse and pericellularly, respectively (63). The collagen content of types I, III, IV, and V, especially type I, is greatly increased in cirrhosis of all etiologies (64, 65). Increased type III is a marker of disease activity (66,67). In addition, fibronectin, a cell surface protein (68), laminin (69), and proteoglycan (70), which are components of the normal extracellular matrix, are all increased. During hepatic fibrogenesis, fibronectin deposition precedes and probably modulates the deposition of collagen (69), but during active hepatic regeneration following subtotal hepatectomy, which greatly stimulates collagen synthesis, fibronectin deposition does not increase and no fibrosis develops (71).

Increased fibrosis is the result of many factors in addition to increased collagen and fibronectin production, including decreased collagenase activity, stimulation of fibroblasts and monocytes (61), and the presence of transforming growth factor, which is derived from hematopoietic cells (72), and of platelet-derived growth factor (73), which are chemoattractants for fibroblasts and monocytes. It is intriguing that collagenase activity increases in the early stages of alcoholic fibrosis in baboons, but decreases when cirrhosis develops (74). Anticipated developments in this rapidly advancing area will provide new insights into fibrogenesis and, perhaps, into its suppression and prevention.

There is increasing evidence that collagen degradation may play an important role in modulating fibrogenesis in both normal and cirrhotic livers. Under experimental conditions, cirrhotic lesions produced by carbon tetrachloride are readily reversible early in the course of their development, but ultimately become irreversible (75). Similarly in humans, complete disappearance of cirrhosis has been reported in rare cases of hemochromatosis and Wilson's disease as a result of therapeutic measures that deplete the excessive iron and copper stores, respectively. Presumably, the degradation of collagen in reversible cirrhosis is attributable to increased activity of the collagenases found in the liver. However, the possibility that lysosomal or other enzymes participate in this process has not been excluded. Current interest is focused on the possibility of retarding or reversing the hepatic fibrosis in cirrhotic lesions by using agents that interfere with collagen synthesis, maturation, or transport, or that enhance collagenase activity. Preliminary results of such therapy with colchicine have been encouraging, both in experimental animals (62) and in humans (76,77). Increased understanding of the biochemical mechanisms of fibrogenesis may result in treatment with α-interferon (78), prostaglandins (79), or other substances.

Methods for quantifying the fibrosis in human liver biopsies are crude. Biochemical and immunologic methods are complex (80) and morphometric methods are arduous (81). Colorimetric methods for use on needle biopsy specimens look promising (92).

Hepatocellular regeneration

Although loss of hepatocytes undoubtedly triggers a regenerative response, the factors involved in the induction and maintenance of hepatic deoll replication are uncertain. Experimental studies strongly suggest that insulin plays an important role in this process (83) as does glucagon (84), and that their effects may be mediated by an insulin-dependent growth-promoting factor produced by regenerating liver (85). However, elimination of the endogenous source of insulin and glucogen, which also plays a role, by evisceration, retards, but does not prevent the regenerative response of the liver following partial hepatectomy in the rat (86). Moreover, although the degradation of insulin in the cirrhotic liver is impaired, resulting in hyperinsulinism (87,88), there is no evidence to indicate that the onset of regeneration in such lesions coincides with an increase in circulating insulin. Other factors such as epidermal growth factor (89) and oncogenes (90) may also participate, but it is clear that regeneration is a most complex phenomenon and that its mechanisms are not yet elucidated.

Regeneration of the liver, particularly in its early stages, involves not only hyperplasia, but also hypertrophy of the hepatocytes, so that enlarged and pleomorphic cells are relatively common in the nodules of active cirrhosis. In addition, the proliferating hepatocytes in the regenerating nodules of active cirrhosis are arranged in the form of irregular, two-cell-thick hepatic plates, rosettes, and pseudoducts, a configuration reminiscent of that in the fetal and neonatal liver. However, once the activity of the cirrhosis abates, the hepatocytes tend to revert to a regular, radiating, one-cell-thick plate pattern, as occurs during maturation of the neonatal liver. The factors that govern these spatial relationships of the hepatocytes during and following their proliferation are not known.

Bile duct epithelium and the mesenchymal elements of the liver, including the Kupffer and endothelial cells, collagen, and reticulin, participate in the regenerative response of hepatic parenchyma, although their proliferation lags behind that of the hepatocytes (90,91). It is not clear whether this asynchrony is attributable to variations in the responsiveness of each of these components to a common stimulus, or whether different stimuli are involved.

Hepatocellular degeneration and necrosis

The character and pathogenesis of the hepatocellular degeneration and necrosis in cirrhosis varies, depending on the underlying etiology, so no generalizations are possible. For that reason, they are discussed in other chapters devoted to individual types of cirrhosis.

Vascular changes

Usually, the fibrosis and nodule formation in cirrhotic lesions are associated with alterations in the intrahepatic vasculature that may contribute to perpetuation of the lesions, the production of portal hypertension, and the development of ascites (92).

Extension of fibrous tissue into the spaces of Disse, often accompanied by the development of a basement membrane on the sinusoidal aspect of the hepatic plates, a process, aptly termed *capillarization of the sinusoids* (93), that occurs in some forms of cirrhosis, probably interferes with the exchange of nutrients and oxygen between the blood and hepatocytes, and, thus, may lead to further cell damage and fibrosis. In addition, capillari-

zation, by increasing the resistance to hepatic blood flow, may contribute to the development of postsinusoidal portal hypertension (94).

Fibrous occlusion of the central veins, a vascular lesion that impedes the outflow of blood form the sinusoids and leads to their congestion and capillarization and, secondarily, to atrophy and loss of the intervening hepatic plates, is seen in forms of cirrhosis attributable to chronic alcoholism (5) and veno-occlusive disease (95).

The fibrous septa in cirrhosis that link portal tracts and central veins contain branches of the portal vein that communicate with arterioles, and drain directly into tributaries of the hepatic veins, thus diverting blood from the hepatic parenchyma. As a result, such *portohepatic venous shunts* may perpetuate hepatocellular destruction and secondary fibrogenesis (96).

As cirrhosis advances, there is progressive *diminution* in the number and caliber of *intrahepatic venous channels* as a result of constriction by fibrous tissue (97) and compression by regenerating nodules of parenchyma (98).

Normally, the portal vein provides two-thirds and the hepatic artery one-third of the blood supply to the liver. However, in advanced cirrhosis, with the reduction in the number of portal vein radicles and the development of portal-hepatic venous shunts that divert blood from the sinusoids, the blood supply to the hepatic parenchyma is predominantly arterial. Although this may suffice to support normal hepatic function for a time, progressive fibrosis may ultimately impinge on the hepatic arterioles and further diminish hepatic blood flow (97).

In the normal liver, the hepatic arterioles drain into the sinusoids via a network of capillaries (99). However, in cirrhosis they communicate directly with portal vein radicles in the septa, producing numerous small *arteriovenous shunts* (100) that may play a role in the pathogenesis of portal hypertension.

Ascites

The elevation of intrasinusoidal pressure in cirrhosis that results from perisinusoidal fibrosis, occlusion of central veins, or compression of hepatic veins by regenerating parenchymal nodules (101) leads to increased filtration of plasma into the spaces of Disse, and, secondarily, to enhanced hepatic and thoracic duct lymph flow (102). Bascd on direct measurements, it has been reported that when the volume of hepatic lymph formation exceeds the drainage capacity of the thoracic duct, edema of the liver and the formation of ascites occur and portal pressure is further increased (102). During ascites formation in cirrhotic patients, the lymphatics in the hilum of the liver are increased in number and caliber (103). Furthermore, in early cirrhosis with postsinusoidal obstruction, the protein concentration of ascitic fluid is relatively high, and may approach that of hepatic lymph (104).

Two major determinants of ascites formation are the hydrostatic pressure in the portal vein and the plasma colloidal osmotic pressure (105). In cirrhosis, both an increase in portal pressure, attributable to the vascular lesions described earlier, and a decrease in plasma osmotic pressure, due to suppressed albumin synthesis, contribute to ascites formation. The relative importance of the two factors varies in different patients. The greater the gradients between the portal and the systemic venous pressure amd the ascitic and systemic oncotic pressure, the greater the propensity to form ascites (106).

Additional factors are involved in the pathogenesis of ascites in cirrhosis. Of these, the most important are the renal retention of sodium and expansion of the plasma volume (107), effects attributable to increased aldosterone secretion in response to the enhanced production of renin provoked by alterations in the renal circulation (108). Reduced levels of atrial natriuretic factor and their increase after expansion of plasma volume indicate that they, too, contribute to the water retention (109).

Ascitic fluid is in dynamic equilibrium with the plasma, entering and leaving the peritoneal cavity at relatively rapid rates (110). Most of the fluid that enters the peritoneal cavity is a transudate from the capillaries of the peritoneal serosa, formed as a result of increased hydrostatic pressure in the hepatic sinusoids (111). However, in some cases, seepage of lymph from distended lymphatics in the capsule and hilum of the liver may contribute. Under both normal and abnormal conditions, fluid, colloids, and even particulate material that enter the peritoneal cavity are drained primarily via lymphatics in the diaphragm (112,113). Obviously, the volume of ascitic fluid that accumulates and is retained in the steady state depends on the relative rates at which fluid enters and leaves the peritoneal cavity. Indeed, only a net 700 to 800 ml of ascitic fluid can be mobilized each day without constricting plasma volume (114,115).

Bile duct alterations

Ductular proliferation is a relatively common finding in cirrhotic lesions. According to most authorities, such proliferation is attributable to hyperplasia of ductal and ductular epithelium (116,117). However, there is suggestive evidence that at least under some conditions, the newly formed ductules are derived from regenerating hepatocytes (118,119).

The factors responsible for ductular proliferation have not been clearly defined. Since it occurs in both hepatocellular and obstructive cholestasis, it has been suggested that the retention or reflux of bile may be the primary stimulus (120). However, this does appear to account for the ductular proliferation found in hepatic disorders like cirrhosis that are unaccompanied by cholestasis. One possible alternative is that the breakdown products of either inflammatory cells or necrotic hepatocytes (117) may play an important role. Certainly, the striking ductular proliferation that accompanies the extensive destruction of hepatocytes and the intense inflammatory reaction in viral submassive hepatic necrosis is consistent with this hypothesis. However, the possibility cannot be excluded that in submassive hepatic necrosis and in cirrhosis, the ductules proliferate in response to the same factors that govern hepatocellular regeneration following the loss of hepatocytes. Obviously, other factors must be involved in those lesions that are unaccompanied by hepatocellular necrosis, such as early extrahepatic biliary obstruction.

It has been suggested that proliferating ductules, by serving as conduits for bile, permit the reflux into the parenchyma of bile constituents that serve as irritants or antigenic stimuli, and, thus, perpetuate inflammation and fibrogenesis. The evidence cited in support of this hypothesis is largely speculative, however.

The interlobular and septal bile ducts in cirrhotic lesions also undergo hyperplasia, resulting in their elongation, dilatation, and reduplication (73). However, these alterations, in contrast to those in the ductules, usually are unaccompanied by an inflammatory or fibrotic reaction.

In primary biliary cirrhosis (121–123) and in some cases of drug-induced, chronic, cholestatic hepatitis that progress to secondary biliary cirrhosis (124,125), the interlobular ducts undergo inflammation, degeneration, and necrosis, which lead to their obliteration. No doubt this biliary injury contributes to the cholestasis and progressive fibrosis that occur in such lesions, but additional factors are probably involved.

Hepatic dysfunction and failure

Active cirrhosis invariably impairs hepatic function, evidenced initially by serologic and biochemical abnormalities and, later, by clinical manifestations, such as jaundice, ascites, and edema, and, ultimately, by hepatic failure and death. Progressive destruction of hepatocytes usually accounts for this sequence of events. However, in some cases, secondary intrahepatic vascular changes, hemorrhage from esophageal or gastric varices, intercurrent infection, or the development of hepatocellular carcinoma plays an important role. Based on morphometric studies, it has been estimated that death from hepatic failure ensues when more than 67% of the hepatocytes are destroyed (126). These studies have also shown that estimates of hepatic parenchymal loss cannot be reliably based on total liver weight.

To a variable extent, the hepatocellular destruction in cirrhosis may be halted, leading to improvement in hepatic function, by measures that (1) eliminate the underlying etiologic factor, such as alcohol in the case of alcoholic cirrhosis; (2) modify metabolic aberrations responsible for hepatocellular injury, such as by depleting the excessive iron stores in hemochromatosis or by eliminating increased copper deposits in Wilson's disease; (3) suppress the inflammatory and immunologic reactions involved by the use of immunosuppressive agents in chronic active hepatitis; and (4) prevent or control variceal hemorrhage and intercurrent infections and other complications of cirrhosis that contribute to hepatic injury.

Occasionally, cirrhosis that develops insidiously may remain inactive for long periods. Such *inactive* lesions, often termed *latent cirrhosis* (127), may produce no signs or symptoms of hepatic dysfunction. However, they may be precipitated at some later date by variceal hemorrhage, intercurrent infection, the development of hepatocellular carcinoma, or slowly progressive loss of parenchyma, the atrophy of advancing age, or the continuing effects of underlying etiologic factors.

Complications

In addition to the signs of hepatic dysfunction and portal hypertension that often appear during the development of progression of cirrhotic lesions, the course of the disease may be complicated by the presence of portal hypertension.

Most of the deaths of cirrhotic patients are caused by the complications of portal hypertension rather than the result of hepatocellular function per se. In order of frequency and fatality rates, these complications are hemorrhage from esophagogastric varices, ascites with its consequences, the hepatorenal syndrome and spontaneous bacterial peritonitis, hepatic encephalopathy, and hypersplenism (128). The nature of the complications depends on the type of cirrhosis, which to a large extent determines the type of portal hypertension. Postsinusoidal portal hypertension, which is found in congestive or veno-occlusive cirrhosis, or the Budd-Chiari syndrome, is usually characterized by intractable ascites, as well as any of the other manifestations of portal hypertension. Alcoholic cirrhosis induces sinusoidal portal hypertension due to obliteration of the intersinusoidal communications, and ascites is a common and often severe sign (129). Virtually all of the other types of cirrhosis including postnecrotic posthepatitic cirrhosis and hemochromatosis, Wilson's disease, and primary biliary cirrhosis all have a mixed type of portal hypertension with both sinusoidal and presinusoidal components. These forms of cirrhosis are characterized by higher portal venous pressure levels measured directly in the portal vein than those measured indirectly by hepatic vein catheterization, thus reflecting the presinusoidal component (130). Ascites is neither frequent nor severe in these forms of nonalcoholic cirrhosis. In pure presinusoidal portal hypertension that is seen with portal or splenic vein thrombosis and with schistosomiasis, which is not a true cirrhosis, ascites is not part of the clinical picture. Esophageal varices and hypersplenism may develop in all types of portal hypertension. Ascites, however, occurs only with intrahepatic portal sinusoidal or postsinusoidal portal hypertension. Occasionally, ascites may develop in patients with ''pipestem'' schistosomiasis when the disease is very advanced, usually in conjunction with HBV chronic hepatitis, and sinusoidal portal hypertension coexists. Other consequences of cirrhosis including hypoxemia (131), cholelithiasis (132), peptic ulcer (133), bacteremia (134), bacterial peritonitis (135), bacteriuria (136) and other bacterial infections, hepatocellular carcinoma (137), and portal vein thrombosis (138) may occur with any type of cirrhosis, although they are more likely to occur in the presence of portal hypertension.

Histopathology

Overall architectural pattern

Although the width and contours of the fibrous septa and the size and shape of the parenchymal nodules may vary, the overall pattern of diffuse fibrosis and nodulation is remarkably similar in all forms of cirrhosis, as illustrated by such diverse lesions as alcoholic cirrhosis (Fig. 50), postnecrotic cirrhosis secondary to chronic active hepatitis (Fig. 57), primary biliary cirrhosis (Fig. 570), genetic hemochromatosis (Fig. 571), Wilson's disease (Fig. 572), and congestive cirrhosis (Fig. 503). The one exception to this generalization is the relatively rare form of ''diffuse interstitial cirrhosis'' that may occasionally be encountered in alcoholic liver disease, congenital syphilis, unresolved neonatal hepatitis, or other disorders. Lesions of this type are characterized by a uniformly distributed, fine perisinusoidal and perihepatocytic cellular fibrosis that destroys the normal lobular architecture, but does not provoke a nodular regenerative response (Figs. 62, 63).

The pattern of small nodules and fibrous septa tends to be relatively uniform in moderately advanced micronodular cirrhosis, so the character of the lesions is readily identified in needle biopsy specimens, as is evident in the section of alcoholic cirrhosis illustrated in Figure 50. However, during the early phases

of cirrhosis, some areas of the section may contain occasional intact lobules, or show only bridging fibrosis, so if the specimen is small or fragmented, the nodularity of the lesion may escape detection. Usually, an unbroken section of at least 10 to 15 mm in length ensures against this type of sampling error. The use of multiple biopsies (139) and larger biopsies (140) can decrease sampling error.

As might be anticipated, macronodular cirrhosis may be difficult to identify in needle biopsy specimens, not only because the diameter of the nodules exceeds the width of sections, but also because relatively normal-appearing areas are more common than in micronodular cirrhosis. Obviously, a nodule significantly larger than the width of the specimen, if sectioned through its center, will present as a relatively long segment of apparently normal parenchyma (Fig. 59), bordered on either side by fibrous bands or nodules (Fig. 57), but giving no indication of its nodular character (Figs. 55, 59). Tangential sections of such large nodules appear as semilunar or hemispheric masses of parenchyma outlined by scalloped bands of fibrous tissue that may suggest a zone of bridging fibrosis (Fig. 58). Fortunately, macronodular lesions usually contain at least a few small nodules (Fig. 53) that are often included in needle biopsy sections, thus obviating errors in interpretation. Moreover, the irregular, thickened hepatic plates (Fig. 59), and the absence or irregular pattern of distribution of portal tracts and central veins in the parenchyma of such incompletely visualized nodules (Fig. 55) serve to differentiate them from islands of intact lobules. Only when most of the nodules are slightly larger than normal lobules (1.5–3.0 mm) can the size of the nodules be accurately recognized (Fig. 57). However, irrespective of nodule size, the typical pattern of fibrosis and nodulation is always evident in surgical wedge biopsy sections (Figs. 52–54).

Unfortunately, aspiration needle biopsy of the cirrhotic liver, particularly of the macronodular type, may yield fragments of parenchyma and fibrous tissue, but no frank nodules or well-defined septa, making identification of cirrhosis exceedingly difficult. Such fragmentation is attributable to failure of the biopsy needle to core out segments of the fibrous septa it traverses, while the softer parenchyma within the nodules is readily aspirated. Use of the Klatskin modified Menghini biopsy needle with a tip that is sharply pointed and with a sharp circumferential cutting edge (Figs. 2, 3) will often avoid this problem. When several passes have failed to obtain an adequate core, a Vin-Silverman or Tru-Cut needle may provide a continuous core of tissue (141). If it fails to do so, careful examination of serial Masson- or reticulin-stained sections of the parenchymal fragments often reveals slender remnants of the septa along their margins that are not evident in routine H & E sections. In addition, if the fragments are sufficiently large, cirrhosis may be suggested by the absence of normal portal tracts and central veins, and the presence of a thickened, irregular hepatic plate pattern.

The distinctive distorted architectural pattern in cirrhosis is best visualized in Masson- or reticulin-stained sections. We prefer the former, since it not only demonstrates the distribution of the fibrous tissue but also permits identification of all other components of the liver. However, reticulin-stained sections may be useful in differentiating between zones of collapsed reticulin (Fig. 68) and bands of collagen [(142); Fig. 572], which are sometimes difficult to differentiate on H & E or Masson-stained sections. The presence of copper-associated protein in hepatocytes near septa in patients without other reasons for copper deposition suggests the diagnosis of cirrhosis (143). Similarly, staining for elastic fibers that are not found in fresh areas of collapse can be used to differentiate acute from chronic lesions (144).

Attempts to make a diagnosis of cirrhosis by ultrasonographic and magnetic resonance imaging have met with variable results (145–147). The unequivocal demonstration of the presence or degree of fibrosis can so far be achieved *in vivo* only by histologic methods.

Parenchymal nodules

The parenchymal nodules in cirrhosis vary not only in size but also in shape. Although some may be symmetric and round or oval in shape (Figs. 57, 570, 572), more often they exhibit irregular contours (Figs. 50, 52, 571), and, when large, may be indented or traversed by fibrous projections from the septa (Figs. 52–54).

In active cirrhotic lesions, the margins of the nodules are irregular and ill-defined, owing to erosion of their limiting plates and extension of inflammatory cells and fibrous tissue from the septa into the parenchyma (Figs. 50, 503). In contrast, the nodules in inactive lesions are sharply defined and enclosed within smooth-contoured septa (Figs. 52–54, 449).

The hepatocytes in most cirrhotic nodules are arranged in the form of irregular hepatic plates that are two or more cells thick (Fig. 51), a feature indicative of their *regenerative activity*. In highly active lesions, the regenerating hepatocytes, particularly in the zones bordering the septa, often exhibit a cylindric configuration in the form of rosettes (Fig. 106) or pseudoducts (Fig. 205) that may contain inspissated bile (Fig. 559). In contrast, the parenchymal nodules in late inactive cirrhosis often show no evidence of regenerative activity, the hepatocytes having reverted to a normal, one-cell-thick, radiating, plate pattern (Fig. 56). However, occasionally, such nodules may contain small foci of proliferating hepatocytes (Fig. 203).

Although some of the central veins and portal tracts found within regenerating nodules are newly formed structures, others may represent remnants of the original lobules. Such central vein remnants are relatively common in cirrhotic lesions that evolve as a result of progressive portal-portal bridging fibrosis, as in the case of primary biliary cirrhosis (Fig. 570). Similarly, in cirrhotic lesions that develop as a consequence of progressive central-central bridging fibrosis, some of the nodules may contain intact portal tracts derived from lobules, as in the case of cardiac cirrhosis (Fig. 505). Finally, in the coarsely macronodular type of cirrhosis that follows healing of submassive hepatic necrosis, some of the large nodules often contain multiple intact lobules that escaped destruction during the acute phase of the disease.

The *activity* of cirrhotic lesions is assessed histologically on the basis of the extent to which the limiting plates are eroded, the prominence of hepatocellular degeneration and necrosis, and the intensity of the accompanying parenchymal, inflammatory reaction. As a rule, the degree of activity parallels the severity of the clinical manifestations and biochemical evidence of hepatic dysfunction, and reflects the potential for further progression of the disease. *Erosion of the limiting plates* is segmental in character and affects only a few of the septa in *mildly active lesions* (Fig. 57), is more extensive and involves many of the septa in *moderately active lesions* (Figs. 50, 450), and tends to be universal in *severely active lesions* (Fig. 461). Usually, the severity of the hepatocellular abnormalities and the intensity of the inflammatory reaction in the parenchyma parallels the extent of the erosions. The hepatocellular changes that may be encountered include rosette formation (Fig. 106), ballooning (Fig. 109), and, in the case of alcoholic cirrhosis, both ballooning and Mallory body formation (Fig. 318), features often accompanied by fine pericellular and perisinusoidal fibrosis (Fig. 106). The character of the parenchymal inflammatory exudate varies, being predominantly lymphocytic and plasmacytic in lesions associated with chronic active hepatitis (Fig. 106) and primary biliary cirrhosis (Fig. 109), and mixed neutrophilic and lymphocytic in alcoholic cirrhosis (Fig. 318) and secondary biliary cirrhosis. Characteristically, in *inactive cirrhotic lesions,* the parenchyma shows no evidence of inflammation, degeneration, or necrosis, and the limiting plates are intact (Figs. 52, 53, 449).

Cholestasis is another feature of cirrhosis that denotes activity relatively early in the course. Usually, however, it is a manifestation of hepatic decompensation in relatively advanced cirrhosis. In contrast, to their usual centrilobular localization in noncirrhotic cholestatic lesions, the bile thrombi in cirrhosis may appear first in periportal or periseptal canaliculi (Fig. 557), and only later extend deeper into the parenchymal nodules.

Other alterations in the hepatocytes, although not necessarily indicative of activity, often provide clues to the etiology and pathogenesis of cirrhotic lesions. Among them are *cytoplasmic deposits* of *triglyceride* in alcoholic cirrhosis (Fig. 49), *hemosiderin* in hemochromatosis (Fig. 161), *copper* in Wilson's disease (Fig. 163), *protoporphyrin* in erythropoietic protoporphyria (Figs. 166–170), *amylopectin* in type IV glycogenosis (Figs. 148, 149), *α-1-antitrypsin* bodies in α-1-antitrypsin deficiency (Figs. 152, 153), *mucopolysaccharides* in Hurler's syndrome (Fig. 186), and *cholesterol esters* in Wolman's disease (Figs. 179, 180).

Other hepatocellular *cytoplasmic inclusions* that may be encountered include *Mallory bodies* in alcoholic cirrhosis (Figs. 130, 318), *orcein-positive ground glass cells* in HBsAg-positive cirrhosis (Figs. 136, 138), mitochondria-filled *oncocytes* in various forms of cirrhosis, but particularly in those attributable to chronic hepatitis B infections (Figs. 124, 125), and *megamitochondria* in alcoholic cirrhosis (Fig. 134). *Hepatocellular dysplasia* (Figs. 195, 196), another feature in some cases of cirrhosis, may be of prognostic significance, since it may be a forerunner of hepatocellular carcinoma. Occasionally, excessive multinucleation of hepatocytes occurs in cirrhosis without the other histologic features of dysplasia (142). Whether this lesion has prognostic significance is not known. In posthepatitic cirrhosis, true dysplasia may be seen (148).

Foci of *ischemic hepatocellular necrosis* of variable size are relatively common findings in some of the parenchymal nodules of cirrhosis following massive gastrointestinal hemorrhage or other causes of severe hypotension (Figs. 99, 100).

Fibrous septa

Since the evolution of cirrhotic lesions entails progressive fibrosis and replacement of normal lobules by nodules of regenerating parenchyma, the extent of fibrosis and nodule formation serves as a simple basis for classifying cirrhotic lesions in terms of their stage of development and degree of activity. *Early cirrhotic lesions* are characterized by relatively slender, fibrous septa that outline a few nodules, bridge adjacent lobules without forming nodules, and, occasionally, spare intact lobules. A lesion of this type in primary biliary cirrhosis is illustrated in Figures 573–575. Shown are well-defined nodules, zones of portal-portal bridging fibrosis, and an occasional intact lobule in three adjacent microscopic fields. In *moderately advanced* lesions, the fibrous septa are thicker and the nodules more numerous, but zones of bridging fibrosis may persist. In *advanced cirrhosis,* nodulation is universal, and the septa are relatively thick (Figs. 50, 53, 57, 58). However, in the advanced lesions of diffuse interstitial cirrhosis, fibrosis is extensive, but the individual fibrous bands are slender and diffusely distributed in a pericellular and perisinusoidal distribution (Figs. 62, 63).

In active cirrhosis, irrespective of its stage of development, the septal collagen bundles are relatively loosely arranged, owing to their separation by inflammatory cells and proliferating ductules (Figs. 50, 58, 450), or, in the case of septa derived from large zones of collapsed reticulin, by persistence of sinusoids, inflammatory cells, and ductules (Fig. 468). As the activity of the lesions abates, the collagen bundles tend to condense, forming dense, relatively avascular, acellular septa (Figs. 53, 449).

Usually, the intensity of the inflammatory reaction in the septa parallels that in the parenchyma (Figs. 450, 461). However, septal inflammatory cells may persist long after the lesions become quiescent (Fig. 576), so they are not a reliable criterion of activity. As in the case of parenchymal exudates, the character of the cells found in the septa varies, depending on the etiology of the cirrhosis. Lymphocytes and plasma cells predominate in postnecrotic cirrhosis secondary to chronic active hepatitis (Fig. 467) and primary biliary cirrhosis (Fig. 342), while numerous neutrophils may be encountered in active alcoholic cirrhosis (Fig. 318) and secondary biliary cirrhosis (Fig. 363). Occasionally, the lymphocytes and plasma cells in postnecrotic cirrhosis (Fig. 467) and primary biliary cirrhosis (Fig. 295) are aggregated in the form of lymphoid follicles. In addition, some of the septa and portal tracts contain epithelioid and giant cell granulomas. These are encountered most frequently in primary biliary cirrhosis (Fig. 342), but may also be seen in chronic active hepatitis (Fig. 371).

Bile duct alterations

Ductular proliferation is a relatively common finding in most forms of *active* cirrhosis (Figs. 359, 360, 462). However, the ductules tend to disappear as the activity of the lesions abates (Figs. 53, 449).

In many cases of primary biliary cirrhosis, some of the interlobular ducts show segmental stratification, vacuolization, lymphocytic infiltration, and necrosis of their epithelial lining cells (Figs. 364–367). Often, such ducts lie in close proximity to granulomas or lymphoid follicles (Fig. 295). Although characteristic of intermediate stage primary biliary cirrhosis, duct lesions of this type are not pathognomonic, and may be encountered in other disorders, such as chronic active hepatitis (Figs. 370, 371). As the lesions of primary biliary cirrhosis progress to the late cirrhotic stage, the affected ducts are obliterated, so, ultimately, many of the fibrous portal tracts completely lack interlobular ducts (Fig. 379). In such late stages peripherally located proliferating ductules are often found (Fig. 359).

Vascular abnormalities

In some cases of cirrhosis, central and sublobular veins incorporated within fibrous septa contain organized thrombi. Vascular lesions of this type are relatively common in the Budd-Chiari syndrome (Figs. 215, 502), and may be encountered occasionally in alcoholic cirrhosis (Fig. 273). The coarse longitudinal bundles of collagen in the walls of central and sublobular veins that give them a beaded appearance in cross-section, a feature best visualized in Masson-stained sections, facilitate their identification and differentiation from portal vein radicles.

Widespread, but irregularly distributed zones of severe sinusoidal congestion are a distinctive feature of congestive cirrhosis attributable to long-standing congestive heart failure (Fig. 577) or the Budd-Chiari syndrome (Fig. 213). Rarely, similar zones of severe congestion limited to only a few nodules may be encountered in alcoholic cirrhotic lesions accompanied by occlusion of central and sublobular veins (Fig. 578). However, not infrequently, some of the parenchymal nodules in other forms of cirrhosis exhibit focal areas of mild to moderate congestion in the apparent absence of venous thrombi (Fig. 579).

Capillarization of the sinusoids, characterized by perisinusoidal fibrosis that may narrow or occlude some of the sinusoidal lumens, is a relatively common feature in alcoholic cirrhosis (Fig. 580), but, occasionally, is found in other forms of cirrhosis (93).

References

1. Millward-Sadler GH: Cirrhosis. *In* Pathology of the Liver, edited by R. N. M. MacSween, P. P. Anthony, P. J. Scheuer. 2nd Edition. Edinburgh, Churchill Livingstone, 1987, pp. 342–363.
2. Simpson GEC, Finckh ES: The pattern of regeneration of rat liver after repeated partial hepatectomies. J Pathol Bacteriol 86:361–370, 1963.
3. Perez-Tamayo R: Diffuse interstitial cirrhosis. Am J Clin Pathol 29:226–235, 1958.
4. Popper H, Szanto PB, Parthasarathy M: Florid cirrhosis. A review of 35 cases. Am J Clin Pathol 25:889–901, 1955.
5. Edmondson H, Peters RL, Reynolds TB, Kuzma OT: Sclerosing hyaline necrosis of the liver in the chronic alcoholic. Ann Intern Med 59:646–673, 1973.
6. Peace R: Fatal hepatitis and cirrhosis in infancy. A critical analysis of thirty-two cases studied at necropsy. Arch Pathol 61:107–119, 1956.
7. Poucell S, Ireton J, Valencia-Mayoral P, Downar E, Larratt L, Patterson J, Blendis L, Phillips MJ: Amiodarone-associated phospholipidosis and fibrosis of the liver. Light, immunohistochemical, and electron microscopic studies. Gastroenterology 86:926–936, 1984.
8. Petrelli M, Scheuer PJ: Variations in subcapsular liver structure and its significance in the interpretation of wedge biopsies. J Clin Pathol 20:743–748, 1967.
9. Lieberman E, Salinas-Madrigal L, Gwinn JL, Brennan LP, Fine RN, Landing BH: Infantile polycystic disease of the kidneys and liver: clinical, pathological and radiological correlations and comparison with congenital hepatic fibrosis. Medicine 50:277–318, 1971.
10. Landing BH, Wells TR, Claireaux AE: Morphometric analysis of liver lesions in cystic diseases of childhood. Hum Pathol 11:549–560, 1980.
11. Kerr DNS, Harrison CV, Sherlock S, Walker RM: Congenital hepatic fibrosis. Q J Med 30:91–117, 1961.
12. Desmet VJ: Intrahepatic bile ducts under the lens. J Hepatol 1:545–559, 1985.
13. Stromeyer FW, Ishak KG: Nodular transformation (nodular regenerative hyperplasia) of the liver. A clinicopathologic study of 30 cases. Hum Pathol 12:60–71, 1981.
14. Wanless IR, Godwin TA, Allen F, Feder A: Nodular regenerative hyperplasia in hematologic disorders: a possible response to portal venopathy. A morphometric study of nine cases with an hypothesis on the pathogenesis. Medicine 59:367–379, 1980.
15. Nakanuma Y, Ohta G: Nodular hyperplasia of the liver in primary

biliary cirrhosis of early histological stages. Am J Gastroenterol 82:8–10, 1987.

16. Wanless IR, Mawdsley C, Adams R: On the pathogenesis of focal nodular hyperplasia of the liver. Hepatology 5:1194–1200, 1985.

17. Wanless IR: Understanding non-cirrhotic portal hypertension: menage a fois. Hepatology 8:192–193, 1988.

18. Ishak KG, Rabin L: Benign tumors of the liver. Med Clin North Am 59;995–1013, 1975.

19. Symmers D, Spain DM: Hepar lobatum. Clinical significance of the anatomic changes. Arch Pathol 42:64–68, 1946.

20. Cooney T, Sweeney EC, Coll R, Greally M: Pseudocirrhosis in hereditary haemorrhagic telangiectasia. J Clin Pathol 30:1134–1141, 1977.

21. Martini GA: The liver in hereditary haemorrhagic telangiectasia: an inborn error of vascular structure with multiple manifestations: a reappraisal. Gut 19:531–537, 1978.

22. Andrade ZA, Santana Filho S, Rubin E: Hepatic changes in advanced schistosomiasis. Gastroenterology 42:393–400, 1962.

23. Al-Nakib B, Al-Nakib W, Bayoumi A, Al-Liddawi H, Bashir AA: Hepatitis B virus (HBV) markers among patients with chronic liver disease in Kuwait. Trans R Soc Trop Med Hyg 76:348–350, 1982.

24. Anthony PP, Ishak KG, Nayak NC, Poulsen H, Scheuer PJ, Sobin LH: The morphology of cirrhosis: definition, nomenclature, and classification. Bull WHO 55:521–540, 1977.

25. Leevy CM, Popper H, Sherlock S: Diseases of the Liver and Biliary Tract. Standardization of Nomenclature, Diagnostic Criteria, and Diagnostic Methodology. DHEW Publication No. (NIH) 76–725. Washington, DC, US Government Printing Office, 1976, p. 18.

26. Fauerholdt L, Schlichting P, Christensen E, Poulsen H, Tygstrup N, Juhl E, and The Copenhagen Study Group for Liver Diseases: Conversion of micronodular cirrhosis into macronodular cirrhosis. Hepatology 3:928–931, 1983.

27. Shikata T: Primary carcinoma and liver cirrhosis. In Hepatocellular Carcinoma, edited by K. Okuda, R. L. Peters. New York, John Wiley & Sons, 1976, pp. 53–71.

28. Ludwig J: Some names hang on like leeches. Dig Dis Sci 24:967–969, 1979.

29. Gall EA: Posthepatitic, postnecrotic and nutritional cirrhosis. A pathologic analysis. Am J Pathol 36:241–271, 1960.

30. Baggenstoss AH: Postnecrotic cirrhosis: morphology, etiology and pathogenesis. In Progress in Liver Diseases, Vol. I, edited by H. Popper, F. Schaffner. New York, Grune & Stratton, 1961, pp. 14–38.

31. Baggenstoss AH, Stauffer MH: Posthepatitic cirrhosis. Proc Staff Meet Mayo Clin 28:320–329, 1953.

32. Popper H, Rubin E, Krus S, Schaffner F: Postnecrotic cirrhosis in alcoholics. Gastroenterology 39:669–685, 1960.

33. Powell LW, Mortimer P, Harris OD: Cirrhosis of the liver. A comparative study of the four major aetiological groups. Med J Austral 1:941–950, 1971.

34. MacSween RNM, Scott AR: Hepatic cirrhosis: a clinicopathological review of 520 cases. J Clin Pathol 26:936–942, 1973.

35. Hasan F, Jeffers LJ, deMedina M, Reddy R, Parker T, Schiff ER, Houghton M, Choo QL, Kuo G: Hepatitis C-associated hepatocellular carcinoma. Hepatology 12:589–591, 1990.

36. Katkov WN, Cody H, Evans AA, Kuo G, Choo QL, Houghton M, Dienstag JL: The role of Hepatitis C virus (HCV) in chronic liver disease. Hepatology 10:644, 1989 (abstract).

37. Hoff RH, Bunker JP, Goodman HI, Gregory PB: Halothane hepatitis in three pairs of closely related women. N Engl J Med 304:1023–1024, 1981.

38. Farrell G, Prendergast D, Murray M: Halothane hepatitis. Detection of a constitutional susceptibility factor. N Engl J Med 313:1310–1314, 1985.

39. Sloan TP, Mahgoub A, Lancaster R, Idle JR, Smith RL: Polymorphism of carbon oxidation of drugs and clinical implications. Br Med J 2:655–657, 1978.

40. Morgan MY, Reshef R, Shah RR, Oates NS, Smith RL, Sherlock S: Impaired oxidation of debrisoquine in patients with perhexiline liver injury. Gut 25:1057–1064, 1984.

41. Pares A, Barrera JM, Caballeria J, Ercilla G. Bruguera M, Caballeria L, Castillo R, Rodes J: Hepatitis C virus antibodies in chronic alcoholic patients: association with severity of liver injury. Hepatology 12:1295–1299, 1990.

42. Minuk GY, Kelly JK, Hwang W-S: Vitamin A hepatotoxicity in multiple family members. Hepatology 8:272–275, 1988.

43. Leo MA, Lieber CS: Hepatic fibrosis after long term administration of ethanol and moderate vitamin A supplementation in the rat. Hepatology 3:1–11, 1983.

44. Popper H, Udenfriend S: Hepatic fibrosis. Am J Med 49:707–721, 1970.

45. Maddrey WC, Iber FL: Familial cirrhosis. A clinical and pathological study. Ann Intern Med 61:667–679, 1964.

46. Boyer JL, Klatskin G: Pattern of necrosis of acute viral hepatitis. Prognostic value of bridging (subacute hepatic necrosis). N Engl J Med 283:1063–1071, 1970.

47. Ware AJ, Cuthbert JA, Shorey J, Gurian LE, Eigenbrodt EH, Combes B: A prospective trial of steroid therapy in severe viral hepatitis. The prognostic significance of bridging necrosis. Gastroenterology 80:219–224, 1980.

48. Castilla A, Prieto J, Fausto N: Transforming growth factors β1 and α in chronic liver disease. Effects of interferon alfa therapy. N Engl J Med 324:933–940, 1991.

49. Popper H, Schaffner F, Barka T: Has proliferation of bile ductules clinical significance? Acta Hepato-Spleno 9:129–139, 1962.

50. Feinman L, Lieber CS: Hepatic collagen metabolism: effect of alcohol consumption in rats and baboons. Science 176:795, 1972.

51. Zern MA, Leo MA, Giambrone M-A: Increased type I procollagen mRNA levels and in vitro protein synthesis in the baboon model of chronic alcoholic liver disease. Gastroenterology 89:1123–1131, 1985.

52. Galambos JT, Hollingsworth MA Jr, Falek A, Warren WD: The rate of synthesis of glycosaminoglycans and collagen by fibroblasts cultured from adult human liver biopsies. J Clin Invest 60:107–114, 1977.

53. Henley KS, Laughrey EG, Appleman HD, Flecker K: Effect of ethanol on collagen formation in dietary cirrhosis in the rat. Gastroenterology 72:502–506, 1977.

54. Brenner DA, Chojkier M: Acetaldehyde increases collagen gene transcription in cultured human fibroblasts. J Biol Chem 262:17690–17695, 1987.

55. Holt K, Bennett M, Chojkier M: Acetaldehyde stimulates collagen and noncollagen protein production by human fibroblasts. Hepatology 4:843–848, 1984.

56. Russell RM, Boyer JL, Bagheri SA, Hruban Z: Hepatic injury from chronic hypervitaminosis A resulting in portal hypertension and ascites. Gastroenterology 291:435–440, 1974.

57. Berk PD, Martin JF, Young RS, Creech J, Selikoff IJ, Falk H, Watanabe P, Popper H, Thomas L: Vinyl chloride-associated liver disease. Ann Intern Med 84:717–731, 1976.

58. Gedigk P, Muller R, Bechtelsheimer H: Morphology of liver damage among polyvinyl chloride production workers. A report of 51 cases. Ann NY Acad Sci 246:278–285, 1975.

59. Popper H, Lieber CS: Histogenesis of alcoholic fibrosis and cirrhosis in the baboon. Am J Pathol 98:695–716, 1980.

60. Nakano M, Worner TM, Lieber CS: Perivenular fibrosis in alcoholic liver injury. Ultrastructure and histologic progression. Gastroenterology 83:777–785, 1982.

61. Wahl SM, Hunt DA, Wakefield LM: Transforming growth factor type B induces monocyte chemotaxis and growth factor production. Proc Natl Acad Sci USA 84:5788–5792, 1987.

62. Rojkind M, Dunn MA: Hepatic fibrosis. Gastroenterology 76:849–863, 1979.

63. Chojkier M, Brenner DA: Therapeutic strategies for hepatic fibrosis. Hepatology 8:176–182, 1988.

64. Sherlock S. Hepatic cirrhosis. In Diseases of the Liver and Biliary System, edited by S. Sherlock. 8th Edition. London, Blackwell Scientific Publications, 1989, pp. 410–424.

65. Seyer JM, Hutchenson ET, Kang AH: Collagen polymorphism in normal and cirrhotic human liver. J Clin Invest 59:241–248, 1977.

66. Babbs C, Smith A, Hunt LP. Type III procollagen peptide: a marker of disease activity and prognosis in primary biliary cirrhosis. Lancet 1:1021–1023, 1988.

67. Malizia G, Giannuoli G, Caltagirone M: Procollagen type I production by hepatocytes: a marker of progressive liver disease? Lancet 2:1055–1058, 1987.

68. Clement B, Grimaud J-A, Campion JP: Cell types involved in collagen and fibronectin production in normal and fibrotic human liver. Hepatology 6:225–234, 1986.

69. Maher JJ, Friedman SL, Roll FJ: Immunolocalisation of laminin in normal rat liver and biosynthesis of laminin by hepatic lipocytes in primary culture. Gastroenterology 94:1053–1058, 1988.

70. Arenson DM, Bissell DM: Glycosaminoglycan, proteoglycan, and hepatic fibrosis. Gastroenterology 92:536–538, 1987.

71. Carlsson R, Engvall E, Freeman A: Laminin and fibronectin in cell

adhesion: enhanced adhesion of cells from regenerating liver to laminin. Proc Natl Acad Sci USA 78:2403–2406, 1981.

72. Roberts AB, Sporn MB, Assoian RK: Transforming growth factor type: rapid induction of fibrosis and angiogenesis *in vitro*. Proc Natl Acad Sci USA 83:4167–4171, 1986.

73. Senior RM, Huang JS, Griffin GL: Dissociation of the chemotactic and mitogenic activities of platelet-derived growth factor by human neutrophil elastase. J Cell Biol 100:351–356, 1985.

74. Maruyama K, Feinman L, Fainsilber Z: Mammalian collagenase increases in early alcoholic liver disease and decreases with cirrhosis. Life Sci 30:1379–1384, 1982.

75. Cameron GR, Karunaratne WAE: Carbon tetrachloride cirrhosis in relation to liver regeneration. J Pathol Bacteriol 42:1–21, 1936.

76. Kershenobich D, Vargas F, Garcia-Tsao G, Tamayo RP, Gent M, Rojkind M: Colchicine in the treatment of cirrhosis of the liver. N Engl J Med 318:1709–1713, 1988.

77. Warnes TW, Smith A, Lee FI, Haboubi NY, Johnson PJ, Hunt L: A controlled trial of colchicine in primary biliary cirrhosis. J Hepatol 5:1–7, 1987.

78. Jimenez SA, Freundlich B, Rosenbloom J: Selective inhibition of human diploid fibroblast collagen synthesis by interferons. J Clin Invest 74:1112–1116, 1984.

79. Ruwart JM, Rush BD, Snyder KF: 16,16-Dimethyl prostaglandin E$_2$ delays collagen formation in nutritional injury in rat liver. Hepatology 8:61–64, 1988.

80. Sakakibara K, Ooshima A, Igarashi S, Sakakibara J: Immunolocalization of type III collagen and procollagen in cirrhotic human liver using monoclonal antibodies. Virchows Arch Pathol Anat 409:37–46, 1986.

81. Morseet AFW, Lesch R, Jobsis AC: Histometry of connective tissue in hepatic fibrosis. Acta Histochemica 20(Suppl):331–338, 1978.

82. Jimenez W, Pares A, Caballeria J, Heredia D, Bruguera M, Torres M, Rojkind M, Rodes J: Measurement of fibrosis in needle liver biopsies: evaluation of a colorimetric method. Hepatology 5:815–818, 1985.

83. Starzl TE, Francavilla A, Halgrimson CG, Francavilla FR, Porter KA, Brown TH, Putnam CW: The origin, hormonal nature, and action of hepatotrophic substances in portal venous blood. Surg Gynecol Obstet 137:179–199, 1973.

84. Starzl TE, Porter KA, Putnam CW: Insulin, glucagon, and the control of hepatic structure, function and capacity for regeneration. Metabolism 25:1429–1434, 1976.

85. Starzl TE, Jones AF, Terblanche J, Usui S, Porter K, Mazzoni G: Growth stimulating factor in regenerating canine liver. Lancet 1:127–130, 1979.

86. Bucher NLR: Regeneration of liver in rats deprived of portal splanchnic organs and a portal blood supply. *In* Liver Regeneration After Experimental Injury, edited by R. Lesch, W. Reutter. New York, Stratton Intercontinental Medical Book Corp., 1975, pp. 180–188.

87. Johnston DG, Alberti KGMM, Faber OK: Hyperinsulinism of hepatic cirrhosis: diminished degradation or hypersecretion? Lancet 1:10–12, 1977.

88. Smith-Laing G, Sherlock S, Faber OK: Effects of spontaneous portal-system shunting on insulin metabolism. Gastroenterology 76:685–690, 1979.

89. Leffert HL, Koch KS, Lad PJ, Skelly H, deHemptinne B: Hepatocyte regeneration, replication and differentiation. *In* The Liver: Biology and Pathobiology, edited by I. M. Arias, H. Popper, D. Schacter, D. A. Shafritz. New York, Raven Press, 1982, pp. 601–604.

90. Fausto N: New perspectives on liver regeneration. Hepatology 6:326–327, 1986.

91. Widman JJ, Fahimi HD: The regenerative response of Kupffer cells and endothelial cells after partial hepatectomy. *In* Liver Regeneration After Experimental Injury, edited by R. Lesch, W. Reutter. New York, Stratton Intercontinental Medical Book Corp., 1975, pp. 89–98.

92. Rappaport AM, MacPhee PJ, Fisher MM, Phillips MJ: The scarring of the liver acini (cirrhosis). Tridimensional and microcirculatory considerations. Virchows Archiv A Pathol Anat Histopathol 402:107–137, 1983.

93. Schaffner F, Popper H: Capillarization of the hepatic sinusoids. Gastroenterology 44:239–242, 1963.

94. Reynolds TB, Hidemura R, Michel H, Peters RL: Portal hypertension in alcoholic liver disease. Ann Intern Med 70:497–506, 1969.

95. Bras G, Brandt K: Vascular disorders. *In* Pathology of the Liver, edited by R. N. M. MacSween, P. P. Anthony, P. J. Scheuer. London, Churchill Livingstone, 1987, pp. 478–502.

96. Popper H, Hutterer F: Hepatic fibrogenesis and disturbance of hepatic circulation. Ann NY Acad Sci 170:88–99, 1970.

97. McIndoe AH; Vascular lesions of portal cirrhosis. Arch Pathol Lab Med 5:23–40, 1928.

98. Kelty RH, Baggenstoss AH, Butt HR: The relation of the regenerating liver nodule to the vascular bed in cirrhosis. Gastroenterology 15:285–295, 1950.

99. Elias H, Sherrick JC: Morphology of the Liver. New York, Academic Press, 1969, pp. 80–81.

100. Popper H, Elias H, Petty DE: Vascular patterns of the cirrhotic liver. Am J Clin Pathol 22:717–729, 1952.

101. Nakanuma Y, Ohta G, Doishita K: Quantitation and serial section observations of focal venocclusive lesions of hepatic veins in liver cirrhosis. Virchow's Arch A Pathol Anat and Histopathol 405:429–438, 1985.

102. Dumont AF, Witte MH: Significance of excess lymph in the thoracic duct in patients with hepatic fibrosis. Am J Surg 112:401–406, 1966.

103. Baggenstoss AH, Cain JC: Further studies of the lymphatic vessels at the hilum of the liver in man: their relation to ascites. Proc Staff Meet Mayo Clin 32:615–627, 1957.

104. Witte CL, Witte MH, Dumont AE, Frist J, Cole WR: Lymph protein in hepatic cirrhosis and experimental hepatic and portal venous hypertension. Trans Am Surg Assoc 86;256–266, 1968.

105. Wood LJ, Colman J, Dudley FJ: The relationship between portal pressure and plasma albumin in the development of cirrhotic ascites. J Gastroenterol Hepatol 2:525–531, 1987.

106. Henriksen JH: Colloid osmotic pressure in decompensated cirrhosis: a "mirror image" of portal venous hypertension. Scand J Gastroenterol 20:170–174, 1985.

107. Levy M: Sodium retention and ascites formation in dogs with portal cirrhosis. Am J Physiol 233:572–585, 1977.

108. Unikowsky B, Wexler MJ, Levy M: Dogs with experimental cirrhosis of the liver but without intrahepatic hypertension do not retain sodium or form ascites. J Clin Invest 72:1594–1604, 1983.

109. Epstein M, Loutzenhiser R, Friedland E: Relationship of increased plasma atrial natriuretic factor and renal sodium handling during immersion-induced central hypervolemia in normal humans. J Clin Invest 79:738–745, 1987.

110. Shear L, Swartz C, Shinaberger JA, Barry KG: Kinetics of peritoneal fluid absorption in adult man. N Engl J Med 272:123–130, 1965.

111. Henriksen JH, Lassen NA, Parving H-H, Winkler K: Filtration as the main transport mechanism of protein exchange between plasma and the peritoneal cavity in hepatic cirrhosis. Scand J Clin Lab Invest 40:503–513, 1980.

112. Parving HH, Ranek L, Lassen NA: Increased transcapillary escape route of albumin in patients with cirrhosis of the liver. Scand J Clin Lab Invest 37:643–648, 1977.

113. LeVeen HH, Piccone VA, Hutto RB: Management of ascites with hydrothorax. Am J Surg 148:210–213, 1984.

114. Shear L, Ching S, Gabuzda GJ: Compartmentalization of ascites and edema in patients with hepatic cirrhosis. N Engl J Med 282:1391–1396, 1970.

115. Pockros PJ, Reynolds TB: Rapid diuresis in patients with ascites from chronic liver disease: the importance of peripheral edema. Gastroenterology 90:1827–1833, 1986.

116. Grisham JW, Porta EA: Origin and fate of proliferated hepatic ductal cells in the rat: electron microscopic and autoradiographic studies. Exp Mol Pathol 3:242–261, 1964.

117. Masuko K, Rubin E, Popper H: Proliferation of bile ducts in cirrhosis. Arch Pathol 78;421–431, 1964.

118. Buyssens N: Ductular proliferation. Gastroenterology 49:702–705, 1965.

119. Jorgensen M: A stereological study of intrahepatic bile ducts. 2. Bile duct proliferation in some pathological conditions. Acta Pathol Microbiol Scand, Sect A 81:663–669, 1973.

120. Desmet VJ: Morphologic and histochemical aspects of cholestasis. *In* Progress in Liver Diseases, Vol. IV, edited by H. Popper, F. Shaffner. New York, Grune & Stratton, 1972, pp. 97–132.

121. Popper H, Rubin E, Schaffner F: The problem of primary biliary cirrhosis. Am J Med 33:807–810, 1962.

122. Williams GEG: Pericholangiolitic biliary cirrhosis. J Pathol Bacteriol 89:23–34, 1965.

123. Baggenstoss AH, Foulk WT, Butt HR, Bahn RC: The pathology of primary biliary cirrhosis with emphasis on histogenesis. Am J Clin Pathol 42:259–276, 1964.

124. Gregory DH, Zaki GF, Sarosi A, Carey JB Jr: Chronic cholestasis

following prolonged tolbutamide administration associated with destructive cholangitis and cholangiolitis. Arch Pathol *84*:194–201, 1967.

125. Ishak KG, Irey NS: Hepatic injury associated with phenothiazines. Clinico-pathologic and follow-up study of 36 patients. Arch Pathol *93*:283–304, 1972.

126. Ludwig J, Elveback LR: Parenchyma weight changes in hepatic cirrhosis. A morphometric study and discussion of the method. Lab Invest *26*:338–343, 1972.

127. Ludwig J, Garrison CO, Baggenstoss AH; Latent cirrhosis. A study of 95 cases. Am J Dig Dis *15*:7–14, 1970.

128. Conn HO, Atterbury CE: Cirrhosis. *In* Diseases of the Liver, edited by L. Schiff, E. R. Schiff. 6th Edition. Philadelphia, Lippincott, 1987, pp. 725–864.

129. Conn HO, Groszmann RJ: The pathophysiology of portal hypertension. *In* The Liver: Biology and Pathobiology, edited by I. Arias, H. Popper, D. Schachter, D. A. Shafritz. New York, Raven Press, 1982, pp. 821–848.

130. Boyer TD, Triger DR, Horisawa M, Redeker AG, Reynolds TB: Direct transhepatic measurement of portal vein pressure using a thin needle. Gastroenterology *72*:584–589, 1977.

131. Rodman T: Arterial oxygen unsaturation and the ventilation-perfusion defect of Laennec's cirrhosis. N Engl J Med *263*:73–81, 1960.

132. Nicholas P, Rinaudo PA, Conn HO: Increased incidence of cholelithiasis in Laennec's cirrhosis. Gastroenterology *63*:112–121, 1972.

133. Kirk AP: Peptic ulceration in patients with chronic liver disease. Dig Dis *25*:756–763, 1980.

134. Graudal N, Milman N, Kirkegaard E: Bacteremia in cirrhosis of the liver. Liver *6*:297–303, 1986.

135. Hoefs JC, Canawati HN, Sapico FL: Spontaneous bacterial peritonitis. Hepatology *2*:399–407, 1982.

136. Burroughs AK, Rosenstein IJ, Epstein O: Bacteriuria and primary biliary cirrhosis. Gut *25*:133–138, 1984.

137. Anthony PP: Tumours and tumour-like lesions of the liver and biliary tract. *In* Pathology of the Liver, edited by R. N. M. MacSween, P. P. Anthony, P. J. Scheuer. Edinburgh, Churchill Livingstone, 1987, pp. 598–600.

138. Belli L, Sansalone CV, Aseni P, Romani F, Rondinara G: Portal thrombosis in cirrhotics. Ann Surg *203*:286–291, 1986.

139. Maharaj B, Maharaj RJ, Leary WP, Cooppan RM, Naran AD, Pirie D, Pudifin DJ: Sampling variability and its influence on the diagnostic yield of percutaneous needle biopsy of the liver. Lancet *1*:523–525, 1986.

140. Holund B, Poulsen H, Schlichting P: Reproducibility of liver biopsy diagnosis in relation to the size of the specimen. Scand J Gastroenterol *15*:329–335, 1980.

141. Colombo M, Del Ninno E, DeFranchis R, DeFazio C, Festorazzi S, Ronchi G, Tommasini MA: Ultrasound-assisted percutaneous liver biopsy: superiority of the tru-cut over the Menghini needle for diagnosis of cirrhosis. Gastroenterology *95*:487–489, 1988.

142. Scheuer PJ: Liver Biopsy Interpretation. London, Bailliere-Tindall, 1988, pp. 135–136.

143. Guarascio P, Yentis F, Cevikbas U, Portmann B, Williams R: Value of copper-associated protein in diagnostic assessment of liver biopsy. J Clin Pathol *36*:18–23, 1983.

144. Scheuer PJ, Maggi G: Hepatic fibrosis and collapse: histological distinction by orcein staining. Histopathology *4*:487–490, 1980.

145. Hoefs JC, Aufrichtig D, Lottenberg S: Non-invasive evaluation of hepatic fibrosis using frequency demodulation of ultra-sound signals. Dig Dis Sci *31*:1046–1051, 1986.

146. Taylor KJW, Riely CA, Hammers L, Flax S, Weltin G, Garcia-Tsao G, Conn HO, Duc R, Barwick KW: Quantitative US attenuation in normal liver and in patients with diffuse liver disease: importance of fat. Radiology *160*:65–71, 1986.

147. Chamuleau RAFM, Creyghton JHN, De Nie I, Moerland MA, Van der Lende OR, Smidt J: Is the magnetic resonance imaging proton spin-lattice relaxation time a reliable noninvasive parameter of developing liver fibrosis? Hepatology *8*:217–221, 1988.

148. Lefkowitch JH, Apfelbaum TF: Liver cell dysplasia and hepatocellular carcinoma in non-A, non-B hepatitis. Arch Pathol Lab Med *111*:170–173, 1987.

Chapter 10
Alcohol-Induced Liver Disease

Excessive consumption of ethanol is one of the major causes of hepatic injury in humans, and may lead to the development of fatty infiltration, alcoholic hepatitis, or cirrhosis, individually or in combination. Although such lesions have been the subject of exhaustive investigation for many years, many aspects of their pathogenesis and interrelationships are still obscure.

Factors in alcohol-induced hepatic injury

Metabolic

Alcohol, which cannot be stored in the body, undergoes obligatory catabolism in the liver, yielding seven calories per gram. Such calories provide a source of energy and, at least in experimental animals, may be utilized for the maintenance of growth (1) although less efficiently than those derived from normal diets. However, it has been suggested that if the capacity of the liver to metabolize alcohol completely is exceeded, alcohol or its metabolite, acetaldehyde, induces hepatotoxicity (2,3). The incidence of cirrhosis in chronic alcoholic patients is highest in those who consume more than 160 to 180 g daily, which approximates the maximal amount metabolized a day by adult men, and increases progressively with the duration of excessive drinking (2,3).

Alcohol is oxidized to acetaldehyde in the cytosol and then to acetate in the mitochondria of the hepatocytes by enzymatic reactions with alcohol dehydrogenase and acetaldehyde dehydrogenase, respectively, in which nicotinamide adenine dinucleotide (NAD) serves as a cofactor. The acetate generated may be further oxidized to carbon dioxide and water, or may enter the citric acid cycle and undergo conversion to other metabolites (4,5).

The enzymatic reactions involved in the oxidation of alcohol and acetaldehyde result in the transfer of hydrogen ions to NAD with the formation of NADH. If the alcohol intake is high, the capacity of the liver to dispose of hydrogen ions may be exceeded, leading to an increase in the NADH:NAD ratio and an alteration in the redox state of the liver. These alterations have a number of secondary effects on carbohydrate, lipid, amino acid, and protein metabolism, resulting in aberrations that may be of importance in the pathogenesis of at least some of the hepatic lesions produced by alcohol (5).

Usually, the acetaldehyde generated during the catabolism of alcohol is promptly oxidized. However, chronic alcoholism may impair the oxidative capacity of hepatic mitochondria, so acetaldehyde accumulates in the liver and blood (5,6). These observations have led to the hypothesis that some of the adverse effects of alcohol on the liver are caused by acetaldehyde-induced injury to hepatocellular membranes. Consistent with this hypothesis is evidence indicating that acetaldehyde interacts with amines, amino acids, and glutathione to produce potentially hepatotoxic compounds, promotes lipid peroxidation, and inhibits protein synthesis and secretion, effects that may result in hepatic injury (5,7–9).

Alcohol can also be metabolized in the hepatic microsomes by a microsomal ethanol-oxidizing system (MEOS). MEOS differs from alcohol dehydrogenase not only in its subcellular localization in the endoplasmic reticulum but also in its oxygen dependence, its requirement of NADPH as a cofactor, its pH optimum of 6.8–7.5, instead of 10.8, and its induction of an ethanol-specific form of cytochrome P450 (10) in an adaptive response to prolonged alcohol administration (11). As in the case of other microsomal, drug-detoxifying enzymes, the induction of MEOS results in the proliferation of smooth endoplasmic reticulum (12), which has the identical histologic appearance as HBV ground glass cytoplasmic inclusions except that they are orcein-negative.

Under experimental conditions, chronic alcohol consumption leads to a hypermetabolic state and an increase in the rate of oxygen consumption by the liver. Based on such observations, it has been proposed that relative hypoxia in the centrilobular zones of the liver may play a role in the pathogenesis of alcohol-induced hepatic injury (13). However, the hepatocellular cytoplasmic vacuolization produced by hypoxia (14) and the centrilobular coagulation necrosis characteristic of severe ischemia bear little resemblance to the lesions of alcoholic liver disease. It is unlikely, therefore, that relative hypoxia is a major determinant of alcohol-induced hepatic injury, although, conceivably, it plays a contributory role by rendering the liver more susceptible to other adverse effects of alcohol.

Toxic

The relationship between alcohol intake and the development of cirrhosis (2,3), fatty infiltration, and ultrastructural changes in the liver following the ingestion of alcohol under conditions of adequate nutrition in humans (12,15,16) provides the basis for considering alcohol to be a hepatotoxin. The induction of alcoholic hepatitis and cirrhosis in baboons maintained for long periods on a nutritionally adequate diet containing 50% of its calories in the form of alcohol (17,18) supports this point of view. However, the fact that alcoholic hepatitis and cirrhosis occur in only a minority of heavy drinkers, and that most attempts to reproduce these lesions in experimental animals have been unsuccessful (19,20) appear to be inconsistent with that concept, and suggest that other factors may be involved. There is little doubt that fatty infiltration is a direct effect of alcohol, related in some way to its metabolism, but not necessarily indicative of a hepatotoxic action. It is possible that alcohol is indirectly toxic, for example, by decreasing hepatic stores of glutathione (7), thus interfering with its protective functions against oxidative damage caused by a variety of other agents (8).

At first sight, the reported reproducibility of alcoholic hepatitis and cirrhosis in baboons appears to provide convincing evidence that alcohol is hepatotoxic. However, the adequacy of the protein and lipotropic content of the diet used in these experiments has been questioned (20) and the possibility suggested that alcohol merely accentuates lesions attributable to borderline choline deficiency, a well-known effect of alcohol in other species (21,22). It is apropos that primates maintained on a liquid diet that contained 40 to 50% of its calories in the form of alcohol, but one richer in protein and lipotropic activity, failed to develop hepatic fibrosis or cirrhosis. Thus, if nutritional factors are not implicated in the pathogenesis of alcoholic cirrhosis, it must be assumed that baboons and humans are uniquely susceptible to the hepatotoxic effects of alcohol. Further studies in the baboon, using diets more richly supplemented with protein and other lipotropes, are needed to exclude the possibility that nutritional factors are involved in the pathogenesis of cirrhosis in animals.

Nutritional

A number of clinical and experimental observations first suggested that malnutrition might be a major factor in the pathogenesis of alcoholic liver disease. However, with the recognition that alcoholic cirrhosis can develop in the apparent absence of malnutrition, and with the increased emphasis on the biochemical, metabolic, and hepatotoxic effects of alcohol, the nutritional theory has fallen in to disfavor.

In support of the nutritional theory may be cited the facts that excessive drinking often is associated with a reduction in food consumption, many chronic alcoholic patients exhibit overt signs of malnutrition, dietary supplements of protein and other lipotropic substances appear to improve hepatic function and prolong survival in patients with alcoholic cirrhosis (23), and diets deficient in protein and other lipotropes induce the development of cirrhosis in experimental animals (24–26).

The occurrence of lesions indistinguishable from those of alcoholic hepatitis and cirrhosis in massively obese patients subjected to jejunoileostomy to induce malabsorption and weight loss (27–30) and their frequent regression following parenteral nutrition appear to support the hypothesis that malnutrition may be a major factor in the pathogenesis of alcoholic liver disease. However, the assumption that malnutrition accounts for the development of hepatitis and cirrhosis following jejunoileostomy may be questioned, since parenteral hyperalimentation does not always reverse such lesions (29). Alternatively, it has been proposed that the hepatic injury seen following jejunoileostomy in dogs is attributable to endotoxin produced by the overgrowth of *Bacteroides* organisms in the blind loop of ileum, and that the appearance of such hepatic lesions can be prevented by the prophylactic administration of doxycycline, which suppresses such organisms. Unfortunately, doxycycline has proved ineffective in protecting against hepatic injury following jejunoileostomy in humans (31), casting doubt on the endotoxin theory. Since ileojejunostomy leads to significant alterations in bile

acid metabolism (32), it has been suggested that bile acids may play a role in the hepatic injury (33), an observation supported by the occasional finding of high serum levels of lithocholic and chenodeoxycholic acids (34).

Since dietary deficiency alone cannot account for the development of hepatic injury under all conditions of alcohol consumption, attention has been focused on the possibility that the adverse effects of alcohol on the liver may be attributable to its interactions with nutrients essential for the maintenance of normal hepatocellular structure and function. In an early study of this possibility, it was found that alcohol increased the choline requirements of the rat (22), an effect later shown to be the result of increased choline oxidase activity (35), and that if the diet was only marginal in choline content, alcohol administration led to the development of cirrhosis (22). The relevance of choline deficiency to hepatic injury in humans has been questioned, since choline oxidase activity and, hence, the choline requirements are significantly lower in primates than in the rat (36). However, the possibility that choline deficiency may play a role in the pathogenesis of hepatic injury in humans cannot be completely discounted, since choline deficiency may lead to the development of cirrhosis in monkeys (25,26).

More recent studies, reviewed elsewhere (37), have demonstrated other interactions between alcohol and essential nutrients that result in alterations in their absorption, storage, release, and degradation, effects that could conceivably affect the liver adversely.

Immunologic

Alterations in both cell-mediated and humoral immunity are demonstrable in many cases of alcoholic liver disease. Since such aberrations occur in alcoholic hepatitis and active cirrhosis, but not in alcohol-induced fatty infiltration or inactive cirrhosis, they appear to be related to the hepatocellular degeneration and necrosis and the inflammatory reaction provoked by alcohol rather than to the direct effects of alcohol or its metabolites. However, the question of whether the immunologic manifestations of alcoholic hepatitis and active cirrhosis are involved in their pathogenesis or are epiphenomena is still unresolved.

Peripheral blood lymphocytes in alcoholic hepatitis exhibit cytotoxicity for a number of target cells, including isolated normal rabbit hepatocytes (38), autologous hepatocytes, and Chang cells (39). Although the antigen responsible for sensitizing such lymphocytes has not been identified, available evidence suggests that it is either alcohol-modified, liver-specific protein (41), or Mallory hyalin (39). Moreover, there is suggestive evidence that the cytotoxic lymphocytes are antibody-dependent K cells (38) and that their cytotoxicity is enhanced by acetaldehyde (39), a feature that may account for the progressive character of the lesions in alcoholic hepatitis when alcohol consumption is continued.

Stimulation of the peripheral lymphocytes in alcoholic hepatitis by either autologous liver or alcohol hyalin results in the release of a factor that increases the incorporation of proline into the collagen produced by cultured fibroblasts (40). This observation has led to the suggestion that an immunologic mechanism may be involved in the fibrogenesis of progressive alcoholic liver disease.

The fact that Mallory hyalin stimulates the transformation and inhibits the migration of cultured lymphocytes in alcoholic hepatitis (40) is consistent with the view that alcohol hyalin may be an antigen in the aberrant, cell-mediated, immune reactions of alcoholic liver disease. However, this interpretation may be open to question, since alcohol and acetaldehyde, which are not antigenic, also stimulate lymphocyte transformation in alcoholic hepatitis (41). Indeed, accumulating evidence indicates that acetaldehyde, which convalently binds to hepatocellular macromolecular proteins, can affect hepatic function and alter hepatic structure, leading to liver cell injury (42). Indeed, such acetaldehyde-generated epitopes are recognized as foreign by the immune system (43).

Alcohol hyalin has also been implicated in abnormal, humoral responses in alcoholic liver disease. Mallory hyalin is detectable in the serum in early alcoholic hepatitis, and later in its course an antibody to Mallory hyalin appears. Furthermore, Mallory hyalin antigen-antibody complexes can be eluted from liver tissue in advanced alcoholic hepatitis and active cirrhosis, even when the antigen and the antibody are no longer detectable in the serum. Although the hypothesis that these alterations in humoral immunity are involved in the pathogenesis of alcoholic hepatitis and cirrhosis merits serious consideration, the alternative possibility that they represent a coincidental response to the presence of alcohol hyalin in the liver cannot be excluded.

A high proportion of patients with active alcoholic liver disease exhibit circulating, immune complexes that contain both IgG and IgA (44). The nature of the antigen in such complexes has not yet been identified, but could be alcohol hyalin, which binds IgA, or, possibly, a protein of intestinal origin. The demonstration of IgA deposition in the sinusoids of the livers of patients with alcoholic, but not nonalcoholic liver disease, has led to the hypothesis that activated, circulating B lymphocytes produce IgA, which may be involved in the pathogenesis of alcoholic-induced liver injury (45). Conceivably, a defect in clearance of this material may be responsible.

Hyperglobulinemia is a well-recognized feature of alcoholic and other types of cirrhosis. At one time it was attributed to hyperreactivity of the humoral, immune system, which resulted in the overproduction of antibodies (46). However, as a result of impaired Kupffer cell function, or diversion of blood via venous collaterals, antigens are not sequestered in Kupffer cells as they are normally, and thus lead to excessive stimulation of antibody production (47). The high titers of antibodies to intestinal bacteria (47) and the impaired reticuloendothelial function in alcoholic cirrhosis (48) are consistent with this interpretation.

Paradoxically, despite some evidence indicating hyperactivity of the immune system, many patients with alcoholic hepatitis and active cirrhosis exhibit signs of impaired cell-mediated immunity. This impairment can be inferred from the reduction in the number of circulating T lymphocytes (49), the failure to develop delayed hypersensitivity to dinitrochlorobenzene (DNCB) (50), reduced skin reactivity to tuberculin purified protein derivative and to other antigens (50,51), a reduced responsiveness of lymphocytes to mitogen stimulation by phytohemagglutinin (52), and decreased responsiveness to vaccination for HBV (53). Neither the explanation for these aberrations, nor their significance in the pathogenesis of alcoholic hepatic injury is known.

A considerable body of experimental evidence indicates that endotoxin, a liposaccharide derived from the cell walls of gram-negative enteric bacteria, is absorbed from the intestinal tract and is detoxified in the liver by the action of reticuloendothelial cells lining the sinusoids. Endotoxin accumulates in the circulation when reticuloendothelial function is impaired, thus lead-

ing to hepatic injury and extrahepatic systemic effects (54). The fact that endotoxin plays a role in the development of the hepatic necrosis induced by hepatotoxins that impair reticuloendothelial function, and that suppression of enteric bacteria by broad-spectrum antibiotics retards or prevents the development of cirrhosis in choline-deficient rats (55) suggest the possibility that endotoxemia may be implicated in the pathogenesis of alcoholic hepatitis and cirrhosis, lesions frequently associated with reticuloendothelial dysfunction. The demonstration of endotoxemia in alcoholic hepatitis and cirrhosis (56) is consistent with this possibility. However, such observations have not been confirmed in all studies, so the role of endotoxin in alcoholic liver disease is still uncertain. The recent demonstration of increased tumor necrosis factor, an immune modulator secreted by monocytes, lymphocytes, and macrophages, in the plasma of patients with severe alcoholic hepatitis gives support to an immunologic pathogenesis (57). However, there is no correlation between levels of plasma necrosis factor and those of endotoxin.

Genetic

Alcoholic hepatitis and cirrhosis develop in only a minority of chronic alcoholic patients, irrespective of their alcohol intake, a fact that is difficult to explain in terms of any of the mechanisms proposed. However, recent studies of histocompatibility antigens in chronic alcoholic patients suggest that individual susceptibility to alcoholic hepatitis and cirrhosis may be genetically determined, possibly by a gene that permits immunologic hyperreactivity, as has been postulated for other, presumed autoimmune hepatic lesions. Thus, an increased prevalence of HLA-B8 in alcoholic hepatitis has been reported from Great Britain (59,60). However, in Norway, alcoholic hepatitis has been associated with HLA-BW40 (61), in Chile, with HLA-B13 (62), in France, with B15 and DR4 (63), and in Japan, with HLA-A2, and HLA-DR3 (64). Moreover, in one of the British studies, the association with HLA-B8 was limited to males (60). Obviously, further studies of this type are needed to explain these apparent discrepancies, to establish whether differences in the distribution of HLA types are indicative of a genetically determined susceptibility to alcoholic hepatitis and cirrhosis, and to define the mechanisms that might be involved in such susceptibility. It seems that genetic associations are even more complex, since there are different types of alcoholism and different genetically determined metabolic pathways (65), each of which may be under genetic control (66). The absence of mitochondrial acetaldehyde dehydrogenase in Asian people (67), which causes flushing and other unpleasant symptoms after alcohol ingestion, diminishes the prevalence of alcohol abuse and alcoholic liver disease in the Far East.

Pathogenesis of alcohol-induced hepatic lesions

1. Fatty infiltration (steatosis) of the liver

Fatty infiltration of the liver occurs in a high proportion of chronic alcoholic patients and is readily reproducible under conditions of adequate dietary intake in both humans (15,16) and animals (15). However, not all heavy drinkers are affected, as is evident from the fact that in one investigation of a consecutive series of 100 chronic alcoholic subjects, fatty infiltration was demonstrable in only 65% of those who had continued to drink heavily to within a week of biopsy (68).

Available evidence indicates that the accumulation of fat in the liver is attributable to the metabolic effects of alcohol, leading to an increase in the uptake and synthesis, and to a decrease in the oxidation and secretion of triglyceride by the hepatocytes (4,5). Often, alcohol-induced fatty infiltration is accompanied by swelling of the hepatocytes due to the retention of protein, an osmotic effect. The increased protein retention is attributed to impairment of protein export, possibly as a result of interference by alcohol with the assembly of tubulin into microtubules (69,70). Proliferation of the smooth endoplasmic reticulum with the formation of orcein-negative ground glass cells (10), another morphologic feature that may be seen in alcoholic fatty liver, has been interpreted as an adaptive response to microsomal oxidation of alcohol [(9,10); Figs. 124, 125]. However, other changes induced by alcohol, including enlargement and distortion of mitochondria (Figs. 134, 135) with disorientation of their cristae, loss of parallel arrays of rough endoplasmic reticulum, and the appearance of autophagic vacuoles containing remnants of degraded organelles, although nonspecific, have been ascribed to the toxic effects of alcohol or acetaldehyde (71).

Usually, fatty infiltration uncomplicated by alcoholic hepatitis, cirrhosis, or pancreatitis, gives rise to no clinical manifestations other than hepatomegaly, and produces little or no biochemical evidence of hepatocellular dysfunction. Serial ultrasonic measurements of the liver have shown, as expected, that the livers of patients with alcoholic liver disease are appreciably larger than those of normal subjects (72). These changes, which are due largely to fatty deposition, diminish with abstention. There is diurnal variation in the hepatic volume of normal subjects. The liver is largest in the morning, falls to its nadir between noon and 2 P.M., and increases again in the afternoon. A similar, more blunted diurnal pattern occurs in patients with alcoholic liver disease.

Rarely, however, when fatty infiltration is excessive, it may be accompanied by cholestasis (73,74). As a rule, such cholestasis abates promptly following the withdrawal of alcohol, but, occasionally, it may progress to hepatic failure and death (74). The pathogenesis of this form of cholestasis is unknown, but has been variously ascribed to compression of ductules by distended hepatocytes—in our opinion, an unlikely possibility—and perhaps to alcoholic pancreatitis (75). It has also been attributed to the hepatotoxic effects of alcohol, leading to increased permeability of ductules, inhibition of essential enzymes involved in bile secretion, and interference with the function of microtubules or microfilaments.

Alcohol-induced liver disease, including fatty infiltration, is associated with increased serum levels of transaminases, particularly aspartate aminotransferase (SGOT). It has been known for years that the ratio of aspartate aminotransferase to alanine aminotransferase in serum (SGOT/SGPT) is elevated in alcoholic liver disease (76,77). This ratio, which is usually >2 in alcoholic hepatitis and active alcoholic cirrhosis and >0.5 in most patients with alcoholic fatty liver, is almost invariably <1.5 and is often <1 in nonalcoholic liver disease. This abnormal ratio appears to reflect a greater decrease in GPT than GOT activity in hepatocytes, thus making relatively more GOT available in the alcoholic liver to "leak" into the serum (78).

SGOT is synthesized in the cytoplasm, and in a slightly lighter form is translocated into the mitochondria (79). Normally about 80% of the SGOT activity in the serum is cytosolic and 20% mitochondrial. In patients with elevated SGOT activity, the mitochondrial isoenzyme is disproportionately increased (80). Mitochondrial SGOT appears to be a reliable indicator of chronic alcoholism (81). The elevated serum levels of mitochondrial SGOT in alcoholic patients appears to represent increased synthesis and increased efflux from the mitochondria (80,82). It is tempting to speculate that the increased SGOT levels are in some way related to the abnormal mitochondria found in alcoholic liver disease (71). Alcoholic fatty infiltration of the liver is a readily reversible lesion that usually resolves, even when severe, within a few weeks following the withdrawal of alcohol. However, the fat tends to clear more slowly when it is associated with alcoholic hepatitis or cirrhosis.

The question of whether persistent fatty infiltration due to continued alcohol consumption can lead to progressive hepatic fibrosis in the absence of complicating alcoholic hepatitis is still a controversial issue. Although there is little doubt that alcoholic cirrhosis follows antecedent alcoholic hepatitis (83,84) and that transitions from uncomplicated fatty infiltration to cirrhosis have only rarely been encountered in humans (85), the possibility cannot be excluded that under some conditions, fatty infiltration can lead directly to hepatic fibrosis. In the baboon, however, progression of fatty infiltration to cirrhosis in the absence of alcoholic hepatitis appears to be the rule (18). Moreover, some degree of hepatic fibrosis is a relatively frequent finding in the uncomplicated alcoholic fatty infiltration seen in humans. Thus, in a consecutive series of 163 such cases in our own unit, mild to moderate fibrosis involving a few portal tracts was present in 53%, mild centrilobular fibrosis in 11%, and focal perisinusoidal fibrosis (capillarization) in 11%, usually in combination, but occasionally alone. Moreover, fibrosis of similar degree and location was demonstrable, although less frequently, in 109 of our patients with fatty infiltration associated with diabetes mellitus or obesity (focal periportal 34%, centrilobular 16%, and perisinusoidal 10%) and in 178 with fatty infiltration of miscellaneous or unknown etiology (periportal 25%, centrilobular 6%, and perisinusoidal 1%). However, in none of these cases have we ever succeeded in documenting a direct transition from fatty infiltration to cirrhosis. In such cases (85), alcoholic hepatitis may have intervened, but not been observed. Frequent biopsies excluded this possibility in the cirrhosis induced by alcohol in the baboon (18). According to some authorities (85), hepatocellular lipid droplets coalesce to form large, extracellular fat cysts that provoke an inflammatory and fibrotic response when they collapse. However, there is no convincing evidence that this accounts for the development of progressive hepatic fibrosis and cirrhosis. Most so-called fat cysts are intracellular, as evidenced by the thin surrounding rim of cytoplasm and the peripherally located, flattened nucleus that usually can be demonstrated in well-fixed, carefully prepared sections, and show no evidence of adjacent inflammation or fibrosis. However, occasionally, large fat globules are extruded from hepatocytes and are encircled by histiocytes to form lipogranulomas (86,87). However, another larger form of lipogranuloma, usually found adjacent or attached to a central vein or, less commonly, within a portal tract, characteristically is composed of a circumscribed mass of lipid-infiltrated macrophages, interspersed with a few lymphocytes and encircled and traversed by fine bands of collagen. Lesions of this type have been attributed to coalescence of small triglyceride-containing lipogranulomas, and it has been suggested that they may be implicated in progressive fibrogenesis (87). However, there is convincing evidence that such granulomas contain saturated hydrocarbons such as mineral oil rather than triglyceride (88,89). Moreover, they occur no more frequently in fatty than in nonfatty livers and show no relationship to the development of hepatic fibrosis.

Based largely on studies of alcohol-induced alterations in collagen metabolism, it has been proposed that alcohol or its metabolites may be directly responsible for fibrogenesis in the alcoholic fatty liver (90–92). However, the stimulatory effect of alcohol on collagen synthesis has not been confirmed in all studies (93,94). Moreover, the fact that fibrosis also occurs in nonalcoholic forms of fatty liver indicates that substances other than alcohol may be operative in this process.

A more convincing case can be made for the role of hepatocellular degeneration and inflammation in the pathogenesis of the fibrosis that may follow alcoholic fatty infiltration. Although hepatocellular necrosis, cell dropout, Mallory body formation, and neutrophilic infiltration, features characteristic of alcoholic hepatitis, are not seen in such lesions, hepatocellular degenerative changes, including ballooning, acidophilic bodies, cytoplasmic clumping, giant mitochondria, infiltrates of lymphocytes, and foci of swollen Kupffer cells, are relatively common. It is conceivable, therefore, that slow loss of hepatocytes or the accompanying mononuclear inflammatory reaction may be responsible for the fibrogenesis in alcoholic fatty livers.

Based on observations in alcohol-induced fatty infiltration in both humans and baboons, it has been suggested that fibrous thickening of the terminal hepatic veins is a forerunner of progressive fibrosis and cirrhosis (95). However, it has been found that fibrous thickening of the terminal hepatic and sublobular veins is no more common in alcoholic fatty livers than in normal livers (96) and has no prognostic significance with respect to the subsequent development of hepatic fibrosis. In contrast, perisinusoidal fibrosis appears to be a marker of potential progression to cirrhosis (96). As a rule, such perisinusoidal fibrosis is the result of antecedent alcoholic hepatitis (97), but, at least in the baboon (18), it appears to develop insidiously in the absence of hepatocellular necrosis, Mallory body formation, or neutrophilic infiltration. Whether it can also occur in humans is still uncertain. Transformation of hepatic sinusoids into conventional vascular channels results from the development of basal laminas and the deposition of collagen (capillarization.) in the spaces of Disse. Recent observations suggest that basal lamina formation on both hepatocytes and endothelial cells and activation of lipocytes in acinar zone 3 precede the deposition of collagen and defenestration of endothelial cells, and may be the first detectable abnormalities of alcoholic liver injury (98,99). Alcohol and vitamin A, both of which can activate Ito cells, may thus potentiate the toxicity of each other (100). Paradoxically, vitamin A levels are decreased in the liver tissue of patients with alcoholic liver disease (100,101). Vitamin A toxicity, which may simulate the hepatic changes of alcoholic fatty liver, may be seen with standard maintenance pharmacologic doses. Microvesicular fatty infiltration may be caused by hyperplasia of *fat storage cells* (Ito cells), which are found primarily in the perisinusoidal areas of zone 3 but are also seen in the portal and septal tissues. When ingestion of vitamin A is large or prolonged, fat storage cells may also be found scattered throughout the lobules (102). Such fatty deposition is probably erroneously attributed to surreptitious alcohol ingestion. These Ito cells, which can be transformed into fibroblast-like cells (103,104), are responsible for perisinusoidal pericellular fibrosis. In experiments in baboons, these myelofibroblasts are found primarily in zone 3 and are not increased in the portal zones (105). In addition, elevation of serum procollagen type III peptide, which correlates closely with prolyl hydroxylase activity in the liver, appears to be an accurate, early marker of alcoholic hepatic fibrogenesis (106,107).

Alcoholic hepatitis

There is general agreement that alcoholic hepatitis, a lesion characterized by hepatocellular degeneration and necrosis, neutrophilic infiltration, and Mallory body formation, affects only a minority of chronic alcoholic patients. In chronic alcoholic patients without overt signs of liver disease, however, histologic evidence of alcoholic hepatitis has been found in from 11% (108) to 38% (109) of cases.

In contrast to fatty infiltration, alcoholic hepatitis has not been successfully reproduced in animals. Although initial reports suggested that baboons were susceptible to experimentally induced alcoholic hepatitis (17), this was not confirmed in a follow-up study reported from the same laboratory (18).

Alcoholic hepatitis is usually defined as a syndrome characterized by jaundice, hepatomegaly, abdominal pain, ascites, fever, and marked leukocytosis (97,110,111), features that may mimic those of acute viral, drug-induced, or toxic hepatitis or extrahepatic biliary obstruction. However, in many cases, the lesions of alcoholic hepatitis are asymptomatic (108,109). It is apparent, therefore, that alcoholic hepatitis is a morphologic rather than a clinical entity, and that its accurate identification requires biopsy documentation. This is borne out by difficulties in making clinical diagnoses of alcoholic liver disease (112).

Following abstinence from alcohol, the lesions of alcoholic hepatitis tend to regress (84). Mild lesions may resolve completely within a few months, but, more commonly, they give rise to varying degrees of residual fibrosis when they heal. Severe lesions may remain active long after the withdrawal of alcohol and may lead to hepatic failure and death. Occasionally, alcoholic hepatitis progresses to cirrhosis despite abstinence (113). In such cases, the mortality rate is very high (about 75%), but in most studies, it has been significantly lower, ranging from 4 to 14% (111,114,115). Serum bilirubin levels appear to be a reliable prognostic index over a wide range of values (116), as are empiric ratios of serum bilirubin and prothrombin values (117,118). The presence of spontaneous encephalopathy in alcoholic hepatitis is another poor prognostic sign (113,118). The progression of alcoholic hepatitis to alcoholic cirrhosis with continued drinking and its reversal with abstinence have been documented by serial liver biopsies (119). In one such series 9 of 26 patients progressed to alcoholic cirrhosis and 5 remained stable with alcoholic hepatitis. Virtually all of the men had continued alcohol abuse, but 4 women developed cirrhosis despite stopping drinking. Improvement was observed only in those who stopped or greatly reduced their alcohol consumption.

In a larger, longer (10–13 years) study of 258 male, noncirrhotic alcohol abusers, it was found that alcoholic hepatitis is a reversible lesion, that the daily volume-duration product is not a reliable predictor of cirrhosis (120). Several investigators have demonstrated that women are at least twice as sensitive to alcohol-induced liver injury as men (119,121).

The bioavailability of alcohol is reduced by alcohol dehydrogenase activity during its first pass through the stomach. Furthermore, women have less gastric alcohol dehydrogenase activity than men and higher blood alcohol levels than men after the oral ingestion of alcohol (122). This phenomenon is even more overt in alcoholic patients, so that in women first pass metabolism of alcohol is virtually absent. Whether this metabolic difference is responsible for the increased susceptibility of women to alcohol, however, remains to be proved.

Under conditions of continued alcohol consumption, the lesions of alcoholic hepatitis remain active, and often progress to cirrhosis. In one carefully studied group of 53 such cases, the lesions progressed to cirrhosis in 21 (40%) and remained active in the remaining 32 (60%) (84). Of particular interest is the fact that 9 of the patients in that series with persistent alcoholic hepatitis showed no evidence of progression over a one-year period.

As indicated by their use of the term "steatonecrosis," some authorities regard fatty infiltration as an essential feature of alcoholic hepatitis (114,123). However, in our own experience and that of others (124), fat may be absent in some cases. The absence of fat may reflect the fact that histologic signs of alcoholic hepatitis persist longer than fatty infiltration.

There is general agreement that alcoholic hepatitis can present without Mallory bodies. Although their presence and number usually correlate with the activity of the lesion, they are of only limited prognostic significance. The degree of hepatocellular necrosis and the intensity of the inflammatory reaction appear to be more important (125,126). Attempts to treat alcoholic hepatitis with corticosteroid therapy, presumably by virtue of its antiinflammatory activity, has given heterogeneous results, but metanalysis of 11 randomized controlled trials suggests that it does reduce mortality, at least in patients with hepatic encephalopathy (127).

Currently, the most widely accepted view is that the development of alcoholic hepatitis is attributable to the hepatotoxic effects of alcohol and its metabolites, or to immunologic reactions that they provoke. However, lesions indistinguishable from those of fatty liver and alcoholic hepatitis occur in nonalcoholic patients with diabetes mellitus (128), obesity (129,130), Indian childhood cirrhosis (131,132), reactions to perhexiline maleate (133) or amiodarone (134), estrogen therapy (135), jejunoileal bypass (27–30), and prolonged fasting in obese individuals (136). This suggests that all such lesions, including those due to alcohol, may share a common, but as yet unidentified pathogenetic mechanism. The demonstration of increased plasma levels of tumor necrosis factor suggests an immunologic mechanism (57). Alternatively, they may represent a similar, but nonspecific reaction to varied etiologic factors.

Alcoholic cirrhosis

The incidence of cirrhosis in chronic alcoholism is surprisingly low, ranging from 2 to 28% (average 18%) in 2178 collected autopsy cases, and from 12 to 31% (average 28%) in 4098 collected biopsied cases (2). Although the development of cirrhosis correlates to some extent with the volume and duration of alcohol consumption, it is noteworthy that in a biopsy study of 526 alcoholic patients, the incidence of cirrhosis, even in

those with a daily intake of over 226 g for at least 11 years, was only 25% (2). This apparent immunity to cirrhosis exhibited by so many heavy drinkers has been attributed by some to the adequacy of their dietary intake (137). However, in our experience and that reported by others, good nutritional intake does not necessarily prevent the development of alcoholic cirrhosis (138). It is evident, therefore, that neither the volume of alcohol consumed nor nutritional factors alone are the determinants of individual susceptibility to such lesions. Genetic factors are probably involved.

The greater susceptibility of women than of men to the development of cirrhosis (139,140) is a prime example of the role of genetics. It has been estimated that more than half of men who consume 200 g of ethanol per day for 15 years will develop chronic alcoholic liver disease (141); i.e. that daily dose of alcohol will cause cirrhosis in 50% of those who consume that amount, the so-called CD_{50}. This rough guideline is the equivalent of one pint of whiskey, 16 cans of beer, or two bottles of wine (142). How much less is required to induce cirrhosis in women is not known. The demonstration that women metabolize alcohol differently from men suggests a pathophysiologic explanation for these observations (143,144). Acetaldehyde metabolism and alcohol elimination have been shown to be greater (144) and alcohol elimination slower (145) in women. The recent demonstration of decreased gastric alcohol dehydrogenase activity in women provides a biochemical basis to integrate these diverse observations. This breakthrough may provide much more important answers about the pathogenesis of alcoholic liver disease than the mere explanation of differences in the response to alcohol by men and women.

Serologic markers of HBV are more frequent in patients with alcoholic liver disease than in nonalcoholic patients (140,146,147), and suggests a potentiating relationship. A similar association between alcoholic liver disease and HCV infection is likely (148).

Circumstantial evidence strongly suggests that alcoholic cirrhosis follows alcoholic hepatitis in most, if not all cases. Thus, serial biopsy studies in patients with alcohol hepatitis have demonstrated progression to cirrhosis within 18 months in 40% of cases (84). Since the hepatitis in the remaining patients in this study who continued to drink was still active, it is probable that some of them would also have developed cirrhosis had they been followed longer. This possibility is supported by our finding of active alcoholic hepatitis, characterized by Mallory hyalin and infiltrating neutrophils, in 384 (62%) of 615 consecutive biopsy-documented cases of alcoholic cirrhosis. In addition, many of the remaining inactive lesions exhibited perisinusoidal fibrosis and fibrotic occlusion of occasional central veins, features suggestive of healed alcoholic hepatitis. Alcoholic hepatitis may progress to cirrhosis despite the cessation of alcohol (113).

Among the most important goals of histologic assessment of hepatic abnormalities is the correlation with clinical signs and laboratory tests. Hepatic and splenic volume increase in parallel with the degree of hepatic fibrosis (149). Several investigators have demonstrated that portal venous pressure correlates closely with the mean hepatocyte volume (150, 151). A subsequent investigation using blind, histologic interpretation in a broad spectrum of alcoholic liver diseases, however, failed to find a correlation between portal venous pressure and the degree of hepatic necrosis, fatty infiltration, inflammation, or hepatocyte volume (152). However, positive correlations were found between effective portal venous pressure and hepatic vascular resistance, fibrosis, the presence of Mallory bodies, and the degree of destruction of the hepatic architecture. In a subsequent, larger study of patients with alcoholic cirrhosis and portal hypertension, the investigators attempted to correlate portal venous pressure with the same five histologic criteria assessed blindly and semiquantitatively (153). They found a positive correlation between portal pressure and the degree of necrosis, of neutrophilic infiltration, and of fibrosis. By stepwise regression analysis, it was shown that the fibrosis was the most important factor. The histologic hepatic lesions of alcoholic hepatitis did correlate with the hepatic venous pressure gradient. The most important finding was the association between portal pressure and architectural distortion, which is best expressed as the degree of fibrosis. Other studies have shown correlations with the amount of collagen in the space of Disse (150,154) and with the thickness of the perivenular rim of fibrosis (155,156). Obviously several factors play a role in the pathogenesis of alcoholic portal hypertension. These include venous outflow obstruction caused by fibrosis and distorted architecture, increased portal blood flow, and increased hepatic vascular resistance, each of which has its histologic correlates.

In a retrospective review of more than 300 patients with alcoholic liver disease, phlebosclerosis of the hepatic venules was found to be a universal lesion in patients with alcoholic hepatitis and cirrhosis (157). Veno-occlusive lesions of the hepatic veins, however, were found in only 20%. Phlebosclerosis, per se, may be the more important lesion.

Collagenization of the space of Disse (158) and defenestration of the sinusoidal epithelium (159,160), both of which are more apparent in the perivenular zone, may interfere with exchange between the sinusoids and hepatocytes and may thus contribute to the hepatic dysfunction in alcoholic cirrhosis.

Withdrawal of alcohol is followed by laboratory and histologic improvement in the lesions of alcoholic cirrhosis, even under conditions of bare maintenance dietary intake (161). Moreover, sustained abstinence from alcohol enhances survival in patients with alcoholic cirrhosis (162,163), although this favorable effect may not be evident in those with severe portal hypertension.

Usually, the nodules in alcoholic cirrhosis are micronodular in character. However, in some cases, they are macronodular, and resemble those of postnecrotic cirrhosis (164,165). In our own series of 615 biopsy-documented cases of alcoholic cirrhosis, macronodularity was encountered in 81 (13%). It is generally agreed that such lesions develop from micronodular cirrhosis as a result of continued hepatocellular regeneration, leading to enlargement of parenchymal nodules, and progressive destruction of parenchyma, leading to the formation of relatively thick fibrous septa (165). We have demonstrated such transitions by serial biopsy in 8 of our 81 cases (10%) of alcoholic cirrhosis with macronodular lesions. Similar transitions from micronodular to macronodular lesions have been demonstrated within individual postmortem specimens of alcoholic cirrhosis (165). Indeed, transition from micronodular to macronodular cirrhosis appears to be the usual pattern (166). Hyperplastic nodules are most likely to develop after the cessation or sharp reduction in alcohol consumption (167).

Although there is a tendency for the lesions in alcoholic cirrhosis to become inactive and macronodular following prolonged abstention from alcohol, in our own group of 81 patients with macronodular alcoholic cirrhosis, 60 (74%) were still drinking to excess at the time of biopsy, and in 37 (46%), the lesions were active, as evidenced by the presence of Mallory

hyalin and fatty infiltration. It is apparent, therefore, that continued active alcohol consumption does not prevent progressive nodular regeneration, even in the face of significant hepatocellular injury.

Not infrequently, inactive cirrhosis with none of the hallmarks of alcoholic liver disease, such as fatty infiltration, Mallory bodies, and neutrophilic infiltration, are encountered in chronic alcoholic patients, particularly following prolonged periods of abstinence. Lesions of this type pose a difficult diagnostic problem, since they are indistinguishable from those in other forms of cirrhosis. Obviously, other etiologic factors must be excluded in such cases, but, even then, the diagnosis of alcoholic cirrhosis must be regarded as presumptive rather than conclusive. On the other hand, when liver biopsies from patients with nonalcoholic cirrhosis are compared by objective histologic analysis, the histologic similarities are greater than the differences, and suggest that a shared pathogenesis may be responsible for the similarities (168).

Hepatocellular carcinoma

The reported incidence of hepatocellular carcinoma as a late complication of alcoholic cirrhosis is highly variable, ranging from 2% (169) to 30% (170). There is general agreement that hepatocellular carcinoma occurs most frequently in alcoholic patients with macronodular cirrhosis, and it has been proposed that it tends to appear following prolonged abstention from alcohol (170). In our own series of 29 cases, the cirrhosis was macronodular in 71%, and in 76% both historical and histologic features were consistent with prolonged abstinence. Of course, alcohol consumption histories in alcoholic patients are notoriously unreliable. The association of abstinence and the appearance of hepatocellular carcinoma requires confirmation.

Little is known about the pathogenesis of hepatocellular carcinoma in alcoholic cirrhosis. The preferential occurrence of such neoplasms in macronodular lesions suggests that neoplasia may be related in some way to hepatocellular regeneration. Alternatively, it has been proposed that the more prolonged survival and advanced age of alcoholic patients with postnecrotic cirrhosis who have given up alcohol may account for their greater susceptibility to hepatocellular carcinoma (170).

It has been reported that there is an increased prevalence of hepatocellular carcinoma in cirrhotic patients with portacaval anastomoses (171), particularly in those who have survived for a year or more after surgery. Our own studies confirm this association and, in addition, show from postmortem studies that the risk of developing hepatocellular carcinoma is proportional to the degree of portal-systemic shunting (172). Nutritional factors had been thought to be important, largely because of the inordinately high frequency of hepatocellular carcinoma in the malnourished natives of Asia and Africa, but it is now clear that chronic HBV, HDV, and HCV infections play important etiologic roles in such series (148,173).

Hemosiderosis and hemochromatosis

Alcoholic patients frequently exhibit hepatocellular hemosiderosis, which, on occasion, is as extensive as in hereditary hemochromatosis. Thus, stainable iron deposits have been encountered in the livers of 59 to 78% of patients with alcoholic cirrhosis, an incidence significantly higher than that found in nonalcoholic forms of chronic liver disease (174,175). The possible effects of chronic alcoholism on the deposition of hemosiderin in the liver in the absence of cirrhosis has received surprisingly little attention. However, as illustrated by the data summarized in Table 10–1, we have found that hemosiderosis is demonstrable as frequently in patients with alcoholic fatty infiltration or hepatitis as it is in alcoholic cirrhosis. Furthermore, the incidence and extent of hemosiderosis in all three forms of alcoholic liver disease are greater than in comparable nonalcoholic disorders such as the fatty infiltration associated with diabetes mellitus or obesity, chronic active hepatitis, or postnecrotic cirrhosis. These observations suggest that alcohol may play a role in the pathogenesis of hepatic hemosiderosis that may not be directly related to the hepatic injury it produces. Unfortunately, biopsy material in chronic alcoholic patients with no histologic evidence of liver disease is not available to confirm this possibility. It should be noted that the frequency of hemosiderosis in our normal subjects and in those with hepatic disease with significantly lower than that previously reported.

It is noteworthy that the Kupffer cells in our cases also contained small amounts of hemosiderin, and this was seen more commonly in alcoholic than in nonalcoholic patients (see Table 10–1). In those alcoholic patients who were adequately investigated, the presence of hemosiderin in the Kupffer cells could not be correlated with the presence of anemia, hemolysis, antecedent transfusions, or the oral use of iron-containing agents.

In 32 of our patients with alcoholic cirrhosis, the deposits of stainable iron in the liver were as heavy and as widely distributed as in primary idiopathic hemochromatosis (graded 3+ in Table 10–1). Moreover, in 3 of those who died, autopsy revealed similar deposits of hemosiderin in the pancreas and other tissues. Although some of the lesions were indistinguishable from those of hereditary hemochromatosis, others showed histologic features indicative of underlying alcoholic liver disease, such as fatty infiltration in 20 (63%), Mallory hyalin in 14 (44%), and neutrophilic infiltrates in 9 (28%). In one of these cases, histocompatibility antigen typing revealed HLA-A3 and HLA-B14, an association often encountered in hereditary hemochromatosis. This is consistent with the view that in some cases, alcohol merely accelerates expression of the gene responsible for the development of hereditary hemochromatosis (176).

The factors responsible for the development of hemosiderosis in alcoholic liver disease have not been identified. Although chronic liver disease may be associated with enhanced iron absorption, the latter does not correlate with the degree of hemosiderosis, and is no greater in alcoholic than in nonalcoholic liver disease (175). Similarly, the suggestion that hemosiderosis in the alcoholic patient is attributable to an excessive intake of iron contained in wine (177) does not account for the fact that hemosiderosis follows the excessive consumption of other alcoholic beverages, and occurs in nonalcoholic chronic liver disease as well. The possibility that the accumulation of iron in the liver is the result of enhanced iron absorption secondary to a defect in pancreatic secretion, a relatively common finding in alcoholic subjects, is supported by a number of studies, which suggest that a factor in pancreatic juice may inhibit iron absorption (178). However, the interpretation of such studies is difficult, since they do not exclude the possibility that the enhanced absorption of iron found in alcoholic cirrhosis is due to hepatic injury rather than to pancreatic insufficiency (179).

There are a number of well-documented cases of alcoholic and other types of cirrhosis in which portacaval shunting has been followed within a few months to years by the development of hemochromatosis (180,181). This suggests that surgical shunting of blood around the liver may lead to alterations in the uptake, utilization, or deposition of iron in the liver, and that spontaneous shunting may have similar effects and may, thus, account for the development of hemochromatosis. However, the mechanisms involved in these alterations in iron metabolism remain to be clarified.

Table 10–1. Incidence of stainable iron in biopsy sections of liver

Lesions	Nonalcoholic				Alcoholic		
	Normal	Steatosis: diabetes, obesity	Chronic active hepatitis[a]	Postnecrotic cirrhosis[b]	Steatosis	Hepatitis	Cirrhosis
Number of patients	344	109	130	275	163	216	615
Stainable Iron	Percent	Percent	Percent	Percent	Percent	Percent	Percent
Hepatocytes							
Trace	5	4	4	4	12	14	8
1+	7	4	8	4	10	10	10
2+	0	0	1	2	5	6	6
3+	0	0	1	0	1	0	5
Total	12	8	14	10	28	30	29
Kupffer Cells							
Trace	1	4	3	2	3	5	8
1+	2	1	3	1	6	5	10
2+	0	1	1	1	1	1	6
3+	0	0	1	0	0	0	5
Total	3	6	8	4	10	11	29

[a] Exclusive of unresolved acute viral or drug-induced hepatitis.
[b] Includes inactive lesions and those accompanied by chronic active hepatitis.

Histopathology of alcohol-induced hepatic lesions

Alcoholic fatty infiltration (steatosis)

Depending on the severity of alcoholic steatosis, the lipid deposits may involve only a few scattered hepatocytes, affect most of the hepatocytes in the centrilobular and midzones (Fig. 173), or show a panlobular distribution (Fig. 175). Only rarely are the lipid deposits limited to the periportal zones (Fig. 174).

Because they are extracted by the solvents used in fixation and embedding, the hepatocellular lipid deposits in routine microscopic sections appear as sharply circumscribed vacuoles. These may present as single large vacuoles in individual hepatocytes, or as multiple small vacuoles. In the *macrovesicular* type, the lipid globule occupies a significant proportion of the affected cell. When large it displaces the cytoplasm and nucleus to the periphery giving rise to the so-called *signet cells* (Fig. 581). Occasionally, the globules distend the hepatocytes to several times their normal size, giving them the appearance of extracellular fat cysts.

Microvesicular fatty infiltration, also called *alcoholic foamy degeneration,* represents a characteristic pattern of acute alcoholic injury of the liver [(173); Fig. 113]. Patients with this pattern often exhibit jaundice and hepatomegaly. The complications associated with portal hypertension such as ascites, bleeding varices, hepatic encephalopathy, and the hepatorenal syndrome, which may be present with severe macrovesicular fatty infiltration, seem less common in the microvesicular type. Serum alkaline phosphatase activity, SGOT, and serum cholesterol levels are transiently elevated, but leukocytosis and cirrhosis are rarely present. The foamy appearance is more prominent in the centrilobular hepatocytes but the periportal hepatocytes may be involved as well. The fatty droplets fill the cytoplasm and often increase the size of the hepatocyte, but they do not displace the nucleus to the periphery. Foci of cell dropout are often present. Megamitochondria are common. Polymorphonuclear neutrophilic infiltration is uncommon unless alcoholic hepatitis is also present. All findings return promptly to normal after the cessation of alcohol [(182); Fig. 172].

Although the lipid deposits in any given case may be exclusively macrovesicular or microvesicular, both types often coexist (Fig. 581).

Lipogranulomas are relatively common findings in all forms of hepatic fatty infiltration. These present as sharply circumscribed, round or oval structures that contain a central, extracellular lipid globule surrounded by macrophages and a few lymphocytes (Fig. 582). Since the central lipid globule may escape detection in tangential sections, and since the macrophages may sometimes resemble epithelioid cells (Fig. 287), serial sections may be required to distinguish lipogranulomas from other types of granulomas. They may contain collagen fibers. As illustrated in Figure 287, lipogranulomas occasionally contain a significant number of eosinophils.

Extensive fatty infiltration distorts the normal contours and pattern of the hepatic plates (Fig. 581), and compresses the sinusoids, making them difficult to identify (Fig. 171).

Often, the unaffected hepatocytes in alcoholic steatosis exhibit some degree of *pleomorphism* (Fig. 581), but, usually, show no other evidence of regenerative activity. Other, relatively common, parenchymal abnormalities include rare acidophilic bodies (Fig. 583) and occasional small foci of proliferating Kupffer cells (Fig. 584).

Occasionally, severe alcoholic fatty infiltration is accompanied by marked cholestasis that may mimic extrahepatic biliary obstruction. In many cases, the cholestasis can be attributed to the presence of alcoholic hepatitis or pancreatitis (75), but in some cases, it appears to be a manifestation of the hepatocellular injury induced by the alcohol itself. The lesions in such cases are characterized by extensive fatty infiltration (Fig. 585), and a variable number of centrilobular, canalicular bile thrombi, often contained within hepatocellular rosettes or pseudoducts (Fig. 586). In addition, hepatocellular degenerative changes (Fig. 586) and alterations in some of the portal tracts, including stellate fibrosis, lymphocytic and neutrophilic infiltration, and ductular proliferation, may be present (Fig. 587). However, minor degrees of portal fibrosis are relatively common (Fig. 588) and occur with regularity in cases of fatty infiltration with cholestasis (Fig. 587).

Fibrous thickening of the central or sublobular veins, replacement or displacement of centrilobular hepatocytes by bands of collagen, or capillarization of the centrilobular sinusoids are encountered in only a small minority of patients with uncomplicated, alcoholic fatty infiltration. An example of such *centrilobular fibrosis* in an otherwise healthy, asymptomatic, chronic alcoholic patient is illustrated in Figure 589. As previously indicated, it is uncertain whether fibrosis of this type is attributable to the fatty infiltration, to some other direct effect of alcohol, as suggested in the case of alcohol-fed baboons (18), or to antecedent unrecognized alcoholic hepatitis. Our own experience suggests that such lesions, whatever their pathogeneses, show no tendency to progress to cirrhosis, unless they are complicated by intercurrent alcoholic hepatitis.

Alcoholic hepatitis

The lesions of alcoholic hepatitis are characterized by *centrilobular,* hepatocellular *degeneration* and *necrosis,* cytoplasmic or extracellular deposits of alcohol hyalin *(Mallory bodies),* and a predominantly *neutrophilic inflammatory reaction,* usually accompanied by a variable degree of fatty infiltration. As a rule, advanced lesions are accompanied by jaundice, and may lead to hepatic failure and death. In many cases, alcoholic hepatitis of mild or moderate severity gives rise to no clinical manifestations. Although alcoholic hepatitis is potentially reversible following abstention from alcohol, particularly when mild, the lesions may extend to adjacent central veins. They may involve whole lobules if alcohol abuse is continued. Moreover, the lesions often give rise to a distinctive type of fibrosis that may progress to cirrhosis.

Figure 590 illustrates the typical, centrilobular distribution of the lesions and the accompanying fatty infiltration in a case of relatively early, moderately severe alcoholic hepatitis. As is evident at higher magnification in Figure 130, numerous hepatocytes are ballooned, and many contain Mallory bodies. Several small foci of cell dropout and collapse of reticulin are present. Although only rare lymphocytes are seen in this field, other areas in the same section (Fig. 591) show the more typical intense neutrophilic response.

In severe lesions, the centrilobular zones of degeneration, necrosis, and inflammation frequently bridge adjacent central veins (Fig. 47) or portal tracts (Fig. 49). As shown in Figure 318, when the lesions extend to the periportal zones, the portal tracts usually contain numerous neutrophils and proliferating ductules. Rarely, the bile ductular cells may contain typical Mallory hyalin (Fig. 133). Histologic evidence of *cholestasis* (Fig. 592) is another relatively common feature of severe alcoholic hepatitis. Other parenchymal changes that may be seen include occasional acidophilic bodies and scattered macrophages, some of which often contain D-PAS-positive ceroid pigments (lipofuscin).

The earliest and most mild lesions of alcoholic hepatitis are characterized by occasional centrilobular ballooned cells, Mallory hyalin, and inflammatory cells, and may be unaccompanied by hepatic functional abnormalities. Often, such lesions are encountered unexpectedly in patients subjected to liver biopsy for other reasons. Figure 593 illustrates a lesion of this type in a woman with biopsy-documented Hodgkin's disease of the cervical lymph nodes who, because of hepatomegaly, was subjected to liver biopsy to exclude lymphomatous infiltration of the liver. In addition to the occasional, centrilobular, ballooned cells, Mallory hyalin, and neutrophils illustrated, some of the hepatocytes in other fields contained megamitochondria and fat. In retrospect, it was learned that the patient was a moderately heavy social drinker. No doubt many such early lesions are overlooked, and may account for the centrilobular fibrosis found in some alcoholic patients with fatty livers who exhibit no histologic evidence and deny symptoms suggestive of antecedent alcoholic hepatitis.

At one time, *Mallory bodies* were regarded as a pathognomonic feature of alcoholic liver disease. However, it is now recognized that such inclusions occur not only in alcoholic liver disease, where they are centrilobular in distribution, but also in a number of other disorders, including primary biliary cirrhosis (183), Wilson's disease (184), Indian childhood cirrhosis (185), chronic cholestasis of varied etiology (186), nonalcoholic hepatic fibrosis associated with diabetes mellitus or obesity (129–130), the postjejunoileal bypass syndrome (27,29), hepatocellular carcinoma (187), focal nodular hyperplasia (188), and the hepatitis and cirrhosis produced by the drug perhexiline maleate (133) or amiodarone (130). In lesions other than alcoholic hepatitis, especially cholestatic disorders, such as primary biliary cirrhosis, the Mallory hyalin is found primarily in periportal areas [(186); Fig. 594]. In addition, Mallory hyalin can be produced experimentally in mice by the administration of griseofulvin and by colchicine in mice previously treated with colchicine (189).

Three types of Mallory body can be identified by electron microscopy: type 1 is composed of filaments in parallel arrays; type 2, the one encountered most frequently, is made up of closely packed, randomly oriented filaments; and type 3 is composed of granular or amorphous material devoid of filaments, except at their periphery (190). None of these inclusions is membrane-bound. There is suggestive evidence that the three types of Mallory bodies may represent successive stages in their aging. In isolated, purified preparations of type 2 hyalin, the filaments exhibit a hollow core and measure 175 to 250 nm in length, and 14 or 20 nm in diameter (191). In many respects, they resemble the intermediate filaments of the cytoskeleton, but differ in being shorter and thicker, and having an outer fimbricated coat. By means of immunofluorescence, using a guinea-pig antibody against purified bovine prekeratin, it has been shown that the filaments in Mallory hyalin contain a prekeratin-like protein (192). Hepatocytes, like many epithelial cells, contain cytokeratins as their intermediate filaments. It has been suggested that the formation of Mallory hyalin may represent a type of abnormal cytokeratin. It is still uncertain whether these

aggregates of cytokeratin represent material specifically synthesized in response to injury, or are derived from normal intermediate filaments. Prekeratin is not the only constituent of Mallory bodies as shown by the histochemical demonstration of protein (193) and phospholipid (194). Moreover, it is apparent from the variability of its staining properties that Mallory hyalin is not uniform in chemical composition.

Clearly Mallory hyalin represents disorganization of the cytoskeleton of the hepatocytes (195). Three hypotheses about the pathogenesis of Mallory bodies exist. First, the "microtubular failure" concept suggests that they result from the proliferation of intermediate filaments following microtubular disassembly, which can be induced by alcohol metabolism or by griseofulvin or colchicine in mice (194). Second, the "vitamin A deficiency" hypothesis is suggested by the occurrence of Mallory hyalin in several conditions in which vitamin A deficiency exists (196) or the fact that vitamin A is decreased after griseofulvin or alcohol abuse (100,101,196,197). Third, the "preneoplasia" hypothesis is suggested by the observations that increased gamma-glutamyltranspeptidase activity, an oncofetal enzyme, is induced by griseofulvin and other carcinogenic substances (198). Mallory hyalin is usually seen in experimental animals and disorders associated with hepatocellular carcinoma, but it may also occur in Wilson's disease, which does not predispose to hepatocellular carcinoma.

On light microscopy, Mallory bodies appear to be groups of sharply defined, irregular globules of variable shape and size, made up of homogeneous, hyalinized material arranged in the form of beaded chains (Fig. 130). Usually, the chains are irregular or serpiginous in contour, but may be horseshoe-shaped or circular, partially or completely encircling the nucleus (Fig. 130). Occasionally, Mallory bodies present as single or multiple large, round, hyaline globules (Fig. 132). These lesions must be differentiated from other circumscribed cytoplasmic inclusions, which, in contrast to Mallory bodies, usually stain with PAS following diastase digestion.

As a rule, Mallory hyalin is acidophilic, and stains a brilliant orange-red in Masson sections (Fig. 130), and a less intense violaceous red in H & E sections (Fig. 131). Variations in the intensity of staining within the same section are relatively common. Occasionally, some of the Mallory bodies in Masson-stained sections are basophilic, appearing light blue in color, or blue with a bright red central core (Fig. 132). Basophilic Mallory bodies are unusual in H & E sections, except in the case of formalin-fixed, postmortem specimens in which they may appear pale, slate-gray in color.

Special stains, such as chromotrope aniline blue (199), have been recommended to confirm the identity or to facilitate the detection of Mallory hyalin. However, we have found them no more sensitive or specific than routine Masson and H & E stains. Recent studies suggest that the immunoperoxidase technique, using a rabbit antibody directed against purified alcoholic hyalin, is highly specific and more sensitive than any of the other staining methods for the detection of Mallory hyalin (200). Moreover, by means of this technique, it has been possible to demonstrate that the Mallory bodies in alcoholic hepatitis share a common antigenic determinant with those in other, nonalcoholic hepatic lesions (200).

The character of the hepatocytes in which Mallory bodies are found varies. The involved cells are often ballooned, or show other evidence of degeneration, but usually they contain intact nuclei, often with prominent nucleoli (Figs. 131, 318). They may also be encountered in enlarged, but otherwise normal-appearing hepatocytes (Fig. 130). Only rarely are they found in cells distended with large lipid globules.

Some otherwise typical lesions in alcoholic hepatitis contain no Mallory bodies. In our own series of 224 cases, alcoholic hyalin was not detectable in 66 (30%). Usually, this occurs in late inactive fibrotic lesions, but, occasionally, is seen in early active lesions, as illustrated in Figure 595. Shown are ballooned hepatocytes, foci of cell dropout, scattered neutrophils and lymphocytes, and extensive fatty infiltration in the absence of Mallory bodies.

It has been suggested that the neutrophilic inflammatory reaction in alcoholic hepatitis is a chemotactic response to alcoholic hyalin, and that in serial sections, neutrophils can almost always be demonstrated surrounding hepatocytes that contain Mallory hyalin (201). Although there can be little doubt that neutrophils often surround or infiltrate such hepatocytes (Figs. 131, 591), similar infiltrates may be found in the absence of Mallory bodies or in zones of cell dropout at some distance from them (Figs. 592, 596). Moreover, as illustrated in Figure 130, extensive deposition of alcoholic hyalin does not always provoke a neutrophilic reaction. Accordingly, it is more likely that hepatocellular necrosis rather than a chemotactic response to alcoholic hyalin accounts for the infiltration of neutrophils in alcoholic hepatitis. T lymphocytes are also found in the inflammatory response in alcoholic hepatitis (202).

Presumably, hepatocytes containing Mallory bodies ultimately undergo destruction, as suggested by the occasional loss of nuclei, disruption and fragmentation of plasma membranes, and the frequent finding in highly active lesions of extracellular alcoholic hyalin surrounded by neutrophils (Fig. 591). The life cycle of Mallory hyalin is not known. It may be found several weeks or months after alcohol ingestion has ceased amd after active necrosis of hepatocytes has disappeared. Whether it had persisted since the acute stage or developed thereafter is not known. Similarly, it is not known whether Mallory body–containing cells can recover or are destined to die promptly.

Ballooned hepatocytes, too, are presumably dying cells, since they are often accompanied by foci of cell dropout in the absence of Mallory bodies (Fig. 595). However, the possibility cannot be excluded that some ballooned hepatocytes recover following abstention from alcohol.

In contrast to acute viral hepatitis, the destruction of parenchyma during the active progressive phase of alcoholic hepatitis, even when extensive, evokes little or no hepatocellular *regenerative response*. However, as the activity of the lesions abates following the withdrawal of alcohol, the hepatocytes proliferate, as evidenced by the appearance of numerous binucleate cells, occasional mitotic figures, thick hepatic plates, and rosettes (Fig. 597).

With continued activity of the lesions, the loss of hepatocytes in alcoholic hepatitis is accompanied by the development of a distinctive type of *centrilobular fibrosis,* characterized by deposition of collagen around individual hepatocytes (Fig. 225) and within the spaces of Disse in a radiating linear pattern (Fig. 598) that may extend deeply into the lobules (Fig. 223). Often, the central and sublobular veins are similarly affected, resulting in fibrous thickening of their intima and narrowing of their lumens (Fig. 599). As the lesions progress, the fibrous tissue may occlude the sinusoids and replace the hepatocytes, forming relatively large stellate scars (Figs. 90, 600). Often, the central veins in some of the scars are similarly obliterated (Fig. 600). There is convincing evidence that such centrilobular fibrotic occlusion of the sinusoids and hepatic vein radicles plays a sig-

nificant role in the pathogenesis of portal hypertension in alcoholic liver disease (203).

Severe alcoholic hepatitis with centrilobular fibrosis has been termed *sclerosing hyalin necrosis* (97). The term, as commonly employed, implies a distinctive clinical syndrome characterized by jaundice, ascites, abdominal pain, fever, and marked leukocytosis (97). However, identical lesions may be seen in the absence of such clinical manifestations, so sclerosing hyalin necrosis should be regarded as a morphologic rather than as a clinical entity. Moreover, it should be noted that in nonfatal cases, the lesions tend to heal with residual scarring but no alcoholic hyalin.

Characteristically, the hepatocellular changes and intralobular inflammatory reaction in alcoholic hepatitis first appear in the centrilobular zones, but, as the lesions advance, they extend peripherally, ultimately to involve the periportal zones. The fibrosis that accompanies or follows such lesions usually shows a similar pattern of progression (204). However, portal inflammation and fibrosis often appear while the parenchymal lesions are still limited to the centrilobular zones. Conceivably, such portal lesions are indicative of a response to intralobular necrosis and inflammation, but other possibilities cannot be excluded.

Patchy *portal fibrosis* is a relatively common feature of alcoholic hepatitis. It occurs most frequently when the centrilobular zones of necrosis and inflammation extend to the portal tracts, as shown in Figure 49. Usually, under such conditions, the portal fibrosis is accompanied by bile ductular proliferation and a predominantly neutrophilic inflammatory reaction (Fig. 318). However, expansion and fibrosis of the portal tracts may also occur in the absence of such central-portal bridging necrosis (Fig. 601). The portal inflammatory cells in such lesions usually are predominantly lymphocytic (Fig. 602).

The hepatic histology in infants and children with the *fetal alcohol syndrome* is similar to that seen in alcoholic adults (205). Fatty infiltration, predominantly macrovesicular and periportal, is typical and may persist for months or years after birth (Fig. 603). Portal vein fibrosis, central vein sclerosis, and bile ductular regeneration are common. Mallory hyalin, however, is not seen. By electron microscopy increased numbers of myelofibroblasts are seen and capillarization of the sinusoids often develops.

As in the case of alcoholic fatty infiltration, the portal fibrosis, inflammation, and bile ductular changes seen in alcoholic hepatitis may be attributable, in some instances, to complicating factors, such as pancreatitis (75). However, in many cases, this possibility can be excluded. It is uncertain whether the portal tract changes in such cases indicate a response to the accompanying centrilobular necrosis and inflammation, or are the result of slow destruction of periportal hepatocytes attributable to some direct effect of alcohol.

Among a group of patients with chronic alcoholic liver disease, most of whom had cirrhosis, half macronodular and half micronodular, blind interpretation of histologic features revealed highly significant correlations between the portal pressure measured by hepatic vein catheterization and the degree of architectural destruction, of fibrosis, and of hepatic vascular resistance and the occurrence of Mallory bodies (206). No such relationship existed with the degree of hepatic necrosis, fatty infiltration, inflammation, or the size of hepatocytes. In alcoholic cirrhosis portal pressure measured by the catheterization technique is identical to that measured directly in the portal vein, but is lower in patients with nonalcoholic cirrhosis (207).

These investigations indicate that the derangements of hepatic architecture induced by scar tissue are responsible for the hemodynamic derangements in alcoholic liver disease.

The possibility has been considered that chronic alcoholism may give rise to *chronic active hepatitis* (208). Although such lesions may be encountered in heavy drinkers, there is no convincing evidence that they are attributable to alcohol, and it is highly probable that they are coincidental findings. However, the portal fibrosis and inflammation commonly found in alcoholic steatosis and inactive alcoholic hepatitis may mimic the lesions of *chronic persistent hepatitis.*

Under conditions of continued alcohol consumption and progression of the lesions in alcoholic hepatitis, not only central-central (Fig. 47) and central-portal (Fig. 49), but also portal-portal (Figs. 49, 601) fibrous bridges are formed. These distort and ultimately destroy the normal lobular architecture, leading to the development of cirrhosis. Although widely disseminated, the lesions of alcoholic hepatitis are not uniformly distributed, so that, occasionally, intact lobules, zones of bridging fibrosis, and discrete nodules may be encountered in the same section. Thus, the transition from alcoholic hepatitis to cirrhosis may be subtle, so the distinction between the two types of lesion may be difficult in some cases.

Rarely, alcoholic hepatitis gives rise to a diffuse, perisinusoidal, and pericellular fibrosis that destroys the normal lobular architecture, but does not provoke a nodular regenerative response. Such lesions are difficult to classify, but despite the absence of regenerating parenchymal nodules, the term *diffuse interstitial cirrhosis* (209) appears appropriate, although it is not accepted by some pathologists who prefer "diffuse interstitial fibrosis." Figures 62 and 63 illustrate a lesion of this type in a middle aged alcoholic woman who six weeks prior to biopsy presented with deep jaundice, ascites, and hepatic encephalopathy. There was marked clinical improvement and ultimate recovery following a course of prednisone and supportive therapy, but, as can be seen in Figure 63, the lesions at six weeks still showed numerous neutrophils and Mallory hyalin, and extensive, diffuse perisinusoidal and pericellular fibrosis.

Alcoholic cirrhosis

Characteristically, alcoholic cirrhosis is of the *micronodular* type (Figs. 50, 576). However, particularly following prolonged abstention from alcohol, the regenerating parenchymal nodules tend to enlarge, ultimately producing a *macronodular* lesion (Figs. 58, 604), often classified as *alcoholic postnecrotic cirrhosis* (158). The nodules may be as large as 1.5 cm in diameter, but never attain the size of the coarse, irregular nodules that produce a small, misshapen liver, such as that seen following recovery from submassive hepatic necrosis.

Initially, the fibrous septa in alcoholic cirrhosis are relatively slender (Fig. 50), but with progressive destruction of parenchyma, they tend to broaden (Fig. 58). However, they seldom exceed a few millimeters in width. Occasionally, the lesions exhibit relatively large zones of collapsed reticulin, in which are embedded compressed, adjacent portal tracts and central veins, and which contain numerous inflammatory cells and bile ductules. A lesion of this type is illustrated in Figure 605. Usually, in nonalcoholic liver disease, such zones of collapse are the result of antecedent acute confluent panlobular parenchymal necrosis. However, collapse of this type is difficult to explain

on this basis in the case of alcoholic cirrhosis, since such lesions are usually characterized by slowly developing necrosis accompanied by active fibrosis rather than by collapse. Conceivably, the collapse can be attributed to extensive ischemic necrosis secondary to severe esophageal bleeding in some cases, but, as a rule, it occurs in the absence of hemorrhage or any other evidence of complicating acute hepatic necrosis.

In *active lesions,* the contours of the fibrous septa are irregular and ill-defined (Fig. 50) owing to erosion of their limiting plates and extension of portal or septal fibrous tissue and inflammatory cells into the parenchyma (Fig. 606), as in other forms of piecemeal necrosis. By contrast, in *inactive cirrhosis,* the septa are smoothly contoured and outlined by intact limiting plates (Figs. 576, 604).

Frequently, the septa in alcoholic cirrhosis contain *inflammatory cells.* These tend to be most numerous in active lesions with significant parenchymal degeneration, necrosis, and inflammation. Under such conditions, neutrophils predominate (Fig. 606), although they are almost always accompanied by lymphocytes, plasma cells, or macrophages. In most inactive lesions, the septa contain few if any inflammatory cells (Fig. 604), but, in some cases, they may be infiltrated by a moderate number of lymphocytes and plasma cells (Fig. 360).

Ductular proliferation is another feature of active alcoholic cirrhosis (Fig. 606). The ductules tend to diminish in number and may disappear when the activity of the lesions abates (Fig. 604). However, in some inactive lesions, proliferated ductules persist (Fig. 360).

Proliferated bile ducts in alcoholic liver disease typically take a linear shape. The epithelial cells often appear intermediate between bile ductal cells and hepatocytes. Such ductular cells appear to be transformed hepatocytes, and their parenchymal origin can be confirmed by the presence of glucose-6-phosphatase and of glycogen demonstrated histochemically. Occasionally, Mallory hyalin can be seen in bile ductular cells. The typical elongated shape of the proliferated bile ducts suggests transformation from hepatic cords.

Not infrequently, in advanced alcoholic cirrhosis, the septa contain partially or completely *occluded central or sublobular veins* (Fig. 273). These are most easily identified in Masson-stained sections, and may be overlooked in those stained with H & E. Characteristically, the lumens of such vessels contain loosely arranged, fibrous tissue perforated by fine vascular channels, suggesting the presence of an organized, recanalized thrombus. However, in some cases, the fibrosis is limited to the intima, resulting in constriction of the venous lumen, a lesion more consistent with some type of phlebosclerosis (Fig. 273). Undoubtedly, both types of vascular lesions are the sequelae of antecedent alcoholic hepatitis, and, hence, are useful diagnostic features. In some cases, occlusion of the central and sublobular veins is accompanied by foci of sinusoidal congestion and atrophy or loss of the intervening hepatocytes (Fig. 578).

Usually, *hepatocellular regeneration* is a feature of the lesions in alcoholic cirrhosis, as evidenced by the arrangement of the hepatocytes in the form of irregular plates, two or more cells thick (Fig. 51). However, as in other types of cirrhosis, the hepatic plates may revert to a normal, one-cell-thick, radiating pattern in late inactive lesions (Fig. 56).

In *active* alcoholic cirrhosis, the parenchyma shows the same type of *hepatocellular degeneration* and *necrosis, Mallory hyalin,* and *neutrophilic infiltration* seen in alcoholic hepatitis. Usually, these features are most prominent in the periportal and periseptal zones, and account for the destruction of their limiting plates (Figs. 606, 607). However, in severe lesions, they may extend to involve most of the parenchyma (Fig. 580). Often, active lesions are classified as *alcoholic cirrhosis with alcoholic hepatitis,* but we prefer the term *active alcoholic cirrhosis* because of its brevity, and especially because it implies that the hepatitis is an essential feature in the pathogenesis of the cirrhosis rather than a complication.

As in other forms of cirrhosis, *ischemic necrosis,* characterized by eosinophilic zones of hepatocellular coagulation necrosis that affect some of the nodules, is a relatively common finding in alcoholic cirrhosis following extensive hemorrhage from esophageal varices (Fig. 99).

Occasionally, foci of *hepatic cell dysplasia* are seen in alcoholic cirrhosis, particularly in the periseptal zones of advanced inactive lesions. Characteristically, the affected hepatocytes are enlarged, and exhibit nuclear pleomorphism, hyperchromatism, and reduplication. These occur more frequently in HBsAg-positive postnecrotic cirrhosis than in alcoholic cirrhosis (Figs. 195, 196), and are thought by some to be premalignant lesions (210).

Aggregates of *oncocytic (oxyphilic) hepatocytes* may be seen in the advanced lesions of alcoholic cirrhosis, but occur more commonly in HbsAg-positive chronic active hepatitis and postnecrotic cirrhosis (211). Characteristically, the cytoplasm of the oncocytic hepatocytes is distended with innumerable mitochondria that present as fine, closely packed granules that appear bright red in routine H & E and Masson sections (Fig. 124), and deep blue in PTAH-stained sections (Fig. 125).

Cholestasis is a relatively common histologic feature in advanced, active, alcoholic cirrhosis. Characteristically, bile thrombi are found within dilated canaliculi, and often are encircled by hepatocytes arranged in the form of rosettes or pseudoducts (Fig. 608). These tend to be most prominent in the periportal and periseptal zones, but, ultimately, may extend throughout the parenchyma. In addition, small bile droplets may be seen within hepatocytes and swollen Kupffer cells. When cholestasis is severe and prolonged, particularly in cases with terminal hepatic failure, the interlobular ducts may be greatly distended with bile, and show atrophy, degeneration, and necrosis of their lining epithelial cells (Fig. 362). Moreover, under such conditions, groups of hepatocytes and Kupffer cells may undergo pseudoxanthomatous degeneration, forming so-called bile infarcts.

Alcoholic hemosiderosis and hemochromatosis

As previously pointed out, almost one-third of alcoholic patients with liver disease exhibit some degree of hemosiderosis. Usually, this is only minimal or mild in those with uncomplicated fatty infiltrations, but may be more extensive in those with alcoholic hepatitis or cirrhosis. Characteristically, the hemosiderin deposits are found in periportal hepatocytes, and, far less commonly, in a few of the Kupffer cells. As an example, Figure 609 illustrates the mild hemosiderosis found in a case of early alcoholic hepatitis.

Occasionally, the cirrhotic lesions in chronic alcoholic patients are extensively infiltrated with hemosiderin, and are indistinguishable from those of hereditary hemochromatosis. In some instances, it can be shown by HLA typing of the patient and the family that the hemochromatosis is of the hereditary type, the development of the lesion presumably having been accelerated by chronic alcoholism. However, in others, transition from nonsiderotic alcoholic cirrhosis can be documented, strongly suggesting that the lesion is acquired. Although such transitions may follow portacaval shunting, they may also occur spontaneously. Figure 610 illustrates a lesion of the latter type found unexpectedly at autopsy in a middle aged black woman who died of hepatic failure. She was a chronic abuser of alcohol who four years previously was found to have severe active alcoholic cirrhosis with no evidence of hepatic hemosiderosis, anemia, or hyperferremia. In the interim, she had continued to drink heavily, but had received no transfusions or iron-containing medications. At autopsy, in addition to the hemochromatotic lesion illustrated in Figure 610, she exhibited significant pancreatic fibrosis and hemosiderosis, and smaller deposits of hemosiderin in many of her other tissues.

Other hepatic markers of chronic alcoholism

Hepatic megamitochondria (71,212,213) and induction cells (12) occur in a significant number of chronic alcoholic patients. Although not pathognomonic, the presence of megamitochondriosis may prove helpful diagnostically by alerting the pathologist to the possibility of underlying chronic alcoholism.

Mitochondriosis, an increase in the number of mitochondria per cell, occurs commonly in alcoholic liver disease, but may be seen in other forms of liver disease as well (211,214,215).

In one reported study of liver biopsy material, *megamitochondria* were found in 72% of heavy drinkers and in only 10% of patients who consumed little or no alcohol (71). In a much larger series, megamitochondria were found in about 20% of patients with alcoholic hepatitis (212). Surprisingly, they occurred almost exclusively in patients with alcoholic hepatitis of mild or moderate severity, for example, in those with prothrombin times of less than four seconds prolonged, and only rarely in those with severe alcoholic hepatitis. Patients with giant mitochondria appear to represent a subgroup of alcoholic hepatitis with mild clinical and laboratory signs of liver disease; fewer episodes of infection, gastrointestinal bleeding, azotemia, diabetes, hepatic encephalopathy, or hepatorenal syndrome; a lower incidence of cirrhosis; and better long-term survival (212).

Different types of megamitochondria can be distinguished on electron microscopy, and one particular type of spherical megamitochondria with a paucity of cristae (type I) may be specific for alcoholic liver disease (213). However, in our experience, the incidence has been significantly lower, less than 10%, a discrepancy that may reflect our failure to have searched diligently for megamitochondria in all cases. Nevertheless, we too regard such cytoplasmic inclusions as presumptive evidence of chronic alcoholism. Thus, of 50 of our patients who exhibited hepatic megamitochondria in our series, 45 (90%) proved to be excessive drinkers.

At the light microscopic level, these *giant mitochondria* present as sharply defined, cytoplasmic inclusions that contain closely packed eosinophilic granules. They are usually found in the pericentral regions of the lobules (213). These may be encountered in otherwise normal-appearing hepatocytes (Fig. 134), or within cells that are ballooned or infiltrated with fat (Fig. 135). Usually, megamitochondria are round in shape, but cigar-shaped structures containing elongated, crystalline inclusions have been reported (71). Megamitochondria vary greatly in size, ranging from barely detectable at the light microscopic level, to structures as large as or even larger than the nuclei of affected cells (Fig. 134). Often, several inclusions are present within a single hepatocyte (Fig. 134). Although they have no predilection for any particular segment of the lobules or parenchymal nodules, they frequently are found in groups of contiguous hepatocytes. Neither their incidence, number, nor size bear any relationship to the character of the hepatic lesions in chronic alcoholic patients, occurring with equal frequency in those with normal livers and those with various forms of alcoholic liver disease. However, there is suggestive evidence that the occurrence of megamitochondria correlates with the magnitude and duration of alcohol consumption, and that they tend to disappear two or three months following abstention (71).

Giant mitochondria can be readily seen on H & E stain, and probably less well with the Masson stain (213,214). Characteristically, megamitochondria fail to stain with PAS following diastase digestion.

In an adaptive response to its prolonged administration, alcohol induces its oxidizing enzyme system, MEOS (10,11), accompanied by the proliferation of the smooth endoplasmic reticulum (12) and the formation of *ground glass (induction) cells* [(12); Figs. 124, 125]. In contrast to HBsAg-positive ground glass cells, induction cells do not stain with orcein, aldehyde fuchsin, or Victoria blue, tend to be slightly more granular and less sharply circumscribed, and are only rarely encircled by a clear halo. Moreover, the lipofuscin granules in the peripherally displaced cytoplasm tend to aggregate along the plasma membranes, particularly around the canaliculi. Figure 142 illustrates several such induction cells in a chronic alcoholic patient with an otherwise normal liver.

Hepatocellular carcinoma

The hepatocellular carcinomas that occur in alcoholic cirrhosis have no distinctive histologic features that differentiate them from similar neoplasms found under other conditions.

Histologic differential diagnosis of alcoholic liver disease

Fatty infiltration

Diabetes mellitus, obesity, and, less commonly, other conditions are associated with fatty infiltration. Although such lesions are virtually indistinguishable histologically from those produced by alcohol, the presence of megamitochondria is almost invariably indicative of an alcoholic etiology (215). Numerous vacuolated, glycogen nuclei are suggestive of underlying diabetes mellitus, but are nonspecific and an unreliable diagnostic criterion.

Alcoholic hepatitis and cirrhosis

Obesity, diabetes mellitus, and *jejunoileal bypass* occasionally give rise to lesions that are indistinguishable from those of al-

coholic hepatitis and cirrhosis. In such cases, differentiation depends on the accompanying *clinical and laboratory features* rather than the histologic findings (215).

In the advanced cirrhotic lesions of *Wilson's disease,* the presence of fatty infiltration and Mallory bodies may suggest alcoholic cirrhosis. However, usually, the lesions resemble those of chronic active hepatitis and cirrhosis more closely, and exhibit hepatocellular deposits of rhodanine-positive, copper-containing granules, and orcein-positive, protein-copper granules.

The rapidly progressive lesions of *Indian childhood cirrhosis* are characterized by marked ballooning of the hepatocytes, the presence of Mallory bodies, and a variable degree of cholestasis. However, in contrast to alcoholic cirrhosis, there is no accompanying fatty infiltration, and the cytoplasm in most of the hepatocytes contains high concentrations of copper distributed both diffusely and in granular form throughout the liver, and numerous granular deposits of orcein-positive granular-deposits of copper-binding protein.

Chronic active hepatitis

Several reports of chronic active hepatitis, in which the only recognized insult to the liver is alcohol, have been published (216,217). This disorder progresses if alcohol consumption continues and improves with abstinence.

Inactive alcoholic postnecrotic cirrhosis

In the absence of a history of antecedent alcohol abuse, the macronodular type of alcoholic cirrhosis in its late inactive phase following prolonged abstention may be difficult to distinguish from other forms of inactive cirrhosis, such as chronic active hepatitis with cirrhosis during remission, the relatively quiescent lesions in some cases of advanced Wilson's disease, and cryptogenic cirrhosis. However, the presence within the septa of central veins occluded by fibrous tissue, prominent foci of perisinusoidal and pericellular fibrosis, and stellate scarring around spared central veins strongly suggest an underlying alcoholic etiology.

Acute viral hepatitis superimposed on alcoholic cirrhosis

Acute viral hepatitis superimposed on alcoholic cirrhosis may induce both a characteristic clinical and histologic picture (218). Clinically the patients exhibit an acute viral hepatitis, usually after blood transfusions, but many of them develop hepatic encephalopathy, and the fatality rate is higher than with acute HBV or NANB hepatitis alone (218,219). Histologically, the changes are similar to those of viral hepatitis in noncirrhotic patients, but are superimposed on patterns of cirrhosis and are accompanied by findings such as fatty infiltration and Mallory bodies. It differs in that the usual regenerative response is meager or absent. It is characterized by the sparsity of doubly nucleated cells, the absence of marked variations in hepatocyte cell size, and the presence of clusters of small, uniform, hydropic hepatocytes.

References

1. Klatskin G, Gewin HM, Krehl WA: Effects of prolonged alcohol ingestion on the liver of the rat under conditions of controlled adequate dietary intake. Yale J Biol Med 23:317–331, 1951.
2. Lelbach WK: Cirrhosis in the alcoholic and its relation to the volume of alcohol abuse. Ann NY Acad Sci 252:85–105, 1975.
3. Grant BF, Defour MC, Harford TC: Epidemiology of alcoholic liver disease. Semin Liver Dis 8:12–25, 1988.
4. Isselbacher KJ: Metabolic and hepatic effects of alcohol. N Engl J Med 296:612–616, 1977.
5. Lieber CS: Biochemical and molecular basis of alcohol-induced injury to liver and other tissues. N Engl J Med 319:1639–1650, 1988.
6. Matthewson K, Mardini H, Barlett K, Record CO: Impaired acetaldehyde metabolism in patients with non-alcoholic liver disorders. Gut 27:756–764, 1986.
7. Jewell SA, DiMonte D, Gentile A, Guglielmi A, Altomare E, Albano O: Decreased hepatic glutathione in chronic alcoholic patients. J Hepatol 3:1–6, 1986.
8. Sies H: Oxidative stress. In Oxidative Stress, edited by H. Sies. London, Academic Press, 1985, pp. 1–8.
9. Brunt P: The liver and alcohol. J Hepatol 7:377–383, 1988.
10. Lieber CS: Metabolic effects of ethanol and its interaction with other drugs, hepatotoxic agents, vitamins and carcinogens: a 1988 update. Semin Liver Dis 8:47–68, 1988.
11. Lieber CS: New pathway of ethanol metabolism in the liver. Gastroenterology 59:930–937, 1970.
12. Lane BP, Lieber CS: Ultrastructural alterations in human hepatocytes following ingestion of ethanol with adequate diets. Am J Pathol 49:593–603, 1966.
13. Orrego H, Kalant H, Israel Y, Blake J, Medline A, Rankin JG, Armstrong A, Kapur B: Effects of short-term therapy with propylthiouracil in patients with alcoholic liver disease. Gastroenterology 76:105–115, 1979.
14. Brewer DB, Heath D: Electron microscopy of anoxic vacuolation in the liver cells and its comparison with sucrose vacuolation. J Pathol Bacteriol 90:437–441, 1965.
15. Lieber CS, Jones DP, De Carli LM: Effects of prolonged ethanol intake: production of fatty liver despite adequate diets. J Clin Invest 44:1009–1021, 1965.
16. Rubin E, Lieber CS: Alcohol-induced hepatic injury in nonalcoholic volunteers. N Engl J Med 278:869–876, 1968.
17. Lieber CS, De Carli LM, Rubin E: Sequential production of fatty liver, hepatitis, and cirrhosis in sub-human primates fed ethanol with adequate diets. Proc Natl Acad Sci 72:437–441, 1975.
18. Popper H, Lieber CS: Histogenesis of alcoholic cirrhosis in the baboon. Am J Pathol 98:695–716, 1980.
19. Patek AJ Jr, Bowry SC, Sabesin SM: Minimal hepatic changes in rats fed alcohol and a high casein diet. Arch Pathol Lab Med 100:19–24, 1976.
20. Rogers AE, Fox JG, Murphy JC: Ethanol and diet interactions in male rhesus monkeys. Drug-Nutr Interact 1:3–14, 1981.
21. Lowry JV, Ashburn LL: Effect of alcohol in experimental liver cirrhosis. Q J Study Alc 3:168–175, 1942.
22. Klatskin G, Krehl WA, Conn HO: The effect of alcohol on the choline requirement. I. Changes in the rat's liver following prolonged ingestion of alcohol. J Exp Med 100:605–614, 1954.
23. Patek AJ Jr, Post J, Ratnoff OD, Mankin H, Hillman RW: Dietary treatment of cirrhosis of the liver. Results in one hundred and twenty-four patients observed during a ten year period. JAMA 138:543–549, 1948.
24. Lillie RD, Ashburn LL, Sebrell WH, Daft FS, Lowry JV: Histogenesis and repair of the hepatic cirrhosis in rats produced with low protein diets and preventable with choline. Public Health Rep 57:502–508, 1942.
25. Wilgram GF: Experimental Laennec type cirrhosis in monkeys. Ann Intern Med 51:1134–1158, 1959.
26. Patek AJ Jr, Bowry S, Hayes KC: Cirrhosis of choline deficiency in the rhesus monkey. Possible role of dietary cholesterol. Proc Soc Exp Biol Med 148:370–374, 1975.
27. Baker AL, Elson CO, Jaspan J, Boyer JL: Liver failure with steatonecrosis after jejunoileal bypass. Recovery with parenteral nutrition and reanastomosis. Arch Intern Med 139:289–292, 1979.
28. Hamilton DL, Vest TK, Brown BS, Shah AN, Menguy RB, Chey WY: Liver injury with alcoholic-like hyalin after gastroplasty for morbid obesity. Gastroenterology 85:722–726, 1983.
29. Haines NW, Baker AL, Boyer JL: Prognostic indicator of hepatic injury following jejunoileal bypass performed for refractory obesity: a prospective study. Hepatology 1:161–167, 1981.
30. Vyberg M, Raun V, Andersen B: Pattern of progression in liver injury following bypass for morbid obesity. Liver 7:271–276, 1987.
31. Yost RL, Duerson MC, Russell WL, O'Leary JP: Doxycycline in the prevention of hepatic dysfunction following jejunoileal bypass in humans. Arch Surg 114:931–934, 1979.
32. Bruusgaard A, Sorensen, TJ, Krag E: Bile acid metabolism after jejunoileal bypass operation for obesity. Scand J Gastroenterol 11:833–838, 1976.
33. Popper H, Schaffner F: Nutritional cirrhosis in man? N Engl J Med 285:577–578, 1974.
34. Moxley RT III, Pozefsky T, Lockwood DH: Protein nutrition and liver disease after jejunoileal bypass for morbid obesity. N Engl J Med 290:921–926, 1974.
35. Carter EA, McCarron MJ, Isselbacher KJ: Chronic ethanol feeding increases choline oxidation in the rat. Unpublished observations, personal communication.
36. Sidransky H, Farber E: Liver choline oxidase activity in man and in several species of animals. Arch Biochem Biophys 87:129–133, 1960.
37. Jacobs RM, Sorrell MF: The role of nutrition in the pathogenesis of alcoholic liver disease. Semin Liver Dis 1:244–253, 1981.
38. Cochrane AMG, Moussouros A, Portmann B, McFarlane IG, Thomson AD, Eddleston ALWF, Williams R: Lymphocyte cytotoxicity for isolated hepatocytes in alcoholic liver disease. Gastroenterology 72:918–923, 1977.
39. Kakumu S, Leevy CM: Lymphocyte cytotoxicity in alcoholic hepatitis. Gastroenterology 72:594–597, 1977.
40. Leevy CM, Chen T, Zetterman R: Alcoholic hepatitis, cirrhosis, and immunologic reactivity. Ann NY Acad Sci 252:106–115, 1975.
41. Sorrell MF, Leevy CM: Lymphocyte transformation and alcoholic liver injury. Gastroenterology 63:1020–1025, 1972.
42. Sorrell MF, Tuma DJ: Hypothesis: alcoholic liver injury and the covalent binding of acetaldehyde. Alcohol Clin Exp Res 9:306–309, 1985.
43. Israel Y, Hurwitz E, Niemela O: Monoclonal and polyclonal antibodies against acetaldehyde-containing epitopes in acetaldehyde protein adducts. Proc Natl Acad Sci USA 83:7923–7927, 1986.
44. Penner E, Albini B, Milgrom F: Detection of circulating immune complexes in alcoholic liver disease. Clin Exp Immunol 34:28–31, 1978.
45. Van de Wiel A, Delacroix DL, Van Hattum J: Characteristics of serum IgA and liver IgA deposits in alcoholic liver disease. Hepatology 7:95–99, 1987.
46. Havens WP Jr, Shaffer JM, Hopke CJ Jr: The production of antibody by patients with chronic hepatic disease. J Immunol 67:347–356, 1951.
47. Triger DR, Wright R: Hyperglobulinemia in liver disease. Lancet 1:1494–1496, 1973.
48. Cooksley WGE, Powell LW, Halliday JW: Reticuloendothelial phagocytic function in human liver disease and its relationship to haemolysis. Br J Haematol 25:147–164, 1973.
49. Bernstein IM, Webster KH, Williams RC Jr, Strickland RG: Reduction in circulating T lymphocytes in alcoholic liver disease. Lancet 2:488–490, 1974.
50. Berenyi MR, Straus B, Cruz D: In vitro and in vivo studies of cellular immunity in alcoholic cirrhosis. Am J Dig Dis 19:199–205, 1974.
51. Snyder N, Bessoff J, Dwyer JM, Conn HO: Depressed delayed cutaneous hypersensitivity in alcoholic hepatitis. Dig Dis 23:353–358, 1978.
52. Chen T, Leevy CM: Lymphocyte proliferation inhibitory factor (PIF) in alcoholic liver disease. Clin Exp Immunol 26:42–45, 1976.
53. Mendenhall C, Roselle GA, Lybecker LA, Marshall LE, Grossman CJ, Myre SA, Weesner RE, Morgan DD: Hepatitis B vaccination. Response of alcoholic with and without liver injury. Dig Dis Sci 33:263–269, 1988.
54. Nolan JP: Endotoxin, reticuloendothelial function, and liver injury. Hepatology 1:458–465, 1981.
55. Salmon WD, Newberne PM: Effect of antibiotics, sulfonamides, and a nitrofuran on development of hepatic cirrhosis in choline-deficient rats. J Nutr 76:483–486, 1962.
56. Tarao K, So K, Moroi T, Ikeuchi T, Suyama T, Endo O, Fukushima K: Detection of endotoxin in plasma and ascitic fluid of patients with cirrhosis: its clinical significance. Gastroenterology 73:539–542, 1977.
57. Bird GLA, Sheron N, Goka AKJ, Alexander GJ, Williams RS: In-

creased plasma tumor necrosis factor in severe alcoholic hepatitis. Ann Intern Med *112:*917–920, 1990.

58. Fulenwider JT, Sibley C, Stein SF, Evatt B, Nordlinger BM, Ivey GL: Endotoxemia of cirrhosis: an observation not substantiated. Gastroenterology *78:*1001–1004, 1980.

59. Bailey RJ, Krasner N, Eddleston ALWF, Williams R, Tee D, Doniach D, Kennedy LA, Batchelor JR: Histocompatibility antigen, autoimmune bodies and immunoglobulins. Br Med J *2:*727–729, 1976.

60. Morgan MY, Ross MGR, Ng CM, Adams DM, Thomas HC, Sherlock S: HLA-B8, immunoglobulins, and antibody responses in alcohol-related liver disease. J Clin Pathol *33:*488–492, 1980.

61. Bell H, Nordhagen R: Association between HLA-BW40 and alcoholic liver diseases with cirrhosis. Br Med J *1:*882, 1978.

62. Melendez M, Vargas-Tank L, Fuentes C, Armas-Merino R, Castillo D, Wolff C, Wegmann ME, Soto J: Distribution of HLA histocompatibility antigens, ABO blood groups and Rh antigens in alcoholic liver disease. Gut *20:*288–290, 1979.

63. Doffoel M, Tongio MM, Gut JP: Relationships between 34 HLA-A, HLA-B and HLA-DR antigens and three serological markers of viral infections in alcoholic cirrhosis. Hepatology *6:*457–463, 1986.

64. Shigeta Y, Ishii H, Takagi S: HLA antigens as immunogenetic markers of alcoholism and alcoholic liver disease. Pharmacol Biochem Behav 13 (Suppl):89–94, 1980.

65. Bosron WF, Li T-K: Genetic polymorphism of human liver alcohol and aldehyde dehydrogenases and their relation to alcohol metabolism and alcoholism. Hepatology *6:*502–510, 1986.

66. Devor EJ, Reich T, Cloninger CR: Genetics of alcoholism and related end-organ damage. Semin Liver Dis *8:*1–11, 1988.

67. Peters TJ, Ward RJ: Role of acetaldehyde in the pathogenesis of alcoholic liver disease. Mol Aspects Med *10:*179–190, 1988.

68. Devenyl P, Rutherdale J, Sereny G, Olin JS: Clinical diagnosis of alcoholic fatty liver. Am J Gastroenterol *54:*597–602, 1970.

69. Baraona E, Leo MA, Borowsky SA, Lieber CS: Pathogenesis of alcohol-induced accumulation of protein in the liver. J Clin Invest *60:*546–554, 1977.

70. Tuma DJ, Jennett RB, Sorrell MF: Effect of ethanol on the synthesis and secretion of hepatic secretory glycoproteins and albumin. Hepatology *1:*590–598, 1981.

71. Bruguera M, Bertran A, Bombi JA, Rodes J: Giant mitochondria in hepatocytes. A diagnostic hint for alcoholic liver disease. Gastroenterology *73:*1383–1387, 1977.

72. Leung NWY, Farrant P, Peters TJ: Liver volume measurement by ultrasonography in normal subjects and alcoholic patients. J Hepatol *2:*157–164, 1986.

73. Ballard H, Bernstein M, Farrar JT: Fatty liver presenting as obstructive jaundice. Am J Med *30:*196–201, 1961.

74. Morgan MY, Sherlock S, Scheuer PJ: Acute cholestasis, hepatic failure, and fatty liver in the alcoholic. Scand J Gastroenterol *13:*299–303, 1978.

75. Afshani P, Littenberg GD, Wollman J, Kaplowitz N: Significance of microscopic cholangitis in alcoholic liver disease. Gastroenterology *75:*1045–1050, 1978.

76. Harinasuta U, Chomet B, Ishak K: Steatonecrosis—Mallory body type. Medicine *46:*141–162, 1967.

77. Cohen JA, Kaplan MM: The SGOT/SGPT ratio: an indicator of alcoholic liver disease. Dig Dis Sci *24:*835–838, 1979.

78. Matloff DS, Selinger MJ, Kaplan MM: Hepatic transaminase activity in alcoholic liver disease. Gastroenterology *78:*1389–1392, 1980.

79. Sakalibara R, Huynh QK, Nishida T: *In vitro* synthesis of glutamic oxaloacetic transaminase isoenzymes of rat liver. Biochem Biophys Res Commun *95:*1781–1788, 1980.

80. Nalpas B, Vassault A, Charpin S, Lacour B, Berthelot P: Serum mitochondrial aspartate aminotransferase as a marker of chronic alcoholism: diagnostic value and interpretation of a liver unit. Hepatology *6:*608–612, 1986.

81. Nalpas B, Vassault A, Le Guillou A, Lesgourgues B, Ferry N, Lacour B, Berthelot P: Serum activity of mitochondrial aspartate aminotransferase: a sensitive marker of alcoholism with or without alcoholic hepatitis. Hepatology *4:*893–896, 1984.

82. Jenkins WJ, Peters TJ: Mitochondrial enzyme activities in liver biopsies from patients with alcoholic liver disease. Gut *19:*341–344, 1978.

83. Galambos J: Alcohol and liver disease. Am J Dig Dis *14:*477–490, 1969.

84. Galambos J: Natural history of alcoholic hepatitis. III. Histological changes. Gastroenterology *63:*1026–1035, 1972.

85. Leevy CM: Fatty liver: a study of 270 patients with biopsy proven fatty liver and a review of the literature. Medicine *41:*249–276, 1962.

86. Christoffersen P, Braendstrup O: Lipogranulomas in human liver biopsies with fatty change. A morphological, biochemical and clinical investigation. Acta Pathol Microbiol Scand (A) *79:*150–158, 1971.

87. Petersen P, Christoffersen P: Ultrastructure of lipogranulomas in human fatty liver. Acta Pathol Microbiol Scand (A) *87:*45–49, 1979.

88. Delladetsima JK, Horn T, Poulsen H: Portal tract lipogranulomas in liver biopsies. Liver *7:*9–17, 1987.

89. Wanless IR, Geddie WR: Mineral oil lipogranulomata in liver and spleen. Arch Pathol Lab Med *109:*283–286, 1985.

90. Feinman L, Lieber CS: Hepatic collagen metabolism: effect of alcohol consumption in rats and baboons. Science *176:*795, 1972.

91. Chen TSN, Leevy CM: Collagen biosynthesis in liver disease of the alcoholic. J Lab Clin Med *85:*103–112, 1975.

92. Mezey E, Potter JJ, Slusser RJ, Abdi W: Changes in hepatic collagen metabolism in rats produced by chronic ethanol feeding. Lab Invest *36:*206–214, 1977.

93. Galambos JT, Hollingsworth MA Jr, Falek A, Warren WD: The rate of synthesis of glycosaminoglycans and collagen by fibroblasts cultured from adult human liver biopsies. J Clin Invest *60:*107–114, 1977.

94. Henley KS, Laughrey EG, Appelman HD, Flecker K: Effect of ethanol on collagen formation in dietary cirrhosis in the rat. Gastroenterology *72:*502–506, 1977.

95. Van Waes L, Lieber CS: Early perivenular sclerosis in alcoholic fatty liver. An index of progressive liver disease. Gastroenterology *73:*646–650, 1977.

96. Nasrallah SM, Nassar VH, Galambos JT: Importance of terminal hepatic venule thickening. Arch Pathol Lab Med *104:*84–86, 1980.

97. Edmondson HA, Peters RL, Reynolds TB, Kuzma OT: Sclerosing hyaline necrosis of the liver in the chronic alcoholic. Ann Intern Med *59:*646–673, 1963.

98. Horn T, Junge J, Christoffersen P: Early alcoholic liver injury: changes of the Disse space in acinar zone 3. Liver *5:*301–310, 1985.

99. Horn T, Junge J, Christoffersen P: Early alcoholic liver injury. Activation of lipocytes in acinar zone 3 and correlation to degree of collagen formation in the Disse space. J Hepatol *3:*333–340, 1986.

100. Leo MA, Lieber CS: Hypervitaminosis A: a liver lover's lament. Hepatology *8:*412–417, 1988.

101. Leo MA, Lieber CS: Hepatic vitamin A depletion in alcoholic liver injury. N Engl J Med *307:*597–601, 1982.

102. Geubel AP, Alves N, Rahier J: Vitamine A hepatotoxicity: diagnosis, prognosis, and dose-effect relationship. A study of 34 consecutive cases. (abstract) J Hepatol 7(Supp 1):535, 1988.

103. Okanue T, Burbige EJ, Franch SW: The role of the Ito cell in perivenular fibrosis and intralobular fibrosis in alcoholic hepatitis. Arch Pathol Lab Med *107:*459–463, 1982.

104. Minato Y, Hasumura Y, Takeuchi J: The role of fat-storing cells in Disse space fibrogenesis in alcoholic liver disease. Hepatology *3:*559–566, 1983.

105. Mak KM, Lieber CS: Portal fibroblasts and myofibroblasts in baboons after long-term alcohol consumption. Arch Pathol Lab Med *110:*513–516, 1986.

106. Torres-Salinas MT, Pares A, Caballeria J, Jimenez W, Heredia D, Bruguera M, Rodes J: Serum procollagen type III peptide as a marker of hepatic fibrogenesis in alcoholic hepatitis. Gastroenterology *90:*1241–1246, 1986.

107. Tanaka Y, Minato Y, Hasumura Y, Takeuchi J: Evaluation of hepatic fibrosis by serum proline and amino-terminal type III procollagen peptide levels in alcoholic patients. Dig Dis Sci *31:*712–717, 1986.

108. Ugarte G, Iturragia H, Insunza I: Some effects of ethanol on normal and pathologic livers. *In* Progress in Liver Diseases, Vol. III, edited by H. Popper, F. Schaffner. New York, Grune & Stratton, 1970, pp. 355–370.

109. Green JR: Subclinical acute liver disease of the alcoholic. Australas Ann Med *14:*111–124, 1965.

110. Phillips GB, Davidson CS: Liver disease of the chronic alcoholic simulating extrahepatic biliary obstruction. Gastroenterology *33:*236–244, 1957.

111. Conn HO, Blei AT, Chojkier M, Schade R, Taggart GJ, Atterbury CE: The naked physician: the blind interpretation of liver function tests in the differential diagnosis of jaundice. *In* The Liver: Quantitative Aspects of Structure and Function, edited by R. Preisig, J. Bircher. Gstaad Symposium, 1978, pp. 386–394.

112. Kryger P, Schlichting P, Dietrichson O, Juhl E: The accuracy of the clinical diagnosis in acute hepatitis and alcoholic liver disease. Clinical versus morphological diagnosis. Scand J Gastroenterol *18:*691–696, 1983.

113. Helman RA, Temko MH, Nye SW, Fallon HJ: Alcoholic hepatitis: natural history and evaluation of prednisolone therapy. Ann Intern Med 74:311–321, 1971.

114. Harinasuta U, Zimmerman HJ: Alcoholic steatonecrosis. I. Relationship between severity of hepatic disease and presence of Mallory bodies in the liver. Gastroenterology 60:1036–1046, 1971.

115. Green J, Mistilis S, Schiff L: Acute alcoholic hepatitis. A clinical study of fifty cases. Arch Intern Med 112:67–78, 1963.

116. Conn HO, Hallak R: Alcoholic hepatitis syndrome: prognosis and course. In Current Perspectives in Hepatology, edited by L.B. Seeff, J.H. Lewis. New York, Plenum Publishing Corp., 1989, pp. 211–218.

117. Maddrey WC, Boitnott JK, Bedine MS: Adrenocorticosteroid therapy of alcoholic hepatitis. Gastroenterology 75:193–199, 1978.

118. Carithers RL Jr, Herlong HF, Diehl AM, Shaw EW, Combes B, Fallon HJ, Maddrey WC: Methylprednisolone therapy in patients with severe alcoholic hepatitis. A randomized multicenter trial. Ann Intern Med 10:685–690, 1989.

119. Pares A. Caballeria J, Bruguera M, Torres M, Rodes J: Histological course of alcoholic hepatitis. Influence of abstinence, sex and extent of hepatic damage. J Hepatol 2:33–42, 1986.

120. Sorensen TIA, Bentsen KD, Eghøje K, Orholm M, Hoybye G, Christoffersen P: Prospective evaluation of alcohol abuse and alcoholic liver injury in men as predictors of development of cirrhosis. Lancet 2:241–244, 1984.

121. Morgan MY, Sherlock S: Sex-related differences among 100 patients with alcoholic liver disease. Br Med J 1:939–942, 1977.

122. Frezza M, di Padova C, Pozzato G, Terpin M, Baraona E, Lieber CS: High blood alcohol levels in women. The role of decreased gastric alcohol dehydrogenase activity and first-pass metabolism. N Engl J Med 322:95–99, 1990.

123. Harinasuta U, Chomet B, Ishak K, Zimmerman HJ: Steatonecrosis-Mallory body type. Medicine 46:141–162, 1967.

124. Lischner MW, Alexander JF, Galambos JT: Natural history of alcoholic hepatitis. I. The acute disease. Am J Dig Dis 16:481–494, 1971.

125. Christoffersen P, Eghøje K, Juhl E: Mallory bodies in liver biopsies from chronic alcoholics. A comparative morphological, biochemical, and clinical study of two groups of chronic alcoholics with and without Mallory bodies. Scand J Gastroenterol 8:341–346, 1973.

126. Birschbach HR, Harinasuta U, Zimmerman HJ: Alcoholic steatonecrosis. II. Prospective study of prevalence of Mallory bodies in biopsy specimens and comparison of severity of hepatic disease in patients with and without this histologic feature. Gastroenterology 66:1195–1202, 1974.

127. Imperiale TF, McCullough AJ: Do corticosteroids reduce mortality from alcoholic hepatitis? A meta-analysis of the randomized trials. Ann Intern Med 113:299–307, 1990.

128. Nagore N, Scheuer PJ: The pathology of diabetic hepatitis. J Pathol 156:155–160, 1988.

129. Adler M, Schaffner F: Fatty liver hepatitis and cirrhosis in obese patients. Am J Med 67:811–816, 1979.

130. Diehl AM, Goodman Z, Ishak KG: Alcohol-like liver disease in non-alcoholics. Gastroenterology 95:1056–1062, 1988.

131. Klass HJ, Kelly JK, Warnes TW: Indian childhood cirrhosis in the United Kingdom. Gut 21:344–350, 1980.

132. Nayak NC: Indian childhood cirrhosis. In Pathology of the Liver, edited by R.N.M. MacSween, P.P. Anthony, P.J. Scheuer. 2nd Edition. Edinburgh, Churchill Livingstone, 1987, pp. 358–360.

133. Pessayre D, Bichara M, Feldmann G, Degott C, Potet F, Benhamou J-P: Perhexilene maleate-induced cirrhosis. Gastroenterology 76:170–177, 1979.

134. Simon JB, Manley PN, Brien JF: Amiodarone hepatotoxicity simulating alcoholic liver disease. N Engl J Med 311:167–172, 1984.

135. Seki K, Minami Y, Nishikawa M, Kawata S, Miyoshi S, Imai Y, Tarui S: 'Nonalcoholic steatohepatitis' induced by massive doses of synthetic estrogen. Gastroenterologica Jpn 18:197–203, 1983.

136. Capron J-P, Delamarre J, Dupas JL, Braillon A, Degott C, Quenum C: Fasting in obesity. Another cause of liver injury with alcoholic hyaline? Dig Dis Sci 27:265–268, 1982.

137. Patek AJ Jr, Toth IG, Saunders MG, Castro GAM, Engel JJ: Alcohol and dietary factors in cirrhosis. An epidemiological study of 304 alcoholic patients. Arch Intern Med 135:1053–1057, 1975.

138. Wilkinson P, Santamaria JN, Rankin JG: Epidemiology of alcoholic cirrhosis. Australas Ann Med 18:222–226, 1969.

139. Saunders JB, Davis M, Williams R: Do women develop alcoholic liver disease more readily than men? Br Med J 282:1140–1143, 1981.

140. Norton R, Batey R, Dwyer T, MacMahon S: Alcohol consumption and the risk of alcohol related cirrhosis in women. Br Med J 295:80–82, 1987.

141. Lelbach WK: Epidemiology of alcoholic liver disease. Vol 5 in Popper H, Schaffner F, eds. Progress in Liver Disease. New York, Grune & Stratton, pp. 494–515, 1976.

142. Conn HO: Alcohol content of various beverages: all booze is created equal. Hepatology 12:1252–1254, 1990.

143. Frezza M, DiPadova C, Pozzato G, Terpin M, Baraona E, Lieber CS: High blood alcohol levels in women: the role of decreased gastric alcohol dehydrogenase activity and first-pass metabolism. N Engl J Med 322:95–99, 1990.

144. Arthur MJ, Lee A, Wright R: Sex differences in the metabolism of ethanol and acetaldehyde in normal subjects. Clin Sci 67:397–401, 1984.

145. Mishra L, Sharma S, Potter JJ, Mezey E: More rapid elimination of alcohol in women as compared to their male siblings. Alcoholism: Clin Exp Res 13:752–754, 1989.

146. Hislop WS, Follett EA, Bouchier IAD. Serological markers of hepatitis B in patients with alcoholic liver disease: a multi-centre survey. J Clin Pathol 34:1017–1023, 1981.

147. Villa E, Rubbiani L, Barchi T: Susceptibility of chronic symptomless HBsAg carriers to ethanol-induced hepatic damage. Lancet 2:1243–1245, 1982.

148. Pares A, Barrera JM, Caballeria J, Ercilla G, Bruguera M, Caballeria L, Castillo R, Rodes J: Hepatitis C virus antibodies in chronic alcoholic patients: association with severity of liver injury. Hepatology 12:1295–1299, 1990.

149. Tarao K, Hishino H, Motohashi I, Iimori K, Tamai S, Ito Y, Takagi S, Oikawa Y, Unayama S, Fujiwara T, Odagiri K, Ikeda T, Hayashi K, Sakurai A, Uchikoshi T: Changes in liver and spleen volume in alcoholic liver fibrosis of man. Hepatology 9:589–593, 1989.

150. Orrego HL, Blendis IR, Crossley A: Correlation of intrahepatic pressure with collagen in the Disse space and hepatomegaly in humans and in the rat. Gastroenterology 80:546–556, 1981.

151. Blendis LM, Orrego H, Crossley IR, Blake JE, Medline A, Israel Y: The role of hepatocyte enlargement in hepatic pressure in cirrhotic and noncirrhotic alcoholic liver disease. Hepatology 2:539–546, 1982.

152. Krogsgaard K, Gluud C, Henriksen JH, Christoffersen P: Correlation between liver morphology and haemodynamics in alcoholic liver disease. Liver 5:173–177, 1985.

153. Poynard T, Degott C, Munoz C, Lebrec D: Relationship between degree of portal hypertension and liver histologic lesions in patients with alcoholic cirrhosis. Effect of acute alcoholic hepatitis on portal hypertension. Dig Dis Sci 32:337–342, 1987.

154. Nataf C, Feldmann G, Lebrec D, Degott C, Descamps J-M, Rueff B, Benhamou J-P: Idiopathic portal hypertension (perisinusoidal fibrosis) after renal transplantation. Gut 20:531–537, 1979.

155. Goodman ZD, Ishak KG: Occlusive venous lesions in alcoholic liver disease. A study of 200 cases. Gastroenterology 83:786–796, 1982.

156. Myakawa H, Iida S, Leo MA, Greenstein RJ, Zimmon Ds, Lieber CS: Pathogenesis of precirrhotic portal hypertension in alcohol-fed baboons. Gastroenterology 88:143–150, 1985.

157. Burt AD, MacSween RNM: Hepatic vein lesions in alcoholic liver disease: retrospective biopsy and necropsy study. J Clin Pathol 39:63–67, 1986.

158. Orrego H, Medline A, Blendis LM: Collagenisation of the Disse space in alcoholic liver disease. Gut 20:673–679, 1979.

159. Horn T, Henriksen JH, Christoffersen P: The sinusoidal lining cells in "normal" human liver. A scanning electron microscopic investigation. Liver 6:98–102, 1986.

160. Horn T, Henriksen JH, Christoffersen P, Henriksen JH: Alcoholic liver injury: defenestration in noncirrhotic livers. A scanning electron microscopic study. Hepatology 7:77–82, 1987.

161. Klatskin G, Yesner R: Factors in the treatment of Laennec's cirrhosis. I. Clinical and histological changes observed during a control period of bed-rest, alcohol withdrawal, and a minimal basic diet. J Clin Invest 28:723–735, 1949.

162. Powell WJ Jr, Klatskin G: Duration of survival in patients with Laennec's cirrhosis. Influence of alcohol withdrawal, and possible effects of recent changes in general management of the disease. Am J Med 44:406–420, 1968.

163. Borowsky SA, Strome S, Lott E: Continued heavy drinking and survival in alcoholic cirrhotics. Gastroenterology 80:1405–1409, 1981.

164. Gluud C, Christoffersen P, Eriksen J, Wantzin P, Knudsen BB, and the Copenhagen Study Group for Liver Diseases: Influence of ethanol on development of hyperplastic nodules in alcoholic men with micronodular cirrhosis. Gastroenterology 93:256–260, 1987.

165. Rubin E, Krus S, Popper H: Pathogenesis of postnecrotic cirrhosis in alcoholics. Arch Pathol 73:288–299, 1962.
166. Fauerholdt L, Schlichting P, Christensen E, Poulsen H, Tygstrup N, Juhl E, and the Copenhagen Study Group for Liver Diseases: Conversion of micronodular cirrhosis into macronodular cirrhosis. Hepatology 3:928–931, 1983.
167. Gluud C, Christoffersen P, Eriksen J, Wantzin P, Knudsen B, and Copenhagen Study Group for Liver Diseases: Influence of ethanol on development of hyperplastic nodules in alcoholic men with micronodular cirrhosis. Gastroenterology 93:256–260, 1987.
168. Diehl AM, Goodman Z, Ishak KG: Alcohol-like liver disease in nonalcoholics. Gastroenterology 95:1056–1062, 1988.
169. MacDonald RA: Cirrhosis and primary carcinoma of the liver. Changes in their occurrence at the Boston City Hospital, 1897–1954. N Engl J Med 255:1179–1183, 1956.
170. Lee FI: Cirrhosis and hepatoma in alcoholics. Gut 7:77–85, 1966.
171. Bjorneboe M, Rikardt Andersen J, Christensen U, Skinhoj P, Moller Jensen O: Does a portal-systemic shunt increase the risk of primary hepatic carcinoma in cirrhosis of the liver? Scand J Gastroenterol 20:59–64, 1985.
172. Rofe S, Schuster M, Conn HO: The relationship between hepatocellular carcinoma and portal-systemic shunting. (Unpublished observations).
173. Beasley RP, Hwang L-Y: Hepatocellular carcinoma and hepatitis B virus. Semin Liver Dis 4:113–121, 1984.
174. Scheuer PJ, Williams R, Muir AR: Hepatic pathology in relatives of patients with haemochromatosis. J Pathol Bacteriol 84:53–64, 1962.
175. Williams R, Williams HS, Scheuer PJ, Pitcher CS, Loiseau E, Sherlock S: Iron absorption and siderosis in chronic liver disease. Q J Med 36:151–166, 1967.
176. Simon M, Bourel M, Genetet B, Fauchet R: Idiopathic hemochromatosis. Demonstration of recessive transmission and early detection by family HLA typing. N Engl J Med 297:1017–1021, 1977.
177. MacDonald RA, Baumslag N: Iron in alcoholic beverages. Possible significance for hemochromatosis. Am J Med Sci 247:649–654, 1964.
178. Murray MJ, Stein N: Does the pancreas influence iron absorption? A critical review of information to date. Gastroenterology 51:694–700, 1966.
179. Tuttle SG, Figueroa WG, Grossman MI: Development of hemochromatosis in a patient with Laennec's cirrhosis. Am J Med 26:655–658, 1959.
180. Ecker JA, Gray PA, McKittrick JE, Dickson DR: The development of postshunt hemochromatosis-parenchymal siderosis in patients with cirrhosis occurring after portasystemic shunt surgery. A review of the literature and report of two additional cases. Am J Gastroenterol 50:13–29, 1968.
181. Conn HO: Portacaval anastomosis and hepatic hemosiderin deposition: a prospective, controlled investigation. Gastroenterology 62:61–72, 1972.
182. Uchida T, Kao H, Quispe-Sjogren M, Peters RL: Alcoholic foamy degeneration: a pattern of acute alcoholic injury of the liver. Gastroenterology 84:683–692, 1983.
183. MacSween RNM: Mallory's ('alcoholic') hyaline in primary biliary cirrhosis. J Clin Pathol 26:340–342, 1973.
184. Levi AJ, Sherlock S, Scheuer PJ, Cumings JN: Presymptomatic Wilson's disease. Lancet 2:575–579, 1967.
185. Nyak NC, Roy S: Morphological types of hepatocellular hyalin in Indian childhood cirrhosis: an ultrastructural study. Gut 17:791–796, 1976.
186. Gerber MA, Orr W, Denk H, Schaffner F, Popper H: Hepatocellular hyalin in cholestasis and cirrhosis: its diagnostic significance. Gastroenterology 64:89–98, 1973.
187. Nakanuma Y, Ohta G: Expression of Mallory bodies in hepatocellular carcinoma in man and its significance. Cancer 57:81–86, 1986.
188. Wetzel WJ, Alexander RW: Focal nodular hyperplasia of the liver with alcoholic hyalin bodies and cytologic atypia. Cancer 4:1322–1326, 1979.
189. Denk H, Gschnait F, Wolff K: Hepatocellular hyalin (Mallory bodies) in long term griseofulvin-treated mice: a new experimental model for the study of hyalin formation. Lab Invest 32:773–776, 1975.
190. Yokoo H, Minick OT, Batti F, Kent G: Morphologic variants of alcoholic hyalin. Am J Pathol 69:25–40, 1972.
191. Franke WW, Denk H, Schmid E, Osborn M, Weber K: Ultrastructural, biochemical, and immunologic characterization of Mallory bodies in griseofulvin-treated mice: fimbricated rods of filaments containing prekeratin-like polypeptides. Lab Invest 40:207–220, 1979.

192. Hazan R, Denk H, Franke WW: Change of cytokeratin organization during development of Mallory bodies as revealed by a monoclonal antibody. Lab Invest 54:543–553, 1986.
193. Katsuma Y, Swierenga SHH, Khettry U, Marceau N, French SW: Changes in the cytokeratin intermediate filament cytoskeleton associated with Mallory body formation in mouse and human liver. Hepatology 7:1215–1223, 1987.
194. French SW, Swierenga SHH, Okanoue T: Cytoskeleton of the liver cell in health and disease. In The Liver, edited by E. Farber, M.J. Phillips. Baltimore, Williams & Wilkins, 1986.
195. Barbatis C, Morton J, Woods JC, Burns J, Bradley J, McGee J O'D: Disorganization of intermediate filament structure in alcoholic and other liver diseases. Gut 27:765–770, 1986.
196. Denk H, Franke WW, Kerjaschki D, Eckerstorfer R: Mallory bodies in experimental animals and man. Int Rev Exp Pathol 20:77–121, 1979.
197. Leo MA, Arai M, Sato M, Lieber CS: Hepatotoxicity of vitamin A and ethanol in the rat. Gastroenterology 82:194–205, 1982.
198. Nakanuma Y, Ohta G: Is Mallory body formation a preneoplastic change: a study of 181 cases of liver bearing hepatocellular carcinoma and 82 cases of cirrhosis. Cancer 55:2400–2404, 1985.
199. Roque AL: Chromotrope aniline blue method of staining Mallory bodies of Laennec's cirrhosis. Lab Invest 2:15–21, 1953.
200. Fleming KA, Morton JA, Barbatis C, Burns J, Canning S, McGee JO'D: Mallory bodies in alcoholic and non-alcoholic liver disease containing a common antigenic determinant. Gut 22:341–344, 1981.
201. Christoffersen P: Light microscopic features in liver biopsies with Mallory bodies. Acta Pathol Scand, Section A, 80:705–712, 1972.
202. Bird GL, Williams R: Factors determining cirrhosis in alcoholic liver disease. Mol Aspects Med 10:97–105, 1988.
203. Reynolds TB, Hidemura R, Michel H, Peters R: Portal hypertension without cirrhosis in alcohol liver disease. Ann Intern Med 70:492–506, 1969.
204. Nakano M, Worner TM, Lieber CS: Perivenular fibrosis in alcoholic liver injury. Ultrastructure and histologic progression. Gastroenterology 83:777–785, 1982.
205. Lefkowitch JH, Rushton AR, Feng-Chen K-C: Hepatic fibrosis in fetal alcohol syndrome. Gastroenterology 85:951–957, 1983.
206. Krogsgaard K, Gluud C, Henriksen JH, Christoffersen P: Correlation between liver morphology and haemodynamics in alcoholic liver disease. Liver 5:173–177, 1985.
207. Boyer TD, Triger DR, Horisawa M: Direct transhepatic measurement of portal vein pressure using a thin needle. Gastroenterology 72:584–589, 1977.
208. Goldberg SJ, Mendenhall CL, Connell AM, Chedid A: "Nonalcoholic" chronic hepatitis in the alcoholic. Gastroenterology 72:598–604, 1977.
209. Perez-Tamayo R: Diffuse interstitial cirrhosis. Am J Clin Pathol 29:226–235, 1958.
210. Anthony PP, Vogel CL, Barker LF: Liver cell dysplasia: a premalignant condition. J Clin Pathol 26:217–223, 1973.
211. Lefkowitch JH, Arborgh BAM, Scheuer PJ: Oxyphilic granular hepatocytes. Mitochondrion-rich liver cells in hepatic disease. Am J Clin Pathol 74:432–441, 1980.
212. Chedid A, Mendenhall CL, Tosch T, Chen T, Rabin L, Garcia-Pont P, Goldberg SJ, Kiernan T, Seeff LB, Sorrell M, Tamburro C, Weesner RE, Zetterman R, and Veterans Administration Cooperative Study of Alcoholic Hepatitis: Significance of megamitochondria in alcoholic liver disease. Gastroenterology 90:1858–1864, 1986.
213. Uchida T, Kronborg I, Peters RL: Giant mitochondria in the alcoholic liver diseases: their identification, frequency and pathologic significance. Liver 4:29–38, 1984.
214. Fleming KA, McGee JO'D: Review article: alcohol induced liver disease. J Clin Pathol 377:721–733, 1984.
215. Desmet VJ: Alcoholic liver disease. Histological features and evolution. Acta Med Scand 703:111–126, 1985.
216. Crapper RM, Bhatal PS, Mackay IR: Chronic active hepatitis in alcoholic patients. Liver 3:327–337, 1983.
217. Nei J, Matsuda Y, Takada A: Chronic hepatitis induced by alcohol. Dig Dis Sci 28:207–215, 1983.
218. Feller A, Uchida F, Rakela J: Acute viral hepatitis superimposed on alcoholic liver cirrhosis: clinical and histopathologic features. Liver 5:239–246, 1985.
219. Theodossi A, Wilkinson SPW, Portmann B: De novo acute infection and reactivation of hepatitis B virus in established cirrhosis. Br Med J 2:893–895, 1979.

Chapter 11
Primary Biliary Cirrhosis

At one time, primary biliary cirrhosis was regarded as a rare disorder that affected middle-aged women exclusively and that invariably proved fatal in five or six years. However, advances over the past 25 years that have facilitated recognition of the disease in its early stages have led to striking changes in our concepts of the prevalence, manifestations, and natural history of primary biliary cirrhosis. These advances include the identification of distinctive histologic features of primary biliary cirrhosis (1–5), the discovery that mitochondrial antibodies appear in a high proportion of cases (6–9), and the widespread use of automated biochemical screening of serum, which has exposed large numbers of asymptomatic cases by the discovery of high serum levels of alkaline phosphatase and the recognition that this disorder has a more benign course in many patients (10).

Since the critical feature of the lesions is destruction of interlobular and septal bile ducts prior to the development of cirrhosis, the lesions are classified by some authorities as *chronic nonsuppurative destructive cholangitis* (4,11).

Increasing evidence suggests that an autoimmune mechanism is involved in the pathogenesis of primary biliary cirrhosis. Nevertheless, the etiology of the disease remains obscure.

Clinical features

Prevalence

The striking increase in the frequency with which primary biliary cirrhosis is being recognized is illustrated by the fact that less than 50 cases had been identified during the 100 years that followed its description in 1851 (12), but at least five series of more than 200 cases each have been reported in the past decade (5,13–16). Based on epidemiologic data, it has been estimated that the prevalence of primary biliary cirrhosis is approximately 54 cases per million (17).

Sex and age distribution

Women predominate; men comprise approximately 10% of the cases. Primarily biliary cirrhosis is usually encountered in individuals ranging in age from 35 to 65 years. However, occasionally, the disease occurs before the age of 30 or after 70. The course and outcome are similar in men and in women (16,18).

Symptomatic primary biliary cirrhosis

Usually, the onset of the disease is insidious, and is characterized by pruritus, fatigue, or malaise. Mild jaundice is an initial complaint in approximately 25% of cases. Other, less common, presenting symptoms include weight loss, anorexia, nausea, vomiting, abdominal pain, or bleeding from varices. In a small minority of cases, the onset is abrupt with overt jaundice, a feature that, in some cases, appears to be provoked by pregnancy or the use of estrogens or oral contraceptive steroids.

At presentation, the physical findings include hepatomegaly, mild jaundice, splenomegaly, or hyperpigmentation in various combinations in half the cases. Xanthomas are encountered in less than one-third of cases, and ascites only rarely. Obviously, the findings in any given case depend on how far the hepatic lesions have advanced before the appearance of symptoms. Once symptoms appear, the course of the disease tends to be progressive. However, the rate of progression is highly variable. In most cases death ensues as a result of hepatic failure or hemorrhage from esophageal varices if hepatic transplantation is not performed (19).

Early reports suggested that the life expectancy in patients with symptomatic primary biliary cirrhosis was between 5 and 6 years. However, in more recent studies, the mean survival time in such individuals was approximately 12 years, and some lived for over 20 years (15). In our 243 cases of symptomatic primary biliary cirrhosis (15)), survival was significantly reduced in patients who presented with jaundice, ascites, splenomegaly, low serum levels of albumin, or high serum concentrations of immunoglobulins compared with those without these abnormalities. Moreover, the duration of survival varied inversely with the degree of fibrosis, the extent of limiting plate erosion and the severity of cholestasis found on biopsy at the time of diagnosis. Although not confirmed in our cases (15) or those of some other authorities (12), it has been reported that the presence of granulomas in the lesions of primary biliary cirrhosis is associated with a better prognosis (20). The presence of severe cholestasis, however, is associated with a poor prognosis (5,14,21,22).

Asymptomatic primary biliary cirrhosis

Most cases of asymptomatic disease are recognized following the unexpected discovery of an otherwise unexplained, elevated level of serum alkaline phosphatase or, less commonly, following the detection of hepatomegaly in the course of a routine physical examination. In most large series of primary biliary cirrhosis collected over two or three decades, asymptomatic cases have ranged from 13% (12) to 37% (14), whereas in series collected since the advent of automated, biochemical screening of serum, the number of asymptomatic cases has tended to be higher (23,24). One-half to two-thirds of patients with asymptomatic primary biliary cirrhosis, who tend to be older than those with symptomatic disease, remain symptom-free (16).

Despite the absence of symptoms, the lesions in such cases do not differ from those in symptomatic cases, and may be in an advanced stage of development. In most studies, the disease has ultimately become symptomatic in from 16% (25) to 78% (14) of cases, usually within 2 or 3 years (15,26), and has proved fatal in up to 30% (26). In our group of 38 asymptomatic primary biliary cirrhosis patients followed for up to 19 years (mean 6.9 years), 14 (38%) ultimately developed signs or symptoms of chronic liver disease, and 4 (11%) died, although liver disease was a contributory factor in only 2 (5%) (10,15). However, the life expectancy in this group of asymptomatic patients did not differ from that in the general population matched for age and sex. Such observations clearly demonstrate that the onset of symptoms in primary biliary cirrhosis may be preceded by a long interval during which the lesions are active and progressive, but inapparent clinically. Moreover, they suggest that in some patients the lesions may not be progressive, and may never give rise to symptoms, a possibility that still requires confirmation.

However, another group of investigators who initiated follow-up at the time of referral of their patients (27), rather than retrospectively as was done in our patients (10,15), found that 89% of the asymptomatic patients developed symptoms and two-thirds of the noncirrhotic patients developed cirrhosis during a median follow-up of 7.6 years. Furthermore, life expectancy was much shorter than we had observed. We conclude that the manner of selection of our patients apparently minimized the apparent progress of the disease and maximized survival. Further investigations will be required to settle this controversy.

Complications

Hepatocellular failure or hemorrhage from esophageal varices secondary to portal hypertension account for most deaths in patients with primary biliary cirrhosis. In approximately 10% of cases, death is attributable to coincidental disease, particularly myocardial infarction, a complication that does not appear to correlate with the alterations in serum cholesterol that may occur in primary biliary cirrhosis (15). Only rarely is the course of primary biliary cirrhosis complicated by the development of hepatocellular carcinoma (28,29). Primary biliary cirrhosis may be associated with an increased prevalence of extrahepatic malignancy, particularly cancer of the breast (30). It is noteworthy that complications of portal hypertension, such as hemorrhage from esophageal varices or ascites, occur as the initial presentation in about 10% of cases (16), but may be encountered during the precirrhotic phase of primary biliary cirrhosis (31). Indeed, many of the intrahepatic portal vein branches have been noted to be narrowed (32). Although it is generally assumed that the portal hypertension in such cases is attributable to presinusoidal obstruction of blood flow secondary to portal fibrosis, this assumption has not been documented by hemodynamic studies.

Nodular regenerative hyperplasia, which is frequently associated with portal hypertension (33), has been thought to be extremely uncommon in primary biliary cirrhosis. Indeed, in one series, no cases of nodular regenerative hyperplasia were reported among more than 200 consecutive patients with primary biliary cirrhosis (5). It has been suggested that this negative association may be a diagnostic artifact (34), since wedge biopsies are usually required to make the diagnosis of nodular regenerative hyperplasia and needle biopsies are performed in the overwhelming majority of patients with primary biliary cirrhosis (35). It has been postulated that the presence of unsuspected nodular regenerative hyperplasia is responsible for the portal hypertension in many patients with primary biliary cirrhosis. To test this hypothesis a series of 26 patients with early primary biliary cirrhosis who had had wedge biopsies of the liver were studied (35). Nine of them (36%) had nodular regenerative hyperplasia and at least two-thirds of these 9 had portal hypertension.

Often, advanced primary biliary cirrhosis gives rise to secondary extrahepatic manifestations. Of these, some of the most important are attributable to the malabsorption of fat and fat-soluble vitamins that results from the reduced biliary excretion of bile acids that accompanies prolonged cholestasis. Deficiencies of all four fat-soluble vitamins have been reported. Bone pain and compression fractures, particularly of the vertebrae due to both osteomalacia and osteoporosis, are among the most disabling complications of the disease (36). The factors involved in the pathogenesis of these lesions include: malabsorption of vitamin D and calcium, aberrations in the hepatic metabolism of vitamin D and its metabolites, alterations in the biliary and urinary excretion of vitamin D and its metabolites, inadequate exposure to sunlight, and prolonged immobilization (37). Fortunately, the osteomalacia that some patients develop can be corrected or prevented by the administration of calcium and vitamin D supplements, particularly in the form of 25 OH-vitamin D (36). However, the osteoporosis is refractory to currently available therapy, although it is reasonable to attempt to retard its development by the avoidance of prolonged immobilization and by adequate protein intake.

Manifestations of malabsorption that may appear as complications of primary biliary cirrhosis include steatorrhea, night blindness, and xerophthalmia of vitamin A deficiency (38,39)), and a hemorrhagic diathesis due to hypoprothrombinemia secondary to vitamin K deficiency (38).

Vitamin E deficiency has also been shown to be common in primary biliary cirrhosis. Pancreatic insufficiency is one of the disorders that may be associated with primary biliary cirrhosis (40).

Gallstones occur with remarkable frequency in primary biliary cirrhosis. In one series investigated by means of endoscopic retrograde cholangiography, the incidence was 39% (27), and in other series studied postmortem, it was more than 30% (41). As in other forms of cirrhosis, most such stones are of the pigment type, suggesting that hemolysis may be a factor in their pathogenesis (42). However, other possible mechanisms for the development of cholelithiasis in primary biliary cirrhosis have not been adequately excluded.

Periostitis of the tibia and fibula or clubbing of the fingers is demonstrable in almost one-third of patients with primary biliary cirrhosis, but is no more common than in other forms of cirrhosis (43). The occurrence of this complication does not correlate with the duration or severity of primary biliary cirrhosis, and is of uncertain pathogenesis.

Associated diseases

Often primary biliary cirrhosis is accompanied by one or more disorders usually regarded as manifestations of autoimmune reactions. These include Sjögren's (sicca) syndrome (44,45), rheumatoid arthritis (46), scleroderma (47), dermatomyositis and mixed connective tissue disease (48), the CRST syndrome (calcinosis cutis, Raynaud's phenomenon, sclerodactyly, and telangiectasia) (45,49), autoimmune thyroiditis (50), systemic lupus erythematosus (51), celiac disease (52), interstitial pulmonary fibrosis (53), polymyalgia rheumatica (54), and retroperitoneal fibrosis (55).

Sometimes, it is almost impossible to differentiate primary biliary cirrhosis from sarcoidosis. Such patients often present with pulmonary symptoms such as pleuritic pain, pulmonary infiltrations, and granulomas that are sometimes preceded or sometimes followed by pruritus (56,57). Histologically, the hepatic lesions are characteristic of primary biliary cirrhosis, and antimitochondrial antibodies are present. Kveim-Siltzbach tests, although rarely performed at present, have usually been negative. Whether these cases are primary biliary cirrhosis, sarcoidosis, both, or a completely separate syndrome is not known.

Renal tubular acidosis, another extrahepatic disorder commonly associated with primary biliary cirrhosis, has been attributed to the retention of copper and its deposition in the distal renal tubules (58). Asymptomatic bacteriuria has been found frequently in primary biliary cirrhosis (59), but this association is unexplained.

Results of therapy

A number of forms of therapy have been reported to induce improvement in clinical and laboratory aspects of primary biliary cirrhosis in randomized clinical trials. Adrenal corticosteroid therapy has been reported to induce hepatic improvement, but also to increase bone loss (60). Ursodeoxycholic acid has also been reported to cause improvement in some of the biochemical abnormalities of primary biliary cirrhosis (61,62). In addition, penicillamine (63,64), chlorambucil (65), and azathioprine (66) have also induced impressive reversal of the histologic abnormalities. In a preliminary report methotrexate has been found to be associated with laboratory and, perhaps, clinical improvement (67).

Laboratory features

Biochemical

The most constant biochemical marker of cholestasis in primary biliary cirrhosis is a raised level of serum alkaline phosphatase (68). Usually, activity is increased 2 to 10 times the upper limit of normal. However, not infrequently, it may be within normal range or only minimally increased (16). As a rule there is a parallel increase in the activities of serum 5'-nucleotidase and gamma-glutamyltranspeptidase.

In a high proportion of cases, the serum bilirubin concentration is increased, but in almost one-third, it is normal. Although the level may fluctuate, it tends to remain relatively low, between 1.5 and 5.0 mg/dl for long periods. Marked hyperbilirubinemia is an ominous sign, since, usually, it signifies the onset of preterminal hepatocellular failure.

Hypercholesterolemia is a relatively common finding in primary biliary cirrhosis. Usually, the concentration ranges between 250 and 600 mg/dl, but, occasionally, it exceeds 1000 mg/dl. With the onset of hepatocellular failure, the serum cholesterol concentration tends to fall, and often reaches subnormal levels terminally.

Hypoalbuminemia is a relatively late manifestation of primary biliary cirrhosis. However, the serum concentrations of immunoglobulins, and especially IgM, are frequently raised, even early in the course of the disease (68,69). Since high levels of IgM are found in at least 70% of cases, they are of particular interest and provide useful confirmatory evidence of the diagnosis in primary biliary cirrhosis.

Impairment of biliary copper excretion is one of the features of the prolonged cholestasis that characterizes primary biliary cirrhosis. As a result, the concentration of copper in the liver, urine, and serum rises and tends to increase with progression of the disease. Since the hepatic levels of copper may reach those found in Wilson's disease, the possibility has been considered that the retention of copper may play an important contributory role in progression of the lesions.

A close positive correlation between the extent of copper accumulation and the degree of bile duct loss has been demonstrated (70). Furthermore, these extensive copper deposits, which are also seen in chronic obstructive jaundice (71), suggest that primary biliary cirrhosis may represent a cholestatic lesion rather than a hepatocellular disorder (72), especially when it occurs prior to the development of cirrhosis. Some authorities believe that the copper deposition, which appears to be due to a combination of diminished biliary secretion and enhanced hepatic uptake (73,74), is not injurious to the liver (71,75).

The demonstration of extensive copper deposition in primary biliary cirrhosis has led to several controlled therapeutic trials of D-penicillamine, which chelates copper (64,76,77). Although such therapy has proved effective in increasing the urinary excretion of copper and reducing its concentration in the liver, and has had a favorable effect on the raised serum levels of alkaline phosphatase, transaminase, and IgM, it has not induced regression of the histologic lesions. If D-penicillamine does have a favorable effect on primary biliary cirrhosis, it is still uncertain whether this effect is attributable to the decrease in hepatic copper concentration or is the result of the other effects of D-penicillamine on collagen maturation and modulation of immune function.

Immunologic

Antimitochondrial antibody is demonstrable in the serum of 85 to 95% of patients with primary biliary cirrhosis (6,8,78). Characteristically, the antibody reacts with antigenic determinant in the inner membranes of mitochondria that is neither organ- nor species-specific (79). Although encountered most frequently in primary biliary cirrhosis, antimitochondrial antibody is not pathognomonic of the disease, being found in a significant fraction of patients with chronic active hepatitis (80,81), cryptogenic cirrhosis (81), and other autoimmune diseases (82). Only rarely is antimitochondrial antibody detectable in cases of extrahepatic biliary obstruction (6,8).

Recent radioimmunoassay (83) and complement fixation (84) studies of the interactions of antimitochondrial antibody with various antigenic determinants in mitochondria have demonstrated that the mitochondrial antibody detectable by indirect immunofluorescence comprises a heterogeneous group of antibodies. Only one of these, an antibody that interacts with a mitochondrial inner membrane antigen (M2) that is susceptible to trypsin degradation, is specific for primary biliary cirrhosis. Although this antibody is also detectable in some patients with cholestatic chronic active hepatitis, the M2 in such cases is usually accompanied by a second antibody that interacts with a trypsin-resistant antigen (M4) derived from the outer membranes of mitochondria (84,85). Studies have suggested that the presence in serum of anti-M8 antibodies, which react with outer mitochondrial membranes and are specific for primary biliary cirrhosis, is found predominantly in patients who have had a very aggressive course (86). Another antimitochondrial antibody, M9, appears to be associated with early primary biliary cirrhosis. Recombinant, cloned autoantigens provide an accurate, simple, rapid means of measuring specific antimitochondrial antibodies (87).

The actual autoantigens responsible for antimitochondrial antibodies consist of two closely related substances, i.e., the E-2 component of mammalian pyruvate dehydrogenase complex (88) and protein X, a distinct polypeptide that possesses cross-reactive antimitochondrial antibody epitopes with pyruvate dehydrogenase complex (89) and that both are always detectable in the antimitochondrial antibody of patients with true primary biliary cirrhosis (90).

One-third to one-half the patients with primary biliary cirrhosis also exhibit other autoimmune antibodies in their serum (81). Most of these, including smooth muscle, antinuclear, gastric parietal cell, and thyroid antibodies are neither tissue- nor species-specific. However, antibodies directed specifically against constituents of liver, namely, ductules (91) and canalicular membranes, (92) have been identified.

Pathogenesis

Although the etiology of primary biliary cirrhosis remains obscure, many of its features suggest that immunologic mechanisms are involved in its pathogenesis. These include abnormalities of humoral and cell-mediated immunity, the frequent association of primary biliary cirrhosis with other autoimmune disorders, and some of the histologic features of the hepatic lesions. The interactions and relative importance of these various immunologic aberrations are still uncertain, but there is increasing evidence that they may reflect an underlying defect in immunoregulation characterized by a deficiency of suppressor T cell function, as in other forms of autoimmune disease (93–95).

Humoral immunity

Indicative of altered humoral immunity in primary biliary cirrhosis is the frequency with which the serum contains raised concentrations of immunoglobulins, and especially IgM (68,69), antimitochondrial (6,8,84–87) and other autoimmune antibodies (81)), antibodies to canalicular (92) and ductular antigens (91), and circulating immune complexes (96,97). However, the possibility that circulating immune complexes may be implicated is suggested by the presence of antigenic determinants derived from the biliary tract (98) and are the occurrence of complement activation, as evidenced by hypercatabolism of C3 and impairment of complement-dependent reticuloendothelial function (99). The observation that IgG can be detected on the surface of isolated hepatocytes in primary biliary cirrhosis (100) is also consistent with the hypothesis that antibody- or immune-complex-mediated cytotoxicity is involved in the pathogenesis of its lesions. In this connection, it is noteworthy that a type of nonsuppurative destructive cholangitis with granuloma formation resembling that of primary biliary cirrhosis has been reported in rabbits immunized with an extract of bovine biliary epithelium (101). Nevertheless, recent data demonstrate convincingly by means of a variety of different techniques that immune complexes are not present in primary biliary cirrhosis (102).

Paradoxically, despite evidence of hyperactivity of the humoral immune system in primary biliary cirrhosis, the antibody response to some antigens, such as hemocyanin, is impaired (103).

Cell-mediated immunity

The interaction of cultured lymphocytes in primary biliary cirrhosis with liver-specific lipoprotein (104) and a protein fraction in bile (105) to produce the lymphokine, migration inhibition factor, is consistent with an underlying cell-mediated, immune response to these antigens. The cytotoxicity of such lymphocytes for hepatocytes (106,107) lends further support to this interpretation. However, the elaboration of migration inhibition factor and the cytotoxicity of the lymphocytes in primary biliary cirrhosis are not specific for the disease, so their role in its pathogenesis is still in doubt. Impairment of cell-mediated immunity (108), abnormalities of T cell subsets (109) and of serum immunoregulatory factors have been reported (110). Several plausible pathogenetic hypotheses have been proposed (111–113).

Skin test anergy to a variety of antigens (103,104) and impairment of mitogen-induced lymphocyte transformation (114,115) are two other abnormalities of cell-mediated immunity in primary biliary cirrhosis.

The occurrence of granulomas in the liver and, occasionally, in extrahepatic tissues as well (116), and the intimate contact between lymphocytes and the epithelial cells of degenerating bile ducts (117) are two histologic features of primary biliary cirrhosis lesions that have been interpreted as evidence of an underlying, cell-mediated, immune mechanism.

Chronic graft-versus-host disease, a disorder that often follows bone marrow transplantation, is characterized by an immunologic reaction of grafted lymphocytes directed against host histocompatibility antigens (HLA), leading to the development of distinctive, disseminated lesions, particularly in tissues containing ductal epithelial cells that are rich in HLA (118). Many features of chronic graft-versus-host disease, such nonsuppurative destructive cholangitis, the sicca syndrome, skin lesions, hypergammaglobulinemia, and circulating immune complexes, closely resemble those in primary biliary cirrhosis. This has led to the suggestion that primary biliary cirrhosis may be a manifestation of chronic graft-versus-host disease in which the patients' lymphocytes react with the HLA in the ductal epithelial cells of the liver, salivary glands, lachrymal glands, and pancreas (44). According to this hypothesis, the failure of T cell self-recognition is attributable to bacterial- or viral-induced alterations in the antigenicity of HLA, or the persistence of maternal lymphocytes that enter the circulation via the placenta during fetal life. Attempts to confirm this hypothesis so far have failed (119).

Genetic factors

The familial occurrence of primary biliary cirrhosis and hyperglobulinemia (120) and the frequency with which seroimmunologic abnormalities and other autoimmune disorders are encountered in relatives of primary biliary cirrhosis (121,122) suggest that susceptibility to the disease may be hereditary. Attempts to demonstrate a distinctive pattern of ABO genetic markers in primary biliary cirrhosis have been unsuccessful (123). However, investigations have shown a sixfold positive association between HLA-DRw8, a class II antigen of the major histocompatibility complex, and primary biliary cirrhosis (124). A negative association between HLA-DR5 and primary biliary cirrhosis was also noted. Furthermore, they found that another class II antigen, HLA-DRw52, was associated with higher serum bilirubin levels, which is an important prognostic indicator in primary biliary cirrhosis, while the HLA-DR2 antigen was associated with lower serum bilirubin concentrations (124).

Miscellaneous factors

The possibility that infection with the respiratory, enteric orphan (REO) virus-3 may predispose to the development of primary biliary cirrhosis, as has been suggested for chronic nonsuppurative destructive cholangitis in infants (125), has been considered (126). However, anti-Reo-3 titers, although higher than in control subjects, do not appear to support such an association (126).

Histopathology

The lesions of primary biliary cirrhosis are characterized by destruction of interlobular and septal bile ducts, accompanied or followed by progressive portal and periportal inflammation, fibrosis, and loss of hepatocytes, leading ultimately, in many cases, to the development of cirrhosis (1–5). Characteristically, the portal and ductal lesions are focal in character and patchy in distribution, so they may escape detection, particularly in small needle biopsy specimens.

There can be little doubt that chronic nonsuppurative destructive cholangitis is an essential feature of the lesions, and that the resulting obliteration of bile ducts and obstruction to bile flow in the liver play an important role in the perpetuation and progression of the disease. However, the widely held view that the interlobular and septal ducts are the initial site of injury and that all other features of the lesions are secondary to the retention and regurgitation of bile is open to question. Portal inflammation, erosion of the limiting plates, portal and periportal fibrosis and intralobular collections of lymphocytes, proliferating Kupffer cells, and granulomas may be encountered in the apparent absence of damaged ducts. Although the failure to detect such ducts may be due to inadequate sampling, the alternative possibility cannot be excluded that the portal and parenchymal lesions are attributable to the same pathogenetic mechanisms responsible for duct injury.

To assess prognosis and to monitor the effects of therapy, attempts have been made to classify the lesions of primary biliary cirrhosis in terms of their stage of development. However, such staging is of only limited value, since sampling errors due to the patchy distribution of the lesions are relatively common, and since biopsy specimens frequently contain variable lesions at different stages of development.

According to the most widely used classification, first proposed by Scheuer (4), stage 1 is characterized by florid duct lesions, stage 2, by ductular proliferation, stage 3, by scarring, and stage 4, by nodular cirrhosis. With minor modifications in terminology, the classification of Popper and Schaffner (127) is virtually identical. In the Scheuer staging system it is assumed that damage to the interlobular and septal ducts is the earliest lesion that occurs in primary biliary cirrhosis. However, ductal lesions may be found at any stage of the disease, although they tend to diminish in number late in its course (96). This suggests that ductal lesions may be a sign of progressive disease activity rather than an early manifestation of primary biliary cirrhosis. Another problem with this staging system is that it is not applicable in the case of lesions characterized by portal inflammation without significant fibrosis, ductular proliferation, or evidence of interlobular duct injury, which are commonly encountered in needle biopsy specimens.

In the alternative staging system (128), stage 1 lesions, classified as portal hepatitis, are characterized by a portal inflammatory reaction unaccompanied by piecemeal necrosis. Stage 2 lesions, classified as periportal hepatitis, are characterized by portal and periportal inflammation with piecemeal necrosis, but no evidence of bridging fibrosis or necrosis. Stage 3 lesions, classified as septal, are characterized by fibrous septa or bridging necrosis, and stage 4 lesions are characterized by overt cirrhosis. In this grading system, the presence or absence of ductal lesions and ductular proliferation is disregarded. Although the classification of lesions in this system is relatively simple and readily applicable in the assessment of needle biopsy specimens, no convincing evidence has been presented to establish that the classification correlates with longevity, the only reliable criterion of how far the disease has advanced.

In our own long-term study of patients with primary biliary cirrhosis (15), we have found that the duration of survival varies inversely with the extent of fibrosis, the degree to which the limiting plates are eroded, and the severity of cholestasis.

Bile duct lesions

Although not pathognomonic, among the most destructive features of the lesions in *active progressive* primary biliary cirrhosis are inflammation, degeneration, and necrosis of the epithelium that lines interlobular and septal ducts that range from 40 to 800 μm in diameter. Characteristically, such lesions affect only a minority of ducts *at any one time* and are segmental in distribution (129), so they seldom are numerous in biopsy sections, and often escape detection in needle biopsy specimens. It is the smallest ducts that are most frequently destroyed (130), although larger ducts may be involved as well (131).

In early duct lesions, the epithelial cells often contain cytoplasmic vacuoles and infiltrating lymphocytes, show reduplication and loss of polarity of their nuclei, and are indistinctly outlined (Fig. 364). Later, the epithelial cells proliferate, leading to their stratification and the formation of papillary projections into the lumen of the duct (Fig. 365). In addition, there may be segmental or complete loss of the basement membrane with foci of epithelial necrosis (Fig. 366) or frank rupture (Fig. 367). Rarely, the necrotic ducts are dilated and contain numerous neutrophils (Fig. 611).

As a result of necrosis, the affected interlobular and septal ducts are obliterated. Since this process continues as long as the lesions remain active, there is a progressive reduction in the number of ducts, an important diagnostic feature in primary biliary cirrhosis. Normally, one or more interlobular or septal ducts can be identified in 85% of portal tracts that contain a hepatic arteriole and portal venule, whereas in the more advanced stages of primary biliary cirrhosis such ducts are present in less than 40% of the portal tracts (2). Typical enlarged fibrotic portal tracts containing an arteriole and portal veins, but devoid of an interlobular or septal duct, are illustrated in Figures 378 and 379. Occasionally, the site of the previously destroyed duct is marked by an aggregation of lymphocytes (Fig. 378) or a granuloma (Fig. 612).

Although inflammation, degeneration, and necrosis of epithelium are most readily identified in interlobular and septal ducts measuring 40 to 80 μ in diameter, they also occur in much smaller ducts (Fig. 368). However, by means of serial sections, it can be demonstrated that, at all stages of primary biliary cirrhosis, small ducts, as small as cholangioles, frequently are obliterated (130).

Despite the fact that ductal epithelial lesions are regarded as pathognomonic of primary biliary cirrhosis by some authorities (131), there is convincing evidence that they also occur, but less commonly, in other conditions, including chronic active hepatitis, acute viral hepatitis, drug-induced hepatitis, some forms of granulomatous hepatitis, "cryptogenic" cirrhosis, sclerosing cholangitis, graft-versus-host disease, and in transplanted livers undergoing chronic rejection reactions. Ductal epithelial lesions in primary biliary cirrhosis may exhibit distinctive histologic features that permit differentiation from those in other diseases (132), but these lesions are not frequently found in our experience.

As the portal tracts expand and undergo fibrosis, ductular proliferation, often accompanied by a neutrophilic infiltration, may occur (Fig. 359). Although emphasized as a distinctive feature of primary biliary cirrhosis following the destruction of interlobular and septal ducts (4), many enlarged fibrotic portal tracts devoid of such ducts show no evidence of ductular proliferation (Fig. 378). Rarely, some of the proliferating ductules contain small bile thrombi (Fig. 379), a finding consistent with the generally held view that the proliferation is attributable to biliary obstruction.

With progression of the lesions and advancing fibrosis, the proliferating ductules tend to disappear, as is evident from their absence in the late cirrhotic lesion illustrated in Figure 613. Occasionally, proliferating ductules are vacuolated and show degenerative changes (Fig. 614). However, it is uncertain whether the loss of most ductules is attributable to such degeneration or is the result of atrophy secondary to compression by fibrous tissue.

Portal inflammation

The portal tracts containing interlobular and septal duct epithelial lesions invariably are infiltrated by numerous inflammatory cells (Figs. 364–368). Lymphocytes predominate, but almost always they are accompanied by numerous plasma cells and occasional histiocytes (Fig. 615). Often, the cells are aggregated in the form of lymph follicles, some of which may contain germinal centers of more loosely arranged cells. Such follicles frequently lie adjacent to or in intimate contact with degenerating ducts (Fig. 295). Eosinophils are relatively common in the portal exudates of primary biliary cirrhosis. Usually, they are few in number, but, in some cases, they are numerous, and may be accompanied by mild to moderate peripheral eosinophilia, as in the case illustrated in Figure 328. Often, the portal exudates include macrophages that contain D-PAS-positive material (Fig. 334). The latter resembles lipofuscin, but it has been suggested that it is a derivative of regurgitated bile (127). When the bile ducts are destroyed and the process is no longer active, the inflammatory changes disappear as well. Although gross extravasation of bile is never evident, the occurrence of foamy histiocytes (pseudoxanthoma cells) in the portal tracts of some cases is consistent with at least a minor degree of bile reflux. Figure 616 illustrates such portal pseudoxanthoma cells in a patient with primary biliary cirrhosis who exhibited no histologic evidence of cholestasis.

A variable number of portal tracts that contain intact interlobular or septal ducts are similarly infiltrated with inflammatory cells (Fig. 617). Such exudates have been attributed to extension of the inflammatory reaction from around damaged ducts lying deeper in the section (133). However, the frequency with which such portal tracts show segmental (Fig. 618) or complete erosion of their limiting plates (Fig. 296) suggests that the inflammatory reaction may be related to the underlying pathogenetic mechanism responsible for both ductal and hepatocellular injury.

Granulomas

Although not pathognomonic, portal granulomas are another distinctive feature of primary biliary cirrhosis encountered in almost half the cases (116). Frequently, the granulomas lie close to degenerating ducts (Fig. 295), but, in some cases, they are associated with intact ducts (Fig. 619), or occur in portal tracts devoid of ducts (Fig. 612), possibly indicating the site of antecedent duct destruction. Moreover, in a small number of cases, the granulomas are found within the lobules or within extrahepatic tissues, such as hepatic, hilar or mediastinal lymph nodes, omentum, or lung (116). Figure 343 illustrates a centrilobular granuloma in a patient with well-documented primary biliary cirrhosis who also exhibited numerous portal and hepatic hilar node granulomas. Sometimes, these granulomas contain foamy macrophages around an injured or ruptured bile duct.

Most of the granulomas in primary biliary cirrhosis resemble those of sarcoidosis, characteristically presenting as sharply circumscribed, compact masses of epithelioid and giant cells, usually surrounded and occasionally infiltrated by lymphocytes, but showing no evidence of necrosis (Figs. 342, 612, 619). These sarcoid-like granulomas tend to occur far from the portal tracts. However, in some cases, the lesions contain loosely arranged, epithelioid and giant cells separated by numerous lymphocytes (Fig. 343), or are characterized by ill-defined collections of histiocytes and lymphocytes (Fig. 620).

Portal fibrosis

As previously indicated, the lesions of primary biliary cirrhosis may be found at all stages of their development in a single section, which is what makes histologic staging of the disease so difficult. This is particularly impressive in the case of portal fibrosis, which may range in degree from its complete absence in one microscopic field to fullblown cirrhosis in adjacent fields. This is illustrated in Figures 573–575, which depict three adjacent microscopic fields in a surgical wedge biopsy section of a patient with advanced primary biliary cirrhosis. The first (Fig. 573) shows typical cirrhosis (stage 4); the second (Fig. 574), bridging fibrosis without nodule formation (stage 3); and the third (Fig. 575), intact lobular architecture with little or no fibrosis. Variations in lobular architecture of this type are more common in primary biliary cirrhosis than in many of the other lesions from which it must be differentiated, so it is a useful diagnostic feature. However, in small needle biopsy specimens, such variations in architecture may be difficult to identify, or may lead to errors in histologic staging.

In early lesions, the portal tracts may be heavily infiltrated with inflammatory cells, but may not show evidence of expansion or fibrosis (Fig. 617). Even when the portal tracts are expanded as a result of periportal, parenchymal destruction, there may be no accompanying fibrosis (Fig. 295). However, ultimately, the inflamed portal tracts undergo scarring. Initially, they appear as enlarged stellate structures that do not distort the normal lobular architecture (Fig. 621) (stage 3), but as the fibrosis advances, it tends to bridge adjacent portal tracts (Fig. 622) (stage 3 or 4), and then extends to encircle nodules of parenchyma, destroying the normal lobular architecture and giving rise to cirrhosis (Fig. 613) (stage 4). As might be anticipated from their development as a result of progressive, portal-portal bridging, some of the cirrhotic nodules in primary biliary cirrhosis often contain intact central veins (Figs. 570, 613). However, portal fibrosis frequently extends to involve the centrilobular zones, so many of the nodules are devoid of central veins (Figs. 573, 613).

Depending on their age, the fibrous septa in primary biliary cirrhosis may be slender (Fig. 613) or relatively broad (Fig. 570). The contours of the fibrotic portal tracts and septa vary with the activity of the lesions, appearing irregular when the limiting plates are eroded during periods of activity (Fig. 296), and smooth-contoured when the lesions are inactive (Fig. 613).

Occasionally, in the late stage of primary biliary cirrhosis, some of the interlobular or septal ducts are encircled by concentric bands of collagen (Fig. 623). Although the occurrence of such lesions in primary sclerosing cholangitis has been emphasized (134), it is important to recognize that they may be encountered under other conditions, and have no diagnostic specificity.

As previously indicated, obstruction to intrahepatic bile flow secondary to destruction of bile ducts plays an important role in the fibrogenesis of primary biliary cirrhosis. However, the prominence of piecemeal necrosis and the occurrence of intralobular inflammatory lesions in the apparent absence of cholestasis in some cases suggest that other factors related to the underlying pathogenesis of the disease may be involved.

Parenchymal lesions

Destruction of the limiting plates and extension of portal inflammatory cells and fibrous tissue into the periportal parenchyma are relatively common features in the active, progressive lesions of primary biliary cirrhosis. However, such piecemeal necrosis tends to be segmental and random in distribution, and only rarely is as extensive as in chronic active hepatitis. In addition to piecemeal necrosis, the fibrous septa in advanced primary biliary cirrhosis frequently are bordered by a band of degenerating, ballooned hepatocytes. This phenomenon is sometimes referred to as biliary piecemeal necrosis. Although such ballooning may be the result of accompanying cholestasis, cells of this type may be found in areas that show no evidence of cholestasis, as illustrated in Figure 109. In fact, it appears that patients with prominent piecemeal necrosis are different from those with predominantly cholestatic lesions (22). Furthermore, the prognosis is better in those with piecemeal necrosis and lymphocytic infiltration than in those with predominantly cholestatic lesions.

Bile thrombi appear in the periportal and periseptal canaliculi relatively late in the course of primary biliary cirrhosis (Fig. 557). Occasionally, however, dilatation of the canaliculi may be detected before the appearance of such cholestasis (Fig. 208). As the lesion advances, bile thrombi often extend deeper into the parenchyma, where they may be found in both dilated canaliculi and swollen, proliferating Küpffer cells (Fig. 624). Rarely, sharply circumscribed groups of pseudoxanthoma cells derived from hepatocytes and Küpffer cells undergoing "feathery" degeneration, are encountered in the periportal or periseptal parenchyma (Fig. 625). Although usually associated with bile thrombi elsewhere in the section and undoubtedly attributable to cholestasis, aggregates of pseudoxanthoma cells often contain no histologically demonstrable bile. Such lesions may be encountered in any form of prolonged, relatively severe cholestasis, and are not necessarily indicative of extrahepatic biliary obstruction, as is commonly believed.

Patients with predominantly cholestatic lesions in general tend to progress more frequently to cirrhosis and to have a worse prognosis than those who do not show this feature (22).

Typical Mallory bodies, characteristically found in periportal or periseptal hepatocytes, are relatively common in the advanced lesions of primary biliary cirrhosis. Although they occur most frequently in lesions containing bile thrombi, and probably are attributable to cholestasis, they often bear no spatial relationship to bile thrombi, and may occur in their absence, as illustrated in Figure 556.

Due to impairment of biliary copper excretion in primary biliary cirrhosis, copper tends to accumulate in the liver. Characteristically, the copper is concentrated in the lysosomes of periportal and periseptal hepatocytes and presents as bright red cytoplasmic granules in rhodanine-stained sections (Fig. 626). With orcein stain copper-associated protein takes on a purplish color (Fig. 627). According to some reports (135), such copper-containing granules occur in a high proportion of patients with primary biliary cirrhosis, and are a useful diagnostic feature. However, in our experience, copper deposits are an inconstant finding but are usually found in advanced lesions. Moreover, similar copper-containing granules, although usually in small numbers, may be encountered in other forms of chronic liver disease, such as chronic active hepatitis, postnecrotic cirrhosis, and alcoholic cirrhosis (Fig. 628), particularly when accompanied by chronic cholestasis. Thus, the presence of rhodanine-positive, cytoplasmic granules is of only limited value in the histologic differential diagnosis of primary biliary cirrhosis.

Under conditions of excessive copper deposition, the cytoplasm of the periportal and periseptal hepatocytes may contain granules that appear dark brown or black in orcein-stained sections. The granules also stain with aldehyde fuchsin, but cannot be visualized in routine H & E or Masson-stained sections, and do not take up D-PAS, iron, bile, or melanin stains (136). Based on their histochemical reactions, the granules appear to be copper-protein complexes linked by sulfhydryl and disulfide bonds, although some contain lipofuscin as well (137). On electron microscopy the granules are found within large lysosomes or autophagic vacuoles (138). Orcein-positive cytoplasmic granules are seen most commonly in primary biliary cirrhosis (135), but also occur in Wilsons' disease (135), Indian childhood cirrhosis (137), and, less frequently, in chronic active hepatitis, postnecrotic cirrhosis, and extrahepatic biliary obstruction (139).

The presence of orcein-positive granules is said to be a useful feature in the histologic differential diagnosis of primary biliary cirrhosis (140). However, while such granules are almost always encountered in advanced lesions, as illustrated in Figure 629, in our experience they occur less frequently than rhodanine-positive granules in early lesions, and are of only limited value diagnostically.

Frequently, in the active lesions of primary biliary cirrhosis, the parenchyma contains a variable number of scattered foci of lymphocytes and swollen, proliferating Kupffer cells that may be accompanied by occasional acidophilic bodies (Fig. 630). Less commonly, there are circumscribed foci of inflammation and hepatocellular degeneration and necrosis indicative of focal hepatitis (Fig. 631). Focal inflammatory and degenerative lesions of this type appear to bear no relationship to cholestasis, and probably are attributable to the same mechanism involved in the pathogenesis of duct injury, destruction of periportal parenchyma, and granuloma formation.

Hepatocellular regeneration, as evidenced by the presence of twin-cell plates and pseudoducts or rosettes (Fig. 205), is a relatively common feature in the active lesions of primary biliary cirrhosis, both in the precirrhotic and cirrhotic phases of the disease. Presumably, such regeneration is the result of biliary obstruction secondary to destruction of interlobular and septal ducts. However, its occurrence in many cases in the absence of histologically demonstrable cholestasis suggests that other factors may be involved as well.

Nodular regenerative hyperplasia is often seen in early precirrhotic primary biliary cirrhosis usually in association with portal hypertension (35). The hyperplastic hepatocytes are arranged concentrically around the portal vein (Figs. 632, 633).

Histologic staging of lesions

Histologic grading of the lesions of primary biliary cirrhosis should reflect the extent to which the disease has advanced and its activity. Based on our observation that survival in primary biliary cirrhosis varies inversely with the extent of fibrosis, the degree to which the limiting plates are eroded, and the severity of cholestasis (15), we grade the degree of fibrosis as follows: stage 1, no fibrosis; stage 2, portal fibrosis without bridging; stage 3, bridging fibrosis; and stage 4, cirrhosis. Each stage is further qualified by the extent to which the limiting plates are eroded (none, mild, moderate, or severe) and the degree of cholestasis (none, mild, moderate, or severe). In the case of lesions that exhibit variations in their stage of development, the most advanced is used for classification.

Although immunotherapy has been shown in randomized clinical trials to induce laboratory and, sometimes, clinical improvement, histologic improvement is less clearcut (63, 65, 66). Anecdotal studies of methotrexate (15 mg per week) have shown similar improvement (140A). The histologic changes induced in a 39-year-old white woman with stage II PBC are documented in Figures 633A, 633B, 633C, and 633D. These histologic improvements, which were observed by blind readings of the before-and-after biopsies by the investigators, were accompanied by disappearance of pruritus, reduction in fatigue, return to normal of the serum alkaline phosphatase, and sustained improvement in the SGPT.

It is unlikely that in stage III or IV PBC, in which bile ducts have been destroyed and cirrhosis has already developed, such therapy can cause significant histologic improvement. In earlier, Stage I or II, precirrhotic PBC, it appears that such therapy can reduce the inflammation, the bile duct degeneration, and piecemeal necrosis. Blind, randomized clinical trials are needed to establish this relationship.

Histologic differential diagnosis

Chronic active hepatitis

The lesions of primary biliary cirrhosis may be difficult to differentiate from those of autoimmune chronic active hepatitis, particularly when the latter are accompanied by inflammation, degeneration, and necrosis of ductal epithelium (141,142) and by the presence of mitochondrial antibody (6,81). This has led to the suggestion that the two diseases may share a common pathogenesis that occasionally leads to the development of overlapping mixed lesions (127,143). However, the striking differences between the responses of primary biliary cirrhosis and chronic active hepatitis to corticosteroid therapy (144) and the fact that the mitochondrial antibodies with which they are associated differ in their antigenic specificities are more consistent with the view that the two diseases are distinct etiologic entities. Different immunologic abnormalities have been found in the two diseases (113).

Although the distinction between the diseases is not always possible on histologic grounds alone (142), the two lesions usually show significant differences: (1) piecemeal necrosis in primary biliary cirrhosis tends to be segmental, and seldom is as widely disseminated or accompanied by as extensive intercellular and perisinusoidal fibrosis as in chronic active hepatitis; (2) ductal epithelial lesions are more numerous, and loss of interlobular and septal ducts is more prominent in primary biliary cirrhosis than in chronic active hepatitis; (3) granulomas are relatively common in primary biliary cirrhosis, but occur only rarely in chronic active hepatitis; and (4) orcein staining for copper-associated protein may be strongly positive in primary biliary cirrhosis but is absent or weakly positive in chronic active hepatitis (140,142).

Primary sclerosing cholangitis

In some cases, the hepatic lesions of primary sclerosing cholangitis exhibit features resembling those of primary biliary cirrhosis. These include interlobular, ductal, epithelial inflammation, degeneration, and necrosis; fibrous obliteration of ducts; ductular proliferation; and, rarely, granulomas. Although in primary sclerosing cholangitis the involved ducts are often encircled by concentric bands of collagen (134), this lesion is an inconstant feature and, as previously indicated, occurs in other conditions. Cholestasis and portal neutrophilic infiltrates appear to be more common than in primary biliary cirrhosis. Both diseases show frequent evidence of subclinical pancreatitis as evidenced by elevated levels of pancreatic isoenzymes, but primary biliary cirrhosis is associated with pancreatic hypofunction, as shown by decreased secretion of pancreatic juice and trypsin, while primary sclerosing cholangitis is not (40). It is postulated that the pancreatic disorder in primary biliary cirrhosis is part of the sicca syndrome (40). However, identification of primary sclerosing cholangitis is rarely possible on the basis of hepatic histologic findings alone. The diagnosis depends on cholangiographic evidence that both the intrahepatic and extrahepatic bile ducts are involved in a characteristic ductal fibrotic process (145,146)

In a possible related disorder, classified as primary intrahepatic obliterating cholangitis (147), the lesions are limited to medium sized intrahepatic bile ducts. Although the hepatic lesions may resemble those of primary biliary cirrhosis superficially, the affected ducts are characteristically replaced by fibrous cords, and none shows the ductular epithelial changes seen in primary biliary cirrhosis.

Sarcoidosis

Occasionally, sarcoidosis may be difficult to distinguish from primary biliary cirrhosis. Sarcoidosis may have most of the clinical, serologic, and histologic features of primary biliary cirrhosis, but, in addition, usually shows extrahepatic manifestations, primarily pulmonary that are more typical of sarcoidosis (56,57).

Drug-induced chronic cholestatic hepatitis

Rarely, idiosyncratic drug reactions give rise to a form of chronic cholestatic hepatitis that may progress to cirrhosis. Lesions of this type may be accompanied by ductal epithelial inflammation, degeneration, and necrosis, as in primary biliary cirrhosis. In addition, loss of interlobular ducts has been reported in prolonged, drug-induced, cholestatic hepatitis (148,149). However, in the few such cases that we have encountered, the interlobular and septal ducts were not reduced in number.

Usually, differentiation between drug-induced chronic cholestatic hepatitis and primary biliary cirrhosis depends on the history of drug intake and the abrupt onset of jaundice after an appropriate interval rather than on the histologic features of the hepatic lesions.

Extrahepatic biliary obstruction

The hepatic lesions of early extrahepatic biliary obstruction, characterized by centrilobular cholestasis and portal edema, neutrophilic infiltration, and ductular proliferation, are readily differentiated from those of primary biliary cirrhosis. However, the secondary biliary cirrhotic lesions that appear following prolonged, unrelieved biliary obstruction may resemble those of advanced primary biliary cirrhosis in its late stages when cholestasis is extensive and ductal epithelial lesions and granulomata are no longer present. The paucity of interlobular and septal ducts in primary biliary cirrhosis and the prominence of portal and septal neutrophils and ductular proliferation in extrahepatic biliary obstruction are the only features that usually serve to distinguish between the two lesions.

References

1. Popper H, Rubin E, Schaffner F: The problem of primary biliary cirrhosis. Am J Med 33:807–810, 1962.
2. Baggenstoss AH, Foulk WT, Butt HR, Bahn RC: The pathology of primary biliary cirrhosis with emphasis on histogenesis. Am J Clin Pathol 42:259–276, 1964.
3. Rubin E, Schaffner F, Popper H: Primary biliary cirrhosis. Chronic non-suppurative destructive cholangitis. Am J Clin Pathol 46:387–407, 1965.
4. Scheuer PJ: Primary biliary cirrhosis. Proc R Soc Med 60:1257–1260, 1967.
5. Portmann B, Popper H, Neuberger J, Williams R: Sequential and diagnostic features in primary biliary cirrhosis based on serial histologic study in 209 patients. Gastroenterology 88:1777–1790, 1985.
6. Walker JG, Doniach D, Roitt IM, Sherlock S: Serological tests in diagnosis of primary biliary cirrhosis. Lancet 1:827–831, 1965.
7. Klatskin G, Kantor FS: Mitochondrial antibody in primary biliary cirrhosis and other diseases. Ann Intern Med 77:533–541, 1972.
8. Avigan MI, Adamson G, Hoofnagle JH, Jones EA: The in vitro production of antibodies to mitochondrial antigens by peripheral blood mononuclear cells from patients with primary biliary cirrhosis. Hepatology 6:999–1004, 1986.
9. Manns M, Gerken G, Kyriatsoulis A, Tranivein C, Reske K, Meyer zum Buschenfelde KHM: Two different subtypes of antimitochondrial antibodies are associated with primary biliary cirrhosis: identification and characterization by radioimmunoassay and immunoblotting. Hepatology 7:893–899, 1987.
10. Beswick DR, Klatskin G, Boyer JL: Asymptomatic primary biliary cirrhosis: long term follow-up and natural history. Gastroenterology 89:267–271, 1985.
11. Sherlock S: The syndrome of disappearing intrahepatic bile ducts. Lancet 2:493–496, 1987.
12. Addison T, Gull W: On a certain affection of the skin, vitiligoidea - α plana, tuberosa. Guy's Hosp Rep 7:265–272, 1851.
13. Christensen E, Crowe J, Doniach D, Popper H, Ranek L, Rodes J, Tygstrup N, Williams R: Clinical patterns and course of disease in primary biliary cirrhosis based on analysis of 236 patients. Gastroenterology 78:236–246, 1980.

14. Kapelman B, Schaffner F: The natural history of primary biliary cirrhosis. Semin Liver Dis *1*:273–281, 1981.

15. Roll J, Boyer JL, Barry D, Klatskin G: The prognostic importance of clinical and histologic features in asymptomatic and symptomatic primary biliary cirrhosis. N Engl J Med *308*:1–7, 1983.

16. Brenard R, Degos F, Degott C, Lassoued K, Benhamou JP: La cirrhose biliaire primitive: modes actuels de presentation. Etude clinique, biochimique, immunologique et histologique de 206 malades observes de 1978 a 1988. Gastroenterol Clin Biol *14*:307–312, 1990.

17. Triger D: Primary biliary cirrhosis: an epidemiological study. Br Med J *281*:772–775, 1980.

18. Rubel LR, Rabin L, Seeff LB, Licht H, Cuccherini BA: Does primary biliary cirrhosis in men differ from primary biliary cirrhosis in women? Hepatology *4*:671–677, 1984.

19. Esquivel CO, Van Thiel DH, Demetris AJ, Bernardos A, Iwatsuki S, Markus B, Gordon RD, Marsh JW, Makowka L, Tzakis AG, Todo S, Gavaler JS, Starzl TE: Transplantation for primary biliary cirrhosis. Gastroenterology *94*:1207–1216, 1988.

20. Lee RG, Epstein O, Jauregui H, Sherlock S, Scheuer PJ: Granulomas in primary biliary cirrhosis: a prognostic feature. Gastroenterology *81*:983–986, 1981.

21. Lefkowitch JH: Bile ductular cholestasis: an ominous histopathologic sign related to sepsis and 'cholangitis lenta.' Hum Pathol *13*:19–24, 1982.

22. Nakanuma Y, Saito K, Unoura M: Semiquantitative assessment of cholestasis and lymphocytic piecemeal necrosis in primary biliary cirrhosis: a histologic and immunohistochemical study. J Clin Gastroenterol *12*:357–362, 1990.

23. Tornay AS Jr: Primary biliary cirrhosis. Natural history. Am J Gastroenterol *73*:223–226, 1980.

24. Hanik L, Eriksson S: Presymptomatic primary biliary cirrhosis. Acta Med Scand *202*:277–281, 1977.

25. James O, Macklon AF, Watson AJ: Primary biliary cirrhosis: a revised clinical spectrum. Lancet *1*:1278–1281, 1981.

26. Long RG, Scheuer PJ, Sherlock S: Presentation and course of asymptomatic primary biliary cirrhosis. Gastroenterology *72*:1204–1207, 1977.

27. Balasubramaniam K, Grambsch PM, Wiesner RH, Lindor KD, Dickson ER: Diminished survival in asymptomatic primary biliary cirrhosis. A prospective study. Gastroenterology *98*:1567–1571, 1990.

28. Krasner H, Johnson PJ, Portmann B, Watkinson G, MacSween RN, Williams R: Hepatocellular carcinoma in primary biliary cirrhosis. Report of four cases. Gut *20*:255–258, 1979.

29. Melia WN, Johnson PJ, Neuberger J, Zaman S, Portmann BC, Williams R: Hepatocellular carcinoma in primary biliary cirrhosis. Detection by α-fetoprotein estimation. Gastroenterology *87*:660–663, 1984.

30. Goudie BM, Burt AD, Macfarlane GJ, Birnie GM, Boyle P, Mills PR: Breast cancer in primary biliary cirrhosis. Br Med J *291*:1597–1598, 1985.

31. Spisni R, Smith-Laing G, Epstein O, Sherlock S: Results of portal decompression in patients with primary biliary cirrhosis. Gut *22*:345–349, 1981.

32. Nakanuma Y, Ohta G, Kobayashi K, Kato Y: Histological and histometric examination of the intrahepatic portal vein branches in primary biliary cirrhosis without regenerative nodules. Am J Gastroenterol *77*:405–413, 1982.

33. Guarda LA, Hales MR: Nodular regenerative hyperplasia of the liver. Report of two cases and review of the literature. J Clin Gastroenterol *3*:157–164, 1981.

34. Arora S, Kaplan M: Portal hypertension in early-stage primary biliary cirrhosis: a possible explanation. Am J Gastroenterol *82*:90–91, 1987.

35. Nakanuma Y, Ohta G: Nodular hyperplasia of the liver in primary biliary cirrhosis of early histological stages. Am J Gastroenterol *82*:8–10, 1987.

36. Matloff DS, Kaplan MM, Neer RM, Goldbert MJ, Bitman W, Wolfe HJ: Osteoporosis in primary biliary cirrhosis: effects of 25-hydroxyvitamin D₃ treatment. Gastroenterology *83*:97–102, 1982.

37. Bloomer FR, Ghent CN: Management of the intractable cholestasis of primary biliary cirrhosis. Semin Liver Dis *1*:345–353, 1981.

38. Munoz SJ, Heubi JE, Balistreri WF, Maddrey WC: Vitamin E deficiency in primary biliary cirrhosis: gastrointestinal malabsorption, frequency and relationship to other lipid-soluble vitamins. Hepatology *4*:525–531, 1989.

39. Herlong HF, Russell RM, Maddrey WC: Vitamin A and zinc therapy in primary biliary cirrhosis. Hepatology *1*:348–351, 1981.

40. Epstein O, Chapman RWG, Lake-Bakaar G: The pancreas in primary biliary cirrhosis and primary sclerosing cholangitis. Gastroenterology *83*:1177–1184, 1982.

41. Bouchier IAD: Postmortem study of the frequency of gallstones in patients with cirrhosis of the liver. Gut *10*:705–710, 1969.

42. Nicholas P, Rinaudo PA, Conn HO: Increased incidence of cholelithiasis in Laennec's cirrhosis. A postmortem evaluation of pathogenesis. Gastroenterology *63*:112–121, 1972.

43. Epstein O, Dick R, Sherlock S: Prospective study of periostitis and finger clubbing in primary biliary cirrhosis and other forms of chronic liver disease. Gut *22*:203–206, 1981.

44. Epstein O, Thomas HC, Sherlock S: Primary biliary cirrhosis is a dry gland syndrome with features of chronic graft-versus-host disease. Lancet *1*:1166–1168, 1980.

45. Culp KS, Fleming Cr, Duffy J, Baldus WP, Dickson ER: Autoimmune associations in primary biliary cirrhosis. Mayo Clinic Proc *57*:365–370, 1982.

46. Marx WJ, O'Connell DJ: Arthritis of primary biliary cirrhosis. Arch Intern Med *139*:213–216, 1979.

47. O'Brien ST, Eddy WM, Krawitt EL: Primary biliary cirrhosis associated with scleroderma. Gastroenterology *62*:118–121, 1972.

48. Epstein O, Burroughs AK, Sherlock S: Polymyositis and acute onset systemic sclerosis in a patient with primary biliary cirrhosis: a clinical syndrome similar to the mixed connective tissue disease. J R Soc Med *74*:456–458, 1981.

49. Reynolds TB, Denison EK, Frankel HD, Lieberman FL, Peters RL: Primary biliary cirrhosis with scleroderma, Raynaud's phenomenon and telangiectasia. New syndrome. Am J Med *50*:302–312, 1971.

50. Elta GH, Sepersky RA, Goldberg MJ, Connors CM, Miller KB, Kaplan MM: Increased incidence of hypothyroidism in primary biliary cirrhosis. Dig Dis Sci *28*:971–975, 1983.

51. Hall S, Axelsen PH, Larson DE, Bunch TW: Systemic lupus erythematosus developing in patients with primary biliary cirrhosis. Ann Intern Med *100*:388–389, 1984.

52. Gabrielsen TO, Hoel PS: Primary biliary cirrhosis associated with coeliac disease and dermatitis herpetiformis. Dermatologica *170*:31–34, 1985.

53. Wallace JG Jr, Tong MJ, Ueki BH: Pulmonary involvement in primary biliary cirrhosis. J Clin Gastroenterol *9*:431–435, 1987.

54. Robertson JC, Batstone GF, Loebl WY: Polymyalgia rheumatica and primary biliary cirrhosis. Br Med J *4*:1128–1130, 1978.

55. Sevenet F, Capron-Chivrac D, Delcenserie R, Lelarge C, Delamarre J, Capron J-P: Idiopathic retroperitoneal fibrosis and primary biliary cirrhosis. A new association? Arch Intern Med *145*:2124–2125, 1985.

56. Keeffe EB: Sarcoidosis and primary biliary cirrhosis. Literature review and illustrative case. Am J Med *83*:977–981, 1987.

57. Maddrey WC: Sarcoidosis and primary biliary cirrhosis: associated disorders? N Engl J Med *308*:588–590, 1983.

58. Pares A, Rimola A, Bruguera M, Mas E, Rodes J: Renal tubular acidosis in primary biliary cirrhosis. Gastroenterology *80*:681–686, 1981.

59. Burroughs AK, Rosenstein JJ, Epstein O: Bacteriuria and primary biliary cirrhosis. Gut *25*:133–138, 1984.

60. Mitchison HC, Bassendine MF, Malcolm AJ, Watson A, Record CO, James GFW: A pilot, double-blind, controlled 1-year trial of prednisolone treatment in primary biliary cirrhosis: hepatic improvement but greater bone loss. Hepatology *10*:420–429, 1989.

61. Leuschner U, Fischer H, Kurtz W, Buldutuna S, Hubner K, Hellstern A: Ursodeoxycholic acid in primary biliary cirrhosis: results of a controlled double-blind trial. Gastroenterology *97*:1268–1274, 1989.

62. Poupon RE, Eschwege E, Poupon R,: Ursodeoxycholic acid for the treatment of primary biliary cirrhosis. Interim analysis of a double-blind multicentre randomized trial. J Hepatol *11*:16–21, 1990.

63. Dickson ER, Fleming TR, Wiesner RH, Baldus WP, Fleming CR, Ludwig J, McCall JT: Trial of penicillamine in advanced primary biliary cirrhosis. N Engl J Med *312*:1011–1015, 1985.

64. Epstein O, Jain S, Lee RG, Cook DG, Boss AM, Scheuer P, Sherlock S: D-penicillamine treatment improves survival in primary biliary cirrhosis. Lancet *1*:1275–1277, 1981.

65. Hoofnagle JH, Davis GL, Schafer DF, Peters M, Avigan MI, Pappas SC, Hanson RG, Minuk GY, Dusheiko MG, Campbell G, MacSween RNM, Jones EA: Randomized trial of chlorambucil for primary biliary cirrhosis. Gastroenterology *91*:1327–1334, 1986.

66. Christensen E, Neuberger J, Crowe J, Altman DG, Popper H, Portmann B, Donisch D, Ranek L, Tygstrup N, Williams R: Beneficial effect of azathioprine and prediction of prognosis in primary biliary cirrhosis: final results of an international trial. Gastroenterology *89*:1084–1091, 1985.

67. Kaplan MM. Methotrexate treatment of chronic cholestatic liver diseases: friend or foe? Q J Med 72:757–761, 1989.
68. Hadziyannis S, Scheuer PJ, Feizi T, Naccarato R, Doniach D, Sherlock S: Immunological and histological studies in primary biliary cirrhosis. J Clin Pathol 23:95–98, 1970.
69. MacSween RNM, Horne CHW, Moffat AJ, Hughes HM: Serum protein levels in primary biliary cirrhosis. J Clin Pathol 25:789–792, 1972.
70. Nakanuma Y, Miyamura H, Ohta G, Kobayashi K, Kato Y, Hattori N: Correlation between disappearance of the intrahepatic bile ducts and histologic changes in the liver in primary biliary cirrhosis. Am J Gastroenterol 76:506–510, 1981.
71. Walshe JM: Copper: its role in the pathogenesis of liver disease. Semin Liver Dis 4:252–263, 1984.
72. Guarascio P, Yentis F, Cevikbas U, Portmann B, Williams R: Value of copper-associated protein in diagnostic assessment of liver biopsy. J Clin Pathol 36:18–23, 1983.
73. Janssens AR, Van Den Hamer CJA: Kinetics of ^{64}copper in primary biliary cirrhosis. Hepatology 2:822–827, 1982.
74. Winge DR: Normal physiology of copper metabolis. Semin Liver Dis 4:239–251, 1984.
75. Epstein O: Liver copper in health and disease. Postgrad Med J 59:88–94, 1983.
76. Fleming CR, Ludwig J, Dickson ER: Asymptomatic primary biliary cirrhosis. Presentation, histology, and results with D-penicillamine. Mayo Clin Proc 53:587–593, 1978.
77. Matloff DS, Alpert E, Resnick RH, Kaplan MM: A prospective trial of D-penicillamine in primary biliary cirrhosis. N Engl J Med 306:319–326, 1982.
78. Gershwin ME, Coppel RL, Mackay IR: Primary biliary cirrhosis and mitochondrial autoantigens—Insights from molecular biology. Hepatology 8:147–151, 1988.
79. Berg PA, Wever P, Oehring J, Lindenborn-Fotinos J, Stechemesser E: Significance of different types of mitochondrial antibodies in primary biliary cirrhosis. In Hepatology. A Festschrift for Hans Popper, edited by H. Brunner, H. Thaler. New York, Raven Press, 1985, pp. 231–242.
80. Kenny RP, Czaja AJ, Ludwig J. Dickson ER: Frequency and significance of antimitochondrial antibodies in severe chronic active hepatitis. Dig Dis Sci 31:705–711, 1986.
81. Doniach D, Roitt IM, Walker JG, Sherlock S: Tissue autoantibodies in primary biliary cirrhosis, active chronic (lupoid) hepatitis, cryptogenic cirrhosis and other liver diseases and their clinical implications. Clin Exper Immunol 1:237–262, 1966.
82. Hodges JR, Hall AJ, Wright R: Primary biliary cirrhosis and antimitochondrial antibodies. Lancet 2:362, 1981.
83. Manns M, Meyer zum Buschenfelde K-H: A mitochondrial antigen-antibody system in cholestatic liver disease detected by radioimmunoassay. Hepatology 2:1–7, 1982.
84. Berg PA, Klein R, Lindenborn-Fotinos J: Antimitochondrial antibodies in primary biliary cirrhosis. J Hepatol 2:123–131, 1986.
85. Berg PA, Klein R: Clinical and prognostic relevance of different mitochondrial antibody profiles in primary biliary cirrhosis (PBC). In Molecular Aspects of Primary Biliary Cirrhosis, edited by O. Epstein. Mol Aspects Med 8:235–247, 1985.
86. Weber P, Brenner J, Stechemesser E, Klein R, Weckenmann U, Kloppel G, Kirchhof M, Fintelmann V, Berg PA: Characterization and clinical relevance of a new complement-fixing antibody—Anti-M8—in patients with primary biliary cirrhosis. Hepatology 6:553–559, 1986.
87. Van de Water J, Cooper A, Surh CD, Coppel R, Danner D, Ansari A, Dickson R, Gershwin E: Detection of autoantibodies to recombinant mitochondrial proteins in patients with primary biliary cirrhosis. N Engl J Med 320:1377–1380, 1989.
88. Yeaman SJ, Fussey SPM, Danner DJ, James OFW, Mutimer DJ, Bassendine MF: Primary biliary cirhosis: identification of two major M2 mitochondrial autoantigens. Lancet 1:1067–1069, 1988.
89. Mutimer DJ, Fussey SPM, Yeaman SJ, Kelly PJ, James OFW, Bassendine MF: Frequency of IgG and IgM autoantibodies to four specific M2 mitochondrial autoantigens in primary biliary cirrhosis. Hepatology 10:403–407, 1989.
90. Surh CD, Roche TE, Danner DJ, Ansari A, Coppel RL, Prindiville T, Dickson ER, Gershwin ME: Antimitochondrial autoantibodies in primary biliary cirrhosis recognize cross-reactive epitopes on protein X and dihydrolipoamide acetyltransferase of pyruvate dehydrogenase complex. Hepatology 10:127–133, 1989.
91. Bernstein RM, Neuberger JM, Bunn CC, Callender ME, Hughes GRV,
92. Williams R: Diversity of autoantibodies in primary biliary cirrhosis and chronic active hepatitis. Clin Exper Immunol 55:553–560, 1984.
92. Ballardini G, Mirakian R, Bianchi FB, Pisi E, Doniach D, Botazzo GF: Aberrant expression of HLA-DR antigens on bile duct epithelium in primary biliary cirrhosis: relevance to pathogenesis. Lancet 2:1009–1013, 1984.
93. James SP, Elson CO, Jones EA, Straber W: Abnormal regulation of immune globulin synthesis in vitro in primary biliary cirrhosis. Gastroenterology 79:242–254, 1980.
94. Dienstag JL, Weake JR, Wands JR: Abnormalities of mononuclear cell regulation in vitro in primary biliary cirrhosis. Liver 1:230–243, 1981.
95. James SP, Vierling JM. Stroben W: The role of the immune response in the pathogenesis of primary biliary cirrhosis. Semin Liver Dis 1:322–337, 1981.
96. Gupta RC, Dickson ER, McDuffie FC, Baggenstoss AH: Circulating IgG complexes in primary biliary cirrhosis. A serial study in forty patients followed for two years. Clin Exp Immunol 34:19–27, 1978.
97. Wands JR, Dienstag JL, Bhan AK, Feller ER, Isselbacker KJ: Circulating immune complexes and complement activation in primary biliary cirrhosis. N Engl J Med 298:233–237, 1978.
98. Amoroso P, Vergagni D, Wojcicka BM, McFarlane IG, Eddleston ALWF, Tee DEH, Williams R: Identification of biliary antigens in circulating immune complexes in primary biliary cirrhosis. Clin Exp Immunol 42:95–98. 1980.
99. Jones EA, Frank MM, Jaffe CJ, Vierling JM: Primary biliary cirrhosis and the complement system. Ann Intern Med 90:72–84, 1979.
100. Krogsgaard K, Tage-Jensen U, Wantzin P, Aldershirle J, Hardt F: Localization of immunoglobulin in the liver cell surface in primary biliary cirrhosis. J Clin Pathol 34:1076–1079, 1981.
101. Kawai K, Kitagawa H, Higashimori T, Matsui T, Fujiyama S, Monna T, Yamamoto S, Morisawa S: Experimental chronic non-suppurative destructive cholangitis in rabbits following immunization with bile duct antigen. Gastroenterol Jpn 15:337–345, 1980.
102. Goldberg MJ, Kaplan MM, Mitamura T, Anderson CL, Matloff DS, Pinn VW, Agnello V: Evidence against an immune complex pathogenesis of primary biliary cirrhosis. Gastroenterology 83:677–683, 1982.
103. Fox RA, Dudley FJ, Sherlock S: The primary immune response to haemocyanin in patients with primary biliary cirrhosis. Clin Exp Immunol 14:473–480, 1973.
104. Miller J, Smith MGM, Mitchell CG, Reed WD, Eddleston ALWF, Williams R: Cell-mediated immunity to a human liver-specific antigen in patients with active chronic hepatitis and primary biliary cirrhosis. Lancet 2:296–297, 1972.
105. Wojcicka-McFarlane BM, McFarlane IG, Amoroso P, Williams R: Differential in vitro immune responses to biliary tract antigens in primary biliary cirrhosis and chronic active hepatitis. Liver 1:268–279, 1981.
106. Geubel AP, Keller RH, Summerskill WHJ, Dickson ER, Tomasi TB, Shorter RG: Lymphocyte cytotoxicity and inhibition studied with autologous liver cells: observations in chronic active liver disease and the primary biliary cirrhosis syndrome. Gastroenterology 71:450–456, 1976.
107. MacSween RNM, Burt AD: The cellular pathology of primary biliary cirrhosis. Mol Aspects Med 8:269–292, 1985.
108. James SP, Vierling JM, Strober W: The role of the immune response in the pathogenesis of primary biliary cirrhosis. Semin Liver Dis 1:322–337, 1981.
109. MacSween RNM, Burt AD: The cellular pathology of primary biliary cirrhosis. Mol Aspects Med 8:269–292, 1985.
110. MacLean CA, Goudie BM, MacSween RNM, Sandiland GP: Scrum Fc receptor-like molecules in primary biliary cirrhosis: a possible immunoregulatory mechanism. Immunology 53:315–324, 1984.
111. Jones EA: Primary biliary cirrhosis: potential pathogenic mechanisms and the effets of therapies on the disease process. In Recent Advances in Hepatology, No. 1, edited by H.C. Thomas, R.N.M. MacSween. Edinburgh, Churchill Livingstone, 1984, pp. 131–151.
112. Vento S, O'Brien CJ, McFarlane BM, McFarlane IG, Eddleston ALWF, Williams R: T-lymphocyte sensitization to hepatocyte antigens in autoimmune chronic active hepatitis and primary biliary cirrhosis: evidence for different underlying mechanisms and different antigenic determinants as targets. Gastroenterology 91:810–817, 1986.
113. Gershwin ME, Mackay IR: Primary biliary cirrhosis: paradigm or paradox for autoimmunity. Gastroenterology 100:822–833, 1991.
114. Fox RA, James DG, Scheuer PJ, Sharma O, Sherlock S: Impaired

delayed hypersensitivity in primary biliary cirrhosis. Lancet *1*:959–962, 1969.

115. James SP, Vierling JM, Strober W: The role of the immune response in the pathogenesis of primary biliary cirrhosis. Semin Liver Dis *1*:322–337, 1981.

116. Fagan EA, Moore-Gillon JC, Turner-Warwick M: Multiorgan granulomas and mitochondrial antibodies. N Engl J Med *308*:572–575, 1983.

117. Bernauu D, Feldmann G, Degott C, Gisselbrecht C: Ultrastructural lesions of bile ducts in primary biliary cirrhosis. A comparison with the lesions observed in graft versus host disease. Hum Pathol *12*;782–793, 1981.

118. Shulman HM, Sullivan KM, Weiden PL, McDonald GB, Striker GE, Sale GE, Hackinan R, Tsoi M-S, Storb R, Thomas ED: Chronic graft-versus-host syndrome in man. A long-term clinicopathologic study of 20 Seattle patients. Am J Med *69*:204–217, 1980.

119. McFarlane IG, McFarlane Bm, Haines AJ, Eddleston ALWF, Williams R: Relationship between primary biliary cirrhosis and chronic graft versus host disease: investigation of histocompatibility (HLA) antigenic determinants in biliary tract antigens. Clin Sci *64*:113–116, 1983.

120. Jaup GH, Zettergren LSW: Familial occurrence of primary biliary cirrhosis associated with hypergammaglobulinemia in descendents: a family study. Gastroenterology *78*:549–555, 1980.

121. Galbraith RM, Smith M, Mackenzie RM, Tee DE, Doniach D, Williams R: High prevalence of seroimmunologic abnormalities in relatives of patients with active chronic hepatitis or primary biliary cirrhosis. N Engl J Med *290*:63–69, 1974.

122. Williams M, Smith PM, Doniach D: Primary biliary cirrhosis and chronic active hepatitis in two sisters. Br Med J *2*:566, 1976.

123. Hamlyn AN, Morris JS, Sherlock S: ABO blood groups, rhesus negativity and primary biliary cirrhosis. Gut *15*:480–481, 1974.

124. Gores GJ, Moore SB, Fisher LD, Powell FC, Dickson ER: Primary biliary cirrhosis: associations with Class II major histocompatibility complex antigens. Hepatology *7*:889–892, 1987.

125. Glaser JH, Balistreri WF, Morecki R: The role of reovirus type 3 in pesistent infantile cholestasis. J Pediatr *105*:912–915, 1984.

126. Minuk GY, Rascanin N, Paul RW, Lee PWK, Buchan K, Kelly JK: Reovirus type 3 infection in patients with primary biliary cirrhosis and primary sclerosing cholangitis. J Hepatol *5*:8–13, 1987.

127. Popper H, Schaffner F: Nonsuppurative destructive cholangitis and chronic hepatitis. In Progress in Liver Diseases, edited by H. Popper, F. Schaffner. 3rd Edition. New York, Grune & Stratton, 1970, pp. 336–354.

128. Ludwig J, Dickson ER, McDonald GSA: Staging of chronic non-suppurative destructive cholangitis (syndrome of primary biliary cirrhosis) Virchow's Arch (Pathol Anat) *379*:103–112, 1978.

129. Williams GEG: Pericholangiolitic biliary cirrhosis. J Pathol Bacteriol *89*:23–34, 1965.

130. Nakanuma Y, Ohta G: Histometric and serial section observations of the intrahepatic bile ducts in primary biliary cirrhosis. Gastroenterology *76*:1325–1332, 1979.

131. Portmann B, MacSween RNM: Diseases of the intrahepatic bile ducts. In Pathology of the Liver, edited by R.N.M. MacSween, P.P. Anthony, P. J. Scheuer. Edinburgh, Churchill Livingstone, 1987, pp. 424–435.

132. Christoffersen P, Poulsen H. Scheuer PJ: Abnormal bile duct epithelium in chronic aggressive hepatitis and primary biliary cirrhosis. Hum Pathol *3*:227–235, 1972.

133. Scheuer PJ: Liver Biopsy Interpretation, 3d Edition. London, Balliere Tindall, 1987, pp. 54–57.

134. Ludwig J. Barham SS, La Russo NF, Elveback LR, Wiesner RH, McCall JT: Morphologic features of chronic hepatitis associated with primary sclerosing cholangitis and chronic ulcerative colitis. Hepatology *1*:632–640, 1981.

135. Ludwig J, McDonald GSA, Dickson ER, Elveback LR, McCall JT: Copper stains and the syndrome of primary biliary cirrhosis. Evaluation of staining methods and their usefulness for diagnosis and trials of penicillamine treatment. Arch Pathol *103*:467–470, 1979.

136. Sipponen P: Orcein-positive hepatocellular meterial in long-standing biliary diseases. I. Histochemical characteristics. Scand J Gastroenterol *11*:545–552, 1976.

137. Popper H, Goldfischer S, Sternlieb I, Nyad NC, Madhavan TV: Cytoplasmic copper and its toxic effects. Studies in Indian childhood cirrhosis. Lancet *1*:1205–1208, 1979.

138. Sipponen P: Orcein positive hepatocellular material in long-standing biliary diseases. II. Ultrastructural studies. Scand J Gastroenterol *11*:553–557, 1976.

139. Salaspuro MP, Sipponen P, Makkonen H: The occurrence of orcein-positive hepatocellular material in various liver diseases. Scand J Gastroenterol *11*:677–681, 1976.

140. Sipponen P, Salaspuro MP, Makkonen HM: Orcein positive hepatocellular material in the histologic diagnosis of primary biliary cirrhosis. Ann Clin Res *7*:274–277, 1975.

140a. Kaplan MM, Knox TA. Treatment of primary biliary cirrhosis with low-dose weekly methotrexate. Gastroenterology *101*:1332–1338, 1991.

141. Poulsen H, Christoffersen P: Abnormal bile duct epithelium in chronic aggressive hepatitis and cirrhosis. A review of morphology and clinical, biochemical and immunologic features. Hum Pathol *3*:217–225, 1972.

142. Williamson JMS, Chalmers DM, Clayden AD, Dixon MF, Ruddell WSJ, Losowsky MS: Primary biliary cirrhosis and chronic active hepatitis: an examination of clinical, biochemical and histopathological features in differential diagnosis. J Clin Pathol *38*:1007–1012, 1985.

143. Doniach D, Walker JG: A unified concept of autoimmune hepatitis. Lancet *1*:813–815, 1969.

144. Geubel AP, Baggenstoss AH, Summerskill WHJ: Response to treatment can differentiate chronic active liver disease with cholangitic features from the primary biliary cirrhosis syndrome. Gastroenterology *71*:444–449, 1976.

145. Chapman RWG, Arborgh BAM, Rhodes JM, Summerfield JA, Dick R, Scheuer PJ, Sherlock S: Primary sclerosing cholangitis: a review of its clinical features, cholangiography, and hepatic histology. Gut *21*:870–877, 1980.

146. Wiesner RH, LaRusso NF, Ludwig J, Dickson ER: Comparison of the clinicopathologic features of primary sclerosing cholangitis and primary biliary cirrhosis. Gastroenterology *88*:108–114, 1985.

147. Bhathal PS, Powell LW: Primary intrahepatic obliterating cholangitis: a possible variant of sclerosing cholangitis. Gut *10*:886–893, 1969.

148. Zelman S: Liver cell necrosis in chlorpromazine jaundice (allergic cholangiolitis). A serial study of twenty-six needle biopsy specimens in nine patients. Am J Med *27*:708–729, 1959.

149. Ishak KG, Ivey NS: Hepatic injury associated with phenothiazines. Clinicopathologic and follow-up study of 36 patients. Arch Pathol *93*:283–304, 1972.

Chapter 12
Hepatic Lesions in Disorders of Iron Metabolism

Introduction

Definitions

The term *hemosiderosis* or *siderosis* refers to any abnormal deposition of stainable iron in the tissues, irrespective of its etiology. Although hemosiderin, which is a denatured form of ferritin, predominates in such deposits, ferritin is also present. Iron deposits may be limited to a single tissue, such as the liver, but they are usually more widely disseminated.

Hemochromatosis is a less easily defined term (1). Although it often is interpreted as a form of hemosiderosis accompanied by evidence of hepatic injury, such as portal fibrosis or cirrhosis, it is also used to define all forms of hemosiderosis encountered in individuals with hereditary iron storage disease (genetic hemochromatosis), irrespective of whether there is accompanying hepatic damage. To complicate the problem of definition further, opinions are divided about how to classify the secondary iron deposition that sometimes occurs in preexisting cirrhosis. For example, should the hemosiderosis that occurs after a portacaval shunt be considered hemochromatosis?

The term *iron overload* refers to any condition in which the total body nonheme tissue iron stores exceeds the normal range of 1 to 1.5 g.

Total body iron

The normal total body content of iron ranges form 3 to 5 g, of which 1.5 to 3.0 g is incorporated in hemoglobin, 100 to 300 mg is complexed with protein in the form of myoglobin, cytochrome, and catalase, 3 to 5 mg is found in the circulation bound to a β_1-globulin, transferrin, and 0.1 to 1 mg as ferritin and from 1.0 to 1.5 g is stored in the tissues in the form of ferritin and hemosiderin (2,3). Under normal conditions, the liver contains the largest fraction of storage iron, approximately 400 mg, one-half to two-thirds in the form of ferritin, the remainder in the form of hemosiderin (4). The two other major sites of iron storage, the bone marrow and spleen, contain approximately 300 mg and 25 mg, respectively (4). Under conditions of abnormally increased iron absorption from the intestinal tract, iron accumulates in the hepatocytes, first as ferritin and, as the amount becomes excessive, i.e., >1000 μg/g, as hemosiderin. As iron stores increase, ferritin concentrations increase, but the high percentage of ferritin at lower levels of iron deposition decreases so that ferritin constitutes less than half the total amount of iron in the liver (5). Ferritin synthesis, which is inducible by iron, is most active in liver, spleen, and bone marrow, but also occurs in most other tissues (3). Ferritin concentration in serum roughly parallels that total content of iron

in the body. When ferritin molecules are fully saturated with iron, they aggregate and are degraded by lysosomal action to form hemosiderin (6). When the storage capacity of the liver is exceeded, iron deposits appear in other tissues, chiefly in the acinar cells of the pancreas and the secretory cells of other exocrine and endocrine glands. Although the Kupffer cells and splenic reticuloendothelium are spared under such conditions, following multiple transfusions, episodes of hemolysis, or the intravenous administration of iron-containing preparations, they often contain large amounts of hemosiderin.

Storage iron

Normal hepatocytes contain iron in the form of *ferritin,* spherical micelles of ferric hydroxyphosphate enclosed within a shell of apoferritin. On electron microscopy, they can be identified as distinctive 50 to 70 Å particles dispersed through the cytosol and lysosomes (7). Because of their small size, ferritin particles cannot be visualized in normal hepatocytes by light microscopy and cannot be identified histochemically. However, when the particles are greatly increased in number under conditions of iron overload, they may react with acidified potassium ferrocyanide imparting a diffuse, pale blue color to the cytoplasm (Fig. 159). Occasionally, swollen Kupffer cells filled with phagocytized ferritin particles derived from adjacent necrotic hepatocytes exhibit a similar diffuse Prussian blue reaction.

The composition of the protein shell of ferritin, which consists of 24 polypeptide subunits, differs in different tissues. Thus, hepatic isoferritin differs from the pulmonary and renal isoferritins in the composition of the component subunits (8). In addition, serum ferritin, which is a hollow sphere capable of containing 4000 molecules of iron, differs from the tissue ferritins.

Hemosiderin granules are aggregates of ferritin particles without their apoferritin coats. Occasionally, these granules are organized in the form of crystalline arrays. In addition, the granules often contain a protein that resembles apoferritin, ferric iron bound to polysaccharide, lipid, and lipofuscin (7). Characteristically, the granules are found in lysosomes and are most numerous in periportal hepatocytes.

Although small amounts of hemosiderin can be detected in the liver in a high proportion of individuals with normal iron stores (4), such pigment is demonstrable by histochemical means or by electron microscopy (9) in only a small minority of cases.

In routine H & E sections, hemosiderin deposits appear as relatively coarse, greenish-brown, pigment granules with sharply defined, refractile edges (Fig. 158). Characteristically, the granules stain deep blue when treated with acidified potassium ferrocyanide (Prussian blue reaction) (Fig. 159). Because of their location in lysosomes, hemosiderin granules tend to aggregate alongside the canaliculi and often outline their course (Fig. 158).

Both ferritin and hemosiderin provide a labile pool of iron that can be mobilized when needed for increased heme synthesis, a feature that permits the removal of excessive iron stores by phlebotomy.

Iron absorption, excretion, and transport

In healthy adults, the absorption and losses of iron are in equilibrium, so the total body stores of iron remain constant.

Under normal conditions, the amount of iron absorbed from the intestinal tract, chiefly in the duodenum, is limited to approximately 1 mg daily, even though the diet usually contains 10 to 25 mg. Before such absorption can occur, the iron must be reduced to its ferrous state. On entering the mucosal cells of duodenum in the ferrious state, the iron is converted to the ferric state to form ferritin. Part of the ferritin releases its iron, again as ferrous iron, which passes into the circulation where it is bound to transferrin. Transferrin binds iron tightly, but reversibly, as does ferritin. A molecule of transferrin, however, binds only 2 atoms of iron compared with the 4000 atoms for a molecule of ferritin (10). Not all of the factors that govern the rate of iron absorption have been identified. However, it is clear that the uptake of iron is increased under conditions of iron deficiency, excessive iron intake, anemia accompanied by ineffective erythropoiesis, and the genetically determined metabolic defect that characterizes idiopathic hemochromatosis. In contrast, suppression of erythropoiesis and the ingestion of agents, such as phosphates, that form insoluble salts of iron in the intestinal tract, inhibit iron absorption.

Losses of iron in healthy adult males approximate 1 mg daily, two-thirds via the intestinal tract in sloughed mucosal cells, traces of blood and bile, the remainder in urine, sweat, and desquamating skin. In women, menstrual loss averages an additional 0.5 mg daily. The losses of iron tend to decrease under conditions of iron deficiency and to increase with iron overload. Such changes, however, are negligible, and have little effect on iron balance, but large losses of hemoglobin that result from hemorrhage or phlebotomy mobilize iron from storage sites for increased heme synthesis. To a lesser extent the administration of chelating agents, such as deferoxamine, that enhance the urinary excretion of iron can reduce iron stores significantly.

Table 12–1. Etiologic types of iron overload

Hereditary hemochromatosis

Secondary iron overload
Anemia with ineffective erythropoiesis
Transfusional iron overload
Dietary and medicinal iron overload
Hemodialysis iron overload
Alcoholic iron overload
Porphyria cutanea tarda
Portacaval anastomosis iron overload
Iron overload in renal transplant recipients

Neonatal iron overload
Idiopathic neonatal hemochromatosis
Zellweger's syndrome
Hypermethioninemia
Congenital atransferrinemia

Except for a minute fraction of ferritin, all the iron that enters the circulation from the intestinal tract or from tissue deposits of ferritin and hemosiderin is transported in the serum bound to transferrin (11). In healthy adults, the concentration of iron in the serum is approximately 125 μg/dl (range 80–200 μg/dl), that of transferrin in terms of serum total iron binding capacity, approximately 360 μg/dl (range 310–430 μg/dl), and the percentage saturation of transferrin with iron, approximately 35% (range 26–49%). When iron stores are depleted, the serum concentration of iron and the percentage saturation of transferrin fall, whereas under conditions of iron overload they rise. However, not all abnormalities of serum iron concentration reflect alterations in body iron stores, since infection not infrequently leads to hypoferremia (11), and liver damage to hyperferremia (12). Transferrin is synthesized in the liver, so reduced levels of total serum iron binding capacity are relatively common in various forms of hepatic disease (13).

Experimental evidence suggests that the uptake of iron by both erythrocytes (14) and hepatocytes (15) is dependent on the binding of iron-transferrin to specific cell surface receptors. Iron is taken up by hepatocytes by endocytosis by three pathways: (1) transferrin-receptor-mediated uptake of transferrin-bound iron; (2) non-receptor-mediated, fluid phase absorption of transferrin-bound iron; and (3) fluid phase endocytosis of non-transferrin-bound iron (15,16). The concentration of transferrin receptors on the surface of hepatocytes, however, is inversely related to the amount of iron available. In genetic hemochromatosis with increased iron stores, transferrin receptors on the surface of hepatocytes are absent (17,18). This down regulation is reversible (19). Thus, non-transferrin-bound iron may play a major role in the absorption of iron in iron storage disease (20). It is postulated that this down regulation is not a primary defect in hemochromatosis, but is secondary to iron overload. This concept is supported by the fact that the hemochromatosis gene is located on chromosome 6 (21), whereas the gene for transferrin receptors is located on chromosome 3 (22). Actually, a gene for the hepatic receptor for ferritin has been located on chromosome 6 (23), which suggests that a structural defect at that site might be a more likely explanation for the primary defect in hemochromatosis.

The serum ferritin concentration correlates directly with the total body iron stores both in healthy individuals and in those with iron deficiency or overload (3). However, the coefficient of correlation is relatively low. In addition to iron storage disease, high serum levels of ferritin are seen in acute and chronic liver disease, as a result of ferritin release from damaged hepatocytes, and in leukemia and Hodgkin's disease, due to increased ferritin synthesis by neoplastic cells (3).

Hepatic injury due to iron overload

A number of observations support the view that chronic iron overload may lead to hepatic damage. Among these may be cited: (1) the frequent occurrence of portal fibrosis and cirrhosis in all forms of hepatocellular hemosiderosis; (2) the reversal of such collagen deposition following the removal of excessive iron stores by phlebotomy (24); and (3) the experimental production in dogs of hemosiderosis and cirrhosis resembling the lesions of idiopathic hemochromatosis by the long-term parenteral administration of iron dextran and iron sorbitol in massive doses (25). Although the mechanisms responsible for hepatic injury and fibrosis in iron overload are still uncertain, several possibilities have been proposed: (1) the deposition of ferritin and hemosiderin increases the fragility and disrupts lysosomes, resulting in the release of acid hydrolases (26,27); (2) the capacity to synthesize hemosiderin and ferritin may be exceeded, leading to the release of free iron that promotes the peroxidation of hepatocyte organelles (28,29); and (3) excessive iron deposits stimulate collagen synthesis (30). Evidence in favor of the peroxidation hypothesis is mounting and many investigators now accept that iron-induced liver injury is mediated by free radicals (31).

Etiologic types of iron overload

In addition to hereditary hemochromatosis, there are a number of secondary types. These disorders may represent enhanced absorption of iron for a variety of reasons. Some are genetically determined disorders, such as *porphyria cutanea tarda* (32), which is usually mild but may be intensified when alcoholic liver disease coexists (33) or when the gene for hemochromatosis is present (33). Other types are acquired, including the form that develops after *portacaval anastomosis* (34), after *hemodialysis* (35), or after *kidney transplantation* (36). Fibrosis has not been reported in the iron overload associated with chronic renal failure (35), but fullblown hemochromatosis has been observed after kidney transplantation (36) (see later). Most of these acquired disorders are exaggerated by the presence of the gene for hemochromatosis.

Hereditary hemochromatosis

Definition

Hereditary hemochromatosis, which is also known as idiopathic, genetic, familial, and primary hemochromatosis, is a hereditary disorder transmitted as an autosomal recessive trait characterized by excessive intestinal absorption of iron starting at birth that results in progressive accumulation of iron in the tissues.

Genetic factors

The incidence of histocompatibility antigens HLA-A3, B7, and B14 is significantly increased in patients with idiopathic hemochromatosis (37–39). About three-fourths of patients with hereditary hemochromatosis have histocompatibility antigen HLA-A3 (38). Other HLA haplotypes of the HLA-A locus have been identified in individual families (40). Family studies of the disease suggest that homozygotes carry two hemochromatosis alleles located on chromosome 6 close to the HLA locus, and that siblings who exhibit identical A and B haplotypes are similarly homozygous, whereas siblings, parents, and offspring who share only one haplotype are heterozygous (37–46). The frequency of the hemochromatosis gene in certain populations is 4.5%, which corresponds to a prevalence of the disease of 0.2% (46).

Although some heterozygotes may exhibit minor degrees of enhanced iron absorption and deposition, full clinical expression of the disease is said to occur exclusively in homozygotes (47).

Pathogenesis

It is apparent that the iron overload in idiopathic hemochromatosis must be attributable to excessive absorption of iron from the intestinal tract. Indeed, as many as 41% of patients with hereditary hemochromatosis have excessively high alcohol consumption (38). However, the mechanisms responsible for the increased iron absorption are uncertain (47). Of several possibilities that have been considered, the most important are (1) a defect in the mucosal control of iron absorption (48); (2) an abnormal affinity of the liver for transferrin iron (49); and (3) an abnormality in the handling of iron by the reticuloendothelial tissues. It has been shown that Kupffer cells may release iron, which is then taken up by hepatocytes (50).

The role of alcohol in the pathogenesis of idiopathic hemochromatosis is still uncertain. The fact that the HLA typing patterns in idiopathic hemochromatosis and alcoholic liver disease differ is consistent with the view that the two diseases are unrelated (44). However, the frequency of chronic alcoholism in some families with idiopathic hemochromatosis has led to the suggestion that alcohol may play a role in expression of the disease, both in homozygotes and heterozygotes (51,52). Indeed, most patients with massive iron accumulation have hereditary hemochromatosis (42,53). Actually the concentration of hepatic iron is lower in alcoholic than in nonalcoholic patients with hereditary hemochromatosis (53).

Clinical manifestations

Since the daily increment in iron stores is only a few milligrams, and overt signs of the disease do not appear until 20 to 60 g have accumulated, the clinical manifestations of idiopathic hemochromatosis usually do not become evident until the age of 40 to 60 years (1). However, in a small minority of cases, overt disease appears in childhood and adolescence (54).

Clinically evident idiopathic hemochromatosis affects males 10 times as frequently as females. Losses of iron due to menstruation, pregnancy, and lactation, which minimize the accumulation of iron in the tissues, probably account for this difference. Consistent with this interpretation is the fact that in half the women affected by the disease, the menses have been absent or scanty. However, overt hemochromatosis has been reported in a small number of premenopausal women who have menstruated normally and borne children (55).

The principal clinical manifestations of hereditary hemochromatosis include weakness and malaise, hepatomegaly, hyperpigmentation, diabetes mellitus, loss of libido, heart failure, arthropathy, peripheral neuritis, and abdominal pain, either singly or, more commonly, in various combinations.

In almost all cases of hemochromatosis, the *liver* is *enlarged* and *indurated* owing to deposition of hemosiderin and varying degrees of fibrosis with or without accompanying cirrhosis. Signs of *hepatocellular failure* are relatively infrequent, except terminally in untreated cases. The hepatomegaly is accompanied by splenomegaly in half the cases, and by other signs of portal hypertension, including esophageal varices and hemorrhage, in almost one-third of cases (56). These features may vary with the manner of case selection. The incidence of complicating hepatocellular carcinoma is relatively high, averaging 14%, and tends to increase with advancing age, reaching 60% of those who survive to the age of 70 (1,57).

Hyperpigmentation of the skin, which occurs in half the patients, is due primarily to deposition of melanin in the basal layers of the epidermis (1). However, in some cases, hemosiderin deposits around the sweat glands in the corium contribute to the dark color of the skin (58).

Diabetes mellitus is demonstrable in almost two-thirds of patients with hemochromatosis (59). Although glucose intolerance may be due to iron-mediated destruction of the islets by hemosiderin deposits in some cases, in others it appears to be a manifestation of familial diabetes (59), or may be attributable to the underlying cirrhosis (60). The view once held that hemochromatotic diabetes does not give rise to the complications of classic diabetes mellitus (61) has changed as recent evidence has shown that it is associated with nephropathy, neuropathy, peripheral vascular disease, or retinopathy in over 20% of cases, (60). However, insulin resistance does appear to occur more frequently in hemochromatotic than in classic, adult-onset diabetes mellitus (60).

Loss of libido, impotence, or *testicular atrophy* are relatively common features in idiopathic hemochromatosis, the reported incidence ranging from approximately 20 to 70% (62). The pathogenesis of such hypogonadism is still uncertain, but has been variously attributed to cirrhosis, hemosiderin-induced testicular atrophy, and hypopituitarism secondary to deposition of hemosiderin in the anterior lobe. The results of some endocrine studies suggest that pituitary insufficiency rather than primary testicular atrophy or cirrhosis accounts for the hypogonadism (63,64). Consistent with this interpretation is the fact that the hypogonadism may be accompanied by evidence of impaired adrenal and thyroid function. However, other endocrine studies have been contradictory, and suggest that the hypogonadism may be attributable to a defect in the responsiveness of the testes to interstitial cell–stimulating hormone, and to an abnormality in the testicular-hypothalamic-pituitary feedback mechanism (62).

Heart failure is the presenting complaint in 15% of patients with hemochromatosis and accounts for death in one-third of such cases (1).

A distinctive type of *arthropathy* is encountered in at least half the patients with hemochromatosis (31,65) and, occasionally, is the presenting complaint that leads to the discovery of the disease (66).

Abdominal pain is a relatively common complaint in hemochromatosis, occurring in one-third of patients during the course of the disease (1). In some, the pain is attributable to complicating peritonitis, pancreatitis, or hepatocellular carcinoma, but, in many cases, the etiology is obscure. Of particular interest are attacks of acute abdominal pain accompanied by circulatory collapse that often proves fatal (67). The pathogenesis of this syndrome is still uncertain, but, on the basis of incomplete studies, it has been suggested that the abdominal pain and shock may be due to extreme hyperferremia (68), the release of large amounts of ferritin (69), or endotoxemia secondary to gram-negative bacteremia (67,70). Of these possibilities, endotoxemia appears most likely, since gram-negative bacteria have

been recovered on culture of the peritoneum or blood in several such cases (67,70).

Prognosis and effects of venesection therapy

Mean survival from the time of diagnosis in patients with hemochromatosis is about 10 to 11 years (57). One-third survive for at least 5 years (71). In individual cases, however, survival for up to 30 years has been reported (1). Life expectancy is reduced in those who present with cirrhosis or diabetes, but is normal in the others. The causes of death include heart failure in 30%, hepatocellular failure in 15%, hematemesis in 15%, hepatocellular carcinoma in 15%, and diabetic coma in 5%. Diagnosis prior to the development of cirrhosis is important because venesection therapy results in normal life expectancy in such patients. Prognosis is not affected by the sex of the patient.

Repeated phlebotomy, which removes about 500 mg of iron per liter of blood and induces the mobilization of iron from tissue deposits of hemosiderin and ferritin for heme synthesis, is an effective method of reducing the excessive iron stores in hemochromatosis (72). Although no randomized controlled trials of venesection therapy have been reported, and it is unlikely that such studies will ever be undertaken, normal life expectancy has been found when therapy was instituted prior to the development of cirrhosis (57). In addition, most of the manifestations of the disease are improved by venesection therapy. Presumably, the prevalence of hepatocellular carcinoma is reduced by venesections performed before the cirrhosis has developed (57). In one series of 28 phlebotomized patients, life expectancy averaged eight years, and the survival rate after five years was 89% (72). Often, venesection therapy is followed by a reduction in the size of the liver, improvement in hepatic function and glucose tolerance, regression of heart failure, and a decrease in hyperpigmentation (73). However, the hypogonadism and arthropathy appear to be irreversible, and the late development of hepatocellular carcinoma is not always prevented. In a few cases, the hepatic fibrosis regresses to some extent, and rarely, cirrhosis appears to resolve (24,57).

Laboratory features

The principal biochemical findings in homozygous hereditary hemochromatosis include: (1) increased serum iron, (2) increased serum ferritin, (3) decreased serum transferrin (iron-binding capacity), and (4) increased saturation of serum transferrin with iron (45). Rarely, the serum ferritin level in such individuals is normal (74). No one of these abnormalities is diagnostic, but in combination they almost always signify iron overload, although they do not distinguish between idiopathic and other forms of hemochromatosis (75). In one study, transferrin saturation levels greater than 62% were found to be the single best indicator of genetic hemochromatosis (76).

Approximately 25% of individuals with heterozygous hemochromatosis exhibit a slight increase in serum iron and transferrin saturation, but usually show normal levels of serum ferritin (45,77).

As a rule, the high levels of serum ferritin in homozygous

hereditary hemochromatosis are associated with large amounts of stainable iron in the liver, and hepatic concentrations of iron in excess of 429 μg/100 mg wet liver (74). The concentrations of serum iron and ferritin, the degree of transferrin saturation, and the amount of iron deposited in the liver are lower in women than in men, probably reflecting the loss of iron during menstruation.

Diagnosis

The diagnosis of hereditary hemochromatosis has undergone a series of changes in the past few years. *Serum iron* concentrations are considered unreliable because they may be elevated in normal individuals. Furthermore, they are frequently normal in patients with increased iron stores (78). *Serum ferritin* levels, however, generally reflect hepatic and total body iron content (79). Serum ferritin concentrations of >1000 μg/ml, five to six times the normal concentration of 150–200 μg/ml, are found in the large majority of patients with genetic hemochromatosis, but normal levels may be found in some patients with precirrhotic hemochromatosis (80). Occasionally, falsely elevated serum ferritin levels may be seen in patients with hepatic necrosis (81).

The most reliable method of establishing the diagnosis of hereditary hemochromatosis is the iron concentration of the liver tissue. Levels greater than 1000 μg/100 mg of dry liver tissue, i.e., more than 10 times the upper limit of normal, are diagnostic of idiopathic hemochromatosis (82) and can differentiate it from the hemosiderosis of alcoholic liver disease. Furthermore, in hereditary hemochromatosis the amount of iron increases linearly with age and the hepatic iron to age ratio has been shown to be a reliable diagnostic index (82). Indeed, the *hepatic iron index,* i.e., hepatic iron concentration μmol/g dry weight divided by the patient's age in years, is a reliable way of differentiating between homozygous and heteroxygous hemochromatosis (83). Homozygotes accrue about 5 μmol (0.3 mg), and heterozygotes about 1 μmol (0.06 mg) per gram dry weight per year. Hepatic iron values <1.9 μmol (0.1 mg) per gram exclude homozygosity and values >1.5 (0.08 mg) exclude heterozygosity. Furthermore, there appears to be a threshold level above which there is a high risk of developing cirrhosis, i.e., >400 μmole/g [24 mg] dry liver weight).

It has been suggested that iron levels may be accurately assessed by the mean linear attenuation coefficient determined during computerized tomography. This CT number, which is based on the radiodensity of iron and other substances in the liver (84–86), is a modification of the Haunsfield quantitative system of expressing radiodensity. It is reduced by fatty infiltration, is unaffected by scar tissue (87) or copper (88), but is increased by iron, which has a high atomic number. Single energy CT scanning may give falsely negative results in patients with increased iron stores (89), probably due to the coexistence of fat, which decreases the mean CT number. Dual or trienergy scanning, which is much more cumbersome (85), however, provides an accurate, noninvasive method of measuring the amount of iron in liver tissue. The CT number correlates with the serum ferritin concentration (90) and the hepatic iron content (91). Objective comparisons of CT and magnetic resonance imaging with serum ferritin and transferrin saturation indicate that although these imaging techniques are diagnostically more

accurate than these biochemical measurements, they are not cost effective in routine evaluations (92).

In screening for hemochromatosis among the families of probands, all first- and second-degree relatives should be tested, including HLA typing for first-degree relatives (93). Transferrin saturation is the most useful test and the serum ferritin level is the next most useful. When these tests are positive or there is clinical or laboratory evidence of liver disease, liver biopsy is indicated. In population screening, transferrin saturation is the most discriminating test, and in those with more than 55% saturation, serum ferritin levels are indicated (93,94).

Histopathology of the liver in hereditary hemochromatosis

In the earliest stages of idiopathic hemochromatosis, the hepatic lesions are characterized by deposition of hemosiderin in the periportal hepatocytes unaccompanied by portal fibrosis or distortion of the lobular architecture (Fig. 634). Such lesions are encountered most frequently in asymptomatic siblings of patients with overt hemochromatosis, and especially in women. Figure 161 illustrates such a lesion in an asymptomatic 40-year-old woman with hepatomegaly and high serum levels of iron, ferritin, and transferrin saturation who was the sister of a man with advanced hemochromatosis. Shown is the periportal distribution and Prussian blue reaction of hemosiderin deposited in hepatocytes. At higher magnification (Fig. 158), it can be seen that the periportal hepatocytes are normal in appearance and arrangement, but contain numerous coarse, brown, refractile hemosiderin granules that outline the course of the canaliculi, owing to their location in pericanalicular lysosomes. The distribution of the granules on either side of the canaliculi outlining their lumens is more clearly visualized in an adjacent section stained for iron (Fig. 159). As illustrated in Figure 160, the hemosiderin granules stain with PAS following diastase digestion, a feature attributable to their content of lipofuscin and polysaccharide.

As the iron stores in hemochromatosis increase and the lesions become symptomatic, the deposits of hemosiderin in the liver extend to involve the midzonal and centrilobular hepatocytes, although they continue to be most prominent around the portal tracts (Fig. 635). In addition, some portal tracts are expanded and fibrotic (Fig. 636), show erosion of their limiting plates (Fig. 637), and contain proliferating ductules, lymphocytes, plasma cells, and macrophages (Fig. 637). Characteristically, most of the portal macrophages and a variable number of ductules contain coarse hemosiderin granules that give a Prussian blue reaction (Fig. 336) and stain bright red with PAS following diastase digestion (Fig. 638). Not infrequently, small foci of cell dropout in which hepatocytes are replaced by clusters of swollen Kupffer cells containing phagocytized hemosiderin can be found in the periportal zones (Fig. 162). Taken together with the erosion of the limiting plates, these foci of cell dropout suggest that expansion and fibrosis of the portal tracts is due to low grade destruction of periportal hepatocytes. Iron-laden Kupffer cells are first seen as fibrous septa develop and as the amount of iron storage increases (95).

With further advance of the lesions in hemochromatosis, the fibrosis extends to bridge adjacent portal tracts (Fig. 639), and, ultimately, to destroy the normal lobular architecture, leading to the development of micronodular cirrhosis (Fig. 571). During its development, the fibrosis often is patchy in distribution, so portal fibrosis, bridging fibrosis, and nodule formation may be encountered in adjacent microscopic fields. As in other forms of cirrhosis, the hepatocytes in the nodules are arranged in an irregular, thickened, plate pattern indicative of regeneration (Fig. 640). Rarely, late in its course, the cirrhosis in hemochromatosis is macronodular in type (Fig. 641).

A number of systems for semiquantitative, histologic grading of the amount of iron in the liver have been reported (47,79, 96–99). These have all used four grade scales. It is even possible to estimate the amount of iron in the liver grossly by inspection of the stained slides with the naked eye (100). Comparisons of the amount of iron estimated histologically with the concentration of iron in the liver determined chemically have shown a good correlation, but the relationship is not linear. This disparity results from the wide range of iron concentrations in livers with grade 3 or 4 hemosiderin. Thus, grade 0 to 1 of iron deposition is seen when the iron concentration ranges from 10 to 150 μg/100 mg dry liver weight. Grade 4 hemosiderin is seen, however, in livers that contain from 1000 to 5000 μg/100 mg dry liver weight. Thus, when the amount of iron deposition becomes excessive, the histologic estimates tend to underestimate the amount of iron by a factor of two or three. From the practical point of view, the precise concentration of iron is not important once it has been shown histologically that excessive hepatic iron stores exist in the liver. However, the amount of iron seen histologically varies widely from nodule to nodule.

The newest and most impressive advance in the quantitation of stainable hepatic iron is the *computerized measurement of iron* in liver biopsies (101). The mean area that stains for iron on histologic sections using a microcomputer image analysis system is expressed as the percentage of the area of the biopsy analyzed. In normal biopsies the percentage is virtually zero, but in hemochromatosis it is about 10% compared with 0.1% in alcoholic cirrhosis and 0.03% in nonalcoholic liver disease. These values correlate well with the hepatic iron concentration, with the hepatic iron index, and with other objective measurements of iron storage (101). Obviously, this new technique requires technologic modifications to differentiate between areas that stain for iron faintly and those that stain densely, since both may be recorded as iron-positive.

Secondary hemosiderosis and hemochromatosis

Anemia and erythropoietic hemochromatosis

Chronic refractory anemias characterized by ineffective erythropoiesis frequently are accompanied by varying degrees of hemosiderosis and fibrosis that mimic the lesions of idiopathic hemochromatosis. Iron overload of this type occurs most frequently in thalassemia major (102–103) and sideroblastic anemia (104), but may be encountered occasionally in congenital spherocytic hemolytic anemia (105), congenital nonspherocytic hemolytic anemia (106), and megaloblastic anemia (107). Indirect evidence suggests that iron overload under such conditions is attributable to increased iron absorption in response to erythropoiesis rather than to anemia per se (108). However, in many cases, multiple transfusions, inappropriate iron therapy,

and hemolysis are important contributory factors responsible for the accumulation of iron. In at least one study, the incidence of HLA-A3 in patients with sideroblastic anemia was found to be as high as in idiopathic hemochromatosis, and led to the conclusion that the presence of this allele of hemochromatosis accounts for the development of iron overloading in some heterologous cases (109).

The distribution of iron in the tissues, the clinical manifestations and the biochemical features of iron overload in erythropoietic hemochromatosis are similar to those in idiopathic hemochromatosis, except that it gives rise to diabetes mellitus less frequently and rarely, if ever, is complicated by hepatocellular carcinoma.

As a rule the hepatic lesions of erythropoietic hemochromatosis are indistinguishable from those of idiopathic hemochromatosis. In some patients, erythropoietic hemochromatosis is characterized by extensive deposits of hemosiderin in the hepatocytes, and by lesser amounts in Kupffer cells, portal macrophages, and bile ducts, as illustrated in the advanced cirrhotic lesion in a case of thalassemia major shown in Figure 642 and 643. However, in most cases, the hemosiderin deposits are particularly prominent in Kupffer cells and portal macrophages, a feature that is more suggestive of erythropoietic than of idiopathic hemochromatosis. An early precirrhotic lesion of this type is illustrated in a six-year-old boy with sideroblastic anemia since birth (Figs. 644, 645). As in idiopathic hemochromatosis, the extent of fibrosis, which is predominantly portal, ranges from minimal or none (Fig. 646), to portal-portal bridging (Fig. 647), and, ultimately, to fullblown cirrhosis (Fig. 648).

Transfusional hemosiderosis and hemochromatosis

Since blood contains 500 mg of iron per liter and the capacity to eliminate such iron is limited to a few milligrams daily at most, multiple transfusions invariably lead to some degree of iron overload with deposition of hemosiderin not only in the liver but also in other tissues as well.

According to some authorities (110–112), the hepatic lesions produced by multiple transfusions are characterized by a type of hemosiderosis that involves the Kupffer cells and portal macrophages predominantly and that may be accompanied by varying degrees of portal fibrosis, but never gives rise to cirrhosis, a feature attributed to the allegedly innocuous behavior of hemosiderin in reticuloendothelial cells (112). Later, however, following multiple transfusions, the hepatocytes often contain large amounts of hemosiderin, as the hemosiderin appears to be redistributed from the reticuloendothelial to the parenchymal cells. In occasional cases of aplastic anemia, such deposits are accompanied by frank cirrhosis and other features resembling those of idiopathic hemochromatosis (113–115). Figure 649 illustrates a lesion of this type in a patient with long-standing aplastic anemic and myelofibrosis. At autopsy the patient exhibited features indistinguishable from those of idiopathic hemochromatosis. As can be seen in Figure 650, most of the hepatocytes, but only some of the Kupffer cells in this case, contained numerous hemosiderin granules.

It has been suggested that, usually, the transfusion of at least 200 units of blood containing 50 g of iron is required to produce the fullblown picture of hemochromatosis, and that this may account for the relative infrequency of cirrhosis in patients with transfusional hemosiderosis who uncommonly receive such large volumes of blood (113).

Usually, the amount of iron found in the tissues following multiple transfusions exceeds that contained in transfused blood (116). This suggests that the hemosiderosis is due, in part at least, to increased iron absorption, possibly of genetic origin, a consequence of the anemia or of ineffective erythropoiesis.

Although hepatocellular carcinoma is a relatively frequent complication of idiopathic hemochromatosis, it is rare in secondary hemochromatosis. It has been reported, however, in a patient with transfusional hemochromatosis associated with congenital hypoplastic anemia (the Blackfan-Diamond syndrome) (115).

Dietary and medicinal iron overload

A high proportion of native blacks in South Africa, especially Bantus, exhibit evidence of iron overload (116–118). As a rule, this is manifested by a mild to moderate degree of hepatic hemosiderosis, portal fibrosis, and, occasionally, cirrhosis. However, in a minority of cases, the deposits of hemosiderin are accompanied by micronodular cirrhosis and other features that resemble those of idiopathic hemochromatosis. Available evidence indicates that the iron overload in the Bantu is attributable to the excessive intake of iron contained in native beer prepared and stored at low pH in iron containers. It is highly probable that alcohol is a contributory factor in the pathogenesis of the cirrhosis in such cases.

Hemochromatosis has been reported as a sequela of prolonged oral administration of iron for therapeutic purposes. Almost without exception, such therapy has been inappropriate, having been prescribed for such disorders as spherocytic hemolytic anemia (119) and hereditary nonspherocytic hemolytic anemia (106). In these cases, factors such as ineffective erythropoiesis and anemia undoubtedly have played a role in enhancing iron absorption.

Hemodialysis iron overload

Hemosiderosis is a relatively common finding in patients with chronic renal disease on long-term maintenance hemodialysis (120). Although the iron deposits occur in many tissues, their distribution differs from that in idiopathic hemochromatosis in that they are prominent in the liver and spleen, but often spare the bone marrow. The hepatic lesions are characterized by hemosiderosis of the hepatocytes and, to a lesser extent, of the Kupffer cells and portal macrophages. When the hemosiderosis is extensive, it may be accompanied by varying degrees of portal fibrosis, but, as a rule, this does not progress to cirrhosis or give rise to clinical manifestations.

Chronic anemia, iron administration, transfusions, and hemolysis probably play an important role in the pathogenesis of this type of hemosiderosis. However, studies of their histocompatibility antigens have demonstrated that hemodialysis patients who exhibit alleles of hemochromatosis, HLA-A3, B7, or B14, show the highest serum levels of ferritin and the greatest transfusion requirements (121). This suggests that susceptibility to iron overload in such individuals may be, at least in part, genetically determined, i.e., hereditary hemochromatosis.

Alcoholic hemochromatosis

About one-third of patients with hemochromatosis give a history of drinking alcohol to excess (1). Histocompatibility antigen typing in such individuals and their close relatives suggests that, in some cases, alcohol may facilitate iron overload in both homozygous and heterozygous carriers of the gene for idiopathic hemochromatosis (52,53). However, there is convincing evidence that chronic alcoholism often is associated with increased deposition of iron in the liver, and that, occasionally, this may progress to an acquired form of hemochromatosis that is indistinguishable from the idiopathic genetic type (see Chapter 10). It has been suggested that, usually, the iron overload in such cases, estimated on the basis of the amount that can be removed by repeated venesection, is significantly less than in idiopathic hemochromatosis, but that when the iron load is excessive, the lesion is probably of genetic origin (82,122).

Iron overload in porphyria cutanea tarda

Porphyria cutanea tarda is a disorder characterized by excessive hepatic synthesis and urinary excretion of uroporphyrin I and to a lesser degree uroporphyrin III associated with photosensitivity that leads to cutaneous fragility, pigmentation, scarring, and hypertrichosis. Often, but not invariably, the hepatocytes and Kupffer cells contain hemosiderin deposits. The disease appears to be attributable to the combined effects of an inherited deficiency of uroporphyrinogen decarboxylase, a hepatic enzyme that normally converts uroporphyrinogen to coproporphyrinogen, and iron overload that further depresses the activity of this enzyme (123–125). Coexistent heterozygous hemochromatosis, is a likely explanation (126).

Frequently, the iron overload is associated with chronic alcoholism, but, in some cases, it is attributable to other causes, such as refractory anemia (127). Occasionally, estrogens induce porphyria cutanea tarda, which is not always accompanied by hemosiderosis (128). Lupus erythematosus is another disorder that may be associated with porphyria cutanea tarda in the absence of iron overload (129).

Of note is the fact that reduction of iron stores by repeated phlebotomy leads to a decrease in hepatic and urinary uroporphyrin and remission of the cutaneous manifestations of porphyria cutanea tarda, even when there is no evidence of iron overload (130). Thus, not only iron but also other factors may be responsible for the appearance of porphyria and cutaneous manifestations in individuals who are genetically predisposed to the disease.

Fatty infiltration, hemosiderosis, and red autofluorescence indicative of uroporphyrin deposition are the principal features of the hepatic lesions in porphyria cutanea tarda. Other less common findings include varying degrees of portal inflammation and fibrosis, foci of parenchymal necrosis, and evidence of hepatocellular regeneration (131,132).

Usually, the fatty infiltration is mild to moderate in extent and patchy in distribution. Although it frequently is associated with alcohol abuse, ballooning of the hepatocytes and Mallory bodies indicative of alcoholic liver disease are rare.

Characteristically, the iron deposition is mild to moderate in extent, and involves the periportal hepatocytes predominantly (Fig. 651). However, often, scattered through the lobules, there are small foci of cell dropout filled with clusters of swollen macrophages that contain both hemosiderin (Fig. 652) and diastase-resistant PAS-positive lipofuscin (Fig. 653).

Invariably, in untreated cases, the cytoplasm of many hepatocytes exhibits the typical, red autofluorescence of uroporphyrin in ultraviolet light (Fig. 654). Since uroporphryin is solubilized in water, it may escape detection in sections that have been washed during routine staining. For that reason, freeze-dried or alcohol-fixed dried sections are recommended for the demonstration of such autofluorescence (133). However, we have found that Carnoy's-fixed, unstained, paraffin-embedded sections serve equally well for this purpose. It should be noted that the sections must be examined promptly, since the red fluorescence tends to fade within a few minutes following exposure to ultraviolet light. During remissions of porphyria cutanea tarda induced by repeated venesection, the fluorescence of uroporphyrin may no longer be demonstrable.

Scattered acidophilic bodies and a thickened, irregular, hepatic plate pattern indicative of regenerative activity (Fig. 653) are other hepatocellular changes seen in some cases.

According to some reports (131,134), the cytoplasm of some hepatocytes in porphyria cutanea tarda invariably contains needle-like crystals of uroporphyrin that can be visualized by both polarization and electron microscopy. This feature is not mentioned in most other reports, an oversight that has been attributed to solubilization of the crystals in the water used to wash sections during routine staining (135). Accordingly, it has been emphasized that fresh frozen sections or unstained, paraffin-embedded sections are required for the demonstration of the crystals. However, in none of our 10 cases of porphyria cutanea tarda have we succeeded in detecting cytoplasmic crystals in Carnoy's-fixed, paraffin-embedded sections, despite the presence of large amounts of uroporphyrin by fluorescence.

In many cases of porphyria cutanea tarda, the portal tracts are enlarged, fibrotic, and infiltrated with lymphocytes, plasma cells, and macrophages that often are aggregated in the form of follicles (Fig. 655). Progression to cirrhosis occurs in approximately one-third of cases (131,132), a feature that correlates with advancing age (131).

A remarkably high incidence of hepatocellular carcinoma (47%) has been encountered at autopsy in patients with porphyria cutanea tarda accompanied by cirrhosis (136). In addition, rare instances of porphyria cutanea tarda have been reported in patients with hepatocellular carcinoma (137) or hepatocellular adenoma (138) in the absence of cirrhosis. In such cases, uroporphyrin fluorescence has been limited to the tumor, and, in one instance, removal of such an adenoma has led to remission of the porphyria cutanea tarda (138). Thus, under some conditions, hepatic neoplastic cells may exhibit the metabolic defect responsible for porphyria cutanea tarda.

The pathogenesis of the hepatic lesions in porphyria cutanea tarda is uncertain. Although chronic alcoholism and hemosiderosis may be contributory factors in some cases, the lesions are not typical of either alcoholic liver disease or hemochromatosis. This has led to the suggestion that the lesions may be unique and attributable to the metabolic defect in porphyria cutanea tarda (131).

Iron overload following portacaval anastomosis

Occasionally, portacaval anastomosis is followed within a few years by the development of hemosiderosis that, in some cases, is sufficiently severe and widely distributed to produce clinical manifestations and alterations in serum iron, ferritin, and transferrin saturation that mimic those of idiopathic hemochromatosis (139–142). However, even under those conditions, the magnitude of the iron overload usually is less than in idiopathic hemochromatosis.

Postshunt hemochromatosis is encountered most frequently in patients with alcoholic cirrhosis, but has also been reported in postnecrotic cirrhosis, Wilson's disease, and primary biliary cirrhosis (142), and has been reproduced experimentally in dogs (143) and rats (144). It has not been reported following portacaval anastomosis in cases of extrahepatic or idiopathic portal hypertension. It has been emphasized that postshunt hemochromatosis occurs more frequently following end-to-side than side-to-side portacaval anastomosis (140,141,144).

Although multiple transfusions, iron administration, anemia, pancreatitis, and chronic alcoholism may be contributory factors in some cases, the basic mechanism responsible for the rapid uptake and deposition of iron following portacaval anastomosis is not known.

Iron overload in renal transplant recipients

After renal transplantation, hemosiderosis may develop [(36, 145); Fig. 656]. The amount of iron stored appears to be more than would be expected from the transfusions received during transplantation (Figs. 657, 658). Most of these patients had had chronic hemodialysis, however, which can be associated with iron overload (120, 121).

Neonatal iron overload

Idiopathic neonatal hemochromatosis

A rare form of neonatal iron overload that appears to be transmitted as an autosomal recessive trait has been reported in siblings and in occasional sporadic cases (146–148). As a rule, the disease proves fatal within a few days or weeks. Noabnormalities of serum iron, ferritin, or transferritin saturation are demonstrable in the parents of affected infants. It isnot yet clear whether idiopathic neonatal hemochromatosis isa single discrete disorder or a spectrum of related syndromes (149).

The disease is characterized by massive deposits of hemosiderin in the lysosomes of hepatocytes (Fig. 659) and pancreatic acinar cells, and lesser amounts in the myocardium and the endocrine and exocrine glands. The Kupffer cells do not accumulate iron. The liver, which is the most severely affected organ, invariably exhibits cirrhosis, giant cell transformation of the hepatocytes, and grossly distorted architecture (Fig. 660).

Clearly, the deposits of hemosiderin in this disease are attributable to excessive transport of iron across the placenta during fetal life. Little is known about the factors responsible for this process, but since there is no evidence of maternal iron overload in such cases, it is highly probable that a fetal defect is involved.

Zellweger's cerebro-hepato-renal syndrome

Zellweger's syndrome, a rare hereditary disorder that is transmitted as an autosomal recessive trait and that invariably proves fatal within a few months, is characterized by widespread gliosis of the brain, hepatic lesions, multiple small renal cortical cysts, and skeletal anomalies, usually accompanied by hemosiderosis of the liver and other tissues (150–153).

In addition to varying degrees of hepatocellular and Kupffer cell hemosiderosis (Fig. 661), the liver usually shows foci of hepatocellular necrosis and mild to severe diffuse fibrosis that often progress to cirrhosis [(150,151); Fig. 662]. Multinucleated giant cells are common (Fig. 663). Cholestasis and anomalies of the intrahepatic bile ducts are less constant features.

The basic metabolic defect in Zellweger's syndrome is uncertain. A block in lysine metabolism, leading to the urinary excretion of pipecolic acid (153), and a block in the synthesis of chenodeoxycholic and cholic acid from cholesterol, resulting in the accumulation and excretion of their metabolic precursors, dihydroxy-, trihydroxy-, and tetrahydroxycoprostanic acids (153), have been reported. In addition, abnormalities of the mitochondria and absence of peroxisomes have been observed in the tissues of patients with Zellweger's syndrome (151). This has led to the suggestion that the increased iron absorption in the disease may be attributable to diminished activity of the iron-containing enzymes normally found in these structures (151).

Hypermethioninemia

A unique type of hereditary hypermethioninemia, possibly related to hereditary tyrosimemia, is characterized by generalized aminoaciduria, markedly increased levels of methionine in the serum and urine, accumulation and excretion of α-ketomethiolbutyric acid, which produces an unusual "boiled-cabbage" urinary odor, and the development of cirrhosis, islet cell hyperplasia, and renal tubular degeneration that usually proves fatal within a few months (154,155).

Usually, the cirrhosis is micronodular in type and is accompanied by both fatty infiltration and hemosiderosis. In contrast to other forms of neonatal iron overload, the hemosiderosis of hypermethioninemia is limited to the liver. The pathogeneis of this disorder is still uncertain, although it is generally assumed that a defect in methionine metabolism is present.

Congenital atransferrinemia

This very rare disorder is characterized by hypochromic anemia, the absence of transferrin in the serum, and pulmonary hemosiderosis (156). In some of these patients, iron absorption is increased. The iron overload appears to arise from two causes: from increased absorption of iron and from blood transfusions, which many of these patients require. The mechanism by which the absence of transferrin leads to the anemia and iron deposition in the lungs is not known.

References

1. Finch SC, Finch CA: Idiopathic hemochromatosis, an iron storage disease. A. Iron metabolism in hemochromatosis. Medicine 34:381–430, 1955.
2. Halliday JW, Powell LW. Serum ferritin and isoferritins in clinical medicine. Prog Hematol 11:229–266, 1979.
3. Jacobs A, Worwood M: Ferritin in serum. Clinical and biochemical implications. N Engl J Med 292:951–956, 1975.
4. Morgan EH, Walters MNI: Iron storage in human disease. Fractionation of hepatic and splenic iron into ferritin and haemosiderin with histochemical correlations. J Clin Pathol 16:101–107, 1963.
5. Zuyderhoudt FMJ, Sindram JW, Marx JJM, Jorning GGA, van Gool J: The amount of ferritin and hemosiderin in the livers of patients with iron-loading diseases. Hepatology 3:232–235, 1983.
6. Hoy TG, Jacobs A: Ferritin polymers and the formation of haemosiderin. Br J Haematol 49:593–602, 1981.
7. Richter GW: The iron-loaded cell: the cytopathology of iron storage. A review. Am J Pathol 91:377–396, 1978.
8. Worwood M: Ferritin in human tissues and serum. Clin Haematol 11:275–307, 1982.
9. Tanikawa K: Ultrastructural Aspects of the Liver and its Disorders, 2nd Edition. New York, Igaku-Shoin, 1979, p. 12.
10. Harrison PM, Clegg GA, May K: Ferritin structure and function. In Iron and Biochemistry and Medicine, II, edited by A. Jacobs, M. Worwood. London, Academic Press, 1980.
11. Cartwright GE, Wintrobe MM: Chemical, clinical, and immunologic studies on the products of human plasma fractionation. XXXIX. The anemia of infection. Studies on the iron-binding capacity of serum. J Clin Invest 28:86–98, 1949.
12. Christian ER: Behavior of serum iron in various diseases of liver. Arch Intern Med 94:22–33, 1954.
13. Gitlow SE, Beyers MR, Colmore JP: Metabolism of iron. II. Intravenous iron tolerance tests in Laennec's cirrhosis. J Lab Clin Med 40:541–549, 1952.
14. Jandl JH, Katz JH: The plasma-to-cell cycle for transferrin. J Clin Invest 42:314–326, 1963.
15. Young SP, Aisen, P: Transferrin receptors and the uptake and release of iron by isolated hepatocytes. Hepatology 1:114–119, 1981.
16. Mortgan EH, Baker E: Role of transferrin receptors and endocytosis in iron uptake by hepatic and erythroid cells. Ann NY Acad Sci 526:65–82, 1988.
17. Sciot R, Paterson AC, Vand Den Ord JJ, Desmet VJ: Lack of hepatic transferrin receptor expression in hemochromatosis. Hepatology 7:831–897, 1987.
18. Anderson GJ, Halliday JW, Powell LW: Transferrin receptors in hemochromatosis. Hepatology 7:967–969, 1987.
19. Lombard M, Nauomov NV, Bomford A: Regulation of the hepatic transferrin receptor in hereditary hemochromatosis. Hepatology 7:1107, 1987 (abstract).
20. Wright TL, Brissot P, Ma WL: Characterization of nontransferrin bound iron clearance by rat liver. J Biol Chem 261:10909–10914, 1986.
21. Simon M, Yaouang J, David V: Genetics of hemochromatosis: HLA association and mode of inheritance. Ann NY Acad Sci 526:11–22, 1987.
22. van de Rijn M, Geurts van Kessel AHM, Kroezen V: Localization of a gene controlling the expression of the human transferrin receptor to the region q12 leads to qter of chromosome 3. Cytogenet Cell Genet 36:525–531, 1983.
23. Munro HN: The ferritin genome: structure, expression and regulation. Ann NY Acad Sci 526:113–123, 1988.
24. Powell LW, Kerr JFR: Reversal of "cirrhosis" in idiopathic haemochromatosis following long-term intensive venesection therapy. Austral Ann Med 19:1–4, 1970.
25. Lisboa PE: Experimental hepatic cirrhosis in dogs caused by chronic massive iron overload. Gut 12:363–368, 1971.
26. Seymour CA, Peters TJ: Organelle pathology in primary and secondary haemochromatosis with special reference to lysosomal changes. Br J Haematol 40:239–253, 1978.
27. Selden C, Own M, Hopkins JMP, Peters TJ: Studies on the concentration and intracellular localization of iron proteins in liver biopsy specimens from patients with iron overload with special reference to their role in lysosomal disruption. Br J Haematol 44:593–603, 1980.
28. Arstila AU, Smith MA, Trump BF: Microsomal lipid peroxidation: morphological characterization. Science 175:530–533, 1972.
29. Bacon BR, Britton RS: The pathology of hepatic iron overload: a free radical-mediated process? Hepatology 11:127–137, 1990.

30. Iancu TC, Neustein HB, Landing BH: The liver iin thalassemia major: Ultrastructural studies: In Iron Metabolism Ciba Foundation Symposium 51 (New Series)). Amsterdam, Elsevier North-Holland, 1977, pp. 293–316.

31. Chojkier M, Houglum K, Solis-Herruzo J, Brenner DA: Stimulation of collagen gene expression by ascorbic acid in cultured human fibroblasts. A role for lipid peroxidation? J Biol Chem 264:16957–16962, 1989.

32. Cortes JM, Oliva H, Paradinas FJ, Hernandez-Guio C: The pathology of the liver in porphyria cutanea tarda. Histopathology 4:471–485, 1980.

33. Pimstone NR: Porphyria cutanea tarda. Semin Liver Dis 2:132–142.

34. Lombard CM, Strauchen JA: Postshunt hemochromatosis with cardiomyopathy. Hum Pathol 12:1149–1151, 1981.

35. Kothari T, Swamy AP, Lee JCK, Mangla JC, Cestero RVM: Hepatic hemosiderosis in maintenance hemodialysis (MHD) patients. Dig Dis Sci 25:363–368, 1980.

36. Rao KV, Anderson WR: Hemosiderosis and hemochromatosis in renal transplant recipients. Clinical and pathological features, diagnostic correlations, predisposing factors, and treatment. Am J Nephrol 5:419–430, 1985.

37. Beaumont C, Simon M, Fauchet R, Hespel JP, Brossot P, Geneter B: Serum ferritin as a possible marker of the hemochromatosis allele. N Engl J Med 301:169–174, 1979.

38. Gollan JL: Diagnosis of hemochromatosis. Gastroenterology 84:418–421, 1983.

39. Ishak KG, Sharp HL: Metabolic errors and liver disease. In Pathology of the Liver, edited by R.N.M. MacSween, P.P. Anthony, P.J. Scheuer. 2nd Edition. Edinburgh, Churchill Livingstone, 1987, pp. 99–180.

40. Askari AD, Muir WA, Rosner IA, Moskowitz RW, McLaren GD, Braun WE: Arthritis of hemochromatosis. Clinical spectrum, relation to histocompatibility antigens and effectiveness of early phlebotomy. Am J Med 75:957–965, 1983.

41. Bassett ML, Halliday JW, Powell JW: HLA typing in idiopathic hemochromatosis: distinction between homozygotes and heterozygotes with biochemical expression. Hepatology 1:120–126, 1981.

42. Bassett ML, Halliday JW, Powell, LW: Genetic hemochromatosis. Semin Liver Dis 4:217–227, 1984.

43. Bomford A, Eddleston ALWF, Kennedy LA, Batchelor JR, Williams R: Histocompatibility antigens as markers of abnormal iron metabolism in patients with idiopathic haemochromatosis and their relatives. Lancet 1:327–329, 1979.

44. Simon M, Fauchet R, Hespel JP, Beaumont C, Brissot P, Hery B, De Nercy YH, Genetet B, Bourel M: Idiopathic hemochromatosis: a study of biochemical expression in 247 heterozygous members of 63 families: evidence for a single major HLA-linked gene. Gastroenterology 78:703–708, 1980.

45. Valberg LS, Lloyd DA, Ghent CN, Flanagan PR, Sinclair NR, Stiller CR, Chamberlain MJ: Clinical and biochemical expression of the genetic abnormality in idiopathic hemochromatosis. Gastroenterology 79:884–892, 1980.

46. Edwards CQ, Dadone MM, Skolnick MH, Kushner JP: Hereditary hemochromatosis. Clin Haematol 11:411–435, 1982.

47. Powell LW, Halliday JW: Iron absorption and iron overload. A comparative study of the four major aetiological groups. Clin Gastroenterol 10:707–736, 1981.

48. Cox TM, Peters TJ: Uptake of iron by duodenal biopsy specimens from patients with iron-deficiency anaemia and primary haemochromatosis. Lancet 1:123–124, 1978.

49. Batey RG, Pettit JE, Nicholas AW, Sherlock S, Hoffbrand AV: Hepatic iron clearance from serum in treated hemochromatosis. Gastroenterology 75:856–859, 1978.

50. Aisen P: Iron metabolism in isolated hepatic cells: interactions between Kupffer cells and hepatocytes. Ann NY Acad Sci 526:93–100, 1988.

51. Simon M, Bourel M, Genetet B, Fauchet R: Idiopathic hemochromatosis. Demonstration of recessive transmission and early detection by family HLA typing. N Engl J Med 297:1017–1021, 1977.

52. Williams R, Scheuer PJ, Sherlock S: The inheritance of idiopathic haemochromatosis. A clinical and liver biopsy study of 16 families. Q J Med 31:249–265, 1962.

53. LeSage GD, Baldus WP, Fairbanks VF, Baggenstoss AH, McCall JT, Moore SB: Hemochromatosis: genetic or alcohol-induced? Gastroenterology 84:1471–1477, 1983.

54. Perkins KW, McInnes IWS, Blackburn CRB, Beal RW: Idiopathic haemochromatosis in children. Report of a family. Am J Med 39:118–126, 1969.

55. Fryd CH, Knobel B: Primary hemochromatosis in a premenopausal woman. Israel J Med Sci 6:44–48, 1970.

56. Farmer RG, Sullivan BH Jr: Portal hypertension in hemochromatosis. Am J Dig Dis 9:56–63, 1964.

57. Niederau C, Fischer R, Sonnenberg A, Stremmel W, Trampisch HJ, Strohmeyer G: Survival and causes of death in cirrhotic and in noncirrhotic patients with primary hemochromatosis. N Engl J Med 313:1256–1262, 1985.

58. Hellier FF: The nature and causation of skin pigmentation in haemochromatosis. Br J Dermatol 47:1–12, 1935.

59. Conn HO, Schreiber W, Elkington SG, Johnson TR: Cirrhosis and diabetes. I. Increased incidence of diabetes in patients with Laennec's cirrhosis. Am J Dig Dis 14:837–852, 1969.

60. Dymock IW, Cassar J, Pyke DA, Oakley WG, Williams R: Observations on the pathogenesis, complications and treatment of diabetes in 115 cases of haemochromatosis. Am J Med 52:203–210, 1972.

61. Krines K, Kim O, Knowles HC Jr: Glomerulosclerosis, hemochromatosis, and diabetes mellitus. Am J Clin Pathol 54:47–52, 1970.

62. Walker RJ, Newton JR, Williams R: Testicular function and pituitary-hypothalamic axis in the hypogonadism of primary idiopathic haemochromatosis. Med Chir Dig 5:67–71, 1976.

63. Stocks AE, Powell LW: Pituitary function in haemochromatosis and cirrhosis of the liver. Lancet 2:298–299, 1972.

64. Walton C, Kelly WF, Laing I, Bu'Lock DE: Endocrine abnormalities in idiopathic haemochromatosis. Q J Med 52:99–110, 1983.

65. Hamilton E, Williams R, Barlow KA, Smith PM: The arthropathy of idiopathic haemochromatosis. Q J Med 37:171–182, 1968.

66. M'Seffar A, Fornasier VL, Fox IH: Arthropathy as the major clinical indication of occult iron storage disease. JAMA 238:1825–1828, 1977.

67. MacSween RNM: Acute abdominal crisis, circulatory collapse and sudden death in haemochromatosis. Q J Med 35:589–598, 1966.

68. Howard RB, Balfour WM, Cullen R: Extreme hyperferremia in two instances of hemochromatosis with notes on the treatment of one patient by means of repeated venesection. J Lab Clin Med 43:848–859, 1954.

69. Taylor HE: The possible role of ferritin in the production of shock in hemochromatosis. Am J Clin Pathol 21:530–535, 1951.

70. Jones NL: Irreversible shock in haemochromatosis. Lancet 1:569–572, 1962.

71. Strohmeyer G, Niederau C, Stremmel W: Survival and causes of death in hemochromatosis: observations in 163 patients. Ann NY Acad Sci 526:245–257, 1988.

72. Williams R, Smith PM, Spicer EJF, Barry M, Sherlock S: Venesection therapy in idiopathic haemochromatosis. An analysis of 40 treated and 14 untreated patients. Q J Med 38:1–16, 1969.

73. Grace ND: Hemochromatosis: clinical aspects and response to therapy. In Current Perspectives in Hepatology, edited by L.B. Seeff, J.H. Lewis. New York, Plenum Medical Book Co., 1989, pp. 287–297.

74. Wands JR, Rowe JA, Mezey SE, Waterbury LA, Wright JR, Halliday JW, Isselbacher KJ, Powell LW: Normal serum ferritin concentrations in precirrhotic hemochromatosis. N Engl J Med 294:302–305, 1976.

75. Valberg LS, Ghent CN, Lloyd DA, Frei JV, Chamberlain MJ: Diagnostic efficiency of tests for detection of iron overload in chronic liver disease. Can Med Assoc J 119:229–236, 1978.

76. Dadone MM, Kushner JP, Edwards CQ, Bishop DT, Skolnick MH: Hereditary hemochromatosis. Analysis of laboratory expression of the disease by genotype in 18 pedigrees. Am J Clin Pathol 78:196–207, 1982.

77. Edwards CQ, Cartwright GE, Skolnick MH, Amos DB: Homozygosity for hemochromatosis: clinical manifestations. Ann Intern Med 93:519–525, 1980.

78. Halliday JW, Cowlishaw JL, Russo AM, Powell LW. Serum ferritin in diagnosis of haemochromatosis. Lancet 2:621–623, 1977.

79. Brissot P, Bourel M, Herry D: Assessment of liver iron content in 271 patients: a reevaluation of direct and indirect methods. Gastroenterology 80:557–565, 1981.

80. Finch CA, Huebers H: Perspectives in iron metabolism. N Engl J Med 306:1520–1528, 1982.

81. Prieto J, Barry M, Sherlock S: Serum ferritin in patients with iron overload and with acute and chronic liver diseases. Gastroenterology 68:525–533, 1975.

82. Bassett ML, Halliday JW, Powell LW: Value of hepatic iron mea-

surements in early hemochromatosis and determination of the critical iron level associated with fibrosis. Hepatology 6:24–29, 1986.

83. Summers KM, Halliday JW, Powell LW: Identification of homozygous hemochromatosis subjects by measurement of hepatic iron index. Hepatology 12:20–24, 1990.

84. Mills SR, Doppman JL, Nienhuis AW: Computed tomography in the diagnosis of disorders of excessive iron storage of the liver. J Comput Assist Tomogr 1:101–104, 1977.

85. Chapman RWG, Williams G, Bydder G: Computed tomography for determining liver iron content in primary haemochromatosis. Br Med J 280:4429–4442, 1980.

86. Roudot-Thoraval F, Halphen M, Larde D, Galliot M, Rymer JC, Galalcteros F, Dhumeaux D: Evaluation of liver iron content by computed tomography: its value in the follow-up of treatment in patients with idiopathic hemochromatosis. Hepatology 3:974–979, 1983.

87. Fawcitt RA, Forbes W ST C, Isherwood I. Computed tomographic scanning in liver disease. Clin Radiol 29:251–254, 1978.

88. Smevik B, Ritland S, Nilsen T, Johansen O: Liver attenuation values at computed tomography related to liver copper content. Scand J Gastroenterol 17:461–463, 1982.

89. Guyader D, Gandon Y, Deugnier Ý, Jouanolle H, Loreal O, Simon M, Bouel M, Carsin M, Brissot P: Evaluation of computed tomography in the assessment of liver iron overload. Gastroenterology 97:737–743, 1989.

90. Howard JM, Ghent CN, Carey LS: Diagnostic efficacy of hepatic computed tomography in the detection of body iron overload. Gastroenterology 84:209–215, 1983.

91. Raudot-Thoroval F, Halphen M, Larade D: Evolution of liver iron content by computed tomography. Hepatology 3:974–978, 1983.

92. Bonkovsky HL, Slaker DP, Bills EB, Wolf DC: Usefulness and limitations of laboratory and hepatic imaging studies in iron-storage disease. Gastroenterology 99:1079–1091, 1990.

93. Bassett ML, Halliday JW, Bryant S, Dent O, Powell LW: Screening for hemochromatosis. Ann NY Acad Sci 526:274–289, 1988.

94. Edwards CQ, Griffen LM, Drummond C, Skolnick MH, Kushner: JP: Screening for hemochromatosis in healthy blood donors: preliminary results. Ann NY Acad Sci 526:258–273, 1988.

95. Scheuer PJ: Liver Biopsy Interpretation, 4th Edition. London, Bailliere Tindall, 1988, pp. 207–217.

96. Conn HO: Portacaval anastomosis and hepatic hemosiderin deposition: a prospective, controlled investigation. Gastroenterology 62:61–72, 1972.

97. Rowe JW, Wands JR, Mezey E, Waterbury LA, Wright JR, Tobin J, Andres R: Familial hemochromatosis: characteristics of the precirrhotic stage in a large kindred. Medicine 56:197–211, 1977.

98. Searle JW, Kerr JFR, Halliday JW, Powell LW: Iron storage disease. In Pathology of the Liver, edited by R.N.M. MacSween, P.P. Anthony, P.J. Scheuer. 2nd Edition. Edinburgh, Churchill Livingstone, 1987, pp. 181–201.

99. van Deursen C, de Metz M, Koudstaal J, Brombacher P: Accumulation of iron and iron compounds in liver tissue: a comparative study of the histological and chemical estimation of liver iron. J Clin Chem Clin Biochem 26:617–622, 1988.

100. Conn HO, Strauss RH, Conn MB: Estimation of hepatic hemosiderin by gross inspection of iron-stained histologic sections. Yale J Biol Med 45:133–138, 1972.

101. Olynyk J, Hall P, Sallie R, Reed W, Shilkin K, Mackinnon M: Computerized measurement of iron in liver biopsies: a comparison with biochemical iron measurement. Hepatology 12:26–30, 1990.

102. Ley TJ, Griffith P, Nienhuis AW: Transfusion haemosiderosis and chelation therapy. Clin Haematol 11:437–464, 1982.

103. Jean G, Terzoli S, Mauri R, Borghetti L, DiPalma A, Piga A, Magliano M, Melevendi M, Cattaneo M: Cirrhosis associated with multiple transfusions in thalassaemia. Arch Dis Child 59:67–70, 1984.

104. Kushner JP, Lee GR, Wintrobe MM, Cartwright GE: Idiopathic refractory sideroblastic anemia. Clinical and laboratory investigation of 17 patients and review of the literature. Medicine 50:139–159, 1971.

105. Barry M, Scheuer PJ, Sherlock S, Ross CF, Williams R: Hereditary spherocytosis with secondary haemochromatosis. Lancet 2:481–485, 1968.

106. Pletcher WD, Brody GL, Meyers MC: Hemochromatosis following prolonged iron therapy in a patient with hereditary nonspherocytic hemolytic anemia. Am J Med Sci 246:27–34, 1963.

107. Granville N, Dameshek W: Hemochromatosis with megaloblastic anemia responding to folic acid. Report of a case. N Engl J Med 258:586–589, 1958.

108. Bothwell TH, Pirzio-Biroli G, Finch CA: Iron absorption. I. Factors influencing absorption. J Lab Clin Med 51:24–36, 1958.

109. Cartwright GE, Edwards CQ, Skolnick MH, Amos DB: Association of HLA-linked hemochromatosis with idiopathic refractory sideroblastic anemia. J Clin Invest 65:989–992, 1980.

110. Dubin IN: Idiopathic hemochromatosis and transfusion siderosis. A review. Am J Clin Pathol 25:514–542, 1955.

111. Kleckner MS Jr, Baggenstoss AH, Weir JF: Hemochromatosis and tranfusional hemosiderosis. A clinical and pathologic study. Am J Med 16:382–394, 1954.

112. Powell LW, Bassett ML, Halliday JW: Hemochromatosis: 1980 update. Gastroenterology 78:374–381, 1980.

113. Morningstar WA: Exogenous hemochromatosis. A report of three cases. Arch Pathol 59:355–362, 1955.

114. Pengelly CDR, Jones P: Acquired haemochromatosis following multiple blood transfusions for hypoplastic anaemia. Lancet 2:445–446, 1956.

115. Steinherz PG, Canale VC, Miller DR: Hepatocellular carcinoma, transfusion induced hemochromatosis and congenital hypoplastic anemia (Blackfan-Diamond syndrome). Am J Med 60:1032–1035, 1976.

116. Bothwell TH, Bradlow BA: Siderosis in the Bantu. A combined histopathological and chemical study. Arch Pathol 70:279–292, 1960.

117. Bothwell TH, Seftel H, Jacobs P, Torrance JD, Baumslag N: Iron overload in Bantu subjects. Studies on the availability of iron in Bantu beer. Am J Clin Nutr 14:47–51, 1964.

118. Higginson J, Keeley KJ: Liver disease in the South African Bantu. A review of liver biopsies from 262 Bantu patients. Gastroenterology 38:332–342, 1960.

119. Wallerstein RO, Robbins SL: Hemochromatosis after prolonged oral iron therapy in a patient with chronic hemolytic anemia. Am J Med 14:256–260, 1953.

120. Ali M, Fayemi O, Rigolosi R, Frascino J, Marsden T, Malcolm D: Hemosiderosis in hemodialysis patients. An autopsy study of 50 patients. JAMA 244:343–345, 1980.

121. Gomez E, Ortega F, Morales J, Gago E, Comas A, Alvarez J: Serum ferritin and HLA antigens in patients on maintenance haemodialysis. Lancet 1:836–837, 1981.

122. Powell LW: Changing concepts of haemochromatosis. Postgrad Med J 46:200–209, 1970.

123. Felsher B, Kushner JP: Hepatic siderosis and porphyria cutanea tarda: relation of iron excess to the metabolic defect. Semin Hematol 14:243–251, 1977.

124. Felsher BF, Carpio NM, Engleking DW, Nunn AT: Decreased hepatic uroporphyrinogen decarboxylase activity in porphyria cutanea tarda. N Engl J Med 306:766–769, 1982.

125. Kushner JP, Steinmuller DP, Lee GR: The role of iron in the pathogenesis of porphyria cutanea tarda. II. Inhibition of uroporphyrinogen decarboxylase. J Clin Invest 56:661–667, 1975.

126. Beaumont C, Fauchet R, Phung ZN: Porphyria cutanea tarda and HLA-linked hemochromatosis: evidence against a systematic association. Gastroenterology 92:1833–1836, 1987.

127. Felsher BM, Redeker AG: Acquired porphyria cutanea tarda, primary refractory anemia and hepatic siderosis. Report of a case. Arch Intern Med 188:163–167, 1966.

128. Vail JT Jr: Porphyria cutanea tarda and estrogens. JAMA 201:671–674, 1967.

129. Hetherington GW, Jetton RL, Knox JM: The association of lupus erythematosus and porphyria. Br J Dermatol 82:118–124, 1970.

130. Epstein JH, Redeker AG: Porphyria cutanea tarda. A study of the effect of phlebotomy. N Engl J Med 279:1301–1304, 1968.

131. Cortes JM, Oliva H, Paradinas JF, Hernandez-Guio C: The pathology of the liver in porphyria cutanea tarda. Histopathology 4:471–485, 1980.

132. Uys CJ, Eales L: The histopathology of the liver in acquired (symptomatic) porphyria. S Afr J Lab Clin Med 9:190–197, 1963.

133. Enterback L, Lundvall O: Properties and distribution of liver fluorescence in porphyria cutanea tarda. Virchows Arch A (Pathol Anat) 350:293–302, 1970.

134. Waldo ED, Tobias H: Needle-like cytoplasmic inclusions in the liver in porphyria cutanea tarda. Arch Pathol 96:368–371, 1973.

135. James KR, Cortes JM, Paradinas FJ: Demonstration of intracytoplasmic needle-like inclusions in hepatocytes of patients with porphyria cutanea tarda. J Clin Pathol 33:899–900, 1980.

136. Kordacv V: Frequency of occurrence of hepatocellular carcinoma in patients with porphyria cutanea tarda in long-term followup. Neoplasma 19:135–139, 1972.

137. Thompson RPH, Nicholson DC, Farnan T, Whitmore DN, Williams

R: Cutaneous porphyria due to a malignant primary hepatoma. Gastroenterology 59:779–783, 1970.

138. Tio TH, Leijnse B, Jarrett A, Rimington C: Acquired porphyria from a liver tumour. Clin Sci 16:517–527, 1957.

139. Tuttle SG, Figueroa WG, Grossman MI: Development of hemochromatosis in a patient with Laennec's cirrhosis. Am J Med 26:655–658, 1959.

140. Grace ND, Balint JA: Hemochromatosis associated with end-to-side portacaval anastomosis. Am J Dig Dis 11:351–358, 1966.

141. Ecker JA, Gray PA, McKittrick JE, Dickson DR: The development of post-shunt hemochromatosis parenchymal siderosis in patients with cirrhosis occurring after portasystemic shunt surgery. A review of the literature and report of two additional cases. Am J Gastroenterol 50:13–29, 1968.

142. Conn HO: Portacaval anastomosis and hepatic hemosiderin deposition: a prospective controlled investigation. Gastroenterology 62:61–72, 1972.

143. Doberneck RC: A comparison of hemosiderosis and hematopoiesis after end-to-side and side-to-side portacaval shunt. Surgery 70:428–432, 1971.

144. Rubin E, Kohan P, Tomita F, Jacobson JH II: Experimental hepatic siderosis following portacaval shunt. Proc Soc Exp Biol Med 115:350–352, 1964.

145. Anderson WR, Rao KV: Hepatic iron overload in renal transplant recipients: ultrastructural observations. Ultrastruct Pathol 10:227–234, 1986.

146. Goldfischer S, Grotsky HW, Chang C-H, Berman EL, Richert RR, Karmarkar SD, Roskamp JO, Morecki R: Idiopathic neonatal iron storage involving the liver, pancreas, heart, and endocrine and exocrine glands. Hepatology 1:58–64, 1981.

147. Blisard KS, Bartow SA: Neonatal hemochromatosis. Hum Pathol 17:376–383, 1986.

148. Witzleben CL, Uri A: Perinatal hemochromatosis: entity or end result? Hum Pathol 20:335–340, 1989.

149. Collins J, Goldfischer S: Perinatal hemochromatosis: one disease, several diseases or a spectrum? Hepatology 12:176–177, 1991.

150. Smith DW, Optiz JM, Inhorn SL: A syndrome of multiple developmental defects including polycystic kidney and intrahepatic biliary dysgenesis in 2 siblings. J Pediatr 67:617–624, 1965.

151. Goldfischer S, Moore CL, Johnson AB, Spiro AJ, Valsamis MP, Wisniewski HK, Ritch RH, Norton WT, Rapin I, Gartner LM: Peroxisomal and mitochondrial defects in the cerebro-hepato-renal syndrome. Science 182:62–64, 1973.

152. Danks DM, Tippett P, Adams C, Campbell P: Cerebro-hepato-renal syndrome of Zellweger. A report of eight cases with comments upon the incidence, the liver lesion, and a fault in pipecolic acid metabolism. J Pediatr 86:382–387, 1975.

153. Hanson RF, Szczepanik-Van Leeuwen P, Williams GC, Grabowski G, Sharp HL: Defects of bile acid synthesis in Zellweger's syndrome. Science 203:1107–1108, 1979.

154. Perry TL, Hardwick DF, Dixon GH, Dolman CL, Hansen S: Hypermethioninemia: a metabolic disorder associated with cirrhosis, islet cell hyperplasia, and renal tubular degeneration. Pediatrics 36:236–250, 1965.

155. Partington MW, Haust MD: A patient with tyrosinemia and hypermethioninemia. Can Med Assoc J 97:1059–1067, 1967.

156. Fairbanks VF, Beutler E: Congenital atransferrinemia and idiopathic pulmonary hemosiderosis. In Hematology, edited by W.J. Williams, E. Beutler, A.J. Erslev. 3rd Edition. New York, McGraw-Hill, 1983.

Chapter 13
Wilson's Disease (Hepatolenticular Degeneration)

Wilson's disease is a hereditary, metabolic disorder transmitted as an autosomal recessive trait and characterized by the accumulation of copper in the tissues, leading to pathologic alterations in the liver, brain, eyes, kidneys, skeletal system, and blood (1). The gene for this disorder is linked to the esterase locus on chromosome 13 (2). It is actually a common disorder in which heterozygous carriers make up almost 1% of the population. The use of proper techniques in the screening of asymptomatic members of the families of patients with Wilson's disease will help identify the disease in its preclinical state (3).

Although some heterozygotes exhibit abnormalities of copper metabolism (4–6) and ultrastructural changes in the liver (7), clinically evident Wilson's disease occurs exclusively in homozygotes.

Pathogenesis

The high concentrations of copper found in the affected tissues and the observation that reducing copper stores by chelation with D-penicillamine, triethylenetetramine dihydrochloride (trientine), and, zinc prevent the development of overt disease in asymptomatic homozygous carriers (8,9). In addition they induce remission of the disease in those already affected (8–10) support the generally accepted view that copper retention plays a major role in the pathogenesis of Wilson's disease. However, it is evident that additonal factors must be involved, since accumulation of copper alone, as in some newborns (11) and in experimental animals (12), does not lead to the typical hepatic and central nervous system signs of Wilson's disease. A hereditary disease in Bedlington terriers is also characterized by the accumulation of copper and the development of cirrhosis and occasionally of neurologic signs, as in Wilson's disease (13).

Absorption, hepatic uptake, and excretion of copper

Approximately 50% of the daily dietary intake of 2 to 5 mg of copper is absorbed in the stomach and proximal duodenum, and enters the circulation loosely bound to albumin. The liver, which has an avidity for the complex, promptly clears the serum of copper, and transfers it to a thiol-rich protein in the cytosol of the hepatocytes. Thereafter, a fraction of this protein-bound copper is utilized in the synthesis of copper proteins, such as cytochrome c oxidase and ceruloplasmin, and some is taken up by lysosomes and then excreted in the bile (8).

Normally, copper balance is maintained by biliary secretion and subsequent fecal excretion of copper (14) in the form of stable complexes that are not reabsorbed in the intestinal tract (15,16), so that the total body copper remains relatively constant at 60 to 100 mg throughout life (17).

Some studies have suggested that enhanced absorption of copper from the intestinal tract accounts for its accumulation in Wilson's disease (18). However, there is more convincing evidence that it is attributable to diminished biliary excretion of copper (19,20) secondary to a defect in lysosomes that serve as the source of biliary copper (20). The possibility that impairment of lysosomal function also accounts for the high concentration of copper found in the liver of newborn infants during the first six months of life is suggested by the predominantly lysosomal localization of such copper (21).

Other mechanisms that have been considered to account for the retention of copper in Wilson's disease include the presence of a genetically determined abnormal protein with an unusual avidity for copper (22), and a defect in copper metabolism attributable to impairment of ceruloplasmin synthesis.

Ceruloplasmin deficiency

Ceruloplasmin is a glycoprotein with oxidase activity, which is synthesized in the liver and which migrates electrophoretically as an α_2-globulin. It contains eight atoms of copper per molecule (0.32% by weight). It normally circulates in the serum at a concentration of 20 to 40 mg/dl, and contains approximately 95% of the copper in the circulation. The copper incorporated into newly synthesized ceruloplasmin, which closely corresponds to the amount absorbed from the diet, remains tightly bound until the ceruloplasmin, which has a half-life of four to five days, is degraded in the liver, resulting in the release of copper, which is excreted into the bile (23).

It has been suggested that nonceruloplasmin copper in the plasma, i.e., the difference between the total plasma copper concentration and the copper in ceruloplasmin, is potentially toxic copper and should be kept as low as possible to minimize tissue toxicity (24).

Impairment of ceruloplasmin synthesis is a distinctive feature of Wilson's disease. Usually, this is manifested by a low level of ceruloplasmin in the serum, but in 5% of cases, the level remains within normal limits (25,26), although it never exceeds 30 mg/dl (25). Moreover, similarly low serum levels may be encountered in the newborn, in some cases of severe hepatocellular disease, malabsorption, protein-losing enteropathy, sprue, and the nephrotic syndrome (27), or, rarely, as a familial trait unrelated to Wilson's disease (28). However, only in Wilson's disease can a defect in synthesis be demonstrated by analysis of copper kinetics (25). Normally, following the oral administration of a tracer dose of ^{64}Cu, there is a prompt rise in serum radioactivity that reaches a peak in 1 to 4 hours. Thereafter, radioactivity declines transiently only to rise again to a secondary peak at 48 hours, indicative of newly synthesized ceruloplasmin entering the circulation. Characteristically, in Wilson's disease, there is no secondary rise in radioactivity, thereby suggesting impairment of ceruloplasmin synthesis.

To account for the occurrence of Wilson's disease in the face of normal serum levels of ceruloplasmin, the possibility has been considered that the ceruloplasmin in Wilson's disease may be structurally abnormal in some patients (29). The amino acid sequence of ceruloplasmin has been completely determined (30), but attempts to confirm such structural abnormalities have been unsuccessful (31).

Since estrogens can raise the serum level of ceruloplasmin (32), it has been suggested that hyperestrogenemia secondary to liver disease may account for the occasional occurrence of normal serum ceruloplasmin concentrations in Wilson's disease (33). However, this appears unlikely, since patients with normal ceruloplasmin's levels may exhibit only trivial hepatic lesions (25).

Although there can be little doubt that impairment of ceruloplasmin synthesis is a distinctive feature of Wilson's disease, its level in the serum does not correlate with the magnitude of copper retention, the severity of the hepatic lesions, or the age of onset of the disease (33). The serum level may be low in heterozygotes who show no tendency to develop overt disease (4). This suggests that a deficiency of ceruloplasmin does not account for the accumulation of copper in Wilson's disease. It has been proposed that the retention of copper may be due to a gene mutation that results in perpetuation of the fetal mode of copper homeostasis, which is characterized by low concentrations of ceruloplasmin in the serum and high concentrations of copper in the liver that normally revert to adult levels within the first six months of life (34).

Distribution and concentration of copper in the tissues

In normal subjects the concentration of copper in the tissues is higher in the liver, brain, heart, and kidneys than in skeletal muscle, spleen, and other tissues (35).

In Wilson's disease, copper accumulates predominantly in the liver. It may reach concentrations 30 to 50 times the normal level, i.e., <50 $\mu g/g$ of dried tissue, before clinical manifestations appear (5). The copper concentrations in the liver may vary from one site in the liver to another (24). As the disease advances and hepatic storage sites are saturated, the liver ultimately loses its capacity to sequester additional copper, so copper is deposited in the brain and other tissues (36).

Early in the course of Wilson's disease, copper is localized in the cytosol of the hepatocytes, but later is found in the lysosomes (37,38), suggesting expansion of a second compartment. Striking alterations in the ultrastructure of the mitochondria and fatty infiltration appear during the phase when the copper is localized in the cytoplasm (5), and tend to disappear in late lesions when the copper is predominantly lysosomal in distribution (37,38). This has led to the suggestion that copper is toxic and accounts for mitochondrial damage and secondary fatty infiltration when it is diffusely distributed through the cytoplasm, but is innocuous when confined to the lysosomes (37,38).

In this connection, it has been emphasized that the high concentration of copper in the lysosomes of newborn infants induces no adverse effects on the liver. However, a pathogenetic role for the lysosomal copper deposits found in the advancing lesions of Wilson's disease and those in a variety of cholestatic disorders (11,39) cannot be excluded with certainty. Another feature of copper metabolism in Wilson's disease that remains to be elucidated is the tendency for the hepatic copper concentration to decline and for copper to shift to other tissues, particularly the central nervous system, as the disease progresses from its early presymptomatic phase to its advanced stage (40). It is generally assumed that this is attributable to the release of copper following hepatocellular necrosis, but the possibility that other factors are involved in the shift of copper cannot be excluded.

Clinical manifestations

Although the accumulation of copper in Wilson's disease begins at birth, clinical manifestations do not appear before the age of 6 years, but are evident in almost half the cases by the age of 15 (8). Only rarely is the onset delayed until as late as the sixth decade (41). Thus, the disease usually is encountered in older children, adolescents, and young adults. The four-step classification of Deiss et al provides a useful guideline for staging the disease (42).

The character of the initial clinical manifestations varies, depending, in part at least, on the age at onset. In one series of 151 symptomatic patients, the initial manifestations were predominantly hepatic in 42%, neurologic in 34%, psychiatric in 10%, and hematologic, endocrine, renal, or other causes in about 14% (1). In 25% of the cases, there was evidence that two or more systems were involved. Usually, the presenting manifestations are hepatic in children, and hepatic or neurologic in adolescents and adults.

Characteristically, the lesions in Wilson's disease are progressive, so, as a rule, late in the course of the disease, the manifestations are multisystemic.

Hepatic manifestations

The hepatic manifestations of Wilson's disease are not distinctive. Recognition that the disease may be present and that copper studies are needed for its confirmation is usually prompted by other features, such as a family history of Wilson's disease, the patient's age, the discovery of Kayser-Fleischer rings, the presence of hemolysis, the finding of low serum levels of uric acid and inorganic phosphorus indicative of renal tubular dysfunction, or the development of neurologic manifestations.

Despite the deposition of large amounts of copper in the liver, there may be no accompanying signs of hepatic dysfunction during the early phase of Wilson's disease (5). However, some asymptomatic patients exhibit hepatomegaly and raised serum levels of transaminase, and on biopsy, are found to have fatty infiltration, varying degrees of fibrosis, or even cirrhosis (43).

As the lesions advance, they often give rise to hepatic manifestations indicative of acute hepatitis, acute hemolytic anemia, or chronic active hepatitis or cirrhosis. Usually, these appear at an earlier age than neurologic signs and symptoms. However, in some cases, the hepatic lesions advance insidiously and do not become clinically apparent until much later. The acute hepatitis, which occurs in about one-fourth of these patients, simulates viral hepatitis, but is associated with a hemolytic component (1). Even when it appears to be fulminant hepatic failure, transaminase values are curiously low, hemolysis predominates, and renal insufficiency is often present (1,44–46).

Acute hemolysis and hepatic failure. Rarely, the onset of Wilson's disease is acute, with fever, jaundice, and malaise, followed by severe intravascular hemolysis, ascites, and hepatic encephalopathy (47–50). In such cases, death from hepatic failure, occasionally accompanied by acute renal failure (49), may ensue within two or three weeks. However, recovery following D-penicillamine therapy has been reported (51,52). Moreover, in some cases, the hemolysis is transient or recurrent, and may be unaccompanied by evidence of hepatic failure (53,54). The clinical features in cases with acute hemolysis suggest some form of fulminant acute hepatitis, but the lesions found at autopsy usually are characterized by cirrhosis with varying degrees of hepatic degeneration, necrosis, and inflammation (44–50).

Almost always, the acute hemolysis of Wilson's disease is accompanied by the excretion of inordinately large amounts of copper in the urine. This feature supports the generally accepted view that the destruction of erythrocytes is attributable to the toxic effects of copper mobilized from the tissues and released into the circulation. This is supported by similar observations in sheep with copper intoxication. Hepatic necrosis probably accounts for the mobilization of copper in some cases, but in others, neither the source nor the factors responsible for the release of copper are known. Equally obscure is the explanation for the development of acute hepatocellular necrosis in previously quiescent cirrhotic lesions. A redistribution of copper from the lysosomes to the cytoplasm of the hepatocytes has been suggested as a possible mechanism (48).

Fulminant hepatitis. Not infrequently, patients with Wilson's disease present with fulminant hepatic failure (54–58). These cases, which are difficult to differentiate from other types of fulminant hepatitis, show the characteristic low ceruloplasmin, elevated urinary copper levels, and low or normal serum copper concentration (55,56). Their serum bilirubin levels are usually higher than in fulminant hepatocytes of other types, probably associated with the hemolytic activity that is usually present (47–50). The correct diagnosis is extremely important in view of the rapid death of untreated patients and the availability of curative therapy by transplantation. Histologically, the hepatitis cannot be differentiated from that of fulminant viral hepatitis except for the presence of extensive copper deposition (55).

Chronic active hepatitis. In some patients with Wilson's disease, the presenting signs and symtpoms closely resemble those of chronic active hepatitis (59,60). As in other forms of chronic active hepatitis, the onset may be acute, with jaundice and fever, suggesting acute viral hepatitis, or insidious. Unless treated with D-penicillamine, the lesions tend to progress, often giving rise to cirrhosis and, occasionally, to hepatic failure.

Usually, Kayser-Fleischer rings are present, but slit-lamp examination may be required for their demonstration early in the course of the disease. At any time, neurologic signs and symp-

toms may appear, but they are not always present, even in terminal hepatic failure due to Wilson's disease.

Cirrhosis. By far the most common hepatic lesion in advanced untreated Wilson's disease is cirrhosis. In some patients, the typical signs and symptoms of cirrhosis appear during the course of clinically overt chronic active hepatitis. However, in others, the development of cirrhosis is insidious. In the absence of neurologic manifestations, such lesions may be erroneously identified as cryptogenic (61) or juvenile cirrhosis (62). Some patients who exhibit no clinical signs of either hepatic or neurologic disease present with splenomegaly, portal hypertension, and hemorrhage from esophageal varices (63,64), or signs of hypersplenism (65). In such cases, the underlying disorder may be misinterpreted as evidence of extrahepatic or idiopathic portal hypertension or Banti's syndrome. In some patients with the predominantly neurologic form of Wilson's disease, there are no clinical signs of hepatic involvement, but cirrhosis is frequently found at autopsy (66).

The cirrhosis is macronodular in most patients, but may be mixed or even micronodular (1). In contrast to other forms of macronodular cirrhosis, Wilson's disease is only rarely complicated by *hepatocellular carcinoma* (1,67–70). Conceivably, copper has an antineoplastic effect (68). The cirrhosis of Wilson's disease, like other cirrhoses, is associated with an increased prevalence of pigmented gallstones, presumably a consequence of chronic hemolysis (71).

Neuropsychiatric manifestations

Due to deposition of copper in the brain, there is widespread loss of nerve cells and hyperplasia of protoplasmic astrocytes. Such changes are most prominent in the basal ganglia, where the lesions may show gray-brown pigmentation and cavitation.

The neurologic manifestations of Wilson's disease tend to be relatively acute and rapidly progressive in children and more chronic in adults. The most common feature is a tremor that is fine initially and coarse and flapping later. Other signs include dystonia with muscular rigidity and contractures, athetosis, a mask-like facies with grimacing and drooling, dysarthria, and slurring of speech (72). Often, as previously indicated, there are no accompanying clinical signs of liver disease.

Psychiatric disorders of various types are relatively common in Wilson's disease (73), and, occasionally, they are the predominant manifestations of the disease (1). Often, in such cases, Kayser-Fleischer rings, which are invariably present, are the only clue to the nature of the underlying disease.

Cranial CT and nuclear magnetic resonance (NMR) scanning can show the existence of abnormalities in the basal ganglia and thalamus prior to the appearance of neurologic symptoms (74,75). The latter method has been shown to be more sensitive (75).

Ocular manifestations

Deposition of copper in Descemet's membrane on the posterior surface of the cornea produces *Kayser-Fleischer rings,* which present as greenish brown bands at the periphery of the corneas close to the limbus. Early in their development, the rings may be incomplete, appearing as pigmented crescents at the upper poles of the corneas, or may require slit-lamp microscopy for their identificatioin.

Kayser-Fleischer rings are encountered in approximately 90% of patients with Wilson's disease, but are not demonstrable during the early, presymptomatic phase of the disease. Following successful decoppering with D-penicillamine therapy, the rings disappear.

Although highly suggestive of Wilson's disease, Kayser-Fleischer rings are not pathognomonic, since they may occur in other hepatic disorders accompanied by chronic cholestasis and copper retention, such as primary biliary cirrhosis, chronic active hepatitis, cryptogenic cirrhosis, and neonatal hepatitis (76,77). Also to be differentiated from the Kayser-Fleischer rings of Wilson's disease are the corneal rings produced by deposition of carotene in arcus senilis (78).

Rarely, Wilson's disease is complicated by the development of *sunflower cataracts* due to deposition of copper on the anterior and posterior surfaces of the lenses, a lesion similar to that produced by embedded copper-containing foreign bodies (79). In some cases, removal of the copper and resolution of the cataracts are induced by D-penicillamine therapy.

Renal manifestations

Although overt kidney disease is relatively rare, many patients with Wilson's disease exhibit laboratory evidence of impaired renal function involving the renal tubules in particular, that is attributable to the toxic effects of copper deposited in the kidneys (80,81). The principal abnormalities that may be encountered include defects in the acidification, dilution, and concentration of the urine; increased urinary excretion of amino acids, uric acid, phosphate, and glucose; proteinuria; and microscopic hematuria, changes that usually revert to normal following D-penicillamine therapy. Occasionally, the low serum levels of uric acid or inorganic phosphorus may be the first clue to the diagnosis of Wilson's disease. Of interest is the fact that heterozygotic patients for Wilson's disease often exhibit similar, but less extensive renal functional abnormalities (82).

Some patients with Wilson's disease exhibit hypercalciuria, which occasionally, is associated with the development of renal stones (83,84). The pathogenesis of this abnormality is uncertain. Although renal tubular acidosis may account for the hypercalciuria and nephrolithiasis in some cases, often it is not present. Hypoparathyroidism, attributed to copper deposition in the parathyroids, may contribute to the skeletal disease (85).

As previously indicated, acute renal failure may complicate the course of Wilson's disease in cases with acute intravascular hemolysis (49,54).

Skeletal manifestations

Abnormalities of the bones and joints can be demonstrated radiographically in a high proportion of patients with Wilson's disease (1,86). These include demineralization, Milkman's pseudofractures, spontaneous fractures, osteomalacia, renal rickets, subchondral fragmentation, and cystic changes in bone, chondrocalcinosis, chondromalacia, and premature degenerative arthritis. The pathogenesis of these skeletal changes is un-

certain, but it is highly probable that multiple factors are involved, including renal tubular acidosis, chronic liver disease, immobilization, and malnutrition.

Cardiac manifestations

Although no clinical cardiac disorders have been reported, cardiac hypertrophy, interstitial fibrosis, and focal myocarditis have been found (87).

Biochemical features

The characteristic biochemical findings in Wilson's disease include low serum levels of ceruloplasmin (less than 20 mg/dl) and copper (less than 100 μg/dl), increased urinary excretion of copper (greater than 100 μg/24 hours), failure to incorporate orally administered radiocopper into ceruloplasmin, and a high concentration of copper in the liver (greater than 250 μg/g dry liver tissue). Measurement of the concentration of copper can differentiate homozygous patients, who have an increased copper concentration starting in infancy, from heterozygous subjects (1). Conversely, low concentrations may be encountered in patients with severe hepatocellular disease and a variety of other disorders. Occasionally, heterozygous carriers of Wilson's disease exhibit low serum levels of ceruloplasmin, depression of radiocopper incorporation into ceruloplasmin, and increased concentrations of copper in the liver. However, the hepatic copper concentration rarely exceeds 250 μg/g of dry liver tissue, an important point in the differentiation between heterozygotes and homozygotes.

High levels of urinary and hepatic copper equal to those in Wilson's disease may be encountered in chronic cholestatic disorders such as primary biliary cirrhosis, neonatal cholestasis, and Indian childhood cirrhosis. However, they are accompanied by normal or raised concentrations of ceruloplasmin. Moreover, in Wilson's disease, high concentrations of urinary and hepatic copper usually occur in the absence of cholestasis.

Histopathology of associated hepatic lesions
Presymptomatic disease

In young children with presymptomatic Wilson's disease, the histologic appearance of the liver may be normal, despite the presence of high concentrations of copper in the cytoplasm of the hepatocytes. Frequently, however, recognition of the disease in presymptomatic cases in delayed sufficiently long to permit the development of structural alterations in the hepatic parenchyma and portal tracts. Although characteristic, none of these alterations is a constant feature or diagnostic of Wilson's disease (1,5,38,43).

1. *Fatty infiltration* of variable extent is the abnormality encountered most frequently. The lipid droplets may be macro-

vesicular or microvesicular and, usually, are randomly distributed (Fig. 664).

2. Often, the periportal hepatocytes contain *glycogen nuclei*. These resemble the vacuolated nuclei seen in diabetes mellitus and other disorders but tend to be more numerous, larger, and more irregular in contour (Fig. 665).

Except for the lipid droplets and glycogen nuclei, the hepatocytes appear normal and are usually arranged in a normal, one-cell-thick, hepatic plate pattern. Lipofuscin pigment is often abundant, and sometimes the granules are larger and more irregular than normal (88). Occasionally, liver cell ballooning or acidophilic bodies may be encountered, unaccompanied by any intralobular inflammatory reaction (Fig. 666). Sometimes Küpffer cells appear enlarged and may contain iron in patients who have had episodes of hemolysis.

3. The large amounts of *copper* that accumulate in the cytoplasm of the hepatocytes in presymptomatic cases of Wilson's disease are not demonstrable histochemically by routine staining with rubeanic acid or rhodanine. However, Timm's silver sulfide method produces diffuse cytoplasmic staining indicative of copper deposition (8,11). Although this reagent reacts with other metals, it is reasonably reliable in the detection of copper when there is no accompanying hemosiderosis.

4. Varying degrees of *portal fibrosis and inflammation* may be seen during the late phase of presymptomatic Wilson's disease. Usually, the affected portal tracts are enlarged and show stellate scarring with slender fibrous septa or without bridging fibrosis (Fig. 667). Occasionally, the fibrosis is extensive and accompanied by nodule formation, giving rise to an inactive form of macronodular cirrhosis. Characteristically, in such presymptomatic lesions, the limiting plates of the portal tracts and septa are intact, the portal exudates are limited to relatively few lymphocytes, and there is no significant ductular proliferation or intralobular inflammation, degeneration, or necrosis.

5. Highly characteristic *ultrastructural alterations* of the hepatocytes are often found during the presymptomatic phase of Wilson's disease (1,38,40). These have been attributed to the toxic effects of the copper that accumulates in the cytoplasm and is thought to play an important role in the pathogenesis of the hepatic lesions. Characteristically, the hepatocellular mitochondria exhibit marked pleomorphism, increased density of their matrix, separation of their normally apposed inner and outer membranes, widening of the intercristal spaces, and crystalline, dense, or vacuolated inclusions. In addition, the peroxisomes tend to be enlarged and misshapen, and contain a granular flocculent matrix of variable electron density.

Symptomatic disease

The hepatic lesions of symptomatic Wilson's disease are highly variable, and differ to some extent, depending on whether the clinical manifestations are predominantly hepatic or extrahepatic. Many of the histologic features are nonspecific in that they mimic those in other disorders, particularly chronic active hepatitis and postnecrotic cirrhosis. Other reported abnormalities such as dense, eosinophilic cytoplasm with areas of rarefaction may be difficult to determine (1,88,89). However, most lesions on liver biopsy show at least some of the structural abnormalities that are more distinctive, although not pathognomonic of Wilson's disease. These include fatty infiltration, gly-

cogen nuclei, stainable copper deposits, increased lipofuscin, and Mallory bodies.

In patients who present with jaundice, ascites, or other evidence of hepatic decompensation, irrespective of whether the onset is acute or insidious, the lesions closely resemble those of classic *chronic active hepatitis*. Often, the lesions have advanced to the stage of cirrhosis, even when they are discovered within a few weeks or months following the appearance of signs and symptoms.

As in classic chronic active hepatitis, the early lesions are characterized by expansion, fibrosis, and infiltration of the portal tracts by numerous lymphocytes and plasma cells, accompanied by erosion of the limiting plates, extension of the fibrous tissue and inflammatory cells into the periportal parenchyma, and, occasionally, by fibrous or necrotic bridging of adjacent portal tracts. Figure 668 illustrates such an early lesion in a 17-year-old girl who presented with fatigability, and was found to have hepatosplenomegaly and raised serum levels of transaminase and gamma globulin, originally interpreted as evidence of chronic active hepatitis. However, an inordinately low serum uric acid level of 1.6 mg/dl found on routine biochemical screening suggested the possibility of Wilson's disease. This diagnosis was subsequently established on laboratory and clinical grounds.

As previously indicated, often, in patients who present with signs of hepatic decompensation, the lesions are characterized by *chronic active hepatitis* that has already progressed to *cirrhosis*. Figure 562 illustrates such an advanced active lesion in an 11-year-old boy who presented at another institution with jaundice, ascites, and edema of one month's duration. Examination revealed an enlarged liver and massive splenomegaly, which were interpreted as evidence of Hodgkin's disease. Exploratory laparotomy carried out for staging purposes unexpectedly revealed a coarsely nodular, cirrhotic liver, and splenomegaly, but no evidence of lymphoma. As illustrated in Figure 562, the normal lobular architecture was replaced by large nodules of regenerating parenchyma encircled by fibrous septa infiltrated with numerous lymphocytes and plasma cells. Everywhere, the septa showed erosion of their limiting plates with extension of fibrous tissue and inflammatory cells into the parenchyma (Fig. 669) and striking alterations in the adjacent hepatocytes, characterized by ballooning, marked pleomorphism, and an irregular, thickened, plate pattern with rosette formation and foci of cell dropout (Fig. 670). Some of the septa contained numerous proliferating ductules (Fig. 671), and in some fields there were occasional, periportal, acidophilic bodies. Initially, these features were considered typical of severe chronic active hepatitis and postnecrotic cirrhosis of unknown etiology. However, the presence of numerous periportal glycogen nuclei (Fig. 156), lipofuscin granules (Fig. 156), rhodanine-positive copper-containing granules (Fig. 163), orcein-positive copper-protein granules (Fig. 164), and numerous Mallory bodies, some of which were surrounded by neutrophils (Fig. 563), suggested Wilson's disease. Subsequently, the diagnosis of Wilson's disease was confirmed by the demonstration of Kayser-Fleischer rings, a low serum ceruloplasmin level, and a high concentration of copper in the liver. Unfortunately, death from hepatic failure ensued a week following laparotomy and before D-penicillamine therapy could be instituted.

The copper can be seen histologically with rubeanic and rhodanine stains, which demonstrate the cupric form (Cu II) [(90); Figs. 163, 672), and by the presence of copper-associated protein by orcein staining [(11); Fig. 164]. Copper-associated protein is probably polymerized metallothionein, which binds copper in the cuprous state (Cu I) in a nontoxic form (91). In Wilson's disease, biopsies may be histochemically negative despite excessive amounts of copper shown by atomic absorption spectrophotometry (11,92). Although no copper-associated protein is seen in normal livers, immunoreactive metallothionein is present in centrilobular hepatocytes. Necrotic periportal hepatocytes, especially in Wilson's disease, stain heavily for metallothionein [(93); Fig. 673].

Patients with Wilson's disease who present with manifestations attributable primarily to *portal hypertension,* such as hemorrhage from esophageal varices, hypersplenism, or massive splenomegaly, may exhibit no clinical or biochemical evidence of hepatic disease. However, invariably in such cases, biopsy reveals an inactive, coarsely nodular postnecrotic cirrhosis with a variable number of histologic features suggestive of Wilson's disease. Figure 671 illustrates a lesion of this type in a 12-year-old boy who presented with a ruptured spleen following blunt abdominal trauma. At laparotomy, the spleen was found to be greatly enlarged and lacerated, and the liver exhibited a previously unrecognized and asymptomatic coarsely nodular cirrhosis. As can be seen in Figure 671, the normal lobular architecture was replaced by large nodules of regenerating parenchyma separated by broad, smooth-contoured bands of fibrous tissue. Although the septa contained a moderate number of lymphocytes and proliferating ductules, the limiting plates were intact, and there was no evidence of parenchymal degeneration, necrosis, or inflammation, features indicative of an inactive lesion. Only a few of the parenchymal nodules contained rhodanine-positive copper-containing granules (Fig. 672), and there were no other histologic features suggestive of Wilson's disease. However, further investigation revealed the presence of Kayser-Fleischer rings, low serum levels of ceruloplasmin and uric acid, and greatly increased urinary excretion of copper, findings that confirmed the diagnosis and led to the institution of D-penicillamine therapy.

Even early in the course of Wilson's disease, the cytoplasm of the hepatocytes invariably contains a high concentration of copper, and, often, there are histologic changes in the liver of the type seen in presymptomatic Wilson's disease. Despite the absence of clinical features indicative of liver disease, the hepatic lesions tend to progress, so, almost always, an inactive macronodular cirrhosis of the type illustrated in Figure 671 is found at autopsy. Occasionally, hepatic decompensation or hemorrhage from esophageal varices is a sudden, unexpected, terminal event.

Although the broad zones of fibrosis found in the type of inactive macronodular cirrhosis illustrated in Figure 671 suggest the possibility of antecedent, clinically inapparent, submassive, acute hepatocellular necrosis. Such acute, necrotic lesions are rarely if ever encountered in Wilson's disease. In some cases, the cirrhosis is the sequela of progressive chronic active hepatitis that has gone into remission, but, in others, it appears to develop insidiously in the absence of overt hepatocellular necrosis or an inflammatory reaction, presumably as a result of fibrogenesis and slow destruction of hepatocytes secondary to the toxic effects of retained copper.

Characteristically, *glycogen nuclei* are found in periportal hepatocytes. In adult patients, they are relatively common, occurring in diabetes mellitus and a wide variety of other disorders, and may even be seen in otherwise normal livers. However, they are far less frequent in children, so their presence, particularly if accompanied by fatty infiltration, portal fibrosis, or

chronic active hepatitis, should draw attention to the possibility of Wilson's disease (Figs. 156, 174).

In contrast to the uniform, finely granular character of the *lipofuscin* granules and their localization in the cytoplasm of centrilobular hepatocytes in the normal liver, those in Wilson's disease are coarse and irregular in contour and are found predominantly in periportal hepatocytes [(88,89); Fig. 156]. The aggregation of these pigment granules along the course of the canaliculi attests to their lysosomal localization.

In the later stages of Wilson's disease, lysosomal deposits of *copper* present as cytoplasmic granules that stain with rubeanic acid and rhodanine. Usually, they are found in periportal hepatocytes (Fig. 163), but in advanced cirrhotic lesions, they may be present in most of the hepatocytes contained within some of the nodules (Fig. 672). In many cases, the distribution of copper-containing granules is not uniform, so they may escape detection in small, needle biopsy specimens. As illustrated in Figure 164, some of the granules often contain copper-binding protein complexes that stain with orcein (94). Deposits of stainable copper and copper-protein complexes are not diagnostic of Wilson's disease, since they may be encountered in other hepatic disorders accompanied by cholestasis and copper retention, such as primary biliary cirrhosis, chronic acitve hepatitis, cirrhosis, neonatal cholestasis, and hepatocellular carcinoma (11,94,95). They are found in hepatocellular carcinoma, but not in metastatic malignancy (96). Nevertheless, their presence is an indication for further studies to exclude Wilson's disease, particularly in children and young adults. Staining for copper is not a routine procedure, but is recommended in all such individuals who present with chronic hepatic disease of unknown etiology. Of the methods available for demonstrating copper-containing granules, we have found rhodanine more reliable and easier to interpret than rubeanic acid staining.

Typical *Mallory bodies,* usually found within ballooned hepatocytes and occasionally surrounded by neutrophils, are an important clue to the diagnosis of Wilson's disease (Fig. 563). Characteristically, they are encountered in advanced active lesions, but not in those that are early or inactive. Although their association with fatty infiltration may suggest underlying alcoholic liver disease, the Mallory bodies in Wilson's disease are characteristically found in hepatocytes located in the periportal or periseptal zones rather than in the centrilobular zones. Similar Mallory bodies may be encountered under a variety of other conditions, often associated with cholestasis. However, those in Wilson's disease frequently are found in the absence of overt cholestasis.

Effect of D-penicillamine therapy in Wilson's disease

Prolonged treatment with D-penicillamine and a diet low in copper and supplemented with potassium sulfide to reduce copper absorption leads to significant reduction in hepatic copper concentration (5,8), decrease in hepatic fatty infiltration and fibrosis (5,8–10), and reversal or improvement in the ultrastructural abnormalities of the hepatic mitochondria (97). In most cases, such improvements are associated with a delay in the onset of overt Wilson's disease or increased survival (98).

New forms of therapy for Wilson's disease are emerging. *Trientine* (triethylenetetramine dihydrochloride), another chelating agent, which was introduced in 1969 (99), is as effective as penicillamine (100,101). Therapy with both penicillamine and trientine has sometimes been associated with progression of the neurologic signs of Wilson's disease despite a reduction in the copper content of the liver (102).

In 1983, zinc sulfate, which inhibits almost completely the absorption of copper (103), was introduced (104). It appears to be as effective as penicillamine or trientine (105–107), especially when taken in the fasting state as zinc acetate, which is almost free of side effects (24). Indeed, when taken with food zinc is less well absorbed and may be less effective clinically (24,108).

When all else fails, liver transplantation has been shown to reverse all of the manifestations of Wilson's disease and to prolong life (109).

Hepatic alterations in heterozygotes

Usually, in heterozygotic carriers of the Wilson's disease gene, the histologic appearance of the liver is normal. However, in a few well-documented cases, we have encountered a significant number of periportal glycogen nuclei. Moreover, it has been reported that some heterozygotes exhibit ultrastructural changes in their hepatocellular mitochondria identical with those found in homozygotes (7).

Differentiation between heterozygous and presymptomatic homozygous carriers of the Wilson's disease gene

Presymptomatic homozygous carriers of the Wilson's disease gene require lifelong D-penicillamine therapy to prevent progression of the disease and the development of overt clinical manifestations (5), whereas heterozygotes are not at risk and require no treatment (4). Therefore, differentiation between these two groups is important. Usually, this poses no problem, but sometimes it may prove difficult (100).

As a rule, presymptomatic homozygotic patients can be identified on the basis of a serum ceruloplasmin level below 20 mg/dl, a daily urinary copper excretion in excess of 100 μg, and a concentration of copper in the liver higher than 250 μg/g of dried tissue (5). In the small number of cases with normal ceruloplasmin levels, a defect in the incorporation of radiocopper into newly synthesized ceruloplasmin can be demonstrated. However, some heterozygotic subjects exhibit similarly low serum concentrations of ceruloplasmin (4), hepatic concentrations in excess of 250 μg/g of dried tissue (7), and impairment of radiocopper incorporation into ceruloplasmin (6), so these criteria do not always distinguish between heterozygous and homozygous individuals. Histologic evidence of significant fatty infiltration in combination with glycogen nuclei and portal fibrosis favors the homozygous state but, often, is absent. In potential cases the demonstration of the characteristic hepatic lesions by CT or NMR may prove to be the most sensitive and the least invasive method of making the diagnosis (74,75). In such cases, a therapeutic trial of D-penicillamine, trientine, or zinc may be indicated.

References

1. Scheinberg IH, Sternlieb I: Wilson's Disease, Philadelphia, W.B. Saunders, 1984.
2. Frydman M, Bonne-Tamir B, Farrer LA, Conneally PM, Magazanik A, Ashbel S, Goldwitch Z. Assignment of the gene for Wilson's disease to chromosome 13: linkage to the esterase D locus. Proc Natl Acad Sci 82:1819–1821, 1985.
3. Lindahl JM, Sharp HL: Screening asymptomatic family members for Wilson's disease. Minn Med 65:473–475, 1982.
4. Sternlieb I, Morrell AG, Bauer CD, Combes B, De Bobes-Sternberg S, Scheinberg IH: Detection of the heterozygous carrier of Wilson's disease gene. J Clin Invest 40:707–715, 1961.
5. Sternlieb I, Scheinberg IH: Prevention of Wilson's disease in asymptomatic patients. N Engl J Med 278:352–359, 1968.
6. Strickland GT, Beckner WM, Leu M-L, O'Reilly S: Turnover studies of copper in homozygotes and heterozygotes for Wilson's disease and controls: isotope tracer studies with ^{67}Cu. Clin Sci 43:605–615, 1972.
7. Lough J, Wiglesworth FW: Wilson's disease. Comparative ultrastructure in a sibship of nine. Arch Pathol 100:659–663, 1976.
8. Sternlieb I: Copper and the liver. Gastroenterology 76:1615–1628, 1980.
9. Walshe JM: Treatment of Wilson's disease with trientine (triethylene tetramine) dihydrochloride. Lancet 1:643–646, 1982.
10. Rossaro L, Sturniolo GC, Giacon G, Montino MC, Lecis PE, Schade RR, Corazza GR, Trevisan C, Naccarato R: Zinc therapy in Wilson's disease: observations in five patients. Am J Gastroenterol 85:665–668, 1990.
11. Goldfischer S, Popper H, Sternlieb I: The significance of variations in the distributions of copper in liver disease. Am J Pathol 99:715–730, 1980.
12. Sternlieb I: Copper and liver injury. In Hepatology: A Festschrift for Hans Popper, edited by H. Brunner, H. Thaler. New York, Raven Press, 1985, pp. 243–253.
13. Owen CA, Ludwig J: Inherited copper toxicosis in Bedlington terriers—Wilson's disease (hepatolenticular degeneration). Am J Pathol 106:432–438, 1982.
14. Van Berge Henegouwen GP, Tangedahl TN, Hofman AF, Northfield TC, La Russo NF, McCall JT: Biliary secretion of copper in healthy man. Quantitation by an intestinal perfusion technique. Gastroenterology 72:1228–1231, 1977.
15. Gollan JL, Deller DJ: Studies on the nature and excretion of biliary copper in man. Clin Sci 44:9–15, 1973.
16. Lewis KO: The nature of the copper complexes in bile and their relationship to the absorption and excretion of copper in normal subjects and in Wilson's disease. Gut 14:221–232, 1973.
17. Sternlieb I: Gastrointestinal copper absorption in man. Gastroenterology 52:1038–1041, 1967.
18. Bush JA, Mahoney JP, Markowitz H, Gubler CJ, Cartwright GE, Wintrobe MM: Studies on copper metabolism. XVI. Radioactive copper studies in normal subjects and in patients with hepatolenticular degeneration. J Clin Invest 34:1766–1778, 1955.
19. Strickland GT, Beckner WM, Leu M-L: Absorption of copper in homozygotes and heterozygotes for Wilson's disease and controls: isotope tracer studies with ^{67}Cu and ^{64}Cu. Clin Sci 43:617–625, 1972.
20. Winge DR: Normal physiology of copper metabolism. Semin Liver Dis 4:239–247, 1984.
21. Goldfischer S, Bernstein J: Lipofuscin (aging) pigment granules of the newborn human liver. J Cell Biol 42:253–261, 1969.
22. Uzman LL, Iber FL, Chalmers TC, Knowlton M: The mechanism of copper deposition in the liver in hepatolenticular degeneration (Wilson's disease). Am J Med Sci 231:511–518, 1956.
23. Sternlieb I, Morell AG, Tucker WD, Greene MW, Scheinberg IH: The incorporation of copper into ceruloplasmin: in vivo: studies with copper^{64} and copper^{67}. J Clin Invest 40:1834–1840, 1961.
24. Brewer GJ: Zinc therapy of Wilson's disease: two views. Hepatology 6:1047–1048, 1986.
25. Sternlieb I, Scheinberg IH: The role of radiocopper in the diagnosis of Wilson's disease. Gastroenterology 77:138–142, 1979.
26. Sass-Kortsak A, Cherniak M, Geiger DW, Slater RJ: Observations on ceruloplasmin in Wilson's disease. J Clin Invest 38:1672–1682, 1959.
27. Gault MH, Stein J, Aronoff A: Serum ceruloplasmin in hepatobiliary and other disorders: significance of abnormal values. Gastroenterology 50:8–18, 1966.
28. Cox DW: Factors influencing serum ceruloplasmin levels in normal individuals. J Lab Clin Med 68:893–904, 1966.
29. Poulik MD, Bearn AG: Heterogeneity of ceruloplasmin. Clin Chim Acta 7:374–382, 1962.
30. Takahashi N, Ortel TL, Putnam FW: Single-chain structure of human

ceruloplasmin: the complete amino acid sequence of the whole molecule. Proc Natl Acad Sci USA *81*:390–395, 1984.

31. Holtzman NA, Naugton MA, Iber FL, Gaumnitz BM: Ceruloplasmin in Wilson's disease. J Clin Invest *46*:993–1002, 1967.

32. Russ EM, Raymunt J: Influence of estrogens on total serum copper and ceruloplasmin. Proc Soc Exp Biol Med *92*:465–466, 1956.

33. Sternlieb I, Scheinberg IH: Ceruloplasmin in health and disease. Ann NY Acad Sci *94*:71–76, 1961.

34. Epstein O, Sherlock S: Is Wilson's disease caused by a controller gene mutation resulting in perpetuation of the fetal mode of copper metabolism into childhood? Lancet *1*:303–305, 1981.

35. Cartwright GE, Wintrobe MM: Copper metabolism in normal subjects. Am J Clin Nutr *14*:224–232, 1964.

36. Osborne SB, Walshe JM: The influence of genetic and acquired liver defects on radio-copper turnover in Wilson's disease. Lancet *2*:17–20, 1969.

37. Goldfischer S, Sternlieb I: Changes in the distribution of hepatic copper in relation to the progression of Wilson's disease (hepatolenticular degeneration). Am J Pathol *53*:883–901, 1968.

38. Sternlieb I: Evolution of the hepatic lesion in Wilson's disease (hepatolenticular degeneration). *In Progress in Liver Diseases,* Vol. IV, edited by H. Popper, F. Schaffner. New York, Grune & Stratton, 1972, pp. 511–525.

39. Smallwood RA, Williams HA, Rosenoer VM, Sherlock S: Liver-copper cells in liver disease. Studies using neutron activation analysis. Lancet *2*:1310–1313, 1968.

40. Sternlieb I: Mitochondrial and fatty changes in hepatocytes of patients with Wilson's disease. Gastroenterology *55*:354–367, 1968.

41. Fitzgerald MA, Gross JB, Goldstein NP, Wahner HW, McCall JT: Wilson's disease (hepatolenticular degeneration) of late adult onset. Report of a case. Mayo Clin Proc *50*:438–442, 1975.

42. Deiss A, Lynch RE, Lee GR, Cartwright GE: Long-term therapy of Wilson's Disease. Ann Intern Med *75*:57–65, 1971.

43. Levi AJ, Sherlock S, Scheuer PJ, Cumings JN: Presymptomatic Wilson's disease. Lancet *2*:575–579, 1967.

44. McCullough AJ, Weisner RH, Fleming CR, Dickson ER: Antemortem diagnosis and short-term survival of a patient with Crohn's disease presenting as fulminant hepatic failure. Dig Dis Sci *29*:862–864, 1984.

45. Rector WG, Uchida T, Kanel GC, Redeker AG, Reynolds TB: Fulminant hepatic and renal failure complicating Wilson's disease. Liver *4*:341–347, 1984.

46. Hartleb M, Zahorska-Markiewicz B, Ciesielski A. Wilson's disease presenting in sisters as fulminant hepatitis with hemolytic episodes. Am J Gastroenterol *82*:549–551, 1987.

47. McIntyre N, Clark HM, Cumings JN, Sherlock S: Hemolytic anemia in Wilson's disease. N Engl J Med *276*:439–444, 1967.

48. Roche-Sicot J, Benhamou J-P: Acute intravascular hemolysis and acute hepatic failure associated as a first manifestation of Wilson's disease. Ann Intern Med *86*:301–303, 1977.

49. Hamlyn AN, Gollan JL, Douglas AP, Sherlock S: Fulminant Wilson's disease with haemolysis and renal failure: copper studies and assessment of dialysis regimens. Br Med J *2*:660–663, 1977.

50. Lehr H, Pauschinger M, Pittke E, Kurrle E, Heimpel H: Haemolytic anaemia as initial manifestation of Wilson's disease. Blut *56*: 45–46, 1988.

51. Iser JH, Stevens BJ, Stening GF, Hurley TH, Smallwood RA: Hemolytic anemia of Wilson's disease. Gastroenterology *67*:290–293, 1974.

52. Robitaille GA, Piscatelli RL, Majeski EJ, Gelehrter TD: Hemolytic anemia in Wilson's disease. A report of three cases with transient increase in hemoglobin A₂. JAMA *237*:2402–2403, 1977.

53. Deiss A, Lee GR, Cartwright GE: Hemolytic anemia in Wilson's disease. Ann Intern Med *73*:413–418, 1970.

54. Gur H, Aderka D, Finkelstein A, Levo Y: Fulminant Wilsonian hepatitis: difficulties in diagnosis and treatment. Am J Gastroenterol *83*:679–681, 1988.

55. McCullough AJ, Fleming CR, Thistle JL, Baldus WP, Ludwig J, McCall JT, Dickson ER: Diagnosis of Wilson's disease presenting as fulminant hepatic failure. Gastroenterology *84*:161–167, 1983.

56. McCullough AJ, Wiesner RH, Fleming CR, Dickson ER: Antemortem diagnosis and short-term survival of a patient with Wilson's disease presenting as fulminant hepatic failure. Dig Dis Sci *29*:862–864, 1984.

57. Adler R, Mahroviski V, Heuser ET: Fulminant hepatitis. A presentation of Wilson's disease. Am J Dis Child *131*:870–872, 1977.

58. Enomoto K, Ishibashi H, Irie K, Okumura Y, Nomura H, Fukushima M, Inaba S, Niho Y: Fulminant hepatic failure without evidence of cirrhosis in a case of Wilson's disease. Jpn J Med *28*:80–84, 1989.

59. Sternlieb IM, Scheinberg IH: Chronic hepatitis as a first manifestation of Wilson's disease. Ann Intern Med *76*:59–64, 1972.

60. Archer GJ, Monie RDH: Wilson's disease and chronic active hepatitis. Lancet *1*:486–587, 1977.

61. Chalmers TC, Iber FL, Uzman LL: Hepatolenticular degeneration (Wilson's disease) as a form of idiopathic cirrhosis. N Engl J Med *256*:235–242, 1957.

62. Lygren T: Hepatolenticular degeneration (Wilson's disease) and juvenile cirrhosis in the same family. Lancet *1*:275–276, 1959.

63. Sternlieb I: The development of cirrhosis in Wilson's disease. Clin Gastroenterol *4*:267–273, 1975.

64. Sternlieb I, Scheinberg IH, Walshe JM: Bleeding esophageal varices in patients with Wilson's disease. Lancet *1*:638–641, 1970.

65. Hoagland HC, Goldstein NP: Hematologic (cytopenic) manifestations of Wilson's disease (hepatolenticular degeneration). Mayo Clin Proc *53*:498–502, 1978.

66. Wilson SAK: Progressive lenticular degeneration: a familial nervous disease associated with cirrhosis of the liver. Brain *34*:295–509, 1911–1912.

67. Kamakura K, Kimura S, Igarashi S, Fujiwara K, Oda T, Yoshitoshi Y, Shoti S: A case of Wilson's disease with hepatoma. J Jpn Soc Intern Med *64*:232–238, 1975.

68. Wilkinson ML, Portmann B, Williams R: Wilson's disease and hepatocellular carcinoma: possible protective role of copper. Gut *24*:767–771, 1983.

69. Madden JW, Ironside JW, Triger DR, Bradshaw JPP: An unusual case of Wilson's disease. Q J Med *55*:63–73, 1985.

70. Polio J, Enriquez RE, Chow A, Wood WM, Atterbury CE: Hepatocellular carcinoma in Wilson's disease. Case report and review of the literature. J Clin Gastroenterol *11*:220–224, 1989.

71. Rosenfield N, Garand RJ, Watkins JB: Cholelithiasis and Wilson's disease. J Pediatr *92*:210–215, 1978.

72. Denny-Brown D: Hepatolenticular degeneration (Wilson's disease). Two different components. N Engl J Med *270*:1149–1156, 1964.

73. Goldstein NP, Ewert JC, Randall RV, Gross JB: Psychiatric aspects of Wilson's disease (hepatolenticular degeneration): results of psychometric tests during long term therapy. Am J Psychiatry *124*:1555–1561, 1968.

74. Kendall BE, Pollock SS, Barr NM: Wilson's disease: clinical correlation with cranial computed tomography. Neuroradiology *22*:1–5, 1981.

75. Lawler GA, Pennock JM, Steiner RE: Nuclear magnetic resonance (NMR) imaging in Wilson disease. J Comput Assist Tomog *7*:1–8, 1983.

76. Fleming CR, Dickson ER, Wahner HW, Hollenhorst RW, McCall JT: Pigmented corneal rings in non-Wilsonian liver disease. Ann Intern Med *86*:285–288, 1977.

77. Frommer, D, Morris J, Sherlock S, Abrams J, Newman S: Kayser-Fleischer-like rings in patients without Wilson's disease. Gastroenterology *72*:1331–1335, 1977.

78. Giorgio AJ, Cartwright GE, Wintrobe MM: Pseudo-Kayser-Fleischer rings. Arch Intern Med *113*:817–818, 1961.

79. Cairns JE, Williams HP, Walshe JM: "Sunflower cataract" in Wilson's disease. Br Med J *3*:95–96, 1969.

80. Bearn AG, Yu TF, Gutman AB: Renal function in Wilson's disease. J Clin Invest *36*:1107–1114, 1957.

81. Danks DM: Disorders of copper transport. In *The Metabolic Basis of Inherited Disease,* edited by CR Scriver, AL Baudet, WS Sly, and D Valle, 6th Edition. New York, McGraw-Hill Book Co., 1989, pp. 1411–1231.

82. Leu M-L, Strickland GT: Renal function in heterozygotes for Wilson's disease. Am J Med Sci *263*:19–24, 1971.

83. Litin RB, Randall RV, Goldstein NP, Power MH, Dressner GR: Hypercalciuria in hepatolenticular degeneration (Wilson's disease). Am J Med Sci *252*:715–720, 1966.

84. Wieber DO, Wilson DM, McLeod RA: Renal stones in Wilson's disease. Am J Med *67*:249–254, 1979.

85. Carpenter TO, Carnes DL Jr, Anast CS: Hypoparathyroidism in Wilson's disease. N Engl J Med *309*:873–877, 1983.

86. McClure J, Smith PS: Calcium pyrophosphate dihydrate deposition in the intervertebral discs in a case of Wilson's disease. J Clin Pathol *36*:764–773, 1983.

87. Factor SM, Cho S, Sternlieb I, Scheinberg, IH, Goldfischer S: The cardiomyopathy of Wilson's disease: myocardial alterations in nine cases. Virch Arch A Pathol Anat *397*:301–311, 1982.

88. Stromeyer FW, Ishak KG: Histology of the liver in Wilson's disease. A study of 34 cases. Am J Clin Pathol *73:*12–24, 1980.
89. Ishak KG, Sharp HL: Metabolic errors and liver disease. *In* Pathology of the Liver, edited by R.N.M MacSween, P.P. Anthony, P.J. Scheuer. 2nd Edition. Edinburgh, Churchill Livingstone, 1987, pp 99–180.
90. Pearse AGE: Inorganic constituents and foreign substances. *In* Histochemistry, Theoretical and Applied, Vol. 2. 4th Edition. Edinburgh, Churchill-Livingstone, 1985, pp. 991–995.
91. Vaux DJT, Watt F, Grime GW, Takacs T: Hepatic copper distribution in primary biliary cirrhosis shown by the scanning proton microprobe. J Clin Pathol *38:*653–658, 1985.
92. Jain S, Scheuer PJ, Archer B, Newman SP, Sherlock S: Histologic demonstration of copper and copper-associated protein in chronic liver diseases. J Clin Pathol *31:*784–790, 1978.
93. Elmes ME, Clarkson JP, Mahy NJ, Jasani B: Metallothionein and copper in liver disease with copper retention: a histopathological study. J Pathol *158:*131–137, 1989.
94. Ludwig J, McDonald GSA, Dickson ER, Elveback LR, McCall JT: Copper stains and the syndrome of primary biliary cirrhosis. Evaluation of staining methods, and their usefulness for diagnosis and trials of penicillamine treatment. Arch Pathol Lab Med *103:* 467–470, 1979.
95. Sumithran E, Looi LM: Copper-binding protein in liver cells. Hum Pathol *16:*677–682, 1985.
96. Guigui B, Mavier P, Lescs M-C, Pinaudeau Y, Dhumeaux D, Zafrani ES: Copper and copper-binding protein in liver tumors. Cancer *61:*1155–1158, 1988.
97. Sternlieb I, Feldmann G: Effects of anticopper therapy on hepatocellular mitochondria in patients with Wilson's disease. An ultrastructural and stereological study. Gastroenterology *71:*457–461, 1976.
98. Sternlieb I, Scheinberg JJ: The prevention of clinical Wilson's disease. J Clin Invest *46:*1120–1128, 1967.
99. Walshe JM: Management of penicillamine nephropathy in Wilson's disease; a new chelating agent. Lancet *2:*1401–1402, 1969.
100. Walshe JM: Diagnosis and treatment of presymptomatic Wilson's disease. Lancet *2:*435–436, 1988.
101. Walshe JM: Treatment of Wilson's disease with trientine (triethylene tetramine) dihydrochloride. Lancet *1:*643–647, 1982.
102. Scheinberg IH, Jaffe ME, Sternlieb I: The use of trientine in preventing the effects of interrupting penicillamine in Wilson's disease. N Engl J Med *317:*209–213, 1987.
103. Van den Hamer CJA, Hoogenraad TU. ^{64}Cu loading tests for monitoring zinc therapy in Wilson's disease. Trace Elements Med *1:*84–87, 1984.
104. Brewer GJ, Hill GM, Prasad AS: A new treatment for Wilson's disease. Ann Intern Med *99:*314–320, 1983.
105. Brewer GJ: Zinc therapy for the treatment of Wilson's disease. Generics *1:*54–55, 1985.
106. Hill GM, Brewer GJ, June JE: Treatment of Wilson's disease with zinc. II. Validation of oral ^{64}copper with copper balance. Am J Med Sci *292:*344–349, 1986.
107. Hoogenraad TU, Van Den Hamer CJA: Three years of continuous oral zinc therapy in 4 patients with Wilson's disease. Acta Neurol Scand *67:*356–364, 1983.
108. Oelshlegel FJ, Brewer GJ: Absorption of pharmacological doses of zinc. *In* Zinc Metabolism: Current Aspects in Health and Disease, edited by A.S. Prasad, G.J. Brewer. New York, Alan R. Liss, 1977, pp. 299–311.
109. Polson RJ, Rolles K, Calne RY, Williams R, Marsden D: Reversal of severe neurological manifestations of Wilson's disease following orthotopic liver transplantation. Q J Med *244:*685–691, 1987.

Chapter 14
Hepatic Lesions in Disorders of Carbohydrate and Glycoprotein Metabolism

Disorders of carbohydrate metabolism

Diabetes mellitus

The liver plays the primary role in normal carbohydrate metabolism (1). It accepts carbohydrates and other glucogenic substances from the digestive tract, converts them to metabolizable monosaccharides, and, in times of plenty, stores the excess as glycogen. It is the largest source of glucose in the body. It provides glucose by glycogenolysis promptly when plasma glucose levels fall and it can maintain plasma glucose levels for long periods by gluconeogenesis from amino acids, glycerol, lactate, and other substrates. It responds to and modulates the effects of insulin, glucagon, catecholamines, and other hormones on carbohydrate metabolism.

In *type I diabetes mellitus,* insulin deficiency leads to increased hepatic gluconeogenesis, reduced utilization of absorbed glucose, and failure of the liver to suppress its output of glucose when hyperglycemia occurs. Insulin deficiency also stimulates ketogenesis as a result of increased lipolysis in adipose tissue, mobilization of free fatty acids to the liver, and enhanced β-oxidation of fatty acids, so that the liver is a key factor in the development of ketoacidosis when type I diabetes mellitus is uncontrolled (2).

Similar abnormalities in hepatic glucose metabolism occur in type II maturity-onset diabetes mellitus, but, usually, these are not accompanied by increased hepatic ketogenesis. The primary metabolic defect appears to be insulin resistance rather than a deficiency of insulin. The resistance to insulin in such cases may be attributable to the obesity that often accompanies the diabetes.

Many cirrhotic patients exhibit impairment of glucose tolerance, which appears to be of hepatogenous origin. Usually, the serum level of insulin in such cases is elevated, so insulin resistance rather than deficiency probably accounts for the defect in glucose homeostasis. Although the mechanism responsible for such insulin resistance is uncertain, several possible factors have been postulated, including portacaval shunting of insulin (3), potassium depletion, and increased secretion of glucagon and growth hormone (2).

A number of hepatic lesions may be encountered in patients with diabetes mellitus (4). These include steatosis, steatonecrosis, and cirrhosis.

Fatty infiltration. Many patients with type II diabetes mellitus exhibit fatty infiltration of the liver (4,5). Fatty infiltration is encountered in over half the patients with type II diabetes, but in only 5% of those with type I diabetes. The adipocytes show reduced responses to insulin (6).

In *type II diabetes,* neither the occurrence nor the extent of fatty infiltration correlates with the degree of control of hyperglycemia. Furthermore, the infiltration is not eradicated by maintaining a normal blood sugar level. This has led to the suggestion that the obesity commonly associated with this type of diabetes is more important than impairment of carbohydrate metabolism in the pathogenesis of fatty infiltration. However, obesity is not present in all cases, so other diabetes-related factors, such as increased mobilization of lipid from the depots, enhanced hepatic synthesis of triglyceride, or a defect in the transport of triglyceride out of the liver, may be implicated. Lesions of this type may be accompanied by mild hepatomegaly and slightly raised serum levels of alkaline phosphatase and transaminase, but do not produce any other clinical or laboratory manifestations.

The fatty infiltration in *type I diabetes* is more clearly related to insulin deficiency, and can be prevented, ameliorated, or abolished by the administration of insulin. Increased mobilization of lipid from the depots, enhanced hepatic triglyceride synthesis, and impairment of triglyceride export are the principal factors responsible for the accumulation of fat in the liver. When the diabetes is poorly controlled, and particularly when it is complicated by ketoacidosis, there may be enlargement of the liver, which is occasionally massive, and sometimes accompanied by the development of jaundice, ascites, and abdominal pain. Usually steatosis is responsible, but in some cases, insulin-induced glycogenosis is an important factor in the development of massive hepatomegaly.

The *histologic features* of diabetic, fatty infiltration are not specific. Frequently, many of the periportal hepatocytes contain glycogen-filled nuclei (Fig. 674). Although glycogen nuclei are suggestive, but not diagnostic of diabetes mellitus, they may also occur in Wilson's disease (Fig. 665), a wide variety of other hepatic disorders, and, often, in otherwise normal livers (Figs. 14, 15). The deposits of lipid are similarly nonspecific and are indistinguishable from those in the fatty infiltration of chronic alcoholism (Fig. 581), obesity, and other disorders. Occasionally, centrilobular hepatocytes are ballooned or show other degenerative changes, and some of the lobules contain rare acidophilic bodies or aggregates of swollen Kupffer cells, macrophages that may enclose lipid globules to form lipogranulomas (Fig. 176). Such changes, sometimes termed "diabetic hepatitis," may precede glucose intolerance (7). In some cases, particularly when fatty infiltration is extensive, the portal tracts and, to a lesser extent, the centrilobular zones show mild stellate fibrosis and lymphocytosis (Fig. 675).

Cirrhosis. The incidence of cirrhosis is two to three times higher in diabetics than in nondiabetic patients (5). However, the role of diabetes mellitus as an etiological factor in the pathogenesis of cirrhosis is still uncertain. In at least half the cases of patients with both diabetes and cirrhosis, the cirrhosis antedates the diabetes, so it is either coincidental or is involved in the pathogenesis of the diabetes. Since a family history of diabetes has been found to be almost three times as common in cirrhotic as in noncirrhotic patients, it is conceivable that cirrhosis precipitates diabetes in genetically predisposed individuals (8). These observations require confirmation. There are reasons to suspect that other etiologic factors, particularly chronic alcoholism and viral hepatitis, especially that caused by HCV, may be implicated in the development of cirrhosis in some diabetic patients (5). In occasional cases, hemochromatosis is responsible. Such observations support the generally accepted view that diabetes mellitus is not a significant etiologic factor in cirrhosis. Nevertheless, it may play a role in some cases. Of particular note in this connection are rare reports of biopsy-documented transitions from diabetic fatty infiltration to cirrhosis (9,10).

Except for hemochromatosis, the cirrhotic lesions associated with diabetes mellitus show no distinctive features. In our experience, most of the lesions are micronodular and often have been accompanied by some degree of fatty infiltration. However, in some published reports, macronodular cirrhosis, classified as postnecrotic, has predominated (11).

Lesions that mimic alcoholic hepatitis and cirrhosis in nonalcoholic patients. A small but significant number of nonalcololic patients present with hepatic lesions that are indistinguishable from those of alcoholic hepatitis and cirrhosis (12–15). Lesions of this type, which have been classified by some as ''nonalcoholic steatohepatitis'' (14), occur predominantly, but not exclusively, in middle-aged or elderly women with type II diabetes mellitus or obesity. Occasionally, this form of diabetic hepatitis may precede the onset of glucose intolerance by several years (7). Although the diabetes is emphasized as an etiologic factor in some reports (13) and the obesity in others (12), it should be noted that the lesions may occur in the absence of either or both, so the relative importance of these factors and their possible interrelationships are not known. However, the possibility that obesity may plan an important role in some cases is suggested by the occurrence of similar lesions resembling alcoholic hepatitis and cirrhosis following jejunoileal bypass for the treatment of massive obesity (16–18).

The clinical and laboratory manifestations of nonalcoholic steatohepatitis are similar to those in alcoholic hepatitis and cirrhosis. However, they tend to be less severe, and appear to progress more slowly. A high proportion of affected individuals exhibit evidence of nonhepatic medical disorders, for which they seek medical advice, after which their hepatic disease is discovered. In our own series of 27 patients, 21 of whom had cirrhosis by biopsy, 22 had other medical problems, of which ischemic heart disease was the most common. Only 12 presented for investigation or treatment of recognized liver disease (19).

The relationship of nonalcoholic steatohepatitis to antecedent fatty infiltration in diabetes mellitus or obesity is uncertain. Although it is conceivable that the steatonecrosis is a consequence of diabetes or obesity, neither we nor others have been able to document progression of fatty infiltration to steatonecrosis in nonalcoholic patients.

Figure 676 illustrates a typical example of nonalcoholic steatohepatitis during its late cirrhotic phase. The lesion is characterized by diffuse fibrosis, micronodule formation, and extensive fatty infiltration. In addition, it shows erosion of the limiting plates and scattered, periseptal, ballooned cells, Mallory bodies, and neutrophils, features indistinguishable from those of alcoholic cirrhosis (Fig. 677).

Insulin-induced glycogenosis. Insulin and hyperglycemia increase glycogen synthesis and inhibit glycogenolysis, resulting in increased deposition of glycogen in the liver. In some cases of type I diabetes mellitus and, occasionally, in type II diabetes that requires large doses of insulin, the deposition of glycogen, often accompanied by hepatic retention of water, produces massive hepatomegaly that may be accompanied by abdominal pain, jaundice, or ascites (20–22). Hepatomegaly of this type may occur acutely during the treatment of ketoacidosis, or insidiously in patients undergoing prolonged therapy with large doses of insulin. Under both conditions, the lesions, which are characterized by excessive deposits of glycogen in most hepatocytes, tend to regress when the dose of insulin is reduced. Characteristically, the affected hepatocytes, which are enlarged and obscure the sinusoids, contain pale, finely vacuolated cytoplasm and small, dark nuclei and are outlined by prominent, relatively straight, and sharply angulated plasma membranes that produce a characteristic, mosaic pattern (Fig. 184).

Occasionally, diabetic patients who receive small or moderate doses of insulin may also exhibit focal glycogenosis characterized by sharply circumscribed groups of enlarged, pale hepatocytes with prominent, straight, sharply angulated plasma membranes (Fig. 185). Such lesions may be single or multiple, but have no clinical significance.

Mauriac's syndrome. Rarely, children with insulin-dependent, poorly controlled diabetes mellitus exhibit retardation of growth and sexual development, obesity, a florid facies, massive hepatomegaly, and hypercholesterolemia, a constellation known as the Mauriac syndrome (23). Characteristically, the liver shows massive deposition of glycogen, only occasionally accompanied by fatty infiltration.

Although the possibility of primary pituitary dysfunction has been considered to explain this disorder, it is more likely that the failure in growth and sexual development is attributable to poorly controlled diabetes, and the hepatic glycogenosis to the large doses of insulin used in therapy.

Hereditary glycogen storage diseases

Ten types of hereditary glycogen storage disease (glycogenosis) have been identified (24–26). Each is characterized by a specific enzyme deficiency that leads to the accumulation of glycogen in the tissues. With the exception of types VI and VIII, they are transmitted as autosomal recessive traits. The sites of the enzymatic defects, the character and distribution of the glycogen deposits, and the nature of the associated lesions differ in each of the glycogenoses, although they overlap to some extent. Only those types that affect the liver are included in the following discussion.

Type I glycogenosis (von Gierke's disease, hepatorenal glycogenosis). Type I glycogenosis is characterized by insufficient hepatic and renal *glucose-6-phosphatase* (G-6-P), which blocks the conversion of glucose-6-phosphate to glucose, resulting in hypoglycemia and the accumulation of glycogen in the liver and kidneys. Type Ia glycogen storage disease is caused by a deficiency of G-6-P, but a clinically indistinguishable variant, Type Ib, has normal G-6-P activity, but does not transport the enzyme normally (27,28). Type Ib may occur in adults (29). Secondarily, the hypoglycemia in both variants leads to increased mobilization of lipid from the depots, giving rise to hyperlipemia, ketosis, and fatty infiltration of the liver.

Usually, the clinical manifestations appear during the neonatal period, and are characterized by hypoglycemic convulsions and hepatomegaly. Later, there is stunting of growth, enlargement of the kidneys, a tendency to obesity, and increased susceptibility to fatal, intercurrent infections during the first two years of life. Other, less common features include xanthomatosis, gouty tophi, and uric acid nephropathy. Frequently, the manifestations abate after the age of six years. The syndrome can appear in adults (30).

Therapy with frequent feeding of glucose and starchy foods has recently been supplemented by the administration of uncooked cornstarch (31) or other carbohydrates that release glucose slowly (32). Portacaval anastomosis has been used successfully in patients not responding to diet therapy (33). Liver transplantation has been reported to prolong survival (34).

The principal biochemical alterations include fasting hypoglycemia that does not respond to glucagon or epinephrine, chronic lactic acidosis, hyperuricemia, and raised serum levels of cholesterol, fatty acids, and triglycerides. Except for slightly increased serum transaminase levels in some cases, there is no other biochemical evidence of hepatocellular dysfunction.

The prominent histologic features of the *hepatic lesions* in type I glycogenosis include excessive deposits of glycogen, a variable degree of fatty infiltration, and, usually, the presence of glycogen nuclei. With the exception of those that contain lipid droplets, most of the hepatocytes are distended by the glycogen deposits. Characteristically, the hepatocytes are greatly enlarged, and appear thereby to compress sinusoids. They contain pale, finely vacuolated cytoplasm and small, centrally located, dark nuclei and are outlined by prominent, relatively straight, angulated plasma membranes that create a characteristic, mosaic pattern (Fig. 678). This pattern may be caused by the straight borders of the distended cells with small, regular central nuclei and inconspicuous, compressed sinusoids. The glycogen nuclei, similar to those seen in diabetes mellitus (Fig. 674) and other disorders (Figs. 14, 15, 665), are often seen. Mallory bodies and centrilobular pericellular fibrosis have been reported (35).

The glycogen and lipid deposits are unaccompanied by hepatocellular degeneration or necrosis, and show no tendency to provoke portal fibrosis or cirrhosis. However, the development of hepatic adenomas has been reported in patients with type I glycogenosis late in the course of the disease (36). Occasionally, hepatocellular carcinoma has been encountered in type I glycogenosis (37,38).

The glycogen deposits in type I glycogenosis are readily demonstrable histochemically in alcohol- or Carnoy's-fixed specimens of liver by means of the PAS or Best's carmine stain, and characteristically are digested by diastase. However, such staining methods are of little value in establishing the increased glycogen content of the liver in type I glycogenosis or in differentiating the latter from other forms of glycogenosis. Reliable identification of the disease depends on the biochemical documentation of glucose-6-phosphatase deficiency in the liver or kidneys.

Type II glycogenosis (Pompe's disease).

Type II glycogenosis, is characterized by a deficiency of lysosomal *acid α-glucosidase* (acid maltase), which leads to an accumulation of glycogen in most tissues, but especially in skeletal muscle, myocardium, and, to a lesser extent, in the liver (39,40).

When the disease presents in infancy, usually at the age of three or four years, the principal clinical manifestations include progressive muscular weakness, respiratory distress, marked cardiomegaly, cardiac arrhythmias, macroglossia, and slight hepatomegaly. As a rule, death from cardiac or respiratory failure ensues within a year.

The form of type II glycogenosis that appears in late childhood or early adult life is characterized by progressive muscular weakness that mimics muscular dystrophy, and usually proves fatal within a decade. There are no accompanying manifestations of cardiac or hepatic involvement.

Hypoglycemia is not a feature of type II glycogenosis, and the blood sugar responses to glucagon and epinephrine administration are normal.

The only histologic feature of the *hepatic lesions* in type II glycogenosis is the presence within the hepatocytes of numerous uniformly distributed, fine, cytoplasmic vacuoles. These vacuoles represent enlarged lysosomes filled with glycogen, as shown by electron microscopy, their reactivity with PAS, and their susceptibility to digestion by diastase. The diagnosis of type II glycogenosis has been made *in utero* by electron microscopic examination of amniotic fluid (41). The hepatocytes are only minimally enlarged, show a normal hepatic plate pattern, and contain no glycogen nuclei or fat droplets. The portal tracts are normal, and the lesions show no tendency to undergo fibrosis. Lymphocytes, both in the circulation and in the bone marrow, contain the same type of fine, PAS-positive, cytoplasmic vacuoles found in the hepatocytes, a feature that is helpful in identifying type II glycogenosis.

Type III glycogenosis (Cori's disease, limit dextrinosis).

The underlying defect in type III glycogenosis is a deficiency of the debranching enzyme, *amylo-1, 6-glucosidase,* which leads to the deposition in the liver, skeletal muscle, and myocardium of an abnormal type of glycogen characterized by excessively long outer branches (42,43).

The clinical manifestations rarely appear before the age of one year and vary, depending on the severity and distribution of the enzyme defect. However, in most cases, the signs and symptoms resemble those of type I glycogenosis, although they may be less severe. The disease tends to abate during puberty, so survival into adulthood is relatively common. In cases with predominantly skeletal muscle and myocardial muscle involvement, the principal manifestations are muscular weakness, hypotonia, and cardiomegaly. Therapy with cornstarch has caused improvement in the hepatic abnormalities and in growth (44).

The *hepatic lesions* closely resemble those in type I glycogenosis, but, in addition, may show a variable degree of portal fibrosis that occasionally progresses to cirrhosis (Fig. 182). Despite their abnormal biochemical structure, the hepatocellular glycogen deposits stain with PAS (Fig. 183) and are readily digested by diastase. Numerous enlarged, vacuolated glycogen nuclei are found in the periportal hepatocytes (Fig. 183). In many cases, some of the portal tracts are enlarged and fibrotic (Fig. 679), and, rarely, there is portal-portal bridging fibrosis and nodule formation, giving rise to macronodular cirrhosis. The cirrhotic lesion illustrated in Figure 680 was encountered in a six-year-old boy with biochemically documented type III glycogenosis who had had recurrent, hypoglycemic convulsions since the age of one year, and who presented with hepatosplenomegaly.

Type IV glycogenosis (Andersen's disease, amylopectinosis). The underlying defect in this very rare disease is a deficiency of the glycogen branching enzyme *amylo-1, 4-1, 6-transglucosidase* (45). As a result, an abnormal glycogen, resembling amylopectin and characterized by few branch points and elongated outer chains, accumulates in the liver and other tissues.

The principal clinical manifestations include hepatosplenomegaly, additional signs of cirrhosis, hypotonia, and failure to thrive. These appear during early childhood and usually prove fatal in 1 to 10 years as a result of hepatic failure. Rarely, death is due to cardiac failure.

The outstanding feature of the *hepatic lesions* is the presence within numerous periportal and periseptal hepatocytes of distinctive cytoplasmic inclusions (46) that closely resemble those in Lafora's disease (47) and the pseudo-Lafora bodies produced by drugs such as disulfiram (48) and cyanamide (49) and a variety of other cytoplasmic inclusions (see Chapter 4). These present as pale, non-membrane-bound, round or kidney-shaped, homogeneous or finely granular, faintly eosinophilic inclusions that displace the nuclei to the periphery of the cells, and often are encircled by a narrow clear halo (Fig. 148). Identical cytoplasmic inclusions are seen in the central nervous system and in other tissues (46). In contrast to HBsAg-positive ground glass cells for which they may be mistaken, Lafora-like bodies do not stain with orcein or aldehyde fuchsin, show a periportal zonal distribution, and are intensely PAS-positive (Fig. 149). Characteristically, PAS reactivity is abolished by pectinase, but not by diastase digestion. On electron microscopy, Lafora bodies appear as non-membrane-bound, globular masses of randomly arranged, branching filaments interspersed with occasional, normal-appearing, glycogen rosettes. Occasionally, some of the Kupffer cells and portal macrophages are enlarged and contain PAS-positive amylopectin-like granular deposits. Fatty infiltration is an inconstant feature.

As the lesions advance, there is progressive enlargement and fibrosis of the portal tracts accompanied by a mononuclear inflammatory reaction and ductular proliferation, ultimately leading to portal-portal bridging fibrosis, nodule formation, and the development of cirrhosis.

Type VI glycogenosis (Hers' disease).

Type VI glycogenosis, is characterized by a deficiency of hepatic *phosphorylase*, which leads to an accumulation of glycogen in the liver (43,50). Muscular phosphorylase is not affected. The mode of transmission is uncertain, but appears to be autosomal dominant with variable penetrance.

Hepatomegaly and growth retardation, which are apparent during early childhood, are the principal clinical manifestations. Hypoglycemia, hyperlipemia, acidosis, and resistance to glucagon-induced hyperglycemia are inconstant features. Survival into adulthood is the rule.

The *hepatic lesions* are similar to those in type I glycogenosis with the following exceptions: (1) the hepatocellular enlargement, mosaic pattern, and glycogen infiltration of the hepatocytes are patchy in distribution; (2) vacuolated glycogen nuclei are absent; and (3) portal fibrosis is encountered in some cases, but cirrhosis has not been reported.

Type VIII glycogenosis.

Type VIII glycogenosis is inherited as an X-linked recessive trait and is characterized by a deficiency of *phosphorylase b kinase*, which leads to the accumulation of glycogen in the liver and central nervous system (43).

Hepatomegaly and progressive degeneration of the central nervous system, which appear in infancy or early childhood, are the principal clinical manifestations. Hypoglycemia and resistance to glucagon-induced hyperglycemia are not features of the disease. Usually, death ensues within a few years.

The *hepatic lesions* are characterized by glycogen-distended hepatocytes with prominent plasma membranes producing a mosaic pattern that is irregular in distribution and most prominent in the periportal zones. There is no accompanying fibrosis or vacuolization of the nuclei.

Type IX glycogenosis.

Two biochemically distinguishable forms of type IX glycogenosis have been identified, one inherited as an autosomal recessive trait (IXa), the other as a sex-linked recessive trait (IXb) (43). In both forms, there is a defect in hepatic phosphorylase activation, resulting in the accumulation of glycogen in the liver.

Hepatomegaly is the principal clinical manifestation of the disease, which tends to run a benign course. Hypoglycemia is not a feature, and the hyperglycemic response to glucagon is normal.

The *hepatic lesions* resemble those in type VIII glycogenosis. Cirrhosis is not a component in the syndrome.

Galactosemia

Congenital galactosemia, an autosomal recessive hereditary disorder (51–53), is characterized by a deficiency of galactose-1-phosphate uridyl transferase that blocks the conversion of galactose-1-phosphate (Gal-1-P) to uridine diphosphogalactose, an essential step in the normal metabolism of galactose (54). As a result, Gal-1-P accumulates in the tissues, leading to hepatic, renal, ocular, and central nervous system damage. Full expression of the disease occurs exclusively in homozygous carriers of the galactosemia gene, which is located on chromosome 3 (55). However, heterozygotes exhibit slightly reduced levels of Gal-1-P uridyl transferase, and may be mildly intolerant of galactose (51,52). The clinical manifestations of galactosemia are provoked by the ingestion of milk or other dietary sources of galactose, and, with the exception of mental retardation, are readily preventable or reversible if the intake of milk and other sources of galactose is promptly discontinued once the disease is recognized (55–58). It has been suggested that in infants with severe disease that appears soon after birth, hepatic injury may begin *in utero* due to transplacental passage of galactose in the case of mothers who exhibits galactosemia during the last week or two of gestation (56).

The clinical manifestations and age at onset in galactosemia may vary (56,57). In classic cases, vomiting, diarrhea, and weight loss appear soon after feeding of milk is begun, usually within the first week or two of life. Unless milk is withdrawn, these are followed over a period of weeks or months by the development of jaundice, hepatosplenomegaly, cataracts, and mental retardation. In such cases, death from hepatic failure, other complications of cirrhosis, or intercurrent infection ensues within a few weeks or months.

The onset of overt disease in less severely affected infants may be delayed for months or even years, the early manifestations being characterized by feeding difficulties, retarded growth, occasional vomiting, and mental retardation. Ultimately, the more distinctive features of the disease, including hepatomegaly, cataracts, and galactosuria, become apparent.

Hereditary galactokinase deficiency is another disorder of galactose metabolism that causes galactosemia and galactosuria (59), but it causes no hepatic lesions.

The principal biochemical abnormalities in fully developed galactosemia include galactosuria, aminoaciduria, proteinuria, and progressive hepatocellular dysfunction. Occasionally, the rise in serum galactose levels following the ingestion of milk or other galactose-containing foods is accompanied by hypoglycemia, which may be symptomatic. Often, the presence of reducing material in the urine provides the first clue to the diagnosis. Although this substance reacts with Benedict's solution or Clini-Test tablets, it fails to react with test strips impregnated with glucose oxidase (Clinistix), features that differentiate galactose from glucose. More precise identification of galactose in urine requires chromatographic analysis. However, the diagnosis of galactosemia should always be confirmed by demonstrating a deficiency of Gal-1-P uridyl transferase. This is carried out most conveniently in a hemolysate of packed red cells, and has the advantage that it is applicable to cord blood, so the disease can be identified at birth, a feature of particular importance in newborns with a family history of galactosemia. In fact, the diagnosis has been established *in utero* (60).

The principal features of the hepatic lesions in galactosemia include fatty infiltration, transformation of the hepatic plates into acinar or duct-like structures, bile stasis, ductular proliferation, and fibrosis that ultimately may progress to cirrhosis. Fatty infiltration is extensive and usually appears early, although it tends to diminish as the lesions advance (Figs. 681, 682). Characteristically, many of the hepatocytes are ballooned and are arranged in the form of acini or pseudoducts, some of which contain lumens filled with inspissated bile (Fig. 682). Giant cell transformation of hepatocytes may be seen (61).

Ductular proliferation is another early feature that is usually accompanied by expansion and fibrosis of the portal tracts and infiltration of the portal zones with neutrophils, lymphocytes, and PAS-positive macrophages (Fig. 683).

As the lesions advance, portal fibrosis increases progressively, leading to the development of portal-portal bridges, distortion of the normal lobular architecture (Fig. 681), and, eventually, cirrhosis. Usually, the septa are relatively slender, but, in some cases, they may be broad.

Rarely, the hepatic lesions are accompanied by hepatocellular adenomas, which are discovered at autopsy (62).

All features of the hepatic lesions, including the fibrosis, tend to regress following the withdrawal of milk and other dietary sources of galactose (58). In at least one reported case with an advanced hepatic lesion, follow-up needle biopsy suggested that cirrhosis had undergone complete resolution within a few months (58). Long-term survival with cirrhosis has been observed occasionally.

Hereditary fructose intolerance

Two types of hereditary fructose intolerance have been identified, the most common attributable to a deficiency of fructose-1-phosphate aldolase, the other to a deficiency of fructose-1,6-diphosphatase.

Fructose-1-phosphate aldolase deficiency. This hereditary disorder, transmitted as an autosomal recessive trait, is charac-

terized by a marked deficiency of hepatic *fructose-1-phosphate aldolase* or a less severe, inconstant deficiency of hepatic *fructose-1,6-diphosphate aldolase* (63–65). The resulting accumulation of fructose-1-phosphate in the former disorder leads to hepatic and renal injury. In addition, due to a secondary deficiency of fructose-1,6-diphosphate and depletion of intracellular ATP and inorganic phosphorus, gluconeogenesis and glycogenolysis are inhibited, resulting in hypoglycemia and increased mobilization of free fatty acids from lipid depots.

Clinical manifestations appear soon after the introduction of fructose into the diet in the form of sucrose or fruit. The severity of the disorder depends on how early in life fructose administration is begun. In infants fed fructose before the age of six months, the onset is abrupt, with abdominal pain, anorexia, vomiting, and weight loss. Soon thereafter, signs of hepatic and renal impairment appear. These include hepatomegaly, jaundice, ascites, lactic acidosis, aminoaciduria, proteinuria, and, sometimes, disseminated intravascular coagulopathy (66). Fructosuria and glycosuria are less constant features. Progression to growth retardation (67), cirrhosis, and death from hepatic failure or intercurrent infection may ensue if the nature of the disease is not recognized and fructose administration is continued. Usually, withdrawal of fructose from the diet leads to a prompt remission in all signs and symptoms of the disease.

If fructose administration is delayed until after the age of six months, the manifestations may be mild or absent. However, a distaste for sweets and hepatomegaly are relatively common. The absence of dental cavities in such patients is a minor beneficial aspect of the syndrome. Growth and development are not affected.

The principal biochemical findings during the acute phase of the disease in young infants are fructosuria, fructosemia, metabolic acidosis, hypoglycemia, and delayed clearance of fructose from the serum following its administration.

The *hepatic lesions* in the early active phase of the disease resemble those of galactosemia and are characterized by fatty infiltration, pseudoacinar arrangement of the hepatocytes, bile stasis, varying degrees of portal fibrosis, and cirrhosis. Occasionally, the lesions present as neonatal hepatitis with giant cell transformation of the parenchyma (68). The cirrhosis in hereditary fructose intolerance is usually described as early or mild (69).

Fructose-1,6-diphosphatase deficiency. This rare autosomal recessive hereditary disorder is characterized by a deficiency of hepatic *fructose-1,6-diphosphatase* (70,71). Its clinical manifestations, recurrent lactic acidosis, hypoglycemia, and hepatomegaly, appear in early infancy following the introduction into the diet of fructose in the form of sucrose or fruit. Withdrawal of fructose leads promptly to remission of all signs and symptoms. Rarely, failure to discontinue the intake of fructose is fatal.

Fructose-1,6-diphosphatase is required for the synthesis of glucose from its precursors, especially lactate and amino acids, such as alanine. Therefore, its absence blocks gluconeogenesis. Following an oral test dose of fructose in affected infants, there is a sharp increase in the serum levels of fructose, lactate, pyruvate, ketones, and free fatty acids, and a marked fall in the concentration of glucose and inorganic phosphorus. These changes are diagnostic of the disorder.

The *hepatic lesions* in this form of fructose intolerance are characterized by fatty infiltration without accompanying hepatocellular degeneration, inflammation, or fibrosis. On direct analysis, the liver shows little or no fructose-1,6-diphosphatase activity, but contains a normal complement of the other enzymes involved in fructose metabolism.

Disorders of glycoprotein metabolism

Mucopolysaccharidoses

A number of hereditary disorders are characterized by a deficiency of specific lysosomal enzymes involved in the catabolism of mucopolysaccharrides (26,71). As a result, there is widespread deposition of mucopolysaccharides in the tissues and excretion of their partially degraded metabolites in the urine. Except for type II (Hunter's syndrome), which is X-linked, all the other mucopolysaccharidoses are transmitted as autosomal recessive traits.

Differentiation between the various forms of mucopolysaccharidosis depends on the clinical manifestations and identification of the specific enzyme deficiency involved by assaying leukocytes or cultured skin fibroblasts. In five of the seven forms of mucopolysaccharidosis that have been identified, the liver and spleen are involved. Only these five are discussed here.

The *hepatic lesions* in all five are remarkably similar, and cannot be differentiated on histologic grounds alone. Due to the deposition of mucopolysaccharide in their lysosomes, both the hepatocytes and Kupffer cells are swollen, and contain pale, vacuolated, and reticulated cytoplasm. This is illustrated in Figure 186, showing the appearance of the hepatic parenchyma in a case of Hurler's syndrome. Histochemical demonstration of mucopolysaccharide may be difficult, since it tends to leach out in most aqueous fixatives. However, fixation in Lindsay's dioxane-picrate followed by staining with colloidal iron are suitable for this purpose. Mucopolysaccharide stains only weakly with PAS and is resistant to diastase digestion. However, it is readily digested by hyaluronidase and reacts metachromatically with toluidine blue.

Varying degrees of fibrosis, both portal and parasinusoidal, are relatively common, particularly in older children, and may progress to either micronodular or macronodular cirrhosis.

Mucopolysaccharidosis, type I (MP I, Hurler's syndrome). MP I, the most common form of mucopolysaccharidosis, is characterized by a deficiency of *α-L-iduronidase*, which blocks the normal degradation of MP, resulting in its accumulation in the tissues, and the urinary excretion of its partially degraded metabolites, dermatan sulfate and heparan sulfate (71,72). Full expression of the disease is limited to homozygous carriers of the MP I gene; heterozygotes may exhibit a similar, but less severe enzyme deficiency. The diagnosis can be made by a deficiency of the enzyme in leukocytes (73).

Clinical manifestations appear during the first year or two of life and include coarsening and distortion of the facial features that produce a gargoyle-like appearance, progressive retardation of growth and mental development, skeletal abnormalities, hepatosplenomegaly, vascular and cardiac anomalies, and clouding of the corneas. Death almost always occurs before the age of 10 years.

Mucopolysaccharidosis, type II (MP II, Hunter's syndrome). The enzyme defect in this disorder is a deficiency of *α-L-iduronidase sulfatase* that leads to the accumulation of MP in the tissues and the urinary excretion of dermatan sulfate and heparan sulfate (71).

The clinical manifestations are similar to those in MP I, except for the absence of corneal opacification.

Mucopolysaccharidosis, type III (MP III, Sanfilippo's syndrome). MP III occurs in four phenotypically identical forms with different enzyme defects: type A, which results from a deficiency of *heparitin sulfatase;* type B, from a deficiency of N-*acetyl-α-D-glucosidase;* and types C and D, in which the precise nature of the defect remains unknown (71). Accumulation of MP in the tissues and urinary excretion of heparan sullate occur in both types. Except for the absence of corneal opacities, the clinical manifestations are similar to those in MP I.

Mucopolysaccharidosis, type IV (MP IV, Morquio's syndrome). MP IV is characterized by a deficiency of *arylsulfatase* and urinary excretion of keratosulfate (71).

The clinical features include severe skeletal deformities, progressive corneal opacification, hepatosplenomegaly, and aortic regurgitation, which appear in late childhood. There is no accompanying mental retardation.

Mucopolysaccharidosis, type VI (MP VI). MP VI results from a deficiency of *arylsulfatase B* (71). Clinically the pattern is similar to that of Hurler's syndrome (MP I) except that mental deterioration is not present early in childhood. The hepatosplenomegaly, skeletal abnormalities, and corneal opacification are less severe than in MP I.

Mucopolysaccharidosis, type VII (MP VII). MP VII is attributable to a deficiency of *β-glucuronidase,* and is characterized by mental retardation, dysostosis multiplex, hepatosplenomegaly, urinary excretion of dermatan sulfate and chondroitin-4,6-sulfate, and susceptibility to recurrent pulmonary infections (71,74).

Mannosidosis

Mannosidosis, a rare autosomal recessive hereditary disorder that resembles mucopolysaccharidosis, is characterized by a deficiency of the lysosomal enzymes *acidic α-mannosidase A and B* (75,76). As a result, mannose-rich oligosaccharides accumulate in the tissues, and are greatly increased in the urine. Assays of leukocytes or cultured skin fibroblasts are used to identify the enzyme deficiency.

The principal clinical features, which usually appear during the second year of life, include retardation of growth and mental development, coarse facial features similar to the gargoylism of Hurler's syndrome, opacification of the corneas and lenticular cataracts, hepatosplenomegaly, x-ray evidence of dysostosis multiplex, deafness, and susceptibility to recurrent infections. Some patients survive into adulthood.

The *hepatic lesions* are characterized by the presence of numerous PAS-negative vacuoles in the cytoplasm of the hepatocytes. On electron microscopy, the vacuoles present as large lysosomes filled with amorphous, filamentous or membranous material (77).

Fucosidosis

Fucosidosis, another autosomal recessive hereditary disorder that resembles mucopolysaccharidosis, is characterized by a severe deficiency or absence in all tissues of the lysosomal enzyme α-1-fucosidase (26,78,79). As a result, fucose-containing glycoproteins, glycolipids, polysaccharides, and oligosaccharides accumulate in the tissues.

The principal clinical manifestations include retardation of growth and mental development, neurologic deficits, skeletal abnormalities, thickening of the skin, gargoyl-like facies, hepatosplenomegaly, and susceptibility to recurrent respiratory infections.

In some cases (type I), the disease is rapidly progressive and proves fatal before the age of six years. In others (type II), the course of the disease is relatively slow, so survival to adolescence or early adulthood is possible. A distinctive feature in such slowly progressive fucosidosis is the occurrence of a generalized skin eruption known as angiokeratoma. There is no apparent difference in the enzyme in the two types of fucosidosis (80).

The *hepatic lesions* in fucosidosis are similar to those in Hurler's syndrome, being characterized by swelling and cytoplasmic vacuolization of the hepatocytes and Kupffer cells.

Mucolipidosis

A group of rare, hereditary, lysosomal storage diseases, classified as mucolipidoses, are characterized by multiple defects in the metabolism of mucopolysaccharides, lipids, and glycoproteins (66,81–83). However, the specific enzyme defects in the various forms of mucolipidosis have not been clearly identified.

Several of the mucolipidoses exhibit clinical features that resemble those of Hurler's syndrome, but are unaccompanied by an increase in the urinary excretion of mucopolysaccharides. The hepatic lesions in such cases are characterized by vacuolization of the cytoplasm of the hepatocytes, Kupffer cells, and portal macrophages.

Alpha-1-antitrypsin deficiency

Alpha-$_1$-antitrypsin (A_1AT), a glycoprotein of relatively low molecular weight (54,000) that inhibits trypsin and other proteases, is synthesized in the liver and secreted into the serum where it circulates at a concentration of 200 to 300 mg/dl (84–86). It comprises approximately 90% of the α-1-globulins.

The gene locus for A_1AT is on chromosome 14 (87). Over 30 alleles of the A_1AT gene have been identified in the protease inhibitor (Pi) system based on their relative electrophoretic mobilities on starch gel followed by immunoelectrophoresis, or by means of isoelectric focusing. The phenotype in all individuals is determined by codominant inheritance of one gene from each parent, and is expressed as Pi followed by two alphabetic letters, their sequence in the alphabet varying inversely with their relative electrophoretic mobility, the A protein migrating most rapidly and Z most slowly. Rarely, a null gene is present, making differentiation between homozygotes and heterozygotes, as in the case of Pi MM and Pi M null, difficult, and requiring special studies for their identification. The use of monoclonal antibodies specific for the mutant α-1-antitrypsin in an ELISA procedure is a relatively simple, precise method for identifying carriers of the Pi Z gene (88).

The A_1AT phenotype in 90 to 95% of normal individuals is Pi MM (89). Such individuals exhibit normal serum levels of A_1AT and no evidence of related hepatic or pulmonary disease.

Usually, A_1AT deficiency is associated with the Pi Z gene, which occurs in approximately 1% of the population. Rarely, similarly low serum levels of A_1AT are attributable to Pi null or Pi PZ A_1AT deficiency. Low levels may also be observed in patients with massive hepatic necrosis or severe protein-losing diseases.

Homozygous Pi ZZ A_1AT deficiency. Characteristically, the serum concentration of A_1AT in Pi ZZ homozygotes is less than 20% of normal, a level sufficiently low to permit its recognition by the absence of an α-1-globulin peak in routine electrophoretic patterns of the serum proteins.

Two-thirds of infants with homozygous Pi ZZ develop hepatic disease (90). It has been estimated that from 10 to 20% of infants with neonatal cholestasis have underlying Pi ZZ A_1AT deficiency. The hepatic lesions in such cases may present as (1) neonatal hepatitis with or without partial giant cell transformation of the liver (91); (2) neonatal cholestasis with or without a paucity of intrahepatic bile ducts (92,93), or (3) progressive, neonatal cholestasis with portal fibrosis and ductular proliferation (92,93). In most infants, the cholestasis tends to regress, but, in about 15%, the hepatic lesions progress to cirrhosis (94).

In both homozygous and heterozygous carriers of the Pi Z gene, the periportal hepatocytes contain distinctive diastase-resistant, PAS-positive, globular, cytoplasmic inclusions of A_1AT, irrespective of whether or not other hepatic lesions are present (Figs. 152,153).

In a small but significant number of older children, homozygous Pi ZZ A_1AT deficiency may be associated with macronodular or mixed micro/macronodular cirrhosis. Usually, the onset in such cases is insidious, and there is no history of antecedent neonatal cholestasis. Rarely, the cirrhosis is accompanied by panlobular emphysema, a complication much more commonly seen in adults than in children.

Adults with homozygous Pi ZZ A_1AT deficiency only occasionally present with cirrhosis, although about 50% of those older than 50 years have cirrhosis (95). It often presents at that age as a cryptogenic cirrhosis (96). More commonly, patients exhibit a panlobular form of emphysema that appears early in adult life and that affects primarily the lower lobes of the lungs. Occasionally, hepatic and pulmonary lesions occur in combination. However, only a minority of adult Pi ZZ carriers exhibit either type of lesion. Men with Pi ZZ A_1AT deficiency have an increased risk of developing hepatocellular carcinoma (97).

Heterozygous A_1AT deficiency. The clinical significance of heterozygous A_1AT deficiency (Pi MZ and Pi SZ), in which serum levels of A_1AT average approximately 60% of normal, in the pathogenesis of hepatic and pulmonary disease is not known. Although there are sporadic reports of cirrhosis and chronic active hepatitis or pulmonary emphysema in some affected individuals, more extensive studies have failed to confirm a relationship between such lesions and heterozygous A_1AT deficiency.

Distinctive Pi Z A_1AT hepatocellular cytoplasmic inclusion. In both homozygous and heterozygous carriers of the Pi Z gene, many of the periportal hepatocytes contain sharply circumscribed, globular cytoplasmic inclusions, some of which may be encircled by a halo, which is an artifact of fixation. These inclusion bodies, which are usually multiple, vary in size from 1 to 30 μm in diameter (98). Except for enlargement of the hepatocytes that contain multiple globules, the cells otherwise appear normal. In routine H & E sections, the inclusions are faintly eosinophilic (Fig. 152), and may be difficult to visualize when small. They stain brilliantly red with PAS and are resistant to diastase digestion (Fig. 153). They tend to show a peripheral ring of positivity with less intense staining in the centers of the globules (98). These globules exhibit autofluorescence under ultraviolet light (99). They appear to be present in greater numbers in homozygous than in heterozygous patients (100). These inclusions represent A_1AT in the dilated cisternae of the smooth and rough endoplasmic reticulum as shown by their appearance on electron microscopy, and by their reactivity with appropriately labeled antibody to A_1AT (88). In some cases, deposits of A_1AT can be detected in the cytoplasm of hepatocytes in the absence of D-PAS-positive globules (101,102).

Similar, PAS-positive, diastase-resistant globules may be seen in conditions other than A_1AT deficiency. They tend to occur in the livers of patients with sinusoidal congestion and centrilobular hypoxia (103). Identical cytoplasmic inclusions are often seen in the neoplastic cells of patients with hepatocellular carcinoma (104,105) and other tumors (106). These pseudo-A_1AT globules tend to be distributed in perivenular or periacinar hepatocytes in contrast to true A_1AT inclusions, which tend to appear in periportal hepatocytes. On the basis of the lobular distribution alone, one can assume with a high degree of certainty that such inclusions in periportal cells represent A_1AT (107). Furthermore, they do not show the characteristic ultraviolet autofluorescence of A_1AT bodies (99). These pseudoglobules may contain a variety of substances, including fibrinogen, gamma globulin, or albumin (98,103).

The A_1AT cytoplasmic inclusions tend to be small in young infants, and may be impossible to identify in D-PAS-stained sections before the age of 12 weeks. Immunofluorescent or immunoperoxidase methods may identify these inclusions (100).

Not all diastase-resistant, PAS-positive, hepatocellular globules are indicative of A_1AT deficiency. The possibility of such deficiency must therefore be confirmed by measurement of serum levels of A_1AT, or by immunologic antibody reactions. We and others (108) have encountered such non-A_1AT, D-PAS-resistant inclusions in a variety of lesions, but most frequently in active alcoholic liver disease (Fig. 154) and in patients with cytoplasmic bile stasis. Sometimes, hepatocellular carcinoma cells contain D-PAS-positive, globular deposits of A_1AT in the absence of similar inclusions in adjacent, non-neoplastic hepatocytes, and in the absence of other evidence of A_1AT deficiency. In such cases, it is presumed that the neoplastic cells synthesize and accumulate A_1AT locally (109).

Pathogenesis of hepatic injury associated with A_1AT deficiency. It has been proposed that the accumulation of Pi ZZ A_1AT injures hepatocytes. Although there is no correlation between the amount deposited in the liver and the degree of injury, patients who have no A_1AT globules do not develop liver disease (110). On the other hand, in some individuals with severe A_1AT deficiency and extensive deposition of the A_1AT in the liver, no hepatic lesions develop. It has been proposed that decreased plasma levels of A_1AT in A_1AT deficiency do not inhibit the proteases released during hepatic injury and inflammation and thus render the liver susceptible to the injurious effects of infections or of other exogenous toxic factors (111).

References

1. Steinberg D: *In* Best and Taylor's Physiological Basis of Medical Practice, edited by J.B. West. 11th Edition, Baltimore, Williams & Wilkins, 1985, pp. 792–804.
2. Felig P, Sherwin R: Carbohydrate homeostasis, liver and diabetes. *In* Progress in Liver Diseases, Vol. V, edited by H. Popper, F. Schaffner. New York, Grune & Stratton, 1976, pp. 149–171.
3. Ohnishi K, Mishira A, Takashi M: Effects of intra- and extrahepatic portal systemic shunts on insulin metabolism. Dig Dis Sci 28:201–207, 1983.
4. Stone BG, van Thiel DH: Diabetes mellitus and the liver. Semin Liver Dis 5:8–28, 1985.
5. Creutzfeldt W, Frerichs H, Sickinger K: Liver disease and diabetes mellitus. *In* Progress in Liver Diseases, Vol. III, edited by H. Popper, F. Schaffner. New York, Grune & Stratton, 1970, pp. 371–407.
6. Taylor R, Heine RJ, Collins J, James OFW, Alberti KGMM: Insulin action in cirrhosis. Hepatology 5:64–70, 1985.
7. Batman PA, Scheuer PJ: Diabetic hepatitis preceding the onset of glucose intolerance. Histopathology 9:237–243, 1985.
8. Conn HO, Schreiber W, Elkington SG, Johnson TR: Cirrhosis and diabetes. I. Increased incidence of diabetes in patients with Laennec's cirrhosis. Am J Dig Dis 14:837–852, 1969.
9. Kalk H: The relationship between fatty liver and diabetes mellitus. Germ Med Month 5:1–13, 1960.
10. Leevy CM: Fatty liver: a study of 270 patients with biopsy proven fatty liver and a review of the literature. Medicine 41:249–276, 1962.
11. MacDonald RA, Mallory GK: The natural history of postnecrotic cirrhosis. A study of 221 autopsy cases. Am J Med 24:334–357, 1958.
12. Adler M, Schaffner F: Fatty liver and cirrhosis in obese patients. Am J Med 67:811–816, 1979.
13. Falchuk KR, Fiske SC, Haggitt RC, Federman M, Trey C: Pericentral hepatic fibrosis and intracellular hyalin in diabetes mellitus. Gastroenterology 78:535–541, 1980.
14. Ludwig J, Viggieno TR, McGill DB, Ott BJ: Nonalcoholic steatohepatitis. Mayo Clinic experience with a hitherto unnamed disease. Mayo Clin Proc 55:434–438, 1980.
15. Latry P, Bioulac-Sage P, Echinard E: Perisinusoidal fibrosis and basement membrane-like material in the livers of diabetic patients. Hum Pathol 18:755–780, 1987.
16. Galambos JT: Jejunal bypass and nutritional liver injury. Arch Pathol Lab Med 100:229–231, 1976.
17. Baker AL, Elson CO, Jaspan J, Boyer JL: Liver failure with steatonecrosis after jejunoileal bypass. Recovery with parenteral nutrition and reanastamosis. Arch Intern Med 139:289–292, 1979.
18. Hocking MP, Duerson MC, O'Leary JP: Jejunoileal bypass for morbid obesity. N Engl J Med 308:995–998, 1983.
19. Miller DJ, Ishimaru H, Klatskin G: Non-alcoholic liver disease mimicking alcoholic hepatitis and cirrhosis. Gastroenterology 77:26, 1979 (Abstract).
20. Marble A, White P, Bogan IK, Smith RM: Enlargement of the liver in diabetic children. I. Its incidence, etiology and nature. Arch Intern Med 62:740–750, 1938.
21. Evans RW, Littler TR, Pemberton HS: Glycogen storage in the liver in diabetes mellitus. J Clin Pathol 8:110–113, 1955.
22. Bronstein HD, Kantrowitz PA, Schaffner F: Marked enlargement of the liver and transient ascites associated with the treatment of diabetic acidosis. N Engl J Med 261:1314–1318, 1959.
23. Mauriac P: Hepatomegalie, nanisme, obesite dans le diabete infantile. Presse Med 54:826–827, 1946.
24. McAdams AJ, Hug G. Bove KE: Glycogen storage disease, types I to X. Hum Pathol 5:463–487, 1974.
25. Hers H-G, Van Hoof F, de Barsy T: Glycogen storage diseases. *In* The Metabolic Basis of Inherited Disease, edited by C.R. Scriber, A.L. Beaudet, W.S. Sly, D. Valle. 6th Edition. New York, McGraw-Hill Inf Svcs Co, 1989, pp. 425–452.
26. Ishak KG, Sharp HL: Metabolic errors and liver disease. *In* Pathology of the Liver, edited by R.N.M. MacSween, P.P. Anthony, P.J. Scheuer. 2nd Edition. Edinburgh, Churchill Livingstone, 1987, pp. 99–180.
27. Narisawa K, Igarashi Y, Otomoto H, Tada K: A new variant of gly-

cogen storage disease type I probably due to a defect in the glucose-6-phosphate transport system. Biochem Biophys Res Commun 83:1360–1364, 1978.

28. Kuzuya T, Matsuda A, Yoshida S, Narisawa K, Tada K, Saito T, Matushita: An adult case of type Ib glugen-storage disease: enzymatic and histochemical studies. N Engl J Med 308:566–569, 1983.

29. Sherlock S: Diseases of the Liver and Biliary System, 8th Edition. London, Blackwell Scientific Publications, 1989, pp. 481–486.

30. Burchell A, Jung RT, Lang CC: Diagnosis of type 1a and 1c glycogen storage diseases in adults. Lancet 1:1059–1962, 1987.

31. Chen Y-T, Cornblath M, Sidbury JB: Cornstarch therapy in type I glycogen storage disease. N Engl J Med 310:171–175, 1984.

32. Smit GPA, Berger R, Potasnick R, Moses SW, Fernandes JC: The dietary treatment of children with type I glycogen storage disease with slow release carbohydrate. Pediatr Res 18:879–881 1984.

33. Starzl TE, Putnam CW: Portal diversion treatment for glycogen storage disease and hyperlipemia. JAMA 233:955–957, 1975.

34. Malatack JJ, Finegold DN, Iwatsuki S, Shaw BW, Gartner JC, Zitelli BJ: Liver transplantation for type I glycogen storage disease. Lancet 1:1073–1075, 1983.

35. Itoh S, Ishida Y, Matsuo S: Mallory bodies in a patient with type 1a glycogen storage disease. Gastroenterology 92:520–526, 1987.

36. Howell RR, Stevenson RE, Ben-Menachem Y, Phyliky RL, Berry DH: Hepatic adenomata with type I glycogen storage disease. JAMA 236:1481–1484, 1976.

37. Grossman H, Ram PC, Coleman RA, Gates G, Rosenberg ER, Bowie JD, Wilkinson RH: Hepatic ultrasonography in type I glycogen storage disease (von Gierke disease): detection of hepatic adenoma and carcinoma. Radiology 141:753–756, 1981.

38. Fink AS, Appleman HD, Thompson NW: Hemorrhage into a hepatic adenoma and type Ia glycogen storage disease: a case report and review of the literature. Surgery 97:117–123, 1985.

39. McAdams AJ, Hug C, Bove KE: Glycogen storage disease, type I to X. Criteria for morphologic diagnosis. Hum Pathol 5:463–487, 1974.

40. Hers HG, DeBarsy T: Type II glycogenosis (acid maltase deficiency). In Lysosomes and Storage Disease, edited by H.G. Hers, F. Van Hoof. New York, Academic Press, 1973, pp. 197–216.

41. Hug G, Soukup S, Ryan M, Chuck G: Rapid prenatal diagnosis of glycogen-storage disease type II by electron microscopy of uncultured amniotic fluid cells. N Engl J Med 310:1018–1022, 1984.

42. Van Hoof F, Hers HG: The subgroups of type III glycogenosis. Eur J Biochem 2:265–270, 1967.

43. Hers HG, Van Hoof F, de Barcy T: Glycogen storage diseases. In: The Metabolic Basis of Inherited Disease, edited by CR Scriver, AL Beaudet, WS Sly, and D Valle, 6th Edition. McGraw-Hill Book Co., New York, 1989, pp. 425–452.

44. Borowitz SM, Greene HL: Cornstarch therapy in a patient with type III glycogen storage disease. Paediatr Gastroenterol Nutr 6:631–638, 1987.

45. Bannayan GA, Dean WJ, Howell RR: Type IV glycogen-storage study. Am J Clin Pathol 66:702–709, 1976.

46. Schochet SS Jr, McCormick WF, Zellweger H: Type IV glycogenosis (amylopectinosis). Light and electron microscopic observations. Arch Pathol 90:354–363, 1970.

47. Nishimura RN, Ishak KG, Reddick R, Porter R, James S, Barranger JA: Lafora's disease: diagnosis by liver biopsy. Ann Neurol 8:409–415, 1980.

48. Vasquez JJ, Guillen FJ, Zozaya J, Lahoz M: Cyanamide-induced liver injury. A predictable lesion. Liver 3:225–230, 1983.

49. Bruguera M, Lamar C, Bernet M, Rodes J: Hepatic disease associated with ground-glass inclusions in hepatocytes after cyanamide therapy. Arch Pathol Lab Med 110:906–910, 1986.

50. Hug G: Nonbilirubin genetic disorders of the liver. In The Liver, edited by E.A. Gall, P.K. Mostofi, Baltimore, Williams & Wilkins, 1973, pp. 21–71.

51. Holzel A, Komrower GM: A study of the genetics of galactosaemia. Arch Dis Child 30:155–159, 1955.

52. Dawson SP, Hickman RO, Kelley VC: Galactosemia. A genetic study of four generations by enzyme assay. Am J Dis Child 100:69–73, 1960.

53. Segal S: Disorders of galactose metabolism. In The Metabolic Basis of Inherited Disease, edited by C.R. Scriber, A.K. Beaudet, W.S. Sly, D. Valle. 6th Edition. New York, McGraw-Hill, 1989, pp. 453–480.

54. Isselbacher KJ, Anderson EP, Kurahashi K, Kalckar HM: Congenital galactosemia, a single enzymatic block in galactose metabolism. Science 123:635–636, 1956.

55. Allerdice PW, Tedesco TA: Localisation of human gene for galactose-1 phosphate-uridyl transferase. Lancet 2:39–40, 1975.

56. Holzel A, Komrower GM, Schwarz V: Galactosemia. Am J Med 22:703–711, 1957.

57. Guest GM: Hereditary galactose disease. JAMA 168:2015–2019, 1958.

58. Applebaum MN, Thaler MM: Reversibility of extensive liver damage in galactosemia. Gastroenterology 69:496–502, 1975.

59. Gitzelman R: Galactosaemia and other inherited disorders of galactose metabolism. In Liver in Metabolic Diseases, edited by L. Bianchi, W. Gerok, L. Landmann, K. Sickinger, G.A. Stalder. Lancaster, MTP Press, 1983, pp. 235–238.

60. Shin YS, Endres W, Reity M, Schaub J: Prenatal diagnosis of galactosemia and properties of galactose-1-phosphate uridyltransferase in erythrocytes of galactosemic variants as well as in human fetal and adult organs. Clin Chim Acta 128:271–281, 1983.

61. Suzuki H, Gilbert EF, Anido V, Jones B, Klingberg WG: Galactosemia. A report of two fatal cases with giant cell transformation of the liver in one. Arch Pathol 82:602–609, 1966.

62. Edmonds AM, Hennigar GR, Crooks R: Galactosemia. Report of a case with autopsy. Pediatrics 10:40–47, 1952.

63. Levin B, Snodgrass GJAI, Oberholzer VG, Burgess EA, Dobbs RH: Fructosemia. Observations on seven cases. Am J Med 45:826–838, 1968.

64. Froesch ER: Metabolic errors of fructose metabolism. In Liver in Metabolic Disease, edited by L. Bianchi, W. Gerok, L. Landmann, K. Sickinger, G.A. Stalder. Lancaster, MTP Press, 1983, pp. 239–248.

65. Gitzelman R, Steinmann B, van den Berghe G: Disorders of fructose metabolism. In The Metabolic Basis of Inherited Disease, edited by C.R. Scriver, A.L. Beaudet, W.S. Sly, D. Valle. 6th Edition. New York, McGraw-Hill Inf Svcs Co, 1989, pp. 399–424.

66. Maggiore G, Borgna-Pignatti C: Disseminated intravascular coagulation associated with hereditary fructose intolerance. Am J Dis Child 136:169–170, 1982.

67. Mock KM, Perman JA, Tahler MM: Chronic fructose intoxication after infancy in children with hereditary fructose intolerance: a cause of growth retardation. N Engl J Med 309:764–767, 1983.

68. Odievre M, Gertil C, Gautier M, Alagille D: Hereditary fructose intolerance in childhood: diagnosis, management and course in 55 patients. Am J Dis Child 132:605–608, 1978.

69. Hardwick DF, Dimmick JE: Metabolic cirrhosis of infancy and early childhood. In Perspectives in Pediatric Pathology, Vol. 3, edited by H.S. Rosenberg, R.P. Bolande. Chicago, Year Book Medical Publishers, 1976, pp. 103–144.

70. Pagliara AS, Karl IE, Keating JP, Brown BI, Kipnis DM: Hepatic fructose-1, 6 diphosphatase deficiency. A cause of lactic acidosis and hypoglycemia. J Clin Invest 51:2115–2123, 1972.

71. Neufeld EF, Muenzer J: The mucopolysaccharidoses. In The Metabolic Basis of Inherited Disease, edited by C.R. Scriver, A.L. Beaudet, W.S. Sly, D. Valle. 6th Edition. New York, McGraw-Hill Inf Svcs Co, 1989, pp. 1565–1587.

72. Van Hoof F: Mucopolysaccharidoses and mucolipidoses. J Clin Pathol 27 (suppl. 8):64–80, 1974.

73. Dulaney JT, Milunsky A, Moser HW: Detection of the carrier state of Hurler's syndrome by assay of alpha-L-iduronidase in leukocytes. Clin Chim Acta 69:305–310, 1976.

74. Sly WS, Quinton BA, McAlister WH, Rimoin DL: Beta glucuronidase deficiency: report of clinical, radiologic, and biochemical features of a new mucopolysaccharidosis. J Pediatr 82:249–257, 1973.

75. Kistler JP, Lott IT, Kolodny EH, Friedman RB, Mersasian R, Schur J: Mannosidosis. New clinical presentation, enzyme studies and carbohydrate analysis. Arch Neurol 34:45–51, 1977.

76. Desnick RJ, Sharp HL, Grabowski GA, Brunning RD, Quie PJ, Sung JH, Gorlin RJ, Ikonne JU: Mannosidosis: clinical, morphologic, and biochemical studies. Pediatr Res 10:985–996, 1976.

77. Gordon BA, Carson R, Haust MD: Unusual clinical and ultrastructural features in a boy with biochemically typical mannosidosis. Acta Paediatr Scand 69:787–792, 1980.

78. Hers HG, Van Hoof E: The genetic pathology of lysosomes. In Progress in Liver Diseases, Vol. III, edited by H. Popper, F. Schaffner. New York, Grune & Stratton, 1970, pp. 185–205.

79. Kornfeld M, Snyder RD, Wenger DA: Fucosidosis with angiokeratoma. Electron microscopic changes in the skin. Arch Pathol Lab Med 101:478–485, 1977.

80. Beratis NG, Turner BM, Labadie G, Hirschorn K: L-fucosidase in cultured skin fibroblasts from normal subjects and fucosidosis patients. Pediatr Res *11*:862–866, 1977.

81. Van Hoof F: Mucopolysaccharidoses and mucolipidoses. J Clin Pathol *27* (suppl 8):64–93, 1974.

82. Legum CP, Schorr S, Berman ER: The genetic mucopolysaccharidoses and mucolipidoses: review and comment. *In* Advances in Pediatrics, Vol. 22, edited by I. Schulman. Chicago, Year Book Medical Publishers, 1976, pp. 305–347.

83. Nolan CM, Sly WS: I-cell disease and pseudo-Hurler polydystrophy: disorders of lysosomal enzyme phosphorylation and localization. *In* The Metabolic Basis of Inherited Disease II, edited by C.R. Scriver, A.L. Beaudet, W.S. Sly, D. Valle. New York, McGraw-Hill Inf Svcs Co, 1989, pp. 1589–1592.

84. Sharp HL, Bridges RA, Krivit W, Freier EF: Cirrhosis associated with α-1 antitrypsin deficiency: a previously unrecognized inherited disorder. J Lab Clin Med *73*:934–939, 1969.

85. Eriksson SG: Liver disease in α_1-antitrypsin deficiency: aspects of incidence and prognosis. Scand J. Gastroenterol *20:* 907–911, 1985.

86. Sharp HL: α-1-antitrypsin: an ignored protein in understanding liver disease. Semin Liver Dis *2*:314–328, 1982.

87. Cox DW, Markovic VD, Teshima IE: Genes for immunoglobulin heavy chains and for 1-antitrypsin are localised to specific regions of chromosome 14Q. Nature *279*:428–430, 1982.

88. Wallmark A, Alm R, Eriksson S: Monoclonocal antibody specific for the mutant α_1-antitrypsin and its application in an ELISA procedure for identification of PiZ gene carriers. Proc Natl Acad Sci *81*:5690–5693, 1984.

89. Fagerhol MK, Cox DW: The Pi polymorphism: genetic, biochemical and clinical aspects of human α_1-antitrypsin. Adv Hum Genet *11*:1–62, 1981.

90. Sveger T, Thelin T: Four year old children with α_1-antitrypsin deficiency: clinical follow-up and parental attitudes towards neonatal screening. Acta Paediatr Scand *70*:1–7, 1981.

91. Psacharopoulos HT, Mowat AP, Cook PJL, Carbile PA, Portmann B, Rodeck CH: Outcome of liver disease associated with α_1-antitrypsin deficiency (PiZ). Arch Dis Child *58*:882–887, 1983.

92. Odievre, Martin JP, Hadchouel M, Alagille D, Thaler MM: α_1-antitrypsin deficiency and liver disease in children. Phenotypes, manifestations, and prognosis. Pediatrics *57*:226–231, 1976.

93. Alagille D: α-1-antitrypsin deficiency. Hepatology *4*:115–120, 1984.

94. Sveger T: Prospective study of children wish α_1-antitrypsin deficiency: eight-year-old follow up. J Pediatr *104*:91–97, 1984.

95. Hodges TR, Millward-Sadler GH, Barbatis C, Wright R: Heterozygous MZ α_{-1}-antitrypsin deficiency in adults with chronic active hepatitis and cryptogenic cirrhosis. N Engl J Med *304*:557–560, 1981.

96. Thatcher BS, Winkelman EI, Tuthill RJ: α-1-antitrypsin deficiency presenting as cryptogenic cirrhosis in adults over 50. J Clin Gastroenterol *7*:405–408, 1985.

97. Eriksson S, Carlson J, Velez R: Risk of cirrhosis and primary liver cancer in α-1-antitrypsin deficiency. N Engl J Med *314*:736–739, 1986.

98. Clausen PP, Lindskov J, Gad I: The diagnostic value of α-1-antitrypsin globules in liver cells as a morphological marker of α-1-antitrypsin deficiency. Liver *4*:353–359, 1984.

99. Wanless IR: α-1-antitrypsin deficiencies. AFIP Postgraduate Course 1988.

100. Rakela J, Goldschmiedt M, Ludwig J: Late manifestation of chronic liver disease in adults with α-1-antitrypsin deficiency. Dig Dis Sci *32*:1358–1362, 1987.

101. Callea F, Fevery J, DeGroote J, Desmet VJ: Detection of PiZ phenotype individuals by α-1-antitrypsin (AAT) immunohistochemistry in paraffin-embedded liver tissue specimens. J. Hepatol *2*:389–401, 1986.

102. Theaker JM, Fleming KA: α-1-antitrypsin and the liver: a routine immunohistological screen. J Clin Pathol *39*:58–62, 1986.

103. Qizilbash A, Young-Pong O: α_1-antitrypsin liver disease. Differential diagnosis of PAS-positive, diastase resistant globules in liver cells. Am J Clin Pathol *79*:697–702, 1983.

104. Phillips MJ, Poucell S, Patterson J, Valencia P: The Liver: An Atlas and Text of Ultrastructural Pathology. New York, Raven Press, 1987.

105. Reintoft I, Hagerstrand I: Demonstration of α_1-antitrypsin in hepatomas. Arch Pathol Lab Med *103*:495–498, 1979.

106. Ordonez NG, Manning JI, Hanssen G. α-1-antitrypsin in islet cell tumors of pancreas. Am J Clin Pathol *80*:277–282, 1983.

107. Triger DR, Millward-Sadler GH: α-1-antitrypsin deficiency and liver disease. *In* Liver and Biliary Disease: Pathophysiology, Diagnosis Management, edited by R. Wright, G.H. Millward-Sadler, K.G.M.M. Alberti, S. Karran. London, Bailliere Tindall, 1985, pp. 983–1001.

108. Pariente EA, Degott C, Marlin J-P, Feldmann G, Potet F, Benhamou J-P: Hepatocytic PAS-positive diastase-resistant inclusions in the absence of α-1-antitrypsin deficiency: high prevalence in alcoholic cirrhosis. Am J Clin Pathol *76*:299–302, 1981.

109. Thung SN, Gerber MA, Popper H: Antigenic expression in hepatocellular carcinoma. Gastroenterology *75*:990, 1978.

110. Muensch H, Naslow W: Liver disease and α-1-antitrypsin deficiency. Lancet *2*:983–984, 1982.

111. Udall JN, Bloch KJ, Walker WA: Transport of proteases across neonatal intestine and development of liver disease in infants with α-1-antitrypsin deficiency. Lancet *1*:1441–1443, 1982.

Chapter 15
Hepatic Lesions in Disorders of Lipid Metabolism

Obesity

Fatty infiltration of the liver

A high proportion of obese individuals exhibit fatty infiltration of the liver (1–3). Usually, the extent of the steatosis parallels the severity and duration of the obesity, but there are many exceptions (see Chapter 15).

The deposition of triglycerides in the liver is attributable to excessive caloric intake, but, in some cases, other complicating factors, particularly type II diabetes mellitus (4), play a contributory role.

The fatty deposition associated with obesity is indistinguishable from that associated with alcohol abuse (Fig. 586). As a rule, the lipid droplets are macrovesicular and randomly distributed. In a small, but significant minority of cases, the lesions show additional features, such as occasional balloon cells, small intralobular collections of lymphocytes and Kupffer cells, occasional lipogranulomas, and mild periportal or central fibrosis.

Such lesions may be accompanied by hepatomegaly, Bromsulphalein (BSP) retention, and minimally raised serum levels of alkaline phosphatase and the transaminases, but show no tendency to progress to cirrhosis.

Nonalcoholic steatonecrosis

Occasionally, nonalcoholic obese individuals exhibit lesions that closely resemble those of alcoholic hepatitis and cirrhosis (5–7). Such lesions are encountered most frequently in women (8), and particularly in those with accompanying diabetes mellitus (9). However, they may be found in men who are neither obese nor diabetic, but who exhibit other extrahepatic disorders (10). The pathogenesis of nonalcoholic steatohepatitis remains obscure.

Hepatic lesions following jejunoileal bypass for massive obesity

During the period of maximum weight loss in the first year following jejunoileal bypass for the treatment of massive obesity, there is a tendency for hepatic fatty infiltration to increase significantly. Usually, as the weight stabilizes, the fat regresses.

In addition, in some cases, the liver shows progressive changes that give rise to lesions that resemble those of alcoholic hepatitis and cirrhosis (11–14). When severe, these may be accompanied by nausea, vomiting, abdominal pain, and signs of hepatic failure, including jaundice, ascites, hepatosplenomegaly,

hepatic encephalopathy, and coagulopathy. Restoration of the normal continuity of the intestinal tract, if carried out promptly, usually leads to recovery, but not always (15). This disorder is also seen after gastroplasty operations (16). In a few instances, recovery has followed parenteral hyperalimentation.

The pathogenesis of this type of hepatic failure is still uncertain. The favorable effects of parenteral hyperalimentation in some cases suggest that protein malnutrition may account for the underlying hepatic injury. However, such therapy is not always effective, so other pathogenetic factors have been invoked. These include endotoxemia secondary to overgrowth of *Bacteroides* or other organisms in the blind loop of intestine, and abnormalities of bile acid metabolism.

Another feature of the hepatic lesions that may follow jejunoileal bypass in almost a quarter of the cases is the occurrence of sarcoid-like, noncaseating, epithelioid granulomas (17).

According to one group of investigators, obese patients who exhibit pericentral hepatic fibrosis preoperatively are particularly susceptible to the development of steatohepatitis and cirrhosis following jejunoileal bypass (18). Indeed, such patients already have obesity-related steatonecrosis. As yet, these observations have not been confirmed by others.

Hepatic lesions associated with parenteral nutrition

Cholestatic jaundice is common in infants being treated with parenteral nutrition. (19–21). If nutritional therapy is continuous and prolonged, fibrosis or cirrhosis may develop (22). In adults, fatty infiltration is common and bile stasis may be present (23).

Lipoprotein disorders

Hyperlipoproteinemias

Normally, the serum lipids, including cholesterol, cholesterol esters, triglycerides, and phospholipids, are bound to specific apoproteins in various combinations to form five types of circulating lipoproteins (24). They can be differentiated on the basis of their lipid components and their behavior on ultracentrifugation and electrophoresis (25).

Most of the hyperlipoproteinemias are hereditary in nature, but the patterns have not all been elucidated.

Type I hyperlipoproteinemia (24,25) is an autosomal recessive disorder that is characterized by lactescent serum caused by the presence of increased chylomicrons. Due to *lipoprotein lipase* deficiency these chylomicrons are not cleared from the plasma. Some patients with the disorder have episodes of abdominal pain with recurrent pancreatitis of unknown cause. Hepatosplenomegaly is usual, but liver function is normal. The liver usually shows macrovesicular fat. Low density lipoprotein (LDL) and very low density lipoprotein (VLDL) levels are low. Xanthomas are often present.

Type II hyperlipoproteinemia (familial hypercholesterolemia) (24,25) is an autosomal dominant disorder that is much more severe in its homozygous state. Patients develop xanthomas and premature atherosclerosis. The serum is clear. LDL levels are increased in some variants and VLDL and LDL in others. The disorder is caused by impaired regulation of cholesterol metabolism apparently related to a deficiency of LDL receptors.

Types III, IV, and V hyperlipoproteinemia are lipemic disorders associated with xanthomas, impaired carbohydrate metabolism, hepatosplenomegaly, and premature atherosclerosis (24–26).

Hepatomegaly and splenomegaly are encountered most frequently in forms of hyperlipoproteinemia accompanied by high serum levels of triglycerides, as in types I, III, IV, and V. In such cases, the principal histologic features of the hepatic lesions include: (1) the presence of numerous scattered Kupffer cells that are enlarged and contain pale, foamy cytoplasm due to the presence of microvesicular lipid droplets, and (2) varying degrees of macrovesicular hepatocellular fatty infiltration (27). Less commonly, the Kupffer cells present as sea-blue histiocytes.

Abetalipoproteinemia (Bassen-Kornsweig syndrome)

Abetalipoproteinemia (26,28), an autosomal recessive disorder, is characterized by an absence of apolipoprotein B accompanied by alterations in the intestinal tract, eyes, central nervous system, red blood cells, and liver. The underlying enzymatic defect responsible for the abetalipoproteinemia and the mechanisms involved in the pathogenesis of the associated tissue lesions are still speculative, but deficiencies of specific apoproteins, which are synthesized in the liver (29,30), have been demonstrated.

Steatorrhea that appears in early infancy is the initial clinical manifestation (30). Later in childhood, the steatorrhea tends to diminish, but the other more distinctive features of the disease appear. These include a neurologic disorder that resembles Friedreich's ataxia, an atypical form of retinitis pigmentosa, and spiculation of the circulating erythrocytes (acanthosis). Characteristically, the serum concentrations of cholesterol, triglyceride, and phospholipid are low. In addition, there is an absence of β-lipoprotein.

Hepatomegaly is often present and the hepatocytes are infiltrated with small lipid droplets (28,31). The fatty infiltration may be accompanied by ballooning necrosis of the hepatocytes, Mallory bodies, increased transaminase levels, and progressive portal fibrosis that leads to the development of micronodular cirrhosis (28,32). Acanthocytes are present in the sinusoids, and phagocytosis of these deformed red blood cells has been demonstrated by electron microscopy (31). This disorder has been seen in patients who are receiving dietary supplements of medium-chain triglycerides (MCT), which tend to reduce the steatorrhea. It is not clear whether the progressive character of such lesions is attributable to abetalipoproteinemia or to the MCT therapy.

Familial high density lipoprotein deficiency (Tangier disease)

Tangier disease, an autosomal recessive inborn error of lipid metabolism, is characterized by a severe deficiency or absence of high density lipoprotein (HDL) in the plasma, associated with widespread deposition of cholesterol esters in the reticuloendothelial cells of numerous tissues (33–35). It has been suggested that the basic defect is abnormal regulation of the synthesis of one of the major apoproteins of α-lipoprotein.

The principal clinical manifestations that may appear at any age include enlargement and orange discoloration of the tonsils, hepatosplenomegaly, lymphoadenopathy, opacification of the corneas, peripheral neuropathy, and focal orange-brown pigment deposits in the rectal mucosa. Both thrombocytopenia and xanthomas have been reported in individual patients.

Although the typical cells of Tangier disease are found in the lymphoid tissues of the body and in the colon, they may be scanty in the liver (36). The hepatic lesions are characterized by the presence of scattered, enlarged Kupffer cells that contain cholesterol, which gives the cytoplasm a pale, foamy appearance (37). In frozen sections, the cytoplasm of such cells is sudanophilic, gives a positive Schultz reaction for cholesterol, and contains birefringent, cleft-like crystals of cholesterol esters in polarized light.

Hereditary lipid storage diseases

Cholesterol, cholesterol esters and triglycerides

Cholesterol ester storage disease. Cholesterol ester storage disease (38–41), an autosomal recessive hereditary disorder, is characterized by a deficiency of the lysosomal enzymes, *acid cholesterol ester hydrolase* and *acid triglyceride lipase* that lead to the accumulation of cholesterol esters and triglycerides in the liver and many other tissues. The disease appears to be a mild variant of Wolman's disease (42).

The onset of the disease is insidious, but usually is recognized in childhood. It may begin *in utero*. Indeed, the diagnosis has been made before birth (43). The principal early manifestations include hepatomegaly and raised serum levels of cholesterol esters and triglycerides. Splenomegaly and signs of portal hypertension are less constant features, and, usually, are encountered relatively late in the course of the disease.

The disease may remain asymptomatic without evidence of hepatic dysfunction. However, in some cases, the lesions are accompanied by fibrosis that progresses to cirrhosis and ultimately to hepatic failure or the complications of portal hypertension.

In most cases, the *hepatic lesions* are characterized by the bright orangish color of the liver biopsy core. The hepatocytes and Kupffer cells are enlarged with pale, foamy, vacuolated cytoplasm and centrally located nuclei [(44,45); Fig. 684]. In frozen sections, the vacuoles stain with oil red 0 and other sudanophilic dyes and in polarized light exhibit birefringent, needle-like arrays of cholesterol ester crystals.

Progressive portal fibrosis with ductular proliferation leads to the development of micronodular cirrhosis in some cases [(40); Fig. 685].

Wolman's disease. The enzymatic defect in Wolman's disease (41,46,47), another autosomal recessive inherited lipidosis, is similar to that in cholesterol ester storage disease (42). However, it appears to be more severe, has its onset during the first few weeks of life, and usually proves fatal within a few months. In addition to more extensive deposition of triglyceride and cholesterol esters in the tissues, the adrenals characteristically are enlarged and are usually calcified. A similar disorder has been reported in fox terriers (48).

The association between Wolman's disease and cholesterol ester storage disease is not known (49), but it has been suggested that the defect in Wolman's disease is in the hepatocytes, and in cholesterol ester storage disease, in the Kupffer cells (50).

The histologic patterns in the two disorders are similar (51). In Wolman's disease the hepatocytes and Kupffer cells, as in cholesterol ester storage disease, contain cholesterol and cholesterol esters that cause foamy cytoplasm in routine sections (Fig. 179), and show arrays of birefringent crystals in polarized light (Fig. 180). Pericellular fibrosis and bile ductular proliferation may be present (52).

Cerebrotendinous xanthomatosis. Cerebrotendinous xanthomatosis (53–55), an autosomal recessive hereditary lipidosis, is characterized by excessive deposits of cholesterol and cholestanol throughout the tissues. The underlying defect is a block in the hepatic biosynthesis of bile acids (56).

The principal manifestations include xanthomatous infiltration of the tendons and lungs, cataracts, premature atherosclerosis, progressive cerebellar ataxia, and dementia. Therapy with chenodeoxycholic acid has been reported to slow the progress of the disease (57).

On electron miroscopy, the cytoplasm of the hepatocytes and Kupffer cells contain electron-dense pigment granules and crystalline bodies thought to represent nonmetabolizable bile alcohols (54). On light microscopy, some of the hepatocytes contain fine, golden brown granules in their cytoplasm. By electron microscopy, perisinusoidal fibrosis and abnormal mitochondria have been demonstrated (58).

Familial fatal neonatal hepatic steatosis. Familial fatal neonatal hepatic steatosis (59–61), a rare familial disorder, is characterized by extensive deposition of triglycerides in the liver and other tissues. It appears shortly after birth and usually proves fatal within a few days to weeks. Survival for as long as two years has been reported, however.

Since the disease occurs primarily in males, inheritance is thought to be sex-linked. However, nothing is yet known about the biochemical defect responsible for the accumulation of triglycerides in the tissues, so the possibility that more than one entity is involved cannot be excluded.

The clinical manifestations are lethargy, hypotonia, hepatomegaly, and failure to thrive. Frequently, jaundice, kernicterus, hypoglycemia, splenomegaly, and a bleeding diathesis are also present.

The principal feature of the *hepatic lesions* is the presence in all hepatocytes of numerous large and small lipid droplets. Swelling of the hepatocytes tends to compress and obliterate the sinusoidal lumens. Occasionally, a few of the Kupffer cells also contain small lipid droplets. In infants who die within a few days or weeks, the portal tracts appear normal. However, in those who survive for several months, portal fibrosis and portal-portal fibrous bridging are frequently present.

Glucocerebroside lipidosis (Gaucher's disease)

Gaucher's disease (62,63), an autosomal recessive hereditary disorder, is characterized by a deficiency of *β-glucocerebrosidase,* a lysosomal enzyme involved in the degeneration of sphingolipids in cell membranes. As a result, glucocerebroside (glucosylceramide), a complex of glucose, sphingosine, and fatty acids derived from the membranes of senescent leukocytes, erythrocytes, platelets, and macrophages, accumulates in the reticuloendothelial cells of the liver, spleen, and bone marrow.

Although a deficiency of glucocerebrosidase and accumulation of glucocerebroside in Kupffer cells are found in all cases of Gaucher's disease, the disease presents in three forms that tend to breed true in affected families: the adult (type 1), the infantile (type 2), and the juvenile (type 3). These three subtypes, which *reflect* the deficiency of different molecular forms of β-glucocerebrosidase, can be differentiated by identification of the phenotypes by means of monoclonal antibodies (64).

The *adult type,* the most common form of Gaucher's disease, affects Ashkenazi Jews predominantly. Usually, it is progressive, but, in some cases, it may remain asymptomatic for many years. In general, the manifestations become apparent by the age of 30 and include in various combinations hepatosplenomegaly, anemia, and thrombocytopenia, erosion and expansion of the cortex of the long bones, brownish pigmentation of the skin over the lower extremities, and, occasionally, distinctive wedge-shaped yellow deposits in the sclerae (pingueculae). Enlargement of lipid-filled cells compresses the sinusoids and may give rise to portal hypertension and cirrhosis (65). Variceal hemorrhage has been reported (66). The thrombocytopenia and anemia, which may be manifestations of hypersplenism, may be reversed by splenectomy (67). Frequently, the serum tartrate–resistant, acid phosphatase level is elevated.

The *infantile form* of Gaucher's disease runs a more acute course, usually appearing within the first few months of life and resulting in death before the age of two years. The principal manifestations are hepatosplenomegaly and evidence of progressive deterioration of the central nervous system, including opisthotonus, hypertonicity, and mental retardation.

In the *juvenile* form of Gaucher's disease, as in the infantile type, central nervous system manifestations predominate. The onset is delayed until later in childhood and the course of the disease is less acute.

Treatment with bisphosphonates has caused improvement in the bone lesions (68). Correction of the enzyme abnormalities by bone marrow transplantation is currently under investigation (69).

The distinctive feature in all forms of Gaucher's disease is the presence of enlarged macrophages that contain deposits of glucocerebroside—the Gaucher cells. Most commonly, these are encountered in the liver, spleen, and bone marrow, but may be found in a variety of other tissues.

In the liver, only the Kupffer cells and occasional portal macrophages show the typical features of Gaucher cells. The affected cells are enlarged, measuring up to 100 μm in diameter, and contain abundant pale cytoplasm and small, dark nuclei. Characteristically, the cytoplasm is filled with numerous thread-like inclusions that give it a crinkled, tissue-paper appearance (Fig. 246). The inclusions are diastase-resistant, PAS-positive (Fig. 247) and show intense acid-phosphatase activity. Due to an increase in ferritin, some of the Gaucher cells stain diffusely in the Prussian blue reaction. In some, but not all cases, the deposits exhibit autofluorescence.

The distinctive cytoplasmic striations in Gaucher cells are best seen in Masson- (Fig. 246) and PAS-D-stained sections (Fig. 247).

Often, as illustrated in Figures 246 and 247, large focal collections of Gaucher cells fill the sinusoids and compress the intervening hepatocytes, leading to their atrophy and ultimate loss and may stimulate collagen deposition (67). Changes of this type may account for the development of the portal hypertension reported in some cases. Hemopoietic cells may also be seen.

On electron microscopy, the cytoplasm of Gaucher cells contains numerous membrane-bound, closely packed tubular structures that represent lysosomal collections of aggregated, glucocerebroside molecules (70).

Gaucher-like cells are found occasionally in patients with chronic myelogenous leukemia (71). In such cases, the accumulation of glucocerebroside is attributable to increased leukocyte turnover rather than to a hereditary defect in its enzymatic degradation.

Rarely, cells that closely resemble Gaucher cells have been found in the bone marrow of patients with multiple myeloma. Although such *pseudo-Gaucher* cells exhibit the typical light microscopic and histochemical features of Gaucher cells, it has been shown by electron microscopy and immunofluorescence that they contain crystalline immunoglobulins rather than glucocerebroside (72).

Sphingomyelin lipidosis (Niemann-Pick disease)

Niemann-Pick disease (73) comprises a group of hereditary disorders characterized by hepatosplenomegaly and the accumulation of sphingomyelin and other lipids in many of the tissues. Of the five types that have been identified, the most common is the acute neuropathic form that affects young infants.

Type A, acute neuropathic, infantile Niemann-Pick disease. Type A, an autosomal recessive hereditary disease that affects Ashkenazi Jews in particular, is characterized by a deficiency of sphingomyelinase, a lysosomal enzyme that normally splits phosphorylcholine from the sphingomyelin released from the subcellular and plasma membranes during the turnover of all cells in the body. Because of this block in its degradation, sphingomyelin accumulates in the reticuloendothelial cells of many tissues and in the ganglion cells of the central nervous system. Often, the sphingomyelin deposits contain other lipids, especially cholesterol and other sphingolipids.

The clinical manifestations appear in early infancy, and are characterized by vomiting, hepatosplenomegaly, retardation of growth and mental development, and the appearance in one-third to one-half the cases of a cherry red spot in the macular region of the eyes, as in Tay-Sachs disease. Usually, death ensues by the third year of life.

In a small minority of cases, the initial features are those of neonatal hepatitis, which usually regresses, but may give rise to an inactive form of cirrhosis.

The distinctive histologic feature of the lesions in Niemann-Pick disease is the presence of large, foamy, reticuloendothelial cells (N-P cells) in the bone marrow, liver, and spleen. In the liver, the N-P cells are limited initially to the Kupffer cells, but

as the disease advances, hepatocytes may be affected as well. Moreover, the number of N-P cells tends to increase with time. Aggregated N-P cells tend to fill the sinusoids in some areas and may lead to focal atrophy and destruction of the hepatic plates.

Characteristically, the affected Kupffer cells are greatly enlarged, measuring 20 to 90 μm in diameter, and, in paraffin-embedded sections, contain pale, finely vacuolated, foamy cytoplasm and small, eccentric, pyknotic nuclei (Fig. 248). Often, in addition to sphingomyelin, the N-P cells contain abundant lipofuscin, so they are PAS-D-positive (Fig. 249). Sea-blue histiocytes are sometimes seen [(14); Fig. 686].

In frozen sections, the cytoplasmic vacuoles stain lightly with oil red 0, and show birefringent crystals in polarized light and react in the Schultz modification of the Lieberman-Burchard reaction, indicating the presence of cholesterol and cholesterol esters.

On electron microscopy, the cytoplasm of the N-P cells contains numerous lysosomal inclusions made up of concentrically arranged, laminated membranes in the form of myelin-like figures.

Type B, non-neuropathic, chronic Niemann-Pick disease. The type B disorder closely resembles type A Niemann-Pick disease, but differs in several ways: (1) the onset is delayed until later in childhood; (2) the central nervous system is spared; (3) pulmonary infiltration with N-P cells and increased susceptibility to pneumonia are relatively common; and (4) the course of the disease is more prolonged.

Type C, subacute, neuropathic Niemann-Pick disease. The features of type C disease are similar to those in type A Niemann-Pick disease, except that, (1) the onset occurs after the first year of life, (2) neurologic manifestations are more severe, and (3) hepatosplenomegaly is a less prominent feature.

Type D, Nova Scotia variant of Niemann-Pick disease. The type D disorder, limited to an inbred group of Acadians of French descent who reside in western Nova Scotia, resembles type C Niemann-Pick disease. However, affected individuals show no deficiency of sphingomyelinase, and the biochemical basis for this accumulation of sphingomyelin remains obscure. The neurologic syndrome, which is characterized by spasticity and seizures, is extremely severe. Macular degeneration does not occur. Transient cholestatic jaundice often occurs in infancy.

Type E, adult, non-neuropathic Niemann-Pick disease. Type E, a relatively benign disorder of adults, is characterized by moderate hepatosplenomegaly, accumulation of sphingomyelin in the liver and spleen, and the presence of N-P cells in the bone marrow.

The biochemical basis for the accumulation of sphingomyelin is not known, and the level of liposomal sphingomyelinase is normal. It has been suggested that this form of the disease may account for some cases of the sea-blue histiocyte syndrome.

GM₁ Gangliosidoses

Type 1, generalized infantile GM₁ gangliosidosis. Type 1 gangliosidosis (65,75), an autosomal recessive hereditary disorder, is characterized by a deficiency of all three isomers (A, B, and C) of *β-galactosidase,* lysosomal enzymes involved in the catabolism of GM_1 ganglioside and keratin-like mucopolysaccharides. As a result, GM_1 ganglioside and mucopolysaccharide accumulate in the lysosomes of neurons and most other tissue cells.

The clinical manifestations appear at birth or shortly thereafter, and are characterized by retardation of growth and mental development, progressive motor dysfunction, hepatosplenomegaly, skeletal abnormalities, the occurrence in half the cases of a cherry red spot in the maculae of the eyes, and coarsening and other abnormalities of the facial features. Death from intercurrent infection occurs by the age of two years.

The *hepatic lesions* are characterized by clusters of enlarged Kupffer cells filled with pale, finely vacuolated, foamy cytoplasm. The vacuoles are weakly PAS-D-positive and contain acid mucopolysaccharide that stains with alcian blue. Some of the hepatocytes contain fine vacuoles that stain with oil red 0 in frozen sections, but are PAS-D-negative.

On electron microscopy, the vacuoles in hepatocytes and Kupffer cells are membrane-bound and contain amorphous and fibrillar material (76).

Type 2, juvenile GM_1 gangliosidosis. Type 2 gangliosidosis closely resembles the infantile type of GM_1 gangliosidosis, but differs in several ways: (1) it is attributable to a deficiency of only the B and C isomers of β-galactosidase; (2) has its onset at the end of the first year of life; (3) runs a more prolonged course; and (4) is accompanied by less extensive deposition of ganglioside in the viscera.

GM_2 gangliosidoses

Type 1, GM_2 gangliosidosis (Tay-Sachs disease). Tay-Sachs disease (77) is an autosomal recessive hereditary disorder that is characterized by a deficiency of type *B hexosaminidase,* a lysosomal enzyme involved in the normal catabolism of GM_2 ganglioside. This leads to the accumulation of GM_2 ganglioside in the lysosomes of neurons, and to a lesser extent in those of visceral cells, and to progressive degeneration of the central nervous system. It occurs 10 times as frequently in Ashkenazi Jews as in non-Jewish individuals.

The clinical manifestations, which appear at three to six months of age, are characterized by progressive motor and mental deterioration, the presence of a cherry red spot in the maculae of the eyes, and blindness. Death from intercurrent infection usually occurs by the age of three years.

The light microscopic appearance of the liver is normal, but, on electron microscopy, the vacuoles in hepatocytes contain amorphous material, and Kupffer cells may contain membrane-bound fibrillary structures (76).

Type 2, GM_2 gangliosidosis (Sandhoff's disease). Type 2 gangliosidosis (77) closely resembles type 1 GM_2 gangliosidosis, except that PAS-D-positive deposits can sometimes be seen in hepatocytes or Kupffer cells by light microscopy. It is attributable to a deficiency of both *type A and type B hexosaminidase.* Askhenazi Jews are not especially susceptible.

Type 3, GM_2 gangliosidosis. In this more mild variant of the disease, which is caused by a *partial deficiency of type B hexosaminidase,* neurologic dysfunction dominates the course. No macular cherry red spots develop and there are no hepatic abnormalities.

Glycosphingolipidosis (Fabry's disease)

Fabry's disease (65,78) is a rare, inborn error of lipid metabolism that is transmitted as an X-linked recessive trait, and is characterized by a deficiency of α-galactosidase A, a lysosomal hydrolase that is required for the degradation of glycosphingolipids. As a result, the glycosphingolipids accumulate in vascular endothelium, reticuloendothelial cells, and the parenchymal cells of most viscera. The principal sites of deposition include the skin, nervous system, eyes, heart, and kidneys. The diagnosis can be made by the immunohistologic demonstration of glycosphinogolipid in the cells of the renal tubules (79).

In hemizygous males, the clinical manifestations appear in late childhood or adolescence, and include generalized vascular skin lesions (angiokeratoma), peripheral neuritis with pain and paresthesias in the extremities, episodic abdominal pain, opacification of the corneas, proteinuria and renal failure, angina pectoris, and heart failure. Usually, death occurs in the fifth decade as a result of cardiac or renal failure.

The disease tends to be mild or asymptomatic in heterozygous females, but corneal opacities are relatively common. Rarely, the disease is as severe in heterozygous women as in homozygous men (80).

In some cases, the liver contains clusters of enlarged Kupffer cells and portal macrophages filled with deposits of glycolipid and cholesterol. The Kupffer cells stain intensely with PAS and are diastase-resistant. In frozen sections, the cholesterol reacts in the Schultz modification of the Lieberman-Burchard reaction and is seen as birefringent, needle-like crystals in polarized light.

On electron microscopy, the cytoplasm of the hepatocytes and Kupffer cells contains enlarged lysosomes filled with dense, parallel, osmiophilic lamellae in a matrix of low electron density (81).

Farber's lipogranulomatosis

Farber's lipogranulomatosis (82–84), an autosomal recessive hereditary disorder, is characterized by a deficiency of *acid ceramidase,* a lysosomal enzyme that catalyzes the hydrolysis of ceramide to sphingosine and fatty acids. As a result, ceramide, a normal product of complex sphingolipid degradation, accumulates in the lysosomes of histiocytes, hepatocytes, and neurons in many tissues. Accumulations near the neurons lead to the formation of foam cells and granulomas.

The principal clinical manifestations that appear in early infancy include painful swelling of the joints, periarticular, subcutaneous nodules, hoarseness with swelling of the larynx and epiglottis, pulmonary infiltration, peripheral neuropathy, mental retardation, hepatomegaly, and, occasionally, splenomegaly.

Although many of the affected tissues show histiocytic, granulomatous reactions with varying degrees of fibrosis late in the course of the disease, such lesions are rare in the liver. Histologic sections usually show fine vacuolization of the cytoplasm in scattered Kupffer cells and occasionally hepatocytes. In frozen sections, the vacuoles are PAS-positive and show birefringence in polarized light.

On electron microscopy, the cytoplasm of the hepatocytes contains large, clear, membrane-bound vacuoles and lysosomes filled with dense, granular matrix. The lysosomes in the Kupffer cells contain small tubular structures in an osmiophilic matrix.

Most affected infants die of intercurrent pulmonary infections by the age of two years, but survival into adolescence has been reported.

Sulfatide lipidosis (metachromatic leukodystrophy)

Metachromatic leukodystrophy (65,85–87), an autosomal recessive hereditary disorder of glycosphingolipid metabolism, is characterized by a deficiency of *arylsulfatase A,* a lysosomal enzyme required for the hydrolysis of cerebroside sulfate (galactosylsulfatide). As a result, there is an accumulation of cerebroside 3-sulfate in the central nervous system, kidneys, gallbladder, and less commonly, in other tissues.

The disease may occur in infancy, adolescence, or in adulthood (86,87). The clinical features are predominantly neurologic and attributable to progressive destruction of myelin. Characteristically, the sites of abnormal lipid deposition contain macrophagic or extracellular metachromatic granules. Sulfatide accumulation is also seen in gallbladders, which tend to be small and fibrotic and to show multiple polyps (88).

In the liver, the granules may be found in portal macrophages, Kupffer cells, bile duct cells, or hepatocytes. In frozen sections they appear to be mahogany red-brown with cresyl violet stain, and deep red in toludine blue–stained sections. In addition, they stain with alcian blue owing to the presence of sulfate groups.

Phytanic acid storage disease (Refsum's syndrome)

Refsum's syndrome (89), an autosomal recessive hereditary disorder, is characterized by a deficiency of the mitochondrial enzyme *phytanic acid α-hydroxylase.* This enzyme is required for the oxidation of phytanic acid to α-hydroxyphytanic acid. The phytanic acid is of dietary origin. The deficiency of phytanic α-hydroxylase leads to an accumulation of phytanic acid in most of the tissues, but especially in the liver and kidneys.

The clinical manifestations usually appear in childhood or adolescence, and uncommonly in adults. They include decreasing vision, ataxia, nerve deafness, and weakness of the extremities caused by retinitis pigmentosa, cataracts, peripheral neuropathy, and cerebellar ataxia. The cerebrospinal fluid protein concentration is usually elevated (90). Skin changes such as palmar hyperkeratosis and icthyosis of the trunk may also occur.

Dietary treatment, which consists of reducing the intake of phytanic acid, has resulted in some improvement in neurologic symptoms and signs (91).

The *hepatic lesions* are characterized by hepatomegaly due to fatty deposition, but show no other distinctive features. On electron microscopy, however, abnormal laminar structures have been noted in the sinusoidal epithelial cells (92,93).

Sea-blue histiocytes

A number of apparently unrelated disorders are associated with the presence in the bone marrow, spleen, and, less commonly, in the liver of large histiocytes containing coarse cytoplasmic granules that appear deep blue in Giemsa- or Wright-stained sections (94,95). Such cells have been encountered in chronic myelogenous leukemia (96), idiopathic thrombocytopenic purpura (97), Neimann-Pick disease (74,98,99), hyperlipoproteinemi (100), cholesterol ester storage disease (101), Tay-Sachs disease, Wolman's disease, Gaucher's disease (102), familial lecithin-cholesterol acyltransferase deficiency, and familial lipochrome histiocytosis.

Figure 686 illustrates the typical sea-blue histiocyte granules in the Kupffer cells of the patient with type V hyperlipoproteinemia associated with hepatosplenomegaly and angina pectoris.

In addition, the sea-blue histiocyte syndrome has been reported as a specific entity characterized by the histiocytic storage of glycosphingolipids and phospholipids (95). However, on histochemical analysis, the granules have proved to be identical with the abnormal lipids found in each of these other lipid disorders, so the existence of a specific storage disease characterized by sea-blue histiocytosis is in doubt.

The granules in sea-blue histiocytes exhibit the properties of lipofuscin (ceroid) (100), including PAS-D-positivity to acid-fast staining and golden yellow autofluorescence.

On electron microscopy, the granules are membrane-bound, electron-dense bodies with whorls of membrane resembling myelin figures. These findings are consistent with the view that the inclusions represent lysosomes that contain phospholipids derived from cell membranes.

References

1. Kern WH, Heger AH, Payne JH, De Wind LT: Fatty metamorphosis of the liver. Arch Pathol 96:342–346, 1973.
2. Nasrallah SM, Wills CE Jr, Galambos JT: Hepatic morphology in obesity. Dig Dis Sci 26:325–327, 1981.
3. Braillon A, Capron JP, Herve MA, Degott C, Zuenum C: Liver in obesity. Gut 26:133–139, 1985.
4. Wanless IR, Albrecht S, Bilbao J, Frei JV, Heathcote EJ, Roberts EA, Chiasson D: Multiple focal nodular hyperplasia of the liver associated with vascular malformations of various organs and neoplasia of the brain: a new syndrome. Mod Pathol 2:456–462, 1989.
5. Adler M, Schaffner F: Fatty liver hepatitis and cirrhosis in obese patients. Am J Med 67:811–816, 1979.
6. Braillon A, Herse MA, Degott C: Liver in obesity. Gut 26:133–139, 1985.
7. Clain JE, Stephens DH, Charboneau JW: Ultrasonography and computed tomography in focal fatty liver. Report of two cases with special emphasis on changing appearance over time. Gastroenterology 87:948–952, 1984.
8. Ludwig J, Viggiano TR, McGill DB, Ott BB: Nonalcoholic steatohepatitis. Mayo Clinic experiences with a hitherto unnamed disease. Mayo Clin Proc 55:434–438, 1980.
9. Falchuk KR, Fiske SC, Haggitt RC, Federman M, Trey C: Pericentral hepatic fibrosis and intracellular hyalin in diabetes mellitus. Gastroenterology 78:535–541, 1980.
10. Schaffner F, Thaler H: Nonalcoholic fatty liver disease. *In* Progress in Liver Diseases, Vol. VIII, edited by H. Popper, F. Schaffer. New York, Grune & Stratton, 1986, pp. 283–298.
11. Baker AL, Elson CO, Jaspan J, Boyer JL: Liver failure with steatonecrosis after jejunoileal bypass. Recovery with parenteral nutrition and reanastamosis. Arch Intern Med 139:289–292, 1979.
12. Galambos JT: Jejunal bypass and nutritional liver injury. Arch Pathol Lab Med 100:229–231, 1976.
13. Peters RL, Gay T, Reynolds TB: Post-jejunoileal-bypass hepatic disease. Its similarity to alcoholic hepatic disease. Am J Clin Pathol 63:318–331, 1975.
14. Hocking MP, Duerson MC, O'Leary JP: Jejunoileal bypass for morbid obesity. N Engl J Med 308:995–999, 1983.
15. Styblo T, Martin S, Kaminski KL. The effects of reversal of jejunoileal bypass operations on hepatic triglyceride content and hepatic morphology. Surgery 96:632–640, 1984.

16. Hamilton DL, Vest TK, Brown BS, Shah AN, Menguy RB, Chey WY: Liver injury with alcoholic-like hyalin after gastroplasty for morbid obesity. Gastroenterology 85:722–726, 1983.

17. Banner BF, Banner AS: Hepatic granulomas following ileal bypass for obesity. Arch Pathol Lab Med 102:655–657, 1978.

18. Haines NW, Baker AL, Boyer JL, Glagov S, Schneir H, Jaspan J, Ferguson DJ: Prognostic indicators of hepatic injury following jejunoileal bypass performed for refractory obesity: a prospective study. Hepatology 1:161–167, 1981.

19. Pereira GR, Sherman MS, DiGiacomo J, Ziegler M, Rother K, Jacobowski P: Hyperalimentation-induced cholestasis. Increased incidence and severity in premature infants. Am J Dis Child 135:842–845, 1981.

20. Hughes CA, Talbot IC, Ducker DA, Harran MJ: Total parenteral nutrition in infancy: effect on the liver and suggested pathogenesis. Gut 24:241–248, 1983.

21. Whitington PF. Cholestasis associated with total parenteral nutrition in infants. Hepatology 5:693–696, 1985.

22. Cohen C, Olsen MM: Pediatric total parenteral nutrition. Arch Pathol Lab Med 105:152–156, 1981.

23. Bower RH: Hepatic complications of parenteral nutrition. Semin Liver Dis 3:216–224, 1983.

24. Schaefer EJ, Levy RI: Pathogenesis and management of lipoprotein disorders. N Engl J Med 312:1300–1310, 1985.

25. Roberts WC, Levy RI, Fredrickson DS: Hyperlipoproteinemia. A review of the five types with first report of necropsy findings in Type 3. Arch Pathol 90:46–56, 1970.

26. Mahley RW, Rall DS Jr: Type III hyperlipoproteinemia: the role of apolipoprotein E in normal and abnormal lipoprotein metabolism. In The Metabolic Basis of Inherited Disease, edited by C.R. Scriver, A.L. Beaudet, W.S. Sly, D. Valle. 6th Edition. New York, McGraw-Hill Book Co., 1989, pp. 1195–1214.

27. De la Iglesia FA, Lewis JE, Buchanan RA, Marcus EL, McMahon G: Light and electron microscopy of liver in hyperlipoproteinemic patients under long-term gemfibrozil treatment. Atherosclerosis 43:19–37, 1982.

28. Partin JS, Partin JC, Schubert WK, McAdams J: Liver ultrastructure in abetalipoproteinemia: evolution of micronodular cirrhosis. Gastroenterology 67:107–118, 1974.

29. Malloy MJ, Kane JP, Hardman DA, Hamilton RL, Dalal KB: Normotriglyceridemic abetalipoproteinemia: absence of the B-100 apolipoprotein. J Clin Invest 67:1441–1450, 1981.

30. Takashima Y, Kodema T, Lida H, Kawamura M, Aburatini H, Itakura H: Normoglyceridemic abetalipoproteinemia in infancy: an isolated abetalipoprotein B-100 deficiency. Pediatrics 75:541–546, 1985.

31. Avigan MI, Ishak KG, Gregg RE, Hoofnagle JH: Morphologic features of the liver in abetalipoproteinemia. Hepatology 4:1223–1226, 1984.

32. Illingworth DR, Connor WE, Miller RG: Abetalipoproteinemia. Report of two cases and review of therapy. Arch Neurol 37:659–667, 1980.

33. Herbert PN, Forte T, Heinen RJ, Fredrickson DS: Tangier disease. One explanation of lipid storage. N Engl J Med 299:519–521, 1978.

34. Dechelotte P, Kantelip B, de Laguillaumie BV, Labbe A, Meyer M: Tangier disease. A histological and ultrastructural study. Pathol Res Pract 180:424–430, 1985.

35. Assman G, Schmitz G, Brewer HB Jr: Familial high density lipoprotein defiency: Tangier disease. In The Metabolic Basis of Inherited Disease, edited by C.R. Scriver, A.L. Beaudet, W.S Sly, D. Valle. 6th Edition. New York, McGraw-Hill Book Co., 1989, pp. 1267–1282.

36. Bale PM, Clifton-Bligh P, Benjamin BNP, Whyte HM: Pathology of Tangier disease. J Clin Pathol 24:609–616, 1971.

37. Brook JG, Lees RS, Yules JH, Cusack B: Tangier disease (α-lipoprotein deficiency). JAMA 238:332–334, 1977.

38. Schiff L, Schubert WK, McAdams AJ, Spiegel EL, O'Donnell JF: Hepatic cholesterol ester storage disease, a familial disease. I. Clinical aspects. Am J Med 44:538–546, 1968.

39. Sloan HR, Fredrickson DS: Enzyme deficiency in cholesterol ester storage disease. J Clin Invest 51:1923–1926, 1972.

40. Beaudet AL, Ferry GD, Nichols BL, Jr., Rosenberg HS: Cholesterol ester storage disease: clinical, biochemical, and pathological studies. J Pediatr 90:910–914, 1977.

41. Schmitz G, Assmann G: Acid lipase deficiency: Wolman disease and cholesterol ester storage disease. In The Metabolic Basis of Inherited Disease, edited by C.R. Scriver, A.L. Beaudet, W.S. Sly, D. Valle.

6th Edition. New York, McGraw-Hill Book Co., 1989, pp. 1623–1644.

42. Barton BK, Remy WT, Rayman L: Cholesterol ester and triglyceride metabolism in intact fibroblasts from patients with Wolman's disease and cholesterol ester storage disease. Pediatr Res 18:1242–1245, 1984.

43. Desai PK, Astrin KH, Thung S, Gordon RE, Short MP, Coates PM, Desnick RJ: Cholesterol ester storage disease: pathologic changes in an affected fetus. Am J Med Genet 26:689–698, 1987.

44. Lageron A, Polonovski J: Histochemical abnormalities in liver and jejunal biopsies from a case of cholesterol ester storage disease. J Inherited Metab Dis 11 (Suppl):139–142, 1988.

45. D'Agostino D, Bay L, Gallo G, Chamoles N: Cholesterol ester storage disease: clinical, biochemical, and pathological studies of four new cases. J Pediatr Gastroenterol Nutr 7:446–450, 1988.

46. Bona G, Bracco G, Gallina MR, Inavarone A, Perona A, Zaffaroni M: Wolman's disease: clinical and biochemical findings of a new case. J Inherited Metab Dis 11:423–424, 1988.

47. Lough J, Fawcett J, Wiegensberg B: Wolman's disease. An electron microscopic, histochemical and biochemical study. Arch Pathol 89:103–110, 1970.

48. von Sandersleben J, Hanichen T, Fiebiger I, Brem G: Lipid storage disease similar to Wolman's disease in humans in the fox terrier. Tierarztl Prax 14:253–263, 1986.

49. Philippart M, Durand P, Borrone C: Neutral lipid storage with acid lipase deficiency: a new variant of Wolman's disease with features of the Senior syndrome. Pediatr Res 16:954–959, 1982.

50. Cutz E, Sondheimer J, Forstner GG, Weber JL: Histochemistry and ultrastructure of liver in cholesterol ester storage disease. Sci Proceed, Pediatr Pathol Club, Toronto, March 20, 1976.

51. Dincsoy HP, Rolfes DB, McGraw CA, Schubert WK: Cholesterol ester storage disease and mesenteric lipodystrophy. Am J Clin Pathol 81:263–269, 1984.

52. Miller R, Bialer MG, Rogers F, Jonsson HT, Allen RV, Hennigar GR: Wolman's disease: report of a case with multiple studies. Arch Pathol Lab Med 106:41–45, 1982.

53. Salen G: Cholesterol deposition in cerebrotendinous xanthomatosis. A possible mechanism. Ann Intern Med 75:843–851, 1971.

54. Salen G, Zaki FG, Sabesin S, Boehme D, Shefer S, Mosbach EH: Intrahepatic pigment and crystal forms in patients with cerebrotendinous xanthomatosis (CTX). Gastroenterology 24:82–89, 1978.

55. Björkem I, Skrede S. Familial disease with storage of sterols other than cholesterol: cerebrotendinous xanthomatosis and phytosterolemia. In The Metabolic Basis of Inherited Disease, edited by C.R. Scriver, A.L. Beaudet, W.S. Sly, D. Valle. 6th Edition. New York, McGraw-Hill Book Co., 1989, pp. 1283–1301.

56. Björkhem I, Fausa O, Hopen G, Oftebro H: Role of 26-hydroxylase in the biosynthesis of bile acids in the normal state and in cerebrotendinous xanthomatosis. J Clin Invest 71:142–148, 1983.

57. Berginer VM, Salen G, Shefer S: Long-term treatment of cerebrotendinous xanthomatosis with chenodeoxycholic acid. N Engl J Med 311:1649–1652, 1984.

58. Boehme DH, Sobel HJ, Marquet E, Salen G: Liver in cerebrotendinous xanthomatosis (CTX): a histochemical and EM study of four cases. Pathol Res Pract 170:192–201, 1980.

59. Peremans J, De Graef PJ, Strubbe G, De Block G: Familial metabolic disorder with fatty metamorphosis of the viscera. J Pediatr 69:1108–1112, 1966.

60. Satran L, Sharp HL, Schenken JR, Krivit W: Fatal neonatal hepatic steatosis: a new familial disorder. J Pediatr 75:39–46, 1969.

61. Wadlington WB, Riley HD: Familial disease characterized by neonatal jaundice, and probable hepatosteatosis and kernicterus: a new syndrome? Pediatrics 51:192–198, 1973.

62. Peters SP, Lee RE, Glew RH: Gaucher's disease, a review. Medicine 56:425–442, 1977.

63. Barranger JA, Ginns EI: Glucosylceramide lipidosis: Gaucher's disease. In The Metabolic Basis of Inherited Disease, edited by C.R. Scriver, A.L. Beaudet, W.S. Sly, D. Valle. 6th Edition. New York, McGraw-Hill Book Co., 1989, pp. 1677–1698.

64. Ginns EI: Determination of Gaucher's disease phenotypes with monoclonal antibody. Clin Chim Acta 131:283–287, 1983.

65. Ishak KG, Sharp HL: Metabolic errors and liver disease. In Pathology of the Liver, edited by R.N.M. MacSween, P.P. Anthony, P.J. Scheuer. 2nd Edition. Edinburgh, Churchill Livingstone, 1987, pp. 99–180.

66. Aderka D, Garfinkel D, Rothem A: Fatal bleeding from esophageal varices in a patient with Gaucher's disease. Am J Gastroenterol 77:838–845, 1982.

67. James SP, Stromeyer FW, Chang C: Liver abnormalities in patients with Gaucher's disease. Gastroenterology *80:*126–133, 1981.

68. Harinck HIJ, Bijvoet OLM, van der Meer JWH, Jones B, Onvlee GJ: Regression of bone lesions in Gaucher's disease during treatment with aminohydroxypropylidene biphosphonate. Lancet *2:*513–515, 1984.

69. Rappeport JM, Ginns EI: Bone-marrow transplantation in severe Gaucher's disease. N Engl J Med *311:*84–88, 1984.

70. Peters SP, Lee RE, Glew RH: Gaucher's disease: a review. Medicine *56:*425–442, 1977.

71. Katlove HE, Williams JC, Gaynor E, Spivack M, Bradley RM, Brady RO: Gaucher cells in chronic myelogenous leukemia: an acquired abnormality. Blood *33:*379–390, 1969.

72. Scullin DC Jr, Shelburne JD, Cohen HJ: Pseudo-Gaucher cells in multiple myeloma. Am J Med *67:*347–352, 1979.

73. Spence MW, Callahan JW: Sphingomyelin-cholesterol lipidoses: the Niemann-Pick group of diseases. *In* The Metabolic Basis of Inherited Disease, edited by C.R. Scriver, A.L. Beaudet, W.S. Sly, D. Valle. 6th Edition. New York, McGraw-Hill Book Co., 1989, pp. 1655–1676.

74. Long RG, Lake BD, Pettit JE: Adult Niemann-Pick disease: its relationship to the syndrome of the sea-blue histiocyte. Am J Med *62:*627–635, 1977.

75. O'Brien JS: β-Galactosidase deficiency; ganglioside sialidase deficiency. *In* The Metabolic Basis of Inherited Disease, edited by C.R. Scriver, A.L. Beaudet, W.S. Sly, D. Valle. 6th Edition. New York, McGraw-Hill Book Co., 1989, pp. 1797–1805.

76. Petrelli M, Blair JD: The liver in GM gangliosidosis types 1 and 2. Arch Pathol *99:*111–116, 1975.

77. Sandhoff K, Conzelmann E, Neufeld EF, Kaback MM, Suzuki K: The GM$_2$ gangliosidoses. *In* The Metabolic Basis of Inherited Disease, edited by C.R. Scriver, A.L. Beaudet, W.S. Sly, D. Valle. 6th Edition. New York, McGraw-Hill Book Co., 1989, pp. 1807–1839.

78. Desnick RJ, Bishop DF: Fabry's disease: α-galactosidase; Schinkler Disease: α-N-acetylgalactosaminidase deficiency. *In* The Metabolic Basis of Inherited Disease, edited by C.R. Scriver, A.L. Beaudet, W.S. Sly, D. Valle. 6th Edition. New York, McGraw-Hill Book Co., 1989, pp. 1751–1796.

79. Chatterjee S, Gupta P, Pyeritz RE, Kwiterovich PO: Immunohistochemical localization of glycosphingolipid in urinary renal tubular cells in Fabry's disease. Am J Clin Pathol *82:*24–28, 1984.

80. Rodriguez FH, Hoffmann EO, Ordinario AT, Baliga M: Fabry's disease in a heterozygous woman. Arch Pathol Lab Med *109:*89–91, 1985.

81. Meuwissen SGM, Dingemans KP, Stryland A, Tager JM, Ooms BCM: Ultrastructural and biochemical liver analyses in Fabry's disease. Hepatology *2:*263–268, 1982.

82. Moser HW, Moser AB, Chen WW, Schram AW: Ceramidase deficiency: Farber's lipogranulomatosis. *In* The Metabolic Basis of Inherited Disease, edited by C.R. Scriver, A.L. Beaudet, W.S. Sly, D. Valle. 6th Edition. New York, McGraw-Hill Book Co., 1989, pp. 1645–1654.

83. Pavone L, Moser HW, Mollica F, Rettino C, Durand P: Farber's lipogranulomatosis: ceramidase deficiency and prolonged survival in three relatives. Johns Hopkins Med J *147:*193–196, 1980.

84. Antonarakis SE, Valle D, Moser HW, Moser A, Qualman SJ, Zinkham WH: Phenotypic variability in siblings with Farber disease. J Pediatr *104:*406–409, 1984.

85. Wolfe HJ, Pietra GG: The visceral lesions of metachromatic leukodystrophy. Am J Pathol *44:*921–930, 1964.

86. MacFaul R, Cavanagh N, Lake BD, Stephens R, Whitfield AE: Metachromatic leukodystrophy: review of 38 cases. Arch Dis Child *57:*168–175, 1982.

87. Kolodny EH: Metachromatic leukodystrophy and multiple sulfatase deficiency: sulfatide lipidosis. *In* The Metabolic Basis of Inherited Disease, edited by C.R. Scriver, A.L. Beaudet, W.S. Sly, D. Valle. 6th Edition. New York, McGraw-Hill Book Co., 1989, pp. 1721–1750.

88. Burgess JH, Kalfayan B, Stungaard RK, Gilbert E: Papillomatosis of the gallbladder associated with metachromatic leukodystrophy. Arch Pathol Lab Med *109:*79–81, 1985.

89. Steinberg D: Refsum disease. *In* The Metabolic Basis of Inherited Disease, edited by C.R. Scriver, A.L. Beaudet, W.S. Sly, D. Valle. 6th Edition. New York, McGraw-Hill Book Co., 1989, pp. 1533–1550.

90. Refsum S: Clinical and genetic aspects of Refsum's disease. *In* Peripheral Neuropathy, Vol. II, edited by P.J. Dyck, P.K. Thomas, E.H. Lambert. Philadelphia, W.B. Saunders, 1975, pp. 868–872.

91. Dry J, Pradalier A, Canny M: Maladie de Refsum: Dix ans de regime dietetique pauvre en acid phytanique et phytol. Ann Med Interne *133:*483–487, 1982.

92. Scotto JM, Hadchouel M, Odievre M, Laudat MH, Saudubray JM, Dulaco O: Infantile phytanic acid storage disease, a possible variant of Refsum's disease. Three cases, including ultrastructural studies of the liver. J Inherited Metab Dis *5:*83–90, 1982.

93. Poulos A, Pollard AC, Mitchell JD, Wise G, Mortimer G: Patterns of Refsum's disease. Phytanic acid oxidase deficiency. Arch Dis Child *59:*222–229, 1984.

94. Kattlove HE, Gaynor E, Spivack M, Gottfied EI: Sea-blue indigestion. N Engl J Med *282:*630–631, 1970.

95. Silverstein MN, Elefson RD, Ahern EJ: The syndrome of the sea-blue histiocyte. N Engl J Med *282:*1–4, 1970.

96. Kelsey PR, Geary CG: Sea-blue histiocytes and Gaucher cells in bone marrow of patients with chronic myeloid leukaemia. J Clin Pathol *41:*960–962, 1988.

97. Rywlin AM, Hernandez JA, Chastain DE, Pardo V: Ceroid histiocytosis of spleen and bone marrow in idiopathic thrombocytopenic purpura (ITP): a contribution to the understanding of the sea-blue histiocyte. Blood *37:*587–593, 1971.

98. Wenger DA, Barth G, Githens JH: Nine cases of sphingomyelin lipidosis, a new variant in Spanish-American children. Juvenile variant of Niemann-Pick disease with foamy and sea-blue histocytes. Am J Dis Child *131:*955–961, 1977.

99. Viana MB, Giugliani R, Leite MH, Barth ML, Lekhwani C, Slade CM, Fensom A: Very low levels of high density lipoprotein cholesterol in four sibs of a family with non-neuropathic Niemann-Pick disease and sea-blue histiocytosis. J Med Genet *27:*499–504, 1990.

100. Rywlin AM, Lopez-Gomez A, Tachmes P, Pardo V: Ceroid histiocytes of the spleen in hyperlipemia: relation to the syndrome of the sea-blue histiocyte. Am J Clin Pathol *56:*572–579, 1971.

101. Besley GT, Broadhead DM, Lawlor E, McCann SR, Dempsey JD, Drury MI, Crowe J: Cholesterol ester storage disease in an adult presenting with sea-blue histiocytosis. Clin Genet 26:195–203, 1984.

102. Lee RE: Histiocytic diseases of bone marrow. Hematol Oncol Clin North Am *2:*657–667, 1988.

Chapter 16
Hepatic Lesions in Disorders of Protein and Amino Acid Metabolism

Protein deficiency

At one time, protein malnutrition was regarded as a major etiologic factor in the pathogenesis of various forms of liver disease in humans, a view based largely on circumstantial evidence, including (a) the prevalence of hepatic disease in areas of the world where dietary protein deficiency is common (1); (b) the frequency of malnutrition in individuals with alcoholic cirrhosis, and their apparent therapeutic response to protein supplementation of their diets (2); (c) the production in experimental animals of fatty infiltration and micronodular cirrhosis by diets deficient in protein and low in lipotropic activity (2–5); and (d) the massive hepatic necrosis and postnecrotic cirrhosis observed in experimental animals maintained on low protein diets deficient in sulfhydryl-containing amino acids (6) or selenium (7). On the basis of a biopsy and postmortem study of malnourished Bantu tribesmen in South Africa it was suggested that although protein deficiency clearly leads to fatty infiltration of the liver in infants with kwashiorkor, it is not responsible for hepatic fibrosis or cirrhosis. Presumably, it may render chronically malnourished individuals especially susceptible to the hepatic injurious effects of viruses, hemosiderosis, toxins, or drugs (8). Subsequent demonstrations of the importance of inapparent hepatitis virus infections including both HBV and HCV, as well as a number of hepatotoxins and drugs, in the pathogenesis of chronic liver disease provide more attractive alternative explanations for the development of cirrhosis (9). Nevertheless, the possibility that protein or other dietary deficiencies may play a contributory role has not yet been excluded with certainty. The association of malnutrition and alcoholic liver disease (10) is discussed more fully in Chapter 10. The simultaneous existence in such patients of vitamin and essential fatty acid and amino acid deficiencies makes it extremely difficult to ascertain their relative roles in the progression to chronic liver disease (11–13).

Reports of the development of hepatic lesions resembling alcoholic hepatitis and cirrhosis following jejunoileal bypass have revived interest in the possibility that nutritional deficiencies may play important roles in the pathogenesis of such lesions (14,15). Although evidence of this type cannot be discounted, it is still open to question, a point still actively debated (16). The enigma is further complicated by the fact that the development of chronic liver disease itself can induce and aggravate malnutrition (17).

Currently, *kwashiorkor* is the only hepatic disease clearly attributable to protein deficiency (18–20). Characteristically, it occurs in infants between the ages of one and three years who have been maintained on diets that are low in protein but relatively high in carbohydrate, so the overall calorie intake is adequate. The principal manifestations include retardation of growth, pellagra-like skin lesions, depigmentation of the hair, hepatomegaly, edema, and anemia. All of these features are readily reversible when the diet is supplemented with protein.

Fatty infiltration of the hepatocytes is the principal feature of the hepatic lesions. Initially, the lipid droplets are microvesicular and periportal in distribution (21,22). As the disease advances, however, the fat droplets assume their more characteristic macrovesicular form and a panlobular distribution (22). Histologically, the appearance is virtually identical to the fatty liver of alcohol (Fig. 175) or obesity (Fig. 675). In a small minority of cases, the portal tracts show fine stellate scarring, lymphocytic infiltration, and occasional eosinophils. Portal inflammation is mild. There is no convincing evidence that such lesions ever progress to cirrhosis (8,18).

When the diet is characterized by a deficiency not only of protein but also of calories and of other essential nutriments, as in marasmus in infancy or prolonged starvation at any age, the liver shows no evidence of fatty infiltration or fibrosis. Under these conditions, the hepatocytes tend to shrink in size owing to reduction in their protein content, and often exhibit an increase in lipofuscin pigmentation (18).

Hereditary amino acid disorders

Hereditary tyrosinemia

Hereditary tyrosinemia (tyrosinemia type I) (23–26), a disorder transmitted as an autosomal recessive trait, is characterized by abnormal tyrosine metabolism manifested by tyrosinemia, the excessive urinary excretion of tyrosine and its metabolites (tyrosyluria), signs of severe hepatic and renal tubular injury, and vitamin D–resistant rickets.

Although most authorities regard an absence of hepatic *p-hydroxyphenyl pyruvic acid oxidase* as the biochemical basis for this inherited disease of tyrosine metabolism, this view has been questioned, and alternative possibilities have been considered (27). The role of the metabolites of tyrosine in the pathogenesis of the hepatic and renal lesions of hereditary tyrosinemia is supported by the therapeutic effectiveness of diets deficient in tryosine and phenylalanine in most cases.

The disease sometimes presents acutely soon after birth, and may lead to death from hepatic failure within a few months, or it may run a more slowly progressive, chronic course that proves fatal during the first decade of life.

When the onset is relatively acute in early infancy, failure to thrive, hepatosplenomegaly, and signs of hepatocellular dysfunction are the principal manifestations. These include hyperbilirubinemia, hypoalbuminemia, and increased levels of the transaminases. In the more chronic form of the disease, features of renal tubular dysfunction that mimic those of the DeToni-Fanconi syndrome, usually accompanied by secondary hypophosphatemic rickets, are more prominent, although evidence of hepatic disease is almost always present.

The *hepatic lesions* in hereditary tyrosinemia are characterized by diffuse, irregularly distributed intralobular and periportal fibrosis that distorts the normal lobular architecture and leads to the formation of nodules of regenerating parenchyma and the development of cirrhosis. As illustrated in Figure 687, progression to cirrhosis occurs relatively early in the acute form of the disease that results in death from hepatic failure within the first few months of life. In such cases, the fibrosis is frequently accompanied by ductular proliferation (Fig. 688), and a number of nonspecific parenchymal changes that resemble those of galactosemia. The latter include transformation of the hepatic plates to pseudoacini or pseudoducts, hepatocellular ballooning, and bile stasis. (Fig. 689). Fatty infiltration in tyrosinemia is a less prominent feature, and, when present, usually is limited to occasional parenchymal nodules (Fig. 690).

In the more chronic form of the disease, fibrosis tends to progress, leading to cirrhosis, which may be micronodular, macronodular, or mixed in type. The distinctive parenchymal changes seen in the acute form of the disease are less prominent or absent.

In almost a third of the infants with tyrosinemia of the chronic type who survive for more than two years, the cirrhosis is complicated terminally by hepatocellular carcinoma (28). Acute, intermittent porphyria (Chapter 18) sometimes occurs in chronic tyrosinemia (29). Liver transplantation has successfully eradicated hereditary tyrosinemia (30).

Cystinosis

Cystinosis (27, 31–33) is an autosomal recessive hereditary disorder characterized by deposition of L-cystine crystals in the eyes and the lysosomes of phagocytic reticuloendothelial cells in many tissues. Although the underlying biochemical defect responsible for cystinosis has not been identified, the primary problem is the impaired transport of cystine out of lysosomes (34).

The disease may present in an infantile, nephropathic, severe form, as an adolescent, more mild form, or in adults as a benign type of cystinosis.

In the *infantile* type, the predominant clinical manifestations, which appear at the age of six to nine months, are attributable to a defect in renal tubular reabsorption that gives rise to the Fanconi syndrome. This disorder is characterized by polyuria, aminoaciduria, excessive loss of inorganic phosphorus that results in vitamin D–resistant rickets, and excessive loss of bicarbonate and potassium that leads to chronic acidosis and hypokalemia. Typical patients are short in stature, have light complexions, and photophobia (35). In addition, the eyes show crystalline deposits of cystine in the corneas and conjunctivae and a retinopathy characterized by peripheral foci of depigmentation and hyperpigmentation. Ultimately, renal failure due to progressive damage to the glomeruli ensues, resulting in death by the age of 10 years. Hypothroidism frequently accompanies this disorder (36).

Late onset cystinosis usually becomes clinically apparent after

the age of five years. The manifestations are similar to those in the infantile form of cystinosis, but are less severe and may be compatible with survival for two decades.

The *benign* form of cystinosis is asymptomatic and is unaccompanied by any evidence of hepatic or renal disease. As a rule, the disease is manifested by crystalline deposits of cystine in the corneas and conjunctivae discovered during the course of a routine slit-lamp examination of the eyes.

The disease can be diagnosed by measuring the amount of cystine in leukocytes or in fibroblasts cultured from the skin and by infrared spectroscopy of hair (37). The diagnosis can be made before birth by the microscopic demonstration of cystine crystals in the fetal tissues (38).

Treatment with cystine-depleting agents such as cysteamine and phosphocysteamine, although poorly tolerated, has induced important therapeutic benefits (39,40).

The *hepatic lesions* in cystinosis are characterized by centrilobular clusters of enlarged Kupffer cells that contain the distinctive hexagonal or rectangular crystals of L-cystine (Fig. 238), which exhibit brilliant birefringence in polarized light (Fig. 239). Less commonly, crystals of the same type are encountered in some portal macrophages. However, despite the deposits of crystals, cystinosis has no other adverse effects on the liver.

Since the crystals of L-cystine are water-soluble, fresh frozen sections or tissue fixed in alcohol or other nonaqueous solutions are required for their demonstration. Although a nonaqueous type of H & E stain is usually recommended, we have found that the crystals may resist dissolution during routine aqueous H & E staining. However, the Masson stain dissolves the crystals, so the affected Küpffer cells appear enlarged and filled with ill-defined granules rather crystals.

Homocystinuria

Homocystinuria (26,41–43) is an autosomal recessive hereditary disorder of methionine metabolism that leads to an accumulation of homocysteine in the tissues, homocystinemia and homocystinuria, and the development of lesions in the eyes, skeleton, blood vessels, and central nervous system. The underlying biochemical defect varies. It may involve a deficiency of either *cystathionine synthetase, 5,10-methylenetetrahydrofolate reductase,* or *N5-methyltetrahydrofolate homocysteine methyltransferase.*

The principal clinical manifestations include ectopia lentis, osteoporosis, kyphoscoliosis, arachnodactyly, arterial and venous thrombosis and embolism, and mental retardation, features that superficially may resemble those of Marfan's syndrome. Hepatomegaly is relatively common, but as a rule, there is no clinical or laboratory evidence of hepatic dysfunction (41).

The *hepatic lesion* is characterized by moderate, nonspecific, centrilobular and midzonal fatty infiltration. Less commonly, sinusoidal congestion, perisinusoidal or central venous fibrosis, intimal thickening, fibrosis of hepatic arterioles, portal fibrosis, or hemosiderosis may be seen individually or in various combinations.

Primary hyperoxaluria

Two types of hereditary hyperoxaluria (hereditary oxalosis) (26,44) have been identified. Both are transmitted as autosomal recessive traits and both are manifested by hyperoxaluria and recurrent nephrolithiasis that appear in childhood. Both are accompanied by progressive deposition of calcium oxalate crystals in the kidneys, nephrocalcinosis, and renal failure that usually proves fatal by the age of 20. The two types differ, however, in pathogenesis of the hyperoxaluria and in some of the other biochemical features.

Type I (glycolic aciduria), the more common of the two, is characterized by a deficiency of α-*ketoglutarate: glyoxylate carboligase,* an enzyme required for the conversion of glyoxylic acid to α-keto-β-hydroxyadipic acid. This deficiency leads to enhanced synthesis of oxalic acid and increased urinary excretion of oxalic glyoxylic, and glycolic acids. Treatment with pyridoxine may prevent or even reverse the renal lesions (45).

Although the enzyme defect responsible for type II hyperoxaluria is less certain, leukocyte studies indicate a deficiency of D-glyceric dehydrogenase, that results in excessive reduction of hydroxypyruvate to L-glyceric acid, increased synthesis of oxalic acid, and increased urinary excretion of oxalic, glyoxylic, and glycolic acids.

In some cases, the deposition of calcium oxalate crystals is not limited to the kidneys, and may be encountered in other tissues, a condition termed *oxalosis*. However, the extrarenal deposits exert no adverse effects on the tissues.

Oxalate crystals are round, globular, or rhomboidal, and may be arranged in the form of sheaves or rosettes. Characteristically, they are colorless or pale yellow, and, in polarized light, exhibit brilliant birefringence. In hepatic oxalosis, the crystals are usually localized to the media of hepatic arterioles (26). Rarely, they are found in the fibrous tissues of portal tracts (46).

Congenital hyperammonemic syndromes

A number of hereditary disorders are characterized by enzyme deficiencies that lead to protein intolerance and episodic hyperammonemia (26,47–49). Although the primary clinical manifestations, protein intolerance and hyperammonemic encephalopathy, are similar in the group as a whole, their mode of onset, severity, and accompanying biochemical findings differ, depending on the specific enzyme deficiency involved. Specific clinical manifestations characterize these diverse disorders, each of which is caused by a specific enzyme defect (49).

By far, the most common congenital hyperammonemic syndromes are attributable to a deficiency of one of the urea cycle enzymes. These include: carbamyl phosphate synthetase (CPS), ornithine transcarbamylase (OTC), arginosuccinate synthetase, arginosuccinase, and arginase (50).

Other less common congenital hyperammonemic disorders include: (1) the syndrome of hyperammonemia, hyperornithemia, and homocitrullinuria; (2) congenital lysine intolerance; (3) lysinuric protein intolerance; (4) citrullinemia; and (5) a variety of rare organic acidemias (51–53).

As a rule, the liver shows no histologic changes, but, in some patients, mild fatty infiltration is present. We have observed essentially normal liver tissue in patients with ornithine transcarbamylase (OTC) and carbamyl phosphate synthetase (CPS) deficiency. In one of the former a mild increase in portal fibrosis was noted (54). Electron microscopic examination showed minimal, nonspecific abnormalities, quite different from the grossly abnormal mitochondrial changes seen in the acquired

OTC and CPS deficiencies of Reye's syndrome (55). In citrullinemia occasional bile plugs have been seen (56).

Parenteral hyperalimentation

Intravenous hyperalimentation has been associated with acalculous cholecystitis, biliary sludge (57), gallstones (58), and abnormalities of liver function such as increased serum alkaline phosphatase and aminotransferase activity (59). In addition, nonspecific histologic abnormalities such as fatty deposition, portal inflammation, and intrahepatic cholestasis have been reported (60–65). Premature and neonatal infants are at particular risk (65). The fatty deposition, which occurs in both adults and children, tends to occur more frequently in children (66). It may be periportal or central in distribution and may be microvesicular or macrovesicular in character. Furthermore, it is not known whether these changes are associated with progression of the liver lesion. These hepatobiliary abnormalities occur less frequently in patients who are receiving oral feedings as well as total parenteral nutrition (TPN) (65).

In a controlled comparison of patients receiving TPN and similar patients not getting TPN, the hepatic histologic findings were similar in the two groups (67). The presence of hepatic lesions appeared to correlate better with the underlying hepatic disorders such as fatty deposition, necrosis, or cholestasis than with the administration of TPN. Furthermore, the presence of Crohn's disease, small bowel resection, or a related disorder, which is often the cause of malnutrition that requires TPN, may itself give rise to similar hepatic lesions.

References

1. Himsworth HP: Lectures on the Liver and its Diseases. Oxford, Blackwell Scientific Publications, 1947, pp. 1–204.
2. Patek AJ Jr, Post J, Ratnoff OD, Mankin H, Hillman RW: Dietary treatment of cirrhosis of the liver. Results in one hundred and twenty-four patients observed during a ten year period. JAMA *138*:543–549, 1948.
3. Lillie RD, Ashburn LL, Sebrell WH, Daft FS, Lowry JV: Histogenesis and repair of the hepatic cirrhosis in rats produced on low protein diets and prevention with choline. Public Health Rep *57*:502–508, 1942.
4. Wilgram GF: Experimental Laennec type of cirrhosis in monkeys. Ann Intern Med *51*:1134–1158, 1959.
5. Glynn LE, Himsworth HP, Lindan O: The experimental production and development of diffuse hepatic fibrosis ("portal cirrhosis"). Br J Exp Pathol *29*:1–9, 1948.
6. Glynn LE, Himsworth HP, Neuberger A: Pathological states due to deficiency of the sulphur containing amino acids. Br J Exp Pathol *26*:326–337, 1945.
7. Schwarz K: Factor 3, selenium and vitamin E. Nutr Rev *18*:193–197, 1960.
8. Higginson J, Grobbelaar BG, Walker ARP: Hepatic fibrosis and cirrhosis in man in relation to malnutrition. Am J Pathol *33*:29–53, 1957.
9. Pares A, Barrera JM, Caballeria J, Ercilla G, Bruguera M, Caballeria L, Castillo R, Rodes J: Hepatitis C virus antibodies in chronic alcoholic patients: association with severity of liver injury. Hepatology *12*:1295–1299, 1990.
10. Sherlock S: Nutrition and the alcoholic. Lancet *1*:436–440, 1984.
11. Morgan AG, Kelleher J, Walker BE, Losowsky MS: Nutrition in cryptogenic cirrhosis and chronic aggressive hepatitis. Gut *17*:113–118, 1976.
12. Morgan MY: Alcohol and nutrition. Br Med Bull *38*:21–29, 1982.
13. Sherlock S, Walshe VM: Hepatic structure and function. *In* Studies of Undernutrition, Wuppertal, Medical Research Council Report, 1946–49, series *275*:111–118, 1951.

14. O'Leary JP: Hepatic complications of jejunoileal bypass. Semin Liver Dis *3*:203–215, 1983.

15. Hocking MP, Diverson MC, O'Leary JP, Woodward ER: Jejunoileal bypass for morbid obesity. Late followup in 100 cases. N Engl J Med *308*:995–999, 1983.

16. Morgan MY: Alcohol and nutrition. Br Med bull *38*:21–29, 1982.

17. Mezey E: Liver disease and nutrition. Gastroenterology *74*:770–783, 1978.

18. Nayak NC: Nutritional liver disease. *In* Pathology of the Liver, edited by R.N.M. MacSween, P.P. Anthony, P.J. Scheuer, 2nd Edition. Edinburgh, Churchill Livingstone, 1987, pp. 265–280.

19. Trowell HC, Davies JNP: Kwashiorkor. I. Nutritional background, history, distribution, and incidence. Br Med *2*:796–798, 1952.

20. Trowell HC, Davies JNP, Dean RFA: Kwashiorkor. II. Clinical picture, pathology, and differential diagnosis. Br Med J *2*:798–801, 1952.

21. Webber BL, Freiman I: The liver in kwashiorkor. Arch Pathol *98*:400–408, 1974.

22. Scheuer PJ: The liver in systemic disease, pregnancy and organ transplantation. *In* Liver Biopsy Interpretation, edited by P.J. Scheuer, 4th Edition London, Bailliere Tindall, 1988, pp. 218–219.

23. Gentz J, Jagenburg R, Zetterstrom R: Tyrosinemia. J Pediatr *66*:670–696, 1965.

24. Carson NAJ, Biggart JD, Bittles AH, Donovan D: Hereditary tyrosinaemia. Clinical, enzymatic and pathological study of an infant with the acute form of the disease. Arch Dis Child *51*:106–113, 1976.

25. Scriver CR, Larochelle J, Silverberg M: Hereditary tyrosinemia and tyrosyluria in a French Canadian geographic isolate. Am J Dis Child *113*:41–46, 1967.

26. Ishak KG, Sharp HL: Metabolic errors and liver disease. *In* Pathology of the Liver, edited by R.N.M. Macsween, P.P. Anthony, P.J. Scheuer. 2nd Edition. Edinburgh, Churchill Livingstone, 1987, pp. 99–180.

27. Goldsmith LA, Laberge C: Tyrosinemia and related disorders. *In* The Metabolic Basis of Inherited Disease, edited by C.R. Scriver, A.L. Beaudet, W.S. Sly, D. Valle. 6th Edition. New York, McGraw-Hill Inf Svcs Co, 1989, pp. 547–562.

28. Weinberg AG, Mize CE, Worthen HG: The occurrence of hepatoma in the chronic form of hereditary tyrosinemia. J Pediatr *88*:434–438, 1976.

29. Strife F: Tyrosinemia with acute intermittent porphyria: aminolevulinic acid dehydratase deficiency related to elevated urinary aminolevulinic acid levels. J Pediatr *90*:400–404, 1977.

30. Van Thiel DH, Gartner LM, Thorp FK: Resolution of the clinical features of tyrosinemia following orthotopic liver transplantation for hepatoma. J Hepatol *3*:42–51, 1986.

31. Russell DS, Barrie HJ: Storage of cystine in the reticuloendothelial system and its association with chronic nephritis and renal rickets. Lancet *2*:899–905, 1936.

32. Schneider JA, Schulman JD: Cystinosis. *In* The Metabolic Basis of Inherited Disease, edited by J.B. Stanbury, J.B. Wyngaarden, D.S. Fredrickson, J.L. Goldstein, M.S. Brown. 5th Edition. New York, McGraw-Hill Book Co., 1983, pp. 1844–1866.

33. Gahl WA, Renlund M, Thoene JG: Lysosomal transport disorders: cystinosis and sialic acid storage disorders. *In* The Metabolic Basis of Inherited Disease, edited by C.R. Scriver, A.L. Beaudet, W.S. Sly, D.L. Valle. 6th Edition. New York, McGraw-Hill Inf Svcs Co, 1989, pp. 2619–2647.

34. Gahl WA, Tietze, F, Bashan N, Steinberz R, Schulman JD: Cystine transport is defective in isolated leukocyte lysosomes from patients with cystinosis. Science *166*:1152–1154, 1969.

35. Gahl WA, Thoene JG, Schneider JA, O'Regan S, Kaiser-Kupfer MI, Kuwabara T: Cystinosis: progress in a prototypic disease. Ann Intern Med *109*:557–569, 1988.

36. Chan AM, Lynch, MJG, Bailey JD. Ezrin C, Fraser D: Hypothyroidism in cystinosis. A clinical, endocrinologic and histologic study involving sixteen patients with cystinosis. Am J Med *48*:678–692, 1970.

37. Lubec G, Nauer G, Pollack A: Non-invasive diagnosis of cystinosis by infra-red spectroscopy of hair. Lancet *1*:623, 1983.

38. Boman H, Schneider JA: Prenatal diagnosis of nephropathic cystinosis. Acta Paediatr Scand *70*:389–393, 1981.

39. Gahl WA, Reed GF, Thoene JG: Cysteamine therapy for children with nephropathic cystinosis. N Engl J Med *316*:971–977, 1987.

40. Smolin LA, Clark KF, Thoene JG, Gahl WA, Schneider JA: A comparison of the effectiveness of cysteamine and phosphocysteamine in elevating free cystine in nephropathic cystinosis. Pediatr Res *23*:616–620, 1988.

41. Schimke RN, McKusick VA, Huang T, Pollack AD: Homocystinuria. Studies of 20 families with 35 affected members. JAMA *193*:711–719, 1965.

42. Gaull G, Sturman JA, Schaffner F: Homocystinuria due to cysthionine synthetase deficiency; enzymatic and ultrastructural studies. J Pediatr *84*:381–390, 1974.

43. Kanwar YS, Manaligod JR, Wong PWK: Morphologic studies in a patient with homocystinuria due to 5,10-methylenetetrahydrofolate reductase deficiency. Pediatr Res *10*:598–609, 1976.

44. Hillman RE: Primary hyperoxalurias. *In* The Metabolic Basis of Inherited Disease, edited by C.R. Scriver, A.L. Beaudet, W.S. Sly, D. Valle. 6th Edition. New York, McGraw-Hill Inf Svcs Co, 1989, pp. 933–944.

45. Alinei P, Guignard JP, Jaeger, P: Pyridoxine treatment of type I hyperoxaluria. N Engl J Med *311*:798–799, 1984.

46. Burke EC, Baggenstoss AH, Owen CA Jr, Power MH, Lohr OW: Oxalosis. Pediatrics *15*:383–391, 1955.

47. Brusilow SW, Horwich AL: Urea cycle enzymes. *In* The Metabolic Basis of Inherited Disease, edited by C.R. Scriver, A.L. Beaudet, W.S. Sly, D. Valle. 6th Edition. New York, McGraw-Hill Inf Svcs Co, 1989, pp. 629–664.

48. Sharp HL: Inherited disorders with metabolic hepatic dysfunction. *In* Bockus Gastroenterology, edited by J.E. Berk. 4th Edition. Philadelphia, W.B. Saunders, 1985, pp. 3236–3258.

49. Flannery DB, Hsia YE, Wolf B: Current status of hyperammonemic syndromes. Hepatology *2*:495–506, 1982.

50. LaBrecque DR, Lathan PS, Riely CA: Heritable urea cycle enzyme deficiency: liver disease in 16 patients. J Pediatr *94*:580–587, 1979.

51. Batshaw ML: Hyperammonemia. Curr Probl Pediatr *14*:1–69, 1984.

52. Rottem M, Statter M, Amit R, Brand N, Bujanover Y, Yatziv S: Clinical and laboratory study in 22 patients with inherited hyperammonemic syndromes Israel J Med Sci *22*:833–836, 1986.

53. Hudak ML, Jones MD, Brusilow SW: Differentiation of transient hyperammonemia of the newborn and urea cycle enzyme defects by clinical presentation. J Med *107*:712–719, 1985.

54. Latham PS, LaBrecque DR, McReynolds JW, Klatskin G: Liver ultrastructure in mitochondrial urea cycle enzyme deficiencies and comparison with Reye's syndrome. Hepatology *4*:404–407, 1984.

55. Partin JC, Schubert WK, Partin JS: Mitochondrial ultrastructure in Reye's syndrome (encephalopathy) and fatty degeneration of the viscera. N Engl J Med *285*:1339–1343, 1971.

56. Wick H, Bachmann C, Baumgartner G, Brechbuler T, Colombo JP, Weimann U: Variants of citrullinemia. Arch Dis Child *48*:636–641, 1973.

57. Messing B, Biries C, Kustlinger F, Bernier JJ: Does total parenteral nutrition induce gallbladder sludge formation and lithiasis? Gastroenterology *84*:1012–1019, 1983.

58. Messing B, Aprahamian M, Rautureau M, Bories C, Bisalli A, Stock-Dawge S: Gallstone formation during total parental nutrition: a prospective study in man. Gastroenterology *86*:1183, 1984 (Abstract).

59. Lindor KD, Fleming R, Abrams A, Hirschkorn MA: Liver function values in adult receiving total parenteral nutrition. JAMA *241*:2398–2400, 1979.

60. Sheldon, GF, Peterson SR, Sanders R: Hepatic dysfunction during hyperalimentation. Arch Surg *113*:504–508, 1978.

61. Dahms BB, Halpin TC: Serial liver biopsies in parenteral nutrition-associated cholestasis of early infancy. Gastroenterology *81*:136–144, 1981.

62. Vileisis RA, Inwood RJ, Hunt CE: Prospective controlled study of parenteral nutrition-associated cholestatic jaundice: effect of protein intake. J Pediatr *96*:893–897, 1980.

63. Baker AL, Rosenberg IH: Hepatic complications of total parenteral nutrition. Am J Med *82*:489–497, 1987.

64. Bowyer BA, Fleming CR, Ludwig J, Petz J, McGill DB: Does long-term home parenteral nutrition in adult patients cause chronic liver disease? JPEN *9*:11–17, 1985.

65. Roy CC, Belli DC: Hepatobiliary complications associated with TPN: an enigma. J Am Coll Nutr *4*:651–660, 1985.

66. Rager R, Finegold MJ: Cholestasis in immature newborn infants: is parenteral alimentation responsible? J Pediatr *86*:264–270, 1975.

67. Wolfe BM, Walker BK, Shaul DB, Wong L, Ruebner BH: Effect of total parenteral nutrition on hepatic histology. Arch Surg *123*:1084–1090, 1988.

Chapter 17
Hepatic Lesions in Disorders of Bilirubin Metabolism

Famililial nonhemolytic unconjugated hyperbilirubinemia

Crigler-Najjar syndrome

The Crigler-Najjar syndrome, first described in 1952 (1,2), is a hereditary disorder attributable to a deficiency of hepatic bilirubin *UDP-glucuronyltransferase*. This deficiency leads to impairment of bilirubin conjugation with glucuronic acid in the liver and its excretion in bile. Relatively deep, persistent acholuric jaundice develops at birth or soon thereafter. Subsequent studies have established that the disease occurs in two forms that differ in several important respects (3).

Type I Crigler-Najjar syndrome is inherited as an autosomal recessive trait, and is caused by the absence of *bilirubin UDP-glucuronyltransferase* activity in the liver (1). It is characterized by high concentrations of unconjugated bilirubin in the serum (>20 mg/dl) that do not decline following the administration of phenobarbital, and by pale bile, which contains little or no conjugated bilirubin. Bilirubin glucuronide is absent in serum (4). Prior to the introduction of phototherapy and albumin exchange, jaundice was complicated by the development of kernicterus, and death usually occurred within the first year or two of life. Several patients have survived into late adolescence. Liver transplantation may be life-saving (5). A phenobarbital-inducing form of UDP-glucuronyltransferase has been sequenced and expressed and suggests the possibility of enzyme replacement in the future (6).

In fatal cases of type I disease, postmortem examination of the liver is usually normal. After patients have received phototherapy, canalicular bile thrombi and mild degrees of portal fibrosis may be present (2). In antemortem biopsy sections stained by the Hall method, the cytoplasm of hepatocytes and Kupffer cells in both type I and type II disease usually exhibits diffuse bile staining (3).

Type II Crigler-Najjar syndrome is a less severe form of the disease, which is transmitted as an autosomal dominant trait (1). Compared with type I, the serum bilirubin concentration tends to be lower and characteristically drops, often to normal levels, following the administration of phenobarbital (7). It is characterized by normal-colored bile that contains bilirubin monoglucuronide (1,8), rarely causes kernicterus, and is compatible with normal survival despite persistence of the jaundice.

Histologically, the liver is normal except for the presence of small amounts of iron (9). There are no characteristic ultrastructural lesions (10).

The homozygous Gunn rat, a mutant strain that is characterized by congenital acholuric jaundice associated with an absence of hepatic bilirubin UDP-glucuronyltransferase activity, exhibits most of the clinical and biochemical features of the Crigler-Najjar syndrome type II (11).

Gilbert's syndrome (constitutional hepatic dysfunction)

Gilbert's syndrome is a relatively common, benign disorder characterized by mild unconjugated hyperbilirubinemia in the absence of overt hemolysis. (1) It exists in 2 or 3% of the population. Only rarely does the serum bilirubin concentration exceed 4 mg/dl, and often it declines spontaneously to the normal range. As a result, jaundice tends to be mild or is present only intermittently and, therefore, is frequently overlooked. Often, the hyperbilirubinemia is discovered unexpectedly on routing examination of the serum. Although the disorder may be encountered at any age, it is most common in adolescents and young adults.

The etiology of Gilbert's syndrome seems variable. The disease is familial in nature and appears to be transmitted as an autosomal dominant hereditary trait (1). Patients with this disorder are heterozygous for a single mutant gene (12). However, hyperbilirubinemia that is attributed to Gilbert's syndrome may be a manifestation of compensated hemolysis, viral hepatitis, or other underlying hepatobiliary disorders (13,14).

The pathogenesis of the hyperbilirubinemia in Gilbert's syndrome is no more uniform than is its etiology. At least two factors, either alone or combined, have been implicated in various studies: deficiency of hepatic *bilirubin UDP glucuronyltransferase* activity (1,15), and a defect in the hepatic uptake of bilirubin by the hepatocytes that is apparently related to altered membrane fluidity (1,16–18). In addition, Gilbert's syndrome and hemolysis may occur together, a combination interpreted as fortuitous rather than etiologically related (12,17,18). However, the concurrence of the two disorders may account for the high levels of serum bilirubin encountered in some cases. A variant of the syndrome, in which indocyanine green, rather than BSP uptake is impaired, appears to involve abnormal porphyrin metabolism (19).

Usually, the liver in cases of Gilbert's syndrome shows no distinctive histologic abnormalities. However, an increase in pericanalicular lipofuscin was an almost constant feature in some studies (20). In our experience in approximately 20 cases, such deposits have been rare by light microscopy. Other inconstant features include occasional cytoplasmic lipid deposits and minimal portal scarring and lymphocytosis.

By electron microscopy there has been controversy about whether there is hypertrophy of the endoplasmic reticulum (21). It has been considered that the presence or absence of this hypertrophy may identify two different metabolic variants of the syndrome (22).

In the absence of unequivocal evidence of nonhemolytic, unconjugated hyperbilirubinemia in other family members, a thorough investigation to exclude other disorders that may mimic Gilbert's syndrome is required to establish the diagnosis. Liver biopsy is only rarely required. A significant rise in the serum bilirubin level following a reduction in the caloric intake to 400 per 24 hours is said to be diagnostic (23). However, a number of studies suggest that the rise in serum bilirubin produced by fasting or reducing the caloric intake may not be specific for Gilbert's syndrome. Similarly, the fall in serum bilirubin levels with phenobarbital is nonspecific (24). Normal or low fasting serum glycocholate levels may be of diagnostic value (25,26). The increase in serum bilirubin levels after intravenous nicotinic acid, which increases the osmotic fragility of erythrocytes, is also nonspecific (27). If necessary, liquid chromatography can establish the diagnosis by demonstrating that unconjugated bilirubin concentrations are higher in Gilbert's syndrome than in chronic hemolysis or chronic hepatitis (28). Despite the opportunities for confusion, the diagnosis is readily made (29). A primate model, the squirrel monkey, has been discovered (30).

Primary shunt hyperbilirubinemia

Another form of nonhemolytic unconjugated hyperbilirubinemia is attributable to an increase in the early-labeled fraction of bilirubin that comprises approximately 10% of the bilirubin produced normally. Bone marrow hemoglobin and other heme compounds serve as the source of this pigment.

Rarely, overproduction of shunt bilirubin is a hereditary disorder (1,31,32), but it is a relatively common finding under a wide variety of other conditions associated with ineffective, secondary erythropiesis (33). As a rule, the hyperbilirubinemia is accompanied by reticulocytosis and increased fecal urobilinogen, but the life span of the circulating erythrocytes is normal.

In the familial (primary) form of the disease, both the periportal hepatocytes and scattered proliferating Küpffer cells may contain hemosiderin granules (31). Similar features are encountered in at least some of the secondary forms of shunt hyperbilirubinemia.

Familial conjugated hyperbilirubinemia (chronic idiopathic jaundice)

Dubin-Johnson syndrome

The Dubin-Johnson syndrome (1,34–37) is a chronic, benign hereditary disorder characterized by a defect in the hepatic excretion of conjugated bilirubin resulting in conjugated hyperbilirubinemia and the appearance of bilirubin in the urine (1). A distinctive feature of the disease is the occurrence within the cytoplasm of the hepatocytes of coarse, dark brown granules that give the liver a dark brown or black color (Fig. 157). The nature of the pigment is still controversial.

In contrast to other forms of conjugated hyperbilirubinemia attributable to hepatocellular disease or biliary obstruction, the Dubin-Johnson syndrome is unaccompanied by an increase in serum bile acid or alkaline phosphatase levels, pruritus, or histologic evidence of cholestasis. Furthermore, the hepatic excretion of conjugated dyes is implied in Dubin-Johnson syndrome. Thus, with few exceptions, the gallbladder fails to visualize on oral cholecystography (34,35). The hepatobiliary tree can be

visualized, however, by ^{99m}Tc-HIDA scans (38). The uptake and conjugation of bromsulphalein (BSP) by the liver are normal, but the hepatic excretion of conjugated BSP into the bile is seriously impaired (22,39). As a result, the clearance of the dye from the serum 45 minutes following an intravenous injection of 5 mg/kg is normal or close to normal. However, there is a secondary rise in the BSP level at 90 to 120 minutes due to regurgitation of its conjugate from the liver, an observation that provides confirmatory evidence of the diagnosis (39).

Another distinctive feature of the Dubin-Johnson syndrome is an increase in the proportion of urinary coproporphyrin excreted as isomer I (65 to 90%) compared with a normal fraction of approximately 25% (40,41). This increment occurs at the expense of isomer III, since total urinary coproporhyrin excretion usually remains normal. Asymptomatic heterozygotes for the abnormal gene excrete isomer I in amounts intermediate between those of homozygotes and normal subjects (41).

Most authorities agree that the Dubin-Johnson syndrome is inherited as an autosomal recessive trait (1,41,42). However, some contradictory evidence has been reported (43).

Usually, jaundice, the principal manifestation of the disease, becomes apparent during the first three decades of life. In most cases, the onset is insidious, but, occasionally, it is acute and may be mistaken for acute viral hepatitis. Although the jaundice tends to persists, it frequently fluctuates in intensity and occasionally is intermittent. Exacerbations may be provoked by intercurrent infections, pregnancy, and the use of oral contraceptives (44). Hepatomegaly or splenomegaly are inconstant features of the disease. For reasons that are not known, some patients complain of intermittent abdominal pain, nausea, anorexia, and weakness. The serum bilirubin concentration varies widely, but usually ranges between 2 and 20 mg/dl, at least half of which is conjugated. The prognosis, however, is excellent (45).

The development of intercurrent viral hepatitis in a patient with the Dubin-Johnson syndrome has been reported to result in the transient mobilization of the pigment from the liver (46).

The outstanding feature of the *hepatic lesions* is the presence within the cytoplasm of the hepatocytes of numerous large, round or irregularly shaped, dark brown granules (Fig. 157). These predominate in the centrilobular zones, but tend to extend to the periphery of the lobules with advancing age of the disorder. Occasionally, similar granules are found within a few of the Kupffer cells and portal macrophages. In older patients, some of the portal tracts may exhibit mild, stellate fibrosis and lymphocytosis, and the parenchyma may contain small foci of hepatocellular necrosis. As previously noted, bile thrombi are not a feature of the syndrome. By electron microscopy these dense pigment bodies are found in lysosomes (47).

Neither the biochemical nature nor the source of the Dubin-Johnson pigment granules is fully understood. Except for their larger size and deeper brown color, the granules closely resemble those of lipofuscin. Both are found within lysosomes (48), and exhibit similar histochemical properties, including inconstant diastase-resistant PAS positivity, acid-fastness, uptake of silver on staining, and insolubility in a wide variety of polar and nonpolar solvents (36). However, differences in ultrastructure (49) and staining reactions (48,49) have been reported. Some investigators suggest that the pigment granules of the Dubin-Johnson syndrome contain melanin (48). The demonstration of persistent melanuria in a reported case (49) lends some support to this possibility. Also, the pigment isolated from the livers of mutant Corriedale sheep with black liver disease, a disorder similar to the Dubin-Johnson syndrome, exhibits physicochemical properties identical with those of melanin (50). Studies in these animals have suggested that the accumulation of the pigment in the liver may be attributable to a defect in the excretion of epinephrine metabolites (51).

Rotor's syndrome

Rotor's syndrome is (1,52–54) is a hereditary form of conjugated hyperbilirubinemia that closely resembles the Dubin-Johnson syndrome except for the absence of pigment in the hepatocytes. Although a number of other differences have been reported, these have not been constant. Moreover, in at least one family with hereditary conjugated hyperbilirubinemia, two members exhibited typical Dubin-Johnson pigment, whereas a third did not (52). Accordingly, the possibility has been considered that the Rotor and Dubin-Johnson syndromes represent variants of the same disorder.

Histologically there are no abnormalities in Rotor's syndrome. The pigment that characterizes the related Dubin-Johnson syndrome is absent. By electron microscopy abnormalities of the mitochondria and peroxisomes are seen (55).

The principal features of Rotor's syndrome usually cited in support of the view that it is a distinct entity unrelated to the Dubin-Johnson syndrome include the following: (1) the gallbladder visualizes normally on oral cholecystography; (2) the uptake of BSP by the liver is impaired, and there is no delayed secondary rise in its serum concentration due to regurgitation of its conjugate from the liver (56); and (3) both total urinary coproporphyrin and its type I isomer are increased (57,58). However, in some cases of the Dubin-Johnson syndrome, the gallbladder visualizes normally on oral cholecystography, and BSP retention is elevated after 45 minutes (34), and, in some studies of Rotor's syndrome, the increase in urinary coproporphyrin involves isomer type I, but is not accompanied by an increase in isomer type III or total coproporphyrin (58).

Available evidence suggests that Rotor's syndrome is inherited as an autosomal recessive trait (1,23).

References

1. Chowdhury JR, Wolkoff AW, Arias IM: Hereditary jaundice and disorders of bilirubin metabolism. *In* The Metabolic Basis of Inherited Disease, edited by C.R. Scriver, A.L. Beaudet, W.S. Sly, D. Valle. 6th Edition. New York, McGraw-Hill Inf Svcs Co, 1989, pp. 1367–1408.
2. Crigler JF Jr, Najjar VA: Congenital familiar nonhemolytic jaundice with kernicterus. Pediatrics *10*:169–180, 1952.
3. Arias IM, Gartner LM, Cohen M, Ben Ezzer J, Levi AJ: Chronic nonhemolytic unconjugated hyperbilirubinemia with glucuronyl transferase deficiency. Clinical, biochemical, pharmacologic and genetic evidence for heterogeneity. Am J Med *47*:395–409, 1969.
4. Muraca M, Fevery J, Blanchaert N: Relationships between serum bilirubins and production and conjugation of bilirubin. Studies in Gilbert's syndrome, Crigler-Najjar disease, hemolytic disorders and rat models. Gastroenterology *92*:309–317, 1987.
5. Kaufman SS, Wood RP, Shaw BW Jr: Orthotopic liver transplantation for type 1 Crigler-Najjar syndrome. Hepatology *6*:1259–1261, 1986.
6. Mackenzie PI. Rat liver UDP-glucuronyltransferase. Sequence and expression of a cDNA encoding a phenobarbital-inducible form. J Biol Chem *261*:6119–6125, 1986.
7. Gollan JL, Dallinger KJC, Billing BH: Excretion of conjugated bilirubin in the isolated perfused rat kidney. Clin Sci Mol Med *54*:381–389, 1978.
8. Fevery J, Blanckaert N, Heirwegh KPM, Preaux A-M, Berthelot P: Unconjugated bilirubin and an increased proportion of bilirubin monoglucuronates in the bile of patients with Gilbert's syndrome and Crigler-Najjar disease. J Clin Invest *60*:970–979, 1977.
9. Scheuer PJ: Hyperbilirubinemias. *In* Liver Biopsy Interpretation, 4th Edition. London, Bailliere Tindall, 1988, pp. 201–206.
10. Desmet VJ: Cholestasis: extrahepatic obstruction and secondary biliary cirrhosis. *In* Pathology of the Liver, edited by R.N. MacSween, P.P. Anthony, P.J. Scheuer, 2nd Edition. Edinburgh, Churchill Livingstone, 1987, pp. 409–423.
11. Schmid R, Axelrod J, Hammaker L, Swarm RL: Congenital jaundice in rats due to a defect in glucuronide formation. J Clin Invest *37*:1123–1130, 1958.
12. Powell LW, Hemingway E, Billing BH, Sherlock S: Idiopathic unconjugated hyperbilirubinemia (Gilbert's syndrome). A study of 42 families. N Engl J Med *277*:1108–1112, 1967.
13. Levine RA, Klatskin G: Unconjugated hyperbilirubinemia in the absence of overt hemolysis. Importance of acquired disease as an etiologic factor in 366 adolescent and adult subjects. Am J Med *36*:541–552, 1964.
14. Arias IM: Chronic unconjugated hyperbilirubinemia without overt signs of hemolysis in adolescents and adults. J Clin Invest *41*:2233–2245, 1962.
15. Black M, Billing BH: Hepatic bilirubin UDP-glucuronyl transferase activity in liver disease and Gilbert's syndrome, N Engl J Med *280*:1266–1271, 1969.
16. Galambos JT, McLaren JR: Hepatic uptake defect in patients with "Gilbert's disease." Arch Intern Med *111*:214–218, 1963.
17. Berk PD, Bloomer JR, Howe RB, Berlin NI: Constitutional hepatic dysfunction (Gilbert's syndrome). A new definition based on kinetic studies with unconjugated radiobilirubin. Am J Med *49*:296–305, 1970.
18. Reichen J: Familial unconjugated hyperbilirubinemia syndromes. Semin Liver Dis *3*:24–45, 1983.
19. McColl KEL, Thompson GG, EL Omar E: Porphyrin metabolism and haem biosynthesis in Gilbert's syndrome. Gut *28*:125–130, 1987.
20. Barth RF, Grimley PM, Berk PD, Bloomer JR, Howe RB: Excess lipofuscin accumulation in constitutional hepatic dysfunction (Gilbert's syndrome). Light and electron microscopic observations. Arch Pathol *91*:41–47, 1971.
21. Jezequel A-M, Mosca PG, Koch MM, Orlandi F: The fine morphology of unconjugated hyperbilirubinemia revisited with stereometry. *In* Familial Hyperbilirubinemia, edited by L. Okolicsanyi. Chichester, John Wiley & Sons, 1981, pp. 69–82.
22. Blanckaert N, Schmid R: Physiology and pathophysiology of bilirubin metabolism. *In* Hepatology, A Textbook of Liver Disease, edited by D. Zakim, T.D. Boyer, Philadelphia, W.B. Saunders, 1990, pp. 254–302.
23. Owens D, Sherlock S: Diagnosis of Gilbert's syndrome: role of reduced caloric intake test. Br Med J *3*:559–563, 1973.
24. Black M, Sherlock S: Treatment of Gilbert's syndrome with phenobarbitone. Lancet *1*:1359–1362, 1970.
25. Roda A, Roda E, Sama C: Serum primary bile acids in Gilbert's syndrome. Gastroenterology *82*:77–83, 1982.
26. Vierling JM, Berk PD, Hofmann AF: Normal fasting-state levels of serum cholylconjugated bile acids in Gilbert's syndrome: an aid to the diagnosis. Hepatology *2*:340–343, 1982.
27. Rollinghoff W, Paumgartner G, Preisig R: Nicotinic acid test in the diagnosis of Gilbert's syndrome: correlation with bilirubin clearance. Gut *22*:663–668, 1981.
28. Sieg A, Stiehl A, Raedsch R, Ullrich D, Messmer B, Kommerell B: Gilbert's syndrome: diagnosis by typical serum bilirubin pattern. Clin Chim Acta *154*:41–47, 1986.
29. Okolicsanyi L, Fevery J, Billing BH: How should mild, isolated unconjugated hyperbilirubinema be investigated? Semin Liver Dis *3*:36–54, 1983.
30. Portman OW, Chowdhury, JR, Chowdhury NR, Alexander M, Cornelius CE, Arias IM: A nonhuman primate model of Gilbert's syndrome. Hepatology *4*:175–179, 1984.
31. Israels LG, Suderman HJ, Ritzmann SE: Hyperbilirubinemia due to an alternate path of bilirubin production. Am J Med *27*:693–702, 1959.
32. Israels LG, Yamamoto T, Skanderbeg J, Zipursky A: Shunt bilirubin: evidence for two components. Science *139*:1054–1055, 1963.
33. Israels LG: The bilirubin shunt and shunt hyperbilirubinemia. *In* Progress in Liver Disease, Vol. III, edited by H Popper and F Schaffner New York, Grune & Stratton, 1970, pp. 1–12.
34. Dubin IN, Johnson FB: Chronic idiopathic jaundice with unidentified

pigment in liver cells. A new clinicopathologic entity with a report of 12 cases. Medicine *33:*155–197, 1954.

35. Sprinz H, Nelson RS: Persistent nonhemolytic hyperbilirubinemia associated with lipochrome-like pigment in liver cells: report of 4 cases. Ann Intern Med *41:*952–962, 1954.

36. Dubin IN: Chronic idiopathic jaundice. A review of fifty cases. Am J Med *24:*268–292, 1958.

37. Arias IM: Studies of chronic familial non-hemolytic jaundice with conjugated bilirubin in the serum with and without an unidentified pigment in the liver cells. Am J Med *31:*510–518, 1961.

38. Bar-Meir S, Bron J, Seligson U, Gottesfeld F, Levy R, Gilat T: ⁹⁹ᵐTc-HIDA cholescintigraphy in Dubin-Johnson and Rotor syndromes. Radiology *142:*743–750, 1982.

39. Mandema E, de Fraiture WH, Nieweg HO, Arends A: Familial chronic idiopathic jaundice (Dubin-Sprinz disease) with a note on bromsulphalein metabolism in the disease. Am J Med *28:*42–50, 1960.

40. Ben-Ezzer J, Rimington C, Shani M, Seligsohn U, Sheba CH, Szeinberg A: Abnormal excretion on the isomers of urinary coproporphyrin by patients with Dubin-Johnson syndrome in Israel. Clin Sci *40:*17–30, 1971.

41. Wolkoff AW, Cohen LE, Arias IM: Inheritance of Dubin-Johnson syndrome. N Engl J Med *288:*113–117, 1973.

42. Edwards RH: Inheritance of the Dubin-Johnson-Sprinz syndrome. Gastroenterology *68:*734–749, 1975.

43. Butt HR, Anderson VE, Foulk WT, Baggenstoss AH, Schoenfield LJ, Dickson ER: Studies of chronic idiopathic jaundice (Dubin-Johnson syndrome). II. Evaluation of a large family with the trait. Gastroenterology *51:*619–630, 1966.

44. Cohen L, Lewis C, Arias IM: Pregnancy, oral contraceptives and chronic familial jaundice with predominantly conjugated hyperbilirubinemia (Dubin-Johnson syndrome). Gastroenterology *62:*1182–1190, 1972.

45. Sherlock S:: Jaundice. *In* Diseases of the Liver and Biliary System, 8th Edition. London, Blackwell Scientific Publications, 1989, pp. 230–247.

46. Varma RR, Grainger JM, Scheuer PJ: A case of the Dubin-Johnson syndrome complicated by acute hepatitis. Gut *11:*817–821, 1970.

47. Seymour CA, Neale G, Peters TJ: Lysosomal changes in liver tissue from a patient with the Dubin-Johnson-Sprinz syndrome. Clin Sci Mol Med *52:*241–250, 1977.

48. Baba N, Ruppert RD: The Dubin-Johnson syndrome: electron microscopic observations of hepatic pigment—a case study. Am J Clin Pathol *57:*306–310, 1972.

49. Ehrlich JC, Novikoff AB, Platt R, Essner E: Hepatocellular lipofuscin and the pigment of chronic idiopathic jaundice. Bull NY Acad Med *36:*488–491, 1960.

50. Cornelius C, Arias IM, Osburn BI: Hepatic pigmentation with photosensitivity: a syndrome in Corriedale sheep resembling Dubin-Johnson Syndrome in man. JAVMA *146:*709–713, 1965.

51. Arias IM: Inheritable and congenital hyperbilirubinemia. Models for the study of drug metabolism. N Engl J Med *285:*1416–1421, 1971.

52. Schiff L, Billing BH, Oikawa Y: Familial nonhemolytic jaundice with conjugated bilirubin in the serum: a case study. N Engl J Med *260:*1315–1318, 1959.

53. Pereira Lima JE, Utz E, Roisenberg I: Hereditary nonhemolytic conjugated hyperbilirubinemia without abnormal liver cell pigmentation. A family study. Am J Med *40:*628–633, 1966.

54. Chowdury JR, Wolkoff AW, Arias IM: Hereditary jaundice and disorders of bilirubin metabolism. *In* the Metabolic Basis of Inherited Disease, edited by C.R. Scriver, A.L. Beaudet, W.S. Sly, D. Valle. 6th Edition. New York, McGraw-Hill Inf Svcs Co, 1989, pp. 1367–1408.

55. Evans J, Lefkowitch J, Lim CK: Fecal porphyrin abnormalities in a patient with features of Rotor's syndrome. Gastroenterology *81:*1125–1130, 1981.

56. Wolpert E, Pascasio FM, Wolkoff AW, Arias IM: Abnormal sulfobromophthalein metabolism in Rotor's syndrome and obligate heterozygotes. N Engl J Med *296:*1099–1101, 1977.

57. Wolkoff AW, Wolpert E, Pascasio FM, Arias IM: Rotor's syndrome. A distinct inheritable pathophysiologic entity. Am J Med *60:*173–179, 1976.

58. Shimizu Y, Naruto H, Ida S, Kohakura M: Urinary coproporphyrin isomers in Rotor's syndrome: a study in eight families. Hepatology *1:*173–178, 1981.

Chapter 18
Hepatic Lesions in Disorders of Porphyrin Metabolism

The porphyrias comprise a group of disorders characterized by defects in the biosynthesis of heme. Depending on the major site of the defect and on its clinical manifestations, it is common practice to classify porphyrias as hemopoietic or hepatic (1–4). However, in some types, the defect in heme synthesis is demonstrable in both the bone marrow and liver, so classification is difficult. Thus, although protoporphyria is frequently designated as erythropoietic, there is evidence that the excessive production of protoporphyrin also occurs in the liver (5). The relationship between porphyrin metabolism and hepatic disorders has been well reviewed (6).

With the exception of *porphyria cutanea tarda,* which may be inherited or acquired, all the other porphyrias to be discussed are hereditary in nature.

Hereditary porphyrias

Congenital erythropoietic porphyria (Gunther's disease)

Gunther's disease (7,8), a rare hereditary disorder, is transmitted as an autosomal recessive trait, and is characterized by a deficiency of *uroporphyrinogen III cosynthase,* chiefly in the erythroid cells of the bone marrow. As a result, uroporphyrin accumulates in the erythroid cells and is excreted in the urine.

The principal manifestations of the disease, which usually appear during infancy, include: (1) photosensitivity of the skin, often with disfigurement; (2) excretion of red urine due to excessive amounts of uroporphyrin; (3) reddish discoloration of the teeth (erythrodentia); (4) hemolytic anemia with bone marrow erythroid hyperplasia and splenomegaly; and (5) red fluorescence of bone marrow normoblasts in ultraviolet light. Activated charcoal, which binds porphyrins, can diminish enteral absorption of endogenous porphyrins excreted into the lumen of the GI tract, and may induce remission (9).

Usually, the liver is normal in appearance and does not exhibit fluorescence in ultraviolet light. However, in one case, death was due to hepatic failure secondary to macronodular cirrhosis (10). In the absence of porphyrin deposition it is highly probable that the cirrhosis in this case was coincidental.

Acute intermittent porphyria

Acute intermittent porphyria (2,8), which is a form of hepatic porphyria inherited as an autosomal dominant trait, is characterized by a block in the conversion of porphobilinogen to uroporphyrin due to a deficiency of *porphobilinogen deaminase.*

At least four mutations have been identified that can cause the acute intermittent porphyria syndrome (6). Secondarily, as a result of the block in porphyrin metabolism, there is an increase in hepatic *delta-aminolevulinic acid* (ALA) synthase activity, leading to excessive hepatic production of ALA and porphobilinogen, which are excreted in the urine.

Usually, the clinical manifestations of acute intermittent porphyria appear during the third decade of life, and are characterized by recurrent attacks of abdominal pain, vomiting, and constipation, neurologic and psychiatric signs, and hypertension. Often, these are inherited or aggravated by the use of drugs such as barbiturates, steroids, and oral contraceptives that induce hepatic microsomal enzymes, by alcohol (11), pregnancy, starvation, or intercurrent infection. Death from respiratory failure may occur during episodes of prominent neurologic manifestations. Photosensitivity is not a feature of the disease. Hepatocellular carcinoma has been reported in association with acute intermittent porphyria (12).

The urine contains high concentrations of porphobilinogen and ALA. On standing, the urine may darken owing to oxidation of porphobilinogen to porphobilin and nonenzymatic conversion to porphyrin.

The livers of patients with acute intermittent porphyria do not fluoresce in ultraviolet light, since neither ALA nor porphobilinogen are fluorescent compounds. Varying degrees of fatty infiltration and hemosiderosis are relatively common features (13). Other nonspecific histologic changes that have been encountered in occasional cases include hepatocellular pleomorphism and regeneration and focal congestion. Electron microscopy shows enlarged, abnormally shaped mitochondria that contain large, electron-dense granules as well as lipofuscin bodies with extensive deposits of ferritin (4).

In some cases, intravenous administration of hematin aborts the acute attacks and reduces the urinary excretion of porphobilinogen and ALA in acute intermittent porphyria (14).

Variegate porphyria (South African mixed porphyria)

Variegate porphyria (8,15), an autosomal dominant hereditary disorder, is characterized by a deficiency of *protoporphyrinogen oxidase,* an enzyme that catalyzes the oxidation of protoporphyrinogen to protoporphyrin (16). High fecal levels of coproporphyrin and protoporphyrin are the principal biochemical findings. Autooxidation of the large amounts of protoporbilinogen excreted in the bile may account for the protoporphyrin that is always present in the feces (16). During acute attacks of abdominal pain or neurologic symptoms, the urine may contain significant amounts of ALA and porphobilinogen.

Variegate porphyria is relatively common in South Africa among the descendents of Dutch immigrants (8). Several large collections of cases have been reported from the United States among family members of Norwegian descent (15,17).

As in the case of acute intermittent porphyria, the clinical manifestations usually appear during the third decade of life and often are characterized by recurrent episodes of abdominal pain, and neuropsychiatric signs. However, in contrast, not infrequently there is evidence of photosensitivity, either alone or in combination with neurologic manifestations. Areas of skin exposed to sunlight are abnormally fragile and often exhibit hyperpigmentation, scarring, and hypertrichosis.

Usually, the liver shows no abnormalities, but slight portal fibrosis and lymphocytosis and cytoplasmic deposits of unidentified pigment have been reported in some cases. Characteristically, the liver does not fluoresce in ultraviolet light.

Hereditary coproporphyria

Hereditary coproporphyria (3,18,19), a disorder transmitted as an autosomal dominant trait, is characterized by a deficiency of *coproporphyrinogen oxidase,* which blocks the conversion of coproporphyrinogen III to protoporphyrinogen IX in the biosynthetic pathway of heme metabolism. This leads to excessive excretion of coproporphyrin III in the feces and the urine. During acute attacks, particularly when complicated by hepatocellular dysfunction, the urine may contain increased amounts of ALA and porphobilinogen.

A high proportion of affected individuals are asymptomatic. However, in about a third of cases, clinical manifestations resembling those of acute intermittent porphyria appear in early adult life. These include intermittent attacks of abdominal pain, vomiting, and obstipation, neurologic signs, psychiatric symptoms, and photosensitivity of the skin. Often, the attacks are precipitated by the use of drugs, particularly barbiturates and steroids, and, occasionally, are associated with pregnancy. Evidence of hepatocellular dysfunction is relatively common during such attacks, and rare instances of overt jaundice have been reported. In cases with marked coproporphyrinuria, the urine may be dark brown in color. Usually, the course of the disease is benign, but rare instances of death from respiratory paralysis have been encountered in patients with severe neurologic manifestations.

No specific *hepatic lesions* have been described in the few cases that have been subjected to biopsy. Rare instances of cholestasis and cirrhosis have been reported, but the relationship of these lesions to the underlying porphyria is in doubt. Occasionally, the hepatocytes exhibit red fluorescence in ultraviolet light (3).

Erythropoietic (erythrohepatic) protoporphyria

Erythropoietic protoporphyria (8,20), a hereditary disorder transmitted as an autosomal dominant trait, is characterized by a deficiency of *heme synthetase (ferrochelatase),* a mitochondrial enzyme that catalyzes the chelation of protoporphyrin with ferrous iron to form heme (21). In affected individuals, the deficiency is demonstrable in the liver (21), bone marrow (22),

and cultured skin fibroblasts (21). Because of this block in the pathway of heme biosynthesis, excessive amounts of protoporphyrin are expected in the bile and feces, and accumulate in the liver, red blood cells, and plasma (23).

Photosensitivity, which appears in childhood and persists, is the principal clinical manifestation of erythropoietic protoporphyria (24). Exposure to sunlight results in itching, burning, and stinging of the skin, followed by the appearance of erythema and edema. Between attacks, exposed areas of skin often exhibit thickening and scarring. In contrast to other forms of porphyric photosensitivity, erythropoietic protoporphyria rarely, if ever, is associated with the formation of vesicles or bullae. Photosensitivity is produced by light in the 400 to 410 nm spectral region and appears to correlate with the plasma protoporphyrin level.

A high proportion of patients with erythropoietic protoporphyria exhibit hepatic lesions on biopsy (25), but in only a small minority of patients are these abnormalities accompanied by clinical or biochemical evidence of hepatic dysfunction (24). Nevertheless, in a small minority of cases, erythropoietic protoporphyria may give rise to progressive hepatic lesions that lead to the development of cirrhosis and hepatic failure that usually prove fatal within a few months (23,24,26). The accumulated protoporphyrin may be directly toxic to hepatocytes (27). Paradoxically, iron therapy, which decreases stool protoporphyrin levels (28), and cholestyramine, which increases fecal excretion (20), both seem to improve liver function. Liver transplantation has been effective in eradication of protoporphyria (6).

The principal laboratory features of erythropoietic protoporphyria include increased concentrations of protoporphyrin in the feces, erythrocytes, and plasma, and red fluorescence of circulating reticulocytes, bone marrow normoblasts, and liver in ultraviolet light. Crystals obtained from the livers of patients have been shown to have the same fluorescence spectrum as protoporphyrin (29). Another hepatobiliary complication of erythropoietic protoporphyria that occurs in approximately 10% of cases is the development of gallstones that contain protoporphyrin (24,25).

The most distinctive feature of the *hepatic lesions* in erythropoietic protoporphyria is the presence of dark brown pigment deposits in the form of granules or globules (Fig. 169). These can be identified as protoporphyrin on the basis of their red fluorescence in ultraviolet light, their birefringence in polarized light, their ultrastructural appearance on electron microscopy (23,30), and by isolation and physicochemical identification (31). The size and location of the pigment deposits and their association with other histologic changes vary with the severity of the hepatic lesions.

Of the methods available for identifying protoporphyrin deposits in the liver, the demonstration of their distinctive birefringence in polarized light is by far the simplest and most rapid (30). The method, which depends on the crystalline structure of the protoporphyrin deposits, is highly specific and sensitive, and has the advantage that it is applicable to routinely prepared, paraffin-embedded sections stained with H & E. In polarized light the scattered cytoplasmic deposits found in the hepatocytes, Kupffer cells, and macrophages appear as brilliantly illuminated red or golden granules (Figs. 168, 341), whereas the large deposits in swollen Kupffer cells, dilated canaliculi, or interlobular ducts present as bright red globules with a dark central Maltese cross (Fig. 170).

Fresh frozen sections are required for the reliable detection of the characteristic red fluorescence of protoporphyrin in ultra-violet light (Fig. 166). Such fluorescence may be generalized when the hepatic concentration of protoporphyrin is high, but often is focal in distribution at lower levels. Characteristically, the fluorescence fades rapidly, usually within a minute or two, when a mercury vapor lamp serves as the light source, but may be sustained for as long as 15 minutes in large deposits when an iodine tungsten quartz lamp is employed (29,32). Moreover, under such conditions, weak, red fluorescence may be detectable in formalin-fixed specimens of liver that contain excessive protoporphyrin.

In the benign asymptomatic hepatic lesions often encountered in erythropoietic protoporphyria, small granular deposits of protoporphyrin pigment are found in scattered Kupffer cells, occasional canaliculi, and portal macrophages (Figs. 340, 341). In addition, a few of the canaliculi may contain nonbirefringent bile thrombi that react with Hall's stain (Fig. 691). Often, inconstant histologic features in such cases include focal portal fibrosis, ductular proliferation, and small foci of hepatocellular degeneration or dropout (23,25).

The hepatic lesions in the relatively rare form of erythropoietic protoporphyria that leads to hepatic failure are characterized by cirrhosis (Fig. 692), massive deposits of protoporphyrin pigment (Figs. 169, 170), and extensive cholestasis, features that may mimic cirrhosis secondary to extrahepatic biliary obstruction (23). Usually, the fibrous septa show erosion of their limiting plates and contain proliferating ductules, inflammatory cells, and pigment deposits, either within macrophages or lying free within the connective tissue (Fig. 693). The largest pigment deposits are globular and lie within greatly enlarged Kupffer cells, dilated canaliculi, or interlobular bile ducts (Figs. 169, 170). Some of the canalicular pigment deposits are mixed with bile and give a positive reaction with Hall's stain, particularly at their periphery. In addition to the large globular deposits, fine granular deposits of protoporphyrin are found within many of the hepatocytes and Kupffer cells (Figs. 167, 168). That the protoporphyrin is more widely distributed through the liver than is evident from the pigment deposits seen in routine H & E-stained sections (Fig. 167) is evident on polarization microscopy (Fig. 168) or fluorescence microscopy (Fig. 166).

The observation that protoporphyrin induces bile salt–independent cholestasis in the isolated perfused rat liver (33) supports the role of cholestasis in the pathogenesis of the hepatic lesions of erythropoietic protoporphyria. However, it is highly probable that the large deposits of protoporphyrin in the cytoplasm of the hepatocytes and Kupffer cells and within the canaliculi and bile ducts contribute significantly to hepatic damage.

Porphyria cutanea tarda

Porphyria cutanea tarda is a hepatic porphyria that is usually inherited as an autosomal disorder of heme synthesis. It can also present as an acquired disorder, occasionally precipitated by chlorinated hydrocarbons. Porphyria cutanea tarda is caused by a deficiency in *uroporphyrinogen decarboxylase* (34) and is characterized by the urinary excretion of uroporphyrin. Alcohol is a precipitating factor that may act as a contributing toxin. Alcohol is not required, however, as severe liver damage may develop in the absence of alcohol abuse. As liver injury in-creases, the porphyrin formed is no longer excreted harmlessly into the bile, and accumulates in the blood. The accumulated porphyrin may itself cause liver damage. Acute attacks are not precipitated by barbiturates or other enzyme-inducing drugs, but sex hormone therapy and chloroquine may induce acute episodes. Hepatic iron accumulation is common in porphyria cutanea tarda, and it has been proposed that a single allele for major histocompatibility-linked, hereditary hemochromatosis may be responsible for the iron (35).

Clinically the disorder is characterized by photosensitivity with vesicle and bulla formation followed by fibrosis, pigmentation, and hypertrichosis.

The hepatic, histopathologic abnormalities of porphyria cutanea tarda are more severe than those seen in acute intermittent porphyria. All show some degree of fatty deposition and hemosiderin accumulation and aggregates of lymphocytes around bile ducts (36). Granuloma-like lesions composed of hypertrophied Kupffer cells, fat droplets, and lymphocytes are often found within the central lobular sinusoids (37). These accumulations, which are found in two-thirds of patients with porphyria cutanea tarda by needle biopsy, do not appear to be associated with hepatocellular carcinoma, which appears to occur in this disorder. Needle-shaped cytoplasmic inclusions can be seen in the hepatocytes of patients with porphyria cutanea tarda by light and fluorescent microscopy. They are best seen in unstained paraffin sections by polarized-light microscopy (36). The disease progresses with age, and in one large series of cases portal fibrosis appeared on average at 48 years of age, cirrhosis at 57 years, and hepatocellular carcinoma, when it was present, appeared at a mean age of 66 years (36). By electron microscopy, the mitochondria show large, electron-dense granules up to 200 μm in diameter. Large lipofuscin bodies are increased in number and contain extensive deposits of ferritin. Myelin figures are common. The fibrosis varies in degree, but eventually one-third of patients with this disorder develop cirrhosis (36,38).

The prevalence of hepatocellular carcinoma in porphyria cutanea tarda ranges from 0% to 47% in different series (39–41). In a recent investigation of 83 patients with porphyria cutanea tarda, the 13 who developed hepatocellular carcinoma (16%) were all cirrhotic men who were older than 50 years of age and had had porphyria cutanea tarda for an average of 20 years (40). Alcohol consumption was not significantly different in the groups with or without hepatocellular carcinoma. However, more than one-half of both groups showed serologic evidence of HBV infection, and 10% were seropositive for HBsAg (6,40). Thus, patients with porphyria cutanea tarda appear to be either especially susceptible to or more frequently exposed to HBV infection. Sometimes, porphyria cutanea tarda develops in patients with hepatic adenomas or hepatocellular carcinomas that contain excessive amounts of porphyrins (42,43).

The cause of the fibrosis in porphyria cutanea tarda is unknown. Conceivably, fibrogenesis can be stimulated by the iron accumulation, but the fibrosis is not invariably associated with hemosiderosis. It has been suggested that mast cells, which are prominently associated with hepatic fibrosis in systemic mastocytosis (13) (Fig. 694) and with fibrosis of many other organs (44), and which are increased in number in the skin of patients with porphyria cutanea tarda (45), might also be increased in their livers (44). In systemic mastocytosis, aggregates of mast cells may invade the parenchyma and replace hepatocytes (Figs. 695, 696) (see Chapter 24).

References

1. Schmid R, Schwartz S, Watson CJ: Porphyrin content of bone marrow and liver in the various forms of porphyria. Arch Intern Med 93:167–190, 1954.
2. Bloomer JR: The hepatic porphyrias. Pathogenesis manifestations, and management. Gastroenterology 71:689–701, 1976.
3. Doss MO: Hepatic porphyrias: pathobiochemical, diagnostic, and therapeutic implications. In Progress in Liver Disease VII, edited by H. Popper, F. Schaffner. New York, Grune & Stratton, 1982, pp. 573–597.
4. Ishak KG, Sharp HL: Metabolic errors and liver disease. In Pathology of the Liver, edited by R.N.M. MacSween, P.P. Anthony, P.J. Scheuer. Edinburgh, Churchill Livingstone, 1987, pp. 101–103.
5. Scholnick P, Marver HS, Schmid R: Erythropoietic protoporphyria: evidence for multiple sites of excess protoporphyrin formation. J Clin Invest 50:203–207, 1971.
6. Rank JM, Straka JG, Bloomer JR: Liver in disorders of porphyrin metabolism. J Gastroenterol Hepatol 5:573–585, 1990.
7. Gellis SS, Feingold M: Congenital erythropoietic porphyria. Am J Dis Child 129:701–702, 1975.
8. Kappas A, Sassa S, Galbraith RA, Nordmann Y: The Metabolic Basis of Inherited Disease, edited by C.R. Scriver, A.L. Beaudet, W.S. Sly, D. Valle. New York, McGraw-Hill, 1989, pp. 1305–1365.
9. Pimstone NR, Gandhi SN, Mukerji SK: Therapeutic efficacy of oral charcoal in congenital erythropoietic porphyria. N Engl J Med 316:390–393, 1987.
10. Kench JE, Langley, FA, Wilkinson JF: Biochemical and pathological studies of congenital porphyria. Q J Med 22:285–294, 1953.
11. Bonkovsky HL, Schned AR: Fatal liver failure in protoporphyria: synergism between ethanol excess and the genetic defect. Gastroenterology 90:191–201, 1986.
12. Lithner F, Wetterberg L: Hepatocellular carcinoma with acute intermittent porphyria. Acta Med Scand 215:271–274, 1984.
13. Biempica L, Kosower N, Ma MH, Goldfischer S: Hepatic porphyrias. Cytochemical and ultrastructural studies of liver in acute intermittent porphyria and porphyria cutanea tarda. Arch Pathol 98:336–343, 1974.
14. Bissell DM: Treatment of acute hepatic porphyria with hematin. J Hepatol 6:1–8, 1988.
15. Fromke VL, Bossenmaier I, Cardinal R, Watson CJ: Porphyria variegata. Study of a large kindred in the United States. Am J Med 65:80–88, 1978.
16. Brenner DA, Bloomer JR: The enzymatic defect in variegate porphyria. Studies with human cultured skin fibroblasts. N Engl J Med 302:765–769, 1980.
17. Muhlbauer JE, Pathak MA, Tishler PV: Variegate prophyria in New England. JAMA 247:3095–3102, 1982.
18. Elder GH, Evans JO, Thomas N, Cox R, Brodie MJ, Moore MR, Goldberg A, Nicholson DC: The primary enzyme defect in hereditary coproporphyria. Lancet 4:1217–1219, 1976.
19. Brodie MJ, Thompson GG, Moore MR, Beattie AD, Goldberg A: Hereditary coproporphyria. Demonstration of the abnormalities in haem biosynthesis in peripheral blood. Q J Med 46:229–241, 1977.
20. McCullough AJ, Barron D, Mullen KD: Fecal protoporphyrin excretion in erythropoietic protoporphyria: effect of cholestyramine and bile acid feeding. Gastroenterology 94:177–181, 1988.
21. Bonkowsky HL, Bloomer JR, Mahoney MJ: Heme synthetase deficiency in human protoporphyria. Demonstration of the defect in liver and cultured skin fibroblasts. J Clin Invest 56:1139–1148, 1975.
22. Bottomley SS, Tanaka M, Everett MA: Diminished erythroid ferrochelatase activity in protoporphyria. J Lab Clin Med 86:126–131, 1975.
23. Bloomer JR, Phillips MJ, Davidson DL, Klatskin G: Hepatic disease in erythropoietic protoporphyria. Am J Med 58:869–882, 1975.
24. De Leo VA, Poh-Fitzpatrick M, Mathews-Roth M, Harber LC: Erythropoietic protoporphyria. 10 years experience. Am J Med 60:8–22, 1976.
25. Cripps DJ, Scheuer PJ: Hepatobiliary changes in erythropoietic protoporphyria. Arch Pathol 80:500–508, 1965.
26. Singer JA, Plaut AG, Kaplan MM: Hepatic failure and death from erythropoietic protoporphyria. Gastroenterology 74:588–591, 1978.
27. Lee RG, Avner DL, Berenson MM: Structure-function relationship of protoporphyrin-induced liver injury. Arch Pathol Lab Med 108:744–746, 1984.
28. Gordeuk VR, Brittenham GM, Hawkins CW: Iron therapy for hepatic dysfunction in erythropoietic protoporphyria. Ann Intern Med 105:27–35, 1986.
29. Bloomer JR, Enriquez R: Evidence that hepatic crytalline deposits in a patient with protoporphyria are composed of protoporphyrin. Gastroenterology 82:569–572, 1982.
30. Klatskin G, Bloomer JR: Birefringence of hepatic pigment deposits in erythropoietic protoporphyria. Specificity and sensitivity of polarization microscopy in the identification of hepatic protoporphyrin deposits. Gastroenterology 67:294–302, 1974.
31. Morton KO, Schneider F, Weimer MK, Straka JG, Bloomer JR: Hepatic and bile porphyrins in patients with protoporphyria and liver failure. Gastroenterology 94:1488–1492, 1988.
32. Cripps DJ, Hawgood RS, Magnus IA: Iodine tungsten fluorescence microscopy for porphyrin fluorescence. A study on erythropoietic protoporphyria. Arch Dermatol 93:129–134, 1966.
33. Avner DL, Berenson MM: Protoporphyrin-induced cholestasis in the isolated in situ perfused rat liver. J Clin Invest 67:385–394, 1981.
34. Kushner JP, Barbuto AJ, Lee GR: An inherited enzymatic defect in porphyria cutanea tarda: decreased uroporphyrinogen decarboxylase activity. J Clin Invest 58:1089–1099, 1976.
35. Kushner JP, Edwards CQ, Dadone MM, Skolnick MH: Heterozygosity for HLA-linked hemochromatosis as a likely cause of the hepatic siderosis associated with sporadic porphyria cutanea tarda. Gastroenterology 88:1232–1238, 1985.
36. Cortes JM, Paradinas FJ, Hernandez-Guio C: The pathology of the liver in porphyria cutanea tarda. Histopathology 4:471–485, 1980.
37. Lefkowitch JH, Grossman ME: Hepatic pathology in porphyria cutanea tarda. Liver 3:19–29, 1983.
38. Turnbull A, Baker H, Vernon-Roberts B, Magnus IA: Iron metabolism in porphyria cutanea tarda and in erythropoietic protoporphyria. Q J Med 166:341–355, 1973.
39. Topi GC, D'Alessandro-Gandolfo L, Griso D, Morini S: Porphyria cutanea tarda and hepatocellular carcinoma. Int J Biochem 12:883–885, 1980.
40. Salata H, Cortes JM, de Salamanca RE, Oliva H, Castro A, Kusak E, Carreno V, Guio CH: Porphyria cutanea tarda and hepatocellular carcinoma: frequency of occurrence and related factors. J Hepatol 1:477–487, 1985.
41. Kordac V: Frequency of occurrence of hepatocellular carcinoma in patients with porphyria cutanea tarda in long-term follow-up. Neoplasia 19:135–139, 1972.
42. Tio TH, Laijnse B, Jarrett A: Acquired porphyria from a liver tumor. Clin Sci 16:517–525, 1957.
43. Thompson RP, Nicholson DC, Farnan T: Cutaneous porphyria due to a malignant primary hematoma. Gastroenterology 59:779–783, 1970.
44. Claman HN: More about mast cells and fibrosis in porphyria cutanea tarda. Hepatology 11:895–896, 1990.
45. Torinuki W, Kudoh K, Tagami H: Increased mast cell numbers in the sclerotic skin of porphyria tarda. Dermatologica 18:75–78, 1989.

Chapter 19
Intrahepatic Cholestasis

Definition

Cholestasis is difficult to define, since the term is used and interpreted differently by different observers. Literally, it means the cessation of bile flow. To most pathologists, however, the term signifies histologic evidence of bile retention in hepatocytes, Kupffer cells, canaliculi, or intrahepatic bile ducts without regard to etiology. Often, the term is used clinically to designate forms of jaundice that are accompanied by pruritus, acholic stools, and high serum levels of conjugated bilirubin, bile acids, cholesterol, and alkaline phosphatase activity. Since these features do not necessarily correlate with the underlying etiology, pathogenesis, or character of the associated hepatic lesions, this classification has little or no clinical significance.

In its broadest sense, the term cholestasis implies impairment of bile flow anywhere along its outflow tract from the hepatocytes to the duodenum, leading to accumulation in the serum of major bile constituents, particularly conjugated bilirubin and bile acids (1,2). A wide variety of etiologic factors that differ in their mode and site of action may be implicated. These include: (1) obstruction of the extrahepatic bile ducts anywhere from their origin in the porta hepatis to the papilla of Vater; (2) widely disseminated injury to the intrahepatic bile ducts, as in primary biliary cirrhosis; (3) diffuse hepatic parenchymal inflammation, degeneration, or necrosis due to viral infection, hepatotoxins, drugs, chronic alcoholism, or a variety of hereditary metabolic disorders; and (4) defects in hepatocellular and canalicular bile secretion unrelated to biliary obstruction or overt hepatocellular damage.

Increasingly, the terms *cholestasis* (3) and *intrahepatic cholestasis* (4) have been adopted as designations for primary defects in canalicular bile flow. It is in this more limited sense that these terms are used in the present chapter.

It should be kept in mind that in addition to jaundice, pruritus, and related clinical manifestations, cholestasis per se may have both hepatic and nonhepatic consequences. Some, such as malabsorption of fat-soluble vitamins, are well known. Others, such as the selective reduction of cytochrome P-450, which may impair microsomal matabolism of drugs (5), are less widely known. The impairment of cardiac function and susceptibility to hypotension are more recently recognized associations (6,7).

Pathogenesis of intrahepatic cholestasis

Experimental studies suggest that under normal conditions, the secretion of bile into the canaliculi is initiated by osmotic forces generated by the active transport of bile acids and other unidentified solutes from the hepatocytes into the canaliculi, and that water and electrolytes enter the bile by passive diffusion through the intervening canalicular and plasma membranes as well as the paracellular pathway (3,4,8,9). The mechanisms for active transport of bile acids and other solutes are independent, and vary in their relative importance as osmotic driving forces in bile secretion in different species. In rodents, bile acids are taken up into the hepatocyte by membrane carriers and are coupled to the inwardly directed chemical gradients for sodium (4). Bile acids appear to be secreted into bile by a membrane carrier, driven largely by the electric membrane potential. By maintaining opposing sodium and potassium high end gradients across the sinusoidal and lateral cell membranes of the liver cell, the sodium pump (Na^+/K^+-ATPase) provides for both chemical and electrical driving forces for the uptake and excretion of bile acids. Less is known about the mechanism involved in generating bile acid–independent flow. However, the biliary excretion of other organic solutes such as glutathione may contribute to the osmotic forces that generate this secretion.

In addition to the osmotic factors that initiate the generation of bile, the numerous actin-containing contractile microfilaments in the ectoplasm and microvilli of the canaliculi appear to play a role in maintaining the tonus and contractility of the canaliculi, thereby facilitating forward propulsion of the bile (10–13).

Experimental studies, mostly in animals, have demonstrated a number of mechanisms that may account for the multiplicity of conditions under which impairment of canalicular bile flow may occur in humans. However, progress in elucidating the pathogenesis of intrahepatic cholestasis has been hampered by a number of factors, including: (1) many of the agents that produce cholestasis in humans fail to do so in animals; (2) cholestasis, particularly when severe or prolonged, induces secondary changes in the hepatocytes, Kupffer cells, and ductules that may contribute to the impairment of bile flow; (3) at least some of the mechanisms proposed to account for impairment of canalicular bile flow may be operative not only at the level of the canaliculi but also elsewhere in the liver; and (4) even the limited evidence currently available suggests that, in many instances, multiple pathogenetic mechanisms are involved.

The principle mechanisms that have been proposed to account for impairment of canalicular bile flow include (1) abnormalities of bile acid metabolism and transport, (2) inhibition of bile acid synthesis, (3) impairment of bile acid–independent bile flow secondary to depression of Na^+/K^+-ATPase activity and other ion transporters, (4) increased permeability of the canalicular membranes, (5) increased leakiness of the paracellular pathway due to injury to the tight junctions, (6) distortion or disruption of the actin-containing, contractile microfilaments in the pericanalicular ectoplasm and canalicular microvilli, and (7) intracanalicular precipitation of bile salts or the metabolites of certain cholestatic agents.

Classification of intrahepatic cholestasis

Intrahepatic cholestasis is caused by a large group of disorders in which either the hepatocytes or canaliculi are injured *(lobular or intra-acinar cholestasis),* or elements of the intrahepatic biliary system are injured. The former category includes congenital cholestatic syndromes, e.g., Alagille's syndrome and tyrosinemia, and acquired disorders, such as viral hepatitis or sarcoidosis. The latter category includes primary biliary cirrhosis and primary sclerosing cholangitis. They will be discussed here in terms of individual types of disorders.

Cholestatic viral hepatitis

Approximately one-third of patients with classic acute viral hepatitis exhibit bile thrombi in their canaliculi. Usually, they are accompanied by parenchymal inflammation, degeneration, and necrosis, which are characteristic of the disease, so such lesions do not qualify as examples of intrahepatic cholestasis, as defined previously. However, in a small minority of cases, jaundice is unusually severe or prolonged, and histologic evidence of cholestasis persists despite resolution of the distinctive inflammatory and hepatocellular abnormalities that were present initially. The degree of histologic severity does not necessarily correlate with the clinical severity. Under such conditions, the clinical, biochemical, and histologic features may be indistinguishable from those in other forms of intrahepatic cholestasis (14,15). However, the canaliculi do not appear to be as dilated as they do in mechanical obstruction (16).

Viral intrahepatic cholestasis has been ascribed by some authorities to specific lesions involving the cholangioles (17). However, this has not been confirmed in most studies of biopsy material (14,15). Acute HAV hepatitis is especially prone to exhibit cholestasis (18–20). Non-A and non-B viral hepatitis may do so also (21).

Drug- and hepatotoxin-induced intrahepatic cholestasis

A wide variety of drugs are capable of inducing cholestasis (Chapter 7). Such reactions are usually classified as idiosyncratic, since they affect only a small minority of exposed individuals, are not dose-dependent, and are not reproducible in animals. The occurrence of fever, rash, and eosinophilia in some cases suggests that reactions of this type may be manifestations of drug sensitization, a possibility considered more fully in Chapter 7. Whatever the pathogenesis of idiosyncratic drug reactions may be, little is known about the mechanisms responsible for the cholestasis they produce. In drug-induced cholestasis the canaliculi appear to be less dilated than in bile duct obstruction (16).

A small number of drugs are unique in that they induce dose-dependent cholestasis in animals with regularity, but do so only sporadically in humans. Included in this group are chlorpromazine and synthetic, C-17-alkylated, androgenic, anabolic and estrogenic steroids (22,23). Under experimental conditions in animals, chlorpromazine impairs the secretion of bile acid–independent bile by inhibiting the activity of Na^+/K^+-ATPase (24). Since the free radicals and metabolites released during the metabolism of chlorpromazine differ with respect to the degree of enzymatic inhibition they induce, it has been proposed that the sporadic susceptibility to cholestasis in humans may depend on individual variations in the metabolism of the drug (25,26).

Ethinyl estradiol, one of the synthetic estrogens, also impairs the flow of bile acid–independent bile in animals (27), but induces overt cholestasis in humans only rarely. Based on studies of women receiving oral contraceptives that contain C-17-alkylated, synthetic, estrogen and progestational steroids, it has been suggested that the occasional occurrence of overt cholestasis in such individuals reflects an exaggerated responsiveness to the normal effects of estrogens on bile flow (28). Such effects may be mediated by reduction in membrane fluidity (29) and may be prevented experimentally by S-adenosylmethionine (30). Such susceptibility may be hereditary in nature, and may be expressed in the same or related individuals as recurrent episodes of intrahepatic cholestasis in pregnancy (31,32).

The jaundice produced by most hepatotoxins is attributable to hepatocellular degeneration or necrosis (22,23). However, a small number of naturally occurring hepatotoxins induce intrahepatic cholestasis in animals. Although their clinical significance in humans is in doubt, these agents have been used extensively in studies of the pathogenesis of intrahepatic cholestasis. Included in this group are (1) lithocholic acid, a metabolite of chenodeoxycholic acid produced in the gut by bacterial action (33); (2) endotoxin, produced by gram-negative bacteria (34); (3) phalloidin, a derivative of th poisonous mushroom *Amanita phalloides* (35); (4) icterogenin, a plant alkaloid that produces jaundice and leads to photosensitization in sheep that feed on *Lippia rhemanni* (36); and (5) sporidesmin, a fungal toxin (37).

Many non-natural, man-made hepatotoxic substances can also cause cholestasis. These include 4,4'-diaminodiphenylmethane (Epping jaundice) (38), paraquat (39), and benoxaprofen (40).

Recurrent (idiopathic) intrahepatic cholestasis of pregnancy

Recurrent intrahepatic cholestasis of pregnancy (41,42) is a disorder characterized by attacks of jaundice and pruritus that recur during successive pregnancies, and resolve promptly without sequelae following delivery. Although worldwide in distribution, the disease is encountered most frequently in Scandinavians (31,32) and other northern Europeans (43) and in Chileans of Indian descent (44). It appears to spare Asian and black women (45). Many familial cases have been reported (46,47), and an association with histocompatibility antigen HLA-BW16 has been demonstrated (48). Factors other than genetic susceptibility may play a role in its expression. In at least one study, the pattern of inheritance suggested that the trait could be transmitted by males as well as by females. Women who have experienced the cholestasis of pregnancy in the past, or have a family history of the disease are unusually susceptible to the type of intrahepatic cholestasis that occasionally follows the use of steroidal oral contraceptives (32,48–50). Indeed, male members of affected families may exhibit cholestasis when taking estrogens (51). These observations are consistent with the view that both types of cholestasis share a common pathogenesis that may be under genetic control.

Occasionally, the episodes of cholestasis are characterized by pruritus unaccompanied by jaundice, a forme fruste of the disease classified as *pruritus gravidarum*. Similar anicteric attacks may recur during subsequent pregnancies, but, more commonly, they alternate with episodes of pruritus accompanied by jaundice.

Usually, the manifestations of recurrent intrahepatic cholestasis of pregnancy appear during the third trimester of pregnancy, but may occur sooner, and have been reported as early as the seventh week of gestation. Often, the initial episode occurs during the first pregnancy, but, in some cases, it follows one or more uncomplicated pregnancies. With rare exceptions, once the disease occurs, it tends to recur in all subsequent pregnancies, although it may vary in time of onset and severity (44).

Characteristically, pruritus is the initial symptom and, usually, is followed within a week or two by the appearance of jaundice. As a rule, the jaundice is mild, the serum bilirubin concentration seldom exceeding 5 mg/dl, and is unaccompanied by hepatomegaly or other clinical manifestations of liver disease. In addition to conjugated hyperbilirubinemia, the serum contains modestly increased levels of alkaline phosphatase, bile acids (52), transaminase, and cholesterol. As further evidence of cholestasis, there is a significant decrease in the transport maximum (Tm) and hepatic storage capacity (S) of BSP (51). Following delivery, pruritus subsides promptly, usually within a few hours to days. Jaundice abates more slowly, but usually clears completely within a week or two.

In addition to occasional postpartum hemorrhage attributable to vitamin K deficiency and hypoprothrombinemia (53), recurrent intrahepatic cholestasis of pregnancy may contribute to maternal morbidity (44). Furthermore, the fetus may be affected adversely, as evidenced by an increased incidence of intrauterine death, fetal distress, and prematurity (43,44,53).

Although the pathogenesis of the disease is still uncertain, available evidence strongly suggests that it is attributable to a genetically determined hyperreactivity to the increased estrogen normally secreted during pregnancy (28) and that estrogenic and progestogenic hormones act synergistically (44). The cholestasis may be reversed by the administration of S-adenosyl-L-methionine (30), a phenomenon also observed in estrogen-induced cholestasis in experimental animals (54).

Benign recurrent intrahepatic cholestasis

Benign recurrent intrahepatic cholestasis (55–64), an uncommon disorder, is characterized by attacks of jaundice and pruritus that recur at intervals over a number of years and alternate with symptom-free periods during which there are no clinical signs of hepatic dysfunction. Although relatively rare, benign recurrent intrahepatic cholestasis has been recognized with increasing frequency since it was first described in 1959, and by now well over 100 cases have been reported. Some investigations during asymptomatic intervals in familial benign recurrent intrahepatic cholestasis, however, have shown abnormal BSP

retention, impaired N-demethylation, and increased plasma concentrations of bile acids (61). This particular kindred may exhibit a specific variant of the disorder that involves the skin.

Usually, the first attack of cholestasis occurs during childhood before the onset of puberty, but, in rare instances, it may not appear until after the age of 30. The onset is characterized by pruritus, which is followed within a week or two by the appearance of jaundice. Both the pruritus and jaundice tend to be relatively severe and usually persist for three or four months, although some attacks of cholestasis may be as brief as two weeks or as long as two years. Other clinical manifestations that occur in some cases include acholic stools, nausea, vomiting, abdominal pain, weight loss, steatorrhea, and rash. Occasionally, the attacks of cholestasis recur seasonally, especially during the autumn, or follow intercurrent, respiratory infections. Characteristically, the cholestasis abates spontaneously and gives rise to no residual hepatic damage even after multiple recurrences over a period of 20 or 30 years. According to some reports, remission may be hastened by the administration of corticosteroids or cholestyramine, but this therapy has not been established. The duration of the symptom-free periods is highly variable, ranging from a few months to several years. Long-term follow-up studies are limited in number, but it is apparent from scattered reports that, in some cases, the recurrences of cholestasis may occur repeatedly over a period of two or three decades. The world's record is 27 episodes over 38 years (22).

The biochemical features of the disease during its active phase resemble those in other forms of intrahepatic cholestasis, and include increased serum levels of bilirubin, most of which is conjugated, bile acids and alkaline phosphatase. However, the serum cholesterol concentration tends to remain within normal limits. Characteristically, no clinical or overt biochemical signs of hepatic dysfunction are present during the symptom-free remissions. However, as noted previously, BSP retention may be abnormal, bile acid levels increased, and N-demethylation impaired in certain kindreds (61).

The etiology of benign recurrent intrahepatic cholestasis is not known. The frequency with which the disease is familial in nature (57) suggests that it may be a genetically determined disorder. Since the onset of the disease usually occurs in childhood and occasionally in early infancy, it is conceivable that it is related to a hereditary form of neonatal cholestasis. That it may have some other genetic basis is suggested by a report of three different forms of cholestasis (benign recurrent intrahepatic cholestasis, recurrent cholestasis of pregnancy, and oral contraceptive–induced cholestasis) in different members of the same family (60). In some families it appears to be inherited as an autosomal recessive (61).

The pathogenesis of the choletasis in benign recurrent intrahepatic cholestasis is equally obscure. Based on observations in individual cases that have not been confirmed in other studies, the cholestasis has been variously ascribed to abnormalities in the metabolism or transport of bile acids (60) or bilirubin (58), occlusion of cholangioles by swelling of their lining epithelial cells, a reduction in the number of intrahepatic bile ducts, or diffuse hepatocellular injury by an unidentified exogenous toxic factor (57).

Considering differences between individual cases of benign recurrent intrahepatic cholestasis with respect to their hereditary pattern, metabolism and transport of bile acids and bilirubin, and the character of their intrahepatic bile ducts, the possibility that the disease comprises an etiologically and pathogenetically heterogeneous group of disorders deserves consideration.

Postoperative intrahepatic cholestasis

Postoperative cholestasis is a relatively common complication of prolonged surgical procedures accompanied by multiple transfusions (65–67). It occurs most frequently when the surgery is prolonged and involves the abdominal or thoracic cavity and when banked rather than fresh blood is used for the transfusions.

Characteristically, the jaundice appears on the first or second postoperative day, reaches a peak in three or four days, and then usually clears within a week or two. Occasionally, the jaundice fails to abate, and death ensues (66,68). However, such fatalities are attributable to other complications, especially hemorrhage, shock, and sepsis, rather than to hepatic failure per se. As a rule, the urine is dark owing to the presence of bile, but in contrast to other forms of cholestasis, the stools are rarely acholic. Only occasionally is the liver enlarged or tender.

Hyperbilirubinemia, predominantly of the conjugated type, is the principal biochemical finding, but in contrast to other forms of cholestasis, the serum levels of alkaline phosphatase and transaminase are either normal or only minimally increased.

Postoperative cholestasis is attributable to the combined effects of a defect in hepatocellular bile secretory function and bilirubin overload. Alterations in the intrahepatic circulation and hypoxemia related to anesthesia, blood loss, and manipulation of the liver during surgery probably account for the hepatic dysfunction. Rapid degradation of erythrocytes that have been stored undoubtedly leads to a large increase in the production of bilirubin that must be cleared by the liver. The fact that postoperative cholestasis is relatively uncommon when fresh blood is employed, that the depth of the jaundice that develops correlates with the volume of transfused blood administered, and that the serum alkaline phosphatase level is often normal suggest that hemolysis or bilirubin overload may be a more important factor than hepatocellular dysfunction in the pathogenesis of postoperative cholestasis. Moreover, these observations suggest that the defect in biliary secretion may be limited to conjugated bilirubin, so postoperative jaundice may not qualify as an example of intrahepatic cholestasis unless further studies demonstrate that the serum contains increased concentrations of other bile constituents, particularly bile acids. Investigations in experimental animals have implicated cardiodepressive effects of bile acids on myocardial contractility (69,70).

Intrahepatic cholestasis in bacterial infections

Severe systemic or extrahepatic infections with a variety of bacteria may be associated with jaundice. Such jaundice is encountered most frequently during early infancy (71–73) but also occurs in adults (74–76). It tends to occur most often in association with gram-negative sepsis (77).

Three types of cholestasis have been recognized in extrahepatic sepsis. The most common is *canalicular cholestasis,* which is most severe in the pericentral zones. It is often associated with portal zone inflammation, Kupffer cell activity, and,

sometimes, fatty infiltration; hepatocellular necrosis is not seen (76,77). The second type is *ductular cholestasis,* in which the bile ductules and canals of Hering in the periportal zones are dilated and filled with deeply staining bile thrombi (16,77–79). Polymorphonuclear leukocytes may infiltrate the area. Interlobular bile ducts are rarely involved (80). The third type is the "nonbacterial" cholangitis of the *toxic shock syndrome* (81,82), which appears to be the result of bacterial toxins, presumably derived from staphylococci.

Based on the occurrence of conjugated hyperbilirubinemia in all cases, raised serum levels of alkaline phosphatase in some, and the character of the hepatic lesions in both light and electron microscopy, most authorities classify the jaundice that accompanies bacterial infection as a form of intrahepatic cholestasis. Because serum levels of alkaline phosphatase and cholesterol are normal or only minimally elevated in many cases of the cholestasis of sepsis, this interpretation has been questioned, and it has been proposed that the secretory defect may be limited to conjugated bilirubin, and therefore, may not qualify as an example of intrahepatic cholestasis (75). Although no data are available to establish whether other constituents of bile, and especially bile acids, accumulate in the serum, at least in the case of gram-negative bacterial infections, it has been demonstrated in the isolated, perfused, rat liver that endotoxin reduces the flow of bile and the excretion of BSP and indocyanine green, features consistent with intrahepatic cholestasis (35).

Intrahepatic cholestasis in extrahepatic Hodgkin's disease

Rarely, Hodgkin's disease is complicated by a form of intrahepatic cholestasis in the absence of lymphomatous infiltration of the liver or bile ducts (83,84). Usually, it is encountered in patients with advanced active disease, but occasionally it occurs before the appearance of overt signs of Hodgkin's disease or in its early stages. As a rule, jaundice and pruritus are intense and persist until death from the lymphoma ensues. However, partial or complete remission of the cholestasis has been reported in patients successfully treated in the early stages of the disease.

The principal biochemical findings include high serum levels of conjugated bilirubin, which may comprise 90% of the total serum bilirubin concentration, and alkaline phosphatase.

Although the pathogenesis of the cholestasis associated with Hodgkin's disease is not known, it is generally assumed that a humoral factor derived from the lymphoma may be responsible for a defect in hepatocellular bile secretory function.

We have observed several patients with alcoholic cirrhosis with the same syndrome in which the conjugated bilirubin fraction was consistently greater than 85% of the total. The cholestasis subsided spontaneously as the alcoholic hepatitis subsided.

Intrahepatic cholestasis secondary to parenteral hyperalimentation

A significant number of adults maintained on total parenteral nutrition exhibit transient elevations of serum bilirubin, alkaline phosphatase, and transaminase, often accompanied by pericentral canalicular cholestasis and periportal fatty infiltration of the liver (85,86). Similar therapy in neonatal infants frequently leads to the development of overt intrahepatic cholestasis.

The histologic picture may occasionally mimic the pattern of extrahepatic biliary obstruction (87). When prolonged, parenteral nutrition may be lead to chronic inflammation and periportal fibrosis (86,87). The pathogenesis of this disease is not known, but it has been suggested that total parenteral nutrition may promote overgrowth of intestinal bacteria, which in turn may give rise to lithocholic acid or endotoxins, both of which are cholestasis-inducing substances (33,34,88,89). It is probable that parenteral nutrition–induced cholestasis may arise in many ways, since many amino acids and synthetic lipid emulsions and carbohydrate preparations and preservative substances are administered simultaneously and in various combinations.

Miscellaneous causes of intrahepatic cholestasis

A variety of heterogeneous disorders may from time to time show intrahepatic cholestasis. They include amyloidosis (90), sickle cell anemia (91), ABO blood type or Rhesus incompatibility or other hemolytic syndromes (92), nephrogenic hepatosplenomegaly (Stouffer's syndrome) (93), and sarcoidosis [(94); Fig. 697].

Neonatal intrahepatic cholestasis

Physiologic jaundice of the newborn results from lack of final development of hepatic functions for the disposal of bile pigment. These functions include uptake by the liver, transport within the hepatocyte, conjugation, and secretion (95)

Histopathology of intrahepatic cholestasis

The histologic features of the hepatic lesions in various forms of intrahepatic cholestasis are remarkably similar. However, they may differ to some extent depending on the duration and severity of the cholestasis. The severity of the histologic lesions does not correlate closely with tests of liver function such as the aminopyrine breath test (96).

Bile canaliculi

Characteristically, in all forms of intrahepatic cholestasis, the centrilobular canaliculi contain bile thrombi and are often dilated (97). Typical examples are illustrated in Figures 443, 493, and 517.

When the cholestasis is severe or prolonged, the bile thrombi may extend to involve midzonal and periportal canaliculi (Fig. 519). In addition, alterations in the hepatocytes, Kupffer cells, and portal tracts may appear. As a rule, these are patchy in distribution, occurring particularly in the areas of most marked

cholestasis, and probably are attributable to the secondary effects of cholestasis.

Hepatocytes

Often in severe cholestasis, the cytoplasm of the centrilobular hepatocytes is bile-stained or contains small bile droplets. These are most readily visualized in sections stained with Hall's bile stain, but also may be seen in sections lightly stained with H & E.

One of the most frequent signs of regenerative activity in cholestasis is the formation of hepatocellular rosettes or pseudoacini that usually contain centrally located bile thrombi (Fig. 110). Other regenerative features may include thickening and irregularity of the hepatic plates (Figs. 443, 519), an increase in the number of binucleated and trinucleated hepatocytes (Fig. 520), and hepatocellular pleomorphism [(98); Fig. 520].

Frequently, the hepatocytes surrounding or adjacent to large bile thrombi show ballooning degeneration of their cytoplasm (Figs. 110, 521). Less commonly, the lobules contain a few scattered acidophilic bodies (Figs. 494, 495, 520). In rare instances of severe or prolonged intrahepatic cholestasis, individual ballooned hepatocytes may contain typical Mallory bodies (Fig. 498), or circumscribed groups of hepatocytes may be the site of pseudoxanthomatous degeneration (Fig. 522).

Small foci of cell dropout leading to focal disruption of the hepatic plates are seen occasionally in areas of marked cholestasis, and often are accompanied by focal proliferation and swelling of Kupffer cells (Fig. 518).

Kupffer cells

Foci of hypertrophied and hyperplastic Kupffer cells are relatively common in prolonged cholestasis (Figs. 443, 495, 518). Usually, they are encountered in the areas of most marked cholestasis, occasionally contain bile droplets (Fig. 518), and may be accompanied by focal infiltrating lymphocytes and neutrophils (Fig. 495). In rare instances of severe or prolonged cholestasis, focal collections of both Kupffer cells and hepatocytes may undergo pseudoxanthomatous degeneration (Fig. 522).

Portal tracts

When intrahepatic cholestasis is prolonged, some of the portal tracts may be expanded by inflammatory cells (Fig. 496) or fibrosis (Figs. 519, 525, 527). They may show segmental erosion of their limiting plates (Figs. 444, 519) and often contain proliferating ductules (Figs. 444, 519). Usually, lymphocytes predominate in the portal exudates (Figs. 496, 519, 523), but, in some cases, these are accompanied by a variable number of neutrophils (Figs. 444, 519) and macrophages. Rarely, in cases of severe prolonged cholestasis, some of the interlobular ducts are widely dilated, contain inspissated bile, and are lined by atrophic, degenerating epithelial cells (Fig. 497).

Chronic cholestasis and cirrhosis induced by idiosyncratic drug reactions

Cases of chronic cholestasis have been reported following idiosyncratic reactions to chlorpromazine (99–102), prochlorperazine (102), organic arsenicals (103), and tolbutamide (104). In several of these patients, progressive portal fibrosis has led to the development of cirrhosis that clinically and histologically resembles primary biliary cirrhosis (99,101,102,104).

Figure 527 illustrates a case of chlorpromazine-induced cholestasis of four years' duration. The lesion shows extensive portal fibrosis and inflammation, erosion of the limiting plates, and portal-portal bridging fibrosis that partially outlines parenchymal nodules.

A more advanced cirrhosis in a patient with chlorpromazine-induced chronic cholestasis of five years' duration is illustrated in Figure 528.

References

1. Desmet VJ: Cholestasis: extrahepatic obstruction and secondary biliary cirrhosis. *In Pathology of the Liver,* edited by R.N.M. MacSween, P.P. Anthony, P.J. Scheuer. 2nd Edition. Edinburgh, Churchill Livingstone, 1983, pp. 364–423.
2. Popper H: Cholestasis: the future of a past and present riddle. Hepatology *1:*187–191, 1981.
3. Erlinger S: What is cholestasis in 1985? J Hepatol *1:*687–690, 1985.
4. Boyer, JL: Mechanisms of bile secretion and hepatic transport. *In* Physiology of Membrane Disorders, edited by T.E. Andreoli, J.F. Hoffman, D.D. Fanestil, S.G. Schultz. New York, Plenum Publishing Corp., 1986, pp. 609–636.
5. Kawata S, Imai Y, Inada M: Selective reduction of hepatic cytochrome P-450 content in patients with intrahepatic cholestasis. A mechanism for impairment of microsomal drug oxidation. Gastroenterology *92:*299–303, 1987.
6. Green J, Beyar R, Sideman S, Mordechovitz D, Better OS: The "jaundiced heart": a possible explanation for postoperative shock in obstructive jaundice. Surgery *100:*14–20, 1986.
7. Deckelbaum L: The jaundiced heart. Hepatology *7:*598–599, 1987.
8. Layden TJ, Elias E, Boyer JL: Bile formation in the rat. The role of the paracellular shunt pathway. J Clin Invest *62:*1375–1385, 1978.
9. Boyer JL: Tight junctions in normal and cholestatic liver: does the paracellular pathway have functional significance? Hepatology *3:*614–617, 1983.
10. Phillips MJ, Oda M, Mak E, Fisher MM, Jeejeebhoy KN: Microfilament dysfunction as a possible cause of intrahepatic cholestasis. Gastroenterology *69:*48–58, 1975.
11. Phillips MJ, Oshio C, Miyairi M: Intrahepatic cholestasis as a canalicular motility disorder: evidence using cytochalasin. Lab Invest *48:*205–211, 1983.
12. Smith CR, Oshio C, Miyairi M, Katz H, Phillips MJ: Coordination of the contractile activity of bile canaliculi. Evidence from spontaneous contractions in vitro. Lab Invest *53:*270–274, 1985.
13. Boyer JL: Contractile activity of bile canaliculi: contraction or collapse? Hepatology *7:*190–192, 1987.
14. Gall EA, Braunstein, H: Hepatitis with manifestations stimulating bile duct obstruction (so-called "cholangiolitic hepatitis"). Am J Clin Pathol *25:*1113–1127, 1955.
15. Dubin IN, Sullivan BH, Le Golvan PC, Murphy LC: The cholestatic form of viral hepatitis. Experience with viral hepatitis at Brooke Army Hospital during the years 1951 to 1953. Am J Med *29:*55–72, 1960.
16. Scheuer PJ: Liver Biopsy Interpretation, 4th Edition. London, Bailliere Tindall, 1988, p. 37.
17. Eliakim M, Rachmilewitz M: Cholangiolitic manifestations in viral hepatitis. Gastroenterology *31:*369–383, 1956.
18. Kryger P, Christoffersen P: Liver histopathology of the hepatitis A virus infection: a comparison with hepatitis type B and non-A, non-B. J Clin Pathol *36:*650–654, 1983.
19. Teixeira MR Jr, Weller IVD, Murray A, Bamber M, Thomas HC, Sherlock S, Scheuer PJ: The pathology of hepatitis A in man. Liver *2:*53–60, 1982.
20. Gordon SC, Reddy KTL, Schiff L, Schiff ER: Prolonged intrahepatic cholestasis secondary to acute hepatitis A. Ann Intern Med *101:*635–637, 1984.
21. Dienes HP, Popper H, Arnold W, Lobeck H: Histologic observations in human hepatitis non-A, non-B. Hepatology *2:*562–517, 1982.
22. Sherlock S: Drugs and the liver. *In* Diseases of the Liver and Biliary System, 8th Edition. Oxford, Blackwell Scientific Publications, 1989, pp. 372–409.
23. Baptista A, Bianchi L, de Groote J, Desmet VJ, Gedigk P, Ishak KG: Histopathology of the intrahepatic biliary tree. Liver *3:*161–175, 1983.
24. Boyer JL: Mechanisms of chlorpromazine cholestasis: hypersensitivity or toxic metabolites? Gastroenterology *74:*1331–1333, 1978.
25. Samuels AM, Carey MC: Effects of chlorpromazine hydrochloride and its metabolites on Mg2+- and Na+, K+-ATPase of canalicular-enriched rat liver membranes. Gastroenterology *74:*1183–1190, 1978.
26. Keefe EB, Blankenship NM, Scharschmidt BF: Alteration of rat plasma membrane fluidity and ATPase activity by chlorpromazine hydrochloride and its metabolites. Gastoenterology *79:*222–231, 1980.
27. Gumucio JJ, Valdivieso VD: Studies on the mechanisms of the ethinylestradiol impairment of bile flow and bile salt excretion in the rat. Gastroenterology *61:*339–344, 1971.
28. Kreek MJ, Sleisinger MH: Estrogen induced cholestasis due to endogenous and exogenous hormones. Scand J Gastroenterol Suppl *7:*123–131, 1970.
29. Blitzer B, Boyer JL: Cellular mechanisms of bile formation. Gastroenterology *82:*346–351, 1982.
30. Frezza M, Surrenti C, Manzillo G, Fiaccadori F, Bortolini M, Di Padova C: Oral S-adenosylmethionine in the symptomatic treatment of intrahepatic cholestasis. A double-blind, placebo-controlled study. Gastroenterology *99:*211–215, 1990.
31. Adlercreutz H, Tenhunen R: Some aspects of the interaction between natural and synthetic female sex hormones and the liver. Am J Med *49:*630–639, 1970.
32. Dalen E, Westerholm B: Occurrence of hepatic impairment in women jaundiced by oral contraceptives and in their mothers and sisters. Acta Med Scand *195:*459–463, 1974.
33. Fisher MM, Magnusson R, Miyai K: Bile acid metabolism in mammals. 1. Bile acid induced intrahepatic cholestasis. Lab Invest *21:*88–91, 1971.
34. Utili R, Abernathy CO, Zimmerman HJ: Cholestatic effects of *Eschericia coli* endotoxin on the isolated perfused rat liver. Gastroenterology *70:*248–253, 1978.
35. Dubin M, Michele M, Feldmann G, Erlinger S: Phalloidin-induced cholestasis in the rat: relation to changes in microfilaments. Gastroenterology *75:*450–455, 1978.
36. Rimington C, Quin JI, Roets GCS: Studies upon the photosensitization in South Africa. I. The icterogenic factor in geel-dikkop. 1. Isolation of active principles from *Lippia rhemanni* pears. Ondersterpoort J Vet Sci *9:*225–255, 1937.
37. Slater TF, Griffiths DB: Effects of sporidesmin on bile flow rate and composition in the rat. Biochem J *88:*60P–61P, 1963.
38. Kopelman H, Scheuer PJ, Williams R: The liver lesion of the Epping jaundice. Q J Med *35:*553–564, 1966.
39. Mullick FG, Ishak KG, Mahabir R, Stromeyer FW: Hepatic injury associated with paraquat toxicity in humans. Liver *1:*209–221, 1981.
40. MacSween RNM, Anthony PP, Scheuer PJ: Pathology of the Liver. Edinburgh, Churchilll Livingstone, 1987, p. 451.
41. Haemmerli VP, Wyss HI: Recurrent intrahepatic cholestasis of pregnancy. Report of six cases and review of the literature. Medicine *46:*299–321, 1967.
42. Mistilis SP: Liver disease in pregnancy, with particular emphasis on the cholestatic syndromes. Austral Ann Med *17:*248–260, 1968.
43. Steven MM: Pregnancy and liver disease. Gut *22:*592–614, 1981.
44. Reyes H: The enigma of intrahepatic cholestasis of pregnancy: lesions from Chile. Hepatology *2:*87–96, 1982.
45. Reyes H, Gonzalez MC, Ribalta J, Aburto H, Matus C, Schramm G, Katz R, Medina E: Prevalence of intrahepatic cholestasis of pregnancy in Chile. Ann Intern Med *88:*487–493, 1978.
46. Holzbach RT, Sivak DA, Braun WE: Familial recurrent intrahepatic cholestasis of pregnancy: a genetic study providing evidence for transmission as a sex-limited, dominant trait. Gastroenterology *85:*175–179, 1983.
47. Reyes H, Ribalta J, Gonzalez-Ceron M: Idiopathic cholestasis of pregnancy in a large kindred. Gut *17:*709–713, 1976.
48. Reyes H, Wegmann ME, Segovia N: HLA in Chileans with intrahepatic cholestasis of pregnancy. Hepatology *2:*463–466, 1982.

49. Orallana-Alcalde JM, Dominguez JP: Jaundice and oral contraceptive drugs. Lancet 2:1278–1280, 1966.

50. Boake WC, Schade SG, Morrissey JF, Schaffner F: Intrahepatic cholestatic jaundice of pregnancy followed by Enovid-induced cholestatic jaundice. Report of a case. Ann Intern Med 63:302–308, 1965.

51. Reyes H, Ribalta J, Gonzalez MC, et al: Sulfobromophthalein clearance tests before and after ethinyl estradiol administration, in women and men with familial history of intrahepatic cholestasis of pregnancy. Gastroenterology 81:226–231, 1981.

52. Lunzer M, Barnes P, Byth K: Serum bile acid concentrations during pregnancy and their relationship to obstetric cholestasis. Gastroenterology 91:825–829, 1986.

53. Reid R, Ivey KJ: Fetal complications of obstetric cholestasis. Br Med J 1:870–872, 1976.

54. Boelsterli UA, Rakhit G, Balazs T: Modulation by S-adenosyl-L-methionine of hepatic Na$^+$, K$^+$-ATPase, membrane fluidity, and bile flow in rats with ethinyl estradiol-induced cholestasis. Hepatology 3:12–17, 1983.

55. Summerskill WHJ, Walshe JM: Benign recurrent intrahepatic "obstructive" jaundice. Lancet 2:686–690, 1959.

56. Schapero RH, Isselbacher KJ: Benign recurrent intrahepatic cholestasis. N Engl J Med 268:708–711, 1963.

57. Williams R, Cartter MA, Sherlock S, Scheuer PJ, Hill KR: Idiopathic recurrent cholestasis: a study of the functional and pathological lesions in four cases. Q J Med 33:387–399, 1964.

58. Brodersen R, Tygstrup N: Serum bilirubin studies in patients with intermittent intrahepatic cholestasis. Gut 8:46–49, 1967.

59. Biempca L, Gutstein S, Arias IM: Morphological and biochemical studies of benign recurrent cholestasis. Gastroenterology 52:521–535, 1967.

60. De Pagter AGF, van Berge Henegouwen GP, Ten Bokkel Huinink JA, Brandt K-H: Familial benign recurrent intrahepatic cholestasis. Interrelation with intrahepatic cholestasis of pregnancy and from oral contraceptives? Gastroenterology 71:202–207, 1976.

61. Eriksson S, Larsson C: Familial benign chronic intrahepatic cholestasis. Hepatology 3:391–398, 1983.

62. Bijleveld CMA, Vonk RJ, Kuipers F, Havinga R, Fernandez J: Benign recurrent intrahepatic cholestasis: a long term follow-up study of two patients. Hepatology 9:532–537, 1989.

63. Putterman C, Keidar S, Brook JG: Benign recurrent intrahepatic cholestasis: 25 years of follow-up. Postgrad Med J 63:295–302, 1987.

64. Minuk GY, Shaffer EA: Benign recurrent intrahepatic cholestasis. Evidence for an intrinsic abnormality in hepatocyte secretion. Gastroenterology 93:1187–1193, 1987.

65. Pichlmayr I, Stich W: Der bilirubinostatische Ikterus, eine neue Ikterusform beim Zusammentreffen von operation Narkose und Bluttransfusion. Klin Wschr 40:665–667, 1962.

66. Kantrowitz PA, Jones WA, Greenberger NJ, Isselbacher KJ: Severe postoperative hyperbilirubinemia simulating obstructive jaundice. N Engl J Med 276:591–598, 1967.

67. Strasberg SM, Silver MD: Postoperative hepatogenic jaundice. Surg Gynecol Obstet 132:81–86, 1971.

68. Dixon JM, Armstrong CP, Duffey SW: Factors affecting morbidity and mortality after surgery for obstructive jaundice: a review of 373 patients. Gut 24:845–850, 1983.

69. Green J, Beyar R, Sideman S: The 'jaundiced heart': a possible explanation for postoperative shock in obstructive jaundice. Surgery 100:14–23, 1986.

70. Heidenreich S, Brinkema E, Martin A: The kidney and cardiovascular system in obstructive jaundice: functional and metabolic studies in conscious rats. Clin Sci 73:5–14, 1987.

71. Bernstein J, Brown AK: Sepsis and jaundice in early infancy. Pediatrics 29:873–882, 1962.

72. Seeler RA, Hahn K: Jaundice in urinary track infection in infancy. Am J Dis Child 118:553–558, 1969.

73. Rooney JC, Hill DJ, Danks DM: Jaundice associated with bacterial infection in the newborn. Am J Dis Child 122:39–41, 1971.

74. Fahrlander H, Huber H, Gloor F: Intrahepatic retention of bile in severe bacterial infections. Gastroenterology 47:590–599, 1964.

75. Miller DJ, Keeton GR, Webber BL, Saunders SJ: Jaundice in severe bacterial infection. Gastroenterology 71:94–97, 1976.

76. Zimmerman HJ, Fang M, Utili R, Seeff LB, Hoofnagle J: Jaundice due to bacterial infection. Gastroenterology 77:362–374, 1979.

77. Banks JG, Foulis AK, Ledingham IMcA, MacSween RNM: Liver function in septic shock. J Clin Pathol 35:1249–1252, 1982.

78. Lefkowitch JH: Bile ductular cholestasis: an ominous histopathologic sign related to sepsis and 'cholangitis lenta'. Hum Pathol 13:19–24, 1982.

79. International Group: Histopathology of the intrahepatic biliary tree. Liver 3:161–175, 1983.

80. Vyberg M, Poulsen H: Abnormal bile duct epithelium accompanying septicaemia. Virchows Arch A. Pathol Anat Histopthol 402:451–458, 1984.

81. Ishak KG, Rogers WA: Cryptogenic acute cholangitis: association with toxic shock syndrome. Am J Clin Pathol 76:619–626, 1981.

82. Gourley GR, Chesney PJ, Davis JP, Odell GB: Acute cholestasis in patients with toxic shock syndrome. Gastroenterology 81:928–931, 1981.

83. Juniper K Jr: Prolonged severe obstructive jaundice in Hodgkin's disease. Gastroenterology 41:199–204, 1963.

84. Perera DR, Greene ML, Fenster LF: Cholestasis associated with extrabiliary Hodgkin's disease. Report of three cases and review of four others. Gastroenterology 67:680–685, 1974.

85. Grant JP, Cox CE, Kleinman LM, Maher MM, Pittman MA, Tangrea JA, Brown JH, Gross E, Beazley RM, Jones RS: Serum hepatic enzyme and bilirubin elevations during parenteral nutrition. Surg Gynecol Obstet 145:573–580, 1977.

86. Bower RH: Hepatic complications of parenteral nutrition. Semin Liver Dis 3:216–224, 1983.

87. Body JJ, Bleiberg H, Bron D, Maurage H, Bigirimana V, Heimann R: Total parenteral nutrition-induced cholestasis mimicking large bile duct obstruction. Histopathology 6:787–792, 1982.

88. Capron JP, Gineston JL, Herve MA, Braillon A: Metronidazole in prevention of cholestasis associated with total parenteral nutrition. Lancet 1:446–447, 1983.

89. Fouin-Fortunet H, LeQuernec L, Erlinger S, Lerebours E, Colin R: Hepatic alterations during total parenteral nutrition in patients with inflammatory bowel disease: a possible consequence of lithocholate toxicity. Gastroenterology 82:932–937, 1982.

90. Pirovino M, Altorfer J, Maranta E, Hammerli UP, Schmid M: Ikterus vom Typ der intrahepatischen Cholestase bei Amyloidose der Leber. Z Gastroenterologie 6:321–331, 1982.

91. Sheehy TW, Law DE, Wade BH: Exchange transfusion for sickle cell intrahepatic cholestasis. Arch Intern Med 140:1364–1366, 1980.

92. Thaler H: Leberkrankheiten. In Histologie Pathophysiologie, Klinik, Berlin, Springer Verlag, 1982.

93. Stauffer MH: Nephrogenic hepatosplenomegaly. Gastroenterology 40:694–699, 1961.

94. Rudzki C, Ishak KG, Zimmerman HJ: Chronic intrahepatic cholestasis of sarcoidosis. Am J Med 59:373–387, 1975.

95. Blanckaert N, Schmid R: Physiology and pathophysiology of bilirubin metabolism. In Hepatology, a Textbook of Liver Disease, edited by D. Zakim, T.D. Boyer. Philadelphia, W.B. Saunders, 1982, p. 246.

96. Baker AL, Krager PS, Kotake AN: The aminopyrine breath test does not correlate with histologic disease severity in patients with cholestasis. Hepatology 7:464–467, 1987.

97. Rolfes DB, Ishak KG: Liver disease in pregnancy. Histopathology 10:555–570, 1986.

98. Spichtin HP, Gudat F, Schmid M, Pirovino M, Altorfer J, Bianchi L: Microtubular aggregates in human chronic non-A, non-B hepatitis with bridging necrosis and multinucleated hepatocytic giant cells. Liver 2:355–360, 1982.

99. Myers JD, Olson RE, Lewis JH, Moran TJ: Xanthomatous biliary cirrhosis following chlorpromazine, with observations indicating overproduction of cholesterol, hyperprothrombinemia, and the development of portal hypertension. Trans Assoc Am Physicians 70:243–260, 1957.

100. Read AE, Harrison CV, Sherlock S: Chronic chlorpromazine jaundice with particular reference to its relation to primary biliary cirrhosis. Am J Med 31:249–258, 1961.

101. Walker CO, Combes B: Biliary cirrhosis induced by chlorpromazine. Gastroenterology 51:631–640, 1966.

102. Ishak KG, Irey NS: Hepatic injury associated with phenothiazines. Clinicopathologic and follow-up study of 36 patients. Arch Pathol 93:283–304, 1972.

103. Stolzer BL, Miller C, White WA, Zuckerbrod M: Postarsenical obstructive jaundice complicated by xanthomatosis and diabetes mellitus. Am J Med 9:124–132, 1950.

104. Gregory DA, Zaki GF, Sarcosi GA, Carey JB Jr: Chronic cholestasis following prolonged tolbutamide administration associated with destructive cholangiolitis. Arch Pathol 84:194–201, 1967.

Chapter 20
Hepatic Lesions In Biliary Tract Disease

Extrahepatic biliary obstruction

The extrahepatic duct system, which drains bile from the liver into the duodenum, extends from the proximal segment of the common hepatic duct at its bifurcation in the porta hepatis to the distal end of the common bile duct in the ampulla of Vater. A wide variety of lesions may affect the ducts anywhere along the course, resulting in partial or complete obstruction to the outflow of bile. Such lesions may be intraluminal, intramural, or extrinsic to the ducts, and may be focal or diffuse in distribution.

Partial obstruction of the extrahepatic bile ducts does not necessarily lead to hyperbilirubinemia because raising the intraductal pressure does not reduce bile flow until the pressure reaches approximately 75% of the maximum bile secretory pressure (P max). As the pressure rises further, bile flow falls rapidly and ultimately ceases when P max is reached (1,2). It has been proposed that canalicular bile secretion continues unabated at P max, but is promptly regurgitated so that bile flow in the common bile duct ceases (1). However, the secretion of bile acids falls more rapidly than the volume of bile flow as intraductal pressure rises (2). This suggests that a concomitant decrease in bile acid–dependent canalicular bile flow contributes to obstructive cholestasis. In the dog, the kidneys can excrete large amounts of bilirubin (3) and may thus prevent the development of hyperbilirubinemia when partial biliary obstruction occurs. However, the renal excretion of bilirubin in humans is so low (4) that it is unlikely to affect the serum bilirubin level significantly under conditions of partial biliary obstruction.

At one time the cholestasis produced by extrahepatic biliary obstruction was attributed exclusively to hydrostatic distension of the canaliculi leading initially to transudation of bile into the lymph of Disse's space and, subsequently, into the blood. It was presumed that with prolongation of the obstruction, canaliculi ultimately ruptured, allowing further escape of bile into both the lymph and blood (5). However, subsequent studies have shown that reflux of bile occurs along the course of most of the distended, intrahepatic, biliary tree and that biliary obstruction leads to changes in the hepatocytes and canaliculi that resemble those of intrahepatic cholestasis. These changes include increased permeability of the tight junctions around the canaliculi, and alterations in the cytoskeleton, plasma membranes and Na^+K^+-ATPase activity of the hepatocytes (6). The relative importance of these factors and the question of whether they are attributable to increased intraductal pressure or to other mechanisms remain to be resolved, so the pathogenesis of extrahepatic obstructive cholestasis is still far from clear.

Etiology and manifestations of extrahepatic biliary obstruction

Choledocholithiasis, benign stricture, and carcinoma are the most frequent causes of extrahepatic biliary obstruction. Other etiologic factors, some of which are relatively common and others rare, include pancreatic disease, acute cholecystitis, primary sclerosing cholangitis, periductal neoplastic, and inflammatory masses, hemobilia, duodenal ulcer, diverticulum, parasitic infestation of the bile ducts and iatrogenic injury of the bile ducts. In infants and older children, the principal causes of extrahepatic biliary obstruction are biliary atresia and choledochal cyst, respectively.

Choledocholithiasis. Most stones in the common bile duct are of the cholesterol type and originate in the gallbladder (7–10). Occasionally, the common bile duct contains pigment stones composed of calcium bilirubinate that form as a result of chronic bile stasis secondary to stricture or sclerosing cholangitis. In the Orient, but only rarely in the United States, pigment stones may arise in the intrahepatic bile ducts and descend into the extrahepatic ducts (11). They form as a result of the action of β-glucuronidase on conjugated bilirubin, which releases conjugated bilirubin, a much less soluble material (12).

From 10 to 20% of individuals over the age of 20 exhibit cholelithiasis, and of these 7 to 20% have stones in the common bile duct (9,10,13). The latter are relatively uncommon below the age of 40, but occur with increasing frequency as age advances, so that the incidence of choledocholithiasis may be as high as 30 to 50% in individuals over the age of 80.

Gallstone obstruction of the biliary tree that occurs soon after gallbladder surgery is usually caused by cholesterol stones that originate in the gallbladder (14). Obstruction that appears long after such surgery tends to be caused by earthy, brown stones that form in the common bile duct (15).

The prevalence of cholelithiasis in patients with all types of cirrhosis is much higher than in noncirrhotic individuals, ranging from 25 to 40% (16–19) and highest in patients with portal hypertension (20). Biliary obstruction, however, is a very uncommon event in cirrhotic patients (16,21). The rarity of extrahepatic obstruction is apparently related to the predominance of bilirubin gallstones in cirrhosis (16,17,19,21), which is the consequence of increased hemolysis (22). The relative rarity of choledocholithiasis in cirrhotic patients compensates for the much higher morbidity and mortality that occurs with biliary surgery in cirrhotic patients (23,24). Extrahepatic biliary obstruction is also relatively uncommon in patients with sickle cell anemia, thalassemia, and other types of chronic hemolysis in which bilirubin stones commonly develop. Conceivably, "nonsurgical" techniques such as lithotripsy, laparoscopy (24A) or percutaneous, nonexcisional cholecystectomy (25) may ultimately be useful in patients who face high risk rates with conventional surgery.

Common duct stones vary in size and number, but often are asymptomatic. However, when impacted at the lower end of the duct, they may cause partial obstruction to bile flow and may lead to the development of jaundice or biliary colic. In addition, choledocholithiasis may give rise to acute cholangitis or pancreatitis with or without accompanying jaundice or colic. Other less common complications include hemobilia (26), secondary sclerosing cholangitis (8), stricture of the sphincter of Oddi (8), or internal bile fistula (27,28).

Obstructive jaundice and colic may subside spontaneously if a stone impacted in the ampulla or Vater passes into the duodenum, or moves up the duct into a more proximal, dilated segment of the duct. However, when cholelithiasis persists, jaundice, colic, or cholangitis tend to recur unless the stones are removed endoscopically, ultrasonically, or surgically (9,10,13,29–31) or are fragmented by lithotripsy (32,33).

Benign strictures. With few exceptions, benign strictures of the extrahepatic bile ducts (34–36) are the sequelae of antecedent biliary tract surgery, particularly cholecystectomy or transplantation (37,38). Occasionally, they follow surgical procedures on the stomach or pancreas, and even less commonly occur as complications of intraabdominal disorders in the absence of surgical intervention. Among the latter are blunt abdominal trauma, large common duct stones, duodenal ulcers or diverticula, subhepatic abscesses, congenital anomalies of the ducts, and chronic pancreatitis (39). Rarely, benign strictures are encountered for which no apparent cause can be found. Such lesions are thought by some to be produced by a localized inflammatory, fibrotic process akin to that seen in the more diffusely distributed lesions of primary sclerosing cholangitis. The existence of "primary benign strictures," as these lesions are designated, as an etiologic entity is still open to question. Fibrosis of the sphincter of Oddi is another form of localized stricture regarded by some as a "primary," inflammatory, fibrotic disorder (40). However, it is so frequently associated with cholelithiasis, choledocholithiasis, or pancreatitis that its primary nature is in doubt.

It is important to recognize that most "benign" strictures often are indistinguishable from neoplasms of the extrahepatic bile ducts, so biopsy at the time of surgical exploration is essential for their differentiation and therapy.

Almost invariably, the strictures that develop following cholecystectomy are the result of trauma to the ducts. However, the predisposing injury is not recognized at the time of surgery in over two-thirds of cases. The types of trauma include inadvertent laceration, ligation of the common bile duct or of an anomalous branch of the hepatic or of the cystic duct stump too close to the common bile duct, crushing of the ducts, rough probing of their lumen, prolonged T-tube drainage and complicating periductal hemorrhage, inflammation, infection, or bile leakage. Such problems occur most frequently when the gallbladder is small and contracted.

Most strictures that follow cholecystectomy measure approximately 2 cm in length, and are found close to the junction of the cystic and common hepatic ducts, affecting the latter alone or in combination with the common bile duct. Occasionally, the cystic duct is adherent to the right hepatic duct and when transected may lead to injury and stricture formation in the right hepatic duct.

Characteristically, strictures attributable to sclerosing chronic pancreatitis affect the distal end of the common bile duct. Rarely, benign strictures of the common hepatic duct have been reported at its bifurcation within the porta hepatis (29). In our experience, such lesions have invariably proved to be carcinomatous (41).

Usually, strictures of the extrahepatic bile ducts produce only partial obstruction to bile flow, and, unless repaired promptly, lead to dilatation and induration of the duct proximal to the stricture and collapse distal to the stricture. When biliary obstruction is prolonged, the major intrahepatic ducts may exhibit similar dilatation and induration, and secondary biliary cirrhosis may develop.

When the common hepatic or common bile duct is inadvertently lacerated or ligated during surgery, jaundice or drainage of bile through the wound may develop during the next few days. However, more commonly, the clinical manifestations of a stricture develop insidiously over a period of weeks, months, or even years.

The principal clinical features in most cases of stricture include recurrent bouts of obstructive jaundice or cholangitis (42). Usually, the liver is enlarged and indurated, and in approximately 20% of cases, there are signs of portal hypertension such as splenomegaly, esophageal varices, or hemorrhage from varices. Often, the attacks of jaundice or cholangitis are accompanied by upper abdominal pain or biliary colic.

The cholangitis is attributable to infection with enteric bacteria, and usually is manifested by fever and leukocytosis, often accompanied by shaking chills, occasionally by bacteremia, and often by septic shock (43). Concomitant jaundice and abdominal pain and tenderness are relatively common, but are not always present. Moreover, such symptoms may occur in the absence of overt clinical signs of cholangitis, although enteric bacteria and evidence of chronic inflammation are almost always demonstrable in the duct proximal to the stricture. Occasionally, acute symptomatic cholangitis responds to antibiotic therapy. However, it invariably recurs unless the stricture is repaired surgically.

Until recently, correction of strictures in the extrahepatic ducts has been difficult even in the hands of the most experienced surgeons (42). Balloon dilatation of biliary strictures (44,45) is the least invasive and one of the most effective therapies available.

Unrelieved strictures may result in the development of secondary biliary cirrhosis, choledocholithiasis, hepatic abscess, external bile fistula, or hemorrhage from esophageal varices. Ultimately, death from hepatic failure or sepsis may ensue.

Neoplasms. Most neoplasms that involve the extrahepatic bile ducts are malignant and show the histologic features of well-differentiated adenocarcinoma, often accompanied by extensive fibrosis. Differential diagnosis by frozen section at surgery is often extremely difficult and is uncertain unless lymphatic or neural invasion is demonstrated. Only rarely are the ducts affected by benign neoplasms, such as adenomas, papillomas, or granular cell tumors.

A number of disorders appear to predispose to the development of bile duct carcinoma, which may be either extrahepatic or intrahepatic. These include ulcerative colitis with or without complicating sclerosing cholangitis (46,48), choledochal cyst, cystic dilatation of the intrahepatic ducts (Caroli syndrome), congenital hepatic fibrosis, polycystic liver, and, in Southeast

Asia, infestation of the ducts by the liver fluke *Clonorchis sinensis* (48).

Carcinoma may occur anywhere along the course of the extrahepatic ducts, but is encountered most frequently in the common bile duct close to the entry of the cystic duct (49,50), in the proximal segment of the common hepatic duct at its bifurcation in the porta hepatis (41,51), or in the ampulla of Vater (52–54). Characteristically, the tumor constricts the duct, leading to partial or complete obstruction of bile flow and dilatation of the ducts proximal to the obstruction. Usually, ductal carcinomas grow slowly, but may extend along the length of the ducts, invade adjacent nerves, or metastasize to regional lymph nodes, the liver, and peritoneum. Distant extra-abdominal metastases are unusual. Cholangitis is a relatively rare presenting manifestation, but is common following surgical exploration of the ducts or palliative procedures to relieve biliary obstruction.

Progressive obstructive jaundice, pruritus, abdominal pain, weight loss, and hepatomegaly are the principal clinical manifestations of extrahepatic ductal carcinoma. The presenting features, prognosis, and differential diagnosis differ to some extent depending on the location of the tumor.

Usually, carcinoma of the common bile duct presents as a firm, circumscribed, annular mass that constricts the duct. Less commonly, it protrudes into the lumen as a polypoid mass. Despite the progressive nature of the lesion, jaundice may fluctuate early in the course of the disease. In only a small minority of cases can the tumor be successfully resected, so, as a rule, only palliative surgery for the relief of biliary obstruction is possible. Death ultimately ensues from hepatic failure or sepsis secondary to unrelieved obstruction and cholangitis. When the tumor extends along the ducts it may be difficult to differentiate from primary sclerosing cholangitis. However, if intrahepatic cholangiography is possible, the intrahepatic bile ducts are uniformly dilated in the former and beaded due to alternating areas of stricture and dilatation in the latter.

Most carcinomas of the common hepatic duct in the porta hepatis resemble small scars that may be overlooked at laparotomy even when accompanied by retrograde, intraoperative cholangiography. Alternatively, they may be mistaken for benign strictures. Frequently, such tumors extend into and may occlude one or both major, tributary hepatic ducts. Indeed, in some cases, the neoplasm appears to start in one of the hepatic ducts and then to extend distally to involve the bifurcation. Occasionally, the tumor at the bifurcation presents as a bulky adenocarcinoma of intrahepatic bile duct origin. Such tumors may be mimicked by metastatic carcinoma or hepatocellular carcinoma. Only rarely are tumors of the bifurcation resectable, so usually only palliative surgery for the relief of biliary obstruction can be performed. Patients with small sclerotic tumors at the bifurcation survive at least twice as long as those with other unresected carcinomas of the bile ducts. Death usually is due to hepatic failure or sepsis, not to metastatic disease.

Symptomatic relief and improved survival may be obtained with nonsurgical biliary drainage (55).

Carcinomas of the ampulla of Vater may present as a polypoid mass that protrudes into the duodenum or as a small, localized nodule. Occasionally, the latter may be so small that it is overlooked at laparotomy, even when duodenostomy is carried out to account for otherwise unexplained obstructive jaundice with dilatation of the extrahepatic ducts. Except in the case of small, localized, ampullary neoplasms, it is rarely possible to identify the site of origin, which may be in the mucosa of the ampulla or papilla of Vater, the distal end of the common

bile or pancreatic duct, or pancreatic acini. Rarely, the tumors are metastatic (56).

In a small number of patients with ampullary carcinoma, the neoplasm can be successfully resected if it is recognized before metastases have occurred.

An unusual clinical feature of ampullary carcinoma that occurs occasionally is spontaneous, transient clearing or regression of obstructive jaundice or intermittent melena or guaiac-positive stools. Usually, this is attributed to necrosis and sloughing of an obstructive polypoid tumor. However, similar remissions may be encountered in patients with small nodular tumors that show no evidence of necrosis. Since the extrahepatic ducts remain dilated during such remissions, it is reasonable to suggest that subsidence of complicating inflammation and edema accounts for the relief of obstruction.

Differentiation between carcinoma of the ampulla and carcinoma in the head of the pancreas may be exceedingly difficult unless the mass can be visualized by ultrasonography or computerized tomography or can be identified at laparotomy.

Pancreatic disease. Pancreatitis, particularly of the alcoholic type, gives rise to obstructive jaundice more frequently than is generally recognized (57–60). In the case of acute pancreatitis, the jaundice tends to be mild and transient, and usually is attributable to compression of the intrapancreatic segment of the common bile duct by the edematous, inflamed head of the pancreas. Occasionally, chronic or recurrent pancreatitis gives rise to persistent, biliary obstruction by inducing fibrotic stenosis of the distal common bile duct or the sphincter of Oddi. Sometimes, the biliary tree is obstructed by gallstone pancreatitis (61), often a difficult diagnosis to make (62). Less commonly, the obstruction is attributable to compression by an adjacent pancreatic pseudocyst.

Carcinoma of the head of the pancreas is a well-recognized, relatively common cause of extrahepatic biliary obstruction (63–65). Usually, it gives rise to progressive jaundice, pruritus, weight loss, and significant hepatomegaly. Despite the traditional view to the contrary, abdominal pain is a feature in almost half the cases. Hydrops of the gallbladder is a relatively common finding. Occasionally, pruritus appears a month or two before the jaundice develops.

Regional and distant metastases are relatively common by the time the disease is recognized, so that life expectancy is brief and successful extirpation of the tumor is possible in only a small number of cases.

Acute cholecystitis. A significant number of patients with acute cholecystitis exhibit jaundice suggestive of extrahepatic biliary obstruction (66–69). Often, the jaundice is attributable to complicating choledocholithiasis, but, in at least half the cases, no stones are found in the common bile duct on surgical exploration or cholangiography. In some of the latter, other causes of biliary obstruction can be demonstrated, such as pancreatitis, a distended gallbladder, stricture of the sphincter of Oddi, or neoplasm. However, in the remainder, the etiology remains obscure (70,71). No doubt, a common duct stone has been passed in some cases, but extension of inflammation and edema from the gallbladder to the extrahepatic bile ducts, spasm of the sphincter of Oddi, and intrahepatic, periductular inflammation and focal, hepatocellular necrosis have been proposed as possible etiologic factors. However, the evidence implicating such factors is far from convincing. The diagnosis of acute acalculous cholecystitis can be made with about equal frequency with infusion cholecystography or HIDA cholescintigraphy (72).

A surprising number of patients with cholelithiasis uncomplicated by acute cholecystitis exhibit histologic changes in the liver, especially mild degrees of portal fibrosis and inflammation, and small foci of degeneration, necrosis, and inflammation in the parenchyma. Except for the more frequent occurrence of dilated canaliculi and bile thrombi, the hepatic lesions in choledocholithiasis are identical (73).

Primary sclerosing cholangitis. (See below.)

Subhepatic periductal neoplastic and inflammatory masses. Enlarged lymph nodes, usually infiltrated with metastatic carcinoma or lymphoma, may impinge upon or encircle the extrahepatic bile ducts, particularly near the porta hepatis. However, the ducts rarely, if ever, are obstructed unless they are invaded by the neoplasm.

Subhepatic abscess of varied etiology is a well-recognized, although relatively rare cause of extrahepatic biliary obstruction.

Hemobilia. Massive hemorrhage into the biliary tract, a relatively rare condition called hemobilia, characteristically gives rise to hematemesis or melena, abdominal pain, and jaundice (26,74–76). The pain and jaundice are attributable to obstruction and distension of the extrahepatic bile ducts by blood and clots. Usually, the bleeding, which may be arterial or venous, is indicative of a relatively large communication between a blood vessel and the biliary tract that may be located in the liver, extrahepatic bile ducts, or gallbladder.

Trauma, either accidental or surgical, that leads to laceration of the liver or injury to the hepatic artery or its branches is the leading cause of hemobilia. Included in this group is needle biopsy of the liver (74). Although less frequent, a wide variety of nontraumatic lesions have been implicated as etiologic factors. Of these, the most common include rupture of a hepatic arterial aneurysm, primary tumors of the liver, especially hepatocellular carcinoma, neoplasms of the bile ducts and gallbladder, and large gallstones. In some parts of the Orient, infestation of the bile ducts with parasites, especially *Ascaris lumbricoides*, is said to be a relatively common cause of hemobilia.

Duodenal ulcer. Despite the intimate anatomic relationship between the lower end of the common bile duct and the duodenum, obstructive jaundice is a relatively rare complication of duodenal ulcer (77). However, it does occur occasionally when the ulcer perforates or penetrates into the pancreas, producing extensive, periduodenal fibrosis. Thus, obstruction of the distal common bile duct may be secondary to complicating pancreatitis or the result of compression by inflammation, edema, or fibrosis.

Duodenal diverticula. Although diverticula of the duodenum are relatively common, and frequently are located close to or actually contain the papilla of Vater, they produce biliary obstruction only rarely (78). In such cases, the obstruction can be due to occlusion of the papilla by the contents of the diverticulum, or to compression of the ampulla of Vater or the distal end of the common bile duct by an adjacent distended diverticulum.

Choledochal cyst. (See below.)

Biliary atresia. Neonatal cholestatic syndromes, which in the past had been described as "atresia" of the bile ducts, are now classified as *infantile obstructive cholangiopathy* (79,80). It has been postulated that the more severe such disorders result from the rapid destruction of bile ducts late during fetal development (81). When all ducts are destroyed, *biliary atresia* results (79); when the injury is incomplete, *hypoplasia of the bile ducts* results in the so-called "paucity of bile ducts" seen in Alagille's syndrome.

Some years ago it was recognized that extrahepatic biliary atresia and neonatal giant cell hepatitis had many features in common (82). More recently, a pathogenetic relationship between these diseases and Reo virus type 3 was suspected on the basis of antibodies to Reo 3 virus in the majority of patients with bilary atresia (83). Subsequently, the finding of virus particles identified as Reo 3 antigens in the necrotic biliary remnants in patients with biliary atresia identified the etiologic agent (84). This relationship is not universally accepted, however (85).

Parasitic biliary obstruction. In the Far East parasitic infestation with *Clonorchis sinensis* is a common cause of biliary obstruction (86) and other biliary disorders (87). In the West, sheep flukes, i.e., *Fasciola hepatis,* can cause similar disease (88). Liver flukes are flat, leaf-shaped worms approximately 20 mm in length, 4 mm in width, and 1 mm in thickness. They use snails and fish as intermediate hosts and are ingested by humans in uncooked fish. The worms migrate through the liver and take up residence in the biliary tree, where they may cause no symptoms or give rise to many biliary disorders. They may cause partial or complete obstruction, bacterial ("oriental") cholangitis (89) or liver abscesses, hemobilia (90), cholelithiasis, and cholangiocarcinoma (91). *Ascaris lumbricoides,* a roundworm, may cause similar problems (92).

These parasites may cause fever with leukocytosis and eosinophilia during their passage through the liver, and any of the signs, symptoms, and laboratory abnormalities of obstructive jaundice. The diagnosis is made by the demonstration of the parasites in the biliary tree by various imaging techniques (88,93) and by the demonstration of the ova in the feces.

Histopathology of hepatic lesions in extrahepatic biliary obstruction

The histologic features of the hepatic lesions in various forms of extrahepatic biliary obstruction are similar, but may differ to some extent depending on the degree and duration of the obstruction, and may be modified by complicating bacterial cholangitis. As a rule, the principal features include cholestasis and secondary changes in the hepatic parenchyma and portal tracts. Although the hepatic lesions of extrahepatic obstruction are characteristic, they are not pathognomonic, since they may be mimicked by those in some forms of intrahepatic cholestasis (Chapter 19).

Cholestasis. In most cases of extrahepatic biliary obstruction, the centrilobular canaliculi are dilated and contain *bile thrombi* (Fig. 698). When the obstruction is of recent origin, and particularly when it is incomplete, such thrombi may be found in only a few of the lobules, or may be absent. However, as the duration or severity of the obstruction increases, the bile thrombi tend to enlarge, are more uniformly distributed in the centrilobular zones, and, ultimately, extend to the midzonal and periportal canaliculi (Fig. 699).

Under conditions of moderate to severe cholestasis, the centrilobular hepatocytes and Kupffer cells frequently are bile-stained or contain cytoplasmic bile droplets. In addition, well-defined, large bile thrombi may be encountered in some of the Kupffer cells and spaces of Disse (Fig. 212). Considering the similarity of their size and shape to the bile thrombi in adjacent dilated canaliculi, it is highly probable that they are derived from ruptured canaliculi.

Hepatic parenchyma. Frequently, the cholestatis in biliary obstruction is associated with alterations in the Kupffer cells and hepatocytes. Usually, these are focal in nature and limited to the zones of cholestasis. However, when biliary obstruction is severe or prolonged, the parenchymal lesions may be prominent and widely distributed.

Swelling, proliferation, and pigmentation of the Kupffer cells with lipofuscin or bile droplets are relatively common findings, even early in the course of the obstruction. In more advanced cases, the Kupffer cells often are aggregated and replace small foci of hepatocytes that have dropped out (Figs. 700, 701). Occasionally, scattered Kupffer cells are swollen and contain pale, foamy cytoplasm, features often classified as *pseudoxanthomatous degeneration,* and interpreted as evidence of bile reflux. Under some conditions, circumscribed collections of both Kupffer cells and hepatocytes are affected by this type of degeneration, giving rise to lesions usually classified as *bile infarcts.*

Not infrequently, the lobules contain small, scattered foci of hepatocellular degeneration or necrosis. Usually, these are found within or adjacent to zones of cholestasis and may present as occasional acidophilic bodies (Fig. 702) or as foci of cell dropout filled with proliferating Kupffer cells (Figs. 700, 701) or neutrophils (Fig. 284).

Under conditions of severe or prolonged biliary obstruction, the parenchyma may contain bile infarcts. Characteristically, such lesions are sharply circumscribed, occur predominantly in the periportal zones (Fig. 298), and contain hepatocytes and Kupffer cells undergoing pseudoxanthomatous degeneration (Fig. 703). In early bile infarcts, the cytoplasm of the affected cells is swollen, pale, and foamy. However, in more advanced lesions, both the hepatocytes and Kupffer cells tend to undergo degeneration and necrosis and contain cytoplasm that appears fibrillar, a feature frequently referred to as *feathery degeneration.* Some bile infarcts contain bile thrombi, extravasated bile, bile-stained macrophages, or other types of inflammatory cells. It is highly probable that bile infarcts, irrespective of whether or not they contain histologically demonstrable bile, are produced by regurgitated constituents of bile, and especially bile acids. Consistent with this view is the observation that adjacent portal tracts occasionally contain degenerating interlobular ducts surrounded by foamy, degenerating macrophages (Fig. 704), or ducts that exhibit necrosis of their walls and extravasation of bile into the surrounding connective tissue (Fig. 361).

Large *bile infarcts* are generally regarded as a pathognomonic feature of extrahepatic biliary obstruction. However, we have encountered such lesions in a number of patients with severe nonobstructive cholestasis, so, in our experience, large bile infarcts have not been reliable histologic criteria of extrahepatic biliary obstruction. With respect to small bile infarcts, there is general agreement that they may occur in any form of severe

cholestasis and, therefore, are of no value to differentiating between obstructive and nonobstructive cholestasis.

Not infrequently, particularly when biliary obstruction is sustained, the hepatocytes show evidence of increased regenerative activity, as indicated by the presence of thick, irregular, hepatic plates (Figs. 202, 284), and rosette formation (Fig. 202) and mitoses.

The nodules of parenchymal tissue tend to be irregular, jigsaw puzzle–shaped islands rather than the spheric nodules seen in most types of cirrhosis (94). Such lesions tend to be associated with portal hypertension. Indeed, the hepatocyte hyperplasia may play an important role in the pathogenesis of portal hypertension (95). These patterns may be reversible when the obstruction is relieved (96).

In prolonged biliary obstruction, as in other forms of chronic cholestasis, copper tends to accumulate in the liver. As a result, the cytoplasm of the periportal hepatocytes may contain rhodamine-positive copper granules (Fig. 561) and orcein-positive granules that contain copper-protein complexes.

Another histologic feature that prolonged biliary obstruction shares with other forms of chronic cholestasis is the occasional occurrence of ballooned periportal hepatocytes that contain Mallory bodies.

Portal tracts. Alterations in the portal tracts are an important feature of the hepatic lesions in extrahepatic biliary obstruction. However, early in the course of the obstruction, the portal changes may be minimal or spotty in distribution and may escape detection in needle biopsy specimens. Under such conditions, histologic differentiation from intrahepatic cholestasis may be impossible if centrilobular canalicular bile thrombi have already appeared. Rarely, alterations in the portal tracts are evident before cholestasis is demonstrable histologically.

In classic cases, at least some of the portal tracts are expanded (Figs. 297, 405). Such expansion is attributable to a number of factors including edema, erosion of the limiting plates, proliferation and elongation of bile ducts, inflammatory reactions, and fibrosis.

Characteristically, the edema is most prominent at the periphery of the portal tract and is evidenced by the loose arrangement of the connective tissue fibers as compared with the more dense, tightly adherent collagen bundles seen at the center of the portal tract (Figs. 297, 405). Erosion of the limiting plates with loss of hepatocytes and collapse of periportal reticulin contributes to this appearance (Figs. 297, 358, 405).

Frequently, the edematous margins of the portal tracts contain proliferating ductules that tend to extend into the periportal parenchyma (Figs. 297, 358). These ductules have detectable lumens, which are lined by cuboidal epithelium with a recognizable basement membrane (97). Such ductules are derived from both active proliferation of ductular cells and by transformation of hepatocyte plates into tubular structures (98). This ductular proliferation has been emphasized as an important diagnostic feature that occurs with regularity (99). However, we have not found marginal ductular proliferation in all needle biopsy specimens of extrahepatic biliary obstruction, and have encountered it in a variety of unrelated lesions associated with erosion of the limiting plates. When the obstruction is severe or prolonged, the epithelial cells of the ductules may be swollen, vacuolated, or show other degenerative changes. Moreover, some of their lumens, which usually are collapsed, may contain bile thrombi.

Often, in sustained biliary obstruction, the interlobular ducts are dilated and elongated (Figs. 314, 315). Due to their tortuosity, they appear to be increased in number in longitudinal sections. In some cases, occasional interlobular ducts are encircled by concentric lamellae of collagen (Fig. 381). As previously indicated, some of the interlobular ducts may show degeneration of their epithelium (Fig. 704) and extravasation of bile (Fig. 361).

As a rule, at least some of the portal tracts contain numerous inflammatory cells, including neutrophils, lymphocytes, and histiocytes. Usually, the neutrophils are most prominent around the ductules and interlobular ducts (Figs. 314, 315, 358), and may infiltrate their walls and lumens (Fig. 315). The presence of numerous neutrophils within the lumens of interlobular ducts does not necessarily imply complicating bacterial cholangitis. This is illustrated in Figure 315, a section obtained from a patient with a carcinoma of the ampulla of Vater, who at laparotomy exhibited no bacteriologic evidence of infection in the biliary tract.

Lymphocytes, occasionally accompanied by plasma cells (Fig. 311), tend to be more numerous than neutrophils, and are found scattered through the portal tract. Histiocytes or macrophages that contain PAS-D-positive lipofuscin are relatively common, particularly following prolonged biliary obstruction. In addition, such cells are also relatively frequent in the region of degenerating interlobular ducts (Fig. 704), and in zones of bile extravasation where they may be accompanied by giant cells.

The portal exudates in extrahepatic biliary obstruction may contain occasional eosinophils, but, rarely, such cells are numerous and may be misinterpreted as evidence of an underlying idiosyncratic drug-induced reaction.

Biliary obstruction stimulates fibrogenesis in the portal tracts and, thus, contributes to their expansion (Fig. 405). In addition, collapse of reticulin and fibrosis may occur in the foci of cell dropout and hepatocellular necrosis found in the zones of maximum cholestasis, resulting in the formation of occasional, centrilobular, stellate scars. Prolonged, unrelieved biliary obstruction may give rise to progressive, portal fibrosis with extension of connective tissue into the parenchyma and the formation of portal-portal and occasional portal-central fibrous bridges (Fig. 705). Occasionally, such fibrosis leads to the destruction of the normal lobular architecture and the replacement of lobules by nodules of regenerating parenchyma, resulting in the development of secondary biliary cirrhosis (Figs. 706, 707). Usually, the lesions of secondary biliary cirrhosis exhibit significant cholestasis, erosion of the limiting plates, and ductular proliferation and follow prolonged, episodic, or persistent obstructive jaundice (100). However, in rare instances of choledocholithiasis or stricture of the common bile duct, secondary biliary cirrhosis may develop insidiously in the absence of jaundice or histologically demonstrable cholestasis. In some cases at least, bacterial cholangitis may play an important role in the pathogenesis of such lesions. Nevertheless, available evidence indicates that biliary obstruction alone can produce secondary biliary cirrhosis. This is best illustrated in the case of biliary atresia or carcinoma at the bifurcation of the common hepatic duct in the porta hepatis that rarely is complicated by bacterial cholangitis unless subjected to surgical manipulation. Often, the parenchymal nodules in secondary biliary cirrhosis are small and monolobular, but large multilobular nodules are not rare. Similarly, the fibrous septa may be slender or broad. Lesions characterized by large nodules and broad septa, particularly when unaccompanied by cholestasis, may closely resemble those of postnecrotic cirrhosis of varied etiology (Fig. 707).

The histopathology of parasitic biliary disease is quite different from that of nonparasitic biliary disease. It is characterized by the presence of dead or disintegrating worms or their ova (Fig. 708), which may injure the epithelium of the biliary tract (Figs. 709, 710). They predispose to bacterial infection (Fig. 711), to stone formation, and to cholangiocarcinoma.

Intrahepatic biliary obstruction

The reserve capacity of the liver to excrete bile is so great that *focal* obstruction of the intrahepatic bile ducts does not produce jaundice, pruritus, or histologic evidence of cholestasis unless both major hepatic ducts are occluded, close to the junction with the common hepatic duct usually by carcinoma (41). In one reported case of bile duct carcinoma, jaundice was attributed to occlusion of the left hepatic duct alone (101). However, the right hepatic duct was dilated, showed carcinoma at its mouth, and was accompanied by cholestasis in the right hepatic lobe, so that bilateral biliary obstruction was almost certainly present in this case (41).

Lesions that injure and occlude widely *disseminated* interlobular or septal bile ducts characteristically give rise to the typical clinical, biochemical, and histologic features of chronic cholestasis, and may lead to the development of biliary cirrhosis. Such lesions include the following disorders:

Primary biliary cirrhosis

Primary biliary cirrhosis, also termed chronic nonsuppurative destructive cholangitis, is the most common cause of chronic cholestasis attributable to destruction of the interlobular bile ducts (Chapter 11).

Primary intrahepatic obliterating cholangitis

Rarely, the hepatic lesions of chronic cholestasis are characterized by the replacement of medium sized intrahepatic bile ducts by fibrous cords (102). It has been suggested that such lesions represent a variant of primary sclerosing cholangitis in which the extrahepatic bile ducts are spared. Although some of the clinical and histologic features, including progression to cirrhosis, resemble those of primary biliary cirrhosis, none of the interlobular ducts show epithelial inflammation, degeneration, or necrosis, there are no accompanying hepatic granulomas, and mitochondrial antibodies are not present.

Intrahepatic biliary atresia

In rare instances of chronic neonatal cholestasis, the lesions are characterized by biliary atresia limited to the intrahepatic ducts.

Idiopathic adulthood ductopenia

Idiopathic adulthood ductopenia is indistinguishable from neonatal, nonsyndromatic paucity of intrahepatic bile ducts, except for its occurrence in adults (103). The disease is characterized by a cholestatic picture, i.e., elevated levels of alkaline phosphatase, sometimes jaundice, normal cholangiography, and the absence of any other cause of nongranulomatous destructive cholangitis, such as primary biliary cirrhosis, sarcoidosis, or primary sclerosing cholangitis. The ductopenia and associated microscopic findings are indistinguishable from those in primary biliary cirrhosis or other diseases of small bile ducts [(104); Figs. 712, 713]. By virtue of the size of the ducts involved, no cholangiographic abnormalities are present. Conceivably, this syndrome may be a delayed manifestation of the infantile syndrome.

Histologically, interlobular bile ducts are absent from more than 50% of small portal tracts (Fig. 712). Nongranulomatous destructive cholangitis and degenerative epithelial changes in interlobular bile ducts are present (Fig. 713).

Sarcoidal intrahepatic cholestasis

It is well recognized that noncaseating epithelioid granulomas are demonstrable in the liver in a high proportion of patients with sarcoidosis (105). In a small minority of cases, such lesions are accompanied by cholestasis (Fig. 697), progressive diminution in the number of interlobular bile ducts, accumulation of copper in the liver, chronic jaundice, pruritus, and progression to cirrhosis (106). It is generally assumed that the loss of ducts is due to their destruction by the granulomatous reaction, although this has not been documented. In two of our own well-documented cases of sarcoidosis, a few of the interlobular ducts showed the same type of epithelial degeneration and inflammation seen in primary biliary cirrhosis (Figs. 376, 377). However, as in previously reported cases, the serum contained no mitochondrial antibodies. Considering the similarity of the hepatic lesions and clinical features of sarcoidal cholestasis to those in primary biliary cirrhosis, and the fact that the latter may be associated with sarcoid-like, extrahepatic granulomas (107), the question arises whether or not the two diseases are related. Usually, the presence of a positive Kveim reaction in sarcoidosis and mitochondrial antibodies in primary biliary cirrhosis has been emphasized as a critical point in their differentiation. However, in at least one reported case, both tests were positive, an observation interpreted as evidence that both diseases were present coincidentally (108). This interpretation is consistent with the generally accepted view that sarcoidosis and primary biliary cirrhosis are unrelated disorders (106), but the evidence on which this is based is inconclusive, so a final conclusion must await elucidation of the etiology of both diseases.

Primary amyloidosis of the liver

Rarely, primary amyloidosis that affects the liver may be accompanied by severe intrahepatic cholestasis (109). This cholestasis has been attributed to deposits of amyloid in the spaces of Disse and the portal tracts that interfere with the outflow of bile from the canaliculi and small interlobular bile ducts (see Chapter 24).

Cholangitis

The morphologic features, etiology, pathogenesis, and clinical manifestations of inflammatory lesions that involve the bile ducts and are classified as cholangitis vary greatly. Such lesions may be acute or chronic, may or may not be attributable to bacterial infection, may be associated with a variety of biliary tract or extrahepatic disorders, and may be symptomatic or asymptomatic. Unfortunately, the microscopic features of the hepatic lesions are of only limited value in distinguishing between the various forms of cholangitis. Usually, such differentiation depends on the clinical and laboratory features, the findings on imaging studies or laparotomy, and the results of bile and blood cultures.

Often, the term cholangitis is used in a limited sense to define a clinical disorder characterized by chills, fever, abdominal pain, and jaundice attributable to biliary obstruction complicated by ascending bacterial infection. However, not all cases are symptomatic or due to biliary obstruction and infection, so it is more rational to regard cholangitis as a morphologic rather than a clinical or etiologic entity.

Although cholangitis occurs most frequently as a complication of extrahepatic biliary obstruction due to choledocholithiasis or benign stricture, it may be encountered in association with acute cholecystitis, acute pancreatitis, and a number of primary disorders of the biliary tract, including primary sclerosing cholangitis, congenital cystic dilatation of the intrahepatic bile ducts, and primary biliary cirrhosis. Rarely, cholangitis is a complication of such extrahepatic diseases as sepsis, pylephlebitis, and ulcerative colitis.

Nonbacterial cholangitis secondary to biliary obstruction

As previously indicated extrahepatic biliary obstruction characteristically provokes an acute, neutrophilic, inflammatory reaction around the proliferating ductules at the margins of the portal tracts. Usually, the neutrophils are most numerous at the periphery of the ductules, but some may invade their walls and lumens, and extend into the remainder of the portal tract. Lesions of this type may produce no symptoms. However, the possibility cannot be excluded that they play a contributory role in the pathogenesis of the accompanying obstructive jaundice.

Bacterial and suppurative cholangitis in biliary obstructive disease

In obstructive jaundice due to choledocholithiasis or benign stricture of the common bile duct, the bile usually contains numerous enteric bacteria (110). Similarly, numerous bacteria of the same type frequently are found in the upper jejunum, presumably as a result of their excretion in bile and subsequent multiplication, leading, in some cases, to a blind loop syndrome (111). For reasons that are not clear, biliary infection is relatively rare in cases of bile duct obstruction due to carcinoma. Although bacterial cholangitis may be asymptomatic, it usually gives rise to attacks of chills, fever, abdominal pain, and jaundice, either alone or in various combinations. These tend to recur and in time may give rise to progressive chronic inflammation and fibrosis of the bile ducts, producing a lesion usually classified as secondary sclerosing cholangitis, or to the development of secondary biliary cirrhosis. Two other complications that may be seen in such cases include multiple liver abscesses and bacteremia.

As a rule, bacterial cholangitis occurs under conditions of partial biliary obstruction. However, bouts of chills, fever, abdominal pain, and jaundice appear to be provoked by an increase in the obstruction resulting from inflammation and edema of the ductal epithelium. Although reduction of mucosal inflammation and edema, either spontaneously or as a result of antibiotic therapy, may lead to a remission of symptoms, the latter tend to recur unless the underlying biliary obstruction can be corrected surgically.

The hepatic lesions are similar to those in extrahepatic biliary obstruction uncomplicated by bacterial cholangitis, although evidence of cholestasis may be absent in some cases. Neutrophilic infiltration of the bile ducts and portal tracts tends to be more extensive when bacterial cholangitis is present, but this is not a reliable criterion for differentiation between patients with and without infected bile ducts (110). Of note is the fact that the liver is often sterile when the bile is infected (110). This suggests that bacteria may not play a significant role in the pathogenesis of the hepatic lesions associated with acute cholangitis.

Septicemia is often associated with a form of cholangitis that affects the canals of Hering, resulting in dilated ducts with inspissated bile thrombi and neutrophilic infiltration (112,113).

Rarely, complete extrahepatic biliary obstruction, most commonly attributable to choledocholithiasis, leads to the development of acute suppurative cholangitis, a condition in which both the extrahepatic and intrahepatic bile ducts are filled with pus under considerable pressure (114–116). Unless the biliary tract is promptly decompressed and drained, death may ensue within a few days. The clinical manifestations are similar to those in other forms of acute bacterial cholangitis, but, in addition, include lethargy, confusion, and septic shock secondary to gram-negative bacteremia. In fatal cases, the principal complications include multiple hepatic abscesses, peritonitis, and renal failure.

Occasionally, suppurative cholangitis is a complication of sepsis of extrahepatic origin. Figure 316 illustrates such a lesion in a patient with *Aerobacter aerogenes* bacteremia secondary to acute pyelonephritis. Laparotomy revealed multiple small hepatic abscesses, but no evidence of extrahepatic biliary obstruction.

Primary sclerosing cholangitis

Primary sclerosing cholangitis (117–121), a disorder of unknown etiology, is characterized by chronic, progressive inflammation and fibrosis of the extrahepatic and intrahepatic bile ducts that lead to thickening and induration of their walls and alternating, segmental constriction and dilatation of their lumens. Frequently, the gallbladder is affected by the inflammatory and fibrotic process. Rarely, the disease is limited to the intrahepatic (102) or extrahepatic bile ducts (119).

In more than half the cases, primary sclerosing cholangitis is associated with ulcerative colitis (117,118,122) and, rarely, with other disorders, such as Crohn's disease (123), retroperitoneal fibrosis (124), orbital fibrosis (125), and Riedel's struma (125). Similar lesions have followed the intraarterial infusions of fluorodeoxyuridine (126). They have also been seen in a variety of immunodeficiency states (127,128), as well as histiocytosis X (129) and autoimmune hemolytic anemia (130). Bile duct abnormalities, including sclerosing cholangitis, have been observed in AIDS (131). It has been suggested that such changes may be the result of opportunistic infections.

The severity of primary sclerosing cholangitis bears no relationship to the extent or activity of the associated ulcerative colitis. Usually, the latter is mild or moderately severe, but may be completely inactive and in remission. Occasionally, the disease precedes the development of overt ulcerative colitis. Based on one large study, it has been estimated that the incidence of sclerosing cholangitis in ulcerative colitis may be as high as 70% (132). More recent estimates are even higher (132A)

Possible pathogenetic factors that have been considered include infection secondary to portal bacteremia or ascending cholangitis, endotoxemia, the reabsorption of toxic, unconjugated bile acids, and an autoimmune reaction possibly triggered by bacterial infection. However, currently available evidence is not consistent with any of these hypotheses.

Primary sclerosing cholangitis affects males twice as frequently as females, and, usually, appears between the ages of 25 and 45 years. Rarely, children younger than 2 years may be affected (133).

Most patients with primary sclerosing cholangitis present with jaundice, pruritus, hepatomegaly, and weight loss, often accompanied by recurrent bouts of acute bacterial cholangitis characterized by chills, fever, abdominal pain, and tenderness. Less often, the disease progresses insidiously and presents as cirrhosis or manifestations of portal hypertension.

A comparison of 60 patients with primary sclerosing cholangitis and 258 with primary biliary cirrhosis revealed a few similarities but many differences. Although both groups showed jaundice, pruritus, and fatigue in most patients, the patients with primary sclerosing cholangitis were younger (mean age 41 versus 53 years), predominantly men (90% versus 63%), and had a higher prevalence of ulcerative colitis (68% versus 1%) (134). Fever and cholangitis were significantly more common in the primary sclerosing cholangitis group while arthritis, thyroid disease, and pigmentation were much more common in primary biliary cirrhosis. Cholestasis is an earlier and more frequent finding in primary sclerosing cholangitis than in primary biliary cirrhosis. In the late stages the characteristic ductular changes make the histologic differentiation easier.

In a minority of cases, the disease is asymptomatic and is discovered in the course of transhepatic or endoscopic retrograde cholangiography carried out to investigate the etiology of otherwise unexplained, increased serum levels of alkaline phosphatase. It is highly probable that asymptomatic cases are more common than is generally appreciated, as evidenced by their frequency in a group of ulcerative colitis patients subjected to routine cholangiography whenever the serum alkaline phosphatase level was increased (132).

The principal biochemical abnormalities in primary sclerosing cholangitis, in order of their frequency, include raised serum levels of alkaline phosphatase, transaminase, bilirubin, and IgM. Liver blood tests including bilirubin, transaminase, alkaline phosphatase, serum albumin, and prothrombin time were similar in the patients with primary sclerosing cholangitis and primary biliary cirrhosis. Mitochondrial antibodies were almost always present in primary biliary cirrhosis, but were rarely so in primary sclerosing cholangitis.

The cholangiographic findings in primary sclerosing cholangitis provide the most reliable criteria for identifying the disease. These are characterized by segmental, alternating areas of stricture and dilatation in the extrahepatic and intrahepatic bile ducts. Usually, the intrahepatic bile ducts appear beaded, attenuated, reduced in number, or difficult to visualize. Although choledocholithiasis, benign strictures, and carcinoma of the extrahepatic bile ducts may give rise to secondary sclerosing cholangitis, the intrahepatic bile ducts tend to be dilated rather than attenuated and beaded. Differentiation between primary sclerosing cholangitis and primary biliary cirrhosis or benign or neoplastic stricture of the extrahepatic bile ducts may be difficult if the intrahepatic bile ducts cannot be visualized on transhepatic or endoscopic retrograde cholangiography (135). In such cases, laparotomy and biopsy of the affected ducts are required to establish the correct diagnosis, although the histologic findings of primary sclerosing cholangitis are nonspecific.

The clinical course in primary sclerosing cholangitis is highly variable. However, in symptomatic cases, the disease tends to be progressive, and frequently gives rise to secondary biliary cirrhosis. Other complications that may occur include the development of biliary pigment stones, suppurative cholangitis, liver abscess, hemorrhage from esophageal varices, and bile duct carcinoma. The latter is a well-known complication of ulcerative colitis alone, so its relationship to primary sclerosing cholangitis when associated with inflammatory bowel disease is uncertain.

Over one-third of patients with clinically overt primary sclerosing cholangitis die of hepatic failure or other complications of their disease over a variable period of time, ranging from six months to 15 years (119). Asymptomatic patients may remain asymptomatic over a period of years (136), but the long-term prognosis in such cases is still uncertain. Cholangiocarcinoma is an occasional complication of primary sclerosing cholangitis in patients with ulcerative colitis (46,47).

The *liver biopsy findings* in primary sclerosing cholangitis are not distinctive, and in the absence of cholangiography may be misinterpreted as evidence of extrahepatic biliary obstruction, chronic active hepatitis, cirrhosis of various types, or portal fibrosis with noncirrhotic presinusoidal portal hypertension. The earliest finding is that of pericholangitis, which is a mild, nonspecific inflammatory reaction around the bile ductules (Fig. 714). The histologic features usually include the following, either alone or in various combinations: (1) portal fibrosis and acute or chronic inflammation with or without accompanying erosion of the limiting plates; (2) alterations in the bile ducts, including ductular proliferation, a reduction in the number of interlobular ducts, concentric, lamellar fibrosis of the interlobular ducts (Figs. 715, 716), which may progress to dense collagenous scars that obliterate the bile ducts (Fig. 717), or degeneration, necrosis, and inflammation of the ductal epithelium (Fig. 718); (3) centrilobular cholestasis; (4) portal-portal fibrous bridging or cirrhosis; (5) accumulation of copper-containing granules in the cytoplasm of periportal hepatocytes (Fig. 719); and (6) a variety of nonspecific parenchymal changes, including small, scattered foci of inflammatory cells, hepatocellular degeneration or necrosis, acidophilic bodies, evidence of hepatocellular regeneration, and occasional fat droplets.

In patients with primary sclerosing cholangitis who present with chronic cholestasis, the hepatic lesions closely resemble those of extrahepatic biliary obstruction. They are characterized by centrilobular, canalicular, and Kupffer cell bile thrombi (Fig. 559) and expanded, fibrotic, and edematous portal tracts containing marginal proliferating ductules surrounded and infiltrated by numerous neutrophils (Fig. 560). Frequently, the more central portions of the portal tracts contain numerous lymphocytes and plasma cells, a variable number of macrophages that often contain lipofuscin, and scattered eosinophils. In about one-third of the cases, some of the large interlobular ducts are surrounded by dense, concentric fibrous lamellae [(137); Fig. 380]. Although this feature is regarded by some as diagnostic of primary sclerosing cholangitis, we have encountered it under a variety of other conditions and consider it a nonspecific finding. Sometimes the ducts disappear entirely leaving the fibrous sheath behind (Fig. 717). The combination of duct atrophy and dense periductular fibrosis is typical of primary sclerosing cholangitis (138). As in other forms of chronic cholestasis, the periportal hepatocytes may contain numerous rhodamine-positive, copper-containing, cytoplasmic granules (Fig. 561) and orcein-positive, granular, copper-protein deposits [(139); Fig. 719]. Taken together with the reduction in the number of interlobular ducts and the presence of occasional ducts that show degeneration or necrosis of their epithelial linings (Fig. 374), such deposits of copper may suggest the possibility of primary biliary cirrhosis. Accordingly, primary sclerosing cholangitis should be excluded by endoscopic retrograde cholangiography in all mitochondrial antibody-negative cases of primary biliary cirrhosis.

Occasionally, the hepatic lesions of primary sclerosing cholangitis mimic those of chronic active hepatitis. These disorders are characterized by (1) expansion and fibrosis of the portal tracts, (2) erosion of the limiting plate, (3) extension of fibrous tissue and inflammatory cells into the parenchyma with the formation of portal-portal bridges, (4) an extensive, predominantly lymphocytic and plasma cell portal inflammatory reaction, and (5) ductular proliferation (Fig. 558).

In approximately one-third of the cases, fibrosis is sufficiently advanced to alter the normal lobular architecture and is often accompanied by nodule formation. Usually, such lesions show the features of secondary biliary cirrhosis, but, as has been pointed out, they may present as cryptogenic cirrhosis (119).

Frequently, the inflammatory and fibrotic lesions that affect the portal tracts and bile ducts in ulcerative colitis are categorized as "pericholangitis" [(140); Fig. 714]. This term is misleading in that the lesions are not necessarily limited to or even predominantly located in the periductular regions, and give no indication that they may be associated with primary sclerosing cholangitis (141). However, some of the lesions classified as "pericholangitis" may represent a nonspecific reaction to ulcerative colitis, since they may be encountered in such cases in the absence of cholangiographic evidence of sclerosing cholangitis. Nevertheless, the possibility that both nonspecific "pericholangitis" and primary sclerosing cholangitis share a common pathogenesis cannot be excluded (142).

Hepatobiliary cystadenoma

Rarely, cystadenomas may cause obstructive jaundice (143). A small fraction of hepatobiliary cystadenomas have a mesenchymal cell layer interposed between an inner epithelial lining and an outer connective tissue layer (144). These rare lesions are known as cystadenomas with mesenchymal stroma or Edmondson's tumor (Fig. 720). They occur almost exclusively in women and may undergo malignant transformation. Histologically they are cysts lined by cuboidal endothelium with a subadjacent layer of mesenchymal stromal cells, under which is found a dense layer of fibrous tissue (143). Cystadenomas without mesenchymal components arise from normal biliary ducts; those with mesenchymal stroma are thought to arise from foci of primitive hepatobiliary and mesenchymal cells (143). These mesenchymal layers may undergo malignant transformation to either carcinoma or sarcoma.

Congenital anomalies of the bile ducts

Congenital choledochal cyst

Congenital choledochal cyst (145–147) is an anomaly characterized by a sharply localized zone of dilatation of the extrahepatic bile ducts apparently due to congenital segmental hypoplasia of the fibromuscular component of the duct wall, often accompanied by distal narrowing of its lumen. It has been suggested that some choledochal cysts may be acquired as a result of the reflux of pancreatic juice into the common bile duct (148).

Choledochal cysts may present as (1) cylindrical or fusiform dilatations centered at the level of the cystic duct and involving both the common hepatic and common bile ducts, (2) cystic diverticula of the common bile duct, or (3) cystic dilatations of the distal intramural segments of the common bile duct within the wall of the duodenum (choledochocele).

Choledochal cysts vary in size from a few centimeters in diameter to massive structures that may contain up to 5 liters of fluid. Although usually single they may be multiple. Often, the cysts are devoid of epithelial linings.

As a rule, a cyst becomes evident clinically during infancy or early childhood, but may be delayed until adult life. Women are affected far more frequently than men. Japanese people appear to be unusually susceptible to the disease.

The principal clinical manifestations include obstructive jaundice, abdominal pain, and a palpable abdominal mass. This classic triad of features is encountered in only a minority of cases, chiefly children. Infants and adults usually present with jaundice, abdominal pain, or a mass, or with combinations thereof. Cholangitis is common in adults (149).

Typically the jaundice is obstructive in type. It is frequently accompanied by pruritus and may be intermittent. The character of the pain varies, but is often colicky in nature. Frequently, palpable abdominal masses fluctuate in size and may be tender.

Complications of choledochal cysts include (1) recurrent acute bacterial cholangitis, (2) the development of pigment stones in the cyst and extrahepatic bile ducts, (3) acute pancreatitis, (4) rupture of the cyst, (5) secondary biliary cirrhosis, and (6) carcinoma of the cyst or adjacent bile ducts.

Occasionally, choledochal cysts are associated with other congenital anomalies of the bile ducts, including congenital hepatic fibrosis, congenital cystic dilatation of the intrahepatic bile ducts (Caroli syndrome) and biliary atresia.

The *liver biopsy findings* in choledochal cyst are not distinctive and vary with the manifestations and duration of activity of the disease. The principal lesions that may be encountered include those of extrahepatic biliary obstruction, acute cholangitis, and secondary biliary cirrhosis, either alone or in various

combinations. Resection of these cysts, rather than bile duct drainage, provides the only long-term cure.

Congenital cystic dilatation of the intrahepatic bile ducts (Caroli syndrome)

Congenital cystic dilatation (150–154) is characterized by segmental, saccular dilatation of the large, intrahepatic bile ducts. Usually, the ductal lesions are bilateral, but rarely they are limited to the right or left lobe of the liver.

Frequently, the Caroli syndrome is associated with congenital hepatic fibrosis, another anomaly that affects small bile ducts, and, rarely, with choledochal cyst. Occasionally, particularly in patients with congenital hepatic fibrosis, the kidneys may show congenital anomalies. Of these the most common is renal tubular ectasia, but rare instances of renal cysts have been reported. Since siblings may be affected, these associated anomalies suggest that the Caroli syndrome may be related to polycystic disease.

Recurrent attacks of acute, suppurative bacterial cholangitis that may be associated with bacteremia and multiple liver abscesses are the principal clinical manifestations of the disease. These bacteriologic complications tend to appear during childhood or early adult life and may lead to death from hepatic failure, sepsis, or even amyloidosis (152). Jaundice is an inconstant feature, but, when present, is recurrent and obstructive in nature, and often is attributable to complicating choledocholithiasis.

In the Caroli syndrome, pigment stones frequently develop in both the intrahepatic and extrahepatic bile ducts. These may give rise to biliary colic and undoubtedly contribute to the recurrent attacks of acute cholangitis and obstructive jaundice characteristic of the disease.

In some cases, congenital cystic dilatation of the bile ducts does not give rise to symptoms. As a rule, such cases are encountered in patients with congenital hepatic fibrosis subjected to routine cholangiographic study to exclude the Caroli syndrome. The clinical features of congenital hepatic fibrosis predominate in such patients, and include hepatosplenomegaly, esophageal varices, or hemorrhage from such varices. The diagnosis can almost always be made relatively noninvasively by intravenous cholangiography, ultrasonography, or computed tomography (155).

In addition to intrahepatic and extrahepatic stones, sepsis, and hepatic abscesses, other less common complications of Caroli's syndrome include secondary biliary cirrhosis, bile duct carcinoma, and amyloidosis.

Depending on the stage of the disease and its activity, the principal *liver biopsy* findings include dilated septal bile ducts, acute or chronic cholangitis and pericholangitis, features of extrahepatic biliary obstruction, including cholestasis and ductular proliferation, and varying degrees of portal fibrosis. In addition, the liver may show the typical features of congenital hepatic fibrosis.

Figures 385 and 386 illustrate the hepatic lesions in a case of Caroli's syndrome associated with congenital hepatic fibrosis. The patient presented at the age of three years with obstructive jaundice, chills, fever, and bacteremia. At laparotomy, cholangiography revealed cystic dilatation of the intrahepatic ducts. In addition, wedge biopsy of the liver showed acute cholangitis and the typical features of congenital hepatic fibrosis. On antibiotic therapy, the cholangitis and bacteremia abated, and, thereafter, the patient remained free of biliary symptoms. However, four years later, at the age of seven, he presented with massive bleeding from esophageal varices, necessitating portacaval anastomosis. Wedge biopsy of the liver at this time exhibited widely dilated septal ducts lined by flattened, cuboidal epithelium embedded in densely collagenized, smoothly-contoured septa, features that are consistent with Caroli's syndrome during its inactive phase (Fig. 385). In adjacent fields, the parenchyma was traversed by numerous smooth-contoured septa containing branched bile ducts typical of congenital hepatic fibrosis (Fig. 386).

Congenital hepatic fibrosis

Congenital hepatic fibrosis (156–159) is a developmental anomaly of the small intrahepatic bile ducts characterized by the presence of numerous widely distributed, dilated, tortuous, and branching ducts within large fibrotic, portal tracts and densely collagenized septa. It is usually accompanied by anomalies of the renal tubules. Available evidence indicates that the disorder is a form of childhood polycystic disease that is hereditary in nature and transmitted as an autosomal recessive trait that often affects siblings. The possibility has been considered that in nonfamilial cases unaccompanied by renal lesions, congenital hepatic fibrosis may not be hereditary in nature. However, the elaborate family studies required to prove this point have not been carried out.

The term "congenital hepatic fibrosis" is an unfortunate choice, since it focuses attention on the fibrotic process and gives no indication of the possible relationship of the disorder to polycystic disease. It is sometimes associated with dilatation of the extrahepatic or intrahepatic bile ducts.

The anomalous ducts in congenital hepatic fibrosis and other forms of polycystic disease represent remnants of embryonal interlobular ducts that normally proliferate in the distal anlage of the liver and then undergo involution (158).

As previously indicated, congenital hepatic fibrosis may be accompanied by other anomalies of the biliary tract, such as Caroli's syndrome and choledochal cyst. Although gross cysts in the liver and kidneys are rarely encountered, they may occur later in life, thereby mimicking adult polycystic disease.

Usually, the clinical manifestations of congenital hepatic fibrosis appear during childhood, but may be delayed until early adult life. Characteristically, the liver is enlarged and firm. Signs or symptoms of portal hypertension, including splenomegaly, esophageal varices, hemorrhage from varices, or evidence of hypersplenism are typically present. Usually, the portal hypertension is of the presinusoidal type and attributable to hypoplasia, compression, or a reduction in the number of small portal vein radicles. Hepatic function is well preserved. However, jaundice, ascites, coma, and other evidence of hepatic failure may follow massive bleeding from esophageal varices.

Ectasia of renal collecting tubules is a common feature of the disease, and radiographically resembles medullary sponge kidney. As a rule, renal function is normal in such cases. However, in adults with congenital hepatic fibrosis, the tubules may distend to form multiple large cysts that resemble those of adult polycystic disease, and may give rise to systemic hypertension and progressive renal failure that ultimately proves fatal. Rarely,

the disease is complicated by the development of bile duct or hepatocellular carcinoma.

As illustrated in Figure 64, the *hepatic lesions* of congenital hepatic fibrosis are characterized by numerous relatively broad, smooth-contoured, densely collagenized septa that contain numerous dilated, branching bile ducts. Although the septa may partially or completely outline nodules of parenchyma and thus mimic cirrhosis, the lobular architecture is intact in many areas and shows no evidence of hepatocellular regeneration. As is evident even at the low magnification of Figure 64, the septa contain few if any inflammatory cells, and there is a striking paucity of small portal vein radicles. In some areas, the portal tracts are completely normal, whereas in others, they are enlarged and fibrotic and contain the same type of dilated, tortuous, branching ducts found in the septa. Such enlarged portal tracts are indistinguishable from von Meyenburg complexes. Except for its distortion by the fibrous septa, the parenchyma is normal in appearance and shows no evidence of cholestasis.

As is evident at higher magnification in Figure 65, most of the anomalous ducts are lined by cuboidal epithelium, and occasionally contain inspissated bile. Not infrequently, however, elongated, slender ducts lined by flattened epithelium and devoid of lumens are found closely adherent to the limiting plates, which invariably are intact.

Childhood polycystic disease

Childhood polycystic disease (160,161) comprises a group of autosomal recessive hereditary disorders characterized by developmental anomalies of the small intrahepatic bile ducts and renal tubules. Each of the four subgroups that have been identified, i.e. perinatal, neonatal, infantile, and juvenile, has a unique genetic basis and breeds true in affected families. The subtypes differ from one another in the age at presentation, in the relative severity and predominance of hepatic and renal lesions, in clinical manifestations, and in prognosis.

Manifestations of childhood polycystic disease

Perinatal type. The perinatal type presents at birth with massive enlargement of the kidneys and respiratory distress, and leads to death within a few hours or days. Renal lesions predominate and are characterized by dilatation and elongation of almost all tubules, producing radially arranged, fusiform cysts throughout the cortex and medulla.

The liver is not enlarged, but usually contains anomalous, dilated and tortuous, small intrahepatic bile ducts, occasionally accompanied by a few small, macroscopic cysts and minimal portal fibrosis.

Neonatal type. The neonatal type presents during the first month of life with massive enlargement of the kidneys and progressive renal failure that results in death within a few weeks or months. As in the perinatal type, renal lesions predominate, but only 60% of the tubules are affected. The hepatic lesions also resemble those in the perinatal type, but often portal fibrosis is a more prominent feature.

Infantile type. Clinical manifestations appear at the age of three to six months and may be predominantly hepatic or renal. In those with predominantly hepatic lesions, both the clinical and histologic features are those of congenital hepatic fibrosis. Portal hypertension and hemorrhage from esophageal varices are relatively common complications of this variant of the disease.

In most cases, approximately 25% of the renal tubules are ectatic, and are accompanied by enlargement of the kidneys. Macroscopic renal cysts may be present in older children. Renal manifestations may predominate in infantile polycystic disease and may lead to death from renal failure before the age of 10 years.

Juvenile type. Hepatic lesions and manifestations typical of congenital hepatic fibrosis predominate in juvenile type polycystic disease. In most instances approximately 10% of the renal tubules are ectatic. This disorder tends to be asymptomatic.

Anomalous bile ducts and renal tubules in other genetic disorders

Adult polycystic disease in children. Rarely, adult polycystic disease, a hereditary disorder that is transmitted as an autosomal dominant trait, affects children, and presents with hepatic and renal lesions that resemble those of childhood polycystic disease. Identification of such cases depends on analysis of the hereditary pattern and manifestations of the disease in the affected family.

Zellweger syndrome (cerebro-hepato-renal syndrome). Zellweger syndrome is characterized by anomalies of the intrahepatic bile ducts, hemosiderosis, hypoplastic kidneys with cortical cysts containing glomeruli in their walls, and cerebral anomalies (see Chapter 12).

Meckel's syndrome. Meckel's syndrome presents with hepatic and renal lesions that resemble those in childhood polycystic disease, but, in addition, is characterized by cerebral malformations and polydactyly.

Ivenmark's familial dysplasia. The principal features of Ivenmark's dysplasia include anomalous intrahepatic bile ducts, hepatic fibrosis, renal dysplasia with cyst formation, and dilatation of the pancreatic ducts accompanied by pancreatic fibrosis.

Adult polycystic disease

Adult polycystic disease (162–164), a hereditary disorder transmitted as an autosomal dominant trait, is characterized by developmental anomalies of the renal tubules and intrahepatic bile ducts. Over a period of years, these ducts distend with fluid to form macroscopic cysts in the kidneys and liver. Occasionally, other anomalies give rise to cysts in the pancreas, spleen, and lungs or to cerebrovascular aneurysms.

Manifestations of adult polycystic disease. With rare exceptions, the clinical manifestations are delayed until the third to fifth decade. Renal cysts are more common and produce symptoms more frequently than hepatic cysts. Nevertheless, in many cases, both types of cyst occur together. It has been estimated that the liver contains cysts in one-third of patients with renal polycystic disease, whereas renal cysts are present in about half those with hepatic polycystic disease.

Renal manifestations. The principal clinical features of adult renal polycystic disease include enlargement of the kidneys, hypertension, hematuria, azotemia, and ultimate death from renal failure or complications of associated cardiovascular disease.

Hepatic manifestations. When the cysts are small and few in number, hepatic polycystic disease gives rise to no clinical manifestations. Usually, in such cases, the cysts are discovered at laparotomy or autopsy, or are detected in the course of scintiscanning.

When the cysts are large and numerous, the liver is enlarged, firm, and nodular. Nevertheless, with few exceptions, hepatic function is well preserved. Rarely, adult polycystic liver disease is complicated by abdominal pain due to hemorrhage into the cysts, jaundice due to compression of major intrahepatic bile ducts by large cysts, portal hypertension, and hemorrhage from esophageal varices and bile duct carcinoma.

Microscopic features of hepatic polycystic disease. The cysts vary in number from a few to innumerable and range in size from a few millimeters to 10 to 15 cm, in diameter. Characteristically they are lined by cuboidal or flattened epithelium and contain no bile, since they do not communicate with actively secreting bile ducts (Fig. 384). Most of the cysts are partially or completely encapsulated by fibrous bands, and, in some cases, are attached to typical von Meyenburg complexes (Fig. 384). The latter are sharply circumscribed collections of dilated, tortuous, branching ducts, some of which may contain bile embedded in dense collagen. Available evidence suggests that these cysts represent remnants of embryonal intralobular bile ducts that failed to undergo normal involution. Moreover, it has been proposed that they are the forerunners of both childhood and adult polycystic liver disease (145). The frequent association in some cases of congenital hepatic fibrosis of von Meyenburg complexes with the cysts in the adult form of the disease, and the occurrence of isolated or bridged groups of such complexes is consistent with this hypothesis.

The parenchyma, portal tracts, and lobular architecture in areas devoid of cysts are normal. Accordingly, polycystic liver disease may escape detection in needle biopsy specimens when the cysts are few in number.

Von Meyenburg complexes (bile duct microhamartomas, cholangiohamartomas)

Von Meyenburg complexes (165,166) are congenital anomalies that are characterized by sharply circumscribed clusters of aberrant bile ducts embedded in dense collagen that are derived from embryonal intralobular bile ducts that fail to undergo normal involution.

As previously indicated, von Meyenburg complexes may be hereditary in some cases and involved in the pathogenesis of congenital hepatic fibrosis, childhood polycystic disease, and adult polycystic disease of the liver. More often, however, they occur sporadically, occasionally in association with a nonparasitic, solitary cyst, but most frequently they are found unexpectedly at laparotomy or autopsy. Rarely, such lesions undergo malignant transformation and give rise to bile duct carcinoma.

Sporadic von Meyenburg complexes may be solitary or multiple. They occur most frequently just beneath Glisson's capsule and present as firm, gray-white, wedge-shaped masses, 5 to 10 mm in diameter, with the base at the surface of the liver. When multiple and deeper in the liver, they may be more irregular in shape and they may be connected to a portal tract, but they are still sharply circumscribed.

Figure 382 illustrates the typical histologic features of a von

Meyenburg complex found beneath Glisson's capsule in the course of a routine cholecystectomy in a patient with cholelithiasis. The lesion is characterized by numerous dilated, tortuous, branching, aberrant bile ducts embedded in densely collagenized stroma. A few of the ducts contain small bits of inspissated bile. Although the lesion superficially resembles a fibrotic portal tract, it contains no portal venous or hepatic arterial radicles and is devoid of inflammatory cells.

Solitary nonparasitic cysts of bile duct origin

Rarely, the liver contains a solitary cyst of variable size lined by cuboidal epithelium and enclosed within a fibrous capsule. Often, the wall contains aberrant bile ducts, or is associated with an adjacent von Meyenburg complex. Such findings suggest that these cysts are congenital in origin and can be attributed to progressive distension of embryonal duct remnants that failed to involute. Although such cysts may be encountered at any age, they occur most frequently during the fourth and fifth decades, and affect women more frequently than men (167–169).

Hepatomegaly or a palpable mass are the principal findings. Mild pain due to distension of the cyst by serous fluid is relatively common. Severe pain is attributed to hemorrhage into the cyst, infection of its contents, or rupture of the cyst into the peritoneum. When the cyst is large, it occasionally compresses major bile ducts and causes obstructive jaundice.

Rarely, blunt trauma that results in parenchymal necrosis and hemorrhage deep within the liver leads to the development of a traumatic cyst (170). Traumatic cysts, which may contain altered blood, bile, or pus, are lined by bile duct epithelium and are not usually enclosed within a well-defined capsule. These cysts may become apparent soon after the trauma, may be recognized after several months, may only be found at laparotomy or autopsy, or may never be found.

References

1. Barber-Riley G: Rat biliary tree during short term periods of obstruction of common duct. Am J Physiol *205*:1127–1131, 1963.
2. Strasberg SM, Dorn BC, Redinger RN, Small DM, Egdahl RH: Effects of alteration of biliary pressure on bile composition: a method for study of primate biliary physiology. Gastroenterology *61*:357–362, 1971.
3. Fulop M, Brazeau P: Impaired renal function exaggerates hyperbilirubinemia in bile duct-ligated dogs. Am J Dig Dis *15*:1067–1072, 1970.
4. Halasz M, Pinter I: Die bilirubinurie beim Menschen und Hunde. Wien Zschf inn Med *6*:252–254, 1949.
5. Rich AR: The pathogenesis of the forms of jaundice. Bull Johns Hopkins Hosp *47*:338–377, 1930.
6. Popper H: Cholestasis: the future of a past and present riddle. Hepatology *1*:187–191, 1981.
7. Strohl EL, Diffenbaugh WG, Gynn V: Symptoms of common duct stones. Analysis of clinical data on one hundred sixty-five patients having exploration of the common duct. Arch Surg *64*:788–793, 1952.
8. Waye LW, Pellegrini CA: Surgery of the Gall Bladder and Biliary Tract. Philadelphia, W.B. Saunders, 1987.
9. Alen B, Shapiro H, Way LW: Management of recurrent and residual common duct stones. Am J Surg *142*:41–49, 1981.
10. Kappas SK, Adams MB, Wilson SD: Intra-operative biliary endoscopy: mandatory for all common duct operations? Arch Surg *117*:604–613, 1982.
11. Wen C-C, Lee H-C: Intrahepatic stones. A clinical study. Ann Surg *175*:166–177, 1972.
12. Neoptolemos JP, Hoffman AF, Moussa AF: Chemical composition of stones in the biliary tree. Br J Surg *73*:515–522, 1981.
13. Matzen P, Malchow-Moller A, Lejerstefte J: Endoscopic retrograde cholangiography in patients with obstructive jaundice: a randomized study. Scand J Gastroenterol *17*:731–740, 1982.
14. Cotton PB: Direct choledochography and related diagnostic methods. Part 1. Direct choledochoscopy. Clin Gastroenterol *12*:101–110, 1983.
15. Bernhoft RA, Pellegrini CA, Motson RW: Composition and morphological and clinical features of common duct stones. Am J Surg *148*:77–86, 1984.
16. Bouchier IAD: Postmortem study of the frequency of gallstones in patients with cirrhosis of the liver. Gut *10*:705–710, 1969.
17. Nicholas P, Rinaudo PA, Conn HO: Increased incidence of cholelithiasis in Laennec's cirrhosis. Gastroenterology *63*:112–121, 1972.
18. Goebee von H, Rudolph HD, Breuer N, Hartmann W, Leder HD: Zum vorkommen von gallensteinen bei leberzirrhose. Z Gastroenterologie *19*:345–355, 1981.
19. Samuel D, Sattouf E, Degott C, Benhamou J-P: Cirrhose et lithiase biliaire en France: une etude necropsique. Gastroenterol Clin Biol *12*:39–42, 1988.
20. Steinberg HV, Beckett WW, Chezmar JL, Torres WE, Murphy FB, Bernardino ME: Incidence of cholelithiasis among patients with cirrhosis and portal hypertension. Gastrointest Radiol *13*:347–350, 1988.
21. Dunnington G, Sampliner R, Kogan F, Alfrey E, Putnam C: Natural history of cholelithiasis in patients with alcoholic cirrhosis. Ann Surg *205*:226–229, 1987.
22. Raedsch R, Stiehl A, Gundert-Remy U, Walker S, Sieg A, Czygan P, Kommerell B: Hepatic secretion of bilirubin and biliary lipids in patients with alcoholic cirrhosis of the liver. Digestion *26*:80–88, 1983.
23. Bloch RS, Allaben RD, Walt AJ: Cholecystectomy in patients with cirrhosis. A surgical challenge. Arch Surg *120*:669–672, 1985.
24. Aranha GV, Kruss D, Greenlee HB: Therapeutic options for biliary tract disease in advanced cirrhosis. Am J Surg *155*:374–377, 1988.
24a. Dubois F: Coelioscopic cholecystectomy: 330 cases. *3*:30–32, 1990.
25. Martin EC: Percutaneous, nonexcisional cholecystectomy. Hepatology *11*:1084–1086, 1990.
26. Bismuth H: Hemobilia. N Engl J Med *288*:617–619, 1973.
27. Piedad OH, Wels PB: Spontaneous internal biliary fistula, obstructive and nonobstructive types: twenty-year review of 55 cases. Ann Surg *175*:75–80, 1972.
28. Haff RC, Wise L, Ballinger W: Biliary-enteric fistulas. Surg Gynecol Obstet *133*:84–88, 1971.
29. Neoptolemos JP, Carr-Locke DL, Fraser I: The management of common bile duct calculi by endoscopic sphincterotomy in patients with gall bladders in situ. Br Med J *71*:69–73, 1984.
30. Staritz M, Ewe K, Meyer Zum Buschenfelde K-H: Endoscopic papillary dilation, a possible alternative to endoscopic papillotomy. Lancet *1*:1306–1310, 1982.
31. Shapero TF, Rosen IE, Wilson SR: Discrepancy between ultrasound and oral cholecystography in the assessment of gallstone dissolution. Hepatology *2*:587–593, 1982.
32. Johlin FC, Lochning SA, Maher JW: Extracorporeal shock wave lithotripsy (ESWL) fragmentation of retained common duct stones. Surgery *104*:192–198, 1988.
33. Taylor MC, Marshall JC, Fried TA: Extracorporeal shock wave lithotripsy (ESWL) in the management of complex biliary tract stone disease. Ann Surg *208*:586–595, 1988.
34. Cole WH, Ireneus C Jr, Reynolds JT: Strictures of the common bile duct. Studies in 122 cases. Ann Surg *142*:537–550, 1955.
35. Tan EGC, Warren KW: Bile duct injuries and stricture. *In* Diseases of the Liver, edited by L. Schiff, E.R. Schiff. 5th Edition. Philadelphia, J.B.Lippincott, 1982, pp. 1543–1547.
36. Way LW: Biliary stricture. *In* Surgery of the Gallbladder and Bile Duct, edited by L.W. Way, C.A. Pellegrini. Philadelphia, W.B. Saunders, 1987.
37. Terblanche J, Allison HF, Northover JMA: An ischemic basis for biliary strictures. Surgery *94*:52–61, 1983.
38. Genest JF, Nanos E, Grundfest-Broniatowski S: Benign biliary strictures: an analytic review (1970–1984). Surgery *99*:409–419, 1986.
39. Lygidakis NJ: Biliary stricture as a complication of chronic relapsing pancreatitis. Am J Surg *145*:804–812, 1983.
40. Cattell RB, Colcock BP: Fibrosis of the sphincter of Oddi. Ann Surg *137*:797–806, 1953.
41. Klatskin G: Adenocarcinoma of the hepatic duct at its bifurcation within the porta hepatis. An unusual tumor with distinctive clinical and pathological features. Am J Med *38*:241–256, 1965.
42. Pelligrini CA, Thomas MJ, Way LW: Recurrent biliary stricture: patterns of recurrence and outcome of surgical therapy. Am J Surg *147*:175–180, 1984.

43. Pitt HA, Postier RG, Cameron JL: Consequences of preoperative cholangitis and its treatment on the outcome of surgery for choledocholithiasis. Surgery 94:447–456, 1983.

44. Shemesh E, Brook O, Bat L: Endoscopic Gruntzig balloon dilation of benign strictures in the biliary system. Isr J Med Sci 21:889–891, 1985.

45. Mueller PR, van Sonnenberg E, Ferrucci JT Jr: Biliary stricture dilation: multicenter review of clinical management in 73 patients. Radiology 160:17–22, 1986.

46. Mir-Madjlessi SH, Farmer RG, Sivak MV Jr: Bile duct carcinoma in patients with ulcerative colitis. Relationship to sclerosing cholangitis: report of six cases and review of the literature. Dig Dis Sci 32:145–154, 1987.

47. Wee A, Ludwig J, Coffey RJ Jr, LaRusso NF, Wiesner RH: Hepatobiliary carcinoma associated with primary sclerosing cholangitis and chronic ulcerative colitis. Hum Pathol 16: 719–726, 1985.

48. Bismuth H, Malt RA: Carcinoma of the biliary tract. N Engl J Med 301:704–708, 1979.

49. Smith VM, Feldman M, Warner CG: Neoplasms of the cystic and hepatic ducts. Am J Dig Dis 7:804–816, 1962.

50. Legge DA, Carlson HC: Cholangiographic appearance of primary carcinoma of the bile ducts. Radiology 102:259–266, 1972.

51. Whelton MJ, Petrelli M, George P, Yong WB, Sherlock S: Carcinoma at the junction of the main hepatic ducts. Q J Med 38:211–230, 1969.

52. Makipour H, Cooperman A, Danzi JT, Farmer RG: Carcinoma of the ampulla of Vater. Review of 38 cases with emphasis on treatment prognostic factors. Ann Surg 183:341–344, 1976.

53. Piorkowski RJ, Blievernight SW, Lawrence W Jr: Pancreatic and periampullary carcinoma: experience with 200 patients over a 12 year period. Am J Surg 143:189–200, 1982.

54. Cooperman A: Periampullary cancer, 1983. Semin Liver Dis 3:181–194, 1983.

55. Hagege H, DeMontigny S, Ink O, Fritsch J, Choury AD, Ligoury C, Etienne JP: Ictere obstructif chez les malades ayant une tumeur hepatique. Resultat du drainage biliaire non chirurgical. Gastroenterol Clin Biol 14:115–119, 1990.

56. Witt PC, Thomas E: Extrahepatic biliary obstruction and small cell lung carcinoma. Ann Intern Med 103:476–482, 1985.

57. Scott J, Summerfield JA, Elias E, Dick R, Sherlock S: Chronic pancreatitis: a cause of cholestasis. Gut 18:196–201, 1977.

58. Sarles H, Sahel J: Cholestasis and lesions of the biliary tract in chronic pancreatitis. Gut 19:851–857, 1978.

59. Aranha GV, Prinz RA, Freeark RJ: The spectrum of biliary tract obstruction from chronic pancreatitis. Arch Surg 119:595–602, 1984.

60. Carter DC: Pancreatitis and the biliary tree: the continuing problem. Am J Surg 155:10–18, 1988.

61. Jones BA, Salsberg BB, Mehta MH: Common pancreatic biliary channels and their relationship to gallstone size in gallstone pancreatitis. Ann Surg 205:123–130, 1987.

62. Neoptolemos JP, Carr-Locke DL, Fraser I: The management of common bile duct calculi by endoscopic sphincterotomy in patients with gallbladder in situ. Br J Surg 71:69–76, 1984.

63. Bell ET: Carcinoma of the pancreas. I. A clinical and pathologic study of 609 necropsied cases. II. The relation of carcinoma of the pancreas to diabetes mellitus. Am J Pathol 33:499–523, 1957.

64. Warren KW, Christophi C, Armendariz R: Current trends in the diagnosis and treatment of carcinoma of the pancreas. Am J Surg 145:813–821, 1983.

65. Mitty HA, Efremidis SC, Yeh H-C: Impact of fine-needle biopsy on management of patients with carcinoma of the pancreas. Am J Roentgenol 137:1119–1128, 1981.

66. Corlette MB, Bismuth H: Acute cholecystitis and jaundice. Arch Surg 106:829–832, 1973.

67. Cheung LY, Maxwell JG: Jaundice in patients with acute cholecystitis: its validity as an indication for common duct exploration. Am J Surg 130:746–748, 1975.

68. Orlando R, Gleason E, Drezner AD: Acute acalculous cholecystitis in the critically ill patient. Am J Surg 145:472–480, 1983.

69. Ullmann M. Hasselgren P-O, Tveit E: Post-traumatic and postoperative acute acalculous cholecystitis. Acta Chir Scand 150:507–512, 1984.

70. Glenn F, Becker CG: Acute acalculous cholecystitis. Ann Surg 195:131–140, 1982

71. Gracie WA, Ransohoff DF: The natural history of silent gallstones. The innocent gallstone is not a myth. N Engl J Med 307:798–803, 1982.

72. Meyers WC, Jones RS: Acalculous cholecystitis and other non neoplastic gall bladder conditions. In Textbook of Liver and Biliary Surgery, edited by R.S. Jones. Philadelphia, J.B. Lippincott, 1990, pp. 295–302.

73. Naccarato R, Rizzo A, Chiaramonte, Farini R, Okoliscanyi L, Parenti A, Lise M, D'Amico D, Pedrazzoli S: Studies of liver structure and function in patients with uncomplicated gallstones. Med Chir Dig 6:65–68, 1977.

74. Seltzer RA, Rossiter SB, Cooperman LR, Liebowitz D: Hemobilia following needle biopsy of the liver. Am J Roentgenol 127:1035–1036, 1976.

75. Sandblom P: Hemobilia. In Diseases of the Liver, edited by L. Schiff, E.R. Schiff. 6th Edition. Philadelphia, J.B. Lippincott, 1987, pp. 1442–1449.

76. Czerniak A, Thompson JN, Hemingway AP: Hemobilia: a disease in evolution. Arch Surg 123:718–725, 1988.

77. Stephenson SL Jr, Rice ML Jr, Rossett NL: Duodenal ulcer producing obstructive jaundice. Gastroenterology 21:584–588, 1952.

78. McSherry CK, Glenn F: Biliary tract obstruction and duodenal diverticuli. Surg Gynecol Obstet 130: 829–836, 1970.

79. Alagille D, Odievre M: Liver and Biliary Tract Disease in Children. New York, John Wiley & Sons 1979.

80. Landing BH: Considerations on the pathogenesis of neonatal hepatitis, biliary atresia and choledochal cyst: the concept of infantile obstructive cholangiopathy. Progr Pediatr Surg 6:113–139, 1974.

81. Desmet VJ: Intrahepatic bile ducts under the lens. J Hepatol 1:545–559, 1985.

82. Morecki R, Glaser J, Cho S: Biliary atresia and reovirus type 3 infection. N Engl J Med 307:481–484, 1982.

83. Glaser JH, Balistreri WF, Morecki R: Role of reovirus type 3 in persistent infantile cholestasis. J Pediatr 6:912–915, 1984.

84. Morecki R, Glaser JH, Johnson AB, Kress Y: Detection of reovirus type 3 in the porta hepatis of an infant with extrahepatic biliary atresia: ultrastructural and immunocytochemial study. Hepatology 6:1137–1142, 1984.

85. Minuk GY, Rascanin N, Paul RW, Lee PWK, Buchan K, Kelly JK: Reovirus type 3 infection in patients with primary biliary cirrhosis and primary sclerosing cholangitis. J Hepatol 5:8–13, 1987.

86. Goldman IS, Brandborg LL: Parasitic diseases of the liver. In Hepatology. A Textbook of Liver Disease, edited by D. Zakin, T.D. Boyer. 2nd Edition. Philadelphia, W.B. Saunders, 1990, pp. 1086–1097.

87. Lin AC, Chapman SW, Turner HR: Clonochiasis: an update. South Med J 80:919–926, 1987.

88. Condomines J, Rene-Espinet JM, Espinos-Perez JC: Percutaneous cholangiography in the diagnosis of hepatic fascioliasis. Am J Gastroenterol 80:384–389, 1985.

89. Bonar S, Burrell IM, West B, Cahow CE: Recurrent cholangitis secondary to oriental cholangiohepatitis. J Clin Gastroenterol 11: 464–468, 1989.

90. Wong RK, Peura DA, Mutter ML: Hemobilia and liver flukes in a patient from Thailand. Gastroenterology 88:1958–1965, 1985.

91. Schwartz D: Cholangiocarcinoma associated with liver fluke infection: a preventable source of morbidity in Asian immigrants. Am J Gastroenterol 81:76–82, 1986.

92. LLoyd DA: Hepatic ascariasis. S Afr J Surg 20:297–304, 1982.

93. Pagola Serrano MA, Vega A, Ortega E: Computed tomography of hepatic fascioliasis. J Comput Assist Tomogr 11:269–278, 1987.

94. Weinbren K, Hadjis NS, Blumgart LH: Structural aspects of the liver in patients with biliary disease and portal hypertension. J Clin Pathol 38:1013–1020, 1985.

95. Hadjis NS, Blumgart LH: Role of liver atrophy, hepatic resection and hepatocyte hyperplasia in the development of portal hypertension in biliary disease. Gut 28:1022–1028, 1987.

96. Yeong ML, Nicholson GI, Lee SP: Regression of biliary cirrhosis following choledochal cyst drainage. Gastroenterology 82:332–335, 1982.

97. Bianchi L: Liver biopsy interpretation in hepatitis. Part I. Presentation of critical morphologic features used in diagnosis (Glossary). Pathol Res Pract 178:2–19, 1983.

98. Vanstapel MJ, Burton M, Desmet VJ: Keratin immunohistochemistry in normal and pathological human liver. Hepatology 4:1037–1043, 1984.

99. Christoffersen P, Hemming P: Histological changes in human liver biopsies following extrahepatic biliary obstruction. Acta Pathol Microbiol Scand Suppl 212:150–157, 1970.

100. Portmann B, Popper H, Neuberger J, Williams R: Sequential and diagnostic features in primary biliary cirrhosis based on serial histologic study in 209 patients. Gastroenterology 88:1777–1790, 1985.

101. Mistilis S, Schiff L: A case of jaundice due to unilateral hepatic duct obstruction with relief after hepatic lobectomy. Gut *4:*13–15, 1963.

102. Bhatal PS, Powell LW: Primary intrahepatic obliterating cholangitis: a possible variant of sclerosing cholangitis. Gut *10:*886–893, 1969.

103. Ludwig J, Wiesner RH, LaRusso NF: Idiopathic adulthood ductopenia. A cause of chronic cholestatic liver disease and biliary cirrhosis. J Hepatol *7:*193–199, 1988.

104. Ludwig J: New concepts in biliary cirrhosis. Semin Liver Dis *7:*293–301, 1987.

105. Klatskin G; Hepatic granulomata: problems in interpretation. Ann NY Acad Sci *278:*427–432, 1976.

106. Rudzki C, Ishak KG, Zimmerman HJ: Chronic intrahepatic cholestasis of sarcoidosis. Am J Med *59:*373–387, 1975.

107. Fox RA, James DG, Scheuer PJ, Sharma O, Sherlock S: Impaired delayed hypersensitivity in primary biliary cirrhosis. Lancet *1:*959–962, 1969.

108. Karlish AJ, Thompson RPH, Williams R: A case of sarcoidosis and primary biliary cirrhosis. Lancet *2:*599–601, 1969.

109. Rubinow A, Koff RS, Cohen AS: Severe intrahepatic cholestasis in primary amyloidosis. A report of four cases and a review of the literature. Am J Med *64:*937–946, 1978.

110. Freedman LR, Goldenberg IS: The relationship between bacterial infection of the hepato-biliary system and common bile duct obstruction in man. Yale J Biol Med *35:* 318–328, 1963.

111. Scott AJ, Khan A: Partial biliary obstruction with cholangitis producing a blind loop syndrome. Gut *9:*187–192, 1968.

112. Ishak KG, Rogers WA: Cryptogenic acute cholangitis: association with toxic shock syndrome. Am J Clin Pathol *76:*619–626, 1981.

113. Lefkowitch JH: Bile ductular cholestasis: an ominous histopathologic sign related to sepsis and 'cholangitis lenta'. Hum Pathol *13:*19–24, 1982.

114. Hinchey EJ, Couper CE: Acute obstructive suppurative cholangitis. Am J Surg *117:*62–68, 1969.

115. Andrew DJ, Johnson SE: Acute suppurative cholangitis. A medical and surgical emergency. Am J Gastroenterol *54:*141–154, 1970.

116. Boey JH, Way LW: Acute cholangitis. Ann Surg *191:*264–271, 1980.

117. Thorpe MEC, Scheuer PJ, Sherlock S: Primary sclerosing cholangitis, the biliary tree, and ulcerative colitis. Gut *8:* 435–448, 1967.

118. Mihas AA, Murad TM, Hirschowitz BI: Sclerosing cholangitis associated with ulcerative colitis. Light and electron microscopic studies. Am J Gastroenterol *70:*614–619, 1978.

119. Chapman RWG, Arborgh BAM, Rhodes JM, Summerfield JA, Dick R, Scheuer PJ, Sherlock S: Primary sclerosing cholangitis: a review of its clinical features, cholangiography and hepatic histology. Gut *21:*870–877, 1980.

120. Wiesner RH, LaRusso NF, Ludwig J: Comparison of the clinicopathologic features of primary sclerosing cholangitis and primary biliary cirrhosis. Gastroenterology *88:*108–116, 1985.

121. Ludwig J, Czaja AJ, Dickson ER: Manifestations of nonsuppurative cholangitis in chronic hepatobiliary disease: morphologic spectrum, clinical correlations and terminology. Liver *4:*105–111, 1984.

122. Barbatis C, Grases P. Shepherd HA, Chapman RW, Trowell J, Jewell DPJ, McGee JO'D: Histological features of sclerosing cholangitis in patients with chronic ulcerative colitis. J Clin Pathol *38:*778–783, 1985.

123. Atkinson AJ: Sclerosing cholangitis: association with regional enteritis. JAMA *188:*183–184, 1964.

124. Bartholomew LG, Cain JC, Woolner LB, Utz DC, Ferris DO: Sclerosing cholangitis. Its possible association with Riedel's struma and fibrous retroperitonitis. N Engl J Med *269:*8–12, 1963.

125. Wenger J, Gingrich GW, Mendeloff J: Sclerosing cholangitis: a manifestation of systemic disease. Increased gamma-globulin, follicular lymph node hyperplasia and orbital pseudotumor. Arch Intern Med *116:*509–514, 1965.

126. Herrmann G, Lorenz M, Kirkowa-Reimann M, Hottenrott C, Hubner K: Morphological changes after intra-arterial chemotherapy of the liver. Hepatogastroenterology *34:*5–9, 1987.

127. Naveh Y, Mendelsohn H, Spira G, Auslaender L, Mandel H, Berant M: Primary sclerosing cholangitis associated with immunodeficiency. Am J Dis Child *137:*114–117, 1983.

128. Bass NM, Chapman RW, O'Reilly A, Sherlock S: Primary sclerosing cholangitis associated with angioimmunoblastic lymphadenopathy. Gastroenterology *85:*420–424, 1983.

129. Thompson HH, Pitt HA, Lewin KJ, Longmire WP Jr: Sclerosing cholangitis and histiocytosis X. Gut *25:*526–530, 1984.

130. Moeller DD: Sclerosing cholangitis associated with autoimmune hemolytic anemia and hyperthyroidism. Am J Gastroenterol *80:*122–125, 1985.

131. Viteri AL, Greene JF Jr: Bile duct abnormalities in the acquired immune deficiency syndrome. Gastroenterology *92:*2014–2018, 1987.

132. Schrumpf E, Fausa O, Kolmannskog F: Sclerosing cholangitis in ulcerative colitis: a follow-up study. Scand J Gastroenterol *17:*33–41, 1982.

132a. La Russo, NF, Wiesner RH, Ludwig J: Sclerosing cholangitis. In Oxford Textbook of Clinical Hepatology, Oxford Medical Publications, 1991, pp. 767–776.

133. El-Shabrawi MH, Wilkinson M, Portmann B, Mieli-Vergani G, Mowat APM: Primary sclerosing cholangitis (PSC) in childhood. J Hepatol *1:*178, 1985.

134. Wiesner RH, LaRusso NF, Ludwig J, Dickson ER: Comparison of the clinicopathologic features of primary sclerosing cholangitis and primary biliary cirrhosis. Gastroenterology *88:*108–114, 1985.

135. MacSween RNM, Burt AD, Haboubi NY: Unusual variant of primary sclerosing cholangitis. J Clin Pathol *40:*541–545, 1987.

136. Helzberg JH, Petersen JM, Boyer JL: Improved survival with primary sclerosing cholangitis. Gastroenterology *92:*1869–1875, 1987.

137. Nakanuma Y, Hirai N, Kono N, Ohta G: Histological and ultrastructural examination of the intrahepatic biliary tree in primary sclerosing cholangitis. Liver *6:*317–325, 1986.

138. Scheuer PJ: Liver Biopsy Interpretation. London, Bailliere Tindall, 1988, p. 51.

139. Guarascio P, Yentis F, Cevikbas U, Portmann B, Williams R: Value of copper-associated protein in diagnostic assessment of liver biopsy. J Clin Pathol *36:*18–23, 1983.

140. Mistilis SP: Pericholangitis and ulcerative colitis. I. Pathology, etiology and pathogenesis. Ann Intern Med *63:*1–16, 1965.

141. Blackstone MO, Nemchausky BA: Cholangiographic abnormalities in ulcerative colitis-associated pericholangitis which resemble sclerosing cholangitis. Am J Dig Dis *23:*579–585, 1978.

142. Ludwig J, Barham SS, LaRusso NF, Elveback LR, Wiesner RH, McCall JT: Morphologic features of chronic hepatitis associated with primary sclerosing cholangitis and chronic ulcerative colitis. Hepatology *1:*632–640, 1981.

143. Akwari OE, Tucker A, Seigler HF, Itani KMF: Hepatobiliary cystadenoma with mesenchymal stroma. Ann Surg *211:*18–27, 1990.

144. Wheeler DA, Edmonson HA: Cystadenoma with mesenchymal stroma (CMS) in the liver and bile ducts. A clinicopathologic study of 17 cases, 4 with malignant change. Cancer *56:*1434–1445, 1985.

145. Yue PCK: Choledochal cyst: a review of 18 cases. Br J Surg *61:*896–900, 1974.

146. Matsumotu Y, Uchida K, Nakase A, Honjo I: Clinicopathologic classification of cystic dilatation of the common bile duct. Am J Surg *134:*569–574, 1977.

147. Komi N, Udaka H, Ikeda N: Congenital study with particular reference to anomalous arrangement of the pancreaticobiliary ducts. Gastroenterol Jpn *12:*293–299, 1977.

148. O'Neill JA, Templeton JM Jr, Schnaufer L: Recent experience with choledochal cysts. Ann Surg *205:*533–541, 1987.

149. Nagorney DM, McIlrath DC, Adson MA: Choledochal cysts in adults: clinical management. Surgery *96:*656–663, 1984.

150. Caroli J, Soupalt R, Kossakowski J, Plocker L, Paradowska M: La dilatation polykystique congenitale des voies biliares intra-hepatiques. Sem Hop Paris *34:*488–495, 1958.

151. Caroli J: Diseases of intrahepatic bile ducts. Is J Med Sci *4:*21–35, 1968.

152. Fevery J, Tanghe W, Kerremans R, Desmet V, DeGroote J: Congenital dilatation of the intrahepatic bile ducts associated with the development of amyloidosis. Gut *13:*604–609, 1972.

153. Murray-Lyon IM, Shelkin DKB, Laws JW, Illing RC, Williams R: Non-obstructive dilatation of the intrahepatic biliary tree with cholangitis. Q J Med *41:* 477–489, 1972.

154. Oguchi Y, Okada A, Nakamura T: Histopathologic studies of congenital dilatation of the bile duct as related to an anomalous junction of the pancreaticobiliary ductal system: clinical and experimental studies. Surgery *103:*168–178, 1988.

155. Moreno AJ, Parker AL, Spicer MJ, Brown TJ: Scintigraphic and radiographic findings in Caroli's disease. Am J Gastroenterol *70:* 299–303, 1984.

156. McCarthy LJ, Baggenstoss AH, Logan GB: Congenital hepatic fibrosis. Gastroenterology *49:*27–36, 1965.

157. Kerr DNS, Okonkwo S, Choa RG: Congenital hepatic fibrosis. Gut *19:*514–521, 1978.

158. Dupond J-L, Miguet JP, Carbillet J-P, Saint-Hillier Y, Prol C, LeConte

des-Floris R: Kidney polycystic disease in adult congenital hepatic fibrosis. Ann Intern Med 88:514–516, 1978.

159. Sherlock S: Cysts and congenital biliary abnormalities. *In* Diseases of the Liver and Biliary System, 8th Edition., Oxford, Blackwell Scientific Publications, 1989, pp. 639–654.

160. Blyth H, Ockenden BG: Polycystic disease of kidneys and liver presenting in childhood. J Med Genet 8:257–284, 1971.

161. Landing BH, Wells TR, Claireaux AE: Morphometric analysis of liver lesions in cystic diseases of childhood. Hum Pathol 11:549–560, 1980.

162. Melnick ZPJ: Polycystic liver. Analysis of seventy cases. Arch Pathol 59:162–172, 1955.

163. Davies CH, Stringer DA, Whyte H: Congenital hepatic fibrosis with saccular dilatation of intrahepatic bile ducts and infantile polycystic kidneys. Pediatr Radiol 16:302–305, 1986.

164. Summerfield JA, Nagafuchi Y, Sherlock S: Hepatobiliary fibropoly-cystic diseases: a clinical and histological review of 51 patients. J Hepatol 2:141–156, 1986.

165. Pollice L, Pagiarulo G: Cholangiohamartomas and congenital hepatic fibrosis. Med Chir Digest 5:19–24, 1976.

166. Homer LW, White HJ, Read RC: Neoplastic transformation of v. Meyenburg complexes of the liver. J. Pathol Bacteriol 96:499–502, 1968.

167. Hudson EK: Obstructive jaundice from solitary hepatic cyst. Am J Gastroenterol 39:161–164, 1963.

168. Ishak KG, Willis GW, Cummins SD, Bullock AA: Biliary cystadenoma and cystadenocarcinoma. Report of 14 cases and review of the literature. Cancer 39:322–338, 1977.

169. Wheeler DA, Edmondson HA: Ciliated hepatic foregut cyst. Am J Surg Pathol 8:467–470, 1984.

170. Jones HV, Harley HRS: Traumatic cyst of the liver. Br J Surg 57:468–470, 1970.

Chapter 21
Circulatory Disorders of the Liver

Sinusoidal disorders

Chronic passive congestion

Any sustained increase in the resistance to the outflow of blood from the liver usually leads to centrilobular sinusoidal congestion, which, if severe or prolonged, may give rise to secondary alterations in the intervening hepatic plates and spaces of Disse.

Chronic passive congestion is encountered most frequently in right ventricular heart failure, but also occurs in constrictive pericarditis, occlusion of the major hepatic veins (Budd-Chiari syndrome), and various forms of veno-occlusive disease that affect small branches of the hepatic veins.

Hepatomegaly and mild hyperbilirubinemia are the principal hepatic manifestations of right ventricular heart failure. Overt jaundice, often accompanied by greatly elevated serum levels of transaminases, usually is indicative of centrilobular ischemic necrosis, often secondary to complicating left ventricular failure (1,2). Less commonly, the sudden appearance of overt jaundice in heart failure is attributable to the bilirubin overload that follows pulmonary infarction.

Splenomegaly, ascites, and other manifestations of portal hypertension are relatively uncommon in right ventricular heart failure, but are frequent findings in constrictive pericarditis, the Budd-Chiari syndrome, and veno-occlusive disease.

The *hepatic lesions* of chronic passive congestion are characterized by dilatation of the centrilobular sinusoids, often accompanied by atrophy of the intervening hepatic plates and occasional small foci of hepatocellular dropout (Fig. 197). In prolonged, moderate, or severe chronic passive congestion, such congestion may extend to the periphery of the lobules or bridge adjacent central zones.

When the congestion is severe, particularly in constrictive pericarditis and the Budd-Chiari syndrome, striking dilatation of the sinusoids may be accompanied by loss of all the centrilobular hepatocytes, giving the appearance of hemorrhagic necrosis [(3); Fig. 213]. However, the outlines of intact sinusoids can still be identified in reticulin-stained sections. Extravasation of blood into the spaces of Disse often contributes to the hemorrhagic appearance of the centrilobular zones (Fig. 214). This is said to be a pathognomonic feature of the Budd-Chiari syndrome (4). However, in our experience and that of others, such extravasation may be encountered in any form of severe sinusoidal congestion or in centrilobular ischemic necrosis (5).

Under conditions of prolonged chronic passive congestion, loss of centrilobular hepatocytes may be followed by collapse of sinusoids and fibrosis (Fig. 215). Occasionally, such foci of fibrosis may bridge adjacent centrilobular zones (Fig. 48), and extend to the portal tracts, which may also show a mild degree of fibrosis. Rarely, the fibrosis is diffuse, giving rise to congestive or cardiac cirrhosis.

Another feature of prolonged congestion is the deposition of collagen in the spaces of Disse surrounding the dilated sinusoids (Fig. 198). By electron microscopy these changes are accompanied by the development of a continuous basement membrane and hypertrophy of the endothelium, thereby converting the fenestrated sinusoids into completely enclosed capillaries, a process, termed capillarization, that may interfere with oxygen and nutrient exchange, and, thus, contribute to the atrophy and loss of hepatocytes (6).

Although the loss of hepatocytes in congestion does not provoke an intense inflammatory reaction, the zones of cell dropout frequently contain swollen, PAS-D-positive, lipofuscin-filled Kupffer cells. Rarely, some of the canaliculi in intact areas contain small bile thrombi.

Congestive ("cardiac") cirrhosis

Prolonged chronic passive congestion may result in centrilobular loss of hepatocytes, collapse of sinusoids and reticulin, and centrilobular fibrosis. The fibrosis may be progressive, leading initially to central-central bridging, later to central-portal bridging, and ultimately to destruction of the normal lobular architecture and its replacement by nodules of regenerating parenchyma, a lesion often called reversed or "cardiac" cirrhosis (7–11). However, "congestive" cirrhosis appears to be a more appropriate designation, since such lesions may occur in forms of chronic passive congestion unrelated to heart disease, as, for example, in the Budd-Chiari syndrome and veno-occlusive disease.

Right ventricular heart failure gives rise to cirrhosis only rarely, but when it does it usually occurs in patients with rheumatic mitral stenosis and tricuspid insufficiency who have experienced recurrent episodes of congestive failure over a period of years. We have encountered, however, numerous cases of congestive cirrhosis as a complication of constrictive pericarditis, the Budd-Chiari syndrome, and veno-occlusive disease.

As in other forms of cirrhosis, the hepatic lesions of congestive cirrhosis are characterized by diffuse fibrosis and the replacement of normal lobules by nodules of regenerating parenchyma (Figs. 503, 516). Early in their development, the nodules are formed by linkage of adjacent central-central fibrous bridges. As a result, the nodules contain a centrally located, intact, portal tract and are enclosed within fibrous septa in which multiple central veins can be identified (Figs. 505, 577), a pattern frequently termed "reversed lobulation." However, as congestion is prolonged, the fibrosis tends to be progressive, leading to fibrotic expansion of the portal tracts and the formation of central-portal fibrous bridges. As a result, the origin of the fibrosis in the central zones is no longer apparent, and nodules showing "reversed lobulation" are reduced in number or disappear (Figs. 503, 516). Sometimes the appearance may be that of nodular regenerative hyperplasia (12).

Characteristically, many of the sinusoids are dilated and show atrophy and loss of hepatocytes from the intervening hepatic plates (Figs. 504, 577), and perisinusoidal fibrosis (Fig. 505). However, often, the congestion is patchy in distribution (Fig. 516), and, occasionally, may escape detection (Fig. 530) unless multiple adjacent sections are examined (Fig. 504).

Frequently, the fibrous septa in congestive cirrhosis contain numerous thin-walled vascular channels of uncertain nature. Some undoubtedly represent greatly dilated sinusoids, but others may be lymphatics, since they often contain no erythrocytes. Usually, they can be differentiated from septal central veins, which tend to have much thicker and often fibrotic walls.

The septa usually contain lymphocytes and proliferating ductules, some of which may extend from the portal tracts to the central veins.

The cirrhotic lesions in the Budd-Chiari syndrome and veno-occlusive disease closely resemble those in heart failure, but, in addition, show fibrotic and thrombotic changes in the hepatic veins.

Periportal sinusoidal congestion

Occasionally, women on prolonged oral contraceptive therapy exhibit hepatomegaly accompanied by congestion of the periportal sinusoids [(13,14); Fig. 216]. When severe, the congestion may extend to the midzones and may be associated with marked atrophy and loss of the intervening hepatocytes, perhaps leading to the formation of relatively large, blood-filled, endothelial-lined cavities suggestive of peliosis hepatis (Fig. 217). The pathogenesis of such lesions is uncertain, but circumstantial evidence suggests that the synthetic estrogens and progestagens in oral contraceptives may exert a toxic effect on the sinusoidal wall.

Based on our experience and that of others, there is suggestive evidence that lesions of this type are reversible following cessation of oral contraceptive therapy.

Noncongestive sinusoidal dilatation

Occasionally, the centrilobular sinusoids are dilated in the absence of congestive heart failure or intrahepatic lesions that impair the outflow of blood from the liver. The etiology and pathogenesis of such lesions are uncertain.

The correlation of noncongestive sinusoidal dilatation with hypoalbuminemia and hypergammaglobulinemia has been attributed to an alteration in hepatic protein synthesis (15), but both are probably nonspecific phenomena. Sinusoidal ectasia was also found to correlate with extrahepatic granulomatous disease, including tuberculosis, brucellosis, and Crohn's disease (16). These findings have led to the suggestion that a humoral factor might be involved, and that the sinusoidal ectasia might represent an early phase of peliosis hepatis.

In our own experience, cryptogenic sinusoidal ectasia has not correlated with the serum levels of albumin or globulin. However, in some cases, the dilatation has occurred in patients with extrahepatic granulomatous disease, Hodgkin's disease, or carcinoma. Although needle biopsy failed to demonstrate the specific lesions of these disorders in the liver, the possibility of hepatic involvement could not be excluded with certainty. New insight into the pathophysiology of the hepatic sinusoidal cells may help explain some of these enigmas (17).

Peliosis hepatis

Peliosis hepatis is characterized by the presence in the liver of multiple, randomly distributed, blood-filled cystic lesions that may range in diameter from a few millimeters to as large as 3 cm. Often, such lesions are accompanied by dilatation of the sinusoids in adjacent areas. Within the past few years the definition of peliosis, which was originally a gross diagnosis, has been expanded to include relatively minor degrees of sinusoidal dilatation (see Chapter 4).

Although the pathogenesis of peliosis hepatis is not known, it is well recognized that it occurs in association with chronic wasting disease, such as tuberculosis and carcinomatosis (18,19), and the prolonged use of synthetic C-17 α-alkyl derivatives of testosterone, including oral contraceptives (20) and androgenic-anabolic steroids (21–23). Peliosis hepatis, usually mild in degree, has also been attributed to the prolonged administration of azathioprine following organ transplantation (24), to AIDS (25), to chronic vitamin A ingestion (26), and to chronic hemodialysis (27), but may be seen in any wasting disease (28). Recognition of a variety of toxic substances, including vinyl chloride, thorium dioxide, adrenal corticosteroids, tamoxifen, and 6-thioguanine (29,30), has led to the hypothesis that peliosis results from a variety of types of injury to endothelial cells (31).

When the peliotic lesions are small and few in number, they give rise to no symptoms, and, often, are discovered unexpectedly at autopsy. However, when large and numerous, they may be associated with hepatomegaly, jaundice, and signs of hepatic failure, or may rupture, resulting in hemoperitoneum and death from hepatic failure or hemorrhage (21). They are usually randomly distributed throughout the hepatic parenchyma without any zonal predominance (29).

Most peliotic lesions present as sharply outlined cystic spaces filled with blood, but unlined by endothelial or Kupffer cells (Fig. 499). Sometimes they may be incompletely lined or lined by damaged endothelial cells (32). Occasionally, some contain remnants of disrupted reticulin and fragments of necrotic hepatocytes (Fig. 500). Lesions of this type undoubtedly are attributable to necrosis of sinusoids, reticulin, and hepatocytes, and, accordingly, have been classified by some authorities as "parenchymal (32)."

In a minority of cases, the peliotic cavities are surrounded by and are in communication with numerous dilated sinusoids (Fig. 217). Since the cavities may be lined by endothelial cells, it is generally assumed that they are derived from dilated sinusoids, and accordingly have been termed "phlebectatic" (32).

Both "parenchymal" and "phlebectatic" peliotic lesions may be encountered in the same liver. This feature is consistent with the view that the injury to the sinusoids and hepatocytes may share a common pathogenesis, i.e., lysis of the reticulin network (28–32). However, the mechanism responsible for such injury remains obscure.

Recently, *bacillary peliosis hepatis* in patients with HIV infection has been reported [(33); Fig. 721] (see Chapter 27). The peliosis in these patients differs from that seen in non-HIV-infected patients by the presence of a fibromyxoid stroma in the former (Fig. 722) that resembles granulation tissue, and the presence of clumps of purple material within this fibromyxoid stroma. They proved to be clumps of bacilli when stained with Warthin-Starry stain and by electron microscopic examination. Erythrocytes extravasate from dilated sinusoids into the spaces of Disse and can actually be seen between hepatocytes (Fig. 723). These peliotic lesions seem identical to *cutaneous bacillary angiomatosis,* a pseudoneoplastic vascular proliferation that contains bacteria (34,35). Indeed, two of eight patients with AIDS-associated bacillary peliosis hepatis had cutaneous bacillary angiomatosis, and the bacilli were morphologically identical to those in the hepatic lesions. The bacilli from the hepatic and the skin lesions have not yet been cultured. These bacilli are very similar to the bacilli that cause cat-scratch disease (36), although it is premature at present to state that this lesion is caused by the cat-scratch bacillus. *Bartonella bacilliformis,* the bacillus that causes bartonellosis, produces lesions like those of cutaneous bacillary angiomatosis, probably by the production of an angiogenic factor that can induce peliotic lesions (37). The bacilli of bacillary peliosis hepatis are sensitive to erythromycin and, probably, doxycycline and antituberculous drugs (35). Treatment results in disappearance of the peliosis.

Disorders of the hepatic veins

Budd-Chiari syndrome

Obstruction to the outflow of blood from the major trunks of the hepatic veins close to or at their ostia or within the inferior vena cava gives rise to the Budd-Chiari syndrome (38–42), a disorder characterized by severe hepatic congestion, ascites, and, ultimately, in most cases, to congestive cirrhosis. The venous obstruction may be due to thrombosis, fibrosis, neoplastic invasion, or a congenital anomaly.

Usually, the thrombi in the Budd-Chiari syndrome occur predominantly in the major trunks of the hepatic veins. However, in most of these cases, organized thrombi are also demonstrable in some of the smaller, more peripheral veins. It is generally assumed that under such conditions, the thrombi extend retrograde from the large to small veins.

Etiology. A wide variety of systemic and local disorders have been implicated as etiologic factors in the pathogenesis of hepatic vein occlusion. However, in at least one-third of the cases, the etiology is unknown. Oral contraceptive steroids have been implicated (43).

Hepatic vein thrombosis. The principal disorders associated with thrombosis of the hepatic veins include polycythemia vera or other myeloproliferative disorders (44), paroxysmal nocturnal hemoglobinuria, ulcerative colitis, pregnancy (postpartum), prolonged use of oral contraceptives or antitumor drugs, and blunt abdominal trauma. Although not documented, the possibility has been considered that some forms of otherwise unexplained hepatic vein thrombosis are attributable to underlying primary phlebitis of the affected vessels. It should be noted that, in some cases, both the hepatic veins and inferior vena cava are involved in the thrombotic process.

Fibrotic occlusion of the hepatic veins. A number of malignant neoplasms may metastasize or extend into the hepatic veins or inferior vena cava to produce the Budd-Chiari syndrome. Of these, the most common are renal cell and hepatocellular carcinomas. Rarely, leiomyosarcoma of the hepatic veins or inferior vena cava is implicated.

Congenital anomalies. Occasionally, the Budd-Chiari syndrome is attributable to a membranous septum or web in the inferior vena cava just above the ostia of the hepatic veins (41). This disorder, which is correctable surgically, occurs most frequently in the Japanese and in South African Bantus. The possibility that such septa are acquired rather than congenital cannot be excluded.

Other presumed congenital anomalies that have been associated with the Budd-Chiari syndrome include: prominence of the Eustachian valve at the junction of the inferior vena cava with the right atrium, agenesis of the hepatic veins, and congenital stenosis of the hepatic veins or inferior vena cava.

Clinical manifestations. Although hepatic congestion, portal hypertension, and congestive cirrhosis are the principal features in most cases of the Budd-Chiari syndrome, the clinical manifestations of the disease differ to some extent depending on whether its onset is acute, subacute, or insidious.

Acute onset. Only rarely is the onset of the disease fulminant (45). In such cases, abdominal pain, sudden ascites, hepatomegaly, and shock are the principal features. Jaundice is either absent or only minimal. As a rule, death from shock or hepatic failure ensues within a few days or weeks.

Subacute onset. In a high proportion of cases, the onset is subacute, with abdominal discomfort and the gradual appearance of ascites and hepatosplenomegaly. The subsequent course of events is highly variable. In some, it is characterized by progressive hepatic failure and jaundice that lead to death within a few months. However, more often, it runs a protracted, fluctuating course characterized by ascites, hepatosplenomegaly, and portal hypertension, which gradually progresses. The partial remissions seen occasionally during the course of the disease are probably due to the recanalization of hepatic vein thrombi and the development of a collateral circulation, whereas extension of thrombi into the smaller, more peripherally located branches of the hepatic veins probably contributes to the progression of the disease.

Insidious onset. The manifestations in this relatively common variant of the disease resemble those in other forms of cirrhosis accompanied by portal hypertension. The caudate lobe of the liver is often hypertrophied, a distinctive feature demonstrable by scintigraphy and attributable to the fact that the veins of the caudate lobe usually drain directly into the inferior vena cava rather than into the hepatic veins. An additional, distinctive feature in cases of Budd-Chiari syndrome accompanied by occlusion of the inferior vena cava is the presence of distended veins over the lower abdomen and edema of the lower extremities. Except in patients with membranous occlusion of the inferior vena cava that can be corrected surgically, or in those successfully subjected to liver transplantation, the Budd-Chiari syndrome usually leads to death from hepatic failure or hemorrhage from esophageal varices. Surgical therapy is effective (42,46,47). Liver transplantation is sometimes curative, although recurrence of the Budd-Chiari syndrome after transplantation has been reported (48). Survival may depend on the development of intrahepatic collaterals (49), which may be demonstrable by computed tomography or by ultrasonography

(50). Rarely, especially in patients with membranous occlusion of the inferior vena cava, the disease may be complicated by the development of hepatocellular carcinoma.

Histologic features of hepatic lesions in the Budd-Chiari syndrome. The *early lesions* of the Budd-Chiari syndrome closely resemble those of severe right ventricular heart failure, and are characterized by marked centrilobular sinusoidal dilatation with atrophy and loss of the intervening hepatocytes. Since the sinusoids are filled with blood, such lesions resemble zones of gross hemorrhage (Figs. 213, 501). However, as is evident in silver-impregnated sections, the reticulin outlining the distended sinusoids is intact. When extensive, such areas of congestion may bridge adjacent central zones, portal zones or both (Fig. 501). It is noteworthy that both the severity and the extent of the congestion may vary from one region to another. Hemorrhage into the spaces of Disse is relatively common, often interrupting the hepatic plates.

One of the most distinctive features of the lesions in the Budd-Chiari syndrome, found in at least half the cases, is the presence of thrombi that usually show evidence of organization or recanalization within the central and sublobular veins (Fig. 215). Some of the central veins show thickening of their intima and fibrosis of their walls.

As in the congestion produced by cardiac failure, the centrilobular zones of hepatocellular atrophy and dropout show minimal or no inflammatory reaction, but often contain lipofuscin-filled, enlarged Kupffer cells.

As a rule, the portal tracts and periportal parenchyma in early lesions are normal.

The *late hepatic lesions* of the Budd-Chiari syndrome are similar to those of congestive ("cardiac") cirrhosis described previously. However, sinusoidal dilatation, hepatocellular atrophy, and cell loss tend to be more severe, but less regular in distribution (Figs. 503, 504). In addition, some of the central and sublobular veins contain organized thrombi, and show intimal thickening and fibrosis. Moreover, hepatocellular nodular transformation is a more prominent feature. As in "cardiac" cirrhosis, occasional nodules show reversal of their lobular pattern with intact centrally located portal tracts (Fig. 505). Acute and organizing thrombi may be bound in the portal veins.

Veno-occlusive disease of the liver

Veno-occlusive disease of the liver (51–58) is customarily attributed to poisoning with one of the pyrrolizidine alkaloids. Other disorders including reactions to bone marrow transplantation (58), renal transplantation (59), and radiotherapy are also characterized by the clinical manifestations of the Budd-Chiari syndrome and widespread occlusion of the central and sublobular veins.

Etiology and epidemiology. Veno-occlusive disease occurs following the ingestion of the pyrrolizidine alkaloids found in plants belonging to the genera *Senecio, Crotalaria,* and *Heliotropium.*

The disease was first recognized in Jamaica, but is now known to be relatively common in South Africa, India, and the Middle East. Rarely, the disease has been reported in the United States. Most sporadic cases follow the use of herbal or bush teas that contain pyrrolizidine or related alkaloids used medicinally. Young, malnourished children appear to be unusually suscep-

tible to this intoxication. The active principle can be transmitted from a pregnant mother to the fetus and it can be found in milk after delivery (60).

Epidemics of veno-occlusive disease that affect individuals at all ages have been reported from South Africa, Afghanistan, and India. In each instance, the ingestion of imperfectly winnowed wheat contaminated with the seeds of *Senecio, Crotalaria,* or *Heliotropium* has been implicated.

Clinical manifestations. Abdominal pain, hepatomegaly, and ascites are the principal features in the acute phase of the disease. Full recovery without significant residuals occurs in about half the cases, but, in the remainder, the disease runs a subacute or chronic course characterized by persistent ascites, hepatomegaly, and signs of cirrhosis and portal hypertension. Death from hepatic failure or hemorrhage from esophageal varices ultimately ensues in a significant number of affected individuals.

In some cases, the disease has a slow, gradual onset and may be confused with chronic hepatitis or cirrhosis accompanied by significant portal hypertension.

Histologic features of hepatic lesions. The most distinctive feature of the hepatic lesions is widespread occlusion of the central and sublobular veins. As in the Budd-Chiari syndrome, this occlusion leads to severe centrilobular sinusoidal congestion, atrophy and loss of the intervening hepatic plates, collapse of the reticulin, and fibrosis. In lesions that fail to resolve, the fibrosis tends to be progressive, ultimately destroying the normal lobular architecture and giving rise to cirrhosis.

Although the lesions resemble those of the Budd-Chiari syndrome, the veins contain no thrombi and the larger hepatic veins are not involved in the occlusive process. Characteristically, the central and sublobular veins in early veno-occlusive disease exhibit intimal edema and hemorrhage that subsequently lead to fibrous thickening of their walls and fibrotic occlusion of their lumens.

Hepatic veno-occlusive lesions unrelated to pyrrolizidine toxicity

Hypervitaminosis A. Large doses of vitamin A, usually in excess of 40,000 units daily, when administered over a period of years produce toxic manifestations in the skin, mucous membranes, bones, and liver (61–63).

Characteristically, the skin is dry and fissured and accompanied by brittle nails, alopecia, cheilosis, and gingivitis. Bone and joint pain associated with periosteal new bone formation is a relatively common feature. Headaches and papilledema (pseudotumor cerebri) may suggest the correct diagnosis (63a).

Early hepatic manifestations include hepatomegaly and impairment of liver function. Rarely, signs of cirrhosis appear, usually accompanied by ascites, splenomegaly, and other evidence of portal hypertension. Esophageal varices and intrapulmonary shunting have been observed in children who have been fed chicken liver pate since infancy (63b).

The *hepatic lesions* early in the course of hypervitaminosis A are characterized by hypertrophy and hyperplasia of the lipocytes (Ito cells) in the spaces of Disse, fibrous thickening and occlusion of the central veins, sinusoidal congestion with atrophy of the intervening hepatic plates, and proliferation of reticulin and collagen within the spaces of Disse. As the lesions advance, there is fibrosis, initially in the centrilobular zones and later in the portal tracts, the formation of central-central and central-portal fibrous bridges, and, ultimately, cirrhosis.

Available evidence suggests that the lipocytes (Ito cells) are precursors of fibroblasts and are responsible for the fibrogenesis in hypervitaminosis A. In routinely stained sections, these appear as large, pale cells with vacuolated cytoplasm in the spaces of Disse (Fig. 259). In fresh frozen sections, lipocytes contain lipid droplets that stain with oil red 0, and exhibit characteristic, transient, green fluorescence under ultraviolet light (Fig. 260)

The deposition of collagen in the spaces of Disse accompanied by atrophy and the loss of intervening hepatocytes in a typical case of hypervitaminosis A are illustrated in Figure 224.

Hepatotoxic chemotherapy. A number of chemotherapeutic or immunosuppressive agents, including azathioprine (59,64) and 6-thioguanine (65), have been implicated as etiologic factors in the development of hepatic veno-occlusive lesions (58,66). The lesions are similar to those produced by pyrrolizidine alkaloids, but, in some instances, are accompanied by hemorrhagic centrilobular hepatocellular necrosis early in their development, as illustrated in a case of 6-thioguanine-induced veno-occlusive disease [(30); Figs. 271, 506].

Graft-versus-host disease. Hepatic veno-occlusive lesions are relatively common following allogeneic bone marrow transplantation (67,68). It has been suggested that such lesions may be manifestations of graft-versus-host disease (67). However, other authorities attribute the veno-occlusive lesions to pretransplant chemotherapy, especially with dimethylbusulfan (67–70).

It is difficult to differentiate the effects of high dose, hepatotoxic, antineoplastic chemotherapy from those of immunosuppression with azathioprine (58,64), which is used in renal transplantation; from those of graft-versus-host disease, which is seen frequently after bone marrow transplantation (58,67); or opportunistic infections such as cytomegalovirus infections (64), which often complicate these procedures in immunocompromised patients.

Familial veno-occlusive disease associated with immune deficiency. Fatal veno-occlusive disease (71) has been reported in three pairs of infant siblings. In two of the three affected families, the parents were consanguineous and of Lebanese descent. The possibility of an underlying immune deficiency state in the affected infants was suggested by the paucity or absence of plasma cells and germinal centers, and evidence of infection with *Pneumocystis carinii*.

Lesions resembling hepatic veno-occlusive disease in myxedema. Ascites in the absence of congestive heart failure is a rare complication of myxedema. In three biopsy-documented cases, the ascites appeared to be related to hepatic lesions resembling those of veno-occlusive disease (72). The lesions were characterized by concentric fibrous thickening and dilatation of the central veins, extension of the fibrosis into the walls of the pericentral sinusoids, and degeneration and loss of the intervening hepatocytes. Thyroid replacement therapy led to clearing of the ascites, but the effects on the hepatic lesions were not investigated.

Radiation hepatitis. Ionizing radiation over the liver in excess of 3,500 rads may produce hepatic lesions that resemble those of veno-occlusive disease (73–75).

The clinical manifestations, which usually appear two to six weeks following completion of radiation therapy, are characterized by ascites, hepatosplenomegaly, and jaundice, but are highly variable in severity.

In some cases, radiation hepatitis proves fatal, but in one-third the lesions may resolve without clinical sequelae within a period of four months. Occasionally, the lesions are progressive and give rise to cirrhosis.

The *earliest lesion* of radiation hepatitis, which is undetectable by light microscopy but can be seen by electron microscopy, is the presence of fibrin in central veins and centrilobular sinusoids (74). Early lesions of radiation hepatitis show intimal thickening and fibrosis of the central and sublobular veins, often accompanied by a meshwork of reticulin fibers with erythrocytes within their lumens. As the lesions, advance, the affected veins undergo progressive fibrosis, leading to obliteration of their lumens, and often encirclement by concentric bands of collagen. Characteristically, the centrilobular sinusoids are dilated and frequently show atrophy and loss of the intervening hepatic plates and perisinusoidal fibrosis, or diffuse centrilobular fibrosis.

Radiation and chemotherapy together may induce acute fatal hepatitis, which cannot be differentiated from viral or drug-induced hepatitis (75).

The *late lesions* of radiation hepatitis, which are irreversible, are characterized by progressive fibrosis that affects both the centrilobular zones and portal tracts, leading to central-central and central-portal bridging fibrosis, and, ultimately, cirrhosis. Sinusoidal congestion is less conspicuous at this stage than in early lesions.

Alcoholic hepatitis and cirrhosis. During the late healing phase of alcoholic hepatitis, the hepatic lesions often show features that resemble those of veno-occlusive disease (76,77). These include stellate, centrilobular, perisinusoidal and pericellular fibrosis, atrophy and loss of the intervening hepatic plates, and narrowing of the sinusoidal lumens (Figs. 223, 225). Occasionally, some of the central and sublobular veins contain organized, partially recanalized thrombi (Fig. 273) accompanied by foci of sinusoidal congestion (Figs. 578, 580). These vascular lesions may play a role in the pathogenesis of portal hypertension in alcoholic liver disease even before the development of cirrhosis (78).

Miscellaneous disorders. Similar lesions may be seen in disseminated intravascular coagulopathy (79), sickle cell disease (80), eclampsia, lipogranulomatosis (81), and other lesions (79,82).

Other disorders of the portal veins and portal hypertension

The pressure in the portal vein, which is normally less 5 mm Hg, depends on the volume of splanchnic blood flow and the resistance to blood flow through the extrahepatic and intrahepatic portal veins, the sinusoids, and the hepatic veins. A number of techniques are available for evaluating the relative importance of each of these factors in the development of portal hypertension. Of these, the most useful are the indirect measurement of portal venous pressure by occluding hepatic venous catheters (83) and the direct measurement by percutaneous transhepatic catheterization of the portal vein (84,85). Visualization of the vessels can also be accomplished by splenic, celiac, or mesenteric arteriography, venacavography, and ultrasonography. The ultrasonographic diagnosis of portal vein patency is fairly accurate and specific (86), but its sensitivity is not well established (87).

Portal hypertension when accompanied by a normal wedged, hepatic vein pressure (WHVP) is classified as *presinusoidal*, and is attributable to extrahepatic obstruction of the portal vein, to a variety of intrahepatic lesions that impede portal blood flow, but do not increase the resistance to flow through the sinusoids or to increased splanchnic blood flow. By convention, portal hypertension accompanied by a raised level of WHVP is classified as *postsinusoidal*. However, it has been pointed out that the WHVP reflects sinusoidal pressure and may rise when the resistance to sinusoidal blood flow is increased (88). Accordingly, *sinusoidal portal hypertension* may be a more appropriate descriptive term in such cases.

Hemorrhage from esophagogastric varices is the most lethal manifestation of portal hypertension. Ascites, spontaneous bacterial peritonitis (89), and the hepatorenal syndrome (90) are other major causes of morbidity and mortality. Portal-systemic encephalopathy is one of the most difficult problems to manage in patients with portal hypertension (91). These problems are usually seen in postsinusoidal portal hypertension, which is almost always accompanied by significant hepatic parenchymal damage.

A small fraction of patients with both noncirrhotic intrahepatic (92) and extrahepatic noncirrhotic portal obstruction exhibit ascites and hepatic encephalopathy, usually after the age of 50 (93).

Extrahepatic presinusoidal portal hypertension

Portal vein thrombosis. Thrombosis of the portal vein, the most common cause of extrahepatic portal hypertension (93–99), affects children more frequently than adults, although it may occur at any age. Usually, the thrombosis occurs silently, so often the appearance of clinical signs of portal hypertension is delayed for months or years. By the time signs appear, the thrombus is organized and the lumen is occluded by fibrous tissue. In some cases the portal vein is converted to a fibrous cord that is difficult to identify, and often is surrounded by numerous parallel collateral veins that form a spongy vascular structure. Radiographically, it is termed *cavernomatous transformation of the portal vein.*

Etiology. A wide variety of etiologic factors have been identified in the pathogenesis of portal vein thrombosis. However, in almost half the cases, the etiology is unknown (100). The principal recognized causes include: (1) *infection and inflammation* including neonatal umbilical sepsis (omphalitis), exchange transfusion via the umbilical vein, septicemia, intraabdominal inflammation (peritonitis, pylephlebitis, pancreatitis, penetrating or perforating duodenal ulcer), and postoperatively following cholecystectomy or splenectomy; (2) *abdominal trauma;* (3) *blood dyscrasias* (polycythemia vera, thrombotic thrombocythemia, myelofibrosis, and leukemia); (4) *pregnancy,* especially during the first two weeks of the puerperium; (5) *neoplasms* (hepatocellular carcinoma and metastatic carcinoma, usually from the breast or pancreas, that invade or com-

press the portal vein; (6) *developmental anomalies* (extension of the normal neonatal obliterative process in the umbilical vein to the portal vein, atresia of the portal vein, and other anomalies of the portal vein); (7) *cirrhosis:* in the West cirrhosis is thought to be a common predisposing factor in portal vein thrombosis, but this association is uncommon in Japan (101); (8) *protein C deficiency:* this new disorder is characterized by a predisposition to develop thromboembolic disease, including portal vein thrombosis (98).

Manifestations. Acute portal vein thrombosis, a rare lesion occasionally encountered during the puerperium, is characterized by abdominal pain and tenderness, ileus, bloody peritoneal fluid, and shock and death.

The clinical manifestations of chronic portal vein thrombosis are those of portal hypertension and its complications, as described previously. Recurrent abdominal pain, especially after meals, is relatively common and has been attributed to postprandial distension of the mesenteric veins. Severe attacks of abdominal pain occur far less frequently and may be due to extension of a portal thrombus to the superior mesenteric vein, a process that usually occurs silently.

Hepatic lesions. Often, the liver appears normal histologically in patients with extrahepatic portal obstruction. However, when large surgical wedge biopsy sections are available, some of the portal tracts are fibrotic (Fig. 391). It has been reported that the fibrosis in such cases is concentric in character and periportal in location. However, in our cases, the fibrosis has appeared to be predominantly periductal. In addition, we have found that, often, the portal vein in the affected portal tract is replaced by numerous fine vascular channels, and that the number of arterioles is increased (Fig. 391).

Splenomegaly and increased portal blood flow. There is convincing evidence that *tropical splenomegaly*, a disorder usually due to chronic malaria, may be accompanied by an increase in splenic and portal blood flow and give rise to portal hypertension. The absence of a significant difference between the portal venous pressure and the wedged hepatic vein pressure indicates increased presinusoidal resistance. In tropical splenomegaly the increase in portal pressure is only slight, and does not usually lead to the development of esophageal varices or hemorrhage. However, in some cases, the portal pressure is high, and may be complicated by esophageal varices. Under such conditions, the portal venous pressure usually is significantly higher than the WHVP, a gradient denoting increased sinusoidal resistance. Portal venograms often demonstrate narrowing and poor filling of the secondary and more distal branches of the portal vein. Some of these patients probably have portal vein thromboses that are clinically and pathologically subtle (101). However, there are no histologic changes in the liver, so the explanation for the increase in intrahepatic presinusoidal resistance remains obscure.

It has been proposed that other forms of splenomegaly associated with various myeloproliferative and reticuloendothelial disorders are also accompanied by increased splenic blood flow that leads to the development of portal hypertension (102). However, investigation of such cases has revealed that the portal hypertension usually is attributable to intrahepatic infiltrates that produce a presinusoidal block to blood flow, or to the development of complicating extrahepatic portal obstruction (103). In addition, it has been shown that in many forms of splenomegaly, such as extramedullary hematopoiesis, the portal venous pressure remains within normal limits (104,105).

Characteristically, large splenic (106,107) or hepatic (106) *arteriovenous fistulae* produce severe portal hypertension in the apparent absence of other complicating factors. However, the latter cannot be excluded with certainty, since simultaneous preoperative measurements of hepatic blood flow, portal pressure, and WHVP are not available in the few cases that have been reported.

Intrahepatic presinusoidal portal hypertension

A number of hepatic lesions that involve the portal tracts lead to the development of presinusoidal portal hypertension as evidenced by raised portal venous pressure and normal wedged hepatic vein pressures. With few exceptions, the hypertension is attributable to increased resistance to the outflow of blood from the distal branches of the portal vein.

Schistosomiasis. Characteristically, in the early active phase of hepatic schistosomiasis, the portal tracts contain granulomas in which schistosomal ova can be identified (Fig. 344) and giant cells are usually present. Early in the course of experimental schistosomiasis, the inflammatory response to the ova induce severe presinusoidal portal hypertension (109). As the lesions advance, there is progressive fibrous obliteration of small portal vein branches (110). Electron microscopic studies indicate that deposition of collagen in the spaces of Disse frequently accompanies these portal changes (111).

In a minority of cases, the portal hypertension in advanced hepatic schistosomiasis appears to be sinusoidal rather than presinusoidal, as evidenced by the fact that wedged hepatic vein pressure equals or exceeds the portal pressure. This has been attributed to hypertrophy of the hepatic arteries and increased arterial blood flow (112).

Sarcoidosis. In a high proportion of patients with sarcoidosis, granulomas are demonstrable in the liver (113). Often, the granulomas are found in the portal tracts (Fig. 345) and may be accompanied by fibrosis and chronic inflammation. However, only rarely are such lesions complicated by the development of clinical presinusoidal portal hypertension (114,115). Presumably, occlusion of distal portal vein radicles accounts for the latter. Although invasion and compression of small portal veins by granulomas can be demonstrated occasionally (Fig. 392), the number of such lesions often appears too small to account for the portal hypertension. Healed fibrotic granulomas can contribute to the portal hypertension.

In some cases of sarcoidal portal hypertension, the wedged hepatic vein pressure is increased significantly (116). Rarely, such postsinusoidal portal hypertension is attributable to the development of sarcoidal cirrhosis. However, in most cases, it occurs in the absence of cirrhosis. It has been suggested that the occurrence of sinusoidal hypertension in sarcoidosis may be due to the development of intrahepatic arteriovenous shunts and increased blood flow (116). Although this hypothesis cannot be excluded, no convincing evidence has been presented in its support.

Congenital hepatic fibrosis. Congenital hepatic fibrosis (117,118), a form of childhood polycystic disease, frequently

is associated with severe presinusoidal portal hypertension. Characteristically, the liver is traversed by numerous broad, relatively smooth-contoured fibrous septa that contain many tortuous, dilated, branching, aberrant bile ducts and a paucity of portal vein radicles (Figs. 64, 65). In many nonfibrotic areas, the lobular architecture is intact. Compression and hypoplasia of the distal portal veins account for the development of presinusoidal portal hypertension.

Toxic hepatic fibrosis. Prolonged use of inorganic *arsenicals* medicinally (119,120) and prolonged exposure to *vinyl chloride* in industry (121) may lead to significant portal fibrosis and the development of presinusoidal portal hypertension. Figure 514 illustrates the extensive portal fibrosis found in a vinyl chloride worker who presented with portal hypertension and bleeding from esophageal varices. Chronic copper intoxication may induce similar lesions (122), as may the toxic oil syndrome (123).

Precirrhotic primary biliary cirrhosis. Occasionally, patients with primary biliary cirrhosis present with hemorrhage from esophageal varices secondary to presinusoidal portal hypertension even before the development of cirrhosis. Although the pathogenesis of such portal hypertension has not been established, it is generally assumed that it is attributable to compression of distal portal vein radicles by the portal fibrosis and inflammation (124,135).

Myeloproliferative and reticuloendothelial disorders. Infiltration of the portal tracts and sinusoids by the abnormal cells of myeloid metaplasia, myelogenous leukemia, Hodgkin's disease, and Letterer-Siwe disease occasionally gives rise to presinusoidal portal hypertension (103).

Intrahepatic sinusoidal and postsinusoidal portal hypertension

Cirrhosis. Cirrhosis, irrespective of its etiology, is the most common cause of portal hypertension and its complications.

Although the character of their lesions vary, as described in previous chapters, all forms of cirrhosis are characterized by increased resistance to the outflow of blood from the liver, enhanced sinusoidal pressure, and significantly increased wedged hepatic vein pressure. A number of factors are responsible for these alterations in the hepatic circulation. These include: (1) obliteration of intersinusoidal communicating vessels; (2) an overall reduction in the volume of the sinusoidal, portal, and hepatic venous vasculature; (3) distortion and compression of the remaining vessels by the nodules of regenerating parenchyma and diffuse fibrosis; and (4) a compensatory increase in the hepatic arterial circulation with the development, in some cases, of arterial-portal venous shunts.

In alcoholic cirrhosis in which the portal hypertension is predominantly sinusoidal without a presinusoidal component, portal venous pressure (PVP) measured directly, e.g., by percutaneous portography, are identical to those measured indirectly by hepatic vein catheterization (84,126). In other types of cirrhosis, in which a presinusoidal component usually exists, the PVP measured directly is almost invariably higher than that measured indirectly (84,126).

Budd-Chiari syndrome and veno-occlusive disease. As previously indicated the sinusoidal portal hypertension in the Budd-

Chiari syndrome and veno-occlusive disease is attributable primarily to an obstruction to the outflow of blood from the hepatic veins or their tributaries. However, as the lesions advance, progressive fibrosis ensues, so many of the factors involved in the pathogenesis of cirrhotic presinusoidal or postsinusoidal portal hypertension play an increasing role.

Other forms of intrahepatic portal hypertension

"Idiopathic" portal hypertension. Portal hypertension in the absence of extrahepatic portal obstruction, cirrhosis, or other obvious intrahepatic lesions known to obstruct hepatic blood flow is generally classified as "idiopathic" (127,136). Other terms applied to this disorder include Banti's syndrome, noncirrhotic portal fibrosis, obliterative portal venopathy, and hepatoportal sclerosis.

The clinical manifestations of idiopathic portal hypertension are similar to those in other forms of presinusoidal portal hypertension. However, except following massive hemorrhage from esophageal varices, hepatic function usually is well preserved, and signs of hepatic failure and encephalopathy are rare. Moreover, sinusoidal pressure is more variable, the wedged hepatic vein pressure being normal in some cases and raised in others. It has been suggested that sinusoidal pressure is normal initially, but tends to rise as a result of a compensatory increase in hepatic arterial blood flow as the disease advances.

The prevalence of idiopathic portal hypertension varies geographically, being relatively common in India, Japan, and other tropical areas, and relatively infrequent in the United States and Europe. It has been estimated that in India 20 to 30% of cases of portal hypertension are idiopathic, whereas in the United States the incidence is only 2 to 3%.

At one time, idiopathic portal hypertension was attributed to the increased splenic arterial blood flow that accompanies splenomegaly. However, as pointed out previously, increased blood flow alone does not produce severe portal hypertension. Moreover, the estimated hepatic blood flow in several cases of idiopathic portal hypertension has been normal.

Largely as a result of extensive studies in India, interest has been focused on the possibility that most, if not all cases of idiopathic portal hypertension are attributable to occlusion of major intrahepatic branches of the portal vein, probably secondary to thrombosis (129–131). In four of our own cases, vinylite-injection corrosion and dissection of the intrahepatic vasculature clearly demonstrated organized thrombi in major branches of the portal vein (132). Splenoportography in these cases had revealed an abrupt cutoff or narrowing at the sites of thrombosis, and attenuation, shortening, or absence of more distal branches of the portal vein. As an alternative, it has been suggested that the occlusions are attributable to a primary form of phlebosclerosis, classified as hepatoportal sclerosis, that may affect both the intrahepatic and extrahepatic portal veins, and may give rise to thrombosis secondarily (133).

Since evidence of intrahepatic portal vein occlusion has not been demonstrable by venography in all cases, other possible mechanisms must be considered. Based on an electron microscopic study, it has been proposed that the primary lesion in idiopathic portal hypertension is a form of perisinusoidal fibrosis of toxic or immunologic origin (134).

Often, the liver appears normal in needle biopsy sections. However, almost always, a significant number of abnormalities are demonstrable in large surgical wedge and postmortem specimens. Occasionally, if multiple blocks of tissue are examined, some of the larger portal veins contain organized, partially recanalized thrombi (Fig. 388). More often, septal portal veins show thickening and fibrosis of their intima (Fig. 389), a lesion generally attributed to incorporation of thrombotic material into the wall of the vessel (129,130). Characteristically, some of the portal tracts are enlarged and fibrotic, contain an increased number of arterioles, and show replacement of normal portal vein radicles by numerous thin-walled vascular channels (Fig. 390). Often, portal fibrosis is most prominent in the subcapsular zone where it may outline small nodules of parenchyma, giving the surface of the liver a fine, granular appearance, or may produce a fine network of fibrous bands. Although this appearance may suggest an underlying cirrhosis, it is important to note that deep in the liver the lobular architecture is normal and septa are absent. Nodular transformation frequently develops (137).

A comparison of autopsy specimens of patients with idiopathic portal hypertension from Japan with specimens from noncirrhotic portal fibrosis of India revealed that pathologically the two disorders were identical (137).

Nodular regenerative hyperplasia of the liver. Rarely, the normal lobules of the liver are replaced by small, widely distributed nodules of regenerating hepatocytes without accompanying septal fibrosis, a lesion classified as nodular regenerative hyperplasia (138–142). As a rule, the nodules range in diameter from 1 to 5 mm, but occasionally are as large as 2 cm, and, characteristically, are outlined by narrow bands of dilated sinusoids and atrophic hepatocytes (Figs. 66, 67) and are encircled by zones of collapsed reticulin. The regenerating hepatocytes in the center of the nodules are enlarged and occasionally are arranged in the form of double hepatic plates. Often, some of the nodules contain a centrally located portal tract and peripherally located central veins, producing the pattern "of reversed lobulation." However, many of the smaller nodules may be devoid of portal tracts and central veins. Less constant histologic features reported in some cases include: (1) expansion and fibrosis of some portal tracts, (2) a reduction in the number and size of small portal vein radicles, (3) small portal vein thrombi, (4) eccentric fibrosis of larger portal veins, possibly indicative of healed thrombi, and (5) moderate portal lymphocytosis. Since the parenchymal nodules may be ill-defined, they often escape detection in needle biopsy specimens, and are best visualized in reticulin-stained, surgical wedge and postmortem sections.

Portal hypertension and its complications, splenomegaly, esophageal varices, and hemorrhage from such varices, occur in some, but not all cases of nodular regenerative hyperplasia. Ascites is uncommon. Based on a small number of reported measurements of wedged hepatic vein pressure in such cases, it is apparent that the hypertension may be either presinusoidal, postsinusoidal, or both.

Hepatomegaly and mild hepatic dysfunction are relatively common in nodular regenerative hyperplasia, but ascites, hepatic encephalopathy, and other signs of hepatic failure are rare. At autopsy, however, the livers are not enlarged.

In a high proportion of cases, nodular regenerative hyperplasia is encountered in patients with a variety of unrelated systemic disorders. This suggests that its pathogenesis may be heterogeneous. Congestive heart failure, rheumatoid arthritis, particularly when accompanied by the Felty syndrome (splenomegaly and leukopenia), and tuberculosis are the most frequently associated disorders. Less commonly, nodular regenerative hyperplasia has been reported in individuals with the CRST syndrome (calcinosis, Raynaud's phenomenon, sclerodactyly, and telangiectasia), subacute bacterial endocarditis, a variety of hematologic disorders, monoclonal IgG immunoglobulinopathy, and macroglobulinemia.

There is no consensus regarding the pathogenesis of nodular regenerative hyperplasia. According to some authorities, atrophy of hepatocytes is the initial event that leads to compensatory hepatocellular hyperplasia, the former being attributable to occlusion of portal veins initiated by thrombosis or by deposits of immune complexes (125,142). Others regard hepatocellular hyperplasia as the primary defect and attribute it to increased portal blood flow secondary to splenomegaly, or to a humoral factor, possibly of immune nature (140,141,143).

The mechanisms responsible for the development of portal hypertension are unknown. Those considered most frequently include increased splenic blood flow, compression and distortion of the intrahepatic vasculature by the nodules of regenerating parenchyma, and thrombotic occlusion of small portal vein radicles.

Partial nodular transformation of the liver. Partial nodular transformation of the liver (144–146), a rare form of portal hypertension, is characterized by the presence of large parenchymal nodules without significant accompanying fibrosis that may occupy up to two-thirds of the liver, located predominantly in the perihilar area. Additional features of the lesion include a reduction in the number of hepatic veins and reversal of the normal lobular architecture within the nodules and conspicuous intimal thickening and fibrosis of the portal vein and its intrahepatic branches.

The portal hypertension, which is of the postsinusoidal type, has been postulated to be caused by increased resistance to the outflow of blood from compression of the hepatic veins by the nodules or a reduction in the number of hepatic veins (144), but this hypothesis is unproven.

The sharp cutoff of the portal vein just beyond its bifurcation within the liver in one case, the difficulty in filling the intrahepatic portal veins in several others, the reversed lobular architecture within the nodules, and the fibrous thickening of the intima of the portal veins described in the original report on this disorder, suggest that partial nodular transformation of the liver may be a form of obliterative portal venopathy ("idiopathic" portal hypertension). Indeed, one of our patients with idiopathic portal hypertension attributable to intrahepatic portal thrombi documented in a postmortem vinylite-injection corrosion cast (119) exhibited coarse perihilar parenchymal nodules identical with those described in partial nodular transformation of the liver. It has been postulated that partial nodular transformation occurs when large portal veins are involved with thrombus, whereas nodular regenerative hyperplasia results from the involvement of small portal veins (147).

Systemic mastocytosis. Systemic mastocytosis (147,148) is a rare disorder characterized by proliferation of atypical mast cells in the bone marrow, liver (Figs. 695, 696), spleen, and skin, often accompanied by hepatic fibrosis [(149); (Fig. 661], splenomegaly, and urticaria pigmentosa. Rarely, the disease is complicated by portal hypertension and bleeding from esophageal varices. In one such case, the hepatic sinusoids were heavily infiltrated with mast cells, and the wedged hepatic vein pressure was increased. Splenectomy led to a reduction in portal pressure and the size of the esophageal varices, and there were

no further bleeding episodes over a period of three years. The portal hypertension was attributed to an increase in splenic blood flow and an increase in the resistance to sinusoidal blood flow due to the infiltration of mast cells. (Figs. 695,696).

Hepatic amyloidosis. Hepatic deposits of amyloid are relatively common in both primary and secondary amyloidosis. Usually, the deposits occur predominantly in arterial walls or the spaces of Disse and lead to compression and occlusion of sinusoids and atrophy of the intervening hepatocellular plates (Figs. 85, 199). Yet, paradoxically, even when the liver and spleen are massively enlarged by the deposits, portal hypertension and esophageal varices are uncommon (150), although they occasionally occur (151). (See Chapter 24.)

Pylephlebitis

Septic thrombosis of the portal vein and its tributaries, termed pylephlebitis, is a relatively infrequent complication of intraabdominal suppuration and, less commonly, of neonatal omphalitis. Before acute appendicitis became a well-recognized entity that required prompt surgical treatment, it was the leading cause of pylephlebitis. However, currently, other intraabdominal suppurative lesions are implicated more frequently. These include cholecystitis, diverticulitis, ulcerative colitis, perforated peptic ulcer, and pancreatic, splenic, and pelvic abscess.

Chills and fever are the principal early manifestations of pylephlebitis, and may be followed by hepatomegaly, tenderness of the liver and mild jaundice, and, occasionally, by splenomegaly. Bacteremia is uncommon at the onset, but is a relatively frequent finding late in the course of the disease when its nature is unrecognized and it is not treated appropriately; multiple liver abscesses may occur in such cases as a result of septic emboli from the portal vein.

In many cases, the manifestations of pylephlebitis are preceded by symptoms referable to the initial intraabdominal septic focus, and suggest the need for exploratory laparotomy. However, in others, the septic focus is silent clinically, so that chills and fever attributable to pylephlebitis are the presenting complaints and give no clue to the nature of the disease.

Successful management of pylephlebitis requires both antibiotic therapy and surgical drainage or removal of the initial septic focus.

The classic type of pylephlebitis is very rarely seen now. However, the syndrome still occurs, often in association with pylethrombosis of diverse etiologies (152). This clinical syndrome is dominated by the presence of progressive ascites and often by variceal hemorrhage, since the septic aspects of the disorder are controlled by antibiotic therapy.

Occasionally, the diagnosis of pylephlebitis can be confirmed by surgical wedge biopsy of the liver obtained at the time of exploratory laparotomy. Figure 387 illustrates a portal vein radicle partially filled with a fibrin thrombus infiltrated and surrounded by neutrophils found in a patient with an appendiceal abscess complicated by pylephlebitis. Such lesions may give rise to multiple hepatic abscesses, as illustrated in Figure 281. Shown is an early periportal abscess in a patient who was found at autopsy to have suppurative pylephlebitis and multiple hepatic abscesses. The primary site of infection seen for the first time late in the course of the disease could not be identified.

Zahn "infarcts" of the liver

Zahn "infarcts" (153,154), also termed atrophic red "infarcts," are uncommon, sharply circumscribed, wedge-shaped zones of marked hepatic hyperemia characterized histologically by striking dilatation of the sinusoids and atrophy of the intervening hepatocellular plates. Almost always they are encountered at autopsy in association with thrombosis of large intrahepatic portal veins or adjacent to neoplasms. In one of our cases, a typical Zahn infarct was associated with occlusion of major hepatic veins by tumor thrombi metastatic from the lung.

Lesions of this type do not qualify as true infarcts in that they do not exhibit evidence of ischemic necrosis.

Hepatic ischemia and disorders of the hepatic arteries

Hepatic ischemia

Centrilobular ischemic necrosis. *Hypotension* and *shock* are accompanied by a reduction in hepatic blood flow, which if of sufficient duration, usually in excess of 24 hours but occasionally as short as 6 hours, leads to centrilobular hypoxia and a characteristic type of centrilobular necrosis.

The most common underlying causes of centrilobular ischemic necrosis include severe hemorrhage, acute myocardial infarction, septic or cardiogenic shock, and surgical or nonsurgical trauma (155,156).

Occasionally, *left ventricular heart failure* leads to centrilobular ischemic necrosis in the absence of myocardial infarction, hypotension, or shock, presumably as a result of reduced hepatic blood flow (157,158).

The severity and character of the clinical manifestations depend on the duration and degree of shock and on the presence of such complicating factors as congestive heart failure and pulmonary edema. Usually, jaundice, hepatomegaly, and high serum transaminase levels, which may exceed 10,000 units, are the principal features that appear within 1 to 10 days from the onset. Extensive necrosis may lead to death from progressive hepatic failure. However, if the underlying cause is brought under control, the lesions tend to heal without significant residuals.

Early in their development, the *hepatic ischemic lesions* are characterized by sharply demarcated centrilobular zones of hepatocytes undergoing coagulation necrosis (Fig. 98). The hepatic plates are intact and there is no early inflammatory reaction. However, the affected hepatocytes contain intensely eosinophilic, relatively dense, homogeneous cytoplasm, and show pyknosis and lysis of their nuclei. When the lesions are severe, the zones of necrosis may involve the midzonal portion of the lobules (zone 2) (159) and may bridge the central veins in adjacent lobules (Fig. 71). It should be noted that the portal tracts and reticulin are intact, features that are unexpected in infarcts.

As the lesions advance, the necrotic, centrilobular hepatocytes undergo lysis, leaving behind dilated sinusoids filled with blood, lipofuscin-filled macrophages, and scattered neutrophils (Fig. 89). In some cases, the canaliculi in the intact midzones contain bile thrombi. Although there is usually little inflammatory response, the portal tracts may contain a variable number of lymphocytes, histiocytes, and occasional neutrophils. Occasionally, large numbers of neutrophils are seen (160). Only rarely

do the centrilobular zones of cell dropout exhibit collapse of their reticulin. As previously noted, in survivors the lesions may result in scarring of the central veins and adjacent sinusoids or may undergo complete resolution without significant residuals.

Hepatic infarction. Hepatic infarcts (159–163) are sharply circumscribed zones of ischemic necrosis that affect all structural components of contiguous lobules. They may range in size from a few millimeters to an entire hepatic lobe. Usually, infarcts are solitary, but occasionally they are multiple. As a rule, hepatic infarction is attributable to occlusion of the hepatic artery or its major branches by ligature, thrombosis, embolism, trauma, or polyarteritis nodosa. Less commonly, it is associated with portal vein thrombosis or occurs in the absence of vascular lesions, particularly following severe shock.

Hepatic infarcts are encountered far less frequently than occlusive hepatic arterial lesions. Several factors account for this discrepancy. Although the hepatic artery contributes 35% of total hepatic blood flow and 50% of the hepatic oxygen requirement, any reduction in its flow leads to an increase in the hepatic extraction of oxygen from the remaining blood circulating through the liver. Occlusion of the hepatic artery close to its origin does not lead to ischemia, since the obstruction is readily bypassed by a collateral circulation via the gastroduodenal and right gastric arteries. Although the right and left hepatic arteries do not communicate with one another normally, ligation of either of these vessels only rarely results in infarction, due, as shown by arteriography, to the rapid development of a translobular collateral circulation following such unilateral arterial ligation.

Occlusion of both the hepatic artery and portal vein invariably leads to massive infarction of the liver.

Often, large hepatic infarcts are manifested by abdominal pain and tenderness, jaundice, and signs of hepatic failure. However, in some cases, manifestations attributable to the underlying disease responsible for the infarction predominate.

Within the first 12 to 24 hours, the lesions present as sharply demarcated, dark red zones of coalescent centrilobular ischemic necrosis. Thereafter, the infarcts are tan or gray in color and are surrounded by a band of hyperemia. Microscopically, the central pale zone exhibits ischemic necrosis of the hepatocytes, central veins, and portal tracts, and is surrounded by infiltrating neutrophils. The parenchyma surrounding the infarct often shows a variable degree of centrilobular ischemic necrosis, infiltration of the portal tracts with lymphocytes, and proliferating ductules.

Ultimately, if the patient survives for several weeks, the ischemic hepatocytes undergo lysis followed by collapse of reticulin and fibrosis, with the formation of a depressed scar.

Disorders of the hepatic arteries

Thrombotic occlusion of the hepatic arteries. Thrombosis of the hepatic artery or its branches is rarely attributable to arteriosclererosis, and is encountered only occasionally as a complication of polyarteritis nodosa. However, it is a relatively common finding following catheterization of the hepatic artery for cancer chemotherapy. Under such conditions, the occlusion is remarkably well tolerated, but may give rise to hepatic infarction if accompanied by thrombosis of the portal vein (164).

Ligation of the hepatic artery. The liver tolerates ligation of the hepatic artery far better than might be anticipated, largely because of its extensive arterial collateral circulation and portal venous supply. Thus, the mortality from hepatic failure and infarction in individuals subjected to this procedure for a wide variety of indications is relatively low, although deaths from other causes related to their underlying disease are relatively common (165,166).

Hepatic artery aneurysm. Most aneurysms of the hepatic artery (167–172) are saccular, but rarely they may be of the dissecting type. Usually, they are extrahepatic, but in approximately 20% of cases they are intrahepatic.

Systemic infection, arteriosclerosis, surgical injury, especially following cholecystectomy, and abdominal trauma, particularly gunshot wounds, are the principal causes of hepatic artery aneurysms. Rarely, they are attributable to polyarteritis nodosa or are of congenital origin.

The clinical manifestations vary, depending on the size and location of the aneurysm and the occurrence of such complicating factors as rupture (168) and dissection (169). The principal features that may present alone or in combination include abdominal pain, jaundice, massive gastrointestinal hemorrhage, and, rarely, acute portal hypertension. When large, a hepatic artery aneurysm may present as a pulsatile epigastric mass with an overlying bruit and thrill. Sometimes it may give rise to abdominal pain by pressure on adjacent viscera, especially the pancreas, and may produce jaundice by compressing the common bile duct. Rupture of the aneurysm, which may occur at any time, may lead to massive hemorrhage into the peritoneum, biliary tract, duodenum, stomach, or portal vein, and fatal outcome. Advances in imaging have made the diagnosis relatively easy and have improved management (173, 174).

Hepatic-portal arteriovenous fistula. A number of etiologic factors have been implicated in the pathogenesis of hepatic-portal arteriovenous fistula (175–177). These include gunshot wounds, blunt trauma to the abdomen, surgical trauma, especially during cholecystectomy, rupture of a congenital or arteriosclerotic aneurysm, intraabdominal inflammatory disease, and congenital anomalies. Such fistulas are far less common than splenic arteriovenous fistulas.

Relatively large hepatic-portal arteriovenous fistulas may be accompanied by an overlying machinery-like murmur, and usually give rise to portal hypertension and its complications (178). The associated hepatic lesions are similar to those encountered in idiopathic portal hypertension. In contrast to other forms of arteriovenous fistula, those that affect the hepatic artery and portal vein rarely give rise to high-output cardiac failure.

Polyarteritis nodosa. Polyarteritis nodosa (179–181) is a systemic disorder characterized by widely disseminated, segmental, inflammatory, and destructive lesions in small and medium sized arteries. As a result, the affected arteries may undergo aneurysmal dilatation, dissection, or rupture, fibrosis, thrombosis, and occlusion, and may lead to ischemia and infarction in various tissues. The arterial lesions may occur anywhere in the body, but are encountered most frequently in the kidneys, liver, gastrointestinal tract, gallbladder, pancreas, myocardium, peripheral nerves, and adrenals. At autopsy, hepatic arterial lesions are demonstrable in at least half the cases (182), but only rarely are they found in liver biopsy sections.

The hepatitis B virus is an important etiologic factor in the pathogenesis of polyarteritis nodosa, and there is convincing evidence that the vascular lesions it produces are attributable to the deposition of immune complexes containing HBs antigen, IgM, and complement (183–187). It is generally assumed that a similar immune mechanism may be involved in other nonviral forms of polyarteritis nodosa, but the evidence for this is less well documented.

As a rule, the clinical manifestations of the disease include fever, anorexia, weight loss, weakness, leukocytosis, and signs or symptoms referrable to ischemia, infarction, or hemorrhage in affected tissues or organs. Of the latter features, the most frequent are hypertension, abdominal pain, and peripheral neuritis.

Although hepatic arterial lesions occur in more than half the cases, in only a minority of patients do hepatic manifestations, such as hepatomegaly or jaundice, predominate. Rarely, the disease presents with the typical features of acute cholecystitis.

Polyarteritis nodosa attributable to infection with the hepatitis B virus has a number of distinctive features. Usually, its onset is characterized by fever, polyarthritis, and a maculopapular or urticarial rash, often followed by the appearance of hypertension and proteinuria (188). In most cases, the accompanying signs and symptoms of viral hepatitis are mild, and may be overlooked until HBs antigenemia is discovered. HBs antigenemia is an invariable finding and may persist.

In HBsAg-positive cases, the *hepatic lesions* usually exhibit the typical features of mild acute viral hepatitis. Less commonly, they resemble those of chronic active or chronic persistent hepatitis, and may be accompanied by typical orcein-positive ground glass cells. Rarely, polyarteritis nodosa occurs in carriers of HBsAg in the absence of hepatic lesions.

A number of hepatic lesions have been reported in nonviral forms of polyarteritis nodosa. These include hepatic infarcts, hepatic arterial aneurysms, occasionally complicated by rupture and hemoperitoneum, and a variety of nonspecific changes, including fibrosis, acute and chronic inflammation and ductular proliferation in the portal tracts, and atrophy and degeneration of the hepatocytes.

As previously indicated, small or medium sized arteries found in liver biopsy sections may show the typical features of polyarteritis nodosa. Early, the lesions are characterized by segmental fibrinoid necrosis of the affected vessel walls (Fig. 399), and later, by edema, acute inflammation, and destruction of the media and internal elastic lamina (Fig. 400). Usually, the inflammatory cells, chiefly neutrophils with a variable number of lymphocytes, plasma cells, and eosinophils, extend through the adventitia into the connective tissue of the portal tract. Some of the affected vessels may undergo aneurysmal dilatation or are occluded by organized thrombi. Healed arterial lesions are characterized by thickening and fibrosis of their intima and media.

Hypersensitivity angiitis. Hypersensitivity angiitis (189), a generalized vasculitis usually due to sensitization to drugs, particularly sulfonamides, often affects the hepatic vasculature. The lesions resemble those of periarteritis nodosa, but affect both portal venous radicles and arterioles, and never become fibrotic.

Giant cell (granulomatous) arteritis. Giant cell arteritis (190–192), a disease of unknown etiology, is associated, in some cases, with the syndrome of polymyalgia rheumatica. Although involvement of the temporal arteries is an important feature in many cases, almost always the disease is generalized, involving both small and large arteries in many parts of the body. Characteristically, the walls of the affected vessels are infiltrated with numerous giant cells and a variable number of other inflammatory cells. Lipocytes may be prominent (192). Rarely, such arterial lesions are encountered in the liver, as illustrated in Figure 401. This lesion was found unexpectedly on needle biopsy of the liver in an elderly woman with prolonged unexplained fever and hepatomegaly. Subsequently, she was found to have biopsy-documented temporal giant cell arteritis that had been previously overlooked.

References

1. Cohen JA, Kaplan MM: Left-sided heart failure presenting as hepatitis. Gastroenterology 74:583–587, 1978.
2. Kubo SH, Walter BA, John DHA, Clark M, Cody RJ: Liver function abnormalities in chronic heart failure. Influence of systemic hemodynamics. Arch Intern Med 147:1227–1233, 1987.
3. Arcidi JM, Moore GW, Hutchins GM: Hepatic morphology in cardiac dysfunction. Am J Pathol 104:159–166, 1981.
4. Leopold JG, Parry TE, Storring FK: A change in the sinusoid-trabecular structure of the liver with hepatic venous outflow block. J Pathol 100:87–98, 1970.
5. Kanel GC, Ucci AA, Kaplan MM, Wolfe HJ: A distinctive perivenular hepatic lesion associated with heart failure. Am J Clin Pathol 73:235–239, 1980.
6. Schaffner F, Popper H: Capillarization of hepatic sinusoids in man. Gastroenterology 44:239–242, 1963.
7. Sherlock S: The liver in heart failure. Relation of anatomical, functional and circulatory changes. Br Heart J 13:273–293, 1951.
8. Dunn GD, Hayes P, Breen KJ, Schenker S: The liver in congestive heart failure: a review. Am J Med Sci 265:174–189, 1973.
9. Ross RM. Hepatic dysfunction secondary to heart failure. Am J Gastroenterol 76:511–518, 1981.
10. Moussavian SN, Dinscoy HP, Goodman S, Helm RA, Bozian RC: Severe hyperbilirubinemia and coma in chronic congestive heart failure. Dig Dis Sci 27:175–180, 1982.
11. Lefkowitch JH, Mendez L: Morphologic features of hepatic injury in cardiac disease and shock. J Hepatol 2:313–327, 1986.
12. Steiner PE: Nodular regenerative hyperplasia of the liver. Am J Pathol 35:943–953, 1959.
13. Winkler K, Poulsen H: Liver disease with periportal sinusoidal dilation. A possible complication to contraceptive steroids. Scand J Gastroenterol 10:699–704, 1975.
14. Skully RE: Case records of the Massachusetts General Hospital: sinusoidal dilatation associated with the oral contraceptive medication. N Engl J Med 307:934–942, 1982.
15. Poulsen H, Winkler K, Christoffersen P: The significance of centrilobular sinusoidal changes in liver biopsies. Scand J Gastroenterol Suppl 7:103–109, 1970.
16. Bruguera M, Aranguibel F, Ros E, Rodes J: Incidence and clinical significance of sinusoidal dilatation in liver biopsies. Gastroenterology 75:474–478, 1978.
17. Summerfield JA, Jones EA: Further progress towards understanding hepatic sinusoidal cells. J Hepatol 3:413–418, 1986.
18. Zak FG: Peliosis hepatis. Am J Pathol 26:1–10, 1950.
19. Kent G, Thompson JR: Peliosis hepatis. Involvement of reticuloendothelial system. Arch Pathol 72:658–664, 1961.
20. Lewis JH, Tice HL, Zimmerman HJ: Budd-Chiari syndrome associated with oral contraceptive steroids. Review of treatment of 47 cases. Dig Dis Sci 28:673–683, 1983.
21. Bagheri SA, Boyer JL: Peliosis hepatis associated with androgenic-anabolic steroid therapy. A severe form of hepatic injury. Ann Intern Med 81:610–618, 1974.
22. Nadell J, Kosek J: Peliosis hepatis. Twelve cases associated with androgen therapy. Arch Pathol Lab Med 101:405–410, 1977.
23. Paradinas FJ, Bull TB, Westaby D, Murray-Lyon IM: Hyperplasia and prolapse of hepatocytes into hepatic veins during long term methyltestosterone therapy, possible relationship of these changes to the development of peliosis hepatis and liver tumours. Histopathology 1:225–246, 1977.
24. Gerlag PGG, Lobatto S, Driessen WMM: Hepatic sinusoidal dilation with portal hypertension during azathioprine treatment after kidney transplantation. J Hepatol 1:339–348, 1985.
25. Czapar CA, Weldon-Linne CM, Moore DM, Rhone DP: Peliosis hepatis in the acquired immunodeficiency syndrome. Arch Pathol Lab Med 110:611–613, 1986.
26. Zafrani ES, Bernuau D, Feldmann G: Peliosis-like ultrastructural changes of the hepatic sinusoids in human chronic hypervitaminosis A: report of three cases. Hum Pathol 15:1166–1170, 1984.
27. Hillion D, deViel E, Bergue A, Bruet A, Dongradi G, Fendler J-P: Peliosis in a chronic hemodialysis patient. Nephron 35:205–206, 1983.
28. Yanoff M, Rawson AJ: Peliosis hepatis. An anatomic study with demonstration of two varieties. Arch Pathol 77:159–165, 1964.
29. Zafrani ES, Feldmann G: Primary lesions of the hepatic sinusoid. In Sinusoids in Human Liver: Health and Disease, edited by P. Bioulac-Sage, C. Balabaud. Rijswijk, The Küpffer Cell Foundation, 1988, pp. 495–502.
30. Larrey D, Freneaux E, Berson A, Babany G, Degott C, Valla D, Pessayre D, Benhamou J-P: Peliosis hepatis induced by 6-thioguanine administration. Gut 29:1265–1269, 1988.
31. Zafrani ES: An additional argument for a toxic mechanism of peliosis hepatis in man. Hepatology 11:322–323, 1990.
32. Wold LE, Ludwig J: Peliosis hepatis: two morphologic variants? Hum Pathol 12:388–389, 1981.
33. Perkocha LA, Geaghan SM, Yen TSB, Nishimura SL, Chan SP, Garcia-Kennedy R, Honda G, Stoloff AC, Klein HZ, Goldman RL, Van Meter S, Ferrell LD, LeBoit PE: Clinical and pathological features of bacillary peliosis hepatis in association with human immunodeficiency virus infection. N Engl J Med 232:1581–1586, 1990.
34. Knobler EH, Silvers DN, Fine KC, Lefkowitch JH, Grossman ME: Unique vascular skin lesions associated with human immunodeficiency virus. JAMA 260:524–527, 1988.
35. LeBoit PE, Berger TG, Egbert BM, Beckstead JH, Yen TSB, Stoler MH: Bacillary angiomatosis: the histopathology and differential diagnosis of a pseudoneoplastic infection in patients with human immunodeficiency virus disease. Am J Surg Pathol 13:909–920, 1989.
36. English CK, Wear KJ, Margileth AM, Lissner CR, Walsh GP: Cat-scratch disease: isolation and culture of the bacterial agent. JAMA 259:1347–1352, 1988.
37. Garcia FU, Wojta J, Broadley KN, Davidson JM, Hoover RL: Bartonella bacilliformis stimulates endothelial cells in vitro and is angiogenic in vivo. Am J Pathol 136:1125–1135, 1990.
38. Budd G: On Diseases of the Liver, 3rd Edition. Philadelphia, Blanchard & Lea, 1857, pp. 38–50.
39. Chiari H: Ueber die selbstandige Phlebitis obliterans der Hauptstamme der Venae hepaticae als Todesurache. Beitr Path Anat 26:1–20, 1899.
40. Parker RGF: Occlusion of the hepatic veins in man. Medicine 38:369–402, 1959.
41. Mitchell MC, Boitnott JK, Kaufman S, Cameron JL, Maddrey WC: Budd-Chiari syndrome: etiology, diagnosis and management. Medicine 61:199–218, 1982.
42. Madanagopalan N, Solomon V, Jayanthi V, Raghuram K, Valakumar M, Kandasamy I, Gajaraj, Panchanadam M: Clinical spectrum of chronic Budd-Chiari syndrome and surgical relief for 'coarctation' of the inferior vena cava. J Gastroenterol Hepatol 1:359–369, 1986.
43. Lewis JH, Tice HL, Zimmerman HJ: Budd-Chiari syndrome associated with oral contraceptive steroids. Review of treatment of 47 cases. Dig Dis Sci 28:673–679, 1983.
44. Valla D, Casadevall N, Lacombe C, Bruno V, Goldwasser E, Franco D, Maillar J-N, Pariente A, Leporrier M, Rueff B, Muller O, Benhamou J-P: Primary myeloproliferative disorder and hepatic vein thrombosis. Ann Intern Med 103:329–334, 1985.
45. Powell-Jackson PR, Ede RJ, Williams R: Budd-Chiari syndrome presenting as fulminant hepatic failure. Gut 27:1101–1105, 1986.
46. Orloff MJ: Portal-systemic shunts for Budd-Chiari syndrome. Hepatology 7:1389–1391, 1987.
47. Furui S, Yamauchi T, Ohtomo K, Tsuchiya K, Makita K, Takenaka E: Hepatic inferior vena cava obstructions: clinical result of treatment with percutaneous transluminal laser-assisted angiography. Radiology 166:673–677, 1988.
48. Seltman HJ, Dekker A, Van Thiel DH, Boggs DR, Starzl TE: Budd-Chiari syndrome recurring in a transplanted liver. Gastroenterology 84:640–643, 1983.
49. Gupta S, Blumgart LH, Hodgson HJF: Budd-Chiari syndrome: long-term survival and factors affecting mortality. Q J Med 60:781–794, 1986.
50. Gupta S, Barter S, Phillips GWL, Gibson RN, Hodgson HJF: Comparison of ultrasonography, computed tomography and 99m-Tc liver scan in diagnosis of Budd-Chiari syndrome. Gut 28:242–247, 1987.

51. Selzer G, Parker RGF: Senecio poisoning exhibiting as Chiari's syndrome. A report on twelve cases. Am J Pathol 27:885–900, 1951.

52. Stuart KL, Bras G: Veno-occlusive disease of the liver. Q J Med 26:291–315, 1957.

53. McLean EK: The toxic actions of pyrrolizidine (senecio) alkaloids. Pharmacol Rev 22:429–483, 1970.

54. Tandon BN, Tandon RK, Tandon HK, Narndranathan M, Joshi YK: An epidemic of veno-occlusive disease of liver in central India. Lancet 2:271–272, 1976.

55. Stillman AE, Huxtable R, Consroe P, Kohner P, Smith S: Hepatic veno-occlusive disease due to pyrrolizidine (senecio) poisoning in Arizona. Gastroenterology 73:349–352, 1977.

56. Ridker PM, Ohkuma S, McDermott WV: Hepatic veno-occlusive disease associated with the consumption of pyrrolizidine-containing dietary supplements. Gastroenterology 88:1050–1054, 1985.

57. Kumana CR, Lin HJ, Ko W, Wu P-C, Todd D: Herbal tea induced hepatic veno-occlusive disease; quantification of toxic alkaloid exposure in adults. Gut 26:101–104, 1985.

58. Rollins BJ: Hepatic veno-occlusive disease. Am J Med 81:297–306, 1986.

59. Marubbio AT, Danielson B: Hepatic veno-occlusive disease in a renal transplant patient receiving azathioprine. Gastroenterology 69:739–743, 1975.

60. Roulet M, Laurini R, Rivier L, Calame A: Hepatic veno-occlusive disease in newborn infant of a woman drinking herbal tea. J Pediatr 112:433–436, 1988.

61. Muenter MD, Perry HO, Ludwig J: Chronic vitamin A intoxication in adults. Hepatic, neurologic and dermatologic complications. Am J Med 50:129–136, 1971.

62. Russell RM, Boyer JL, Bagheri SA, Hruban Z: Hepatic injury from chronic hypervitaminosis A resulting in portal hypertension and ascites. N Engl J Med 291:435–440, 1984.

63. Jacques EA, Buschmann RJ, Layden TJ: The histopathologic progression of vitamin A-induced hepatic injury. Gastroenterology 76:599–602, 1979.

63a. Carpenter TA, Pettifor JM, Russell RN, Pitha J, Mobartrans Ossip MS, Warner S, Anast CS: Severe hypervitaminosis A in siblings: Evidence of variable tolerance to retinol intake. J. Pediatr 111: 507–512, 1987.

64. Read AE, Wiesner RH, LaBrecque DR, Tifft JG, Mullen KD, Sheer RL, Petrelli M, Ricanati ES, McCullough AJ: Hepatic veno-occlusive disease associated with renal transplantation and azathioprine therapy. Ann Intern Med 104:651–655, 1986.

65. Griner PF, Elbadawi A, Packman CH: Veno-occlusive disease of the liver after chemotherapy of acute leukemia. Report of two cases. Ann Intern Med 85:578–582, 1976.

66. Erichsen C, Jonsson P-E: Veno-occlusive liver disease after dacarbazine therapy (DTIC) for melanoma. J Surg Oncol 27:268–270, 1984.

67. Berk PD, Popper H, Krueger GRF, Decter J, Herzig G, Graw RG Jr: Veno-occlusive disease of the liver after allogeneic bone marrow transplantation. Possible association with graft-versus-host disease. Ann Intern Med 90:158–164, 1979.

68. Shulman HM, McDonald GB, Matthews D, Doney KC, Kopecky KJ, Gauvreau JM, Thomas ED: An analysis of hepatic veno-occlusive disease and centrilobular hepatic degeneration following bone marrow transplantation. Gastroenterology 79:1178–1191, 1980.

69. McDonald GB, Sharma P, Matthews DE, Shulman HM, Thomas ED: The clinical course of 53 patients with veno-occlusive disease of the liver after marrow transplantation. Transplantation 39:603–608, 1985.

70. Shulman HM, Sharma P, Amos D, Fenster LF, McDonald GB: A coded histologic study of hepatic graft-versus-host disease after human bone transplantation. Hepatology 8:463–470, 1988.

71. Mellis C, Bale PM: Familial hepatic veno-occlusive disease with probable immune deficiency. J Pediatr 88:236–242, 1976.

72. Baker A, Kaplan M, Wolfe H: Central congestive fibrosis of the liver in myxedema ascites. Ann Intern Med 77:927–929, 1972.

73. Ingold JA, Reed GB, Kaplan HS, Bagshaw MA: Radiation hepatitis. Am J Roentgenol 93:200–208, 1965.

74. Fajardo LF, Colby TV: Pathogenesis of veno-occlusive liver disease after radiation. Arch Pathol Lab Med 104:584–588, 1988.

75. Hansen MM, Ranek L, Walbom S, Nissen NI: Fatal hepatitis following irradiation and vincristine. Acta Med Scand 212:171–174, 1982.

76. Nakanuma Y, Ohta G, Doishita K: Quantitation and serial section observations of focal veno-occlusive lesions of hepatic veins in liver cirrhosis. Virchows Arch (Pathol Anat) 405:429–438, 1985.

77. Goodman ZD, Ishak KG: Occlusive venous lesions in alcoholic liver disease. Gastroenterology 83:786–796, 1982.

78. Reynolds TB, Hidemura R, Michel H, Peters R: Portal hypertension without cirrhosis in alcoholic liver disease. Ann Intern Med 70:497–506, 1969.

79. Shiamura K, Oka K, Nakazawa M, Kojima M: Distribution patterns of microthrombi in disseminated intravascular coagulation. Arch Pathol Lab Med 107:543–547, 1983.

80. Omata M, Johnson CS, Tong M, Tatter D: Pathological spectrum of liver diseases in sickle cell disease. Dig Dis Sci 31:247–256, 1986.

81. Keen ME, Engstrand DA, Hafez G: Hepatic lipogranulomatosis simulating veno-occlusive disease of the liver. Arch Pathol Lab Med 109:70–72, 1985.

82. Scheuer PJ: Liver Biopsy Interpretation, 4th Edition. London, Bailliere Tindall, 1988, pp. 177–178.

83. Groszmann RJ, Glickman M, Blei AT, Storer E, Conn HO: Wedged and free hepatic venous pressure measured with a balloon catheter. Gastroenterology 76:254–258, 1979.

84. Boyer TD, Triger DR, Horisawa M, Redeker AG, Reynolds TB: Direct transhepatic measurement of portal vein pressure using a thin needle. Gastroenterology 72:584–589, 1977.

85. Staritz V, Poralla T, Meyer zum Buchsenfelde KH: Intravascular oesophageal variceal pressure (IOVP) assessed by endoscopic fine needle puncture after basal conditions, Valsalva manoeuvre and after glyceryl trinitrate application. Gut 26:525–530, 1985.

86. Raby N, Karanj J, Powell-Jackson P, Meire H, Williams R: Assessment of portal vein patency: comparison of arterial portography and ultrasound scanning. Clin Radiol 39:381–385, 1988.

87. Taylor CR: Assessment of portal vein patency: pitfalls and problems in diagnostic comparative studies. Hepatology 10:117–118, 1989.

88. Conn HO, Groszmann RJ: The pathophysiology of portal hypertension. In The Liver, Biology and Pathobiology, edited by I. Arias, H. Popper, D. Schacter, D.A. Shafritz. New York, Raven Press, 1982, pp. 821–848.

89. Conn HO: Spontaneous bacterial peritonitis: variant syndromes. South Med J 80:1343–1346, 1987.

90. Epstein M: The Kidney in Liver Disease, 3rd Edition. Baltimore, Williams & Wilkins, 1988.

91. Conn HO: The hepatic encephalopathies. In Hepatic Encephalopathy: Management with Lactulose and Related Carbohydrates, edited by H.O. Conn, J. Bircher. East Lansing, Medi-Ed Press, 1988, pp. 3–14.

92. Kiire CR: Controlled trial of propranolol to prevent recurrent variceal bleeding in patients with noncirrhotic portal fibrosis. Br Med J 298:1363–1365, 1989.

93. Sherlock S: Extrahepatic portal venous hypertension in adults. Clin Gastroenterol 14:1–7, 1985.

94. Baggenstoss AH, Wollaeger EE: Portal hypertension due to chronic occlusion of the extrahepatic portion of the portal vein: its relation to ascites. Am J Med 21:16–25, 1956.

95. Maddrey WC, Mallik KCB, Iber FL, Basu AK: Extrahepatic obstruction of the portal venous system. Surg Gynecol Obstet 127:989–998, 1968.

96. Webb LJ, Sherlock S: The aetiology, presentation and natural history of extra-hepatic portal venus obstruction. Q J Med 192:627–639, 1979.

97. Sarfeh IJ: Portal vein thrombosis associated with cirrhosis. Clinical importance. Arch Surg 114:902–905, 1979.

98. Orozco H, Guraieb E, Takahashi T, Garcia-Tso G, Hurtado R, Anaya R, Ruiz-Arguelles G, Hernandez-Ortiz J, Casillas MA, Guevara L: Deficiency of protein C in patients with portal vein thrombosis. Hepatology 8:1110–1111, 1988.

99. Capron JP, LeMay JL, Muir JF: Portal vein thrombosis and fatal pulmonary thromboembolism associated with oral contraceptive treatment. J Clin Gastroenterol 3:295–300, 1981.

100. Wanless IR: The pathophysiology of noncirrhotic portal hypertension: a pathologist's perspective. In Liver Cirrhosis. Proceedings of the 44th Falk Symposium, VIIth International Congress of Liver Diseases. Editors J. Boyer, L. Bianchi. Basel, MTP Press Limited, 1986, pp. 293–311.

101. Okuda K, Ohnishi K, Kimura K: Incidence of portal vein thrombosis in liver cirrhosis. An angiographic study of 708 patients. Gastroenterology 89:279–286, 1985.

102. Hunt AH: A Contribution to the Study of Portal Hypertension. Edinburgh, E & S Livingstone Ltd, 1958, pp. 64–65.

103. Shaldon S, Sherlock S: Portal hypertension in the myeloproliferative syndrome and the reticuloses. Am J Med 32:758–764, 1962.

104. Atkinson M, Sherlock S: Intrasplenic pressure as index of portal venous pressure. Lancet 1:1325–1327, 1954.

105. Wanless IR, Albrecht S, Bilbao J, Frei JV, Heathcote EJ, Roberts EA, Chiasson D: Multiple focal nodular hyperplasia of the liver associated with vascular malformations of various organs and neoplasia of the brain: a new syndrome. Mod Pathol 2:456–462, 1989.

106. Johnston GW, Gibson JB: Portal hypertension resulting from splenic arteriovenous fistulae. Gut 6:500–502, 1965.

107. Nissan S, Bar-Maor JA: Bleeding esophageal varices due to splenic arteriovenous fistula. Am J Gastroenterol 55:379–382, 1971.

108. Madding GF, Smith WL, Hershberger LR: Hepatoportal arteriovenous fistula. JAMA 156:593–596, 1954.

109. Dunn MA, Kamel R: Hepatic schistosomiasis. Hepatology 1:653–661, 1981.

110. Andrade ZA, Cheever AW: Alterations of the intrahepatic vasculature in hepatosplenic schistosomiasis mansoni. Am J Trop Med Hyg 20:425–432, 1971.

111. Grimaud J-A, Borojevic R: Chronic human Schistosomiasis mansoni. Pathology of the Disse's space. Lab Invest 36:268–273, 1977.

112. Alves CAP, Alves AR, Abreu WN, Andrade ZA: Hepatic artery hypertrophy and sinusoidal hypertension in advanced schistosomiasis. Gastroenterology 72:126–128, 1977.

113. Klatskin G: Hepatic granulomata: problems in interpretation. Ann NY Acad Sci 278:427–432, 1976.

114. Berger I, Katz M: Portal hypertension due to hepatic sarcoidosis. Am J Gastroenterol 59:147–151, 1973.

115. Tekeste H, Latour F, Levitt RE: Portal hypertension complicating sarcoid liver disease. Am J Gastroenterol 79:389–396, 1984.

116. Maddrey WC, Johns CJ, Boitnott JK, Iber FL: Sarcoidosis and chronic hepatic disease: a clinical and pathologic study of 20 patients. Medicine 49:375–395, 1970.

117. Kerr DNS, Harrison CV, Sherlock S, Walker RM: Congenital hepatic fibrosis. Q J Med 30:91–117, 1960.

118. Landing BH, Wells TR, Claireaux AE: Morphometric analysis of liver lesions in cystic diseases of childhood. Hum Pathol 11:549–560, 1980.

119. Morris JS, Schmid M, Sherlock S: Arsenic and noncirrhotic portal hypertension. Gastroenterology 64:86–94, 1974.

120. Huet P-M, Guillaume E, Cote J, Legare A, Lavoie P, Viallet A: Noncirrhotic presinusoidal portal hypertension associated with chronic arsenical intoxication. Gastroenterology 68:1270–1277, 1975.

121. Blendis LM, Smith PM, Lawrie BW, Stephens MR, Evans WD: Portal hypertension in vinyl chloride monomer workers. A hemodynamic study. Gastroenterology 75:206–211, 1978.

122. Pimentel JC, Menezes AP: Liver disease in vineyard sprayers. Gastroenterology 72:275–283, 1977.

123. Solis-Herruzo JA, Vidal JV, Colina F, Santalla F, Castellano G: Nodular regenerative hyperplasia of the liver associated with the toxic oil syndrome: report of five cases. Hepatology 6:687–693, 1986.

124. Nakanuma UY, Ohta G: Nodular hyperplasia of the liver in primary biliary cirrhosis of early histological stages. Am J Gastroenterol 82:8–10, 1987.

125. Wanless IR: Understanding noncirrhotic portal hypertension: menage a fois. Hepatology 8:192–193, 1988.

126. Pomier-Layrargues G, Kusielewicz D, Willems B, Villeneuve J-P, Marleau D, Cote J, Huet P-M: Presinusoidal portal hypertension in non-alcoholic cirrhosis. Hepatology 5:415–418, 1985.

127. Polish E, Christie J, Cohen A, Sullivan B Jr: Idiopathic presinusoidal portal hypertension (Banti's syndrome). Ann Intern Med 56:624–627, 1962.

128. Mikkelsen WP, Edmondson HA, Peters RL, Redeker AG, Reynolds TB: Extra- and intrahepatic portal hypertension without cirrhosis (hepatoportal sclerosis). Ann Surg 162:602–618, 1965.

129. Boyer JL, Sen Gupta KP, Biswas SK, Pal NC, Mallick KCB, Iber FL, Basu AK: Idiopathic portal hypertension. Comparison with the portal hypertension of cirrhosis and extrahepatic portal vein obstruction. Ann Intern Med 65:41–68, 1967.

130. Nayak AC, Ramalingaswami V. Obliterative portal venopathy of the liver associated with so-called idiopathic portal hypertension or tropical splenomegaly. Arch Pathol 87:359–369, 1969.

131. Iber FL: Portal hypertension in the presence of normal liver morphology. Ann NY Acad Sci 170:115–126, 1970.

132. Boyer JL, Hales MR, Klatskin G: ''Idiopathic'' portal hypertension due to occlusion of intrahepatic portal veins by organized thrombi. A study based on postmortem vinylite-injection corrosion and dissection of the intrahepatic vasculature in 4 cases. Medicine 53:77–91, 1974.

133. Villeneuve JP, Huet RM, Joly J-G, Marleau D, Legare A, Lafortune M, Lavoie P, Viallet A: Idiopathic portal hypertension. Am J Med 61:459–464, 1976.

134. Nataf C, Feldmann G, Lebrec D, Degott G, Descamps J-M, Rueff B, Benhamou J-P: Idiopathic portal hypertension (perisinusoidal fibrosis) after renal transplantation. Gut 20:531–537, 1979.

135. Kingham JGC, Levison DA, Stansfeld AG, Dawson AM: Noncirrhotic intrahepatic portal hypertension. A long-term follow-up study. Q J Med 50:259–268, 1981.

136. Okuda K, Kono K. Ohnishi K, Kimura K, Omata M, Koen H, Nakajima Y, Musha H, Hirashima T, Takashi M, Takayasu K: Clinical study of eighty-six cases of idiopathic portal hypertension and comparison with cirrhosis with splenomegaly. Gastroenterology 86:600–610, 1984.

137. Okuda K, Nakashima T, Okudaira M, Kage M, Aida Y, Omata M, Sugiura M, Kameda H, Inokuchi K, Bhusnurmath SR, Aikat BA: Liver pathology of idiopathic portal hypertension. Comparison with non-cirrhotic portal fibrosis of India. Liver 2:176–192, 1982.

138. Steiner PE: Nodular regenerative hyperplasia of the liver. Am J Pathol 35:943–953, 1959.

139. Lurie B, Novis B, Bank S, Silber W, Botha JBC, Marks IN: CRST syndrome and nodular transformation of the liver. A case report. Gastroenterology 64:457–461, 1973.

140. Blendis LM, Parkinson MC, Shilkin KB, Williams R: Nodular regenerative hyperplasia of the liver in Felty's syndrome. Q J Med 43:25–32, 1974.

141. Rougier P, Degott C, Rueff B, Benhamou J-P: Nodular regenerative hyperplasia of the liver. Report of six cases and review of the literature. Gastroenterology 75:169–172, 1978.

142. Wanless IR, Godwin TA, Allen F, Feder A: Nodular regenerative hyperplasia of the liver in hematologic disorders: a possible response to obliterative portal venopathy. A morphometric study of nine cases with an hypothesis on the pathogenesis. Medicine 59:367–379, 1980.

143. Stromeyer FW, Ishak KG: Nodular transformation (nodular regenerative hyperplasia) of the liver. Hum Pathol 12:60–71, 1981.

144. Sherlock S, Feldman CA, Moran B, Scheuer PJ: Partial nodular transformation of the liver with portal hypertension. Am J Med 40:195–203, 1966.

145. Dick AP, Gresham GA: Partial nodular transformation of the liver presenting with ascites. Gut 13:289–292, 1972.

146. Wanless IR, Mawdsley C, Adams R: On the pathogenesis of focal nodular hyperplasia of the liver. Hepatology 5:1194–1200, 1985.

147. Grundfest S, Cooperman AM, Ferguson R, Benjamin S: Portal hypertension associated with systemic mastocytosis and splenomegaly. Gastroenterology 78:370–373, 1980.

148. Ghandur-Mnaymneh L, Gould E: Systemic mastocytosis with portal hypertension. Autopsy findings and ultrastructural study of the liver. Arch Pathol Lab Med 109:76–78, 1985.

149. Claman, HM: More about mast cells and fibrosis in porphyria cutanea tarda. Hepatology 11:895–896, 1990.

150. Kapp JP: Hepatic amyloidosis with portal hypertension. JAMA 191:497–499, 1965.

151. Finkelstein SD, Fornasier VL, Pruzanski W: Intrahepatic cholestasis with predominant pericentral deposition in systemic amyloidosis. Hum Pathol 13:662–665, 1982.

152. Witte CL, Brewer ML, Witte MH, Pond GB: Protean manifestations of pylethrombosis. Ann Surg 202:191–202, 1985.

153. Horrocks P, Tapp E: Zahn's 'infarcts' of the liver. J Clin Pathol 19:475–478, 1966.

154. Scheuer PJ: Liver Biopsy Interpretation, 4th Edition. London, Bailliere Tindall, 1988, p. 175.

155. Ellenberg M, Osserman KE: The role of shock in the production of central liver cell necrosis. Am J Med 11:170–178, 1951.

156. Killip T III, Payne MA: High serum transaminase activity disease. Circulatory failure and hepatic necrosis. Circulation 21:646–660, 1960.

157. Logan RG, Mowry FM, Judge RD: Cardiac failure simulating viral hepatitis. Three cases with serum transaminase levels above 1,000. Ann Intern Med 56:784–788, 1962.

158. Cohen JA, Kaplan MM: Left-sided heart failure presenting as hepatitis. Gastroenterology 74:583–587, 1978.

159. de la Monte SM, Arcidi JM, Moore GW, Hutchins GM: Midzonal necrosis as a pattern of hepatocellular injury after shock. Gastroenterology 86:627–631, 1984.

160. Lefkowitch JH, Mendez L: Morphologic features of hepatic injury in cardiac disease and shock. J Hepatol 2:313–327, 1986.

161. Zimmerman HM: Infarcts of the liver and the mechanism of their production. Arch Pathol 10:66–78, 1930.

162. Wooling KR, Baggenstoss AH, Weir JF: Infarcts of the liver. Gastroenterology 17:479–493, 1951.

163. Chen V, Hamilton J, Qizilbash A: Hepatic infarction. A clinicopathologic study of seven cases. Arch Pathol Lab Med *100*:32–36, 1976.
164. Lucas RJ, Tumacder O, Wilson GS: Hepatic artery occlusion following hepatic artery catheterization. Ann Surg *173*:238–243, 1971.
165. Berman JK, Fields DC: Advanced atrophic cirrhosis. Present status of hepatic, splenic, and left gastric arterial occlusion as an aid in the control of its complications. Arch Surg *68*:432–441, 1954.
166. Kim DK, Kinne DW, Fortner JG: Occlusion of the hepatic artery in man. Surg Gynecol Obstet *136*:966–968, 1973.
167. Barnett WO, Wagner JA: Aneurysm of the hepatic artery: a cause of obscure abdominal hemorrhage. Ann Surg *137*:561–564, 1953.
168. Croom RD, Frantz PT, Thomas CG, Hothem AL: Aneurysms of the hepatic artery. South Med J *69*:1013–1016, 1976.
169. Hill DE, Lobell M, Edwards JE: Primary dissecting aneurysm of the hepatic artery. Arch Intern Med *133*:471–474, 1974.
170. Bristol R, Gonzales P, Chassin JL: Aneurysm of the hepatic artery. Am J Surg *120*:97–98, 1970.
171. Winchester DP, Seed RW, Bergan JJ, Conn J Jr: Jaundice, hemobilia, and hemoperitoneum. Consequences of rupture of hepatic artery aneurysm. Am J Surg *120*:384–387, 1970.
172. Guerrero EC: Primary dissecting aneurysm of the hepatic artery. Arch Pathol *89*:569–573, 1970.
173. Athey PA, Sax SL, Lamki N: Sonography in the diagnosis of hepatic artery aneurysms. Am J Roentgenol *147*:725–730, 1986.
174. Kibbler CC, Cohen DL, Cruickshank JK, Kushwaha SS, Morgan MY, Dick RD: Use of CAT scanning in the diagnosis and management of hepatic artery aneurysm. Gut *26*:752–756, 1985.
175. Martin LW, Benzing G, Kaplan S: Congenital intrahepatic arteriovenous fistula. Report of a successfully treated case. Ann Surg *161*:209–212, 1965.
176. Donovan AJ, Reynolds TB, Mikkelsen WP, Peters RL: Systemic-portal arteriovenous fistulas: pathological and hemodynamic observations in two patients. Surgery *66*:474–482, 1969.
177. Fulton RL, Wolfel DA: Hepatic artery-portal vein arteriovenous fistula. Report of a case with notes on the pathophysiology of this condition. Arch Surg *100*:307–309, 1970.
178. Inon AE, D'Agostino D: Portal hypertension secondary to congenital arterioportal fistula. J Pediatr Gastroenterol Nutr *6*:471–481, 1987.
179. Mowrey FH, Lundberg EA: The clinical manifestations of essential polyangiitis (periarteritis nodosa), with emphasis on the hepatic manifestations. Ann Intern Med *40*:1145–1164, 1954.
180. Glassman E, Skerrett PV: Rupture of an intrahepatic aneurysm due to polyarteritis nodosa. Am J Med *28*:143–146, 1960.
181. LiVolsi VA, Perzin KH, Porter M: Polyarteritis nodosa of the gallbladder, presenting as acute cholecystitis. Gastroenterology *65*:115–123, 1973.
182. Weinblatt ME, Teser JRP, Gilliam JH III: The liver in rheumatic diseases. Semin Arthritis Rheum *11*:399–408, 1982.
183. Gocke DJ, Hsu K, Morgan C, Bombardieri S, Lockshin M, Christian CL: Association between polyarteritis and Australia antigen. Lancet *2*:1149–1153, 1970.
184. Prince AM, Trepo C: Role of immune complexes involving SH antigen in pathogenesis of chronic active hepatitis and polyarteritis nodosa. Lancet *2*:1309–1312, 1971.
185. Trepo CG, Zuckerman AJ, Bird RC, Prince AM: The role of circulating hepatitis B antigen/antibody immune complexes in the pathogenesis of vascular and hepatic manifestations in polyarteritis nodosa. J Clin Pathol *27*:863–868, 1974.
186. Michalak T: Immune complexes of hepatitis B surface antigen in the pathogenesis of polyarteritis nodosa. A study of seven necropsy cases. Am J Pathol *90*:619–632, 1978.
187. Drueke T, Barbanel C, Jungers P: Hepatitis B antigen-associated periarteritis nodosa in patients undergoing long-term hemodialysis. Am J Med *68*:86–90, 1980.
188. Mihas AA, Kirby D, Kens P: Hepatitis B antigen and polyositis. JAMA *239*:221–222, 1978.
189. Zeek PM, Smith CC, Weeter JC: Studies on periarteritis nodosa. III. The differentiations between the vascular lesions of periarteritis nodosa and of hypersensitivity. Am J Pathol *24*:889–917, 1948.
190. Hamilton CR Jr, Shelley WM, Tumullty PA: Giant cell arteritis: including temporal arteritis and polymyalgia rheumatica. Medicine *50*:1–27, 1971.
191. McCormack LR, Astarita RW, Foroozan P: Liver involvement in giant cell arteritis. Am J Dig Dis *23*:72s–74s, 1978.
192. Leong AS-Y, Alp MH: Hepatocellular disease in the giant-cell arteritis polymyalgia rheumatica syndrome. Ann Rheum Dis *40*:92–95, 1981.

Chapter 22
Hepatic Granulomas

Granulomas are circumscribed, compact masses of epithelioid cells, often interspersed with multinucleated giant cells and lymphocytes. The epithelioid cells are modified phagocytic histiocytes derived probably from circulating monocytes that originate in the bone marrow. Fusion of adjacent epithelioid cells accounts for the development of the giant cells (1).

Early in their development, granulomas contain a network of randomly distributed reticulin fibers, but as the lesions mature, either spontaneously or as a result of therapy, the lesions tend to undergo progressive fibrosis, and, ultimately, may be replaced by a sharply circumscribed, hyalinized scar. However, granulomas may resolve without residual scarring.

Depending on their etiology, active granulomas may coalesce to form large lesions or may exhibit foci of fibrinoid or caseation necrosis. Granulomas vary from 50 to 300 μm, i.e., from half to six times the diameter of a liver biopsy core (2).

A wide variety of etiologic factors have been implicated in the pathogenesis of granulomas. Available evidence suggests that in most, but not all instances, an underlying, cell-mediated, immunologic reaction is involved.

Granulomatous reactions may be limited to a single tissue or organ, but, more commonly, are disseminated. Such lesions are encountered in the liver with remarkable frequency, usually in association with systemic or other extrahepatic disease (3,4).

In our own experience, 689 of 7183 patients (10%) subjected to liver biopsy exhibited hepatic granulomas. Of the 689, 455 (66%) occurred in the 907 patients with systemic or extrahepatic disorders, 190 (28%) in the 5581 with "primary" diseases of the liver, and 44 (6%) in the 695 with no evidence of systemic extrahepatic or primary hepatic disease. It is noteworthy that not all of the systemic and extrahepatic disorders accompanied by granulomas in the liver are known to produce a granulomatous reaction in other tissues. Similarly, with the exception of primary biliary cirrhosis, none of the primary hepatic diseases in which we have encountered granulomas is known to produce similar lesions in non-hepatic tissues. This raises the question whether, under such conditions, the granulomas found in the liver are coincidental and attributable to unrecognized systemic granulomatous disease, a possibility that will be discussed further.

Although the structures of hepatic granulomas may differ, depending on their etiology, relatively few granulomas exhibit histologic features sufficiently distinctive to permit identification of their etiology (5,6). Accordingly, in most cases, the etiologic diagnosis depends on a consideration of the history and clinical features, the results of skin tests and serologic and cultural studies, and the character of the accompanying hepatic lesions.

The discovery of a granuloma in the liver usually suggests the possibility of sarcoidosis or tuberculosis, the two most common causes of such lesions. However, taken together both these diseases accounted for less than half (45%) of the hepatic granulomas encountered in our series of 689 cases. Moreover, since sarcoidal and tuberculous granulomas can seldom be differentiated from others on histologic grounds alone, it is apparent that their identification must be based on strict diagnostic criteria, including the exclusion of other known causes of such lesions.

Even after the most exhaustive investigation, the etiology of hepatic granulomas remains obscure in 20 to 30% of cases (7). The incidence of such lesions in our own series was 6%. However, this may be an underestimate, since some of the granulomas ascribed to "primary" disorders of the liver could conceivably have been due to unrecognized coincidental systemic or extrahepatic disease (Table 22–1). The primary disorders of the liver in which granulomas occur are listed in Table 22–2.

Hepatic granulomas in systemic and extrahepatic diseases

Table 22–1 lists the principal systemic and extrahepatic diseases known to be associated with hepatic granulomas, and gives the incidence of such hepatic lesions in the Yale series of cases.

Sarcoidosis

Sarcoidosis (8,9) is a disease of unknown etiology characterized by widely disseminated, noncaseating, epithelioid granulomas. The principal tissues involved in the order of their frequency include lymph nodes, lungs, liver, spleen, eyes, skin, salivary glands, muscles, joints, kidneys, and central nervous system.

The signs and symptoms of the disease depend on the tissues affected by the granulomatous process. A relatively common, but insufficiently emphasized feature is fever, the incidence of which in some studies has been as high as 41% (10). Usually, the fever is low grade, but, occasionally, it is high and may be accompanied by chills, findings that may be misinterpreted as evidence of tuberculosis. Liver biopsy is very helpful in the diagnosis of patients with prolonged fever (11).

Sarcoidal granulomas are demonstrable in the liver by needle biopsy in at least two-thirds of the cases (11). In our own series of 247 cases, the incidence was 94%, a higher percentage than previously reported. We attribute our high incidence to the relatively large size of our biopsy specimens and to the routine use of serial sections.

Table 22–1. Hepatic granulomas in systemic and other extrahepatic diseases: reported etiologic factors and incidence in Yale series

DISEASE	NO. PATIENTS WITH DISEASE	NO. PATIENTS WITH GRANULOMAS	% PATIENTS WITH GRANULOMAS
Sarcoidosis:	247	231	94
Infection: mycobacterial			
Tuberculosis:	174	76	44
BCG vaccination:	2	2	100
Atypical mycobacteria:	1	1	100
Infection: bacterial			
Brucellosis:	6	5	83
Infection: spirochetal			
Syphilis			
Early acquired:	1	0	0
Late gummatous:	1	1	100
Infection: rickettsial			
Q fever:	8	7	88
Infection: chlamydial			
Psittacosis:	1	1	100
Infection: viral			
Cytomegalovirus:	9	5	56
Infectious mononucleosis:	21	10	48
Infection: protozoal			
Toxoplasmosis:	4	2	50
Infection: mycotic			
Coccidioidomycosis:	1	1	100
Cryptococcosis:	1	0	0
Histoplasmosis:	5	4	80
Infection: parasitic			
Schistosomiasis:	27	20	74
Visceral larva migrans:	2	2	100
Collagen-vascular disease			
Giant cell arteritis:	2	2	100
Polymyalgia rheumatica:	1	1	100
Juvenile rheumatoid arthritis:	12	4	33
Gastrointestinal disease			
Ulcerative colitis:	32	2	6
Crohn's disease:	13	2	15
Histiocytic disease			
Eosinophilic granuloma of lung:	2	1	50
Immunologic disorders			
Chronic granulomatous disease:	1	1	100
Erythema nodosum:	41	37	90
Industrial and environmental disorders			
Berylliosis:	3	3	100
Neoplasms			
Extrahepatic Hodgkin's disease:	?	14	?
Extrahepatic carcinoma:	?	11	?
Psoriasis:	98	11	11
Reactions to foreign bodies			
Starch:	?	1	?
Talc (i.v. drug addicts):	190	1	1

Despite the presence of numerous granulomas in the liver, as evidenced by the frequency with which they can be detected by needle biopsy, most cases of hepatic sarcoidosis are asymptomatic, and less than a quarter exhibit hepatomegaly or mild functional abnormalities. However, occasionally, the lesions give rise to jaundice (12), other signs of hepatic failure, portal hypertension (13), or progress to cirrhosis (14).

The Kveim reaction is positive in approximately 85% of patients with sarcoidosis, and is generally regarded as diagnostic of the disease (15). However, reliable antigen is no longer

Table 22-2. Hepatic granulomas in "primary" liver disease: incidence in Yale series

DISEASE	NO. PATIENTS WITH DISEASE	NO. PATIENTS WITH GRANULOMAS	% PATIENTS WITH GRANULOMAS
Cirrhosis			
Primary biliary:	178	73	41
Alcoholic:	778	38	5
Postnecrotic:	258	7	3
Other types:	226	11	5
Hepatitis			
Drug-induced:	205	17	4
Chronic, unknown etiology:	94	4	4
Viral, acute and chronic:	712	13	2
Toxic:	49	0	0
Other types:	151	0	0
Biliary tract disease			
Pericholangitis, acute or chronic:	172	12	7
Extrahepatic obstruction:	366	9	2
Intrahepatic neoplasms			
Carcinoma, primary or metastatic:	445	2	<1
Lymphoma:	69	1	1
Miscellaneous hepatic lesions:	1878	3	<1

available, produces false-positive reactions in 1 to 2% of non-sarcoidal controls, and tends to lose its reactivity late in the course of sarcoidosis, even when the disease is still active.

Most patients with sarcoidosis exhibit some degree of anergy, as evidenced by failure of the skin to react to tuberculin, mumps or trichophyton antigen. Although a weakly positive tuberculin reaction may be seen in some cases, a strongly positive reaction makes sarcoidosis highly improbable (16,17).

A high proportion of patients with active sarcoidosis exhibit raised serum levels of angiotensin-converting enzyme (ACE) (18). The level tends to parallel the activity of the disease, the total body granuloma load, and the activity of the disease (19). Although a high serum ACE level tends to support a diagnosis of sarcoidosis, it may be encountered in other forms of liver disease (20), and, therefore, is not a reliable diagnostic criterion (21).

Histologic features. Most of the hepatic granulomas found in sarcoidosis are round or oval in shape, and are made up of a sharply circumscribed, compact mass of epithelioid cells interspersed with occasional giant cells and few or no inflammatory cells (Fig. 345). However, not infrequently, some of the lesions are less well defined and contain loosely arranged epithelioid cells infiltrated and surrounded by numerous lymphocytes and a smaller but variable number of histiocytes and plasma cells (Fig. 346).

Although most of the granulomas are found in portal tracts (Figs. 345, 346), they may occur anywhere within the lobules. Rarely, they are encountered within the walls of central or portal veins, compressing and partially occluding their lumens (Fig. 392). Such vascular lesions may contribute to the development of the portal hypertension reported in some cases (14).

Usually, the giant cells are of the Langhans type, but occasionally, they are filled with innumerable nuclei (Fig. 345), a feature more common in sarcoidosis than in other granulomatous diseases. Often, the cytoplasm of the giant cells contains numerous vacuoles, and, rarely, asteroid bodies, stellate crystalline inclusions that have no diagnositic significance. Schau-

mann bodies, concentric laminated calcific inclusions that are occasionally found in sarcoidal lymph nodes, have not been reported in the liver. None was present in any of our own 231 cases.

Most sarcoidal hepatic granulomas contain a fine meshwork of randomly distributed reticulin fibers that tends to be condensed around the periphery of the lesions. However, in some, reticulin fibers are absent, presumably having been destroyed. In our opinion this pattern has no diagnostic significance, although others regard it as a feature more consistent with tuberculosis than sarcoidosis.

Sarcoidal lesions never exhibit caseation necrosis, but, particularly when large, often contain foci of fibrinoid necrosis (Fig. 347).

As the granulomas grow older, they tend to undergo fibrosis, and may ultimately be replaced by circumscribed, hyalinized scars. However, more often, small lesions are encircled by a band of collagen, while larger lesions show fibrosis that is patchy and irregular in distribution (Fig. 347). Although the evidence is not conclusive, our own experience with serial biopsies in a few cases suggests that some small granulomas in sarcoidosis resolve without residual scarring.

When the lesions are extensive, adjacent portal tracts may be expanded and bridged by granulomatous and fibrous tissue (Figs 83, 84). Rarely, in such cases, the lesions may be progressive and lead to the development of cirrhosis, as reported by others (14,22) and seen in 7 of our 231 cases (3%) (Fig. 724). In one reported case (22), a patient with chronic intrahepatic cholestasis, the cirrhosis was biliary in type and attributed to destruction of intrahepatic bile ducts by granulomas. A paucity of intrahepatic bile ducts was not noted in the other cases of cirrhosis, all of which were classified as postnecrotic.

Two of our patients with sarcoidosis and hepatic granulomas exhibited abnormalities in the epithelium lining one of their interlobular ducts identical with those described in primary biliary cirrhosis (Fig. 376). In neither case were these abnormalities associated with chronic cholestasis, cirrhosis, or the presence of mitochondrial antibody. One of the abnormal ducts was in contact with a large granuloma (Fig. 376), but the other was found in a portal tract free of granulomas (Fig. 377). This suggests that the ductal changes in sarcoidosis are not necessarily the result of granulomatous invasion, but may be attributable to some other facet of its pathogenesis similar to that in primary biliary cirrhosis.

In addition to granulomas, the liver in sarcoidosis frequently exhibits a number of nonspecific abnormalities, including foci of hypertrophied, proliferating Kupffer cells, scattered intralobular collections of lymphocytes, occasional degenerating or necrotic hepatocytes, and varying degrees of fibrosis and infiltrating lymphocytes and histiocytes in some of the portal tracts.

Diagnostic criteria in sarcoidosis of the liver. Hepatic granulomas in sarcoidosis exhibit no distinctive features that permit identification of their etiology on histologic grounds alone. Accordingly, in all cases, other known causes of noncaseating granulomas, especially tuberculosis, brucellosis, histoplasmosis, and berylliosis, must be excluded. In addition, consideration must be given to the accompanying clinical and laboratory features that tend to support the diagnosis. The differentiation between sarcoidosis and primary biliary cirrhosis may be especially difficult (23,24). The investigation should include:

1. Ziehl-Neelsen and Grocott (silver methenamine) staining of the biopsy specimen to ensure the absence of acid-fast bacilli and fungi; 2. in appropriate febrile cases, blood cultures to exclude brucellosis; 3. a careful occupational and environmental history to exclude exposure to beryllium compounds; 4. a search for evidence that some of the other tissues commonly affected in sarcoidosis are involved, in particular, hilar adenopathy or pulmonary infiltration in a roentgenogram of the chest, peripheral lymphadenopathy, skin lesions, enlargement of the salivary or lachrymal glands, and signs of iridocyclitis or keratoconjunctivitis on ophthalmoscopic and slit-lamp examination; 5. skin tests with tuberculin, mumps or trichophyton antigen for evidence of anergy. Although a weakly positive tuberculin reaction may be encountered in sarcoidosis, a strongly positive reaction is inconsistent with the diagnosis.; 6. measurement of the serum level of angiotensin-converting enzyme, which, if elevated, supports but does not establish the diagnosis; 7. a Kveim test, if reliable antigen is available.

As a rule, granulomas limited to the liver are not regarded as acceptable evidence of sarcoidosis, unless accompanied by a positive Kveim reaction. However, it has been found that in some Kveim-negative patients with granulomas apparently limited to the liver, typical sarcoidal lesions can be demonstrated by laparotomy in mesenteric nodes or the spleen. Thus, failure to demonstrate involvement of other tissues on routine examination does not exclude the possibility that some granulomas apparently limited to the liver may occasionally be found in true sarcoidosis, even if the Kveim reaction is negative. (Since specific Kveim antigen is rarely available at present, these points are primarily of historic interest.)

A familial form of granulomatous hepatitis of unknown etiology has been reported (25). The authors believe that it probably represents sarcoidosis, which may also be familial.

Mycobacterial infections

Tuberculosis. Hepatic granulomas are relatively common in all forms of tuberculosis (26), presumably as a result of hematogenous spread of tubercle bacilli. In our own series of 174 cases,

granulomas were demonstrable in the liver by needle biopsy in 76 (44%). The highest incidence was found in acute disseminated (miliary) tuberculosis (18/20, 90%) and in "primary" miliary tuberculosis of the liver (7/7, 100%); and the lowest in tuberculous meningitis (1/9, 11%). As might be anticipated, hepatic granulomas were encountered more frequently in patients with clinical evidence of multiple tissue involvement (36/42, 86%) than in those with solitary tissue involvement (40/132, 30%). Similarly, the frequency of hepatic granulomas was higher in patients with active pulmonary tuberculosis (30/79, 38%) than in those with arrested pulmonary lesions (4/32, 13%).

Except in the case of miliary tuberculosis and primary miliary tuberculosis of the liver, most tuberculous hepatic granulomas are asymptomatic, although some may be accompanied by hepatomegaly and mild functional abnormalities if complicated by fatty infiltration, congestion, or amyloidosis.

In addition to fever, sweats, weight loss, and radiologic evidence of disseminated pulmonary infiltration, hepatomegaly and jaundice are relatively common features in acute disseminated tuberculosis.

Primary miliary tuberculosis of the liver is a disorder characterized by massive seeding of the liver by tubercle bacilli in the absence of clinical evidence of a primary focus of infection or apparent involvement of other tissues, although such foci are almost always easily demonstrable at autopsy, particularly in the spleen and intraabdominal lymph nodes. Except for the absence of miliary pulmonary lesions and the more frequent occurrence of splenomegaly, the clinical manifestations are similar to those in acute disseminated miliary tuberculosis. If left untreated, the infection tends to spread and frequently gives rise to miliary tubercles in the lungs, [pleurae lymph glands or meningitis.

Although there are occasional exceptions, most hepatic granulomas attributable to tuberculosis are accompanied by a strongly positive tuberculin reaction.

The *histologic features* of tuberculous hepatic granulomas are remarkably similar to those of sarcoidosis. Although *caseation necrosis* is generally regarded as a hallmark of tuberculous involvement in other tissues, it occurs only rarely in the liver. Indeed, it was encountered only once in the numerous granulomas found in our 76 patients with well-documented tuberculosis (Fig. 348). Occasionally, some of the lesions contain foci of fibrinoid necrosis of variable size (Fig. 349) that are indistinguishable from those of sarcoidosis, or are devoid of necrotic areas (Fig. 350).

Acid-fast bacilli demonstrable on Ziehl-Neelsen staining are virtually diagnostic of tuberculosis. The epidemic of AIDS, however, has changed this long-held criterion, since atypical tuberculosis caused by *M. avium intracellulare* and othr mycobacteria frequently shows mayriads of acid-fast bacilli (see Chapter 27). However, they are detectable in a small minority of cases, and in only 10% in our own series. Culture of the biopsy specimen for tubercle bacilli may be a more effective method for documenting the etiology. However, in the small number of our own cases in which both methods were performed, culture was no more successful than staining for this purpose. Unfortunately, tuberculous hepatic lesions often are encountered unexpectedly in fixed sections, so the opportunity to carry out cultural studies has been lost. As a result, adequate data on the relative efficacy of the staining and cultural methods for detecting tubercle bacilli in liver biopsy specimens are not available. However, experience with other tissues and body fluids suggest that the cultural method is superior.

According to some authorities, other features that favor a tuberculous etiology over a sarcoidal etiology in hepatic granulomas include a predominantly intralobular location, ill-defined irregular contours, an intense lymphocytic inflammatory reaction, many foci of degeneration and necrosis, and destruction of reticulin. In our own experience, none of these criteria is reliable for differentiating tuberculous from sarcoidal hepatic lesions.

Except in the case of granulomas that contain acid-fast bacilli, the diagnosis of tuberculosis depends on the demonstration of tubercle bacilli in other tissues, a strongly positive tuberculin reaction, and clinical features, including the response to specific therapy, that are consistent with the disease.

As in sarcoidosis, the liver in tuberculosis frequently exhibits nonspecific changes, including foci of enlarged, proliferating Kupffer cells, scattered groups of parenchymal and portal lymphocytes, and occasional degenerating or necrotic hepatocytes. In addition, when the disease is advanced, it frequently is accompanied by fatty infiltration and congestion, and, rarely, by amyloidosis.

Bacillus Calmette-Guérin (BCG). Vaccination with the live, attenuated strain of mycobacteria known as BCG (26) for prophylaxis against tuberculosis or, more commonly, in immunotherapy of melanoma, often leads to dissemination of the organisms and the development of granulomas in various tissues, including the liver. Occasionally, it gives rise to granulomatous hepatitis (27).

Most of the hepatic granulomas resemble those of sarcoidosis. However, occasionally, some of the lesions exhibit central caseation necrosis or contain mycobacteria that can be demonstrated by acid-fast staining or recovered on culture.

Atypical (unclassified, anonymous) mycobacteria. Rarely, atypical mycobacteria, particularly the photochromagens *M. kansasii* and *M. avium-intracellulare* (Battey), give rise to disseminated infections that produce granulomas in many tissues, including the liver (28,29). Most reported cases have occurred in young children, and only occasionally in adults, except in AIDS (see Chapter 27).

Atypical mycobacteria, especially *M. avium-intracellulare,* are commonly recovered from granulomas in the acquired immune deficiency syndrome (AIDS) (30). The hepatic granulomas caused by atypical mycobacteria are said to resemble those of tuberculosis. However, while the lesions often contain small foci of necrosis, they rarely exhibit caseation and usually resemble sarcoidal granulomas. In atypical mycobacterial infection the clinical features and the hepatic granulomas are similar to those of sarcoidosis (see Chapter 27).

Leprosy. Hematogenous spread of *Mycobacterium leprae* is relatively common, and frequently leads to the development of hepatic granulomas (31–33). Such lesions are demonstrable by liver biopsy in most cases of lepromatous leprosy, but in only 20% of those with the tuberculoid form of the disease. The higher incidence of hepatic granulomas in patients with lepromatous disease is attributable to their lack of immunity to infection with *M. leprae,* which permits unlimited growth of the organisms, and their tendency to enter the circulation more frequently and in larger numbers.

The hepatic granulomas in tuberculoid leprosy closely resemble those of sarcoidosis, and are made up of compact masses of epithelioid and giant cells that contain few if any acid-fast bacilli. In contrast, the granulomas in lepromatous leprosy are characterized by aggregates of large, pale, foamy histiocytes (lepra cells) that contain numerous acid-fast bacilli. Often, such histiocytic granulomas are accompanied by lepra cells and swollen Kupffer cells that contain *M. leprae* scattered through the lobules. Viable *M. leprae* may persist in the liver long after they have disappeared from the skin lesions following prolonged therapy with dapsone, and may account for relapses of the disease after treatment is stopped.

Secondary amyloidosis is an occasional finding at autopsy in cases of leprosy.

In addition to granulomas, the liver in leprosy often exhibits nonspecific changes, usually due to intercurrent, unrelated diseases. In Taiwan, for example, where the HBsAg-carrier rate is very high (34), it is even higher in patients with leprosy. It has been postulated that leprosy may suppress immunologic reactivity.

The hepatic granulomas in leprosy produce no clinical manifestations, but may give rise to mild degrees of hepatic dysfunction.

Other bacterial infections

Brucellosis. *Brucella abortus* infections (35–38) frequently affect the liver, and may be manifested by hepatomegaly, splenomegaly, hepatic dysfunction, and, rarely, by jaundice and ascites. In chronic infections, cultures of the liver yield *B. abortus* when the organisms are no longer demonstrable in the blood.

In most *B. abortus* infections, the liver contains granulomas that resemble sarcoidal or tuberculous lesions. They may present as sharply circumscribed, compact masses of epithelioid and giant cells (Fig. 725), or as larger, irregular lesions that exhibit central zones of necrosis surrounded by epithelioid and giant cells and a variable number of other inflammatory cells (Fig. 726). In addition to, and, occasionally, instead of granulomas, the lesions may be characterized by a number of nonspecific changes, including scattered foci of hepatocellular necrosis, proliferation of Kupffer cells, intralobular and portal lymphocytic infiltrates, and a variable degree of portal fibrosis. Usually these granulomas are noncaseating (37), especially when the disease is less than three months in duration (38).

Usually, following recovery, the hepatic lesions of brucellosis resolve without significant residuals. However, in rare instances, prolonged or recurrent *B. abortus* infection may lead to progressive fibrosis and the development of cirrhosis.

B. suis is a more invasive organism than *B. abortus,* and only rarely provokes a granulomatous reaction in the liver (39). Occasionally, however, it gives rise to abscesses in the liver and spleen that tend to undergo calcification (40).

The hepatic lesions in *B. melitensis* infections are characterized by scattered foci of inflammatory cells and necrotic hepatocytes, but contain no granulomas (41).

Tularemia. Dissemination of *Franciscella tularensis,* previously known as *Pasteurella,* leads to injury in many tissues, including the liver (42–44). Hepatic lesions are demonstrable at autopsy in most fatal cases of tularemia. The incidence of such lesions in nonfatal infections is not known, but is probably low, since overt manifestations of liver disease, such as jaundice, hepatomegaly, and ascites, are relatively uncommon in survivors.

Early hepatic lesions, encountered during the first two weeks of infection, are characterized by foci of hepatocellular necrosis infiltrated with large mononuclear cells and, occasionally, by neutrophils. Later, they present as granulomas that contain a central zone of necrosis surrounded by radially arranged epithelioid cells and fibroblasts enclosed with a collar of lymphocytes and Langhans giant cells. In some lesions, the zones of necrosis are caseating in character.

Granuloma inguinale. Rarely, the gram-negative bacillus *Donovania granulomatis* (Donovan body), responsible for the venereal disease granuloma inguinale, may induce a fatal disseminated infection that affects many tissues, including the liver (45,46). In such cases, the hepatic lesions are characterized by multiple microabscesses filled with foamy macrophages that contain Donovan bodies.

Donovan bodies are difficult to visualize in formalin-fixed H & E-stained sections, but are readily identified in Warthin-Sperry silver-stained sections *or* in unfixed crushed sections stained by the Wright-Giemsa method. Characteristically, the organisms are approximately 1 μm in length and show bipolar staining, giving them the appearance of safety pins.

Listeriosis. As a rule, infections with *Listeria monocytogenes* present as a febrile illness with signs of meningitis, encephalitis or sepsis, and only rarely as a syndrome that resembles infectious mononucleosis (47–49).

The neonatal form of septicemic listeriosis, acquired either transplacentally or in the birth canal, often presents with jaundice and hepatosplenomegaly, and invariably proves fatal. Characteristically, many of the tissues, including the liver, contain numerous miliary lesions that resemble tubercles, so the disease is commonly termed "granulomatosis infantiseptica." However, many of the "tubercles" represent microabscesses rather than granulomas, although some do contain necrotizing granulomas (50,51). Occasionally, large hepatic abscesses develop (52).

Rarely, in adults, chronic *L. monocytogenes* sepsis gives rise to splenic and hepatic caseating granulomas that are indistinguishable from those of tuberculosis (51,53).

Spirochetal infection: syphilis

Granulomas may be encountered in the liver at any stage of active syphilis. In some cases, the etiology of such lesions can be identified by the demonstration of *Treponema pallidum* in silver-stained sections, but more often this is unsuccessful, so that usually the diagnosis depends on the results of serologic tests or the detection of *Treponema pallidum* by dark-field examination of aspirates from lesions in the skin or mucous membranes.

Congenital syphilis. Intrauterine *Treponema pallidum* infections of the fetus tend to be severe and frequently lead to abortion or stillbirth (54,55).

Severely infected newborns who survive may appear normal at birth, but usually exhibit evidence of widespread syphilitic involvement of the tissues within a few weeks. In those with less severe infections, manifestations of congenital syphilis, usually of more limited distribution, may not appear until several years later. Many infants with congenital syphilis exhibit

hepatosplenomegaly. Overt jaundice is relatively uncommon, but occasionally it is intense and suggests some form of neonatal hepatitis.

In fatal cases of congenital hepatic syphilis, the liver shows fine, diffuse fibrosis that extends from the portal tracts into the lobules, disrupting the hepatic plates and encircling individual or groups of hepatocytes, producing a type of interstitial cirrhosis. The fibrous tissue is infiltrated with numerous lymphocytes and plasma cells and usually contains multiple small, necrotizing granulomas, often classified as gummas. In addition to their dissociation by fibrous bands, the hepatocytes show atrophy and degeneration in some areas and foci of cell dropout. Occasionally, some of the hepatocytes are transformed into multinucleated giant cells as in other forms of neonatal hepatitis. In some cases, the arterioles in the portal tracts show a chronic inflammatory reaction in their walls. Characteristically, in silver-stained sections, numerous spirochetes are demonstrable in the fibrous septa, walls of blood vessels, and hepatocytes.

In less severely infected infants who present with features of neonatal hepatitis, jaundice and hepatosplenomegaly recede following penicillin therapy. The character of the hepatic lesions in such cases and their residuals following therapy, if any, have not been reported.

Occasionally, untreated, asymptomatic, congenital syphilis gives rise to hepatic gummas that are discovered only after a delay of many years.

Early acquired (secondary) syphilis. Occasionally, the rash, mucosal lesions, and lymphadenopathy of secondary syphilis are accompanied by an acute hepatitis with or without jaundice (56). In many respects, the clinical and biochemical features resemble those of acute viral hepatitis. However, the serum levels of alkaline phosphatase tend to be significantly higher and those of transaminase lower in syphilitic than in viral hepatitis of comparable severity.

The hepatic lesions in acute syphilitic hepatitis are nonspecific and variable in character. Usually, they exhibit the following features in various combinations: (1) infiltration of the portal tracts with lymphocytes, histiocytes, neutrophils, and a few eosinophils; (2) foci of hepatocellular necrosis and cell dropout that contain similar inflammatory cells and are most prominent in the centrilobular zones; (3) focal destruction of reticulin in some of the zones of necrosis; (4) acute and chronic inflammation that involves the walls of arterioles and veins (57); (5) swelling and proliferation of Kupffer cells; and (6) sarcoid-like epithelioid granulomas (58,59). Although such granulomas are relatively common in the skin lesions of secondary syphilis (60) and may be more widely disseminated, they have been encountered only rarely in biopsy specimens of liver in cases of acute syphilitic hepatitis (61). Usually, spirochetes are scanty or absent in silver-stained sections. However, in one report, they were demonstrable in 7 out of 15 cases (56). They may be seen more readily by means of flourescent treponemal antibody absorbtion staining (56a).

Characteristically, the lesions of syphilitic hepatitis are rapidly reversible following penicillin therapy.

Syphilitic hepatitis was reported 16 months after kidney transplantation in a patient who was receiving cyclosporine, azathioprine, and prednisone (62). The patient exhibited mild jaundice and fever, hepatosplenomegaly, hepatic tenderness, greatly elevated serum alkaline phosphatase levels, and mild increments in transaminase activity. Serologic tests for syphilis (rapid plasma reagin and a microhemoagglutination assay for

T. pallidum) were positive. There were no skin lesions except for a healing chancre. There were no hepatic granulomas. The degree of inflammation in this patient appeared to be less severe than one would expect in a nonimmunocompromised patient (Fig. 727). Conceivably, the immunosuppression may have suppressed both dermatologic lesions and granuloma formation. Spirochetes were seen by dark-field examination of his liver tissue and confirmed by immunofluorescence staining (Fig. 728) using a specific antiserum for *T. pallidum.* The patient responded to penicillin therapy with a Jarisch-Herxheimer reaction and disappearance of his hepatic disease.

Late (tertiary) syphilis. The characteristic hepatic lesion of late, untreated syphilis (63,64) is the gumma of a focal granuloma that tends to undergo central caseation necrosis followed by fibrous encapsulation and diffuse fibrosis, ultimately giving rise to a depressed, contracted, stellate scar. The lesions vary in size from microscopic to grossly visible, large nodules, and usually are multiple in number and irregular in distribution. When the gummas are numerous and widely distributed, they distort the contours of the liver as they undergo fibrosis, forming coarse, irregular nodules of parenchyma separated by broad, deeply depressed scars, a lesion usually classified as *hepar lobatum.*

In most cases, hepatic gummas are asymptomatic. Occasionally, however, they give rise to abdominal pain and fever, which abate following antiluetic therapy. Rarely, hepar lobatum is complicated by jaundice, ascites, and signs of portal hypertension.

Early gummas are characterized by a central zone of necrosis surrounded by a dense infiltrate of lymphocytes, plasma cells, histiocytes, and a variable number of epithelioid and giant cells. As the lesions undergo progressive fibrosis, they are replaced by relatively broad scars that contain fewer inflammatory cells (Fig. 566). However, even in late hepar lobatum, occasional ill-defined granulomas may still be demonstrable (Fig. 567)).

Rickettsial infection: Q fever

Rickettsial infections due to *Coxiella burnetii,* or Q fever, usually present as an acute, febrile illness with signs of pneumonitis. However, in many cases, the liver is affected, giving rise to hepatosplenomegaly, alterations in hepatic structure and function, and, occasionally, to overt jaundice (65–68a), features that may occur with or without accompanying pneumonitis. The hepatic manifestations of Q fever may be mistaken for those of acute viral hepatitis, particularly in the absence of pneumonitis, unless tests for complement-fixing or agglutinating antibodies to *C. burnetii* are carried out. In some cases, the correct diagnosis may be suggested by the liver biopsy findings, but these always require serologic confirmation, since they are not pathognomonic.

The principal features of the hepatic lesions in Q fever hepatitis include: (1) granulomas; (2) scattered foci of hepatocellular necrosis infiltrated with neutrophils, mononuclear cells, histiocytes, and proliferating Kupffer cells; (3) occasional acidophilic bodies; (4) mild to moderate fatty infiltration; and (5) infiltration of the portal tracts with a variable number of neutrophils, lymphocytes, eosinophils, and histiocytes.

Hepatic granulomas are relatively common in Q fever, and often exhibit features that suggest the diagnosis, although they are not necessarily pathognomonic (68–71). Such distinctive granulomas, termed *ring lesions,* are characterized by a central, lipid-filled vacuole surrounded by a collar of histiocytic, epithelioid, or giant cells, occasionally interspersed with other inflammatory cells, and enclosed within a sharply defined, round or oval-shaped ring of fragmented fibrinoid material (Fig. 221). The fibrinoid ring may be difficult to visualize in routine H & E sections, but appears bright red in Masson-stained sections. Occasionally, serial sections are required to demonstrate the central lipid vacuole. In one reported series based on a study of serial sections, typical *"ring lesions"* were demonstrated in 14 of 17 cases of well-documented Q fever (68). By contrast, in the absence of serial sections, they were encountered in only 2 of the 8 cases submitted to us for review.

In addition to, or instead of ring lesions, the liver in Q fever may contain less distinctive granulomas made up of epithelioid and giant cells, occasionally interspersed with other inflammatory cells and fragments of fibrinoid material (Fig. 729). These may resemble sarcoidal or tuberculous lesions.

While highly suggestive of Q fever, typical ring lesions are not pathognomonic. They have been reported in Hodgkin's disease (68), in infectious mononucleosis, in Epstein-Barr virus infection (72), in visceral leishmaniasis (73), and in allopurinol-induced hepatotoxicity (74). Attempts to confirm the occurrence of fibrin rings in allopurinol-induced hepatic injury failed to show such lesions (75). We have encountered them in six patients with fatty infiltration of the liver associated with chronic alcoholism in three, and in one patient each with erythema nodosum, giant cell arteritis, and tuberculosis. Although all six of these patients were febrile, serial serologic studies failed to demonstrate evidence of *Coxiella burnetii* infection in any. Figure 222 illustrates one of these nonspecific ring lesions in a chronic alcoholic with fatty infiltration of the liver.

Although rickettsia cannot be identified in the hepatic lesions of Q fever on routine microscopy, they may be demonstrable by direct immunofluorescent antibody microscopy (75a).

Chlamydial infections

Lymphogranuloma venereum. Lymphogranuloma venereum, a venereal disease due to infection with one of the subtypes of *Chlamydia trachomatis* (76), is characterized by granulomatous inflammatory lesions that involve the genitalia and perirectal region and granulomatous destruction of the inguinal lymph nodes. There is no convincing evidence of liver involvement with granulomas in patients with lymphogranuloma venereum.

These organisms sometimes cause peritonitis and perihepatitis known as the Fitz-Hugh-Curtis syndrome (77,78), which is generally considered to be a sexually transmitted disease. This syndrome is more common in women and has been attributed to transfallopian passage of the parasites (79), but this pathogenesis is not an acceptable explanation for its occurrence in men (80).

Hepatic granulomas have been reported in two cases of lymphogranuloma venereum (62). However, the relationship of these granulomas to chlamydial infections is in doubt, since one of the patients had Hodgkin's disease and the other had brucellosis. Moreover, in another study, biopsy of the liver in four patients with lymphogranuloma venereum failed to demonstrate granulomas (81).

Psittacosis. Psittacosis, an infection due to *Chlamydia psittaci,* is characterized by high fever, severe constitutional symptoms, and an interstitial pneumonitis. Occasionally, the liver is involved, as evidenced by hepatomegaly, functional impairment, and, rarely, by overt jaundice (82).

As a rule, the hepatic lesions are characterized by scattered, small foci of hepatocellular necrosis, Kupffer cell proliferation, and portal lymphocytosis. In addition, the liver may contain granulomas (83). In the only well-documented case that we have seen, liver biopsy revealed a large, poorly circumscribed granuloma that showed extensive, central, fibrinoid necrosis surrounded by a zone of loosely arranged epithelioid cells, histiocytes, lymphocytes, and occasional giant cells. In many respects, the granuloma resembled a tuberculous lesion.

Viral infections

Cytomegalovirus (CMV) mononucleosis. One type of cytomegalovirus infection in adults produces an acute, febrile illness with lymphocytosis and numerous atypical lymphocytes. In many cases, the fever is accompanied by splenomegaly and, less commonly, by hepatomegaly, mild jaundice, lymphadenopathy, pharyngitis, or rash. Except for the failure of the heterophil antibody titer to rise, the clinical and laboratory features resemble those of infectious mononucleosis so closely that the disorder is commonly termed *cytomegalovirus mononucleosis* (84,85). Most cases are encountered in previously healthy adults or in patients who have recently undergone cardiopulmonary bypass for cardiac surgery. However, a few have been reported following transfusion for other purposes and in leukemic patients during remission. The fever tends to be high and often is prolonged, but usually subsides spontaneously in two to six weeks.

With rare exceptions, the liver is affected in cytomegalovirus mononucleosis. As a rule, there is a slight to moderate increase in serum transaminase activity, and, in some cases, this is accompanied by slightly raised serum levels of alkaline phosphatase and bilirubin. Frequently, the liver is slightly enlarged, but hepatic tenderness and overt jaundice are relatively rare.

Usually, the hepatic lesions in cytomegalovirus mononucleosis are characterized by a prominent, diffuse, mononuclear inflammatory reaction and reticuloendothelial hyperplasia with only minimal hepatocellular necrosis. Many of the sinusoids contain clusters of lymphocytes, plasma cells, large monocytes, and swollen, proliferating Kupffer cells. In some cases, the monocytes are epithelioid in character and are aggregated in the form of circumscribed granulomas that resemble sarcoidal lesions (Fig. 730). These may or may not contain giant cells. Occasional acidophilic bodies and a few small foci of hepatocellular dropout may be found scattered through the lobules. Often, the portal tracts are infiltrated with a variable number of lymphocytes, plasma cells, and histiocytes.

Cytomegalic nuclear inclusions, which are diagnostic of cytomegalovirus infection and may be found in many tissues, particularly at autopsy, are relatively uncommon in the hepatic lesions of cytomegalovirus mononucleosis. When present, such inclusions may be found in an occasional hepatocyte (Fig. 190), bile duct epithelial cell (Fig. 191), or, rarely, in a Kupffer cell. Characteristically, the involved cell is enlarged and contains within its nucleus a large, reddish blue inclusion surrounded by a clear halo.

The clinical features and liver biopsy findings in cytomegalovirus mononucleosis, except for the occasional presence of cytomegalic nuclear inclusions, are similar to those in infectious mononucleosis and toxoplasmosis mononucleosis. In addition, particularly when atypical lymphocytosis is not a prominent feature or the hepatic lesions show more extensive necrosis than is usual, the disease may be mistaken for acute viral hepatitis. Differentiation between these disorders usually depends on appropriate serologic or cultural studies. In the case of cytomegalovirus infection, these entail the demonstration of a rising titer of specific complement-fixing or immunofluorescent IgM antibody, or isolation in cultures of human embryonic fibroblasts of the virus from urine, throat washing, or livers biopsy material.

Infectious mononucleosis. Infectious mononucleosis (86–89), an acute, febrile illness due to infection with the Epstein-Barr virus, is manifested clinically by pharyngitis, lymphadenopathy, and splenomegaly. Characteristically, it is accompanied by lymphocytosis with a high proportion of distinctive atypical lymphocytes and the appearance in the serum of heterophil agglutinin and specific IgM antibodies to the Epstein-Barr virus. The liver is affected in most infections of this type, as evidenced by alterations in hepatic function and structure. However, jaundice, hepatomegaly, and other features suggestive of an acute hepatitis occur in only 10% of cases. Usually, the unfection is self-limited, but rare instances of fatal, massive hepatic necrosis have been reported.

The outstanding feature of the hepatic lesions in infectious mononucleosis is an extensive, intense, mononuclear inflammatory reaction that involves both the parenchyma and portal tracts, and is out of proportion to the degree of hepatocellular necrosis. Characteristically, the sinusoids contain numerous large mononuclear cells, foci of swollen, proliferating Kupffer cells, and a variable number of lymphocytes and plasma cells. As shown in Figure 218, the monocytes and Kupffer cells may distend the lumens of the sinusoids in some areas, leading to atrophy and interruption of the intervening hepatic plates. Scattered through the lobules are occasional acidophilic bodies and small foci of hepatocellular dropout, usually filled with proliferating Kupffer cells. Although seldom mentioned in published reports (71), small, sharply circumscribed epithelioid cell granulomas may be encountered within the lobules in the majority of the cases (5). Lesions of this type, which resemble sarcoidal granulomas, were found in 10 of our 21 cases (Fig. 731). Another feature of note is the prominence of hepatocellular regenerative activity, as evidenced by the presence of numerous mitotic figures and binucleate cells and prominent pleomorphism, out of proportion to the degree of necrosis. Canalicular bile thrombi are unusual, but may be encountered in cases with overt jaundice.

Usually, the portal tracts are densely infiltrated with lymphocytes, monocytes, and histiocytes, occasionally interspersed with a variable number of plasma cells, eosinophils, and epithelioid cells. In severe lesions, some of the portal tracts may be expanded, contain proliferating ductules, and show erosion of their limiting plates.

In some cases, differentiation between the hepatic lesions of infectious mononucleosis and acute viral hepatitis may be difficult. Usually, however, the striking diffuse mononuclear inflammatory reaction and the prominence of hepatocellular mitotic activity and Kupffer cell hyperplasia out of proportion to the extent of hepatic necrosis favor infectious mononucleosis.

Similarly, as previously indicated, the lesions may closely

resemble those produced by some forms of cytomegalovirus infection and toxoplasmosis.

In the last analysis, identification of infectious mononucleosis depends on the demonstration of a rising titer of heterophil agglutinin or specific IgM antibodies to the Epstein-Barr virus.

Varicella. Hepatic granulomas have been reported in a nonfatal case of varicella in an adult (91). The infection was accompanied by fever, hepatic tenderness, and minimally raised serum levels of bilirubin, alkaline phosphatase, and transaminase. Liver biopsy revealed two granulomas, one made up of epithelioid cells interspersed with a few eosinophils and neutrophils, the other composed of both epithelioid and giant cells and showing a central zone of necrosis. There was no evidence of parenchymal necrosis or inflammation, and no nuclear inclusions could be identified.

Protozoal infection: (Toxoplasmosis)

Toxoplasma gondii infections acquired during adult life frequently produce an acute, febrile illness with atypical lymphocytosis and other clinical features that resemble those of infectious mononucleosis, except for the absence of heterophil (Epstein-Barr) antibody (92). Less commonly, the illness is associated with jaundice and other manifestations suggestive of acute viral hepatitis (93). Occasionally, it may present as cholestatic jaundice (94).

Usually, the hepatic lesions in acquired toxoplasmosis resemble those of infectious mononucleosis and may include small, sharply circumscribed, epithelioid granulomas scattered through the lobules. Such granulomas were present in two of our four cases, and have been reported by others (95). Occasionally, in cases with overt jaundice, hepatocellular necrosis may be more prominent. In such cases the lesions resemble those of acute viral hepatitis (93).

Only scant numbers of toxoplasma organisms are found in the hepatic lesions, and they are difficult to identify in routinely stained sections. However, they are readily demonstrable by immunofluorescence. In one of our cases, rare *T. gondii* were found in Kupffer cells in an H & E-stained section of liver (Fig. 253). Their identity was confirmed in a Giemsa-stained smear of the peritoneal exudate of a mouse injected intraperitoneally with a fragment of the same liver biopsy specimen (Fig. 254). For a more detailed description and illustrations of *T. gondii,* the reader is referred to a classic monograph on tropical diseases (96).

Since the organism may be difficult to identify and tissue is often not available for inoculation into mice, the diagnosis of toxoplasmosis usually depends on the demonstration of a rising titer of antibody to *T. gondii.*

Mycotic infections

Blastomycosis

North American blastomycosis (Gilchrist's disease). The primary lesions in *Blastomyces dermatiditis* infections are found in the skin or lungs (97). Dissemination of the infection to other tissues, including the liver, is relatively common in the pulmonary type.

The hepatic lesions are characterized by multiple caseating granulomas that resemble those of tuberculosis. Often, they undergo suppuration, forming abscesses with giant cells in their walls.

The infecting organisms, which can be found in both the granulomas and abscesses, are well visualized in silver methenamine (Grocott)–stained sections. These present as round or oval cells, 7 to 20 μm in diameter, enclosed within thick membranes that are highly refractile, giving the appearance of double-contoured capsules. Often, some of the organisms show budding.

Brazilian blastomycosis (paracoccidioidomycosis). Infections with *Paracoccidioides brasiliensis* start in the oral mucosa, spread to regional lymph nodes, and, in some cases, are disseminated to other tissues, including the liver (98). The hepatic lesions are characterized by granulomas composed of epithelioid and foreign body giant cells that contain the infecting organisms and that are predominantly portal in distribution. Occasionally, the portal tracts contain numerous lymphocytes and eosinophils, and may show progressive fibrosis.

The organisms are readily demonstrable in silver methenamine (Grocott)–stained sections. They present as round structures, 5 to 20 μm in diameter, enclosed within thick, double-contoured membranes. Usually, they show budding or are surrounded by a ring of small, spheric daughter cells.

Coccidioidomycosis. In the Southwest of the United States, and in some parts of South America, *Coccidioides immitis* infections are relatively common, usually presenting as a self-limited, benign, febrile illness characterized by pneumonitis, often accompanied by hilar adenopathy and erythema nodosum, a disorder first recognized in California and termed San Joaquin valley fever (99, 100).

Dissemination of *C. immitis* from its primary focus in the lung provokes a granulomatous reaction in many tissues, including the liver, and may prove fatal.

The hepatic granulomas resemble those of sarcoidosis, but may be encircled by numerous eosinophils, and often contain PAS-positive, *C. immitis* spherules, round structures, 10 to 80 μm in diameter, with thick, double-contoured walls and filled with numerous small spores. In some cases, similar spherules and spores are found within parenchymal microabscesses.

Cryptococcosis (torulosis). *Cryptococcus neoformans,* a yeast-like fungus frequently found in the excreta of pigeons and, less commonly, of other birds, is pathogenic for humans (101–104). Inhalation of dust containing the organisms leads to an infection of the lungs that usually is self-limited and may be asymptomatic. In a minority of individuals, particularly those with diabetes mellitus, lymphomatous disease, or undergoing prolonged corticosteroid or other immunosuppressive therapy, the infection spreads hematogenously to other tissues, including the meninges, brain, bones, skin, and liver. Although amphotericin B therapy is effective in some cases, the mortality rate in prolonged, disseminated infections is relatively high.

Usually, the lesions produced by *C. neoformans* are characterized by circumscribed, noncaseating epithelioid and giant cell granulomas that resemble those of sarcoidosis, except for the presence in some lesions of the infecting organisms.

Primary hepatic cryptococcosis has rarely been observed (102,103). Cryptococcal hepatitis may be cholestatic, and may simulate primary sclerosing cholangitis (104).

Hepatic enlargement and functional abnormalities are relatively common in disseminated cryptococcosis, but overt jaundice or other signs of severe liver injury are infrequent. Both a mild diffuse hepatitis and fatal submassive hepatic necrosis have been reported in icteric cases. Although *C. neoformans* can be demonstrated in such lesions, the possibility of a double infection with the hepatitis virus or an underlying drug reaction could not be excluded.

Usually, cryptococci are found within epithelioid or giant cells and, less commonly, in Kupffer cells. They present as yeast-like organisms, 7 to 15 μm in diameter, enclosed within thick, doubly-refractile capsules that stain intensely with mucicarmine, Gridley's stain, or silver methenamine (Grocott) (Fig. 256). They may be difficult to identify in H & E sections, but, occasionally, as illustrated in Figure 255, are well seen. Budding forms of the organism are infrequent.

Histoplasmosis. Histoplasmosis (105–108), a granulomatous disease caused by *Histoplasma capsulatum,* a fungus found in the soil, is worldwide in distribution, but is most prevalent in the east-central region of the United States. Epidemiologic studies based on histoplasmin skin testing indicate that from 40 to 90% of individuals in the general population of endemic areas are infected, but that only a small minority of these exhibit clinical evidence of active disease.

Infection with *H. capsulatum* follows inhalation of dust containing spores of the organism. In some individuals, the onset of infection is manifested clinically by a flu-like, febrile illness accompanied by evidence of pulmonary infiltration of variable severity, distribution, and character, a syndrome usually classified as *primary acute pulmonary histoplasmosis.* Characteristically, the symptoms abate spontaneously within a few weeks or months, and the disease shows no tendency to progress. Although the pulmonary infiltrates tend to regress, residuals of the primary complexes are relatively common. These may present as calcific deposits in healed lesions that appear two or three years after the onset of infection, or as focal pulmonary lesions that still contain viable *H. capsulatum* when examined postmortem. Despite the benign course of primary pulmonary histoplasmosis, dissemination of the infection to other tissues is not rare. This is evidenced by the frequent occurrence of hilar adenopathy and the occasional recovery of *H. capsulatum* on culture of urine, blood, or bone marrow during the acute phase of the disease, and the delayed appearance of calcific deposits in healed splenic or hepatic granulomas.

Most primary infections with *H. capsulatum* are not recognized clinically at their onset, either because they are asymptomatic or because they are misinterpreted as evidence of other diseases. Usually, in such cases, the diagnosis is made retrospectively on the basis of a positive histoplasmin skin test, the presence of specific complement-fixing antibodies, or the discovery on roentgenography of residuals of primary complexes in the lungs or calcific deposits in the liver or spleen. Rarely, patients with infections of insidious onset present with one of the chronic progressive forms of histoplasmosis.

Progressive disseminated histoplasmosis, a relatively rare disorder that predominantly affects infants and young children of both sexes and men over the age of 40 years, is characterized by constitutional symptoms and a granulomatous reaction in a wide variety of tissues especially the lungs, but also lymph nodes, liver, spleen, bone marrow, adrenals, and the mucosa of the oral cavity, larynx, and gastrointestinal tract. The disease tends to be progressive, and at one time invariably proved fatal, often as a result of complicating Addison's disease secondary

to granulomatous destruction of the adrenals. However, amphotericin B therapy has proved effective in controlling the disease in most patients, although relapses of the infection are relatively common, and a significant number of treated patients still die of their disease.

The similarities between disseminated histoplasmosis and sarcoidosis have been emphasized. However, the age and sex distribution and the frequency of adrenal insufficiency and mucosal ulceration in histoplasmosis serve, in part, to differentiate it from sarcoidosis.

Chronic pulmonary histoplasmosis, another uncommon form of histoplasmosis, affects middle-aged men predominantly and closely resembles cavitary pulmonary tuberculosis both clinically and morphologically. Unless treated, the pulmonary lesions tend to progress and frequently lead to death. However, amphotericin B therapy has proved effective in controlling the disease.

Histologic evidence of hepatic involvement may be encountered in any form of active or inactive histoplasmosis. In at least half the patients with the progressive, disseminated form of the disease, the liver is enlarged and exhibits impairment of function. However, in most cases, the hepatic lesions usually produce no clinical manifestations. Jaundice and ascites are rare, even when the hepatic lesions are extensive.

Several types of hepatic lesions that often occur together in various combinations may be found in histoplasmosis. Except for those that contain histologically demonstrable spores of *H. capsulatum,* none of these lesions is diagnostic of the disease. The principal features of the lesions may include: (1) scattered, sarcoid-like, compact, circumscribed, epithelioid granulomas with or without interspersed giant cells (Fig. 732); (2) caseating granulomas that resemble those of tuberculosis (Fig. 733); (3) healed granulomas that present as sharply circumscribed, globular masses of hyalinized collagen that may contain small calcific deposits; (4) swelling and proliferation of Kupffer cells, which, in some cases, are extensive and lead to atrophy or necrosis of the intervening hepatic plates; and (5) infiltration of the portal tracts with a variable number of lymphocytes, plasma cells, and macrophages.

The spores of *H. capsulatum* present as groups of round or ovoid cells of relatively uniform size, 1 to 5 μm in diameter, that are found within Kupffer cells, giant cells, epithelioid cells, or portal macrophages. Occasionally, in large necrotic lesions, they may be extracellular in location. Numerous organisms are found in severe infections with extensive Kupffer cell hyperplasia or large necrotizing granulomas, but are rare or absent in noncaseating sarcoid-like epithelioid granulomas, and may be difficult to find in many other hepatic lesions of histoplasmosis.

The spores of *H. capsulatum* are difficult to identify and may be overlooked in H & E sections, but may present as groups of fine, red dots each encircled by a clear halo (Fig. 257). The organisms are best visualized as black or dark brown rings when stained with silver methenamine (Fig. 258). Other reagents that stain the outer membranes of *H. capsulatum* and facilitate identification include PAS and Gridley's stain.

Since the hepatic lesions in histoplasmosis are not pathognomonic and may contain no histologically demonstrable organisms, confirmation of the diagnosis usually depends on other criteria. The most reliable test is a positive culture of *H. capsulatum* from blood, bone marrow, sputum, scrapings of ulcers in the oral or laryngeal mucosa, or biopsy material from involved tissues, including the liver. If such cultures are unsuccessful, the diagnosis may depend on the demonstration of a positive histoplasmin skin test or the presence of specific complement-fixing antibody. In individuals from endemic areas, the presence of antibody may be indicative of antecedent, rather than current, infection.

Cat-scratch disease

Cat-scratch disease is a self-limited bacterial infection that can cause hepatic and splenic granulomas (109). The disease is characterized by lymphadenopathy, fever, and constitutional symptoms. It is diagnosed by a history of contact with a cat, a positive skin test, and the demonstration of characteristic histopathologic features in the absence of any other explanation.

The hepatic granulomas show central suppuration [(109,110); Fig. 734]. The organisms, which are argyrophilic, pleomorphic bacilli, 0.2 to 0.5 μm wide, and 0.8 to 2.0 μm long, can be demonstrated by Warthin-Starry stain (Fig. 735). The demonstration of the characteristic cat-scratch disease bacillus in the involved tissues is diagnostic. Although culture is possible (111), the organism is fastidious and cannot be routinely cultured.

Parasitic infections

Schistosomiasis. Schistosomiasis (108,112–115), a parasitic disease due to infection with the trematodes (blood flukes) *Schistosoma mansoni, S. japonicum, S. mekongi, S. intercalculatum,* or *S. haematobium,* is extremely common and poses a serious health problem in many parts of the world where these parasites are prevalent. Although these parasites share a similar life cycle, they differ in their geographic distribution and, to some extent, in the clinical manifestations they produce.

S. mansoni occurs in Central and South America, especially in Brazil, the Caribbean area, particularly in Puerto Rico, the Middle East, and parts of tropical and subtropical Africa. *S. intercalculatum* is found only in central Africa. The distribution of *S. japonicum* and *S. mekongi* is limited to the Far East and to Southeast Asia, respectively. *S. haematobium* is prevalent in Egypt, around the great lakes of central and East Africa, and in many islands of the Indian Ocean. Most cases of schistosomiasis in the United States are encountered in Puerto Rican immigrants with *S. mansoni* infections.

S. mansoni and *S. japonicum* affect the colon and liver, whereas *S. haematobium* involves the bladder predominantly. However, some *S. haematobium* infections also produce lesions in the colon and liver, although, usually, these are mild and asymptomatic.

Following their excretion into fresh water, each of the schistosome ova in infected feces or urine releases its enclosed miracidium, which then enters a specific snail host. In the snail, the miracidium undergoes further development, producing thousands of cercariae, fork-tailed, motile forms that are discharged into the water. Infection occurs when the cercariae penetrate the intact skin or mucous membranes of an exposed individual and enter the circulation. After passing through the lungs, the cercariae ultimately lodge in the fine intrahepatic branches of the portal vein where they undergo maturation to adult worms. On reaching maturity, paired male and female schistosomes migrate upstream through the portal vein into the inferior mesenteric vein. *S. mansoni* and *S. japonicum* continue

their migration into the submucosal plexus of veins in the colon and rectum where the females extrude their ova into terminal venules. Ultimately, many of the ova erode through the mucosa and are excreted in the feces. However, a significant number of ova are swept back into the portal vein and reach the liver where they produce hepatic lesions. Occasionally, adult *S. mansoni* worms may be found in the intrahepatic branches of the portal vein. It is not clear whether these represent worms that failed to migrate to or were swept back from the inferior mesenteric vein.

In contrast to *S. mansoni* and *S. japonicum, S. haematobium* worms in the inferior mesenteric vein migrate through venous collaterals and ultimately lodge in the submucosal plexus of veins in the bladder where the females deposit their ova. Most of the ova erode through the mucosa and are excreted in the urine.

Except for the occasional occurrence of pruritus when cercariae penetrate the skin, most cases of schistosomiasis are insidious. Usually schistosomiasis is the result of repeated, antecedent exposures to the parasites. In a small minority of cases, the initial exposure leads to an acute illness that appears to be allergic in nature. This allergic response, which is especially severe with *S. japonicum,* is known as the *Katayama syndrome* (116). The illness, which appears three to six weeks following the exposure and at a time when the young adult worms are migrating and beginning to deposit ova, is characterized by fever, severe constitutional symptoms, cough or asthma, hepatosplenomegaly, generalized lymphadenopathy, and marked eosinophilia. Usually, ova are demonstrable in the feces. Early in the course of illness, the liver exhibits extensive infiltration of eosinophils, and, later, granulomas.

The parasite may involve the majority of the population in endemic areas. Three-fourths of the inhabitants of an Egyptian village were shown to be infested, and more than one-third had hepatosplenic schistosomiasis (117).

There is convincing experimental evidence to indicate that a cell-mediated and humoral immunologic response to an antigen in schistosome ova is a major factor in the pathogenesis of the hepatic lesions in both acute and chronic schistosomiasis (114,115). The severity and extent of such lesions vary greatly and are dependent, in part at least, on the load of ova entrapped in the liver, the population of viable mature worms in the tributaries of the portal vein, and the duration of the infection.

Studies of the experimental infection of mice with schistosomal cercariae demonstrate that cyclosporin A can prevent infestation entirely or can decrease the number of surviving worms (118). Furthermore, cyclosporin A diminishes the granulomatous inflammatory response to the eggs of the parasite in the mouse liver, an effect that appears to be independent of the suppression of T cell function (119), the mechanism by which cyclosporin suppresses graft rejection.

In many cases, the hepatic lesions are few in number and limited in distribution, so they produce no clinical manifestations of liver disease. However, when the lesions are extensive, they may give rise to hepatomegaly, splenomegaly, portal hypertension, and esophageal varices that often bleed, a form of the disease usually classified as hepatosplenic schistosomiasis. Characteristically, in such cases, hepatocellular function is well preserved or only minimally impaired (120). Usually, the portal hypertension is presinusoidal in type and attributable to compression and obliteration of intrahepatic portal vein radicles by fibrosis. Studies in mice suggest that small branches of the portal veins at the periphery of the liver are the first vessels to be obliterated (121). However, in a small minority of cases, the wedged hepatic vein pressure is increased, indicative of complicating sinusoidal hypertension, a feature variously ascribed to perisinusoidal fibrosis and enhanced hepatic arterial blood flow (122,123). Although portal and periportal fibrosis may be extensive in hepatosplenic schistosomiasis, and may be accompanied by irregular, densely collagenized septa that distort the lobular architecture of the liver, giving rise to so-called clay pipestem fibrosis, it does not lead to the development of cirrhosis. When cirrhosis is encountered in patients with schistosomiasis, it usually is attributable to such complicating factors as chronic alcoholism, malnutrition, or antecedent viral hepatitis. Based on studies in Brazil, it has been found that hepatosplenic schistosomiasis is associated with a high incidence of chronic HBs antigenemia (124,125). This has led to the suggestion that the parasitic disease renders patients unusually susceptible to chronic hepatitis B infection, and that such infections may play a role in the pathogenesis of complicating chronic active hepatitis and cirrhosis. In the absence of complicating cirrhosis, jaundice, ascites, and hepatic encephalopathy are rare, even following severe hemorrhage from esophageal varices. However, encephalopathy is relatively common following surgically induced portacaval anastomosis.

The *hepatic lesions* of schistosomiasis exhibit a number of characteristic features that vary to some extent depending on the severity of the infection and the size of the biopsy specimen. However, only the presence of granulomas that contain schistosome ova is diagnostic of the disease. Unfortunately, these may escape detection, particularly in mild infections and small biopsy specimens. In such cases, serial sections occasionally facilitate the demonstration of granulomas or ova.

Most of the granulomas are found within portal tracts or the periportal parenchyma, but in severe infestations may be encountered elsewhere in the lobules. As a rule, they are round and sharply circumscribed, often encircled by slender, concentric rings of collagen, and are made up of a compact mass of epithelioid cells and a centrally located multinucleated giant cell that often contains an ovum (Fig. 344). In some cases, the epithelioid cells are interspersed with or surrounded by a variety of inflammatory cells, including lymphocytes, histiocytes, eosinophils, plasma cells, and neutrophils. The ova are characterized by a chitinous shell with a distal, lateral spike in the case of *S. mansoni* (Fig. 736) and a small, distal, lateral knob in the case of *S. japonicum*. The shell of *S. haematobium*, which is encountered in the liver only rarely, is characterized by a terminal spine. Some of the ova contain a viable miracidium, as evidenced by a large, compact collection of intact nuclei within the shell, whereas others contain a degenerating miracidium or are collapsed or fragmented. Occasionally, degenerating ova undergo calcification. Late in their development, the granulomas undergo progressive fibrosis and may present as circumscribed, acellular fibrous nodules. Rarely, a schistosome worm will be seen (Fig. 737).

Often the portal tracts are enlarged, fibrotic, and contain a variable number of lymphocytes, plasma cells, and histiocytes. Such lesions are not limited to portal tracts that contain granulomas, and may represent an independent response to the immunologic reaction provoked by the schistosomes. In some cases, the limiting plates of the portal tracts are eroded, and there is extension of fibrous tissue and inflammatory cells into the periportal parenchyma, producing lesions indistinguishable from those of chronic active hepatitis. As previously indicated, such lesions may, in some instances, be attributable to complicating chronic hepatitis B viral infection.

The irregular, densely collagenized septa characteristic of clay pipestem fibrosis are rarely encountered in needle biopsy specimens, but may be seen in surgical wedge biopsies and are found with regularity at autopsy in cases of advanced hepatosplenic schistosomiasis. Although irregular in shape and distribution, some of these septa, particularly late in the course of the disease, may be smooth-contoured and show no inflammatory reaction. However, in many cases, segments of the septa are bordered by epithelioid cells, giant cells that contain ova, and a variety of inflammatory cells.

Frequently, fine or coarse, dark brown granules of schistosomal pigment are found within groups of Kupffer cells and portal macrophages (Fig. 241). Characteristically, these fail to react with stains for iron or melanin, and are PAS-negative. The pigment is derived from the hemoglobin of host erythrocytes that have been ingested, degraded, and then excreted by the adult schistosomes. In many respects, the pigment resembles that found in malaria. However, the granules in schistosomiasis and malaria differ in their ultrastructure.

In experimental murine schistosomiasis, early treatment with praziquantel, i.e., within eight weeks of infestation, results in a decrease in the size of granulomas and reduction in the amount of collagen deposition (126).

As a result of the granulomatous reaction and fibrosis in the portal tracts, many of the portal vein radicles are compressed, occluded, or obliterated. In addition, the larger septal portal veins may exhibit intimal thickening, inflammation, and fibrosis of their walls, and thrombosis during the active phase of severe hepatosplenic schistosomiasis.

In many cases, the fibrotic portal tracts, especially at their periphery, contain numerous closely packed, thin-walled, vascular channels and an increased number of arterioles, giving them an angiomatous appearance. However, in our experience, such vascular lesions have been rare in needle biopsy specimens.

Often, the spaces of Disse contain an increased number of reticulin fibers. In relatively advanced lesions, these may be readily apparent in sections stained for reticulin, but in early lesions, electron microscopy may be required for their demonstration. When the reticulin fibers in the spaces of Disse are numerous, they may be accompanied by the formation of a basement membrane and deposition of collagen, resulting in capillarization of the sinusoids.

Although the parenchyma usually is spared, except for the formation of granulomas, it occasionally contains small foci of Kupffer cell hyperplasia, infiltrating lymphocytes, or small areas of hepatocellular dropout.

As a rule, hepatocellular regeneration is not a feature of hepatic schistosomiasis. However, in advanced clay pipestem fibrosis, the liver occasionally contains a variable number of regenerating parenchymal nodules limited to the subcapsular zone. As previously noted, this does not progress to classic cirrhosis unless the disease is complicated by other etiologic factors known to produce such lesions.

Following treatment of schistosomiasis, eosinophilic, granulomatous hepatitis has been observed. The eosinophilia is thought to represent the eosinophilic response to the dead worms or ova (127).

Echinococcosis. Granulomas are not observed in hydatid disease caused by *E. granulosus*. With *E. multilocularis* infestation, however, granulomatous reactions around echinococcal lesions are typical. These lesions are characterized by multiple small cystic structures. A chitinous cuticle, often ribbon-like in appearance, outlines the cysts and is surrounded by a rim of hepatocellular necrosis. Radially arranged around these lesions are palisades of epithelioid cells that are infiltrated with and surrounded by histiocytes and lymphocytes (Fig. 738) (see Chapter 23).

Ascariasis. Adult *Ascaris lumbricoides* are nematodes that frequently reside in the lumen of the small intestine in humans (129–133). Most often they remain in the duodenum, but the bile ducts, gallbladder, liver, and pancreas may be involved (131). Usually, these round worms produce no symptoms, but, occasionally, they migrate through the ampulla of Vater into the bile ducts, giving rise to obstructive jaundice, suppurative cholangitis, often known as Oriental cholangitis, or liver abscess (Figs. 708, 709). The worms entrapped in the liver ultimately die and release their content of ova. They may serve as the nidus for gallstone formation (132). The latter may lead to the development of granulomas in the liver or the formation of stones in the intrahepatic bile ducts. The adult worms may be encysted in dense fibrosis, which sometimes breaks down and gives rise to pulmonary emboli (133).

When fertilized ascaris ova are ingested and reach the small intestine, they release larvae that penetrate the mucosa and enter the circulation. On reaching the lungs, the larvae molt, penetrate into the tracheobronchial tree, migrate to the pharynx, and then pass down into the intestinal tract where they mature into adult worms. In the lungs they may incite an eosinophilic inflammatory reaction, but usually produce no adverse effects in other tissues. Rarely, however, the larvae give rise to granulomas in the liver and other tissues. Such lesions are characterized by circumscribed collections of histiocytes and eosinophils that surround the larvae.

Usually, the larvae, which measure approximately 350μm in length and 20 μm in width, and stain deep red with PAS, are difficult to find, largely because most have undergone degeneration and necrosis. In such cases, serial sectioning may be useful in demonstrating one of the larvae.

Visceral larva migrans (toxocariasis). The ingestion of ova of animal helminths that cannot complete their life cycle in humans frequently gives rise to the syndrome of visceral larva migrans (134,135). With few exceptions, the disease affects young children between the ages of one and four years who eat dirt contaminated with the ova of the dog ascarid, *Toxocara canis*, or, less commonly, the ova of the cat ascarid, *Toxocara catis*.

When the embryonated eggs reach the intestine, they hatch and release larvae that penetrate the mucosa and enter portal vessels, lymphatics, and tissue spaces in which they migrate to the liver, lungs, and, less commonly, to the central nervous system, eye, and other tissues.

Characteristically, visceral larva migrans gives rise to marked and prolonged leukocytosis and eosinophilia, which are often accompanied by hepatomegaly, signs of pneumonitis, and hypergammaglobulinemia. Less constant features include fever, constitutional symptoms, anemia, splenomegaly, and convulsions. However, in mild infections, the eosinophilia may be unaccompanied by symptoms. Rarely, the larvae may invade an eye, producing lesions that have been mistaken for retinoblastomas. Usually, the symptoms subside spontaneously over a period of weeks, but the eosinophilia and residual lesions produced by the larvae may persist for many months. As a rule, visceral larva migrans is a self-limited disease in which the

granulomas heal by scarring. However, it occasionally proves fatal.

The *hepatic lesions* are relatively large, ranging from 1 to 10 mm in diameter, and may be visible to the naked eye at laparotomy or autopsy. When fully developed, the lesions are characterized histologically by a large central zone of necrosis surrounded by epithelioid and giant cells interspersed and encircled by numerous eosinophils and plasma cells (Figs. 288, 289). The zones of necrosis resemble pyogenic abscesses, but are filled with eosinophils (Fig. 290). Often, the sinusoids and portal tracts are heavily infiltrated with eosinophils and plasma cells (Figs. 290, 291).

Hepatic capillariasis. Rodents are the natural hosts of *Capillaria hepatica,* a nematode that resembles the common whipworm of humans, *Trichiuris trichiura* (136,137). Characteristically, the mature worms and their ova live in the liver.

Rarely, humans are infected with capillaria by ingesting embryonated ova in dirt or food contaminated by the feces of rats or other animals that have recently eaten liver that contains the parasites, or by eating raw or inadequately cooked, infected liver of squirrels, beavers, or muskrats.

On reaching the intestine, the ova hatch and release larvae that penetrate the mucosa, enter the portal circulation, and are carried to the liver where they undergo maturation to adult worms.

The worms and their ova provoke a necrotizing, granulomatous, fibrotic reaction in the liver (138) that usually is manifested clinically by fever, nausea, vomiting, hepatosplenomegaly, marked leukocytosis and eosinophilia, anemia, and hyperglobulinemia, features that resemble those of visceral larva migrans. Often, the disease proves fatal.

The *hepatic lesions* are characterized by large, widely scattered granulomas that contain centrally located, viable worms filled with ova or a mixture of degenerating or necrotic worms and free ova. Characteristically the worms and ova are surrounded by necrotic material and an outer zone of eosinophils, epithelioid cells, and multinucleated giant cells. The ova, which resemble those of *Trichiuris trichiura,* are barrel-shaped and enclosed within a double-contoured shell with a plug at each end.

In the late stages of the disease, the granulomas tend to undergo scarring, which may lead to extensive fibrosis and distortion of the lobular architecture, producing a cirrhosis-like picture. In addition, some of the granulomas may exhibit areas of calcification.

Tongue worm. The adult form of *Lingulata serrata*, commonly termed tongue worm, is a worm-like arthropod that frequently inhabits the nasal cavity and paranasal sinuses of the dog, and discharges its ova in the nasal secretions (139,140). Occasionally, humans are infected by ingesting such ova. On reaching the intestine, the ova hatch and release larvae that penetrate the mucosa and enter the portal circulation. Usually, these lodge in the liver and, less commonly, in other tissues, where they provoke an indolent, granulomatous reaction and then die.

As a rule, the granulomas produce no signs or symptoms, and are discovered unexpectedly at laparotomy or autopsy. Since they usually are found late in their development, they present as small, firm nodules that may be mistaken for metastases.

Characteristically, many of the hepatic granulomas on sectioning exhibit a central crescentic cavity that contains the remnants of a dead larva, including nondescript debris, body rings,

spines, and curved hooklets, all or some of which may be calcified. Surrounding the cavity, there are occasional foreign body
giant cells and occasional eosinophils enclosed within an outer
capsule of dense, laminated collagen fibers.

Oxyuriasis. Pinworms *(Enterobius vermicularis)* have a simple
life cycle. Humans are the only host, albeit very frequent ones.
One-third of children and one-sixth of adults develop the infestation, which results from the ingestion of the ova deposited in
the perineal area (141). These eggs hatch and release larvae in
the cecum or appendix. Occasionally, the larvae escape from
the intestinal tract via perforations or neoplasms, and subsequently involve the peritoneum and the surface of the liver where
they may form large granulomas [(141–143); Fig. 739]. It is
not clear whether extrahepatic granulomas, which may contain
the nematode itself (Fig. 740), penetrate the liver capsule or
are disseminated hematogenously.

Giardiasis. Giardiasis rarely exhibits any hepatic manifestations. However, it has been reported in association with granulomatous hepatitis and cholangitis (144).

Collagen-vascular diseases

Giant cell arteritis. Giant cell arteritis (145,146), a disorder of
unknown etiology, is characterized by a segmental, subacute,
or chronic granulomatous reaction with numerous giant cells
that involves widely disseminated medium sized and large arteries, leading to thrombosis and, ultimately, to fibrous occlusion. The disease rarely occurs before the age of 55, and affects
women more frequently than men. Since the temporal artery is
affected most frequently, or at least is most readily recognized
clinically, the disease often is classified as *temporal arteritis*.
This term has the disadvantage that it gives no indication of the
systemic nature of the vasculitis. There is increasing evidence
that giant cell arteritis is closely related to, if not identical with,
the syndrome of *polymyalgia rheumatica*.

The clinical manifestations of giant cell arteritis include fever, weakness, anorexia, weight loss, anemia, leukocytosis, and
focal signs and symptoms that are dependent on the particular
vessels affected. Temporal arteritis is characterized by severe
headache and localized tenderness and induration of the involved vessel. Ophthalmic arteritis may present as sudden
blindness that often is bilateral; coronary arteritis by myocardial
infarction; and intracranial arteritis by diverse neurologic disorders. When large peripheral arteries are affected, they may
give rise to intermittent claudication or Raynaud's phenomenon, and may exhibit a decrease in pulsation, an overlying bruit,
or narrowing of their lumens on angiography. Rarely, involvement of the aorta leads to dissection and rupture.

Characteristically, corticosteroid therapy induces healing of
the vascular lesions and prevents progression of the disease.
Accordingly, such therapy is always indicated as soon as the
diagnosis is established to prevent further complications, particularly sudden blindness and myocardial infarction.

Minor abnormalities of hepatic function that may include
bromsulphalein retention, slightly elevated serum levels of alkaline phosphatase and transaminase, and prolongation of the
prothrombin time are relatively common in giant cell arteritis,
but are not accompanied by other clinical signs of liver disease.
Since these abnormalities are readily reversible following cor-

ticosteroid therapy and do not correlate with the presence of
hepatic arterial lesions, it is highly probable that they are attributable to the systemic effects of extrahepatic vascular disease.

Rarely, a few of the hepatic arteries exhibit a giant cell granulomatous reaction in their walls. Most such lesions are encountered at autopsy, but in two of our own cases, they were
demonstrable in needle biopsy sections (Fig. 401). In both instances, the arterial lesions were found unexpectedly and led to
the correct diagnosis, which subsequently was confirmed by biopsy of a temporal artery. In at least one reported case, liver
biopsy revealed a nonspecific epithelioid granuloma in the parenchyma (148).

Polymyalgia rheumatica. Elderly individuals, usually women,
are subject to polymyalgia rheumatica, a disorder of unknown
etiology characterized by stiffness and pain in the muscles around
the shoulder and pelvic girdles, low grade fever, sweats, fatigue, weight loss, and anemia (145,146,149–151). Available
evidence, based on autopsy studies and the biopsy findings in
the temporal artery even when asymptomatic, is consistent with
the widely held view that, in most, if not all cases, the syndrome is a manifestation of underlying, systemic giant cell
arteritis, and, hence, might more appropriately be termed
"polymyalgia arterica."

Corticosteroid therapy is effective in inducing remission of
the disease, and in preventing complications attributable to vascular occlusion, especially sudden blindness.

Frequently, the disease is accompanied by minor alterations
in hepatic function. A number of structural abnormalities of the
liver have been reported in some cases. These have included
small epithelioid granulomas, focal lymphocytic infiltration of
the portal triads and parenchyma, rare foci of hepatocellular
necrosis, and prominence of the Kupffer cells.

Juvenile rheumatoid arthritis. Juvenile rheumatoid arthritis (152–
155), a disease of unknown etiology, is characterized by recurrent bouts of high fever, acute arthritis, transient rash, lymphadenopathy, hepatosplenomegaly, pericarditis, pleurisy, or
pneumonia in various combinations, and often is classified as
Still's disease. As a rule, the disease occurs before the age of
15 years, but it may be seen in adults.

Hepatic involvement, as evidenced by hepatomegaly, elevated levels of serum alkaline phosphatase and aminotransferases, and, rarely, by jaundice, is relatively common in juvenile
rheumatic arthritis. However, in some cases, the hepatic lesions
are attributable to drug therapy, especially to large doses of
aspirin, or to intercurrent infections, such as viral hepatitis or
infectious mononucleosis.

The most frequently reported feature of the *hepatic lesions*
in juvenile rheumatoid arthritis is a lymphocytic portal inflammatory reaction. However, in our experience with adult cases,
a mild focal hepatitis, as evidenced by small foci of hepatocellular necrosis, occasional acidophilic bodies, small intralobular
collections of lymphocytes, and Kupffer cell hyperplasia, has
been relatively common. In addition, we have encountered small,
circumscribed epithelioid granulomas in about one-third of our
cases. Rarely, in cases of juvenile rheumatoid arthritis with extensive prolonged arthritis, the liver may be infiltrated with
amyloid.

Wegener's granulomatosis. Wegener's granulomatosis, a disorder of unknown etiology, is characterized by necrotizing
granulomas that predominantly involve the upper respiratory tract

and lungs along with segmental necrosis of small arteries and veins and focal necrotizing glomerulonephritis. Rarely, necrotizing granulomas may be encountered in the liver (156).

Granulomatous venulitis. Granulomatous venulitis is a disorder of unknown etiology that involves the venous portions of the hepatic circulation. It can give rise to the Budd-Chiari syndrome, which may be rapidly reversed by corticosteroid therapy (157). Sarcoidosis can also result in the Budd-Chiari syndrome (158).

Gastrointestinal diseases

Ulcerative colitis. A wide variety of hepatobiliary lesions may be encountered in ulcerative colitis. These include fatty infiltration, "pericholangitis" (159), primary sclerosing cholangitis, chronic active hepatitis, cirrhosis, pylephlebitis, the Budd-Chiari syndrome, amyloidosis, and bile duct carcinoma (160).

Occasionally, such lesions are accompanied by sarcoid-like epithelioid granulomas with or without interspersed giant cells. Usually, these are few in number and located in the portal tracts or periportal zones. Granulomas of this type were demonstrable by liver biopsy in only 2 (6%) of our 32 patients with ulcerative colitis (Fig. 741).

Crohn's disease. The frequency and character of the hepatic lesions in Crohn's disease are similar to those in ulcerative colitis. In our own series of 13 patients with Crohn's disease subjected to liver biopsy, 2 (15%) exhibited sarcoid-like hepatic granulomas.

Jejunoileal bypass for obesity. In some cases, jejunoileal bypass for massive obesity is followed by an increase in hepatic fatty infiltration and fibrosis and the development of a lesion that resembles alcoholic hepatitis and may progress to cirrhosis. It has been reported that such lesions may be accompanied by the appearance of hepatic granulomas composed of epithelioid cells, lymphocytes, and fibroblasts with occasional, multinucleated giant cells, neutrophils, and eosinophils (161).

Biliopancreatic diversion, a procedure similar in concept to jejunoileal bypass, was devised to avoid the blind loop syndrome postulated to be responsible for the hepatic lesion (161a). Nevertheless, an identical hepatic lesion has been reported after biliopancreatic diversion (161b; see Fig. 779D).

Eosinophilic gastroenteritis. Eosinophilic gastroenteritis, a poorly understood syndrome that often manifests itself by obstruction of the small intestine or stomach, by ascites, or by abdominal pain, may present as low grade hepatitis (162). It has also been reported in association with hepatic granulomas (163,164). In one such patient, who survived for more than 30 years, 62% of 49,000 leukocytes per mm^3 in the peripheral blood were eosinophilic leukocytes (164). The granuloma consisted of epithelioid macrophages and giant cells surrounded by lymphocytes, plasma cells, and many mature eosinophils (Fig. 742). The cause of this syndrome is not known.

Whipple's disease. Hepatic epithelioid granulomas have been reported in several patients with Whipple's disease (165,166). The granulomas were negative for the PAS-diastase-positive granules seen in the characteristic macrophages of Whipple's disease (167).

Histiocytic disease

Pulmonary eosinophilic granuloma. Eosinophilic granuloma, a disorder of unknown etiology, usually presents as a localized, lytic lesion in bone in which osseous tissue is replaced by infiltrating histiocytes and eosinophils. Rarely, multiple eosinophilic granulomas are found in the lungs in the absence of similar lesions in the bones or other tissues (168,169). Liver biopsy in two well-documented cases of eosinophilic granuloma limited to the lung revealed multiple noncaseating epithelioid granulomas in one. In neither case was there evidence of infiltrating histiocytes or eosinophils.

Available evidence suggests that eosinophilic granuloma is related to the group of disorders classified as histiocytosis X and characterized by histiocytic infiltration, not only of bone and lung, but other tissues as well.

Immunologic disorders

Chronic granulomatous disease of children. Chronic granulomatous disease (170–174) is a hereditary disease of young children transmitted as an X-linked recessive trait in boys and as an autosomal recessive trait in girls and some boys. It is characterized by chronic recurrent bacterial infections due to a defect in the bactericidal activity of the polymorphonuclear leukocytes.

Although the affected leukocytes phagocytize bacteria normally, they fail to destroy those that do not produce hydrogen peroxide following phagocytosis. Such organisms include, in particular, staphylococci, *Serratia marcescens,* and certain gram-negative, enteric bacteria.

In vitro studies of the affected leukocytes have demonstrated that following phagocytosis of bacteria they fail to stimulate oxygen consumption, NADH oxidase activity, hydrogen peroxide production, or the reduction of nitroblue tetrazolium. The basic genetic defect is still uncertain. However, it has been suggested that it may be an absence of cytochrome b in the X-linked form of the disease, and a deficiency of glutathione peroxidase activity in the autosomal recessive type.

Usually, the onset of chronic granulomatous disease is in infancy, by the age of two years, and is manifested by recurrent and chronic suppurative lymphadenitis, pneumonitis, and dermatitis. As the disease advances, infections may involve other tissues, including the liver. Hepatomegaly and hyperglobulinemia are present in most cases. Characteristically, the lesions in affected tissues exhibit suppuration, granuloma formation, and the presence of numerous pigmented macrophages. The pigment, which may be diffusely distributed in the cytoplasm as granules, is a lipochrome that resembles lipofuscin. It sometimes accumulates in portal macrophages and in Kupffer cells (175).

The disease leads to death by the age of 10 years, although a few patients survive until early adult life. Fungal infections with *Aspergillus fumigatus, Nocardia asteroidea,* and *Candida albicans* are relatively common terminal complications of the disease.

The *hepatic lesions* in chronic granulomatous disease usually exhibit granulomas that contain a central zone of necrosis surrounded by epithelioid cells, numerous plasma cells, neutrophils, pigmented macrophages, and occasional giant cells. In some cases, multiple granulomas coalesce to form frank abscesses that may be sufficiently large to require surgical drainage.

The previously described lipochrome-filled macrophages, which are PAS-D-positive and exhibit golden autofluorescence, are found in groups scattered through the parenchyma and portal tracts.

Many of the portal tracts are enlarged and fibrotic, and contain numerous inflammatory cells, especially plasma cells, lymphocytes, eosinophils, and pigmented macrophages. In some cases, the limiting plates are eroded, leading to bridging of adjacent portal tracts. Rarely, the fibrosis is sufficiently extensive to destroy the normal lobular architecture with the development of cirrhosis.

Erythema nodosum. Although the pathogenesis of erythema nodosum (176–178) is uncertain, circumstantial evidence suggests that it may represent an immunologic response to a wide variety of etiologic factors, including bacterial, mycotic, and viral infections, drug reactions, and certain other systemic diseases.

In a significant number of cases, the skin lesions are accompanied by bilateral hilar adenopathy. This is encountered most frequently in patients with underlying sarcoidosis, but may occur in tuberculosis, histoplasmosis, and coccidioidomycosis. As might be anticipated, granulomas are demonstrable in the liver in a high proportion of cases. In our experience with 41 patients with erythema nodosum, liver biopsy revealed epithelioid granulomas in 37 of the 38 with bilateral hilar adenopathy, due to sarcoidosis in 36 and tuberculosis in 1. Of note, hepatic granulomas were not found in any of our 3 patients with erythema nodosum unaccompanied by hilar adenopathy who exhibited evidence of streptococcal infection, ulcerative colitis, or a drug reaction.

The skin lesions of erythema nodosum are characterized by a nonspecific inflammatory reaction with no granulomatous features, even when granulomas are present in the liver.

Immunodeficiency syndromes. A variety of hepatic lesions, usually ascribed to recurrent or chronic bacterial or viral infection, have been reported in both congenital and acquired forms of immunodeficiency (179–184). These include: (1) reticuloendothelial hyperplasia, (2) sinusoidal congestion, (3) portal fibrosis, (4) submassive hepatic necrosis, chronic active hepatitis, or postnecrotic cirrhosis, presumably of viral origin, (5) sclerosing cholangitis, and (6) noncaseating epithelioid granulomas.

In some cases, the hepatic granulomas have been attributed to complicating sarcoidosis (179), tuberculosis, or histoplasmosis (181). However, in others, such lesions have been interpreted as a nonspecific response to chronic infection (180).

The single, most common, hepatic, granuloma-inducing disease is the passive congestion related to cor pulmonale and heart failure. Rarely, foci of centrilobular and midzonal necrosis and fibrosis are found in the liver. These too may be related to congestive heart failure or anoxemia, but their pathogenesis is uncertain.

Vineyard sprayers' disease. Vineyard workers who spray grapevines with a mixture of copper sulfate and lime (Bordeaux mixture) over a number of years are subject to the development of distinctive pulmonary and hepatic lesions (188).

The pulmonary lesions are characterized by histiocytic granulomas, hyalinized fibrous nodules, and deposits of copper-containing granules.

The hepatic lesions in such cases vary, but usually exhibit: (1) swelling and proliferation of the Kupffer cells, (2) epithelioid or histiocytic granulomas, (3) granular deposits or copper in the Kupffer cells, histiocytes, and epithelioid cells, and (4) portal and perisinusoidal fibrosis accompanied by "idiopathic" portal hypertension. Rarely, the lesions are characterized by cirrhosis or angiosarcoma.

It has been pointed out that except for the occurrence of copper deposits and granulomas, the hepatic lesions resemble those produced by vinyl chloride and inorganic arsenic, suggesting that the hepatic and pulmonary lesions of vineyard sprayers' disease are attributable to the toxic effects of inhaled copper compounds.

Drug-induced granulomas

Drug-induced hepatic injury may be expressed as granulomatous hepatitis (Chapter 8). Since it is not possible to prove unequivocally the etiology of most granulomas, it has been suggested that the drug-induced nature of many hepatic granulomas is overlooked (189).

The only histologic clue to drug-induced hepatic granulomas may be the *acquired immunodeficiency syndrome (AIDS)*. AIDS is discussed in detail in Chapter 27.

Industrial and environmental disorders

Berylliosis. Inhalation of most beryllium dusts and fumes encountered in industry may give rise after a relatively brief latent period to *acute berylliosis* (185–187), a disorder characterized by an acute pneumonitis that usually resolves spontaneously over a period of several months. Occasionally, however, the disease proves fatal. At autopsy in such cases, the liver often shows centrilobular necrosis, a lesion probably due to chronic passive congestion and anoxemia rather than to the toxic effects of beryllium.

Occasionally, inhalation of dust containing beryllium oxide is followed after a relatively long incubation period, ranging from a month to several years, by the development of *chronic berylliosis*. This disorder is characterized by a chronic, progressive, granulomatous pneumonitis that often leads to death as a result of cor pulmonale and cardiac or respiratory failure. The granulomas, which closely resemble those of sarcoidosis, are found not only in the lungs but also in other tissues, especially the hilar lymph nodes and the liver. Available evidence suggests that the granulomas are manifestations of a cell-mediated sensitization reaction to beryllium.

As illustrated in Figure 515, the hepatic granulomas in chronic berylliosis are characterized by sharply circumscribed collections of epithelioid and giant cells that show no evidence of necrosis. Differentiation of such lesions from those of sarcoidosis is not possible on histologic grounds, and usually depends on a history of exposure to beryllium or a positive skin patch test with 1% beryllium sulfate or nitrate.

In addition to granulomas, liver biopsy frequently reveals the presence of many eosinophils that are common in both tuberculosis and sarcoidal granulomas (189).

Sometimes clinical evidence such as a characteristic syndrome and typical histologic findings can make a most compelling case for drug-induced granulomatosis (75). Allopurinol has been reported in six patients to induce a hypersensitivity reaction characterized by fever, rash, arthralgia, and eosinophilia, with epithelioid granulomas (75).

Neoplastic disease (extrahepatic)

Intraabdominal carcinoma. Regional lymph nodes draining malignant neoplasms in various tissues may contain sarcoid-like epithelioid and giant cell granulomas in the absence of metastatic tumor cells (190,191). We have encountered similar granulomas in the livers of seven patients with intraabdominal carcinoma in whom no hepatic metastases were found on biopsy or at laparotomy. Moreover, none had clinical or laboratory evidence of sarcoidosis or other diseases known to produce hepatic granulomas, so it was assumed that the granulomas were related to the underlying carcinoma.

Extrahepatic Hodgkin's disease. A number of patients with Hodgkin's disease exhibit sarcoid-like epithelioid granulomas in the liver or other tissues, particularly the spleen, abdominal lymph nodes, and bone marrow. Often, these granulomas are unaccompanied by lymphomatous infiltrates (192–194).

Fourteen patients with Hodgkin's disease subjected to liver biopsy in our series exhibited hepatic granulomas without accompanying lymphomatous infiltration. Figure 743 illustrates a granuloma of this type found in an elderly woman who presented with fever, hepatosplenomegaly, and pulmonary infiltration. These findings were initially interpreted as evidence of sarcoidosis, but subsequent autopsy revealed Hodgkin's disease. A postmortem specimen of liver tissue also contained granulomas without lymphomatous infiltrates. It is noteworthy that 1 of the 13 patients reported as examples of "granulomatous hepatitis and prolonged fever of unknown origin," an allegedly distinctive disease that responds to large doses of prednisone, proved to have Hodgkin's disease of the iliac and retroperitoneal lymph nodes at laparotomy (195). The liver in this case contained noncaseating epithelioid granulomas, but no lymphomatous infiltrates.

It has been suggested that the prognosis of Hodgkin's disease may be better in patients with granulomas in the liver or spleen than in those without such lesions (193). This report still requires confirmation.

Hypernephroma. Hepatic granulomas have been seen in hypernephroma and have been considered to represent a paraneoplastic manifestation of the neoplasm (196).

Miscellaneous

Psoriasis. Approximately half the patients with psoriasis show histologic abnormalities in the liver, especially fatty infiltration, nonspecific reactive hepatitis, and portal fibrosis. Such findings usually are attributed to age, obesity, and the use of alcohol rather than to the presence, severity, or duration of the skin lesions. In addition, in our series of 98 psoriatic patients who had liver biopsies, 11 (11%) showed sarcoid-like epithelioid

and giant cell granulomas (Fig. 513). Such lesions have rarely been reported by others (197).

The pathogenesis and significance of the hepatic granulomas in psoriasis are obscure. Our initial impression was that these lesions were indicative of sarcoidosis (198). However, in retrospect, this explanation appears unlikely, since none of the patients had the usual clinical manifestations of the disease and only one had a weakly positive Kveim reaction. It is conceivable that in the latter case, psoriasis and sarcoidosis were coincidental, as has been previously reported (199). None of the patients with granulomas had been treated with methotrexate, so a reaction to this agent can be excluded. However, all had been treated on one or more occasions with topical applications of tar and salicylate ointment and radiation with ultraviolet light (the Goeckerman regimen). Since salicylates are not known to produce granulomas, it is conceivable that the granulomas represented a reaction to absorbed tar, a possibility that merits further investigation.

Idiopathic granulomatous hepatitis. The finding of hepatic granulomas in association with prolonged fever in the absence of other explanations for the syndrome is tentatively termed granulomatous hepatitis. These patients, who often present with fevers of unknown origin (200–202), may eventually be found to have lymphoma, tuberculosis, rickettsial disease, etc., but in some no explanation is ever found (203). Liver functional abnormalities are mild to moderate in severity. Many resolve spontaneously (201), some respond to adrenocorticosteroid or to other antiinflammatory therapy, and some remain unsolved mysteries.

Reactions to foreign bodies

Starch. Starch that is used to powder surgical gloves may give rise to a granulomatous inflammatory reaction in the serosa of any of the body cavities or in surgical wounds (204–206). When the peritoneum is affected, some of the granulomas may be found in the capsule of the liver or, as in one of our cases, in the subcapsular parenchyma. Characteristically, the granulomas are made up of foreign body giant cells, epithelioid cells, and other inflammatory cells. When large, they may show a central zone of caseation necrosis. The lesions tend to heal spontaneously with residual scarring. A distinctive feature of the granulomas is the presence of starch granules. These are difficult to recognize on routine microscopy of H & E sections, but are readily identified in polarized light by their birefringence with a dark, central Maltese cross. In addition, the granules are PAS-positive and react with Lugol's iodine solution.

The patient with hepatic parenchymal starch granulomas mentioned previously was a young woman referred for investigation of recurrent attacks of abdominal pain of three years' duration. At exploratory laparotomy a year after the onset of her pain, she was found to have multiple caseating granulomas that involved the peritoneum, Glisson's capsule, and the subcapsular hepatic parenchyma. Although no acid-fast bacilli were demonstrable in stained sections or on culture, it was assumed that the lesions were indicative of tuberculous peritonitis. Accordingly, she was given a full course of isoniazid and rifampicin therapy, but this had no effect on the symptoms. Reexamination of the original surgical wedge biopsy sections of liver confirmed the presence of old caseating granulomas in Glisson's capsule and the subcapsular hepatic parenchyma. As shown in Figure 744, the lesions contained a large, central core of hyalinizing caseation surrounded by a narrow band of foreign body giant cells, plasma cells, and lymphocytes. Scattered through the lesions were occasional intra- and extracellular, faintly outlined vacuoles that contained a small, central, dark spot. In polarized light, these were birefringent and showed the typical, dark, central Maltese cross of starch granules (Fig. 745). Moreover, the granules reacted with Lugol's solution and PAS, so there was no doubt that the lesions were starch granulomas. It is highly probable that these were attributable to contamination of the peritoneum by glove powder during a cholecystectomy performed two years prior to the onset of recurrent abdominal pain and three years before the discovery of the granulomas at exploratory laparotomy. Although starch-induced granulomatous peritonitis may give rise to abdominal pain, it usually does so within a few weeks of its onset. Further investigation by retrograde pyelography revealed a small stone embedded in the right ureter close to its junction with the renal pelvis. Subsequent surgical removal of the stone led to disappearance of the pain. It was apparent, therefore, that the attacks of abdominal pain in this case were not attributable to the granulomas.

Available evidence suggests that the formation of starch granulomas may be the result of a cell-mediated, immune response to starch.

Talc. Because talc was shown to produce peritoneal granulomas and adhesions, it was abandoned as a powdering agent for surgical gloves more than 25 years ago. However, it has been demonstrated by electron microscopy that many allegedly talc-free gloves are contaminated with talc crystals, and that such crystals may be found within granulomas (207).

More commonly, talc is found in the livers of drug addicts who have injected intravenously agents that contain talc filler. Usually, the talc, which presents as colorless, refractile, birefringent, needle-shaped crystals, is found within Kupffer cells and portal macrophages (208). Occasionally, the crystals give rise to foreign body granulomas (110). In our series talc-containing granulomas of this type were encountered in 1 of 190 liver biopsies from intravenous drug abusers.

Multiple hepatic, splenic, and lymph node granulomas have been reported in patients who had been on long-term hemodialysis and who had hyperaluminumemia (209). Aluminum was demonstrated histochemically in the cytoplasm of macrophages from the granulomas. The patients had no clinical or laboratory evidence of disease related to the liver or to the granulomatous disorder.

Hepatic granulomas in "primary" liver diseases

A significant number of patients with well-defined diseases of the liver, exclusive of those associated with the systemic and extrahepatic disorders discussed in the first section of this chapter, exhibit hepatic granulomas. Such lesions were encountered in 190 (3.4%) of the 5,581 cases of "primary" liver disease in our own series. Their incidence was highest in primary biliary cirrhosis (41%) and ranged from less than 1% to 8% in most other disorders (Table II).

Pathogenesis

The hepatic granulomas found in patients with "primary" liver diseases may be attributable to (1) the same pathogenetic mechanism responsible for the underlying hepatic disorder, (2) unrecognized, coincidental, systemic, or extrahepatic disease (Table 22–1), or (3) a nonspecific response to hepatic injury.

Immunologic factors. A number of studies support the widely held view that nonsuppurative inflammation, degeneration, and destruction of the interlobular bile ducts and the formation of granulomas in primary biliary cirrhosis are the result of an immunologic reaction (Chapter 11). As indicated in Chapter 7, circumstantial evidence suggests that immunologic factors may be implicated in the pathogenesis of the hepatic lesions and granulomas that may be seen in idiosyncratic drug reactions. The possible importance of immunologic reactions in the development of the hepatic lesions in acute and chronic viral hepatitis (Chapter 6), chronic hepatitis of unknown etiology (Chapter 8), and alcoholic liver disease (Chapter 10) has been emphasized. However, there is no convincing evidence that such reactions account for the occasional occurrence of hepatic granulomas in these diseases.

Coincidental systemic or extrahepatic disease. Except in the case of well-documented primary biliary cirrhosis and certain idiosyncratic, drug-induced reactions known to produce granulomas (Chapter 7), the discovery of such lesions in patients with primary diseases of the liver is an indication for further studies to exclude coincidental systemic and extrahepatic disorders that may give rise to hepatic granulomas (see Table 22–1). Usually, such studies prove unrevealing. However, in 2 of our 190 cases of intravenous drug addicts with acute viral hepatitis, the granulomas were shown to be due to sarcoidosis in one and to talc in the other.

Nonspecific granulomatous reactions. It is conceivable that some of the granulomas found in patients with primary diseases of the liver are the consequences of nonspecific responses to hepatic injury of various etiologies.

Histopathology of granulomas in "primary" liver disease

As a rule, these lesions resemble those of sarcoidosis, being made up of circumscribed collections of epithelioid cells interspersed with giant cells and other inflammatory cells or encircled by a slender cuff of collagen fibers. They never exhibit caseation, but may contain foci of fibrinoid necrosis.

The following figures illustrate representative granulomas encountered in primary diseases of the liver: (1) Figure 612 and 619 primary biliary cirrhosis; (2) Figure 746, alcoholic cirrhosis; (3) Figure 747, HBsAg-positive acute viral hepatitis; (4) Figure 526, drug-induced (Diazepam) cholestasis; and (5) Figures 231 and 537, drug-induced (halothane) hepatitis.

Hepatic granulomas of unknown etiology

The etiology of hepatic granulomas cannot be determined in 13 to 36% of cases (210). In our own group of 689 patients with hepatic granulomas, 44 (6%) had no systemic or extrahepatic disorders (see Table 22–1) or primary disease of the liver (see Table 22–2), so no cause for the hepatic granulomas was found in these cases.

Granulomatous hepatitis and prolonged fever of unknown origin is a syndrome characterized by noncaseating hepatic granulomas and sustained and intermittent fever of many months' or years' duration that responds to corticosteroid therapy (195). Although it is generally considered to be a specific etiologic entity, in many instances the disease may be a manifestation of sarcoidosis despite the usual absence of hilar adenopathy, pulmonary infiltration, or a positive Kveim reaction (16). In a group of 30 patients with hepatic granulomas, prolonged fever that responded to corticosteroids, and normal roentgenograms of the chest, more than half exhibited granulomas in extraabdominal tissues, mesenteric lymph nodes, or the spleen, or had a history of antecedent hilar adenopathy. Although the diagnosis of sarcoidosis in such cases has been disputed (211), observations in one of our own cases were consistent with this diagnosis. The patient, a young, black woman with no symptoms, was found to have bilateral hilar adenopathy on routine roentgenography of the chest. She was anergic, and biopsies of a prescalene node and the liver demonstrated the presence of noncaseating epithelioid granulomas, features considered typical of sarcoidosis. Four months later, fever and progressive weight loss appeared. Because these failed to abate spontaneously, she was given a course of antituberculous therapy followed later by small doses of prednisone. Since neither of these therapies proved effective, she was referred to our unit for investigation of relatively high fever and weight loss. Hepatomegaly and splenomegaly were her only abnormal physical findings. Hilar adenopathy was no longer demonstrable. She was still anergic, and a second biopsy of the liver again showed the presence of numerous noncaseating granulomas. Serologic and cultural studies, bone marrow examination, and a Kveim test all yielded negative results. Since Hodgkin's disease could not be excluded with certainty, exploratory laparotomy was carried out. This operation revealed numerous large and small nodules in the liver and spleen and many enlarged mesenteric lymph nodes. Multiple biopsy sections of the liver, spleen, and lymph nodes revealed numerous large, noncaseating granulomas, some of which contained central zones of fibrinoid necrosis. Stained sections and cultures for acid-fast bacilli, mycotic and other organisms were negative. The dosage of prednisone was increased to 40 mg daily. The temperature promptly dropped to normal and she gained weight; both benefits were sustained over a period of at least seven years. Although it was possible to reduce the dose of prednisone to 15 or 20 mg daily, any further reduction invariably led to a recurrence of fever. In this case, we concluded that the granulomatous hepatitis and fever were attributable to sarcoidosis.

It is unlikely that all cases of granulomatous hepatitis with prolonged fever of unknown origin are attributable to sarcoidosis. In this connection, it is noteworthy that of the 13 originally reported cases, 1 ultimately proved to have underlying Hodgkin's disease (195) and in several other cases antituberculous therapy alone led to recovery (211). It is apparent, therefore, that even the most exhaustive investigation may fail to detect evidence of tuberculosis or Hodgkin's disease. Accordingly, a therapeutic trial of antituberculous therapy for two or three months and long-term follow-up studies are indicated in all cases of granulomatous hepatitis with prolonged fever of undetermined etiology.

Noncaseating hepatic epithelioid granulomas have been reported in a number of patients with fever of two to six weeks' duration accompanied by heterophilic antibody-negative lymphocytosis (212,213). In retrospect, it is highly probable that these cases were examples of cytomegalovirus or toxoplasmosis mononucleosis, possibilities that were not excluded by appropriate serologic studies.

Of our 44 patients with hepatic granulomas of unknown etiology, 22 had self-limited, febrile episodes that lasted from a few weeks to four months. Although no patient exhibited lymphocytosis, tests to exclude cytomegalovirus infection and toxoplasmosis were not available early in our experience with such cases. Considering that approximately 40% of patients with classic sarcoidosis exhibit fever that is self-limited (5), it is conceivable that at least some of the hepatic granulomas in this group were attributable to sarcoidosis despite the absence of hilar adenopathy or pulmonary infiltration. However, other possibilities cannot be excluded (214). Of these, inactive tuberculosis merits special consideration. Healed or healing granulomas were found in the liver, spleen, or kidneys in 20% of 452 consecutive autopsies. In 3 of 14 cases, inoculation of the granulomatous tissue into guinea pigs yielded tubercle bacilli. The authors suggested that the granulomas were probably attributable to the dissemination of tubercle bacilli that often occurs at the time of primary infections.

Lipogranulomas

Lipogranulomas differ in many respects from the epithelioid granulomas discussed previously. Characteristically, such lesions exhibit histologic features that are easily identified in microscopic sections. They are derived from globules of extracellular triglyceride extruded from lipid-filled hepatocytes or from droplets of mineral oil absorbed from the intestinal tract, and have no clinical or diagnostic significance.

Triglyceride-induced lipogranulomas in fatty livers

Electron microscopic studies have demonstrated that the development of lipogranulomas in various forms of hepatic fatty infiltration is provoked by the extrusion of lipid, predominantly triglyceride in nature, from infiltrated hepatocytes (215). The reported incidence of such lesions in hepatic steatosis varies greatly, ranging from approximately 10% in our own series to as high as 64% in others (216).

Usually, the lesions are characterized by a centrally located lipid globule surrounded by a circumscribed cuff of histiocytes and lymphocytes (Fig. 176). Less commonly, the exudate includes eosinophils and numerous histiocytes that resemble epithelioid cells (Fig. 287). Tangential sections of such lesions that fail to demonstrate lipid inclusions may lead to the erroneous conclusion that the granulomas are of the epithelioid type. Fatty infiltration of the hepatocytes or the presence of finely vacuolated histiocytes compatible with lipid in the granulomas suggest that serial sections be examined to exclude lipogranulomas. Although we have never encountered them, giant cells are said to occur occasionally in such lesions (216).

It has been reported that lipogranulomas, when numerous,

may coalesce and, ultimately, may give rise to hepatic fibrosis (216). However, we have not been able to confirm this observation in any of our cases in the absence of complicating factors, such as alcoholic hepatitis. Indeed, we have found that the granulomas tend to disappear without a trace as the fatty infiltration of the liver clears.

Mineral oil–induced hepatic lipogranulomas

There is convincing evidence that a mixture of saturated hydrocarbons with the typical mass spectrometric and chemical properties of mineral oil are absorbed from the intestinal tract and frequently appear as lipid droplets in the liver, spleen, and hepatic hilar lymph nodes (216,217). The source of this lipid is the mineral oil widely used in commercial food processing (217, 218) or in radiocontrast medium (219).

In the liver, mineral oil droplets frequently give rise to a distinctive type of lipogranuloma that may be solitary or multiple. They may be encountered in otherwise normal livers or in association with other types of liver disease (219). In our own series of 206 cases, hepatocellular fatty infiltration was present in less than half, and often was only minimal in extent.

The lipogranulomas tend to be found in the centrilobular zones attached or close to central veins, especially near their points of bifurcation. They present as circumscribed collections of vacuolated macrophages (lipophages) interspersed with lymphocytes and strands of collagen (Fig. 177). The lesions tend to persist, but never give rise to progressive fibrosis or capillarization of the surrounding sinusoids. Occasionally, however, the accumulation of collagen within the lesion obliterates its content of lipophages and lymphocytes and produces a circumscribed, solid, fibrous nodule.

In a small minority of cases, the lipogranulomas are located in portal tracts [(219–221); Fig. 178]. Usually, such lesions are larger and less well circumscribed than those in the centrilobular parenchyma, and, frequently, are accompanied by significant portal fibrosis and mononuclear cell infiltration. As in the case of the intralobular lesions, they show no tendency to produce progressive fibrosis.

References

1. Adams DO: The granulomatous inflammatory response. A review. Am J Pathol 84:164–191, 1976.
2. Sherlock S: Hepatic granulomas. In The Liver in Systemic Disease. Blackwell, London, 1989, pp. 535–540.
3. Guckian JC, Perry JE: Granulomatous hepatitis. An analysis of 63 cases and review of the literature. Ann Intern Med 65:1081–1100, 1966.
4. Klatskin G: Hepatic granulomata: problems in interpretation. Mount Sinai J Med 44:798–812, 1977.
5. Ishak KG: Granulomas of the liver. In Pathology of Granulomas, edited by H. L. Ioachim. New York, Raven Press, 1983, pp. 307–369.
6. Scheuer PJ: Hepatic granulomas. Br Med J 285:833–834, 1982.
7. Cunningham D, Mills PR, Quigley EMM, Patrick RS, Watkinson G, Mackenzie JF, Russell RI: Hepatic granulomas: experience over a 10 year period in the West of Scotland. Q J Med 202:162–170, 1982.
8. James DG, Jones-Williams W: Sarcoidosis and Other Granulomatous Disorders. Philadelphia, W. B. Saunders, 1985.
9. Valla D, Pessegueiro-Miranda H, Degott C: Hepatic sarcoidosis with portal hypertension. A report of seven cases with a review of the literature. Q J Med 63:531–540, 1987.
10. Nolan JP, Klatskin G: The fever of sarcoidosis. Ann Intern Med 61:455–461, 1964.
11. Hercules H, Bethlehem NM: Value of liver biopsy in sarcoidosis. Arch Pathol Lab Med 108:831–834, 1984.
12. Bass NM, Burroughs AK, Scheuer PJ, James DG, Sherlock S: Chronic intrahepatic cholestasis due to sarcoidosis. Gut 23:417–421, 1982.
13. Tekeste H, Latour F, Levitt RE: Portal hypertension complicating sarcoid liver disease: case report and review of the literature. Am J Gastroenterol 79:389–396, 1984.
14. Maddrey WC, Johns CJ, Boitnott JK, Iber FL: Sarcoidosis and chronic hepatic disease: a clinical and pathologic study of 20 patients. Medicine 49:375–394, 1970.
15. Siltzbach LE: The Kveim test in sarcoidosis. A study of 750 patients. JAMA 178:476–482, 1961.
16. Israel HL, Sones M: Immunologic defect in patients recovered from sarcoidosis. N Engl J Med 273:1003–1006, 1965.
17. Israel HL, Margolis ML, Rose LJ: Hepatic granulomatosis and sarcoidosis. Further observations. Dig Dis Sci 29:353–356, 1984.
18. Nosal A, Schleissner LA, Mishkin FS, Lieberman J: Angiotensin-1-converting enzyme and gallium scan in noninvasive evaluation of sarcoidosis. Ann Intern Med 90:328–331, 1979.
19. Muthuswamy PP, Lopez-Majano V, Ranginwala M, Trainor WD: Serum angiotensin-converting enzyme (SACE) activity as an indicator of total body granuloma load and prognosis in sarcoidosis. Sarcoidosis 4:142–148, 1987.
20. Schweisfurth H, Wernze H: Changes of serum angiotensin/converting enzyme in patients with viral hepatitis and liver cirrhosis. Acta Hepato-Gastroenterol 26:207–210, 1979.
21. Studdy PR, Bird R: Serum angiotensin converting enzyme in sarcoidosis—its value in present clinical practice. Ann Clin Biochem 26:13–18, 1989.
22. Rudzki C, Ishak KG, Zimmerman HJ: Chronic intrahepatic cholestasis of sarcoidosis. Am J Med 59:373–387, 1975.
23. Fagan EA, Moore-Gillon JC, Turner-Warwick M: Multiorgan granulomas and mitochondrial antibodies. N Engl J Med 308:572–575, 1983.
24. Maddrey WC: Sarcoidosis and primary biliary cirrhosis. Associated disorders? N Engl J Med 308:588–590, 1983.
25. Mahida Y, Palmer KR, Lovell D, Silk DBA: Familial granulomatous hepatitis: a hitherto unrecognized entity. Am J Gastroenterol 83:42–45, 1988.
26. Klatskin G: Mycobacterial infections. In Diseases of the Liver, edited by L. Schiff. 4th Edition. Philadelphia, J. B. Lippincott 1975, pp. 718–722.
27. Flipping T, Mukherji B, Dayal Y: Granulomatous hepatitis as a late complication of BCG immunotherapy. Cancer 46:1759–1766, 1983.
28. Bretza J, Mayfield JD: Mycobacterium intracellulare presenting as a sarcoid-like illness. South Med J 71:872–874, 1978.
29. Wayne LG: The 'atypical' mycobacteria: recognition and disease association. CRC Crit Rev Microbiol 12:185–222, 1985.
30. Kahn SA, Saltzman BR, Klein RS, Mahadevia PS, Friedland GH, Brandt LJ: Hepatic disorders in the acquired immune deficiency syndrome: a clinical and pathological study. Am J Gastroenterol 81:1145–1148, 1986.
31. Karat ABA, Job CK, Rao PSS: Liver in leprosy: histological and biochemical findings. Br Med J 1:307–310, 1971.
32. Chen TSN, Drutz DJ, Whelan GE: Hepatic granulomas in leprosy. Their relation to bacteremia. Arch Pathol Lab Med 100:182–185, 1976.
33. Zawar PB, Holla VV, Patil SM, Zawar MP, Chawan RN: Bacillaemia in lepra reaction: its correlation with liver pathology. Lepr India 55:570–575, 1983.
34. Beasley RP, Hwang L-Y, Lin CC: Incidence of hepatitis among students at a university in Taiwan. Am J Epidemiol 117:213–222, 1983.
35. Spink WW, Hoffbauer FW, Walker WW, Green RA: Histopathology of the liver in human brucellosis. J Clin Lab Med 34:40–58, 1949.
36. Cohen FB, Robins B, Lipstein W: Isolation of Brucella abortus by percutaneous liver biopsy. N Engl J Med 257:228–230, 1957.
37. Williams PK, Crossley K: Acute and chronic hepatic involvement in brucellosis. Gastroenterology 83:455–458, 1982.
38. Cervantes F, Bruguera M, Carbonell J, Force L, Webb S: Liver disease in brucellosis. A clinical and pathological study of 40 cases. Postgrad Med J 58:346–350, 1982.
39. Osmundson PJ, Martin WJ, Stroebel CF: Brucellosis: report of an unusual case. Proc Staff Meet Mayo Clinic 32:58–64, 1957.
40. Spink WW: Host-parasite relationship in human brucellosis with prolonged illness due to suppuration of the liver and spleen. Am J Med Sci 247:129–136, 1964.
41. Young EJ: Brucella militensis hepatitis: the absence of granulomas. Ann Intern Med 91:414–415, 1979.

42. Foshay L: Tularemia: a summary of certain aspects of the disease including methods for early diagnosis and the results of serum treatment in 600 patients. Medicine *19*:1–83, 1940.

43. Pullen RL, Stuart BM: Tularemia: analysis of 225 cases. JAMA *129*:495–500, 1945.

44. Penn RL, Kenasewitz GT: Factors associated with a poor outcome in tularemia. Arch Intern Med *147*:265–268, 1987.

45. Lyford J III, Johnson RW Jr, Blackman S, Scott RB: Pathologic findings in a fatal case of disseminated granuloma inguinale with miliary bone and joint involvement. Bull Johns Hopkins Hosp *79*:349–357, 1946.

46. Sehgal VN, Shyamprasad AL, Beshar PC: The histopathological diagnosis of donovanosis. Br J Vener Dis *60*:45–47, 1984.

47. Nieman RE, Lorber B: Listeriosis in adults: a changing pattern. Report of eight cases and review of the literature, 1968–1978. Rev Infect Dis *2*:207–227, 1980.

48. Ciesielski CA, Hightower AW, Parsons SK, Broome CV: Listeriosis in the United States: 1980–1982. Arch Intern Med *148*:1416–1419, 1988.

49. Buchner LH, Schneierson SS: Clinical and laboratory aspects of *Listeria monocytogenes* infections. With a report of ten cases. Am J Med *45*:904–921, 1968.

50. Ray CG, Wedgwood RJ: Neonatal listeriosis: six case reports and a review of the literature. Pediatrics *34*:378–392, 1964.

51. Yu VL, Miller WP, Wing EJ, Romano JM, Ruiz CA, Bruns FJ: Disseminated listeriosis presenting as acute hepatitis. Case reports and review of hepatic involvement in listeriosis. Am J Med *73*:773–777, 1982.

52. Al-Dajani O, Khatib R: Cryptogenic liver abscess due to *Listeria monocytogenes*. J Infect Dis *147*:961–969, 1983.

53. Inhorn SL, Smits RL, Christenson E: Listeria as a cause of splenic granulomas in a patient with Felty's syndrome. Am J Clin Pathol *33*:330–338, 1960.

54. McIntosh J: The occurrence and distribution of *Spirochaeta pallida* in congenital syphilis. J Pathol Bacteriol *13*:239–245, 1909.

55. Stokes JH: Modern Clinical Syphilology. Philadelphia, W. B. Saunders, 1927, pp. 993–1067.

56. Campisi D, Whitcomb C: Liver disease in early syphilis. Arch Intern Med *139*:365–366, 1979.

56a. Sequira PJL: Syphilis. In Sexually Transmitted Diseases: A Rational Approach to Their Diagnosis, edited by A.E. Jephcott, London, PHLS, 1987.

57. Romeu J, Rybak B, Dave P, Coven R: Spirochetal vasculitis and bile ductular damage in early hepatic syphilis. Am J Gastroenterol *74*:352–354, 1980.

58. Veeravahu M: Diagnosis of liver involvement in early syphilis. A critical review. Arch Intern Med *145*:132–134, 1985.

59. Scully RE, Mark EJ, McNeedley BU: Case records of the Massachusetts General Hospital. N Engl J Med *309*:35–43, 1983.

60. Kahn LB, Gordon W: Sarcoid-like granulomas in secondary syphilis. A clinical and histopathologic study of five cases. Arch Pathol *92*:334–337, 1971.

61. Wagoner GP, Anton AT, Gall EA, Schiff L: Needle biopsy of the liver. VIII. Experiences with hepatic granulomas. Gastroenterology *25*:487–493, 1953.

62. Johnson J: Early syphilitic hepatitis after renal transplantation. J Infect Dis *158*:236–238, 1988.

63. Hahn RD: Syphilis of the liver. Am J Syphilis *27*:529–562, 1943.

64. Symmers D, Spain DM; Hepar lobatum. Clinical significance of the anatomic changes. Arch Pathol *42*:64–68, 1946.

65. Picchi J, Nelson AR, Waller EE, Razavi M, Clizer EE: Q fever associated with granulomatous hepatitis. Ann Intern Med *53*:1065–1074, 1960.

66. Bernstein M, Edmondson HA, Barbour BH: The liver lesion in Q fever. Clinical and pathologic features. Arch Intern Med *116*:491–498, 1965.

67. Dupont HL, Hornick RB, Levin HS, Rapoport MI, Woodward TE: Q fever hepatitis. Ann Intern Med *74*:198–206, 1971.

68. Pellegrin M, Delsol G, Auvergnat C, Familiades J, Faure H, Guiu M, Boigt JJ: Granulomatous hepatitis in Q fever. Hum Pathol *11*:51–57, 1980.

68a. Sawyer LA, Fishbein DB, McDade JE: Q fever: current concepts. Rev Infec Dis *9*:9935–946, 1987.

69. Hofmann CE, Heaton JW: Q fever hepatitis. Clinical manifestations and pathological findings. Gastroenterology *83*:474–479, 1982.

70. Qizilbash AA: The pathology of Q fever as seen on liver biopsy. Arch Pathol Lab Med *107*:364–367, 1983.

71. Voight JJ, Delsol G, Fabre J: Liver and bone marrow granulomas in Q fever. Gastroenterology *84*:887–888, 1983.

72. Nenert M, Mavier P, Dubuc N, Deforges L, Zafrani ES: Epstein-Barr virus infection and hepatic fibrin-ring granulomas. Hum Pathol *19*:608–610, 1988.

73. Moreno A, Marazuela M, Yebra M, Hernandez MJ, Hellin T, Montalban C, Vargas JA: Hepatic fibrin-ring granulomas in visceral leishmaniasis. Gastroenterology *95*:1123–1126, 1988.

74. Vanderstigel M, Zafrani ES, Lejong JL, Schaeffer A, Portos JL: Allopurinol hypersensitivity syndrome as a cause of hepatic fibrin-ring granulomas. Gastroenterology *90*:188–190, 1986.

75. Stricker BHC, Blok APR, Babany G, Benhamou J-P: Fibrin ring granulomas and allopurinol. Gastroenterology *96*:1199–1203, 1989.

75a. Powell OW: Liver involvement in Q fever: Aust Ann Med *10*:52–58, 1961.

76. Schachter J: Chlamydial infections. N Engl J Med *298*:428–434, 1978.

77. Wolmer-Hanssen P, Westrom L, Mardh P-A: Perihepatitis and chlamydial salpingitis. Lancet *1*:901–904, 1980.

78. Wood JJ, Bolton JP, Cannon S, Allan A, O'Connor BH, Daronger S: Biliary-type pain as a manifestation of genital tract infection: the Curtis-Fitz-Hugh syndrome. Br J Surg *69*:251–253, 1982.

79. Shabot JM, Roark GD, Truant AL: *Chlamydia trachomatis* in the ascitic fluid of patients with chronic liver disease. Am J Gastroenterol *78*:291–293, 1983.

80. Francis TI, Osoba AO: Gonococcal hepatitis (Fitz-Hugh-Curtis syndrome) in a male patient. Br J Vener Dis *48*:187–188, 1972.

81. Stineman RS, Korn RJ, Zimmerman JH: Hepatic function studies in lympho-granuloma vernereum. Arch Intern Med *96*:799–803, 1955.

82. Yow EM, Brennan JC, Preston J, Levy S: The pathology of psittacosis. A report of two cases with hepatitis. Am J Med *27*:739–749, 1959.

83. Cornog JL Jr, Hanson CW: Psittacosis as a cause of miliary infiltrates of the lung and hepatic granulomas. Am Rev Respir Dis *98*:1033–1036, 1968.

84. Reller LB: Granulomatous hepatitis associated with acute cytomegalovirus infection. Lancet *1*:20–22, 1973.

85. Bonkowsky HL, Lee RV, Klatskin G: Acute granulomatous hepatitis: Occurrence in cytomegalovirus mononucleosis. JAMA *233*:1284–1288, 1975.

86. Bang J, Wanscher O: The histopathology of the liver in infectious mononucleosis. Acta Med Scand *120*:437–446, 1945.

87. Wadsworth RC, Keil PG: Biopsy of the liver in infectious mononucleosis. Am J Pathol *28*:1003–1016, 1952.

88. Hoagland RJ, McCluskey RT: Hepatitis in mononucleosis. Ann Intern Med *43*:1019–1030, 1955.

89. Finkel M, Parker GW, Fanselau HA: The hepatitis of infectious mononucleosis: experience with 235 cases. Military Med *129*:533–538, 1964.

90. Ross JS, Lee Fanning W, Beautyman W, Craighead JE: Fatal massive hepatic necrosis from varicella-zoster hepatitis. Am J Gastroenterol *74*:423–427, 1980.

91. Eschar J, Reif L, Waron M, Alkan WJ: Hepatic lesion in chickenpox. A case report. Gastroenterology *64*:462–466, 1973.

92. Kean BH, Kimball AC, Christenson WN: An epidemic of acute toxoplasmosis. JAMA *208*:1002–1004, 1969.

93. Vischer TL, Bernheim C, Engelbrecht E: Two cases of hepatitis due to *Toxoplasma gondii*. Lancet *2*:919–921, 1967.

94. Tiwari I, Rolland C-F, Popple AW: Cholestatic jaundice due to toxoplasma hepatitis. Postgrad Med J *58*:299–300, 1982.

95. Martinez-Vazquez JM, Guardia J, Pahissa A, Morgas A, Mirada A, Tornos J, Bacardi R: Hepatite granulomateuse dans la toxoplasmose acquise de l'adulte. Sem Hop Paris *51*:963–965, 1975.

96. Frenkel JK: Toxoplasmosis. *In* Pathology of Tropical and Extraordinary Diseases, Vol. 1, edited by C. H. Binford, D. H. Connor. Washington, Armed Forces Institute of Pathology, 1976, pp. 284–300.

97. Witorsch P, Utz JP: North American blastomycosis. A study of 40 patients. Medicine *47*:169–200, 1968.

98. Londero AT: Paracoccidioidomycosis. *In* Infectious Diseases, edited by P. D. Hoeprich, M. C. Jordan. Philadelphia, J. B. Lippincott, 1989, pp. 502–510.

99. Bacharach T, Zalis EG: Sarcoid syndrome associated with coccidioidomycosis. Am Rev Respir Dis *88*:248–251, 1963.

100. Hoeprich PD: Coccidioidomycosis. *In* Infectious Diseases, edited by P. D. Hoeprich, M. C. Jordan. Philadelphia, J. B. Lippincott, 1989, pp. 489–502.

101. Shields LH: Disseminated cryptococcosis producing a sarcoid type reaction. The report of a case treated with amphotericin B. Arch Intern Med *104*:763–770, 1959.

102. Lefton HB, Farmer RG, Buchwald R, Haselby R: Cryptococcal hepatitis mimicking primary sclerosing cholangitis. A case report. Gastroenterology 67:511–515, 1974.

103. Symmers W St C: Primary hepatic cryptococcosis. Br Med J 287:909–911, 1983.

104. Das BC, Haynes I, Weaver RM, Ackland PR: Primary hepatic cryptococcosis. Br Med J 287:464–466, 1983.

105. Lanza FL, Nelson RS, Somayaji BN: Acute granulomatous hepatitis due to histoplasmosis. Gastroenterology 58:392–396, 1970.

106. Sarosi GA, Voth DW, Dahl BA, Doto IL, Tosh FE: Disseminated histoplasmosis: results of long-term follow-up. A Center for Disease Control cooperative mycosis study. Ann Intern Med 75:511–516, 1971.

107. Smith JW, Utz JP: Progressive disseminated histoplasmosis. A prospective study of 26 patients. Ann Intern Med 76:557–565, 1972.

108. Ishak KG: Granulomas of the liver. In Pathology of Granulomas, edited by H. L. Ioachim. New York, Raven Press, 1983, pp. 307–369.

109. Delahoussaye PM, Osborne BM: Cat-scratch disease presenting as abdominal visceral granulomas. J Infect Dis 161:71–78, 1990.

110. Lenoir AA, Storch GA, DeSchryver-Kecksemeti K, Shackelford GD, Rothbaum RJ, Wear DJ, Rosenblum JL: Granulomatous hepatitis associated with cat scratch disease. Lancet 1:1132–1136, 1988.

111. English CK, Wear DJ, Margileth AM, Lissner CR, Walsh GP: Cat-scratch disease: isolation and culture of the bacterial agent. JAMA 259:1347–1352, 1988.

112. Andrade ZA: Hepatic schistosomiasis. Morphological aspects. In Progress in Liver Diseases, Vol. 2, edited by H. Popper, F. Schaffner. New York, Grune & Stratton, 1965, pp. 228–252.

113. Andrade ZA, Cheever AW: Alterations of the intrahepatic vasculature in hepatosplenic schistosomiasis. Am J Trop Med Hyg 20:425–432, 1971.

114. Warren KS: Hepatosplenic schistosomiasis mansoni: an immunologic disease. Bull NY Acad Med 51:545–550, 1975.

115. Dunn MA, Kamel R: Hepatic schistosomiasis. Hepatology 1:653–661, 1981.

116. Simson IW, Gear JHS: Other viral and infectious diseases. In Pathology of the Liver, edited by R. N. M. MacSween, P. P. Anthony, P. J. Scheuer. 2nd Edition. Edinburgh, Churchill Livingston, 1987, pp. 249–252.

117. Abdel-Wahab MF, Strickland GT, El-Sahly A, Ahmed L, Zakaria S, El-Kady N: Schistosomiasis mansoni in an Egyptian village in the Nile Delta. Am J Trop Med Hyg 29:868–874, 1980.

118. Smith SWG, Chappell LH, Thomson AW, MacGowan AG, Simpson JG: Prophylactic and therapeutic effects of Ciclosporin A in murine Schistosomiasis mansoni: studies on bisexual and unisexual infections and the hepatic inflammatory response. Int Arch Allergy Appl Immunol 85:174–179, 1988.

119. Dunn MA: Suppressive effects of cyclosporin A in murine schistosomiasis. Hepatology 9:339–340, 1989.

120. Warren KS, Reboucas G: Blood ammonia during bleeding from esophageal varices in patients with hepatosplenic schistosomiasis. N Engl J Med 271:921–926, 1964.

121. Andrade ZA, Brito PA: Evolution of schistosomal hepatic vascular lesions after specific chemotherapy. Am J Trop Med Hyg 30:1223–1227, 1981.

122. Grimaud J-A, Borojevic R: Chronic human schistosomiasis mansoni. Pathology of the Disse's space. Lab Invest 36:268–273, 1977.

123. Alves CAP, Alves AR, Abreu WN, Andrade ZA: Hepatic artery hypertrophy and sinusoidal hypertension in advanced schistosomiasis. Gastroenterology 72:126–128, 1977.

124. Lyra LG, Reboucas G. Hepatitis B surface antigen carrier state in hepatosplenic schistosomiasis. Gastroenterology 71:641–645, 1976.

125. Al-Nakib B, Al-Nakib W, Bayoumi A, Al-Liddawi H, Bashir AA: Hepatitis B virus (HBV) markers among patients with chronic liver disease in Kuwait. Trans R Soc Trop Med Hyg 76:348–350, 1982.

126. El-Badrawy NM, Hassanein HI, Botros SS, Nagy FM, Abdallah NM, Herbage D: Effect of praziquantel on hepatic fibrosis in experimental Schistosomiasis mansoni. Exp Mol Pathol 49:151–160, 1988.

127. Penalba C, Marche C, Charmot G, Coulaud J-P, Saimot AG: Eosinophilic granulomatous hepatitis. A propos of 3 cases. Bull Soc Pathol Exot Filiales 80:100–104, 1987.

128. Miguet JP, Bresson-Hadni S: Alveolar echinococcosis of the liver. J Hepatol 8:373–379, 1989.

129. Khaleque KA, Alam KS: Hepatic granuloma caused by Ascaris ova. J Trop Med Hyg 66:249–251, 1963.

130. Neafie RC, Connor DH: Ascariasis. In Pathology of Tropical and Extraordinary Diseases. Washington, Armed Forces Institute of Pathology, 1976, pp. 460–467.

131. Khuroo MS, Zargar SA, Mahajan R: Hepatobiliary and pancreatic ascariasis in India. Lancet 335:1503–1506, 1990.

132. Raney R, Lilly J, McHardy G: Biliary calculus of roundworm origin. Ann Intern Med 72:405–407, 1970.

133. Daya H, Allie A, McCarthy R: Disseminated ascariasis: a case report. S Afr Med J 62:820–822, 1982.

134. Snyder CH: Visceral larva migrans. Ten years' experience. Pediatrics 28:85–91, 1961.

135. Huntley CC, Costas MC, Lyerly A: Visceral larva migrans syndrome: clinical characteristics and immunologic studies in 51 patients. Pediatrics 36:523–536, 1965.

136. Otto GF, Berthrong M, Appleby RE, Rawlins JC, Wilbur O: Eosinophilia and hepatomegaly due to Capillaria hepatica infection. Bull Johns Hopkins Hosp 94:319–336, 1954.

137. Cislaghi F, Radice C: Infection by Capillaria hepatica. First case report in Italy. Helvet Paediatr 25:647–654, 1970.

138. Attah EB, Nagarajan S, Obineche EN, Gera SC: Hepatic capillariasis. Am J Clin Pathol 79:127–130, 1983.

139. Drury RAB: Larval granulomata in the liver. Gut 3:289–294, 1962.

140. Mendeloff J: Healed granulomas of the liver due to tongue worm infection. Am J Clin Pathol 43:433–437, 1965.

141. Smith JW, Gutierrez Y: Medical parasitology. In Clinical Diagnosis and Management by Laboratory Methods, edited by J. B. Henry. Philadelphia, W. B. Saunders, 1984, pp. 1245–1247.

142. Daly JJ, Baker GF: Pinworm granuloma of the liver. Am J Trop Med Hyg 33:62–64, 1984.

143. Mondou EN, Gnepp DR: Hepatic granuloma resulting from Enterobius vermicularis. Am J Clin Pathol 91:97–100, 1989.

144. Roberts-Thompson IC, Anders RF, Bhathal PS: Granulomatous hepatitis and cholangitis associated with giardiasis. Gastroenterology 83:480–483, 1982.

145. Hamilton CR Jr, Shelley WM, Tumulty PA: Giant cell arteritis: including temporal arteritis and polymyalgia rheumatica. Medicine 50:1–27, 1971.

146. Dickson ER, Maldonado JE, Sheps SG, Cain JA Jr: Systemic giant-cell arteritis with polymyalgia rheumatica. Reversible abnormalities of liver function. JAMA 224:1496–1498, 1973.

147. Klein RG, Hunder GG, Stanson AW, Sheps SG: Large artery involvement in giant cell (temporal) arteritis. Ann Intern Med 83:806–812, 1975.

148. McCormack LR, Astarita RW, Foroozan P: Liver involvement in giant cell arteritis. Am J Dig Dis 23 (Suppl): 72–74, 1978.

149. Hamrin B, Jonsson N, Hellsten S: "Polymyalgia arterica." Further clinical and histopathological studies with a report of six autopsy cases. Ann Rheum Dis 27:397–405, 1968.

150. Long R, James O: Polymyalgia rheumatica and liver disease. Lancet 1:77–79, 1974.

151. Gibbs P: Polymyalgia rheumatica and liver disease. Lancet 1:351–352, 1974.

152. Strauss RG, Schubert WK, McAdams AJ: Anyloidosis in childhood. J Pediatr 74:272–282, 1969.

153. Kornreich H, Malouf NN, Hanson V: Acute hepatic dysfunction in juvenile rheumatoid arthritis. J Pediatr 79:27–35, 1971.

154. Bujak JS, Aptekar RG, Decker JL, Wolff SM: Juvenile rheumatoid arthritis presenting in the adult as fever of unknown origin. Medicine 52:431–444, 1973.

155. Rachelefsky GS, Kar NC, Coulson A, Sarkissian E, Stiehm ER, Paulus HE: Serum enzyme abnormalities in juvenile rheumatoid arthritis. Pediatrics 58:730–736, 1976.

156. Godman GC, Churg J: Wegener's granulomatosis. Pathology and review of the literature. Arch Pathol 58:533–553, 1954.

157. Young ID, Clark RN, Manley PN: Response to steroids in Budd-Chiari syndrome caused by idiopathic granulomatous venulitis. Gastroenterology 94:503–509, 1988.

158. Russe EW, Bansky G, Pfaltz M: Budd-Chiari syndrome in sarcoidosis. Am J Gastroenterol 81:71–78, 1986.

159. Mistilis SP, Skyring AP, Goulston SJM: Pericholangitis and ulcerative colitis. II. Clinical aspects. Ann Intern Med 63:17–26, 1965.

160. Kern F: Hepatobiliary disorders in inflammatory bowel disease. In Diseases of the Liver, edited by L. Schiff, E. R. Schiff. 5th Edition. Philadelphia, J. B. Lippincott, 1982, pp. 1603–1614.

161. Banner BF, Banner AS: Hepatic granulomas following ileal bypass for obesity. Arch Pathol Lab Med 102:655–657, 1978.

161a. Holian DK: Biliopancreatic bypass. In Surgery for the Morbidly Obese Patient, edited by M. Deitel. Philadelphia, Lea & Febiger, 1989, pp. 105–111.

161b. Grimm IS, Schindler W, Haluszka O: Steatohepatitis and fatal hepatic failure after biliopancreatic diversion. Am J. Gastroenterol 1992 (in press).

162. Robert F, Omura RF, Durant JR: Mucosal eosinophilic gastroenteritis with systemic involvement. Am J Med 62:139–143, 1977.

163. Weisberg SC, Crosson JT: Eosinophilic gastroenteritis. Report of a case of thirty-two years' duration. Am J Dig Dis 18:1005–1014, 1973.

164. Everett GD, Mitros FA: Eosinophilic gastroenteritis with hepatic eosinophilic granulomas. Report of a case with 30 year follow-up. Am J Gastroenterol 74:519–521, 1980.

165. Girardin M-F S-M, Zafrani ES, Chaumette M-T, Delchier J-C, Metreau J-M, Chumeaux D: Hepatic granulomas in Whipple's disease. Gastroenterology 86:753–756, 1984.

166. Pequignot H, Morin Y, Grandjouan S. Sarcoidose et maladie de Whipple. Association? relation? Ann Med Interne 127:797–806, 1976.

167. Haubrich WS, Watson JHL, Sieracki JC: Unique morphologic features of Whipple's disease. A study by light and electron microscopy. Gastroenterology 39:454–468, 1960.

168. Mazzitello WF: Eosinophilic granuloma of the lung. N Engl J Med 250:804–809, 1954.

169. Livingston HJ: Eosinophilic granuloma of the lung. N Engl J Med 259:959–963, 1958.

170. Carson MJ, Chadwick DL, Brubaker CA, Cleland RS, Landing BH: Thirteen boys with progressive septic granulomatosis. Pediatrics 35:405–412, 1965.

171. Quie PG, Kaplan EL, Page AR, Gruskay FL, Malawista SE: Defective polymorphonuclear-leukocyte function and chronic granulomatous disease in two female children. N Engl J Med 278:976–980, 1968.

172. Holmes B, Park BH, Malawista SE, Quie PG, Nelson DL, Good RA: Chronic granulomatous disease in females. A deficiency of leukocyte glutathione peroxidase. N Engl J Med 283:217–221, 1970.

173. Borregaard N, Johansen KS: Cytochrome b is present in neutrophils from patients with chronic granulomatous disease. Lancet 1:949–951, 1979.

174. Segal AW, Jones OTG: Neutrophil cytochrome b in chronic granulomatous disease. Lancet 1:1036–1037, 1979.

175. Ishak KG, Sharp HL: Metabolic errors and liver disease. In Pathology of the Liver, edited by R. N. M. MacSween, P. P. Anthony, P. J. Scheuer. 2nd Edition. Edinburgh, Churchill Livingstone, 1987, pp. 99–180.

176. Lofgren S: Erythema nodosum. Studies on etiology and pathogenesis. Acta Med Scand 124 (Suppl 174):1–197, 1946.

177. Mather G, Dawson J, Hoyle C: Liver biopsy in sarcoidosis. Q J Med 24:331–350, 1955.

178. James DG: Erythema nodosum. Br Med J 1:853–857, 1961.

179. Zinneman HH, Hall WH, Heller BI: Acquired agammaglobulinemia. Report of three cases. JAMA 156:1390–1393, 1954.

180. Prasad AS, Reiner E, Watson CJ: Syndrome of hypogammaglobulinemia, splenomegaly and hypersplenism. Blood 12:926–932, 1957.

181. Kushner DS, Dubin A, Donlon WP, Bronsky D: Familial hypogammaglobulinemia, splenomegaly and leukopenia with a review of the etiologic factors of the hypogammaglobulinemias. Am J Med 29:33–42, 1960.

182. Good RA, Page AR: Fatal complications of virus hepatitis in two patients with agammaglobulinemia. Am J Med 29:804–810, 1960.

183. Record CO, Eddleston ALWF, Williams R: Intrahepatic sclerosing cholangitis associated with a familial immunodeficiency syndrome. Lancet 2:18–20, 1973.

184. Thomas IT, Ochs HD, Wedgwood RJ: Liver disease and immunodeficiency syndromes. Lancet 1:311, 1974.

185. Dutra FR: The pneumonitis and granulomatosis peculiar to beryllium workers. Am J Pathol 24:1131–1165, 1948.

186. Chesner C: Chronic pulmonary granulomatosis in residents of a community near a beryllium plant: three autopsied cases. Ann Intern Med 32:1028–1048, 1950.

187. Stoeckle JD, Hardy HL, Weber AL: Chronic beryllium disease. Long-term follow-up of sixty cases and selective review of the literature. Am J Med 46:545–561, 1969.

188. Pimentel JC, Menezes AP: Liver disease in vineyard sprayers. Gastroenterology 72:275–283, 1977.

189. McMaster KR, Hennigar GR: Drug-induced granulomatous hepatitis. Lab Invest 44:61–73, 1981.

190. Nadel EM, Ackerman LV: Lesions resembling Boeck's sarcoid in lymph nodes draining an area containing a malignant neoplasm. Am J Clin Pathol 20:952–956, 1950.

191. Gregorie HB Jr. Othersen HB Jr, Moore MP Jr: The significance of sarcoid-like lesions in association with malignant neoplasms. Am J Surg 104:577–586, 1962.

192. Kadin ME, Donaldson SS, Dougman RF: Isolated granulomas in Hodgkin's disease. N Engl J Med 283:859–861, 1970.

193. O'Connell MJ, Schimpff SC, Kirschner RH, Aft AB, Wiernik PH: Epithelioid granulomas in Hodgkin's disease. A favorable prognostic sign? JAMA 233:886–889, 1975.

194. Aderka D, Kraus M, Avidor I, Sidi Y, Weinberger A, Pinkhas J: Hodgkin's and non-Hodgkin's lymphomas masquerading as 'idiopathic' liver granulomas. Am J Gastroenterol 79:642–644, 1984.

195. Simon HB, Wolff SM; Granulomatous hepatitis and prolonged fever of unknown origin: a study of 13 patients. Medicine 52:1–21, 1973.

196. Chagnac A, Gal R, Kimchi D, Zevin D, Machtey I, Levi J: Liver granulomas: a possible paraneoplastic manifestion of hypernephroma. Am J Gastroenterol 80:989–992, 1985.

197. Nyfors A, Poulsen H: Liver biopsies from psoriatics related to methotrexate therapy. I. Findings in 123 consecutive non-methotrexate treated patients. Acta Pathol Microbiol Scand, Sect A, 84:253–261, 1976.

198. Kaplan H, Klatskin G: Sarcoidosis, psoriasis and gout: syndrome or coincidence? Yale J Biol Med 32:335–352, 1960.

199. Farmer JL, Winkelmann RK: Psoriasis in association with sarcoidosis. Report of a case. Arch Dermatol 81:983–986, 1960.

200. Simon HB, Wolff SM: Granulomatous hepatitis and prolonged fever of unknown origin: a study of 13 patients. Medicine 52:1–21, 1973.

201. Zoutman DE, Ralph ED, Frei JV: Granulomatous hepatitis and fever of unknown origin. An 11-year experience of 23 cases with three years' follow-up. J Clin Gastroenterol 13:69–75, 1991.

202. Larson EB, Featherstone HJ, Petersdorf RG: Fever of undetermined origin: diagnosis and follow-up of 105 cases, 1970–1980. Medicine 61:269–292, 1982.

203. Williams GT, Williams WJ: Granulomatous inflammation: a review. J Clin Pathol 36:723–733, 1983.

204. Taft DA, Lasersohn JT, Hill LD: Glove starch granulomatous peritonitis. Am J Surg 120:231–236, 1970.

205. Sobel HJ, Schiffman RJ, Schwarz R, Albert WS: Granulomas and peritonitis due to starch glove powder. Arch Pathol 91:559–568, 1971.

206. Aarons I, Fitzgerald N: The persisting hazards of surgical glove powder. Surg Gynecol Obstet 138:385–390, 1974.

207. Henderson WJ, Melville-Jones C, Griffiths K: Talc contamination of surgical gloves. Lancet 1:1419, 1975.

208. Ishak BW, Ishak KG: Foreign-body reaction in the liver of a drug addict. J Forensic Sci 14:515–520, 1969.

209. Kurumaya H, Kono N, Nakanuma Y, Tomoda F, Takazakura E: Hepatic granulomata in long-term hemodialysis patients with hyperaluminumemia. 113:1132–1134, 1989.

210. Fauci AS, Wolff SM: Granulomatous hepatitis. In Progress in Liver Diseases, Vol. V, edited by H. Popper, F. Schaffner. New York, Grune & Stratton, 1976, pp. 609–621.

211. Simon HB, Wolff SM: Sarcoidosis and granulomatous hepatitis. Ann Intern Med 80:560–561, 1974.

212. Eliakim M, Eisenberg S, Levy IS, Sacks TG: Granulomatous hepatitis accompanying a self-limited febrile ddsease. Lancet 1:1348–1352, 1968.

213. Gelb AM, Brazenas N, Sussman H, Wallach R: Acute granulomatous disease of the liver. Am J Dig Dis 15:842–847, 1970.

214. Reichle HS, Work JL: Incidence and significance of healed tubercles in the liver, spleen and kidneys. Arch Pathol 28:331–339, 1939.

215. Petersen P, Christoffersen P: Ultrastructure of lipogranulomas in human fatty liver. Acta Pathol Microbiol Scand, Sect A, 87:45–49, 1979.

216. Christoffersen P, Braendstrup O, Juhl E, Poulsen H: Lipogranulomas in human liver biopsies with fatty change. A morphological, biochemical and clinical investigation. Acta Pathol Microbiol Scand, Sect A, 79:150–158, 1971.

217. Boitnott JK, Margolis S: Saturated hydrocarbons in human tissues. III. Oil droplets in the liver and spleen. Johns Hopkins Med J 127:65–78, 1970.

218. Boitnott JK, Margolis S: Mineral oil in human tissues. II. Oil droplets in lymph nodes of the porta hepatitis. Bull Johns Hopkins Hosp 118:414–422, 1966.

219. Wanless IR, Geddie WR: Mineral oil lipogranulomta in liver and spleen. Pathol Lab Med 109:283–286, 1985.

220. Cruickshank B, Thomas MJ: Mineral oil (follicular) lipidosis: II. Histologic studies of spleen, liver, lymph nodes and bone marrow. Hum Pathol 15:731–737, 1984.

221. Dinscoy HP, Weesner RE, MacGee J: Lipogranulomas in non-fatty human liver. A mineral oil-induced environmental disease. Am J Clin Pathol 78:35–41, 1982.

Chapter 23
Hepatic Injury in Infection

Many infections of varied etiology and distribution lead to abnormalities of hepatic function and structure that may be accompanied by jaundice. In some cases, such hepatic injury is attributable to spread of the infection to the liver; in others, it appears to be related to the toxic effects of the infection or to such complicating factors as hyperpyrexia, hypoxemia, circulatory failure, malnutrition, or hemolysis.

The hepatic lesions produced by infection are highly variable and depend on the nature of the infecting organisms involved. They include several types of hepatitis, cholestasis, suppurative cholangitis, and portal fibrosis. Except in cases in which the infecting agent can be identified histologically, few of the hepatic lesions are pathognomonic for the specific infection responsible.

Infections known to produce hepatic injury are briefly summarized in this chapter. For further details and references, the reader is referred to more comprehensive reviews of the subject (1–3).

Bacterial infections

Pneumococcus

Most patients with pneumococcal lobar pneumonia exhibit impairment of hepatic function, and in up to one-quarter of such cases there is accompanying jaundice. Although the pathogenesis of the jaundice has not been established, ultrastructural studies suggest that toxic injury to the hepatocytes leads to cholestasis. As an alternative, it has been proposed that hemolysis plays an important role. This view is based to a large extent on the observation that in patients with lobar pneumonia, the occurrence of jaundice appears to correlate with deficiency of glucose-6-phosphate-dehydrogenase (4). Recent reports suggest that black men with lobar pneumonia are particularly susceptible to the development of jaundice, but reasons for such an association are not known (5).

The hepatic lesions in lobar pneumonia with jaundice vary, but usually exhibit swelling of hepatocytes, hyperplasia of the Kupffer cells, foci of necrosis, hepatocellular pleomorphism, and canalicular bile thrombi (5).

Staphylococcus

The liver is seldom involved in staphylococcal bacteremia, although rare instances of hepatic abscess with jaundice have been reported (6). Abscess formation undoubtedly is attributable to

seeding of the liver by staphylococci, but other factors must be involved to account for its low incidence in bacteremia. The hepatic lesions in cases of staphylococcal bacteremia with jaundice have not been described, so the pathogenesis of this complication is uncertain. Hepatocellular injury secondary to the toxic effects of the infection may be the underlying mechanism. However, the frequent occurrence of severe anemia in staphylococcal sepsis suggests that hemolysis may play a role as a contributory factor.

Staphylococcal infections, primarily pneumonitis, are extremely common in fulminant hepatic failure that follows acetaminophen overdosage or viral hepatitis, accounting for about one-half of the bacterial infections that occur so commonly in this syndrome (7). The liver, however, is rarely the site of infection in such patients.

Streptococcus

Jaundice occurs in only a small minority of patients with hemolytic streptococcal bacteremia (8). It has also been reported as an early manifestation of scarlet fever in the absence of bacteremia (9), and, rarely, it is a complication of anaerobic streptococcal sepsis.

The hepatic lesions associated with streptococcal infections, which are highly variable, may be attributable to hepatocellular injury secondary to the toxic effects of the infection or to invasion of the liver by the organisms themselves (10). Histologic features that have been reported include nonspecific reactive hepatitis, foci of parenchymal necrosis, portal inflammatory reactions, and multiple abscesses (11–13).

Prolonged fever of unknown origin was attributed to *Streptococcus viridans* infection of the liver in the absence of bacteremia, biliary tract disease, or any extrahepatic source of infection (14). Liver biopsy showed lymphocytic inflammation of the portal tracts and the loss of periportal hepatocytes. Penicillin therapy led to complete recovery in that case.

Gonococcus

Occasionally, the gonococcus produces an acute perihepatitis in women with pelvic inflammatory disease, leading to the development of a disorder commonly termed the *Fitz-Hugh-Curtis syndrome* (15–17). Characteristically, the onset is abrupt, with severe, right upper quadrant abdominal pain, tenderness, and spasm, fever, and leukocytosis that may be accompanied by a friction rub over the liver. The disease may be mistaken for acute cholecystitis. In patients subjected to laparotomy, the principal findings are a fibrinous peritonitis localized to the surface of the liver and acute inflammation of Glisson's capsule. Occasionally, gonococci can be successfully cultured from the perihepatic exudate or from liver biopsy material. Often, the correct diagnosis is suggested by a history of antecedent lower abdominal pain, fever, physical findings consistent with pelvic inflammatory disease, and the recovery of gonococci from the cervix.

The symptoms of perihepatitis tend to abate spontaneously, but recovery is hastened by antibiotic therapy. In many cases, the acute, inflammatory reaction is followed by the development of "violin-string" adhesions between the anterior surface of the liver and the abdominal wall. Usually they are asymptomatic, but, occasionally, they give rise to chronic or intermittent pain. Lysis of such adhesions at laparoscopy usually relieves the symptoms. It is generally assumed that gonococcal perihepatitis is attributable to the entry of the organisms through the fallopian tubes. However, occasional reports of the Fitz-Hugh-Curtis syndrome in males (18) suggest that the hematogenous spread of gonococci is an alternative mode of transmission.

Rarely, gonococcal infection gives rise to acute endocarditis and septicemia. In most such cases, jaundice is a prominent feature and may be associated with foci of hepatocellular necrosis and neutrophilic infiltration of the liver (19).

Escherichia coli

E. coli infections, particularly those accompanied by bacteremia, may give rise to jaundice (20). This combination is relatively common in young infants with severe E. coli urinary tract infections, but it occurs infrequently in adults (20). The mortality rate in such infants is high, particularly when the infection occurs during the first week of life (21). Prompt recognition of the etiology of infections in newborn infants and administration of appropriate antibiotics usually lead to full recovery. Although sepsis is the principal cause of death, hepatic failure may play an important contributory role in some cases. At portmorten examination, the liver usually shows centrilobular bile stasis, focal parenchymal necrosis, hepatocellular regeneration including giant cell transformation, and minimal portal inflammatory reactions. Occasionally, however, no hepatic lesions can be demonstrated. Almost certainly, toxic hepatocellular injury accounts for the jaundice, although hemolysis may be a contributory factor in some cases.

Spontaneous bacterial peritonitis, often accompanied by bacteremia, is a well-recognized complication of decompensated cirrhosis (22–25). Usually, the infection is due to E. coli or other enteric bacteria, but all types of nonenteric bacteria have been isolated (26). Despite appropriate antibiotic therapy that suppresses the infection, this syndrome often causes or contributes to death (23–25). In spontaneous bacterial peritonitis the primary abnormality is a decreased concentration of complement in ascitic fluid (27) and, therefore, in opsonic activity (28). Bacteremia of any source can result in the entry of organisms into the ascitic fluid (22,29,30). Use of more sensitive bacteriologic techniques suggests that bacterial peritonitis probably occurs twice as frequently as has been reported (31).

In patients with ulcerative colitis, portal vein bacteremia is common. E. coli can be cultured from portal venous blood and from the liver of almost 25% of cases with severe ulcerative colitis (32). This constant seeding of the liver may play a role in the pathogenesis of the sclerosing cholangitis seen so frequently in patients with inflammatory bowel disease (33).

E. coli are the predominant bacteria in both the bacteremias and the suppurative lesions that affect the liver and biliary tract, such as pyogenic abscess, suppurative cholangitis, and pylephlebitis (34). The recent introduction of treatment with monoclonal antibody to endotoxin has greatly improved the prognosis of patients with bacteremia and gram-negative shock (35).

In the toxic shock syndrome, which is characterized by sudden fever and profound hypotension in young, previously healthy individuals, about one-half of the patients are jaundiced (36). It has been postulated that toxins arising in infected vaginal tampons are responsible (37). This pathogenesis is supported by the negative blood cultures and hepatic histologic findings of acute polymorphonuclear inflammation of the portal tracts, microvesicular fat deposition, and little or no cholestasis (38).

Salmonella

Numerous salmonella subtypes have been identified as pathogens in humans but only a few are encountered with any degree of frequency. They include: (1) S. typhimurium, S. enteritidis, and S. heidelberg, the principal causes of acute enterocolitis ("food-poisoning") (39); (2) S. typhi, the agent responsible for typhoid fever; (3) S. paratyphi A, the principal etiologic factor in paratyphoid fever; and (4) S. cholerae suis, an invasive organism that tends to produce bacteremia and septic foci in a number of tissues (40).

Typhoid fever. It has been thought for many years that approximately 25% of patients with typhoid fever exhibit evidence of hepatic injury (41), but more recent reports indicate that serum SGOT activity is increased in virtually all patients (42) and that hepatomegaly is present in at least one-half (43). Jaundice, however, is a relatively infrequent finding, occurring in less than 5% of patients in various series (44). About one-third of cases show pure cholestatic hepatocellular injury (45). Fever is the hallmark of the disease, and blood cultures are almost always positive early in the course (42). Endotoxemia is present in most patients with typhoid fever (46).

Treatment with ampicillin appears to be effective in eradicating the infection and in preventing relapses (41).

The liver biopsy findings in typhoid fever are nonspecific, and are usually characterized by small, scattered foci of hepatocellular necrosis, aggregates of swollen proliferating Kupffer cells, the so-called typhoid nodules, dilatation and congestion of the sinusoids, and infiltration of the parenchyma and portal tracts with lymphocytes and histiocytes (41,44,45). Rarely, a few of the centrilobular canaliculi contain bile thrombi. Fatty infiltration may be present (45).

Occasionally, S. typhi infections produce acute cholecystitis, a complication of typhoid fever that probably occurs more frequently than is recognized clinically. Indeed, it may be responsible for the occasional development of chronic cholecystitis and for the S. typhi carrier state. In addition, rare instances of suppurative cholangitis, pyogenic liver abscess, and suppurative pylephlebitis have been reported as complications of typhoid fever (47), but not in recent years.

Usually, the typhoid carrier state is attributable to chronic infection of the gallbladder, which can be cured by cholecystectomy (48). However, there is evidence that in some cases, the infection involves the intrahepatic bile ducts and does not respond to cholecystectomy or antibiotic therapy (49). Cholecystectomy or T-tube drainage appears to be effective in such cases. Lactulose has been reported to eliminate the typhoid carrier state (50). Carriers with infections of the intrahepatic bile ducts may experience recurrent bouts of cholangitis with jaundice. Although many carriers have a history of antecedent typhoid fever, some do not (48).

Paratyphoid fever. The clinical manifestations and morphologic features of the hepatic lesions in paratyphoid fever are similar to those in typhoid fever (41,51), but are less severe (43).

Other forms of salmonellosis. During World War I, outbreaks of jaundice were attributed to infections with various subtypes of salmonella. However, it is now believed that such epidemics were probably due to concurrent infections with the hepatitis B virus (52). No retrospective studies, such as those performed on the sera of patients involved in outbreaks of HBV hepatitis in World War II (53), have yet been reported to establish the etiology.

Shigella

Sporadic shigella infections that produce acute bacillary dysentery rarely affect the liver. However, in at least one well-documented case subjected to liver biopsy, both the clinical and histologic findings were consistent with a mild cholestatic hepatitis (54). The hepatic lesions in this case were characterized by a few foci of hepatocellular necrosis, canalicular bile thrombi, and a predominantly neutrophilic inflammatory reaction in the portal tracts and ductules.

In epidemics of acute bacillary dysentery, the disease may be complicated by jaundice in a significant number of cases. Epidemiologic evidence suggests that the coincidence of dysentery and jaundice in such epidemics is due to simultaneous infections with shigella bacilli and the hepatitis A virus.

Melioidosis

Pseudomonas pseudomallei, a gram-negative bacillus that is widely distributed in the soil and water of Southeast Asia and other tropical areas, is the cause of melioidosis (55). Infections with this organism are sometimes asymptomatic and, usually, respiratory. Occasionally, they cause septicemia. In the septicemic form of the disease, the liver often develops multiple microabscesses in which many organisms are seen on Giemsa stain (56).

Mild or inapparent infections that are acquired in an endemic area may present as a fulminant illness months or even years after the infected individual has left the endemic area (57). Accordingly, the possibility of melioidosis must be considered in patients with fever of unknown origin who have previously lived or traveled in Southeast Asia or other tropical areas known to be endemic for the disease.

Clostridia

A significant number of patients with *Clostridia perfringens* infections exhibit jaundice. Often, the jaundice in such cases is attributable to hemolysis induced by the release of an exotoxin. However, under some conditions, particularly when the infection is accompanied by bacteremia, clostridia may invade the liver and lead to severe hepatocellular necrosis or abscess formation often accompanied by gas formation in the liver (58). Infections of this type, which may follow acute cholecystitis or biliary tract surgery, tend to be resistant to nonspecific antibiotic therapy and are frequently fatal.

Cat-scratch disease

Granulomas of the lymph nodes, liver, and spleen may occur, and tend to undergo necrosis (see Chapter 22).

Hepatic lesions in *brucellosis, tularemia, granuloma inguinale,* and *listeriosis* are discussed in Chapter 22.

Mycobacterial infections

The hepatic lesions of mycobacterial infections are discussed in Chapter 22.

Viral infections

Many viral infections lead to hepatic injury of several types. Of the agents involved, the most important, in terms of prevalence and geographic distribution, are the hepatitis A, B, D, and the non-A, non-B viruses described in Chapter 6. In this section, discussion will be limited to viruses that produce hepatic lesions less frequently.

Adenovirus

Over 30 serotypes of adenovirus have been identified in humans. Adenoviruses can often be recovered in cultures of lymphoid tissue or of feces of infants and children even in the absence of symptoms. The prevalence of such latent infections makes it difficult to interpret the significance of the adenovirus as an etiologic factor in liver disease. However, there is convincing evidence that the adenovirus can produce fatal, massive, hepatic necrosis in immunocompromised patients (59–61). The hepatic lesions in such cases are characterized by extensive, confluent, hepatocellular necrosis and the presence within surviving hepatocytes of intranuclear viral inclusions.

Adenovirus infections, particularly type 3, have been associated with Reye's syndrome (62,63).

Coxsackie B virus

Epidemic myalgia, myocarditis, pericarditis, and aseptic meningitis are the principal manifestations of infection with group B strains of the Coxsackie virus. Rarely, such enteroviral infections produce an acute hepatitis, frequently associated with myocarditis (64,65). Liver biopsies may show expansion of the portal tracts and erosion of their limiting plates, intense mononuclear and neutrophilic inflammation that involves the portal tracts, blood vessels, and bile ducts, small periportal foci of neutrophils, prominent Kupffer cells, some of which contain bile pigment, and swelling and bile pigmentation of the centrilobular hepatocytes.

Echovirus

Like the Coxsackie viruses, echoviruses are members of the enterovirus group and produce a variety of febrile illnesses that may present with diverse manifestations such as aseptic meningitis, pneumonitis, encephalitis, myocarditis, pericarditis, or enterocolitis. Hepatic involvement is rare in adults, but may be encountered occasionally in young infants and children. Occasionally, an adult may show clinical and biochemical features consistent with a mild acute hepatitis (66), but the histologic characteristics of the hepatic lesions are not known. However, in the overwhelming infections occasionally encountered during the neonatal period, the liver usually shows extensive, nonspecific, hemorrhagic necrosis (67).

Herpes simplex

As a rule, active infections with the type 1 strain of *Herpes virus hominis* (HSV-1) are manifested by herpetic lesions localized in the mucocutaneous junction of the buccal mucosa, whereas those due to the type 2 strain (HSV-2) are accompanied by similar lesions limited to the genital mucosa. However, under some conditions, both strains may produce disseminated infections that involve multiple tissues, including the liver. Although uncommon at all ages, disseminated infections are encountered most frequently in newborn infants with HSV-2 infections acquired during passage through the birth canal (68,69). Most generalized infections in older infants, children, and adults are due to HSV-1, and occur predominantly in individuals with impaired immunity related to therapy or concurrent disease (70,71) or pregnancy (72). However, such infections have been reported in previously healthy adults with no evidence of immunodeficiency (73,74). Indeed, anicteric asymptomatic mild hepatitis occurs in many patients with genital herpes (HSV-1) (74).

Disseminated HSV infections are accompanied by severe hepatitis that often proves fatal. The clinical manifestations in such cases include high fever, jaundice, and progressive hepatic failure, often complicated by terminal, disseminated, intravascular coagulation. Mucocutaneous lesions are an inconstant feature of the disease. In one such case, treatment with acyclovir resulted in dramatic improvement (75).

The *hepatic lesions* of herpes simplex hepatitis are characterized by: (1) irregular zones of confluent, hemorrhagic necrosis in the parenchyma (Fig. 748) that may show bridging, (2) a few scattered acidophilic bodies, (3) destruction of reticulin in some zones of necrosis (Fig. 749), (4) giant cell transformation of the hepatocytes in some neonatal cases, (5) sparse, predominantly mononuclear inflammatory cells in the parenchyma and portal tracts, and (6) intranuclear inclusions (Fig. 192). Patchy areas of coagulation necrosis have been found in some cases (73). Some hepatocytes show these nuclear inclusions adjacent to the zones of necrosis. The intranuclear inclusions are the most distinctive feature of the lesions. However, they are not pathognomonic, since similar inclusions may be encountered in varicella-zoster and cytomegalovirus infections. Characteristically, the affected nucleus is enlarged, shows margination of chromatin along the inner surface of the nuclear membrane, and contains a large, homogeneous or finely granular eosinophilic or amphophilic inclusion encircled by a clear halo (Fig. 192).

Varicella-herpes-zoster

Infections with *Herpes virus varicellae* produce chickenpox in children and herpes zoster in adults. Rarely chickenpox is complicated by dissemination of the virus, which often proves fatal in normal children and in immunocompromised adults (76). In such cases, the liver shows foci of parenchymal necrosis and intranuclear inclusions within the hepatocytes, Kupffer cells, bile duct epithelium, or endothelium (77,78). In addition, destruction of the bile duct epithelium (77) has been observed. In adults with nonfatal varicella, liver biopsy shows epithelioid and giant cell granulomas in the absence of intranuclear inclusions (79). Varicella frequently precedes Reye's syndrome (80).

Lassa fever

Outbreaks of Lassa fever (81,82), an infection caused by an arenavirus, have been reported from various parts of West Africa. In Sierra Leone, where the disease is endemic, 15% of hospital admissions and 30% of deaths in the hospital are due to Lassa fever (83). All of these outbreaks have been characterized by a high case mortality rate, ranging from 30 to 65%. However, serologic evidence suggests that mild and inapparent infections are relatively common in endemic areas. The infection may be transmitted from rodents to humans, or from human to human. Medical personnel who come in close contact with patients, and laboratory workers who handle the patient's body fluids or tissues may occasionally acquire the infection, but casual person-to-person transmission is uncommon (84,85). It is seen in the United States in people returning from Africa (85). Many organs and tissues, especially the liver, are affected in Lassa fever. Although hepatic enlargement and tenderness are frequent findings, overt jaundice is uncommon. Thus, in addition to fever, the clinical manifestations may include an exudative pharyngitis, pneumonitis myositis, myocarditis, and a hemorrhagic diathesis. Death is usually due to sudden cardiovascular collapse. The diagnosis can be established by the demonstration of Lassa fever antigens by monoclonal IgM antibodies in serum and liver tissue (85). Ribavirin therapy appears to be effective (86).

The histopathologic *hepatic lesions* of Lassa fever are not unique. They are characterized by (1) numerous acidophilic bodies, (2) randomly distributed zones of hepatocellular necrosis of variable size that may coalesce to produce portal-portal or portal-central bridging, (3) acidophilic degeneration of perinecrotic hepatocytes, (4) Kupffer cell hyperplasia, (5) a sparse inflammatory exudate (87,88), and (6) occasionally, fatty deposition (88). The reticulin network remains intact. Although fat deposition is not a prominent feature of Lassa hepatitis among the few cases reported, clear vacuoles have been noted in the injured hepatocytes. In the case depicted (Figs. 750, 751), steatonecrosis was limited to the subcapsular area. Conceivably, this finding may not necessarily have been a consequence of the Lassa infection per se.

Marburg virus disease

In 1967, there were outbreaks in Germany and Yugoslavia of a severe, febrile illness that proved fatal in over 20% of cases (89,90). Of those affected, most were laboratory workers who had handled the blood and tissues of vervet monkeys imported from East Africa. The remainder were medical personnel and others who had been in close contact with infected patients. Investigation at the time established that the disease was due to infection with a new virus that was readily transmissible to guinea pigs. Additional epidemics have been reported from South Africa (90) and Kenya (92).

The principal clinical manifestations of Marburg virus disease include high fever, myalgia, conjunctival infection and photophobia, nausea, vomiting and diarrhea, a generalized rash, and evidence of hepatitis, characterized by mild jaundice and elevated serum levels of transaminase. In fatal cases, myocarditis, encephalitis, and disseminated intravascular coagulation may be present. Hepatic lesions are the major finding at autopsy both in humans and in experimentally infected guinea pigs.

Early in their development, the *hepatic lesions* are characterized by the formation of numerous scattered acidophilic bodies and proliferation of the Kupffer cells. As the lesions advance, foci of necrosis appear around the acidophilic bodies and extend into the lobules (93). Often, some of the hepatocytes contain eosinophilic cytoplasmic inclusions. Also, many of the necrotic zones contain basophilic inclusions derived from disrupted nuclei. In late lesions, the hepatocytes may be infiltrated with fat droplets, and the portal tracts may contain lymphocytes and histiocytes. Ultimately, in nonfatal cases, the foci of necrosis are replaced by regenerating hepatocytes, and there are no residuals.

Congenital rubella syndrome

Approximately 20% of infants born of mothers infected with the rubella virus during the first trimester of pregnancy exhibit a syndrome characterized by cataracts, deafness, congenital anomalies of the heart, and mental retardation, often accompanied by microcephaly (94,95). Disorders of the liver, blood, bone, lungs, and blood vessels are common, but less frequent manifestations. The rubella virus, which remains viable for several months in such infants, can be readily recovered on culture of the nasopharynx, body fluids, and tissues.

A high proportion of infants with the congenital rubella syndrome exhibit hepatosplenomegaly (95). Usually, it disappears in a few days, but may persist for several weeks. In some cases, hepatomegaly is accompanied by jaundice and other manifestations of acute hepatitis or biliary obstruction. The hepatic lesions in such infants vary in severity, ranging from fatal giant cell hepatitis to a mild hepatitis characterized by cholestasis, periportal inflammation, and minimal hepatocellular necrosis (96). Occasionally, the hepatitis may give rise to cirrhosis (95). In some cases, the infection involves the biliary tract, leading to atresia or hypoplasia of the extrahepatic or intrahepatic bile ducts (97). The rubella virus can almost always be recovered from the liver in cases with hepatic or biliary tract involvement (97,98).

Rubella

Adults with rubella may develop mild hepatitis characterized by increased transaminase activity (99,100). Histologically, the hepatitis is indistinguishable from that seen in other types of acute viral hepatitis.

Yellow fever

The agent responsible for yellow fever (101,102), a group B arbovirus, is transmitted by *Aedes* mosquitoes from person to person in the urban form of the disease, and from wild monkeys to humans in the sylvatic form. The disease is endemic in South and Central America and in equatorial Africa.

The severity of the infection varies greatly, ranging from mild to fulminant hepatitis. Although the mortality rate in large epidemics has been reported to be as high as 20%, it is usually less than 5%.

In classic cases, after a three to six day incubation period, the onset is abrupt, with fever, headache, and myalgia. After a brief remission in three or four days, the fever recurs and is accompanied by nausea, vomiting, jaundice, proteinuria, azotemia, a bleeding diathesis, and hypotension. Leukopenia is common. In fulminant infections, death from hepatic failure may occur in from three to seven days. Renal failure accounts for most deaths that occur after the 10th day of disease.

The principal features of the *hepatic lesions* in yellow fever include midzonal hepatocellular necrosis and degeneration, fatty infiltration, and a sparse lymphocytic-histiocytic inflammatory reaction. Initially, the necrosis involves individual hepatocytes. However, as the lesions advance, the foci of necrosis tend to coalesce, and, in severe cases, may extend into the centrilobular and periportal zones. Characteristically, a rim of intact hepatocytes around the central veins and portal tracts is spared. Acidophilic degeneration affects individual hepatocytes, and, to a lesser extent, occasional Kupffer cells, leading to the formation of acidophilic bodies, commonly termed Councilman bodies (103). They differ slightly from the acidophilic bodies found in other hepatic lesions (Figs. 94, 218, 422, 454, 666). They occur in relatively large numbers rather than one or two per lobule as is seen in acute viral hepatitis (Fig. 752). They frequently contain ceroid pigment, which is not seen in the more common type of eosinophilic body, and which gives rise to *ochre bodies* (Fig. 753). Finally, Councilman bodies tend to occur in the midzonal portion of the lobules and to cluster together (Fig. 754), while Councilman-like bodies are usually found around the terminal hepatic venules. Often, the nucleoli in intact hepatocytes are enlarged and eosinophilic, and, occasionally, the nuclei contain eosinophilic inclusions. Small collections of histiocytes may be found in the parenchyma adjacent to the foci of degeneration and necrosis. Moreover, the portal tracts may contain mononuclear cells and histiocytes. Characteristically, however, the inflammatory reaction is never prominent, even when parenchymal necrosis is extensive. Invariably, at least some of the hepatocytes show microvesicular fatty infiltration, the extent of which does not correlate with the degree of hepatocellular necrosis nor acidophilic degeneration.

Cytomegalovirus

Infectious mononucleosis hepatitis is discussed in Chapter 22.

Chlamydial infections

The hepatic pathology in *Lymphogranuloma venereum* and *Psittacosis* infections are presented in Chapter 22.

Rickettsial infections

Q fever

Q fever is discussed in Chapter 22.

Rocky Mountain spotted fever

Rickettsia rickettsi, the cause of Rocky Mountain spotted fever, is transmitted to humans by ticks. The illness is characterized by fever, headache, myalgia, and a rash, and proves fatal in approximately 20% of cases, particularly in those over the age of 40. Raised serum levels of bilirubin and transaminase, overt jaundice, and azotemia may be seen in severe infections (104).

The most striking feature of the *hepatic lesions* is an intense, major mononuclear and neutrophilic inflammatory reaction in the portal tracts that involves the walls of the portal vasculature and compresses the interlobular bile ducts (105). Other findings include Kupffer cell erythrophagocytosis and occasional small foci of hepatocellular necrosis. By direct immunofluorescence, rickettsia can be identified in the endothelium of the portal vessels and, less commonly, in the lining cells of the sinusoids.

Spirochetal infections

Leptospirosis

Leptospiral infections in humans invariably are acquired as a consequence of direct or indirect contact with urine or, less commonly, the tissues of animals that harbor leptospira (106–109). The portal of entry for such infections is abraded skin or the intact mucosa of the oropharynx, respiratory tract, or conjunctivae. Over 100 serotypes of leptospira are known to be pathogenic for humans. Of these, the ones encountered most frequently in the United States include *L. icterohemorrhagiae,* usually carried by rats; *L. canicola,* carried by dogs; and *L. pomona,* carried by cattle and swine.

The manifestations of leptospirosis depend not only on the serotype of the organism involved but also on the severity of the infection and the host response. However, most infections are characterized by an abrupt onset of fever and constitutional symptoms associated with leptospiremia that last four to seven days. With the development of antibodies during the second week, the fever abates and the blood is cleared of leptospira. In many infections, dissemination of the organisms to various tissues leads to signs of leptospiral injury of the liver, kidneys, meninges, skeletal muscles, myocardium, eyes, or blood vessels, either alone or in combination. Such localized manifestations may appear during the leptospiremic phase, but usually are more prominent in the afebrile, immune phase of the disease.

By tradition, *L. icterohemorrhagiae* infections accompanied by jaundice and renal failure are classified as Weil's disease. However, most authorities include anicteric *L. icterohemorrhagiae* infections in this category. Others use the term to designate leptospiral infections of any serotype that produce jaundice. To avoid confusion in classification, we prefer to use the term leptospirosis qualified by the serotype of the organism involved.

Typical *L. icterohemorrhagiae* infections are characterized by an abrupt onset of high fever, occasionally accompanied by chills, severe prostration, myalgia, frontal headache, and conjunctival suffusion. These manifestations coincide with the invasion of the blood and cerebrospinal fluid by leptospira and the dissemination of the organisms throughout the body that occurs 6 to 15 days following exposure. In severe infections, the incubation period may be as short as 3 days. Nausea, vomiting, and severe abdominal pain are prominent features in some cases, and may be misinterpreted as signs of an acute abdomen requiring surgical intervention. Others exhibit nuchal rigidity and an increase in the protein content and number of lymphocytes in the spinal fluid, indicative of an aseptic meningitis. If jaundice is present, even when mild, the spinal fluid characteristically shows xanthochromia. In 60 to 80% of cases, jaundice, hepatomegaly, and elevated levels of serum bilirubin, alkaline phosphatase, and transaminase appear between the fourth and seventh day of illness, and usually signify a severe infection. Transaminase values in leptospirosis are not nearly so high as they are in viral hepatitis (109). Other features commonly encountered during the leptospiremic phase of the disease include proteinuria, leukocytosis with an increase in the proportion of neutrophils, and thrombocytopenia. Sometimes, the disease acts like a flu-like illness without involving the liver or kidneys.

Specific complement-fixing and agglutinating antibodies and lysins begin to appear in the serum early in the second week, but do not reach diagnostic titers of 1:300 until a week later. With the onset of the immune response, the temperature drops to normal by lysis and the blood is cleared of leptospira. However, the patient remains ill and leptospira begin to appear in the urine. Characteristically, the jaundice deepens and is accompanied by increasing signs of renal, cardiac, and vascular damage. The urinary findings include significant proteinuria, casts, leukocytes and erythrocytes, fixation of specific gravity at 1.010, and oliguria. In severe infections, the oliguria leads to azotemia and may progress to anuria and death. The principal cardiovascular manifestations include hypotension, cardiac dilatation, arrhythmias, conduction defects, pericarditis, endocarditis, and cardiac failure that may lead to death. A hemorrhagic diathesis due to vascular injury is relatively common in *L. icterohemorrhagiae* infection. In many cases, this is manifested by the occurrence of epistaxis and small petechiae in the conjunctivae. However, in severe infections, the hemorrhagic tendency is more extensive and may present as melena, hematemesis, hemoptysis, hematuria, or purpura in the skin and mucous membranes.

The mortality rate in *L. icterohemorrhagiae* infections ranges from 15 to 25%. Most deaths occur in the second or third week of the disease, and are due to renal failure or, less commonly, to cardiovascular collapse, hemorrhage, or complicating pneumonia. Penicillin is effective therapy (110).

In nonfatal cases, convalescence and full recovery occur between the third and fifth weeks. However, in 20% of cases there is a brief recurrence of fever and constitutional symptoms during this period. Moreover, in 10% of cases, leptospiral iridocyclitis may appear during convalescence or following what appears to be complete recovery.

L. canicola infections produce manifestations similar to those in *L. icterohemorrhagiae* infections. However, they tend to be less severe, produce jaundice less frequently, and rarely cause death.

L. pomona infections cause a self-limited, febrile illness that may be accompanied by iridocyclitis or aseptic meningitis (111).

The other serotypes of leptospira produce relatively mild, influenza-like illnesses that only rarely are accompanied by jaundice or signs of renal injury.

Traditionally, identification of the etiology during the first week of leptospirosis has depended on the detection of leptospira in the blood or spinal fluid by direct, dark-field, or immunofluorescence microscopy, culture on special media, or by inoculation into susceptible animals, such as young guinea-pigs, hamsters, or mice. The organisms are long, slender structures, 6 to 9 μm in length and 0.25 μm in breadth, with sharp, hooked, pointed ends. Tightly coiled, minute spirals that run the length of the spirochete give them a beaded appearance in dark-field illumination. Despite the absence of flagellae or an undulation membrane, they are capable of undulating, twisting, and propulsive movements. At present, leptospiral antigen can be identified in tissues by immunoperoxidase staining (112). The diagnosis can be established rapidly and accurately with the IgM specific dot-ELISA assay (113).

During the second and third weeks of disease, the diagnosis can be established by the demonstration of a rising titer of specific complement-fixing antibodies, agglutinins, and lysins. In addition, leptospira may be found in the urine by dark-field microscopy or in liver tissue by culture or by light microscopy of silver-impregnated sections. Although antibodies begin to appear early in the second week, they do not reach a diagnostic titer until the third week, and reach peak values by the fourth week. Thereafter, the titer may remain high for months or years.

The pathogenesis of the jaundice in leptospirosis is uncertain. Although the clinical and biochemical features of the jaundice suggest that hepatocellular injury is the principal factor involved, neither the occurrence nor the depth of jaundice can be correlated with the degree of hepatic damage demonstrable histologically. Indeed, in some cases, moderately severe jaundice may occur in the absence of obvious hepatic lesions. On the basis of electron microscopic studies, it has been proposed that toxic injury to the organelles accounts for the development of jaundice. Circumstantial evidence suggests that hemolysis may play a contributory role in some cases. Histochemical demonstration of subcellular hepatic injury, as evidenced by reduced glutamic, lactic, and succinic dehydrogenase, may help explain this paradox (111).

It has been postulated that toxins, presumably endotoxins, are responsible for functional and histologic changes in both the liver and kidneys. However, no such toxins have as yet been identified in human infections. It is proposed that the lesions of leptospirosis result from injury of the endothelial lining of the capillaries.

The principal histologic features of the *hepatic lesions* usually found in icteric leptospirosis include centrilobular canalicular bile thrombi, hypertrophy of the Kupffer cells, some of which may contain phagocytosed bile or erythrocytes, scattered acidophilic bodies, and prominent, hepatocellular regeneration, i.e., numerous mitotic figures, binucleate cells, and pleomorphism of hepatocytes and their nuclei. Canalicular bile stasis is seen in icteric cases (114). Often, the sinusoids are dilated and contain neutrophils. Some of the portal tracts may be infiltrated by neutrophils and lymphocytes. Despite jaundice and elevated transaminase levels, hepatic necrosis is virtually invisible. Rarely, however, small foci of necrosis infiltrated with lymphocytes, plasma cells, and histiocytes may be found scattered through the parenchyma. In approximately 25% of cases, leptospira are demonstrable in the liver by the Warthin-Starry silver impregnation method.

The *renal lesions* of leptospirosis, which are more impressive than the hepatic lesions, are characterized by (1) degeneration, necrosis, or regeneration of the epithelium lining the proximal convoluted tubules, (2) infiltration of the interstitial tissue with lymphocytes and plasma cells, (3) bile-stained casts in the lumens of the tubules, and (4) numerous leptospira in the epithelial cells and lumens of the tubules.

Another distinctive lesion of leptospirosis is focal necrosis of individual skeletal muscle fibers, particularly in the legs. The affected fibers are vacuolated, show loss of their striations, undergo hyalinization and are infiltrated with neutrophils and plasma cells, or are replaced by proliferating sarcolemma nuclei or blood. Leptospira are only rarely found in rhabdomyolytic lesions (115).

Relapsing fever

Spirochetes of the genus *Borrelia* produce infections characterized by recurrent bouts of fever over a period of several weeks (116–118). Such infections may be transmitted from person to person by the body louse *(Pediculus humanis corporis)*, or from small mammalian animal to human by ticks of the *Ornithodorus* species. Most louse-borne infections are caused by *B. recurrentis* and occur in epidemics under conditions of overcrowding, poor sanitation, and warfare. However, the disease may be endemic, as it is in Ethiopia. Tick-borne infections occur sporadically and are due to several species of *Borrelia* that differ antigenically from *B. recurrentis,* but are indistinguishable from the latter both in clinical behavior and morphologically.

Borrelia are helical structures with 3 to 19 coarse, irregular coils and a length of 3 to 20 μm with a width of 0.2 to 0.5 μm. During the febrile phase of severe infections, the organisms can be identified in thick or thin smears of blood stained by the Wright or Giemsa method. With defervescence between febrile episodes, most of the organisms are cleared from the blood and appear in the reticuloendothelium, particularly of the spleen and, less commonly, of the liver, where they can be identified in Warthin-Starry silver-impregnated sections. When *Borrelia* are not detectable in blood smears, inoculation of blood into young mice that are highly susceptible to *Borrelia* infection may prove useful in establishing an antemortem diagnosis of relapsing fever.

Characteristically, after an incubation period of approximately seven days, there is an abrupt onset of high fever, chills, prostration, myalgia, and arthralgia. In two-thirds of the cases the liver and spleen are enlarged and tender, and in one-third there is accompanying jaundice. Other less constant features include a transient rash, signs of myocardial injury such as gallop rhythm, conduction defects, and cardiac dilatation, and a hemorrhagic diathesis. The initial, febrile episode usually lasts for six to nine days.

Frequently, spontaneous remission, or one induced by tetracycline, streptomycin, or chloramphenicol therapy, is ushered in by a febrile crisis that resembles a Jarisch-Herxheimer reaction and is thought to be due to the release of endotoxin following the destruction of *Borrelia* organisms. The crisis is characterized by a transient, sharp rise in temperature, chills, profuse sweating, and hypertension followed by severe, prolonged hypothermia, hypotension, and bradycardia. Death from cardiac failure may occur during this period. However, many patients recover only to suffer one or more febrile relapses at four to six-day intervals. In addition to heart failure, other causes of death in relapsing fever include hepatic failure, hyperpyrexic convulsions, hemorrhagic complications, and intercurrent bacterial infection. In some epidemics of louse-borne relapsing fever, the mortality rate has ranged as high as 70%. However, the rate is about 5% in the endemic infections encountered in Ethiopia.

The *hepatic lesions* in icteric relapsing fever are characterized by (1) midzonal and central foci of parenchymal necrosis surrounded by hemorrhage and infiltrated with a variable number of lymphocytes and neutrophils, (2) congestion of the sinusoids, (3) hypertrophy and proliferation of Kupffer cells, some of which contain engulfed erythrocytes and debris, and (4) infiltration of the portal tracts with lymphocytes and monocytes. These findings do not differ from similar, histologic abnormalities in a variety of other disorders of diverse etiology.

Lyme disease

Lyme disease is a generalized disorder caused by another *Borrelia* species, *Borrelia burgdorferi,* a tick-borne spirochete (119). It is characterized by a rash (erythema chronicum migrans), by constitutional symptoms, such as fever, malaise, headache, and, usually, by arthralgia, myalgia, and lymphadenopathy, nausea or vomiting with right upper quadrant pain, hepatomegaly, and increased serum transaminase activity in about one-fifth of the cases (120). Hepatic histology in this early stage has not been studied except for one case in which granulomatous hepatitis

was found (121). However, chronic hepatitis developing six years after the apparent onset of the disease and confirmed by rising titers of fluorescent antibody to *B. burgdorferi* has been reported in one well-studied case (122). Ballooning of hepatocytes, Kupffer cell hyperplasia, microvesicular fat, and neutrophilic infiltration of portal areas was found (Fig. 755). A characteristic finding in Lyme hepatitis is the frequent occurrence of hepatocytes in mitosis, usually metaphase. This finding, which is not often seen normally, is shown in Figure 755. Spirochetes were identified in liver tissue. Whether this case crepresents chronic recurrent hepatitis or reinfection is not clear. Both cases responded promptly to treatment with tetracycline.

Syphilis

(See Chapter 22.)

Protozoal infections

Amebiasis

Entameba histolytica, a relatively common pathogenic protozoan of worldwide distribution, characteristically invades the colonic mucosa where it produces distinctive, flask-shaped ulcers. In some cases, the organisms enter the circulation and are spread to the liver, or, less commonly, to the lungs or brain where they may produce abscesses (123–126).

Infection follows the ingestion of food or water contaminated with the cysts of *E. histolytica* of fecal origin. The cysts, which resist digestion in the stomach, pass into the intestine where they excyst, divide, and give rise to trophozoites, the vegetative form of the parasite that are motile and contain proteolytic enzymes capable of destroying tissue. On reaching the colon, the trophozoites penetrate the mucosa and lead to its ulceration.

The trophozoites, which multiply within the mucosa and on its surface, are shed into the lumen of the colon and are excreted in the feces, usually in the form of cysts. However, when the ulceration is extensive and active, trophozoites may be found in the stools as well as cysts. The cysts tolerate drying after they are excreted and resist destruction in the low pH of the stomach, but trophozoites do not tolerate either drying or low pH. Consequently, only the cysts are infectious.

In many cases of amebic colitis, the mucosal ulcers are small and few in number, so the presence of cysts in the stools may be the only manifestation of the disease. However, under some conditions, the ulcers increase in size and number and coalesce, causing abdominal cramps, loose stools, and, sometimes, frank dysentery.

Amebae that originate in the colonic mucosa can be disseminated to the liver via the portal vein and there give rise to a distinctive form of hepatic abscess. Often, there is a long, latent period between the original amebic infection of the colon and the development of the hepatic abscess. In more than one-half the cases of amebic abscess, the stools no longer contain amebae and there are no clinical signs of symptoms of amebic colitis. The frequency with which amebae spread to the liver and produce abscesses is uncertain. In autopsy studies of fatal amebic infections, the incidence of hepatic abscess has been as high as 80%. However, clinical studies suggest that the true incidence is closer to 3 to 9%. Even this may be an overestimate, since such studies seldom take into account the large number of asymptomatic, amebic, colonic infections.

Occasionally, amebae that spread to the liver traverse the hepatic sinusoids and enter the systemic circulation, leading to the development of amebic abscesses in the lungs or, rarely, in the brain. These metastatic infections occur as complications of hepatic abscesses. Extremely rarely, instances of brain abscesses in the absence of hepatic abscess have been reported.

The factors that predispose to the development of hepatic amebic abscess are uncertain. They affect adult males predominantly, and occur much more frequently in tropical and subtropical areas where amebiasis is endemic than in the temperate zones.

Usually, the onset of clinical manifestations in hepatic amebic abscess is insidious, with dull pain in the right upper quadrant of the abdomen, malaise, low grade fever, and weight loss; with progression of the lesion, the pain increases in severity, may become pleuritic in character, and often radiates to the right shoulder or chest. The fever also increases, and may be intermittent or remittent in character. Occasionally, the onset of the disease is abrupt, with high fever, chills, sweats, and sharp abdominal pain. Cholestasis is common, occurring in almost one-third of patients (127,128). Anorexia, nausea, and cough are other relatively common symptoms.

The liver is almost always enlarged and tender, and is frequently accompanied by elevation and fixation of the right leaf of the diaphragm with overlying signs of atelectasis or fluid. When the right lobe of the liver contains a large, expanding abscess, a mass may be palpable below the right costal margin, or there may be bulging of the intercostal spaces on the right. Abscesses of the left lobe of the liver, which are uncommon, frequently present with a palpable mass in the epigastrium. Jaundice is relatively uncommon, and, when present, is usually mild. However, rare instances of severe obstructive jaundice and hepatocellular failure have been reported.

The principal laboratory findings in most cases of hepatic amebic abscess include moderate leukocytosis, mild normocytic anemia, hypoalbuminemia, moderate elevations of serum alkaline phosphatase and transaminase activity, and slight increments in serum bilirubin concentration (127).

Characteristically, amebic abscesses present as defects in scintiscans, ultrasonograms, CT, and nuclear magnetic scans that demonstrate the precise size and location of the lesion (129). Ultrasonic guidance permits easy aspiration of these abscesses when indicated.

Serologic tests of various types almost always show antibodies to *E. histolytica*. Recent advances include immunofluorescent detection of the cysts in the pus of amebic abscesses (130), identification of the antigen by immune sera (131), and detection of antibody in sera by ELISA assay (132).

Except for some microabscesses that heal spontaneously, most untreated amebic abscesses of the liver tend to enlarge progressively. They may prove fatal as a result of rupture into the peritoneum, pleura, or pericardium, the development of metastatic amebic abscesses, or the development of superimposed, pyogenic, bacterial infection of the abscess. Occasionally, hepatic amebic abscesses extend into the lung and may drain externally via a hepatobronchial fistula, a complication that often

leads to spontaneous recovery. Other rare complications include rupture of the abscess into the gastrointestinal tract, biliary tree, or portal vein, or through the abdominal or thoracic wall.

Several drugs have proved effective in curing amebic abscess of the liver. Of these, metronidazole and tinidazole are the drugs of choice (133). In unresponsive cases, emetine or dehydroemetine plus chloroquine usually prove effective. Needle aspiration of the abscess may be required when the abscess is large and fails to respond promptly to drug therapy. Usually, surgical drainage and appropriate antibiotic therapy are required in the management of amebic abscesses complicated by pyogenic bacterial infection (134,135).

Amebic abscesses vary greatly in size, ranging from a few millimeters to 10 to 15 cm in diameter. Usually, they are solitary and unilocular, and occur predominantly in the right lobe of the liver. Occasionally, however, they are multiple, multilocular, or occur in the left lobe. Characteristically, the abscess is sharply circumscribed, enclosed within a relatively slender membrane, and is filled with liquefied or semisolid, reddish brown material that resembles anchovy paste or chocolate sauce. The outer membrane is lined by a narrow band of coagulative necrosis, and is surrounded by a zone of granulation tissue and an outer ring of compressed and atrophic hepatocytes. The liquefied material at the center of the abscess is made up of amorphous debris, cell fragments, and erythrocytes. Characteristically, there are few or no accompanying inflammatory cells. As a rule, the wall of the abscess contains few collagen fibers. However, in some chronic abscesses, fibrosis may be a prominent feature. When amebic abscesses are complicated by superimposed pyogenic bacterial infections, they usually run a more fulminant course. Such abscesses are filled with foul-smelling, yellow or green pus that may contain innumerable neutrophils and bacteria. Usually, it is difficult to identify amebae in such lesions.

Frequently, *E. histolytica* trophozoites can be demonstrated within the wall of the abscess. These present as round or oval structures 30 to 60 μm in diameter. The nucleus, which occupies approximately one-fifth of the cell, contains a small central karyosome and finely beaded chromatin on the inner surface of the nuclear membrane. The cytoplasm is heavily laden with glycogen and stains deeply with PAS. In addition, some of the trophozoites contain cytoplasmic inclusions of erythrocytes and amorphous debris. The details of the trophozoites are best visualized in sections stained with Heidenhain's iron hematoxylin.

Autopsy studies suggest that *E. histolytica* may multiply in and occlude distal branches of the portal vein, leading to the development of small, periportal foci of infarction. Subsequently, proteolytic enzymes released from the amebae induce progressive lytic necrosis and expansion of these foci with the ultimate development of a frank abscess. There is suggestive evidence that some of the small necrotic foci heal spontaneously with or without residual scarring.

Occasionally, amebic colitis is accompanied by enlargement and tenderness of the liver, abdominal pain, and low grade fever in the absence of overt signs of a hepatic amebic abscess. Since these manifestations frequently abate following a course of antiamebic therapy, the syndrome is considered by some to be a form of *acute amebic hepatitis*. However, liver biopsy in such cases fails to confirm the presence of an acute diffuse hepatitis. The lesions found in such cases are usually focal and nonspecific. Accordingly, it has been proposed that the syndrome is attributable to the nonspecific effects of the colonic infection. In some cases, the manifestations may be attributable to scattered microabscesses that are too small to detect clinically.

Sometimes, *E. histolytica* can produce a nonsuppurative form of *chronic amebic hepatitis* (124). The hepatic lesions in such cases are said to be characterized by chronic inflammation and fibrosis of the portal tracts, and the presence of *E. histolytica* in the portal tracts or parenchyma. The clinical manifestations, which are nonspecific, include malaise, fatigue, anorexia, and right upper abdominal discomfort that may be accompanied by enlargement and tenderness of the liver. Allegedly, the symptoms abate following a course of antiamebic therapy.

Visceral leishmaniasis (kala-azar)

Visceral leishmaniasis (136,137), a protozoal infection due to *Leishmania donovani,* is transmitted to humans by the bites of bloodsucking sandflies of the genus *Phlebotomus* in the Old World and genus *Lutzomyia* in the New World. The disease, which is characterized by extensive invasion of the reticuloendothelial system, is endemic in several areas of the world, the most important being eastern India, northern China, East Africa, the Mediterranean basin, and Brazil. In India, the infection is transmitted from person to person by the sandfly. However, in other parts of the world, domestic or wild dogs or grass rats may serve as intermediate host reservoirs. Patients with AIDS exhibit greatly increased susceptibility (138).

Usually, the onset of clinical manifestations in visceral leishmaniasis is insidious and occurs after a latent period of several months. Low grade fever, malaise, and lassitude are the initial features, but they are followed by intermittent high fever, progressive hepatosplenomegaly, lymphadenopathy, and wasting. Pancytopenia and hypergammaglobulinemia are characteristic. If left untreated, the disease usually proves fatal as a result of cachexia or intercurrent infection. Several drugs have proved effective in the treatment of visceral leishmaniasis. Of these, the most important are the pentavalent antimonials (sodium antimony gluconate and antimony-*N*-methyl-glutamine), and non-metal-containing aromatic diamadines (hydroxystilbamidine isthionate). In addition, amphotericin B has proved useful in some cases that are refractory to other forms of therapy.

Months or even years following apparent recovery from visceral leishmaniasis, some patients develop disfiguring nodules in the skin due to proliferation and infiltration of histiocytes that contain numerous Leishman-Donovan bodies. This syndrome, classified as *post-kala-azar, dermal leishmaniasis,* is thought to be a manifestation of impaired cell-mediated immunity. As a rule, such skin lesions are resistant to therapy.

The principal features of the *hepatic lesions* of visceral leishmaniasis (139) include hyperplasia and hypertrophy of the Kupffer cells (Fig. 756), most of which contain Leishman-Donovan (L-D) bodies within the cytoplasm (Fig. 252). L-D bodies are small, oval-shaped cells, 2×3 μm in diameter, that are enclosed within a thin plasma membrane and contain a relatively large round nucleus and a rod-shaped kinetoplast. The L-D bodies are readily identified in H & E- and Giemsa-stained sections. In addition, some L-D bodies may be found in portal tract histiocytes. In some cases, the hyperplastic, hypertrophied Kupffer cells that contain L-D bodies are aggregated to form small nodules that may be interspersed with lymphocytes and plasma cells. In addition, some of the portal tracts may be infiltrated with similar inflammatory cells and histiocytes, and may show stellate scarring. Fibrin ring granulomas have been reported (140).

Malaria

Four species of protozoa belonging to the genus *Plasmodium* are transmitted to humans by anopheline mosquitoes and produce malaria (141–145). These include *P. vivax* and *P. ovale,* the causes of benign tertian malaria; *P. malariae,* the cause of quartan malaria; and *P. falciparum,* the cause of malignant tertian malaria.

The life cycle of the plasmodium is complex, and involves both a sexual cycle (sporogony) in the mosquito and an asexual cycle (schizogeny) in humans. Infection of the mosquito occurs when it feeds on human blood that contains gametocytes of the parasite. These undergo maturation, fertilization, and multiplication, leading to the development of innumerable sporozoites that disseminate through the body cavity of the mosquito and infiltrate its salivary glands. When the infected mosquito bites a human, it injects a number of sporozoites. These enter the circulation and are transported to the liver where they invade hepatocytes. In the hepatocytes, the sporozoites mature and multiply, leading to the formation of schizonts that contain numerous exoerythrocytic merozoites. Ultimately, the infected hepatocytes release their content of merozoites into the circulation where they promptly invade erythrocytes. In relapsing forms of malaria due to *P. vivax, P. ovale,* and *P. malariae,* some of the merozoites released into the circulation invade new groups of hepatocytes and thus restart the exoerythrocytic cycle of the parasite. Secondary invasion of the hepatocytes and relapses do not occur in *P. falciparum* infections.

As the erythrocytic merozoites mature, they enlarge, metabolize hemoglobin, and undergo several nuclear divisions, leading to the development of a schizont that contains numerous merozoites. Ultimately, the infected erythrocyte ruptures and releases its content of merozoites, which are promptly taken up by other erythrocytes. After several such cycles, some of the merozoites are converted to gametocytes, thus completing the life cycle of the parasite.

Usually, attacks of acute malaria are characterized by bouts of intermittent chills and fever that recur at intervals of 48 hours in the case of tertian malaria and 72 hours in the case of quartan malaria. Each of the febrile paroxysms, which last from 8 to 12 hours, coincides with the rupture of erythrocytes and release of merozoites. Often, the fever is accompanied by splenomegaly, hepatomegaly, and slight impairment of hepatocellular function. Jaundice is relatively uncommon, and, when present, usually is mild and hemolytic in character. However, significant hepatocellular jaundice may be encountered, particularly in *P. falciparum* infections. Indeed, a malarial syndrome of acute hepatic failure simulates fulminant viral hepatitis (146).

The *hepatic lesions* of acute malaria are variable, but usually affect the reticuloendothelium more than the hepatocytes. The features that may be encountered in biopsy sections include: focal Kupffer cell hypertrophy and hyperplasia, deposits of coarse, dark brown granules of malarial pigment (hemozoin) within Kupffer cells or portal macrophages (147), lymphocytic infiltration of the sinusoids and portal tracts, sinusoidal congestion and hepatocellular swelling, pleomorphism, anisonucleosis, and increased mitotic activity. Malarial pigment is a derivative of host hemoglobin that has been altered by plasmodia and released into the blood. Characteristically, the granules exhibit yellow-orange birefringence in polarized light (Fig. 242), and fail to give a Prussian blue reaction for iron. In fatal *P. falciparum* infections, the liver may show extensive centrilobular necrosis (146).

Tropical splenomegaly is a syndrome characterized by persistent hypersplenism, i.e., enlargement of the spleen, anemia, thrombocytopenia, lymphocytosis, and increased serum IgM (147). Since the disorder is encountered most frequently in endemic malarial areas and often is accompanied by a high titer of malaria antibody, most cases are generally attributed to low grade chronic or recurrent malaria. A defect in suppressor T cell function may be in part responsible (148). The hepatic lesions in such cases characteristically exhibit lymphocytic infiltration of the sinusoids and portal tracts that must be distinguished from infectious mononucleosis and other diseases (147). The other characteristic finding is Kupffer cell hyperplasia.

Toxoplasmosis

(See Chapter 22.)

Mycotic infections

Actinomycosis

By tradition, actinomycosis (149–153) is usually classified as a mycotic infection. However, the organism responsible for most such infections in humans, *Actinomyces israelii*, has been identified as an anaerobic or microaerophilic, gram-positive bacillus. Usually, *A. israelii* is a normal inhabitant of the oral cavity. However, under some conditions, including bacterial infection, inflammation, or trauma, the organism may become pathogenic, giving rise to chronic, suppurative lesions in the maxillary-facial, gastrointestinal, or thoracic regions. Actinomycosis may involve any part of the gastrointestinal tract, but affects the appendix, cecum, and liver most frequently.

Hepatic actinomycosis almost invariably follows spread of the infection from a focus in the intestinal tract by direct extension or via the portal vein. However, the intestinal focus may be so inconspicuous that the hepatic lesion appears to be "primary." The diagnosis can be suspected on the basis of imaging studies (154–156), but aspiration is necessary to prove it.

The principal clinical features of hepatic actinomycotic lesions include fever, hepatomegaly, abdominal pain, and wasting (152). Liver "function" tests may be normal despite hepatic abscesses (154). The diagnosis of abscesses can be established by various imaging techniques (155,156). Since none of these findings is pathognomonic, the diagnosis depends on the demonstration of typical sulfur granules in pus (157) or the recovery of *A. israelii* in cultures of such material.

When fully developed, actinomycotic lesions of the liver present as solitary or multiple, firm, multiloculated abscesses that appear honeycombed on section. They are encircled and traversed by bands of collagenized granulation tissue that contain numerous lipid-laden, foamy macrophages, lymphocytes, plasma cells, and fibroblasts. Characteristically, the purulent areas are filled with neutrophils and contain colonies of *A. israelii*. In wet coverslip preparations of aspirated pus, the colonies present as firm, yellow, 1 to 2 mm granules commonly termed sulfur granules. Figure 757 illustrates a group of such granules surrounded by neutrophils in a stained smear of pus aspirated from an actinomycotic liver abscess. As shown in Figure 758, the bulk of the granule is made up of a compact mass of gram-positive filaments, and is surrounded peripherally by a narrow band of short, radiating, clubbed structures. In H & E sections, the granules are stained purple, except for the peripheral clubs, which stain pink. Occasionally, sulfur granules are difficult to find in the suppurative lesions of actinomycosis. However, in such cases, the organisms frequently can be recovered in anaerobic cultures of the pus.

Prolonged administration of penicillin in large doses is highly effective in the treatment of actinomycosis, and leads to cure in approximately 90% of cases (158). Untreated lesions tend to expand and adhere to adjacent viscera and the abdominal wall, and often lead to the development of sinus tracts that drain pus.

Aspergillosis

Rarely, *Aspergillus fumigatus* gives rise to disseminated infections that may involve the liver. In at least two reported cases, the organisms invaded the hepatic veins and led to the development of an acute Budd-Chiari syndrome (159). Although these fungi may escape detection in routine H & E sections, they are readily demonstrable in sections stained with Gridley's or Grocott's stain. Rarely, they invade the common bile duct and form fungus balls that produce biliary obstruction.

Although hepatic aspergillosis is seldom recognized antemortem, available evidence suggests that the diagnosis can be established by needle biopsy of the liver in a high proportion of cases. Since such hepatic lesions frequently occur in the absence of organisms in the blood or signs of aspergillosis in other tissues, the biopsy findings may provide the first evidence of disseminated organisms producing multiple microabscesses in the liver (160,161). Aspergillosis is sometimes a complication of severe hepatic injury (162,163), rather than its cause.

Blastomycosis

(See Chapter 22.)

Candidiasis

Disseminated infections with *Candida albicans* occur predominantly in patients with AIDS or in immunocompromised patients with leukemia or lymphoma who have been treated with corticosteroids and antibiotics (164). In a high proportion of cases, such infections affect the liver, leading to the development of multiple microabscesses or granulomas. Other hepatic lesions that may be encountered include fatty infiltration, sinusoidal congestion, centrilobular necrosis, bile stasis, or nonspecific focal inflammation (165). Characteristically, the combination of microabscesses and granulomas suggests candidiasis, and thus facilitates prompt treatment with amphotericin B and 5-fluocytosine, agents that may prolong survival if administered sufficiently early in the course of the infection.

Coccidioidomycosis, cryptococcosis, and *histoplasmosis* are discussed in Chapter 22.

Helminthic infections

Echinococcosis (hydatid disease)

Hydatid disease (166,168) is an infection caused by the larvae of animal tapeworms belonging to the genus *Echinococcus.* The three species responsible are *E. granulosus, E. multilocularis,* and *E. oligoarthrus.*

Echinococcus granulosus. E. granulosus is endemic in many parts of the world, particularly where sheep-raising is common. At one time, the disease was most prevalent in Australia, New Zealand, and Iceland. Currently, however, it is encountered most frequently in East Africa, and is relatively common in South America, Greece, Spain, and the Middle and Far East. Most cases in the United States are encountered in immigrants from endemic areas. However, occasionally, the infection is acquired locally.

Echinococcosis granulosus, caused by *E. granulosus,* a small, 3 to 6 mm tapeworm that inhabits the small intestine of the dog, is the most common of the three. Ingestion of ova passed in the feces of infected dogs, the definitive hosts of *E. granulosus,* leads to the development of hydatid disease in sheep, cattle, and humans, the intermediate hosts of the parasite. When the viscera of infected sheep or cattle are eaten by dogs, scolices in the cysts are released in the stomach and undergo maturation to adult worms in the small intestine. The life cycles of *E. multilocularis* and *E. oligoarthrus* are similar to that of *E. granulosus,* but the definitive hosts in alveolar echinococcosis are foxes and cats and the intermediate hosts, rodents and humans.

Following its ingestion by an intermediate host, the chitinous envelope of the *E. granulosus* ovum is digested by the gastric juice, releasing the embryo it contains. On reaching the duodenum, these embryos penetrate the mucosa, enter the portal circulation, and are transported to the liver where they mature and produce hydatid cysts. In a minority of cases, the embryos pass through the liver and give rise to cysts in extrahepatic tissues, such as the lungs, kidneys, spleen, brain, or bone.

As the embryo of *E. granulosus* matures in the liver or other tissues, it undergoes vacuolization, and is converted to a complex, encapsulated structure. The capsule comprises a thick, outer, fibrous coat, the adventitia, which is derived from the tissues of the host; a middle layer of acellular, hyalinized material, the laminated membrane; and an inner lining of epithelial cells, the germinal layer. Proliferation and vacuolization of the germinal layer results in the formation of multiple brood capsules, thin-walled cystic structures in which multiple scolices develop (Fig. 759). Characteristically, the scolices contain suckers and a double row of refractile hooklets (Fig. 760). The brood capsules tend to expand progressively and ultimately burst, releasing scolices that settle to the bottom of the cyst where they constitute so-called hydatid sand. As the hydatid cyst grows in size, its germinal layer frequently invaginates to form daughter

cysts (Fig. 761). In a similar manner, they may in turn give rise to granddaughter cysts. Another feature of the cyst capsule in advanced lesions is its tendency to undergo calcification.

E. granulosus hydatids of the liver grow slowly at an estimated rate of 1 mm per month, so they may not become evident clinically for many years following the onset of infection. Many cysts remain asymptomatic unless complicated by rupture or intercurrent, pyogenic infection. However, when large, they may be palpable below the costal margin as firm, smooth, nontender masses, or may give rise to hepatosplenomegaly. Rarely, hydatids near or in the porta hepatis compress the portal vein and produce portal hypertension, or occlude major bile ducts, leading to obstructive jaundice (169).

Rupture of a hydatid cyst into the peritoneum is a serious complication that may prove fatal or result in dissemination of the disease throughout the abdomen. In such cases, severe abdominal pain, anaphylaxis or other features of an allergic reaction, and eosinophilia are the principal clinical manifestations. Rupture of the cyst into the biliary tree is a less serious complication, since much of the discharge ultimately is excreted. It frequently results in recurrent attacks of cholangitis and biliary obstruction due to the blockage of daughter cysts. Less commonly, hydatid cysts rupture into the pleura, lungs, or colon.

Secondary infection of the cyst with pyogenic bacteria may lead to the development of a pyogenic abscess in the liver. Usually, such infections occur in patients with a fistulous tract between the cyst and the biliary tree.

Hydatid cyst fluid contains specific echinococcus antigens. Frequently, they may induce an immunologic response in the host, as evidenced by intradermal skin reactivity, complement fixation, and indirect hemagglutination reactions to the antigens. However, the results of all such tests may be negative if the cyst has never leaked or no longer contains viable parasites. Usually, the preoperative diagnosis of hydatid disease is suggested by roentgenography, ultrasonography, or computerized tomography. Ultrasonographic investigations have identified a number of new reliable diagnostic signs (170,171). The diagnosis can be confirmed in approximately 85% of cases by a positive echinococcus complement fixation, indirect hemagglutination test, immunoelectrophoresis, or ELISA (172,173). Percutaneous aspiration and needle biopsy of the cyst have been contraindicated for diagnostic purposes, since they may result in rupture of the cyst or leakage of cyst fluid and can lead to fatal anaphylaxis or dissemination of the disease, but current management is more aggressive (174,175). Microscopic examination of the hydatid sand may show identifiable scolices (Fig. 762) that can establish the diagnosis, or even the presence of a few hooklets (Fig. 763) that may be virtually diagnostic.

Medical therapy with mebendazole (176) or albendazole (177) offers some hope, but these agents are neither curative nor free of serious side effects. They are especially toxic to the bile ducts, often giving rise to bile duct injury (178) and even sclerosing cholangitis (179).

Alveolar echinococcosis. Alveolar echinococcosis of the liver is an extremely aggressive variant of the more common form of hydatid disease caused by *E. granulosus* (180–182). Indeed, it is often described as ''malignant'' because of its appearance, frequently being mistaken for carcinoma of the liver, and because of its terrible prognosis. It is almost invariably fatal unless completely resected.

It differs from the more common variety of echinococcosis in its etiologic agents *(E. multilocularis versus E. granulosus),* in its life cycle and definitive hosts (foxes instead of dogs, although other carnivores, such as dogs and cats, may become definitive hosts), in its intermediate hosts (rodents instead of sheep and, accidentally, in both disorders, humans), in its gross hepatic appearance, (microvesicular instead of macrovesicular), and in its much more grim prognosis (181). It differs histologically as well.

Ova are excreted in the stools of the definitive hosts and are ingested by intermediate hosts including humans who eat wild, contaminated fruits or who come in contact with the foxes, dogs, or cats, who have ingested rodents infested with the larval form of the cestode.

The disease is found endemically around the Alps in central Europe, in Alaska, in northern Canada, and Japan, and in foci in the USSR, Turkey, and China, always in the habitats of foxes. A few cases have been reported in the northcentral portions of the United States (183).

While *E. granulosus* can be eradicated by careful control of dogs and periodic deworming, *E. multilocularis* cannot, because both the definitive and intermediate hosts are wild. Treatment is inefficient. Chemotherapeutic agents such as albendazol and mebendazol are only modestly effective at best (184). Surgical resection of localized areas of involvement may be effective (182,185), as may portal-systemic anastomoses when portal hypertension develops, or pulmonary resections when pulmonary metastases occur (175). The most recent and most effective form of therapy is orthotopic liver transplantation (186,187).

Clinical signs of disease develop 5 to 20 years after infestation. Upper abdominal discomfort is a common complaint. Some patients develop obstructive jaundice, often with pruritus. Others present with an irregular, enlarged, nodular liver. Biopsy is necessary to differentiate echinococcosis from malignancy. Needle biopsy is rarely, if ever, associated with anaphylactic shock, as it may be when the fluid from *E. granulosus* cysts is spilled. The blood tests tend to be cholestatic with increased serum alkaline phosphatase and gamma-glutamyl transpeptidase activity and normal transaminase values. Eosinophilia is common.

At present, ultrasonography permits a relatively early diagnosis characterized by an irregular, ill-defined hepatic mass. The echinococcal cavities are small, so the tissue appears by ultrasonic examination to be fibrotic, rather than cystic, as it does with *E. granulosus*.

The hepatic lesions of alveolar echinococcosis are characterized by masses of fibrous tissue that are honeycombed with cavities that range from 1 or 2 mm in diameter to several centimeters. Unlike *E. granulosus*, in *E. multilocularis* the daughter cysts, which arise from the germinal membrane, develop on the outside of the original cysts, thus invading the hepatic parenchyma. These lesions tend to grow indefinitely to produce hepatic necrosis in compressed areas around the vesicles, and to stimulate a vigorous granulomatous reaction. This aspect also differentiates *E. multilocularis* from *E. granulosus*, which does not induce a granulomatous reaction. The cystic lesions may cause biliary obstruction or portal hypertension. These parasitic lesions may undergo necrosis and become cavitary. They may become infected, giving rise to hepatic abscesses, cholangitis, and, often, to septicemia.

Histologically, the lesions show hydatid cysts of the liver that are characterized by a thick, laminated layer (Fig. 764). The host reaction is characterized by adjacent, pericystic necrosis and dense bundles of collagen. The parasitic vesicles may be individual or contiguous (Fig. 765). Sometimes the lesions are not cystic, but solid, in which case the laminated layer appears as a contiguous, ribbon-like structure (Fig. 766) around which there is an intense granulomatous reaction characterized by epithelioid cells that are often arranged radially around the lesion, multinucleated giant cells, concentric layers of fibrosis, and a heavy infiltration of lymphocytes (Fig. 767). Protoscoleces develop within the cysts (Fig. 768).

The lesions may rapidly recur after liver transplantation [(186,187); Fig. 769].

Other helminthic diseases including *ascariasis, visceral larva migrans, capillaria hepatica,* and *schistosomiasis* are discussed in Chapter 22.

References

1. Klatskin G: Hepatitis associated with systemic infections. *In* Diseases of the Liver, edited by L. Schiff. 4th Edition. Philadelphia, J.B. Lippincott, 1975, pp. 711–753.
2. Holdstock G, Balasegaram M, Millwood-Sadler GH, Wright R: The liver in infection. *In* Liver and Biliary Disease, edited by R. Wright, K.G.M.M. Alberti, S. Karran, G.H. Millward-Sadler. 2nd Edition. Philadelphia, W.B. Saunders, 1987, pp. 1077–1119.
3. Brandborg LL, Goldman IS: Bacterial and miscellaneous infections of the liver. *In* Hepatology. A Textbook of Liver Disease, edited by D. Zakim, T.D. Boyer. 2nd Edition. Philadelphia, W.B. Saunders, 1990, pp. 1086–1098.
4. Williams AO, Tugwell P, Edington GM: Glucose-6-phosphate dehydrogenase deficiency and lobar pneumonia. Arch Pathol Lab Med *100*:25–31, 1976.
5. Zimmerman HJ, Fang M, Utili R, Seeff LB, Hoofnagle J: Jaundice due to bacterial infection. Gastroenterology *77*:362–374, 1979.
6. Skinner D, Keefer CS: Significance of bacteremia caused by *Staphylococcus aureus:* a study of one hundred and twenty-two cases and a review of the literature concerned with experimental infection in animals. Arch Intern Med *68*:851–875, 1941.
7. Rolando N, Harvey F, Brahm J, Philpott-Howard J, Alexander G, Gimson A, Casewell M, Fagan E, Williams R: Prospective study of bacterial infection in acute liver failure: an analysis of fifty patients. Hepatology *11*:49–53, 1990.
8. Keefer CS, Ingelfinger FJ, Spink WW: Significance of hemolytic streptococcic bacteremia: a study of two hundred and forty-six patients. Arch Intern Med *60*:1084–1097, 1937.
9. Fishbein WN: Jaundice as an early manifestation of scarlet fever. Report of three cases in adults and review of the literature. Ann Intern Med *57*:60–72, 1962.
10. Moore-Gillon JC, Eykyn SJ, Phillips I: Microbiology of pyogenic liver abscess. Br Med J *283*:819–826, 1981.
11. Kotin P, Butt FN: Streptococcal hepatitis. Arch Pathol *52*:288–292, 1951.
12. Sabbaj J, Sutter VL, Finegold SM: Anaerobic pyogenic liver abscess. Ann Intern Med *77*:629–638, 1972.
13. Gleeson DC, Fielding J, Heath DA: *Streptococcus milleri* liver abscesses associated with leiomyosarcoma. Postgrad Med J *59*:323–330, 1983.
14. Weinstein L: Bacterial hepatitis: a case report on an unrecognized cause of fever of unknown origin. N Engl J Med *299*:1052–1054, 1978.
15. Stanley MM: Gonococcic peritonitis of the upper part of the abdomen in young women (phrenic reaction, or subcostal syndrome of Stajano; Fitz-Hugh-Curtis syndrome). Report of cases of three patients treated successfully with penicillin and a summary of the literature. Arch Intern Med *78*:1–13, 1946.
16. Bolton JP, Darougar S: Perihepatitis. Br Med Bull *39*:159–164, 1983.
17. Reichert JA, Valle RF: Fitz-Hugh-Curtis syndrome. A laparoscopic approach. JAMA *236*:266–268, 1976.
18. Kimball MW, Knee S: Gonococcal perihepatitis in a male. The Fitz-Hugh-Curtis syndrome. N Engl J Med *282*:1082–1084, 1970.
19. Brooks GF, Donegan EA: Gonococcal Infection. London, Edward Arnold, Ltd., 1985, p. 239.
20. Banks JG, Foulis AK, Ledingham IMcA, MacSween RNM: Liver function in septic shock. J Clin Pathol *35*:1249–1252, 1982.
21. Rooney JC, Hill DJ, Danks DM: Jaundice associated with bacterial infection in the newborn. Am J Dis Child *122*:39–41, 1971.
22. Conn HO, Fessel JM: Spontaneous bacterial peritonitis in cirrhosis: variations on a theme. Medicine *50*:161–197, 1971.

23. Hoefs JC, Runyon BA. Spontaneous bacterial peritonitis. Disease-a-Month *31*:1–48, 1985.
24. Pinzello G, Simonetta RG, Craxi A: Spontaneous bacterial peritonitis: a prospective investigation in predominantly nonalcoholic cirrhotic patients. Hepatology *3*:545–549, 1983.
25. Crossley IR, Williams R: Spontaneous bacterial peritonitis. Gut *26*:325–331, 1985.
26. Conn HO: Bacterial peritonitis: variant syndromes. South Med J *80*:1343–1346, 1987.
27. Runyon BA: Low-protein-concentration ascitic fluid is predisposed to spontaneous bacterial peritonitis. Gastroenterology *91*:1343–1346, 1986.
28. Akalin G, Lalei Y, Telatar H: Bactericidal and opsonic activity of ascitic fluid from cirrhotic and non-cirrhotic patients. J Infect Dis *147*:1011–1017, 1983.
29. Brayko CM, Kozarek RA, Sanowski Ra: Bacteremia during esophageal variceal sclerotherapy: its cause and prevention. Gastrointest Endosc *31*:10–12, 1985.
30. Gerhartz HH, Sauerbruch T, Weinzieri M: Nosocomial septicemia in patients undergoing sclerotherapy for variceal hemorrhage. Endoscopy *16*:129–130, 1983.
31. Runyon BA, Umland ET, Merlin T: Inoculations of blood culture bottles with ascitic fluid. Arch Intern Med *147*:73–75, 1987.
32. Eade MN, Brooke BN: Portal bacteraemia in cases of ulcerative colitis submitted to colectomy. Lancet *1*:1008–1009, 1969.
33. Wee A, Ludwig J: Pericholangitis in chronic ulcerative colitis: primary sclerosing cholangitis of the small bile ducts? Ann Intern Med *102*:581–587, 1985.
34. Perera MR, Kirk A, Noone P: Presentation, diagnosis and management of liver abscess. Lancet *2*:629–632, 1980.
35. Ziegler EJ, Fisher CJ Jr, Sprung CL, Straube RC, Sadoff JC, Foulke GE, Wortel CH, Fink MP, Dellinger P, Teng NNH, Allen IE, Berger HJ, Knatterud GL, LoBuglio AJ, Smith CR: Treatment of gram-negative bacteremia and septic shock with HA-1A human monoclonal antibody against endotoxin. A randomized, double-blind, placebo-controlled trial. N Engl J Med *324*:429–436, 1991.
36. Shands KN, Dan BB, Schmid GP: Toxic shock syndrome: the emerging picture. Ann Intern Med *94*:264–266, 1981.
37. Larkin SM, Williams DN, Osterholm MT, Tofter RW, Posalsky Z: Toxic shock syndrome: clinical, laboratory and pathological findings in nine fatal cases. Ann Intern Med *96*:858–964, 1982.
38. Ishak KG, Rogers WA: Cryptogenic acute cholangitis: association with toxic shock syndrome. Am J Clin Pathol *76*:619–626, 1981.
39. Dammin GJ: Salmonellosis. *In* Pathology of Tropical and Extraordinary Disease, edited by C.H. Binford, D.H. Connor. Washington, Armed Forces Institute of Pathology, 1976, pp. 150–154.
40. Black PH, Kunz KJ, Swartz MN: Salmonellosis: a review of some unusual aspects. N Engl J Med *262*:811–817; 864–870; 921–927, 1960.
41. Ramachandran S, Godfrey JJ, Perera MVF: Typhoid hepatitis. JAMA *230*:236–240, 1974.
42. Finkelstein R, Markel A, Putterman C, Lerman A, Hashman N, Merzbach D: Waterborne typhoid fever in Haifa, Israel: clinical, microbiologic, and therapeutic aspects of a major outbreak. Am J Med Sci *296*:27–32, 1988.
43. Khosla SN, Singh R, Singh GP, Trehan VK: The spectrum of hepatic injury in enteric fever. Am J Gastroenterol *83*:413–416, 1988.
44. de Brito T, Viera WT, Dias MD: Jaundice in typhoid hepatitis: a light and electron microscopy study based on liver biopsies. Acta Hepato-Gastroenterol *24*:426–433, 1977.
45. Pais P: A hepatitis like picture in typhoid fever. Br Med J *289*:225–226, 1984.
46. Adinolfi LE, Utili R, Gaeta GB, Perna P, Ruggiero G: Presence of endotoxemia and its relationship to liver dysfunction in patients with typhoid fever. Infection *15*:359–362, 1987.
47. Osler W: Hepatic complications of typhoid fever. Johns Hopkins Hosp Rep *8*:373–385, 1899–1900.
48. Freitag JL: Treatment of chronic typhoid carriers by cholecystectomy. Pub Health Rep *79*:567–570, 1964.
49. McFadzean AJS, Ong GB: Intrahepatic typhoid carriers. Br Med J *1*:1567–1571, 1966.
50. Hoffman KL: Treatment of healthy salmonella carriers with lactulose. (Beta-galactosido-fructose). Dtsch Med Wochenschr *100*:1429–1431, 1975.
51. Meals RA: Paratyphoid fever. Arch Intern Med *136*:1422–1428, 1976.
52. Havens WP Jr, Wenner HA: Infectious hepatitis complicated by secondary invasion with salmonella. J Clin Invest *25*:45–52, 1946.
53. Seeff L, Beebe GW, Hoofnagle JH, Norman JE, Buskell-Bales Z, Waggoner JG, Kaplowitz N, Koff RS, Petrini JL, Schiff ER, Shorey J, Stanley MM: Serologic follow-up of the 1942 epidemic of post-vaccination hepatitis in the United States Army. N Engl J Med *316*:965–970, 1987.
54. Horney JT, Schwarzmann SW, Galambos JT: Shigella hepatitis. Am J Gastroenterol *66*:146–149, 1976.
55. Piggott JA: Melioidosis. *In* Pathology of Tropical and Extraordinary Diseases, edited by C.H. Binford, D.H. Connor. Washington, Armed Forces Institute of Pathology, 1976, pp. 169–174.
56. Vainrub B: Bacterical infections of the liver and biliary tract: laboratory studies to determine etiology. Lab Res Methods Bio Med *7*:119–130, 1983.
57. Brundage WG, Thuss CJ, Walden DC: Four fatal cases of meliodosis in U.S. soldiers in Vietnam. Am J Trop Med Hyg *17*:183–191, 1968.
58. Danke SG, King AM, Slack WK: Gas gangrene and related infection: classification, clinical features and etiology, management and mortality: a report of 88 cases. Br J Surg *64*:104–111, 1977.
59. Zuckerman AJ: Virus Diseases of the Liver. London, Butterworths, 1970, pp. 98–109.
60. Carmichael GP Jr, Zahradnik JM, Moyer GH, Porter DD: Adenovirus hepatitis in an immunosuppressed adult patient. Am J Clin Pathol *71*:352–355, 1979.
61. Ohbu M, Sasaki K, Okudaira M, Iidaka K, Aoyama Y: Adenovirus hepatitis in a patient with severe combined immunodeficiency. Acta Pathol Jpn *37*:655–664, 1987.
62. Levy Y, Nitzan M, Beharab A, Zeharia A, Schoenfeld T, Nutman J, Rannon L, Steinherz R: Adenovirus type 3 infection with systemic manifestations in apparently normal children. Isr J Med Sci *22*:774–778, 1986.
63. Edwards KM, Bennett SR, Garner WL, Bratton DL, Glick AD, Greene HL, Wright PF: Reye's syndrome associated with adenovirus infections in infants. Am J Dis Child *139*:343–346, 1985.
64. Sun NC, Smith VC: Hepatitis associated with myocarditis. Unusual manifestation of infection with coxsackie group B, type 3. N Engl J Med *274*:190–193, 1966.
65. Gregor GR, Geller SA, Walker GF, Campomanes BA: Coxsackie hepatitis in an adult with ultrastructural demonstration of the virus. Mount Sinai J Med *12*:575–580, 1975.
66. Schleissner LA, Portnoy B: Hepatitis and pneumonia associated with ECHO virus, type 9 infection in two adult siblings. Ann Intern Med *68*:1315–1319, 1968.
67. Krous HF, Dietzman D, Ray CG: Fatal infections with echovirus types 6 and 11 in early infancy. Am J Dis Child *126*:842–846, 1973.
68. Zuelzer WW, Stulberg CS: Herpes simplex virus as the cause of fulminating visceral disease and hepatitis in infancy. Report of eight cases and isolation of the virus in one case. Am J Dis Child *83*:421–439, 1952.
69. Bird T, Ennis JE, Wort AJ, Gardner PS: Disseminated herpes simplex in newborn infants. J Clin Pathol *16*:423–431, 1963.
70. Chase RA, Pottage JC Jr, Haber MH, Kistler G, Jensen D, Levin S: *Herpes simplex* viral hepatitis in adults: two case reports and review of the literature. Rev Infect Dis *9*:329–333, 1987.
71. Haagsma EB, Klompmaker IJ, Grond J, Bijleveld CM, The TH, Schirm J, Gips CH, Slooff MJ: Herpes virus infections after orthotopic liver transplantation. Transplant Proc *19*:4054–4056, 1987.
72. Goyert GL, Bottoms SF, Sokol RJ: Anicteric presentation of fatal herpetic hepatitis in pregnancy. Obstet Gynecol *65*:585–588, 1985.
73. Goodman ZD, Ishak KG, Sesterhenn IA: *Herpes simplex* hepatitis in apparently immunocompetent adults. Am J Clin Pathol *85*:694–699, 1986.
74. Minuk GY, Nicolle LE: Genital herpes and hepatitis in healthy young adults. J Med Virol *19*:269–275, 1986.
75. Baxter RP, Phillips LE, Faro S, Hoffman L: Hepatitis due to *Herpes simplex* virus in a nonpregnant patient: treatment with acyclovir. Sex Transm Dis *13*:174–176, 1986.
76. Myers MC: Hepatic cellular injury during varicella. Arch Dis Child *57*:317–319, 1982.
77. Johnson HN: Visceral lesions associated with varicella. Arch Pathol *30*:292–307, 1940.
78. Cheatham WJ, Weller TH, Dolan TF Jr, Dower JC: Varicella: report of two fatal cases: necropsy, virus isolation and serologic studies. Am J Pathol *32*:1015–1036, 1956.
79. Eschar J, Reif L, Waron M, Alkan WJ: Hepatic lesion in chicken pox: a case report. Gastroenterology *64*:462–466, 1973.
80. Hurwitz ES, Barrett JJ, Bregman D, Gunn WJ, Pinsky P, Schonverger LB, Drage JS, Kaslow RA, Burlington DB, Quinnan GV: Public

Health Service study of Reye's syndrome and medications. Report of the main study. JAMA *257:*1905–1911, 1987.

81. Casals J: Arenaviruses. Yale J Biol Med *48:*115–140, 1975.
82. Zuckerman AJ, Simpson DH: Exotic virus infections of the liver. *In* Progress in Liver Diseases, Vol. VI, edited by H. Popper, F. Schaffner. New York, Grune & Stratton, 1979, pp. 425–438.
83. McCormick JB, King IJ, Webb PA, Johnson KM, O'Sullivan R, Smith ES, Trippel S, Tong TC: A case-control study of the clinical diagnosis and course of Lassa fever. J Infect Dis *155:*445–455, 1987.
84. Zweighaft RM, Fraser DW, Hattwick MAW, Winkler WG, Jordan WC, Alter M, Wolfe M, Wulff H, Johnson KM: Lassa fever: response to an imported case. N Engl J Med *297:*803–807, 1977.
85. Holmes GP, McCormick JB, Trock SC, Chase RA, Lewis SM, Mason CA, Hall PA, Brammer LS, Perez-Oronoz GI, McDonnell MK, Paulissen JP, Schonberger LB, Fisher-Hoch SP: Lassa fever in the United States. Investigation of a case and new guidelines for management. N Engl J Med *323:*1120–1123, 1990.
86. McCormick JB, King IJ, Webb PA: Lassa fever: effective therapy with ribavirin. N Engl J Med *314:*20–26, 1986.
87. Winn WC Jr, Walker DH: The pathology of human Lassa fever. Bull WHO *52:*535–545, 1975.
88. McCormick JB, Walker DH, King IJ, Webb PA, Elliott LH, Whitfield SG, Johnson KM: Lassa virus hepatitis: a study of fatal Lassa fever in humans. Am J Trop Med Hyg *35:*401–407, 1986.
89. Smith CEG, Simpson DIH, Bowen ETW, Zlotnik I: Fatal human disease from vervet monkeys. Lancet *2:*1119–1121, 1967.
90. Bechtelsheimer H, Korb G, Gedigk P: The morphology and pathogenesis of "Marburg Virus" hepatitis. Hum Pathol *3:*255–264 1972.
91. Gear JSS, Cassel GA, Gear AJ, Trappler B, Clausera L, Meyers AM, Kew MC, Bothwell TH, Sher R, Miller GB, Schneider J, Koornhof HJ, Gomperts ED, Isaacson M, Gear JHS. Outbreak of Marburg virus disease in Johannesburg. Br Med J *4:*489–493, 1975.
92. Smith DH, Johnson BK, Isaacson M, Swanepoel R, Johnson KM, Killey M: Marburg virus disease in Kenya. Lancet *1:*816–820, 1982.
93. Rippey JJ, Schepers NJ, Gear JH: The pathology of Marburg virus disease. S Afr Med J *66:*50–54, 1984.
94. Plotkin SA, Cochran W, Lindquist JM, Cochran GG, Schaffer DB, Scheie HG, Furukawa T: Congenital rubella syyndrome in late infancy. JAMA *200:*435–441, 1967.
95. Korones SB: Congenital rubella syndrome: advances and new concepts. G.P. *35:*78–86, 1967.
96. Esterly JR, Slusser RJ, Ruebner BH: Hepatic lesions in the congenital rubella syndrome. J Pediatr *71:*676–685, 1967.
97. Strauss L, Bernstein J: Neonatal hepatitis in congenital rubella. A histopathological study. Arch Pathol *86:*317–328, 1968.
98. Stern H, Williams BM: Isolation of rubella virus in a case of neonatal giant-cell hepatitis. Lancet *1:*293–295, 1966.
99. Zeldis JB, Miller JG, Dienstag JL: Hepatitis in an adult with rubella. Am J Med *79:*515–516, 1985.
100. Onji M, Kumon I, Kanaoka M, Miyaoka H, Ohta Y: Intrahepatic lymphocyte subpopulations in acute hepatitis in an adult with rubella. Am J Gastroenterol *83:*320–322, 1988.
101. Strano AJ: Yellow fever. *In* Pathology of Tropical and Extraordinary Diseases, edited by C.H. Binford, D.H. Connor. Washington, Armed Forces Institute of Pathology, 1976, pp. 1–4.
102. Moneth TP: Yellow fever, a medically neglected disease. Rev Infect Dis *9:*165–175, 1987.
103. Vieira WT, Gayotto LC, deLima CP, deBrito T: Histopathology of the human liver in yellow fever with special emphasis on the diagnostic role of the Councilman body. Histopathology *7:*195–208, 1983.
104. Helmick CG, Bernard KW, D'Angelo LJ: Rocky mountain spotted fever: clinical, laboratory and epidemiological features of 262 cases. J Infect Dis *150:*480–488, 1984.
105. Adams JS, Walker DH: The liver in Rocky Mountain spotted fever. Am J Clin Pathol *75:*156–161, 1981.
106. Klatskin G: Leptospirosis. Yale J Biol Med *27:*243–266, 1955.
107. Heath CW Jr, Alexander AD, Galton MM: Leptospirosis in the United States. Analysis of 483 cases in man, 1949–1961. N Engl J Med *273:*857–864, 915–922, 1965.
108. Dooley JR, Ishak KG: Leptospirosis. *In* Pathology of Tropical and Extraordinary Diseases, edited by C.H. Binford, D.H. Connor. Washington, Armed Forces Institutes of Pathology, 1976, pp. 101–106.
109. Shenberg E, Gerichter CB, Lindenbaum I: Leptospirosis in man 1970–1979. Am J Epidemiol *115:*352–358, 1982.
110. Watt G, Padre LP, Tuazon ML: Placebo-controlled trial of intrave-

nous penicillin for severe and late leptospirosis. Lancet *1:*433–436, 1988.
111. Schmidt DR, Winn RE, Keefe TJ: Leptospirosis. Arch Intern Med *149:*1878–1880, 1989.
112. Ferreira-Alves VA, Vianna MR, Yasuda PH, DeBrito T: Detection of leptospiral antigen in the human liver and kidney using an immunoperoxidase staining procedure. J Pathol *151:*125–131, 1987.
113. Pappas MG, Ballou WR, Gray MR: Rapid serodiagnosis of leptospirosis using the IgM-specific Dot-ELISA. Comparison with the microscopic agglutination test. Am J Trop Med Hyg *34:*346–354, 1985.
114. Alexander AD: Leptospirosis. *In* Infectious Disease, edited by P.D. Hoeprich, M.C. Jordan. 4th Edition. Philadelphia, J.B. Lippincott, 1989, pp. 812–819.
115. Solbrig MV, Sher JH, Kula RW. Rhabdomyolysis in leptospirosis (Weil's Disease). J Infect Dis *156:*692–693, 1987.
116. Judge DM, Samuel I, Perine PL, Vukotic D: Louse-borne relapsing fever in man. Arch Pathol *97:*136–140, 1974.
117. Gillum RL: Relapsing fever. *In* Pathology of Tropical and Extraordinary Diseases, edited by C.H. Binford, D.H. Connor. Washington, Armed Forces Institute of Pathology 197, 106–110.
118. Horton JM, Blaser MJ: The spectrum of relapsing fever. Arch Intern Med *145:*871–875, 1984.
119. Steere AC, Grodzicki RL, Kornblatt AN, Craft JE, Barbour AG, Burgdorfer W, Schmid GP, Johnson E, Malawista SE: The spirochetal etiology of Lyme disease. N Engl J Med *308:*723–740, 1983.
120. Steere AC, Bartenhagen NH, Craft JE, Hutchinson GJ, Newman JH, Rahn DW, Sigal LH, Spieler PN, Stenn KS, Malawista SE: The early clinical manifestations of Lyme disease. Ann Intern Med *99:*76–82, 1983.
121. Chavanet P, Pillon D, Lancon JP, Waldner-Combernoux A, Maringe E, Portier H: Granulomatous hepatitis associated with Lyme disease (Correspondence). Lancet *2:*623–624, 1987.
122. Goellner MH, Agger WA, Burgess JH, Duray PH: Hepatitis due to recurrent Lyme disease. Ann Intern Med *108:*707–708, 1988.
123. Lamont N McE, Pooler NR: Hepatic amoebiasis. A study of 250 cases. Q J Med *27:*389–412, 1958.
124. Doxiades T, Candreviotis N, Yiotsas ZD, Smyrniotis FE: Chronic amebic hepatitis. Clinical and experimental observations. Arch Intern Med *111:*219–225, 1963.
125. Barbour GI, Juniper K Jr: A clinical comparison of amebic and pyogenic abscess of the liver in sixty-six patients. Am J Med *53:*323–334, 1972.
126. Adams EB, MacLoed IN: Invasive amebiasis. II. Amebic liver abscess and its complications. Medicine *56:*324–334, 1977.
127. Nigam P, Gupta AK, Kapoor KK, Sharan GR, Goyal BM, Joshi LD: Cholestasis in amoebic liver abscess. Gut *26:*140–145, 1985.
128. Knight R: Hepatic amebiasis. Semin Liver Dis *4:*277–302, 1984.
129. Ralls PW, Henley DS, Colletti PM, Benson R, Raval JK, Radin DR, Boswell WD Jr, Halls JM: Amebic liver abscess: MR imaging. Radiology *165:*801–804, 1987.
130. Irshad M, Gandhi BM, Chaudhuri G, Tandon BN: Detection of *Entamoeba histolytica* in the pus of amoebic liver abscess by immunofluorescent technique. Indian J Med Res *81:*575–579, 1985.
131. Joyce MP, Ravdin JI: Antigens of *Entamoeba histolytica* recognized by immune sera from liver abscess patients. Am J Trop Med Hyg *38:*74–80, 1988.
132. Gandhi BM, Irshad M, Chawla TC, Tandon BN: Enzyme linked protein-A: an ELISA for detection of amoebic antibody. Trans R Soc Trop Med Hyg *81:*183–185, 1987.
133. Simjee AE, Gathiram V, Jackson TF, Khan BF: A comparative trial of metronidazole v. tinidazole in the treatment of amoebic liver abscess. S Afr Med J *68:*923–924, 1985.
134. Elechi EN: Experience with percutaneous aspiration of amoebic liver abscesses. Br J Surg *75:*582–583, 1988.
135. Bergamini TM, Larson GM, Malangoni MA, Richardson JD: Liver abscess. Review of a 12-year experience. Am Surg *53:*596–599, 1987.
136. Neafie RC, Connor DH: Visceral leishmaniasis. *In* Pathology of Tropical and Extraordinary Diseases, edited by C.H. Binford, D.H. Connor. Washington, Armed Forces Institute of Pathology, 1976, pp. 265–272.
137. Peters W, Killick-Kendrick R: Leishmaniasis in Biology and Medicine. London, Academic Press, 1986.
138. Falk S, Helm EB, Hubner K, Stutte HJ: Disseminated visceral leishmaniasis (kala azar) in acquired immunodeficiency syndrome (AIDS). Pathol Res Pract *183:*253–255, 1988.
139. Duarte MI, Corbett CE: Histopathological patterns of the liver in-

volvement in visceral leishmaniasis. Rev Inst Med Trop Sao Paulo *29*:131–136, 1987.

140. Moreno AA, Marazuela M, Yebra M, Hernandez MJ, Hellin T, Montalban C, Vargas JA: Hepatic fibrin-ring granulomas in visceral leishmaniasis. Gastroenterology *95*:1123–1126, 1988.

141. Corcoran TE, Hegstrom GJ, Zoeckler SJ, Keil PG: Liver structure in nonfatal malaria. Gastroenterology *24*:53–62, 1953.

142. DeBrito T, Barone AA, Faria RM: Human liver biopsy in *P. falciparum* and *P.vivax*. A light and electron microscopy study. Virchows Arch Pathol Anat *348*:220–229, 1969.

143. Connor DH, Neafie RC, Hockmeyer WT: Malaria. *In* Pathology of Tropical and Extraordinary Diseases, edited by C.H. Binford, D.H. Connor. Washington, Armed Forces Institute of Pathology, 1976, pp. 273–283.

144. Ramachandran S, Perera MVF: Jaundice and hepatomegaly in primary malaria. J Trop Med Hyg *79*:207–210, 1976.

145. Hollingdale MR: Malaria and the liver. Hepatology *5*:327–335, 1985.

146. Joshi YK, Tandon BN, Acharta SK, Babu S, Tandon M: Acute hepatic failure due to *Plasmodium falciparum* liver injury. Liver *6*:357–360, 1986.

147. Fakunle YM: Tropical splenomegaly. Part 1: Tropical Africa. Clin Haematol *10*:963–975, 1981.

148. Fakunle, YM, Greenwood BM: A suppressor T-cell defect in tropical splenomegaly syndrome. Lancet *2*:608–609, 1976.

149. Weese WC, Smith IM: A study of 57 cases of actinomycosis over a 36-year period. A diagnostic failure with good prognosis after treatment. Arch Intern Med *135*:1562–1568, 1975.

150. Chandarlapaty SKC, Dusol M Jr, Edwards R, Pereiras R Jr, Clark R, Schiff ER: [67]Gallium accumulation in Gepatic actinomycosis. Gastroenterology *69*:752–755, 1975.

151. Binford CH, Dooley JR: Diseases caused by fungi and actinomycetes. Deep mycoses. *In* Pathology of Tropical and Extraordinary Diseases, edited by C.H. Binford, D.H. Connor. Washington, Armed Forces Institute of Pathology, 1976, pp. 551–554.

152. Meade RH III: Primary hepatic actinomycosis. Gastroenterology *78*:335–359, 1980.

153. Brown JR: Human actinomycosis: a study of 181 subjects. Hum Pathol *4*:319–330, 1973.

154. Jonas RB, Brasitus TA, Chowdhury L: Actinomycotic liver abscess. Case report and literature review. Dig Dis Sci *32*:1435–1437, 1987.

155. Mongiardo N, DeRienzo B, Zanchetta G, Lami G, Pellegrino F, Squadrini F: Primary hepatic actinomycosis. J Infect *12*:65–69, 1986.

156. Roesler PJ Jr, Wills JS: Hepatic actinomycosis: CT features. J Comput Assist Tomogr *10*:335–337, 1986.

157. Shurbaji MS, Gupta PK, Newman MM: Hepatic actinomycosis diagnosed by fine needle aspiration. A case report. Acta Cytol *31*:751–755, 1987.

158. Harvey JC, Cantrell J, Fisher AM: Actinomycosis: its recognition and treatment. Ann Intern Med *46*:868–885, 1957.

159. Young RC: The Budd-Chiari syndrome caused by aspergillus. Two patients with vascular invasion of the hepatic veins. Arch Intern Med *124*:754–757, 1969.

160. Young RC, Bennet JE, Vogel CL, Carbone PP, DeVita VT: Aspergillosis. The spectrum of the disease in 98 patients. Medicine *49*:147–173, 1970.

161. Rinaldi MG. Invasive aspergillosis. Rev Infect Dis *5*:1061–1077, 1983.

162. Park GR, Drummond GB, Lamb D: Disseminated aspergillosis occurring in patients with respiratory, renal and hepatic failure. Lancet *1*:179–182, 1979.

163. Walsh TJ, Hamilton SR: Disseminated aspergillosis complicating hepatic failure. Arch Intern Med *143*:1189–1191, 1983.

164. Lewis JH, Patel HR, Zimmerman HJ: The spectrum of hepatic candidiasis. Hepatology *2*:479–487, 1982.

165. Moseley RH, Kris MG, Einzig A, West R, Gee TS, Armstrong D: Respiratory alkalosis and abdominal pain heralding Candida hepatitis.

Occurrence in patients with acute leukemia in remission. Arch Intern Med *142*:1495–1497, 1982.

166. Sparks AK, Connor DH, Neafie RC: Echinococcosis. *In* Pathology of Tropical and Extraordinary Diseases, edited by C.H. Binford, D.H. Connor. Washington, Armed Forces Institute of Pathology, 1976, pp. 530–533.

167. Pitts HA, Korzelius J, Tompkins RK: Management of hepatic echinococcosis in Southern California. Am J Surg *152*:110–115, 1986.

168. Gemmell MA, Lawson JR, Roberts MG: Control of echinococcosis-hydatidosis: present status of worldwide progress. Bull WHO *64*:333–343, 1986.

169. McCorkell SJ: Echinococcal cysts in the common bile duct: an uncommon cause of obstruction. Gastrointest Radiol *10*:390–393, 1985.

170. Esfahani F, Rooholamini SA, Vessal K: Ultrasonography of hepatic hydatid cysts: new diagnostic signs. J Ultrasound Med *7*:443–450, 1988.

171. Hoff FL, Aisen AM, Walden ME: MR imaging in hydatid disease of the liver. Gastrointest Radiol *12*:39–47, 1987.

172. Rausch RL, Wilson JF, Schantz PM, McMahon BJ: Spontaneous death of *Echinococcus multilocularis:* cases diagnosed by EM2 ELISA and clinical significance. Am J Trop Med Hyg *36*:576–585, 1987.

173. Macpherson CNL, Romig R, Zeyhle E: Portable ultrasound scanner versus serology in screening for hydatid cysts in a nomadic population. Lancet *2*:259–262, 1987.

174. Bret PM, Fond A, Bretagnolle M, Valette PJ, Thiesse P, Lambert R, Labadie M: Percutaneous aspiration and drainage of hydatid cysts in the liver. Radiology *168*:617–629, 1988.

175. Langer B: Surgical treatment of hydatid disease of the liver. Br J Surg *74*:237–247, 1987.

176. Luder PJ, Witassek F, Weigand K: Treatment of cystic echinococcosis *(Echinococcus granulosus)* with mebendazole: assessment of bound and free drug levels in cyst fluid and of parasite vitality in operative specimens. Eur J Clin Pharmacol *28*:279–287, 1985.

177. Morris DL, Chinnery JB, Georgiou G: Penetration of albendazole sulphoxide into hydatid cysts. Gut *28*:75–82, 1987.

178. Manivel JC, Bloomer JR, Snover DC: Progressive bile duct injury after thiabendazole administration. Gastroenterology *93*:245–251, 1987.

179. Teres J, Gomez-Moli J, Bruguera M: Sclerosing cholangitis after surgical treatment of hepatic echinococcal cysts: report of three cases. Am J Surg *148*:694–701, 1984.

180. Miguet JP, Bresson-Hadni S. Alveolar echinococcosis of the liver. J Hepatol *8*:373–379, 1989.

181. Miguet JP, Bresson-Hadni S, Vuitton D: Echinococcosis of the liver. *In* Oxford Textbook of Clinical Hepatology, edited by N. McIntyre, J-P. Benhamou, J. Bircher, M. Rizzetto. New York, Oxford University Press, 1991, pp. 721–730.

182. Bresson-Hadni S, Miguet JP, Vuitton D, Meyer JP, Becker MC, Didier D, Coche G: L'echinococcose alveolaire hepatique humaine. Revue Generale a propos de 80 cas. Sem Hop Paris *64*:2691–2701, 1988.

183. Gottstein B, Eckert J, Fey H: Serological differentiation between *Echinococcus granulosus* and *Echinococcus multilocularis* infections in man. Z. Parazitkend *69*:347–356, 1983.

184. Taylor DH, Morris DL, Reffin D, Richards KS: Comparison of albendazole, mebendazole and praziquantel chemotherapy of *Echinococcus multilocularis* in a gerbil model. Gut *30*:1401–1405, 1989.

185. Bresson-Hadni S, Vuitton D, Didier D, Etievent JP, Mantion G, Miguet JP, Gillet M: Metastases pulmonaires de l'echinococcose alveolaire. Frequence et mecanisme de survenue. Presse Med *18*:83–88, 1989.

186. Bresson-Hadni S, Franza A, Miguet JP, Vuitton DA, Lenys D, Monnet E, Landecy G, Paintaud G, Rohmer P, Becker MC, Christophe JL, Mantion G, Gillet M: Orthotopic liver transplantation for incurable alveolar echinococcosis of the liver: report of 17 cases. Hepatology *13*:1061–1070, 1991.

187. Vuitton D: Alveolar echinococcosis of the liver: a parasitic disease still in search of a treatment. Hepatology *12*:617–618, 1990.

Chapter 24
Hepatic Lesions in Systemic Diseases

Amyloidosis

Amyloidosis comprises a group of disorders characterized by the deposition in various tissues of a fibrillar protein with distinctive histologic features, staining properties, and ultrastructure. The term amyloid, which means starch-like, was chosen by Virchow because of the similarity of its staining characteristics to those of the corpora amylacea of the brain (1).

Amyloidosis has been recognized for almost a century and a half, during which most writing on the subject has been clinical and descriptive. Only recently have modern biochemical and biophysical methods been utilized with revolutionary results to study the broad array of disorders that constitute amyloidosis.

Classification of amyloidosis

A number of classifications including primary versus secondary, typical versus atypical, systemic versus focal, perireticular versus pericollagenous, and classification by the site of deposition have been proposed. None completely satisfies all situations. Most widely used was the primary versus secondary classification. Patients without any predisposing lesion developed primary (idiopathic) amyloidosis. The amyloid tended to be deposited in the mesenchymal tissues—the cardiovascular system, especially small blood vessels, the alimentary tract, and peripheral nerves—and to a much lesser degree the parenchymatous organs. In secondary amyloidosis the deposition of amyloid was largely in the parenchymal organs—spleen, liver, kidney, and adrenal glands—and involved the mesenchymal tissues to a much lesser extent. Staining characteristics were thought to be more variable in the primary form. The amyloidosis associated with multiple myeloma was generally considered primary because of the distribution of the amyloid. The heredofamilial amyloidoses, which comprise a broad variety of syndromes, were usually classified separately.

This clinical classification has been replaced by a system based on the physicochemical properties of the amyloid (2–4) that in effect is not very different from the clinical one. Indeed, some authorities still employ the primary-secondary terminology (3). The new nomenclature uses an A to designate the protein of amyloid fibrils and a second letter to indicate the nature of the protein or its origin. L, for example, indicates the immunoglobulin light chains that characterize the amyloid seen in patients with plasmacytic or primary amyloid. A is used to represent the specific serum amyloid protein seen in secondary amyloidosis. Serum amyloid A is derived from an acute phase reactant (5). Polymorphic forms of serum amyloid A have been identi-

fied in the same individual (6). It is not clear which specific form of amyloid A is deposited in amyloidosis. F is reserved for those seen in familial, polyneuropathic amyloid, S for the senile amyloid syndromes, and E for those associated with endocrine-associated amyloid (3). Not included in the classification is another amyloid protein, the P component known as AP, which is a unique, pentagonal protein found in all types of amyloid. It is identical to an α-globulin of serum and is related to C reactive protein (7). It has been shown that ^{123}I-labeled serum amyloid P component can be used to identify and locate deposits of amyloid (8).

Primary (systemic) amyloidosis. Primary amyloidosis is characterized by the presence of amyloid protein that consists of immunoglobulin light chains (AL). It is seen rarely in patients with primary amyloidosis (3,4,9) and more frequently in patients with multiple myeloma and other plasma cell dyscrasias (10–22) (Table 24–1). Immunoglobulin heavy chains have been noted in primary amyloidosis (AH) (58a, 58b). Pimary amyloidosis (AL) has been shown to be associated with breast masses in patients with and without multiple myeloma (23).

Secondary amyloidosis. Secondary amyloidosis is characterized by the presence of serum amyloid A protein (AA). It occurs in patients with long-standing disease such as tuberculosis, leprosy, pleuropulmonary suppuration, rheumatoid arthritis, and inflammatory bowel disease (24–38), and in patients with familial Mediterranean fever (FMF) (39,40) (see Table 24–1).

Hereditary amyloidosis. Some types of hereditary amyloidosis, an uncommon form of amyloid, are characterized by the presence of prealbumin (AFp). In other types the protein has not yet been identified. Included in this form are diverse, neuropathic, cardiac, and cutaneous amyloidoses (41–49) (see Table 24–1).

Acquired, nonfamilial amyloidosis. Each type of amyloidosis is characterized by a specific protein, some of which have been identified. Included are senile cardiac and cerebral amyloidosis (AS) (50–55) and some that occur in patients with various types of endocrine tumors (AE) (56,57) (see Table 24–1).

An ancillary classification of amyloidosis is based on the observation that amyloid fibrils are deposited along preexisting collagen (pericollagen amyloidosis) or reticulin fibers (perireticulin amyloidosis) (58). In the perireticular type the amyloid tends to be deposited in small blood vessels, including capillaries and sinusoids. The pericollagenous type also affects blood vessels and, in addition, the stroma of parenchymal organs and the sheaths of muscles and nerves. Pericollagen deposition is seen predominantly in systemic amyloidosis, while

Table 24–1. Classification of amyloidosis

Clinical disorder	Major type amyloid in fibril[a]	Amyloidogenic protein
Systemic amyloidosis		
Idiopathic (primary) amyloidosis	AL	Light Chain
Plasma cell dyscrasias		
Multiple myeloma	AL	Light Chain
Monoclonal gammopathy	AL	Light Chain
Primary macroglobulinemia (Waldenstrom's)	AL	Light Chain
Heavy chain disease	AH	Light Chain
Agammaglobulinemia	AL	Light Chain
Localized plasmacytomas	AL	Light Chain
Secondary amyloidosis		
Chronic granulomatous diseases	AA	Unknown
Tuberculosis		
Leprosy		
Syphilis		
Chronic suppurative diseases	AA	Unknown
Osteomyelitis		
Bronchiectasis		
Paraplegia with chronic infection		
Chronic inflammatory diseases	AA	Unknown
Rheumatoid arthritis		
Ulcerative colitis	AA	Unknown
Regional enteritis (Crohn's)		
Other		
Tumors		
Malignant		
Hodgkins's disease		
Nonlymphoid solid tumors	AA	Unknown
Renal adenocarcinoma		
Medullary thyroid adenocarcinoma		
Malherbe's epithelioma		
Benign		
Hepatic adenoma	AA	Unknown
Familial Mediterranean fever	AA	Unknown
Heredofamilial amyloidosis	AF	Varied
Familial neuropathic		
Portuguese	AFp	Prealbumin
Other		Unknown
Familial cardiac amyloidosis	AF	Unknown
Familial cutaneous amyloidosis	AF	Unknown
Familial urticarial otorenal	AF	Unknown
Familial medullary thyroid carcinoma	AF	Unknown
Acquired nonfamilial amyloidosis		
Senile cardiac amyloidosis	AS	Unknown
Senile cerebral amyloidosis	AS	Unknown
Medullary carcinoma of thyroid	AEt	Thyroid (Calcitonin)
Insulinoma	AEi	Insulin
Other endocrine tumors	AE	Unknown

[a] Other symbols have been employed for some of the rare familial and nonfamilial types of amyloidosis in which specific types of amyloid fibrils have been identified (58b).

perireticulin deposition usually occurs in secondary amyloidosis.

Although the primary-secondary pattern holds true in general, overlapping of clinical features, of the distribution of organs involved, and of biochemical and histologic characteristics blur the boundaries. Indeed, the similarities between primary and secondary amyloidosis are much greater than the differences.

Ultrastructure of amyloid

Amyloid has been shown by electron microscopy to be an array of 70 to 100 nm rigid, parallel, nonbranching, hollow fibrils with a 25 A° core (2–4). It has been shown by x-ray diffraction and infrared spectroscopy to be composed of polypeptide chains that run perpendicular to the axis of the fibrils, having the conformation of a twisted, β-pleated sheet. Recent investigations of the physicochemical nature of the fibrils by fractionation of purified fibrils and identification of fibrillar protein components permits, for the first time, a classification based on the actual composition of the amyloid.

Clinically, *systemic amyloidosis* can be seen in any of the settings seen in primary amyloidosis or in the plasmacytic diseases, which can present in protean ways. The diagnosis of AL amyloidosis can be established by the electrophoretic demonstration in serum of a monoclonal peak, which is present in almost 90% of such patients (59).

Occasionally, localized amyloid deposits in the respiratory or urinary tracts arise in extramedullary plasmacytomas (20,23). The AL type of amyloidosis is often called immunocytic amyloidosis (2). Indeed, this relationship supports the clinical dictum that when primary amyloidosis is found, myeloma must be excluded.

In *secondary amyloidosis*, the clinical syndrome is largely determined by the organs in which the deposition of amyloid is greatest. The kidney, spleen, liver, and adrenal glands are the major organs in which amyloid is found, but other tissues may be involved as well. Patients usually present with hepatomegaly or may have the nephrotic syndrome. Historically, *tuberculosis, leprosy,* and *syphilis* were the *chronic granulomatous infections* that stimulated the development of amyloidosis, but all are now relatively uncommon. Chronic infections of the urinary tract and decubitus ulcers of paraplegic patients now account for an increasingly large fraction of the cases. *Chronic inflammatory diseases* of unknown etiology, such as *rheumatoid arthritis, scleroderma,* and *disseminated lupus erythematosus,* the so-called connective tissue or collagen vascular diseases, also give rise to amyloidosis. *Regional enteritis* has been found to be associated with amyloid with surprising frequency—up to 30%. Amyloidosis is much less common in *ulcerative colitis* (28,29). Some *malignant tumors* such as Hodgkin's disease, occasionally, and hypernephroma, frequently, are associated with secondary amyloidosis.

Although the N-terminal fragments of the light chain are relatively homogeneous, the C-terminal regions are heterogeneous. This suggests that the proteins may vary slightly in different patients or in different sites in the same patient. Small amounts of light chains of the lambda variety have been identified in some patients, suggesting a close linkage with immunoglobulins.

Surprisingly, *familial Mediterranean fever,* an autosomal recessive heredofamilial type of amyloidosis, has also been shown to have type AA amyloid. This disease, which is seen in patients from the Mediterranean basin, especially Jews and Armenians, causes recurrent fever and abdominal pain in childhood and usually terminates with renal failure secondary to renal amyloidosis. Amyloid is deposited widely in the blood vessels. The absence of amyloid in the parenchyma of the liver is striking. It is interesting that this pattern of amyloidosis, which is quite different from the usual secondary amyloidosis, appears chemically similar to the other diverse types of secondary amyloidosis.

Hereditary amyloidosis. The heredofamilial amyloidoses constitute a number of diverse syndromes, which have been described during the past 40 years. They include *familial amyloidosis with polyneuropathy* (Portuguese type) (39,41) and other autosomal dominant neuropathic syndromes (44,45) and *familial cardiac amyloidosis* (46). Other familial amyloidoses are listed in Table 24-1. In none of them has the amyloid protein yet been identified.

Miscellaneous amyloidosis. Several other types of amyloidosis have been recognized. The syndrome of *senile cardiac amyloidosis* is sufficiently frequent and serious to be considered in any elderly patient with idiopathic heart failure (50). It is surprisingly common, occurring at autopsy in 10% of patients over 80 years of age and 50% of those over 90 (48). It is often associated with senile plaques on the surface of the brain, and sometimes with senile dementia. The presence of amyloid with typical staining characteristics (50) and an indistinguishable ultrastructure (52) in these plaques has led to the diagnostic term *senile cerebral amyloidosis* (AS) (54,55).

The major amyloid fibril protein from two patients with senile cardiovascular amyloidosis has been isolated. It has been described as chemically and immunochemically unique, and no amyloidogenic substance has yet been identified (50,51). The protein has been designated ASc1. A second amyloid protein, ASc2, has been isolated from the atria of patients with focal atrial amyloid disease (53).

Localized deposits of amyloid have been associated with a variety of endocrine neoplasms (56). A protein with the identical sequence as part of the thyrocalcitonin molecule (AEt) has been isolated from the amyloid of a patient with *medullary carcinoma of the thyroid* (57). It is presumed that insulin and other specific hormones will be found as the fibrillar protein in specific endocrine types of amyloid (56,57).

Pathogenesis of amyloidosis

The demonstration of segments of light immunoglobulin chains, usually the N-terminal portion of the light chains as the major protein of amyloid fibrils (AL) from patients with plasmacytic disorders, suggests an immunocytic origin of this type amyloid. Proteolytic activity liberates fragments of polypeptide chains, which can form β-pleated fibrils. Indeed, such synthesis occurs *in vitro* after the degradation of Bence-Jones proteins, which are light chains (59), and explains the presence of amyloid in the tubular casts of patients with Bence-Jones proteinuria (60). Bence-Jones proteins very chemically one from the other, and only a few of them have an amino acid sequence that can form

β-pleated sheet fibrils. Thus, some light chains appear to be amyloidogenic.

Interleukin 1, which is produced by macrophages as part of the acute phase response and which stimulates the production of acute phase proteins, have been implicated in the pathogenesis of amyloidosis (61,62). This acute phase protein is presumed to be synthesized by hepatocytes in humans as it is in experimental animals (63,64).

Presumably, amyloid can be derived from a variety of amyloidogenic polypeptides that have structures compatible with β-pleating. These include, of course, polypeptides formed by abnormal plasma cells. They also include polypeptides such as prealbumin and calcitonin that are found in serum. Theoretically, they might include amyloidogenic polypeptides synthesized in other abnormal states. Any of these serum proteins could be taken up, cleaved in lysosomes, and excreted by phagocytes. The proximity of early amyloid deposits to Kupffer cells and phagocytic cells in other tissues tends to support such a site of synthesis.

Pathologic features of amyloid

Grossly, amyloid is an amorphous, hyaline, translucent substance that can be found anywhere in the body. When large amounts of amyloid are present, the organs have a firm, rubbery consistency. The deposits of amyloid give a waxy pink, yellow, or gray appearance. Such deposits take a purple-blue color with iodine and dilute sulfuric acid.

Histologically, amyloid is a homogenous, eosinophilic, extracellular substance that is deposited beneath the endothelium of capillaries or sinusoids or in the walls of arteries and veins, usually in association with connective tissue, and often, in close proximity to Kupffer or other reticuloendothelial cells. It may involve any organ, appearing characteristically in the glomeruli of the kidney, perivascularly in the gastrointestinal tract, and in the spaces of Disse in the liver.

By electron microscopy amyloid consists of fine, parallel, nonbranching, rigid, hollow fibrils. Each fibril is made up of spirals composed of protofibrils. Amyloid is always accompanied by P component, a pentagonal, nonfibrillar glycoprotein that is identical with an α-1-globulin found in serum. It represents about 10% of amyloid deposits by weight, but is not a constituent of the amyloid fibrils themselves. It appears to be adsorbed on the fibrils. Its carbohydrate portion is responsible for the positive, violaceous, periodic acid–Schiff stain that gives amyloid its name.

Histologic features of amyloid

By light microscopy amyloid appears as deposits of amorphic, mildly eosinophilic, translucent, hyaline material. It is pink when stained with *hematoxylin and eosin* (Fig. 770) and blue when stained by the *Masson method* (Figs. 85, 199). With crystal violet or methyl violet stain, it shows red metachromasia.

Alkaline Congo red, which stains amyloid red, is the most useful stain for amyloid. It is highly sensitive for amyloid, but it is not completely specific. Molecules of Congo red are bound to the amyloid parallel to the fibrils. It also stains elastic tissue and dense bundles of collagen, especially when decolorization is incomplete.

When amyloid stained with Congo red is examined between crossed polarizers in a polarizing microscope, a striking green birefringence is seen [(65); Fig. 227]. The specificity of the green birefringence depends on the β-pleated sheet conformation of the polypeptides in the amyloid fibrils and the parallel arrangement of the Congo red molecules to the fibrils. Since the birefringence is related to the orientation of the molecules of dye, as the histologic section is rotated 360° the color changes twice from yellow to green. It is necessary, therefore, to rotate the histologic section on the microscope stage through a 90 to 180% arc to detect small amyloid deposits. Even when deposits of amyloid are extensive, the green birefringence may appear patchy in distribution and varies as the slide is rotated. Green birefringence is not demonstrable in very thin sections (3 μm) or very thick ones (20 μm). In addition, by varying the conditions of fixation, staining, illumination, and orientation, the green birefringence can be abolished. It can be induced in the connective tissues or blood vessels of virtually all normal and diseased organs in both humans and rats (66).

Thioflavin-T staining of amyloid provides a sensitive method of confirming the presence of amyloid (67). With fluorescence microscopy amyloid demonstrates light green fluorescence (Figs. 396, 397). Although thioflavin-T staining itself is not specific for amyloid (68), it is more sensitive than the green birefringence of Congo red. The green fluorescence with thioflavin-T in sections that show green birefringence with Congo red virtually proves the material to be amyloid.

Toluidine blue is another very useful stain for amyloid. When viewed between crossed polarizers, amyloid shows bright red birefringence [(69); Fig. 398]. It is simple, reproducible, and is not affected by the thickness of the section, the type of fixation, or imperfect optics. It is less sensitive than Congo red–green birefringence or thioflavin-T fluorescence in the detection of minute deposits of amyloid.

Although specific antibodies against AL and AM fibrillar amyloid components have been developed (70), they are not widely available. AL and AM amyloid may be differentiated on the basis of their physicochemical composition. Potassium permanganate treatment denatures AA protein by altering the β-pleated conformation, thus abolishing its affinity for Congo red, its red color, and its green birefringence (71). AL amyloid, however, is not denatured by potassium permanganate. Trypsin digestion also abolishes the affinity of AA protein for Congo red, but it is more complicated to perform, and it destroys histologic features.

Clinical manifestations of amyloidosis

Amyloid deposition produces structural and functional disorders by replacing or displacing normal components and by interfering with the normal functions of various tissues. In the liver the deposition of amyloid impairs blood flow and interferes with the exchange of oxygen and nutrients, resulting in atrophy and loss of hepatocytes (Figs. 199, 770). Clinically, it is manifested by fatigue, weakness, and weight loss (72).

The principal organs involved are the kidneys, liver, spleen, and gastrointestinal tract. Deposition of amyloid in mesenchymal tissues favors blood vessels, collagen, and myocardium. Older observations indicated that in secondary amyloidosis the

amyloid was deposited mainly in the kidneys, liver, and spleen (73,74), while in primary amyloidosis the favored sites were blood vessels, collagen, and the gastrointestinal tract (74,75). More recent observations have shown that although these trends tend to persist, these patterns may be less clear-cut or reversed for the two types of amyloidosis (7,76,77). It has been suggested that in patients with primary systemic amyloidosis without multiple myeloma, the presence of increased β-2-microglobulin in serum means a much poorer prognosis than in those with normal levels (78).

Sometimes the clinical presentation is dominated by massive hepatomegaly (79,80), which sometimes may mimic hepatic malignancy (81).

Hepatic manifestations of amyloid

The clinical presentation of amyloid liver disease is usually nonspecific; occasionally there are vague abdominal complaints. Hepatomegaly, however, is characteristic of amyloid. It is present in 50 to 100% of patients in whom the liver is involved (9). Indeed, there is a positive correlation between the weight of the liver and the amount of deposition of amyloid and the extent of atrophy of hepatocytes (9). The spleen is enlarged in from 10 to 50% of patients. More specific signs of liver disease such as spider angiomas, gynecomastia, or abdominal collateral veins are very common. Jaundice occurs uncommonly (82–84), and hepatic failure is extremely rare (9). Portal hypertension occurs in less than 20%, ascites is infrequent (10–15%) and is often associated with congestive heart failure, and variceal hemorrhage and hepatic encephalopathy are rare (85). Portal hypertension in one patient with primary amyloidosis was proved to have been caused by an atrioportal fistula (86). The symptoms and signs reported are dominated by the underlying disease and by the sites of amyloid deposition.

Hepatic dysfunction is mild, inconstant, and nonspecific (83,87). it is characterized by hypoalbuminemia and elevation of serum alkaline phosphatase levels, all of which are nonspecific abnormalities. Cholestasis, however, carries a more serious prognosis (88,89).

Histologic features of hepatic lesions

Amyloid deposits may be interlobular, periportal, or perivascular or a mixture of these three distributions (9,86,90). The typical site of amyloid deposition is the space of Disse, between the endothelium of the sinusoids and the hepatic parenchymal cells (Figs. 85, 199, 770). In the early phases of amyloid deposition, it appears first between the Kupffer cells and the hepatocytes and tends to be heaviest there. As the deposits increase in volume, the hepatic plates undergo atrophy and the sinusoids are compressed, thus destroying the normal architecture (Figs. 85, 199, 770). In such cases portal hypertension may develop (85). According to some reports, amyloid deposition is heavier in the portal areas than in the centrilobular zones (3,9), but this is not true in our experience.

In one large series of hepatic amyloidosis, the amyloid was found exclusively in blood vessels in one-third of the patients and exclusively in the parenchyma of one-fourth (9). When blood vessels are involved, amyloid is found most often in the hepatic arteries and arterioles. When arterial deposition is extensive, the arterial walls are thickened, nuclei are infrequent, and the structure of the wall appears homogenous and smudged (Fig. 396). Veins are similarly involved but less frequently and less severely. Amyloid is also deposited in and around collagen, particularly in the portal areas (Fig. 396). Sometimes, amyloid is seen as deposits of round, amyloid bodies within or between hepatocytes (91,92). Rarely, extensive systemic amyloid is found in patients with such globular hepatic deposits of amyloid (93).

Globular hepatic amyloid presents a uniquely different morphologic pattern from the typical, sinusoidal, portal or arterial deposition. It is not deposited in the usual perireticular pattern. The acellular globules, which may be round, oval, or irregular, range in size from 5 to 40 μm in diameter. They may be deposited in portal tracts (Fig. 771) or in sinusoids (Fig. 772). They sometimes have a laminated appearance. They are most frequently seen in the portal tracts but they may appear in the parenchyma. They may be adjacent to each other but they do not merge. They are deposited in the space of Disse, as shown by the projection of Kupffer cells into the sinusoids (Fig. 773), but they do not cause hepatic cord atrophy as is often seen in conventional amyloid deposition. The amyloid stains with Congo red stain and shows green birefringence under polarized light. Like typical amyloid, the globules stain with thioflavin-T. By virtue of their extracellular deposition they should not be confused with the Shikata bodies of HBV infection, with Lafora bodies, or with the intracytoplasmic inclusion bodies seen in fibrolamellar hepatocellular carcinoma or other malignant lesions or other intracellular or extracellular inclusions.

Objective, histologic comparison of primary and secondary amyloidosis does not support the traditional beliefs. One group "blindly" compared liver tissue from 25 patients with primary (AL) amyloidosis, i.e., patients without a predisposing disease and who had plasmacytosis and light chains in the sera or urine, with liver tissue from 13 patients with secondary (AA) amyloidosis, i.e., patients with tuberculosis, rheumatoid arthritis, osteomyelitis, paraplegia, or familial Mediterranean fever (77). They found that all patients with AL had amyloid deposited in the hepatic parenchyma compared with 77% of the patients with AA amyloidosis. Neither the amount of amyloid, the lobular distribution, the degree of atrophy or regeneration of the hepatocytes, nor the reactivity of the Kupffer cells differed in the two groups. Equally surprising was the observation that amyloid deposition in the blood vessel walls and in the portal tissues was found in all of the AA and in two-thirds of the patients with AL amyloid. Whether these more recent findings reflect better classification of amyloidosis, more objective assessment of the amyloid, or a change in the disease itself is not known. It may well be another example of the "emperor's new clothes" syndrome.

Amorphous, perisinusoidal deposits similar in many ways to amyloid are sometimes seen in patients with *nonamyloid light chain disease* [(94,95); Fig. 774]. About half the patients have a lymphoplasmacytic malignancy but the other half do not. The patients show hepatomegaly and, sometimes, ascites. Serum alkaline phosphatase levels are usually elevated. They differ in that the green birefringence seen with Congo red stain is not present. Kappa or lambda light chains can usually be identified by immunochemical techniques (Fig. 775). The difference between the two disorders can be shown dramatically in patients in whom both amyloid and light chain deposits are present (95,96).

Diagnosis of amyloidosis

The diagnosis of amyloidosis is suggested more by the clinical setting than by any specific amyloid syndrome. About 10 to 15% of patients with plasma cell dyscrasias can be expected to develop amyloidosis, while deposits of amyloid can be demonstrated in a higher percentage of those with familial Mediterranean fever. The development of amyloidosis in patients with chronic infectious and inflammatory disorders should be anticipated.

The diagnosis is established by the histologic demonstration of amyloid using specific histologic or immunocytologic staining methods (70). It is most productive to biopsy involved organs such as liver, tongue, kidney, or skin. In the absence of such obvious sites, biopsy of the rectal (97) or gingival mucosa (98) or fine needle biopsy of the abdominal fat pad (99) can often establish the diagnosis.

Liver biopsy sites have been reported to bleed after needle biopsy in patients with hepatic amyloidosis (100,101). Actually, the dangers are exaggerated, and stories of livers rupturing after liver biopsy have not been documented. Spontaneous rupture of the liver in patients with amyloidosis has been observed (102). Liver biopsies are usually well tolerated when conventional criteria of safety are employed. However, amyloidosis may be associated with factor X deficiency (103). Certainly, when other equally rewarding, more accessible sites of amyloid deposition are available, they should be used. However, when liver biopsies are performed, discretion is advised. The use of needles 1.2 to 1.4 mm in diameter is probably safer than those 1.6 or 2.0 mm in diameter (104).

Globular amyloidosis is seen in patients whose clinical presentation of amyloidosis does not differ in any noticeable way from those of other patients with amyloidosis (93). The underlying disease in the patients with globular amyloid deposits varies widely, including viral hepatitis, pericarditis, cardiomyopathy, chronic pulmonary or renal disease, non-Hodgkin's lymphoma, cirrhosis, congestive heart failure, and benign monoclonal gammopathy (93). Serum electrophoresis is usually normal, but monoclonal gamma globulin peaks are occasionally present. Although amyloid can be found in many organs in these patients, it is seen in its globular form only in the liver. Globular amyloid deposits have also been seen in the lungs, larynx, prostate (106), and thyroid (107).

Some patients with amyloidosis exhibit increased uptake of bone-scanning radionuclides over the liver or other amyloid-containing organs (106). This nonspecific finding is suggestive of, but not diagnostic for amyloidosis.

Treatment with melphalan and prednisone appears superior to colchicine (108).

Collagen vascular disorders

Rheumatoid arthritis

Rheumatoid arthritis, the most common of the systemic collagen disorders, causes its major clinical manifestations in the joints. Mild hepatomegaly and minor abnormalities of hepatic blood tests sometimes occur, but usually the liver is not involved (109,110) except in Felty's (111–113) or Sjögren's syndromes (110). Spontaneous rupture of the liver has been reported in rheumatoid arthritis (114).

The most commonly abnormal blood tests include increased serum alkaline phosphatase activity, which appears to parallel the activity of the arthritis. Analysis of the isoenzymes of alkaline phosphatase in rheumatoid arthritis indicates that the elevations are usually caused by bone isoenzyme, which is proportional to the degree of activity of the arthritis or ankylosing spondylitis (115). Elevations of serum transaminase activity may also occur (110), but they may actually be induced by the administration of salicylate (116), other nonsteroidal, antiinflammatory drugs, methotrexate (117–119), gold (120,121), or other therapeutic agents (122,123) rather than by the arthritis itself.

Mild, nonspecific changes, such as fatty infiltration, portal fibrosis, or mononuclear portal inflammation or sinusoidal dilatation may be seen (110,125). Occasionally, in long-standing severe rheumatoid arthritis, amyloidosis may be present (3,4). In one instance, rheumatoid nodules in the liver have been reported (126). Occasionally, severe arthritis of long duration may be associated with clinically significant liver disease such as chronic active hepatitis or primary biliary cirrhosis (126,127). It is never clear, however, whether the coexistence of such diseases is coincidental or consequential.

Nodular regenerative hyperplasia (see Chapters 3 and 25) is sometimes seen in patients with Felty's syndrome (112,128,129), the severe form of rheumatoid arthritis that is associated with splenomegaly and hypersplenism. Occasionally, portal hypertension occurs, probably as a consequence of the increased splenic blood flow and splenomegaly. Lymphocytic infiltration of the sinusoids may be present in this syndrome. It has been postulated that the arteritis of small, intrahepatic arteries may be responsible for the nodular regenerative hyperplasia (129). Four patients with rheumatoid arthritis who developed malignant histiocytosis have been reported (130). The causes of these associations are not known.

Juvenile rheumatoid arthritis

Still's disease, or juvenile rheumatoid arthritis, is a disorder of unknown etiology characterized by recurrent bouts of high fever, evanescent rash, pleurisy, pneumonia, and arthritis. It usually appears before the age of 15 years, but may occasionally affect adults.

The hepatic abnormalities are similar to those seen in maturity onset rheumatoid arthritis, but occur more commonly and tend to be more severe. Although these hepatic abnormalities are probably related to the underlying immunologic disorder, they may be caused by intercurrent viral infection or the results of aspirin or other therapy (116–123).

One case of chronic active hepatitis with juvenile arthritis and rheumatoid nodules has been reported (131). It is not known which comes first, the hepatitis or the arthritis.

The hepatic manifestations are hepatomegaly and mild hepatic dysfunction and are characterized by elevated serum alkaline phosphatase or transaminase activity. Occasionally, there is hyperbilirubinemia and, rarely, a patient may exhibit overt jaundice.

Histologically, the changes are similar to those of adult rheumatoid arthritis, i.e., fatty deposition, lymphocytic infiltration, and, occasionally, portal fibrosis.

Patients with Still's disease on aspirin therapy, which has been implicated in the pathogenesis of Reye's syndrome (132), are likely candidates to develop Reye's syndrome (133).

Our own experience consists of seven adult patients referred to us with a diagnosis of juvenile rheumatoid arthritis for evaluation of hepatic histopathology. All seven exhibited mild focal hepatitis with lymphocytic and plasmacytic portal inflammation. Neutrophilic infiltration was also present in several patients. The parenchyma showed small foci of cell dropout and acidophilic bodies. Kupffer cell hyperplasia (134,135) and increased mitotic activity were present (136). Small epithelioid granulomas were present in four of the seven. Intralobular infiltration of lymphocytes with occasional neutrophils was common. Whether this relatively homogeneous but nonspecific, histopathologic picture is characteristic of juvenile rheumatoid arthritis, especially in adults, is uncertain, since the cases were quite complex and the diagnosis of juvenile rheumatoid arthritis is a clinical one that cannot be established unequivocally.

Systemic lupus erythematosus

Systemic lupus erythematosus is an immunopathic disorder of unknown cause that involves many organs including the heart, kidneys, lungs, arteries, and liver. The liver is involved relatively frequently, but the primary hepatic manifestations are not usually severe. Three-fourths of patients with systemic lupus erythematosus have no clinical or laboratory manifestations of liver disease (137). Secondary hepatic abnormalities may arise from congestive heart failure or other underlying complications of the systemic lupus erythematosus itself. Some hepatic abnormalities may result from intercurrent disease such as viral hepatitis, or may be consequences of treatment with salicylates or other agents. Reye's syndrome, often in association with aspirin administration, has also been reported in systemic lupus erythematosus (138).

Hepatomegaly, the most common clinical sign, occurs in one-third of patients with systemic lupus erythematosus, and splenomegaly is found in about one-fifth (139). Rare instances of spontaneous rupture of the liver or spleen in patients with lupus have been reported and indicate severe organ involvement (140). Jaundice is uncommon, occurring in only 3% (139), but cholestasis is common (141). It tends to be caused by hemolysis, which is not usually attributed to congestive heart failure. Occasionally, ascites is a complication of chronic hepatitis secondary to viral hepatitis. Furthermore, spontaneous bacterial peritonitis is a surprisingly common complication (142). The Budd-Chiari syndrome is relatively common in systemic lupus erythematosus, presumably as a consequence of the lupus coagulopathy (111,143).

Abnormal liver function tests include increased serum transaminase or alkaline phosphatase levels, hypoalbuminemia, and hyperglobulinemia (141).

The most frequent hepatic histologic lesions are fatty infiltration and portal lymphocytic infiltration (144,145). Intralobular focal necrosis and mononuclear infiltration occur occasionally, but may be secondary to salicylate therapy. Patients with systemic lupus erythematosus may be unusually susceptible to this form of hepatotoxicity (116). Arteritis occurs occasionally, as do small, periportal epithelioid granulomas (141). Primary biliary cirrhosis (146), granulomatous hepatitis (147), and nodular regenerative hyperplasia (148) have all been reported in association with systemic lupus erythematosus.

Viral hepatitis occurs frequently in patients with systemic lupus erythematosus. Usually the infection runs a short, self-limited course, but, occasionally, it is prolonged and may lead to chronic active hepatitis or cirrhosis. We have observed such cases in which the early histopathologic lesion was extensive bridging necrosis.

One of the most intriguing aspects of systemic lupus erythematosus is its relationship to chronic liver disease. The "lupoid" form of chronic hepatitis appears to be chronic active hepatitis in patients with positive LE tests (144,145). The chronic active hepatitis may be a consequence of acute HBV infection accompanied by persistent HBs antigenemia. Indeed, we have observed the systemic lupus erythematosus syndrome develop following an episode of acute HBV hepatitis with bridging hepatic necrosis. Polyarteritis nodosa is considered to be an immunologic consequence of the HBV infection in some instances of periarteritis (149,150). No such relationship appears to exist between HBV and systemic lupus erythematosus (151,152), except for the case we have cited above.

The relationship between systemic lupus erythematosus and chronic active hepatitis has been interpreted in different ways. Some believe that lupoid chronic active hepatitis is identical to classic chronic active hepatitis, that lupoid hepatitis is unrelated to systemic lupus erythematosus, and that the LE phenomenon is merely common to both. Others believe that lupoid hepatitis is usually a manifestation of systemic lupus erythematosus. We find little evidence to support this view. We believe that lupoid hepatitis probably reflects an unusual immunologic response to a hepatotoxic agent such as a virus or drug, just as systemic lupus erythematosus is probably the consequence of a similar, abnormal, immunologic response to an unknown stimulus. We agree that autoimmune chronic active hepatitis and systemic lupus erythematosus are immunologically distinct disorders (153).

Postnecrotic cirrhosis is an occasional finding in systemic lupus erythematosus, but its significance is not clear. It is assumed to be the end stage of an asymptomatic HCV or toxin-induced hepatic injury. It is not known whether the underlying systemic lupus erythematosus predisposes to the development of such lesions or not.

Scleroderma (progressive systemic sclerosis)

Scleroderma is a generalized collagen disorder of unknown etiology that is characterized by induration and fibrosis of the dermis and many of the viscera including the gastrointestinal tract, heart, lungs, and kidneys. It does not often involve the liver. In fact, in a controlled comparison, hepatic abnormalities occurred less commonly in scleroderma than in a control group (154).

Some of the hepatic changes reported appear to be related to complicating congestive heart failure or to anoxia secondary to pulmonary fibrosis, which is a frequent component of the scleroderma syndrome. Other abnormalities, usually in hepatic function tests, may be related to intercurrent hepatic disorders such as acute viral or toxic hepatitis or chronic hepatitis.

The closest relationship between scleroderma and liver disease is the recognition that scleroderma or a variant of scleroderma, the CRST syndrome (calcinosis cutis, Raynaud's phe-

nomenon, sclerodactyly, and telangiectasia), is sometimes associated with primary biliary cirrhosis (155–157) (see Chapter 11). An etiologic relationship between them is unlikely, although scleroderma patients have antimitochondrial antibodies almost identical to those of primary biliary cirrhosis (158) as well as antinuclear antibody and rheumatoid factor in their sera. Systemic sclerosis has been reported in a patient with Wilson's disease after long-term therapy with penicillamine (159).

The signs of hepatic involvement in scleroderma are nonspecific and may include hepatomegaly and splenomegaly. Jaundice and portal hypertension and the consequences of the latter are rare. Similarly, laboratory abnormalities are mild and relatively nonspecific and include hypoalbuminemia, hyperglobulinemia, and increased serum alkaline phosphatase or transaminase levels.

The histologic lesions include focal hepatic necrosis, portal fibrosis, and, rarely, micronodular cirrhosis with patchy, fine septa. Sinusoidal congestion is sometimes seen, usually in patients with congestive heart failure.

Giant cell arteritis

Giant cell arteritis is a disorder of unknown etiology characterized by a segmental subacute or chronic, granulomatous, inflammatory reaction that involves widely distributed medium and large sized arteries. Thrombosis and, ultimately, fibrous occlusion of these vessels may occur. This variable syndrome is rarely seen before age 55 and affects women more frequently than men.

Its constitutional manifestations include fever, weakness, anorexia, weight loss, anemia, and leukocytosis. It is sometimes associated with polymyalgia rheumatica. Its clinical manifestations depend on the distribution of the individual vessels involved. Temporal arteritis, for example, usually causes severe headaches and induration and tenderness of the temporal artery, but may present as a fever of unknown origin. Ophthalmic arteritis presents as sudden blindness, which is sometimes bilateral. Coronary arteritis causes myocardial infarction. Intracranial arteritis may give rise to variable neurologic disorders depending on the arteries involved.

The hepatic manifestations of giant cell arteritis are variable. Rarely, arteritis involving the common hepatic artery or a major branch of the hepatic artery may cause hepatic infarction (160). This syndrome is usually discovered at autopsy. Usually, however, the changes are less dramatic and are reflected by abnormal liver function tests such as elevations of serum alkaline phosphatase and the aminotransferases, prolongation of the prothrombin time, impaired bromsulphalein (BSP) clearance, and hypoalbuminemia (161). These changes are more likely to be consequences of systemic effects of the disease rather than evidence of hepatic arteritis or hepatic arterial insufficiency. However, abnormal radionuclide liver scans have been attributed to arteritis of hepatic vessels (162). These abnormalities tend to respond rapidly, as do the constitutional and focal signs, to adrenocorticosteroid therapy.

The hepatic histology is variable, ranging from normal liver, to fatty infiltration, focal necrosis, lymphocytic infiltration of the portal zones, and granulomatous arteritis, often with giant cells (161). In two of our cases such hepatic arterial lesions were demonstrated in needle biopsy specimens (Fig. 371).

Polymyalgia rheumatica

Polymyalgia rheumatica is a disorder of elderly individuals, especially women, that is characterized by muscular stiffness and pain, low grade fever, sweating, fatigue, weight loss, and anemia. In many cases this syndrome is a manifestation of underlying systemic giant cell arteritis.

Although the hepatic manifestations, such as hepatomegaly, are common, few signs of serious liver disease occur (113,139). Mild abnormalities of liver function tests, especially elevations of serum alkaline phosphatase, occur (113,163), as they do in giant cell arteritis. Polyarteritis in association with primary biliary cirrhosis has been reported (164).

The hepatic lesions are minimal and variable. In many patients the liver is normal. In some there are mononuclear cell infiltrates in the portal zones and parenchyma (165). Fatty infiltration is common (166). Focal hepatic necrosis may be present. Kupffer cells are prominent. Small epithelioid granulomas occur occasionally (161,167).

Both the laboratory and histologic abnormalities tend to respond dramatically to adrenocorticosteroid therapy (160,161).

Polymyalgia rheumatica has been thought to be related to HBV infection because of a high incidence of immunologic markers of HBV in the serum found by some investigators (168), but this relationship has not been confirmed by others (169).

Polyarteritis nodosa

Polyarteritis nodosa is a systemic collagen-vascular disorder that is characterized by inflammatory, destructive lesions of medium and small sized arteries throughout the body. These arteries may develop aneurysms, dissections, or thrombosis and may lead to infarction of almost any organ or tissue. The disease may present as an obscure disorder of any organ system, as fever of unknown origin, or as acute viral hepatitis.

The hepatic manifestations may predominate, since an episode of acute HBV hepatitis may progress into fullblown periarteritis nodosa. It has been demonstrated that HBV infection may cause polyarteritis nodosa by the deposition of immune complexes containing HBs antigen, IgM, and complement in arterial walls (149,150,170,171). HBV is not responsible for all cases of polyarteritis, but the mechanism by which it induces periarteritis nodosa suggests a pathogenetic template for other viruses or toxins (see Chapters 5 and 6). HBV does not appear to be an etiologic agent in other rheumatoid diseases (172), but individual families have shown a high incidence of HBV infection and multiple collagen-vascular disease (173).

Chronic active hepatitis may be part of the polyarteritis syndrome. Often, the liver is normal, although at autopsy, hepatic arterial lesions are found in about half the patients (174). Rupture or dissection of aneurysms may induce abdominal pain and shock, and occlusion of vessels may cause hepatic hematoma, hemorrhage, or infarction (175–178). Indeed, except for the accidental ligation of hepatic arteries, polyarteritis nodosa is probably the most common cause of hepatic infarction.

Except for the finding of an involved artery (Figs. 399,400) or the consequences of arterial occlusion, there are no characteristic hepatic lesions (111).

Wegener's granulomatosis

Wegener's granulomatosis is a rare disorder of unknown cause that is characterized by widely disseminated, necrotizing granulomas and segmental necrosis of small arteries and arterioles. Its clinical features vary depending on the location of the lesions, but destructive ulcerations of the upper respiratory tract, pulmonary infiltrations, and focal glomerulonephritis are almost always present. The discovery of anticytoplasmic antibodies in Wegner's granulomatosis helps differentiate it from other disorders that may mimic it (179). Clinical hepatic manifestations of this disease are rare (180).

Hepatic lesions may be demonstrated in about 15% of cases, but these include granulomas that contain epithelioid and Langhans giant cells interspersed with lymphocytes, plasma cells, neutrophils, and eosinophils. These granulomas, which may show central necrosis, are rare, however (171). Involved arteries show fibrinoid necrosis of all layers of the arterial wall, with neutrophilic infiltration and, often, with mural thrombi, but such lesions rarely occur in the liver. Sometimes, thrombosed, occluded arteries undergo organization and recanalization of the vessel wall and thrombi. Rarely, such lesions have been found in the liver (181).

Familial Mediterranean fever (periodic polyserositis)

Familial polyserositis is a hereditary disorder of Jews, Armenians, and Arabs from the Mediterranean basin that is transmitted as an autosomal recessive trait. One clinical type is characterized by recurrent bouts of fever and abdominal pain, and, sometimes, by acute pleuritis or arthritis. There is little or no amyloid deposition in this form of the disease. The second type, which is common in Israel, is characterized by renal amyloidosis, and patients with this type of familial Mediterranean fever often die of renal failure at an early age (39,40).

This disease has few hepatic manifestations. Except for the renal lesions, amyloid deposition is found almost exclusively in blood vessels. The hepatic sinusoids rarely show amyloid deposition although some amyloid can be found in hepatic arterioles.

Endocrine and metabolic disorders

Acromegaly

Growth hormone binds to somatogenic and lactogenic receptors on hepatocytes to induce the many metabolic effects of growth hormone and prolactin (182). The actual hepatologic effects of acromegaly in humans have not been studied. Much more is known about the effects of liver disease on plasma growth hormone levels and insulin resistance, which are increased (183,184) and somatomedin levels, which are decreased (185).

In patients with acromegaly, however, the liver and spleen are often enlarged. Hepatomegaly is found at autopsy in a large majority and splenomegaly in about half (186), and these findings are confirmed by liver scans and other imaging techniques.

The organomegaly is thought to be a manifestation of generalized organ enlargement in response to increased growth hormone secretion. There is, however, no close correlation between the size of the liver and plasma concentrations of growth hormone (186).

When detected clinically, hepatomegaly, which is found in 15 to 20% of acromegalic patients, usually indicates the presence of other hepatic disorders, especially congestive heart failure. Splenomegaly is clinically detectable in about 5% of patients with acromegaly, but when present it is usually associated with hepatic or hematologic disorders.

Liver function tests are almost always normal in acromegaly except when coincidental hepatic diseases are present. It is known that the BSP transport maximum (Tm) is increased and that the hepatic storage capacity is normal in acromegaly (187).

Hepatic histology is almost always normal, except when other hepatic disorders, such as acute or chronic hepatitis, cirrhosis, or heart failure, are superimposed. Indeed, chronic sinusoidal congestion is the most common hepatic histologic abnormality in acromegaly.

Diabetes mellitus

Hepatic abnormalities in diabetes mellitus are discussed in detail in Chapter 14.

Hyperthyroidism

Although a high proportion of patients with hyperthyroidism have been reported to show evidence of hepatic injury, these observations are based largely on relatively old, postmortem evaluations (188,189). More recent reports of patients with mild hyperthyroidism indicate relatively few clinical signs of hepatic involvement, although liver function tests are sometimes abnormal (190,191). Serum transaminase and alkaline phosphatase activity may be increased. The alkaline phosphatase, however, is derived from both liver and bone (192). Indeed, in such cases the hyperthyroidism may mimic hepatobiliary disease (192). Cholestatic jaundice has been observed (193). In thyroid crisis, however, jaundice occurs frequently, and is found in 20% of fatal cases (194). Rarely, hyperthyroidism has been reported to give rise to bleeding varices (195).

The pathogenesis of hyperthyroid liver disease is not known. It has been suggested that thyrotoxin itself is hepatotoxic and in high concentrations may itself be responsible for liver injury. Hyperthyroid disease that is associated with increased cardiac output without a proportional increase in hepatic blood flow and increased hepatic oxygen consumption (196) may render the liver more susceptible to injury by anoxia, infection, or hepatotoxic agents. Whether the jaundice of thyroid storm is related to congestive heart failure, which occurs commonly (194), to the unmasking of underlying defects in bilirubin metabolism such as Gilbert's disease (197), or to a postulated hepatotoxic action of thyroxin is unclear, but the jaundice disappears when the thyrotoxicosis is successfully treated. Insulin antagonism has been noted in hyperthyroidism (198).

Liver histology in uncomplicated thyrotoxicosis is usually normal (190,191), but fatty infiltration may occur. Nonspecific changes, such as variation in nuclear size, hyperchromatism, and cytoplasmic vacuolation, have been reported (199). In severe thyrotoxicosis, hepatocellular necrosis is often present. It is usually focal and centrilobular in distribution, but in thyroid storm the necrosis may be massive (194). In patients with complicating heart failure, passive congestion is present. Lymphocytosis, portal fibrosis, and cirrhosis occur occasionally. Chronic active hepatitis (200) and sclerosing cholangitis (201) occur more commonly than would be expected by chance.

Sometimes, hepatic abnormalities are the result of hepatotoxic side effects of therapy with propylthiouracil (202) or methimazol (203), and in one instance the simultaneous induction of hyperthyroidism and hepatitis by amiodarone has been reported (204). Hyperthyroidism has been induced by the inappropriate production of thyroid-stimulating hormone by a hepatocellular carcinoma (205).

Hypothyroidism

The liver is not obviously abnormal in adult hypothyroidism, and no consistent or specific abnormalities of liver blood tests have been reported (186,206). Serum transaminase and lactic dehydrogenase activity have been reported to be increased, but these may be the result of altered metabolism of the enzymes rather than of hepatic injury per se (196).

Ascites, which is occasionally found in myxedema, is exudative in character (207,208), and differs from the transudative ascitic fluid of cirrhosis.

Histologic examinations of the liver have shown no hepatic abnormalities (208,210), as is true in one of our cases.

Hyperpyrexia

Hyperpyrexia is defined as an elevation of body temperature above 41°C (106°F) (211), whether related to heat stroke, febrile diseases, or, rarely, to delirium tremens, intracerebral hemorrhage, or malignant hyperthermia (212). Heat stroke, the most common type, is characterized by disturbances of consciousness and, often, by convulsions (213). It is commonly seen in patients who are susceptible to malignant hyperthermia, which develops in patients with an autosomal dominant disorder of muscle membranes (214). It may occur after prolonged exposure to intense sunlight or to elevated temperatures as occurs in deep mines (215). It is characterized by circulatory, renal, metabolic, and coagulatory dysfunction and by injury to muscle and to liver.

Clinically, overt liver disease with jaundice is uncommon, but increased serum transaminase and alkaline phosphatase activity are frequent (216). Elevations of serum transaminase and alkaline phosphatase activities are almost invariable (215). A case of heat stroke following vigorous exercise manifested by fulminant hepatic failure with rhabdomyolysis has been reported (216). In a large series of miners who developed heat stroke in South African gold mines, jaundice was present in the patients who died (215). All patients with heatstroke, however, whose temperatures ranged from 105° to 115°F, had elevations of SGOT (mean 1005 IU) and almost all had elevated SGPT levels (mean 644 IU). Some of these enzymes were derived from muscle tissue, as suggested by simultaneous elevations in serum creatinine phosphokinase activity. There was good correlation between the clinicals signs and the liver function tests. In patients in whom SGOT levels exceed 1000 units during the first 24 hours, severe renal and cerebral damage as well as hepatic injury are common and death is frequent. In those in whom the SGOT is <100 units, the course is usually benign and rarely fatal.

The hepatic histologic abnormalities are suggestive of congestive anoxia. In fatal cases, severe dilatation of central veins and centrilobular necrosis and cholestasis are common (217,218). In more mild cases, small foci of necrosis, dilatation of the central veins and centrilobular sinusoids, and regenerative changes are present. Bile duct proliferation and cholangitis have sometimes been reported. The hepatic histology returns to normal within six to eight weeks.

Malignant hyperthermia is thought to represent hypersensitivity to suxamethonium (219), halothane, or other substances (220) in patients with a hereditary, underlying predisposition to rhabdomyolysis (221). Substances such as phencyclidine, known on the street as angel dust, can induce malignant hyperthermia and submassive hepatic necrosis (220). Unfortunately, it is not clear whether, as in heat stroke, the hepatocellular injury is caused by the hyperthermia, the hypotension associated with the hyperpyrexia, or whether the hepatic injury is caused by the phencyclidine itself.

Gastrointestinal disorders

Celiac sprue (gluten-induced enteropathy)

Celiac sprue is a disease that is characterized by intestinal malabsorption of all nutriments, a characteristic mucosal lesion of the small intestine, and a prompt clinical response to removal from the diet of gluten-containing grains (222). The mucosal surface is flat and free of villi; the intestinal crypts are elongated and hypertrophied. The disease is estimated to occur in about 0.03% of the population.

It has traditionally been divided into childhood and adult celiac disease, but since both are similar clinically, pathogenetically, and therapeutically, we shall discuss celiac sprue as a single entity.

Celiac sprue, which is also known as nontropical sprue, is characterized by diarrhea, malabsorption, steatorrhea, malnutrition, and constitutional symptoms, and, sometimes, by abdominal neurologic or hematologic disorders. It is caused by sensitivity to gluten, which causes injury to the jejunal mucosa with characteristic histologic and functional abnormalities, and responds to the withdrawal of gluten from the diet. Hepatic dysfunction, which is characterized by increased serum levels of SGOT and SGPT, occurs in more than half the patients in some series with this syndrome (222–224). Serum albumin levels are decreased, as in other types of malnutrition (224). Vitamin D deficiency in sprue patients may result in increased serum alkaline phosphatase activity. The return to normal of these abnormalities after institution of a gluten-free diet demonstrates that the gastrointestinal lesion was the cause of the hepatic abnormalities.

Sometimes, splenomegaly without hepatomegaly is found in patients with celiac disease. Hypersplenism has also been described (225) and has been shown to be present in three-fourths of patients with celiac disease (226). Other signs of overt liver disease such as jaundice are rare, and when they occur, are probably related to intercurrent liver disease.

No reports of hepatic histologic lesions in the childhood form of the disorder have been published to our knowledge. In adults, the hepatic lesions are variable in type and nonspecific and do not suggest liver injury of any specific type. Hypoalbuminemia and fatty deposition may be consequences of malnutrition. Nonspecific reactive hepatitis is the most common abnormality (223,227). As might be expected, fatty infiltration is frequently found, as it is in other nutritional disorders (223), and, sometimes, it is massive (228). Portal fibrosis is sometimes seen. Rarely, celiac disease is complicated by chronic active hepatitis (223), micronodular cirrhosis (229), primary biliary cirrhosis (230,231), or hepatocellular carcinoma (223). Sclerosing cholangitis has been reported in patients with celiac disease (226,232), but several also had ulcerative colitis, which is often found in association with sclerosing cholangitis (227).

The pathogenesis of the hepatic lesions in patients with celiac disease is not known. Because celiac disease represents intolerance to a specific protein, the possibility of an immune reaction to explain the liver lesions has been considered (233). This possibility is supported by the finding that HLA-DW3 and B8 phenotypes, which are common in patients with chronic liver disease (223), are frequently seen in celiac disease. There is no direct evidence, however, to support this hypothesis.

Tropical sprue

Tropical sprue is a disease characterized by diarrhea, malabsorption of carbohydrates and fats, and hematologic factors, as well as malnutrition, glossitis, and macrocytic anemia. It occurs in natives or visitors to the tropics. Its cause is unknown, but it may have multiple etiologies. It does not respond to the removal of gluten from the diet.

In the older literature, abnormalities of liver blood tests have been reported to occur commonly in cases of tropical sprue (234), and no later studies are available. These abnormalities may reflect other concurrent disorders. Hypoalbuminemia is seen in one-half and appears to reflect malnutrition. Infrequent elevations of serum bilirubin and transaminase activity probably reflect the existence of intercurrent disorders (235).

Aside from the hepatomegaly and splenomegaly, which are often associated with coincidental disorders, there are no physical signs of liver disease.

The hepatic histologic abnormalities are minimal. Fat is usually not present in tropical sprue in contrast to nontropical sprue in which it is common. The most constant finding is the presence of hemosiderin in periportal hepatocytes and Kupffer cells and of lipofuscin in centrilobular hepatocytes and Kupffer cells (235). The explanation for the iron deposition is not clear.

Whipple's disease (intestinal lipodystrophy)

Whipple's disease is a rare systemic disorder that is characterized by weight loss, diarrhea, malabsorption, fever, and lymphadenopathy, and may show hyperpigmentation of the skin, arthralgia or arthritis, serositis, and central nervous system symptoms (236). Anemia is often present. Weight loss, hypotension, lymphadenopathy, abdominal tenderness, and increased pigmentation of the skin are the most common physical findings. Hepatomegaly is rare and splenomegaly uncommon. Ascites is seen only in the presence of severe hypoalbuminemia. Liver function tests are rarely abnormal.

The lamina propria of the small intestine, the mesenteric lymph nodes, and virtually all other organs including the liver may be infiltrated by large, glycoprotein-containing granules in macrophages accompanied by small gram-positive, rod-shaped bacilli (237). The precise nature of the bacillus is uncertain, but *Hemophilus* species, *Brucella,* and l-form streptococci have been implicated (238). With a PCR-based technique, the Whipple bacillus has been identified in formalin-fixed, paraffin-embedded, extraintestinal tissue from several cases of Whipple's disease as a "novel gram-positive organism related to the actinomycetes, most closely to *Dermatophilus congolensis* and *Arthrobacter globliformis* (238a)." The diagnosis of Whipple's disease is established by the presence of these granules, which stain a brilliant magenta color with periodic acid–Schiff (239). It can be established using a recently reported, specific single 821 base 16S rRNA sequence (238a).

The hepatic histologic changes are restricted to the portal areas and consist of the presence of the typical, large macrophages in the portal tracts that are filled with foamy cytoplasm (240) and contain diastase-resistant, PAS-positive, granular, glycoprotein particles or sickle-shaped inclusions (239). These granules can also be found in the Kupffer cells. Sometimes, periportal fatty deposition and mononuclear infiltration of the portal tracts is present (239). The presence on electron microscopy of tiny bacilli, which are 1 to 2 μm long and 0.25 μm wide, some of which are undergoing degeneration, have been found in the cytoplasm of Kupffer cells (241). The PAS-positive granules in the macrophages and Kupffer cells are derived from the walls of the bacteria. Granulomas have been reported (242). Chronic passive congestion is occasionally present, but it is almost always related to the coexistence of congestive heart failure. Focal hepatitis, which is nonspecific, is occasionally found. Amyloidosis occurs rarely in this disorder.

The disease has been successfully treated with penicillin, erythromycin, tetracycline, chloramphenicol, or trimethoprim-sulfamethoxazole, but no uniformly optimal therapeutic protocol has been established (236).

Eosinophilic gastroenteropathy

Eosinophilic gastroenteritis is an uncommon disease that can cause abdominal pain, nausea, vomiting, diarrhea, gastrointestinal bleeding, protein-losing enteropathy, and malabsorption (243). It is characterized by extensive eosinophilic infiltration of the gastrointestinal tract, which is usually accompanied by striking eosinophilia of the peripheral blood. Eosinophilic infiltration of the mucosa predominates, but deeper layers of the gut wall may be involved. When the eosinophilic infiltration is predominantly mucosal, the major manifestations are malabsorption and enteric protein and blood loss. When the eosinophilic infiltration is primarily in the muscle layer, pain and obstructive symptoms occur. When the eosinophilic infiltration is subserosal, eosinophilic ascites may abruptly appear and just as dramatically disappear, often after steroid therapy. The eosinophilia also involves lymph nodes draining the diseased areas. Occasionally, the liver may be involved.

The disease appears to be immunologically mediated. In children, food allergy appears to play a role. Parasitic infestations have been implicated in some cases. Usually, however, no etiology is evident and no likely causes can be demon-

strated. Antecedent symptoms of allergy are common. Except for the ascites, there are few signs of hepatic involvement.

Histologically, the hepatic lesions most commonly reported are eosinophilic infiltration of the portal areas (244) and the presence of large numbers of eosinophils in the sinusoids, a finding that may reflect the eosinophilia in the peripheral blood. We studied the hepatic lesions in two well-documented cases. In both patients, the portal tracts were enlarged and edematous and were heavily infiltrated with eosinophilic leukocytes and lymphocytes and a few plasma cells. The interlobular ducts were frequently reduplicated and some showed degenerative epithelial changes. Some ducts showed concentric fibrosis. Erosion of the limiting plate was present in both patients. The parenchyma showed focal hepatic necrosis, and in one of these patients a striking, parenchymal eosinophilic infiltration was seen. This patient, who had diarrhea for several months, peripheral eosinophilia (17%), and a vague history of allergy to "starchy foods," showed infiltration of portal tracts with eosinophils, lymphocytes, and occasional plasma cells, and degeneration of interlobular bile ducts (Fig. 776). The symptoms and hepatic lesions regressed over four months on a starch-free diet. Eosinophilic granulomas have been described (245).

Ulcerative colitis

The reported incidence of hepatic findings in ulcerative colitis varies greatly. It depends largely on the method of case selection. Elevated levels of serum alkaline phosphatase and BSP retention, and, less commonly, of the aminotransferases and bilirubin may be anticipated in 10 to 30% of cases (246–248). The true prevalence of hepatic histologic lesions is difficult to determine because liver biopsies have been almost exclusively performed in patients with hepatic dysfunction or in those undergoing colectomy for advanced or complicated disease. This selection of patients skews the material. Furthermore, there are discrepancies between hepatic dysfunction as indicated by abnormal liver function tests and by liver biopsy findings. Often, the biopsies are normal in patients with abnormal blood tests, and, sometimes, the reverse is true. Moreover, there is no close correlation between the prevalence or severity of hepatic lesions and the extent, duration, or severity of colonic lesions (248). Occasionally, hepatic lesions are present in patients before the onset of overt colitis. It is probable that subclinical ulcerative colitis is present in such cases. More to the point, however, only a minority of patients with evidence of hepatic injury exhibit overt signs of liver disease (246,249).

Several types of hepatic lesions are encountered in ulcerative colitis. Some of these lesions, such as fatty infiltration (250), are nonspecific in nature and some are coincidental lesions not directly related to the inflammatory bowel disease. Sometimes, they may occur together. Consequently, the frequency and significance of these associations are uncertain.

The histologic syndrome of *periocholangitis*, which was consolidated in 1965 (249) from earlier descriptions (250–252), was widely accepted but poorly understood. Indeed, the term "pericholangitis" is, in part, a misnomer, since the histologic changes are neither limited to the ductules nor to the periductular zones. The process may involve the portal lymphatics, portal vein radicals, and hepatic parenchymal cells, sometimes extending to the centrilobular area. In the acute phase, the portal tracts are swollen with inflammatory exudate, edema, and cellular infiltrates (Fig. 718). Small and medium sized perilobular bile ducts are affected predominantly, but perilymphangitis and endophlebitis may be present as well as centrilobular bile stasis, Kupffer cell prominence, and focal parenchymal inflammation or necrosis. As the process progresses, the inflammatory response decreases and fibrosis begins to appear. In the chronic phase, the portal structures may be encased in concentric, onion skin collagen. These lesions may be seen in patients with or without primary sclerosing cholangitis (253).

This process, which progresses to *cirrhosis* in from 10 to 20% of patients, may be macronodular (247,249,250,254), micronodular (255), or biliary in type (252,256).

Recognition that sclerosing cholangitis is present in an extremely high percentage of patients with ulcerative colitis (257,258) and that it is similar in its cholangiographic (259) and histologic features (260,261) to sclerosing cholangitis has led to the conclusion that pericholangitis is, in fact, incipient sclerosing cholangitis. However, the pattern of intrahepatic and extrahepatic bile duct involvement occurs more frequently in patients with inflammatory bowel disease, while extrahepatic involvement tends to occur in those without inflammatory disease (262).

Sclerosing cholangitis, a disorder of segmental inflammation, fibrosis, and stricture of intrahepatic and extrahepatic bile ducts, occurs with increased frequency in ulcerative colitis (257,258), but is less commonly seen in regional enteritis (261). The sclerosing cholangitis seen in ulcerative colitis appears in every way to be identical to the primary sclerosing cholangitis that occurs spontaneously in healthy individuals or in patients with disorders such as thyroiditis, retroperitoneal fibrosis, mediastinal fibrosis, or porphyria cutanea tarda. Sclerosing cholangitis in its early stages may be difficult to identify definitively, especially in needle biopsy specimens. At least half of all cases of sclerosing cholangitis occur in patients with ulcerative colitis (259,261,263). Conversely, the incidence of sclerosing cholangitis in unselected groups of patients with ulcerative colitis appears to range from 1 to 4% (261,264). However, in patients with ulcerative colitis in whom there is laboratory evidence of hepatic dysfunction, such as increased serum alkaline phosphatase levels, sclerosing cholangitis may be present in from 50 to 90% of patients with ulcerative colitis (258,261). This very high incidence largely reflects the recent availability of endoscopic retrograde cholangiography, which can demonstrate sclerosing cholangitis that is not evident clinically. The lesions of pericholangitis, however, are not limited to, nor even predominantly located in the periductular regions (259), and may be present in the absence of angiographic evidence of sclerosing cholangitis (261).

Primary sclerosing cholangitis appears to be associated with HLA DR2 and DR3 (265), but this association is unrelated to any such association of these haplotypes with ulcerative colitis.

Histologically, primary sclerosing cholangitis is a very variable lesion (266–268) characterized by segmental stenosis of the intrahepatic ducts, with fibrotic thickening (Figs. 715–717) and infiltration of submucosal and subserosal areas with mononuclear cells (Fig. 718). Hepatocellular atrophy is an occasional finding (269). Features of extrahepatic biliary obstruction or even of secondary biliary cirrhosis may develop, and copper deposition may be present (Fig. 719).

As a consequence of the successful fortuitous therapy of a patient with primary sclerosing cholangitis (269a) and the surprisingly good clinical responsese to methotrexate in primary biliary cirrhosis (269b), studies of methotrexate in primary sclerosing cholagitis were initiated. The clinical and laboratory responses so far have been encouraging (269c). Histologic im-

provement has been demonstrated in a woman after long-term treatment with methotrexate (Figs. 719A, 719B, 719C, 719D). Such instances of beneficial results are anecdotal and will require objective, prospective investigations to establish the value of such therapy. These changes are even more impressive than those shown after methotrexate therapy of primary biliary cirrhosis (Figs. 633A, 633B, 633C, 633D).

Hepatic vein thrombosis, the Budd-Chiari syndrome, has been considered to be an occasional complication of ulcerative colitis (270). The pathogenesis of this relationship is unknown.

Pylephlebitis and *hepatic abscess* are rare complications of ulcerative colitis, which are seen only when the colitis is severe. They have been attributed to the portal vein bacteremia. The fact that they have not been reported as frequently in recent years has been attributed to the widespread use of broad-spectrum antibiotic therapy. There is no direct evidence to support these speculations, however.

Biliary tract carcinoma has been estimated to occur 10 times more frequently in patients with ulcerative colitis than it does in patients without colitis (271–274). It is rarely seen in regional enteritis (276). It usually occurs in patients with ulcerative colitis of long duration (271,272), although it may appear years after proctocolectomy has rid the patient of the clinical manifestations of the colitis.

Atrophy of the lobes in the hilum of the liver is common in patients with primary sclerosing cholangitis (275).

Other hepatic lesions are attributable to systemic effects of the ulcerative colitis such as fatty infiltration (260). Fatty liver occurs in up to one-third of patients with inflammatory bowel disease, and appears to reflect the severity of the underlying colitis, the degree of debilitation, and the nutritional state.

Amyloidosis of the liver, a rare complication of inflammatory bowel disease, tends to occur less commonly in ulcerative colitis than in Crohn's disease (247,276,277).

Some hepatic lesions such as *chronic active hepatitis* and *postnecrotic cirrhosis* seem to show a common pathogenesis with ulcerative colitis. Although specific, autoimmune features such as glomerulonephritis, polyarteritis, thyroiditis, and thrombocytopenic purpura often accompany chronic hepatitis and ulcerative colitis (278), there is no direct evidence that the concurrence of these disorders is a consequence of abnormal autoimmune responsiveness. Actually, the incidence of chronic active hepatitis in ulcerative colitis varies from 1 to 16% (249,256) and of ulcerative colitis in chronic active hepatitis from 4 to 28% (279,280). The latter association seems more common in young patients. Furthermore, chronic active hepatitis is rare in regional enteritis (248,281). The exact prevalence of chronic active hepatitis in ulcerative colitis is not known, since chronic active hepatitis and sclerosing cholangitis may be difficult to differentiate histologically. The reported series suggest that the coexistence of chronic active hepatitis and ulcerative colitis is increased. Inactive postnecrotic cirrhosis also occurs with increased frequency in ulcerative colitis (250,256). Again, it is not clear how often the cirrhosis is a consequence of chronic active hepatitis, sclerosing cholangitis, or intercurrent hepatic disorders, or how often it shares a common pathogenetic mechanism with the ulcerative colitis, but it seems to be closely related to the existence of sclerosing cholangitis (282).

Some hepatic lesions are caused by intercurrent disorders that are not directly related to the ulcerative colitis. *Viral hepatitis* of any type may occur in ulcerative colitis; the course of such infections does not differ from that in otherwise healthy subjects or in patients with other diseases. The increased exposure of patients with ulcerative colitis to blood transfusions, medical procedures, and to the hospital environment increases the risks of developing viral hepatitis. Similarly, exposure to a variety of medications is increased in ulcerative colitis, and the risks of developing *drug-induced hepatic injury* are increased.

The pathogenesis of the hepatic lesions encountered in ulcerative colitis cannot be attributed to any one mechanism, and, therefore, multiple factors have been proposed to explain the variety of hepatic lesions.

The seeding of the liver by portal-borne bacteria has been a popular hypothesis that may account for "pericholangitis." It was postulated that enteric bacteria enter the intestinal lymphatics and portal venous blood through the ulcerated mucosa. The high incidence of *portal vein bacteremia* (24%) and the occasional recovery of bacteria from the livers (11%) of patients with advanced ulcerative colitis at surgery just before colectomy (283) indicate that portal bacteremia is a real threat. If one-fourth of the patients have bacteremia at the time of culture, it is probable that the total prevalence of bacteremia is much higher and that the portal bacterial burden is very high. In the large majority of patients with ulcerative colitis who do not have advanced liver disease, the liver promptly filters the bacteria from the blood. The hepatic abnormalities may represent a reaction to the bacteria rather than to bacterial infection per se. A number of investigators have shown that injections of a variety of enteric organisms into several species of experimental animals can induce hepatic lesions similar to those seen in pericholangitis (284–286). Some investigators, however, have failed to confirm the frequent portal bacteremia or the recovery of bacteria from the liver (286,287).

Against the portal bacterial hypothesis are the dissociation between the presence and severity of the hepatic lesions and of the colitis. The liver lesions may precede the intestinal disease, they show little correlation with the extent or severity of the colitis, and they may persist long after the diseased colon has been surgically removed. Furthermore, the hepatic lesions are independent of the presence or absence of portal vein bacteremia (283). Moreover, antibiotics do not alter the presence or severity of the hepatic abnormalities.

Other pathogenetic mechanisms, including absorption of toxins, the presence of abnormal toxic bile acids, viral infection, injury to arteries, and genetic predisposition, have been suggested (288).

Crohn's disease

Regional enteritis is a segmental, granulomatous, ulcerative, inflammatory disease of unknown cause that involves the terminal ileum and, less frequently, other parts of the gastrointestinal tract. As in ulcerative colitis, hepatic functional abnormalities and histologic lesions are relatively common and relatively nonspecific (261,281).

Liver abscesses are relatively common complications of Crohn's disease with a prevalence 10 to 30 times more frequent than in patients without inflammatory bowel disease (289). They tend to occur as multiple rather than as solitary abscesses, and, often, are the consequences of intraabdominal foci of infection. They appear to represent metastatic infectious manifestations of portal-borne bacteria.

The abnormalities of liver function tests consist mainly of elevations of alkaline phosphatase activity, usually associated with an increase in 5′-nucleotidase activity, which confirms the hepatic origin of this abnormality in most cases (261,281). BSP retention is increased in 15 to 20% of patients. Neither the frequency nor the severity of these abnormalities appears to parallel the extent of the bowel involvement. Serum albumin levels are decreased in one-third the patients. This nonspecific change can be caused by poor nutrition and chronic systemic illness as well as by hepatic injury per se. Serum transaminase levels are increased in 5 to 10% of patients. Serum bilirubin levels are rarely increased except in the presence of complicating or intercurrent hepatobiliary disease.

The hepatic histologic lesions of regional enteritis are similar to those of ulcerative colitis, and may include fatty infiltration, portal fibrosis, portal inflammation, and bile duct proliferation, all of which occur commonly. Focal necrosis occurs occasionally.

"Pericholangitis" is seen in Crohn's disease as well as in ulcerative colitis. The recognition that sclerosing cholangitis is frequently present in Crohn's disease and that sclerosing cholangitis may give rise to the changes of pericholangitis suggests a relationship between Crohn's disease and sclerosing cholangitis as well. In general, sclerosing cholangitis has been thought to be uncommon in regional enteritis (260). In one investigation of the association of primary sclerosing cholangitis in a series of 414 cases of inflammatory bowel disease, 10 patients were found to have otherwise unexplained, elevated serum alkaline phosphatase levels. Eight of these patients had ulcerative colitis and 2 had Crohn's disease. All 10 patients were proved to have sclerosing cholangitis. Histologically, one of the cases of Crohn's disease showed the nonspecific changes of "pericholangitis" and the other the characteristic abnormalities of sclerosing cholangitis with cirrhosis. It seems clear that "pericholangitis" is neither a specific histologic lesion nor a clinical entity. These histologic abnormalities may be seen in primary biliary cirrhosis, obstruction of the biliary tree, and cholangitis, as well as in sclerosing cholangitis. The term "pericholangitis" can best be abandoned. The unexplained findings of "portal triaditis, interlobular hepatitis, and intralobular cholangitic hepatitis," as "pericholangitis" is also known, however, demands investigation of the biliary tree and of the large bowel.

In patients in whom Crohn's disease involves the colon, more systemic complications are seen than in those in whom the disease is restricted to the small intestine (260,281), including the presence of hepatic granulomas and amyloidosis. Hepatic epithelioid giant cell granulomas occur occasionally in regional enteritis, more commonly than in ulcerative colitis (260,281,290). Figure 375 shows such a portal granuloma in a 40-year-old woman with long-standing Crohn's disease. Hepatic amyloidosis occurs more frequently in regional enteritis than in ulcerative colitis and appears to occur more frequently in those with extensive, severe disease especially when it involves the colon and requires colectomy (291).

Cholelithiasis occurs more frequently in patients with regional enteritis than in those with ulcerative colitis and especially in those with extensive or long-standing ileal involvement. One-third of such patients form gallstones (292). The incidence of cholesterol gallstones is also increased in patients who have had ileal resection. The cholelithiasis appears to be related to decreased absorption of bile acids from the ileum. This blockage of the enterohepatic circulation may result in insufficient amounts of bile acids to solubilize cholesterol in bile acid-lecithin micelles, and favors the formation of cholesterol gallstones.

Melanosis coli

Melanosis coli is an asymptomatic, reversible condition in which the mucosa of the colon has become brown-black in color from the use of anthracene cathartic agents such as cascara, sagrada, or senna. Rarely, it is seen in patients who give no history of taking such laxatives, however.

The most frequent sites of pigment deposition are in the cecum and in the rectosigmoid portions of the colon. Occasionally, the ileum is involved (293). The pigment, which by differential staining appears to be melanin-like, fills clusters of macrophages in the lamina propria of the colon and, sometimes, the ileum.

The extracolonic manifestations of melanosis coli are rare, but this pigment has been found in lymph nodes in the mesocolon (294,295) and, very rarely, in the liver (296). Usually, there are no clinical or laboratory manifestations of hepatic involvement. In one reported case, however, abnormalities of serum bilirubin, transaminase, and alkaline phosphatase were reported, but it is not clear that they were attributable to the pigmentation, since the patient had a prior history of excessive alcohol consumption. In that patient the liver was jet black and a gross diagnosis of the Dubin-Johnson syndrome had been made (296). On histologic examination, large amounts of a finely granular, brown pigment filled hypertrophied Kupffer cells and spared the hepatocytes. This pigment was also found in portal macrophages. After the cathartic had been stopped, the pigment gradually disappeared from the liver over a four-year period.

In two biopsy specimens observed by us the liver tissue was grossly black. One patient, who died of coronary artery disease and who had no known hepatic disease, was found at autopsy to have melanosis coli and melanosis hepatis. History related to cathartic usage was unavailable. The other patient, who had taken anthracene carthartic agents, exhibited pink skin and deep red plasma, but was otherwise asymptomatic (297). The pigment consists of coarse, intracellular granules that resemble the pigment seen in the Dubin-Johnson syndrome (Fig. 777) and is usually PAS-D positive. Iron stains of the pigment are negative. However, it reacts with the Fontana-Masson silver stain to show brown-black, melanin-like granules (Fig. 778). In both our patients the pigment was found almost exclusively in the cytoplasm of the hepatocytes, but rare granules were found in the Kupffer cells. The pigment is distributed predominantly in the pericentral and midzonal cells, but is also present in lesser amounts in periportal parenchymal cells (Fig. 779).

The patient with red plasma was followed carefully after she had stopped the cascara cathartic agent. The anthroquinone in her plasma decreased slowly until it and the red color of the plasma had disappeared after four years. After another three years, during which the patient showed no evidence of hepatic disease or laboratory abnormalities, mild melanosis coli persisted and the liver biopsy was repeated. Neither the amount nor the distribution of the pigment had changed (Figs. 799A, 799B, 799C) (Personal communication, S. S. Bottomley).

It is not clear why melanosis coli is an uncommon consequence of common cathartic usage, why the hepatic deposition of the pigment is an extremely rare occurrence, or why in some patients the pigment is found in the parenchymal cells but not in the reticuloendothelial cells and in other cases in the Kupffer cells, but not in the hepatocytes.

Biliopancreatic diversion

Biliopancreatic diversion, a variant of jejunoileal bypass that was recently introduced for the treatment of massive obesity, had been devised in an attempt to avoid the hepatic lesions seen after jejunoileal bypass (297a). This procedure is a complex operation that consists of (a) cholecystectomy, (b) a three-fourths distal gastrectomy with closure of the duodenal stump, (c) a distal iliogastric anastomosis, and (d) a lateral anastomosis between the proximal small bowel and the terminal ileum (297b). The biliopancreatic tract thus created diverts the digestive juices to the distal ileum and avoids the blind loop postulated to be responsible for the characteristic, post-jejuneoileal bypass-induced hepatic injury. Serious hepatic lesions were not reported after this procedure until the recent publication of an article (297c) that describes an acute alcoholic-hepatitis–like lesion (Fig. 779D).

Hematopoietic, lymphoproliferative, and histiocytic disorders

Leukemia

Hepatic involvement is relatively common in all types of leukemia, both acute and chronic. Leukemic infiltration of any organ can occur, and the liver by virtue of its constituent cell types and size is frequently involved.

Hepatomegaly is very common. Almost three-fourths of cases examined at autopsy have livers that weigh more than normal, and in about one-half, the livers are palpable or grossly enlarged (298). Although the livers tend to be largest in chronic myelogenous leukemia, liver size is not helpful in differentiating myelogenous from lymphocytic or monocytic leukemia. *Splenomegaly* is even more common than hepatomegaly. At autopsy, 90% of spleens are enlarged and 70% are grossly so, i.e., >300 g (298). Chronic myelogenous leukemia appears to be associated with the largest spleens, but, as with hepatomegaly, the size of the organ is not a discriminating factor. Jaundice is uncommon; when it occurs it is usually caused by coincidental hepatobiliary disease. Ascites is rare; when it occurs it is probably related to obstruction of vascular or lymphatic vessels.

The hepatic lesions in leukemia involve both the portal tracts and the parenchyma. The *portal tracts* are usually infiltrated and expanded by leukemic cells of the specific type of leukemia [(299); Fig. 277]. The cells tend to be relatively uniform in their stage of maturation (Fig. 352). Portal fibrosis is common in all types of leukemia, but is usually mild in degree. In patients treated with folic acid antagonists, however, the degree of fibrosis appears to be more severe than in those treated in other ways, despite equivalent degrees of leukemic infiltration of the portal tracts (300). The stimulation of the deposition of portal fibrosis by methotrexate in nonleukemic diseases is well known [(301); Fig. 512]. When hepatic disorders such as chronic hepatitis occur in patients with leukemia, the portal infiltrate usually assumes the cell type of the leukemia, as if the leukotactic response is determined by the type of leukocytes most readily available. Intense leukemic infiltration, however, may destroy portal collagen (Fig. 352), reticulin (Fig. 780), and elastic fibers (Fig. 781).

Hepatic parenchymal involvement is characterized by leukemic infiltration and dilatation of the sinusoids (Fig. 268). The leukemic cells are, of course, of the cell line of the specific leukemia, and the cell types are more readily identifiable in the parenchymal tissues than in the portal tracts. Chronic lymphocytic leukemia tends to cause sinusoidal infiltration least commonly and least extensively, and is more likely to show portal infiltration. It may not be possible to differentiate the leukemic cells infiltrating the sinusoids from those in the peripheral blood just passing through the sinusoids. In acute forms of leukemia, blast cells are usually present, often in profusion. Megakaryocytes may be seen in the sinusoids (Fig. 268), but are much more common in the acute forms of leukemia. The hepatic histologic picture in "aleukemic" forms of leukemia does not differ from that in fully developed leukemias (298). Atrophy of hepatocytes occurs in areas of extensive sinusoidal infiltration as it does in severe sinusoidal congestion (Figs. 268, 277). Parenchymal or Kupffer cell hemosiderosis is occasionally seen in leukemia.

Hairy cell leukemia (leukemic reticuloendotheliosis). Hairy cell leukemia gives rise to a discrete clinical syndrome characterized by hypersplenism, pancytopenia, and the presence of "hairy" monocytes in the peripheral blood, and is thought to be of monocytic or lymphocytic origin (302). Frequently, the liver shows sinusoidal and portal infiltration of hairy mononuclear cells. Hairy cells are characterized by abundant cytoplasm with fine, stellate extensions into the space of Disse and into the lumen of the sinusoids (Fig. 266). These filamentous, cytoplasmic projections, which are characteristic of monocytes by scanning electron microscopy, permit differentiation of hairy cell from lymphocytic leukemia (303). The cytoplasm may contain diastase-resistant, PAS-D-positive granules. These leukemic cells can often be identified by a halo of clear cytoplasm around the nuclei (304,305). The diagnosis may be aided by the demonstration of tartrate-resistant, acid phosphatase in the leukemia cells in liver sections (306). The cells appear to contain reticulin fibers, which can be seen on silver staining (Fig. 267). It has been demonstrated that in hairy cell leukemia the spleen contains blood-filled pseudosinuses that are lined by hairy cells, rather than by endothelial cells (307). Similar hepatic angiomatous lesions are found in more than half the cases. They occur in multifocal clusters that resemble hemangiomas (290).

Remission of hairy cell leukemia seems to follow recovery from posttransfusional hepatitis (308). Conversely, HBV infection in patients with acute lymphoblastic leukemia seems to have adverse prognostic influence (309), and chronic hepatitis is a common consequence (310).

The differential diagnosis of leukemia on the basis of hepatic findings may be difficult. Infectious mononucleosis may be especially difficult to differentiate from lymphocytic leukemia. The Epstein-Barr virus (EBV) invades B lymphocytes and elicits a vigorous T cell and antibody response that gives rise to atypical lymphocytes in the peripheral blood and in the portal tracts of the liver (311). Early in the course of infectious mononucleosis, these lymphoid cells, which are EBV-infected, B lymphoblasts, have a lymphoblastoid appearance and many features of malignant proliferation (312). In acute lymphocytic leukemia, the infiltrating cells tend to be more pleomorphic than in infectious mononucleosis. In addition, hepatic necrosis, hyperplasia of Kupffer cells, and polymorphonuclear infiltrates fa-

vor the diagnosis of infectious mononucleosis. Later in the course of infectious mononucleosis, the lymphocytes, which are then reactive T lymphoblasts, appear somewhat more mature and may resemble the cells seen in chronic lymphocytic lymphoma.

Similarly, myeloid metaplasia may mimic myelogenous leukemia. It may not be possible to differentiate the normal leukocyte precursor cells that develop in the hepatic sinusoids of patients with extramedullary hematopoiesis from the malignant caricatures of the leukocytes that infiltrate the liver in leukemia. The presence of numerous megakaryoctyes, erythroblasts, and normoblasts in myeloid metaplasia may help differentiate it from the myelogenous precursors in leukemic infiltrations.

Lymphocytic infiltration of the portal tracts that occurs in a variety of disorders such as chronic hepatitis may resemble lymphocytic leukemia, but the presence of plasma cells, polymorphonuclear cells, and lymphocytic pleomorphism may help differentiate portal exudates from the mature, monotonous lymphocytes typical of chronic lymphocytic leukemia.

Histiocytic medullary reticulosis may be difficult to differentiate from hairy cell leukemia (Fig. 266). Since both malignant disorders are derived from reticulum cells, it is difficult to distinguish these two varieties of abnormal reticulum cells from each other when they infiltrate the liver. Phagocytosis of red cells, leukocytes, and platelets, which is characteristic of histiocytic reticulosis, may differentiate this disorder from hairy cell leukemia. Unfortunately, the phagocytosis is not always demonstrable in the liver. The final diagnosis may depend on electron microscopic examination (311).

Lymphocytic lymphoma may not be differentiable from lymphocytic leukemia. The portal infiltrates are identical in the two types of malignancy. Sinusoidal infiltration is common in lymphocytic leukemia, but lymphocytic lymphomas usually do not extend into the lobules.

Extramedullary hematopoiesis (myeloid metaplasia)

Undifferentiated mesenchymal cells of the liver retain into adulthood the capacity to mature into erythrocytes, leukocytes, and platelets when the stimulus to regenerate blood is sufficiently strong. During fetal life, the liver is the primary site of hematopoiesis, which may persist into the first few months of infancy, especially after premature birth. Hematopoiesis in infancy represents primarily erythrocyte formation, and foci of hematopoiesis contain almost exclusively erythroblasts and normoblasts (Fig. 43), plus a few myeloid elements and rare megakaryocytes. Furthermore, the hematopoiesis is not usually extensive, occurring in only small, scattered, intralobular foci. The spleen, however, is usually enlarged.

Myeloid metaplasia, however, is not physiologic. It represents an attempt of the liver to make blood when the bone marrow is unable to do so, and occurs in disorders in which the bone marrow has been injured by toxins, such as benzene, by irradiation, or by infections, such as tuberculosis or syphilis. This secondary type of myeloid metaplasia is often characterized by hepatomegaly in the absence of splenomegaly. Extramedullary hematopoiesis is also seen when the bone marrow has been replaced by medullary metastases, myelogenous or monocytic leukemia, or multiple myeloma (313). Sometimes, it occurs in disorders of unknown etiology such as myelofibrosis, osteosclerosis, and osteoporosis and, occasionally, after polycythemia vera. The course in the postpolycythemic type is more rapid and lethal, and may terminate in monocytic leuke-mia or malignant lymphoma (314). Sometimes, myeloid meta-plasia occurs in the absence of a recognizable underlying cause, the so-called agnogenic myeloid metaplasia. This form of the disease appears to be relatively benign and slowly progressive.

Hepatic hematopoiesis is almost invariably associated with splenic hematopoiesis, and both the liver and spleen are en-larged. The liver and spleen tend to enlarge progressively the longer the disease lasts. If splenectomy is performed, the liver increases its metaplasia and may become truly massive in size (315,316). When jaundice and hepatic failure occur, coinciden-tal diseases are usually responsible. Portal hypertension may develop and may be manifested by ascites or by hemorrhage from esophagogastric varices (317). Sometimes, the metaplasia may mimic metastatic hepatic malignancy (318). Liver function tests are characterized by increased serum alkaline phosphatase in at least 50% of patients. Only 30% of patients with myeloid metaplasia show an increase in serum bilirubin levels and in only 10% do these levels exceed 2 mg/dl. Serum albumin con-centrations are frequently decreased. Transaminase activity is usually normal.

Extramedullary hematopoiesis of various types can occur. Sometimes occasional megakaryocytes are seen in the liver without other evidence of myeloid metaplasia [(319); Fig. 17]. Such megakaryocytes have been found in less than 2% of our own series of more than 7000 liver biopsies in the absence of any other evidence of myeloid metaplasia. They occur almost exclusively in the sinusoids, but in one case they were seen in portal tracts. They do not appear to occur in any specific he-matologic or hepatic disorder. Such sinusoidal megakaryocytes may not indicate disease per se, but may represent normal, cir-culating megakaryocytes in the peripheral blood.

More typically, however, hepatic hematopoiesis involves both the sinusoids and the portal areas. The amount of myeloid metaplasia generally appears to be proportionately greater than the degree of anemia would require. The basic architecture of the liver is preserved even though 30% of the liver mass may be involved (Fig. 782). This disorder is characterized by the presence of immature, erythropoietic and leukopoietic precur-sor cells and megakaryocytes, primarily in the sinusoids (Fig. 783). Normoblasts usually appear as clusters of dark-staining nuclei with a thin rim of cytoplasm, and are appreciably smaller than lymphocytes, for which they are sometimes mistaken (Fig. 783). Other bone marrow cells may be more difficult to identify in the liver than in bone marrow smears or sections. Some-times, the developing cells may be misinterpreted to be reticu-loendothelial cells. The portal zones may be infiltrated and ex-panded by the precursor blood cells (Fig. 784), which when extensive, may erode the limiting plate of hepatocytes. Portal fibrosis occurs in some cases, but cirrhosis is rare. Portal or hepatic venous thrombosis may ensue.

In addition to sinusoidal infiltration of myeloid elements, collagenization of the space of Disse and capillarization of the sinusoids may occur (317). When the amount of hematopoiesis in the sinusoids and spaces of Disse are extensive, atrophy of the intervening hepatic plates may occur (Fig. 785).

Hemosiderosis often occurs due to increased iron absorption and the rapid turnover of erythroid elements. The frequent pres-ence of immature red and white blood cells in the peripheral blood reflects the lack in the liver and spleen of regulatory fac-tors found in the bone marrow that prevent the escape of these immature forms into the bloodstream.

Several problems in differential diagnosis may occur. Usu-ally the megakaryocytes are easily identified as such, but, sometimes, deformed or shrunken megakaryocytes may be mis-taken for Reed-Sternberg cells. In contrast to Reed-Sternberg cells, however, megakaryocytes are usually diastase-resistant, PAS-positive (Fig. 786), but not always (Fig. 787). The pleo-morphism of hematopoiesis may help differentiate it from leu-kemic and other infiltrations (320).

Portal hypertension of several types may develop. Occasion-ally, it is associated with portal or hepatic venous thrombosis, which is characterized by normal wedged hepatic venous pres-sure (presinusoidal portal hypertension) or elevated wedged he-patic venous pressure (postsinusoidal portal hypertension), re-spectively. Usually, however, the portal hypertension is caused by hematopoietic tissue that obstructs the sinusoids and inter-sinusoidal communications. This type of portal hypertension, which is termed sinusoidal, is characterized by an increased hepatic venous wedged pressure. Sometimes, the portal hyper-tension is thought to be the consequence of greatly increased spleen size and splenic blood flow. Increased hepatic resis-tance, which permits the flow of normal amounts of portal blood, may be too high for an increased amount of splenic blood to flow through the liver. Occasionally, myeloid metaplasia forms masses in the liver, abdomen, lung (321), or virtually anywhere else in the body.

It has been suggested that in patients with myeloid metapla-sia the risks of hemorrhage after liver biopsy are increased. In our experience, postbiopsy bleeding in patients with myeloid metaplasia who satisfy our standard criteria for liver biopsy is extremely uncommon.

Thrombocytopenic purpura

Thrombocytopenia purpura, which is characterized by platelet deficiencies and splenomegaly and is cured by splenectomy, has been found at the time of splenectomy to exhibit perisinus-oidal fibrosis (322).

Multiple myeloma

Myelomatosis is a neoplastic disorder characterized by prolif-eration of plasma cells in the bone marrow with the formation of osteolytic bone lesions and the synthesis of abnormal, mono-clonal, serum globulins or fragments of serum globulins. The disease is characterized by anemia, pathologic fractures, and weight loss. The precipitation of these proteins in the renal tub-ules may give rise to renal failure. These proteins, or part thereof, may be incorporated into amyloid.

Hypatic involvement in multiple myeloma is relatively un-common, although in the late stages hepatomegaly is common (303,304). Hepatomegaly is found in over one-half and spleno-megaly in one-fourth of cases, but portal hypertension is ex-tremely rare. Jaundice and ascites are very uncommon and are usually caused by intercurrent hepatic disorders. Hepatic dys-function is found in about half the patients with myelomatosis (304). Increased BSP retention, hypoalbuminemia, and pro-longed prothrombin times are the most common abnormalities. Increased serum alkaline phosphatase activity is seen in patients with extensive hepatic involvement. The alkaline phosphatase is of hepatic origin as shown by isoenzyme analysis or by confirmation by increased 5′-nucleotidase activity. This differentiation is important, since the bone lesions of multiple myeloma, which are characterized by the absence of osteoblastic activity, are associated with *normal* osteogenic alkaline phosphatase levels. Transaminase activity is occasionally increased. Albumin is often decreased, probably as a consequence of the excessive production of homogeneous plasma globulins. Abnormalities of liver function may be related to intercurrent viral hepatitis, tuberculosis, or drug hepatotoxicity.

The hepatic lesions are characterized by infiltration of the sinusoids (Figs. 788, 789) and portal tracts (Figs. 280, 790), by increased numbers of variably differentiated plasma cells. Identification of the plasma cells and their precursors can be facilitated by staining with methylpyronine green, which stains the cytoplasm a reddish pink color. Occasionally, the infiltrations with plasma cells may be sufficiently great to form tumors (325). Nonspecific, noncaseating epithelioid granulomas have been reported, but are rare.

Amyloidosis is often found in small amounts in the livers of patients with multiple myeloma (326). It occurs more often than myelomatous infiltrations of the liver. Usually it is found in small amounts in intrahepatic arteries (Fig. 396), but, rarely, it is deposited in large amounts in the spaces of Disse, resulting in extensive atrophy of hepatic parenchymal cells (Fig. 199). Extramedullary hematopoiesis of modest proportions occurs occasionally when the bone marrow has been replaced by the neoplastic myelomatous tissue.

Waldenstrom's macroglobulinemia

Waldenstrom's macroglobulinemia, a neoplastic disorder of elderly individuals, is characterized by the proliferation of distinctive plasmacytoid lymphocytes (or lymphocytic plasmacytes) in the bone marrow, lymph nodes, liver, and spleen, and is almost invariably accompanied by the appearance in the serum of an abnormal monoclonal macroglobulin (327). The manifestations of this disease are primarily constitutional—weight loss, anemia, lymphadenopathy, a bleeding diathesis—or related to the physical properties of the abnormal paraproteins in the serum—Raynaud's phenomenon, visual disturbances, neurologic and dermatologic abnormalities.

The liver and spleen are often enlarged. Otherwise, clinical evidence of liver disease is rare. The primary hepatic lesion is the infiltration of portal tracts with plasmacytoid lymphocytes. The deposition of amyloid and of macroglobulins in the space of Disse has been observed (328).

Light chain disease has been reported in Waldenstrom's macroglobulinemia as well as in myelomatosis in association with peliosis hepatis and nodular regenerative hyperplasia (329). It has been postulated that the peliosis and nodular hyperplasia may be consequences of disordered intrahepatic circulation caused by the perisinusoidal deposits. A relationship between light chain and AL-type amyloid deposition has been demonstrated (330).

Sickle cell anemia

The liver is affected in a high proportion of patients with homozygous sickle cell anemia (331,332). This association is characterized by hepatomegaly, which may be present in 90% (333),

and hepatic functional abnormalities (334). In additional to unconjugated hyperbilirubinemia, an almost universal phenomenon that is related to hemolysis (335), bouts of hepatocellular cholestasis with overt jaundice are relatively common (333–336). These episodes of jaundice, which usually occur during sickle cell crises, may be difficult to differentiate from biliary obstruction. Cholelithiasis, which is secondary to the precipitation of excess bilirubin excreted as a result of hemolysis, occurs commonly (337,338). It may be complicated by acute cholecystitis, but extrahepatic biliary obstruction is rare (334). In patients with sickle cell disease who develop coincidental liver disease, such as viral hepatitis or obstructive jaundice, extremely high serum bilirubin levels, often in excess of 50 mg/dl, may occur (339). The surgical therapy of hepatobiliary problems in patients with sickle cell anemia is often difficult and is frequently followed by postoperative complications (340). The abdominal pain that is associated with the sickle cell disease may be caused by a variety of other lesions, and computerized tomography may be helpful in the differential diagnosis (341). Sudden massive enlargement of the liver associated with abdominal pain and a dramatic decrease in hemoglobin concentration has been attributed to intrahepatic sequestration of sickled erythrocytes (342).

The variants of sickle cell anemia such as sickle cell trait (SA), sickle cell-hemoglobin C disease (SC), and sickle cell-thalassemia disease (SFA) induce similar but more mild symptoms, signs, and laboratory abnormalities than sickle cell anemia. Sickle cell crises rarely occur in these variants except in sickle cell-thalassemia. When they do they are much less severe. Patients with these variations of sickle cell anemia, especially SA, may develop splenic infarction at high altitudes or when flying in unpressurized airplanes (343).

The hepatic injury in sickle cell crisis is due primarily to anoxia secondary to decreased sinusoidal blood flow and impaired sinusoidal perfusion as a result of the aggregation of sickled erythrocytes, of Kupffer cells that are swollen by erythrophagocytosis, and of the increased viscosity of the blood (333,344). Anemia contributes to the anoxia (334). In some cases, deposition of fibrin and collagen in the spaces of Disse further impairs the transport of oxygen to the hepatocytes (335). The process of capillarization of the hepatic sinusoids with the development of basement membranes may further impede the transport of nutrients (345). Hepatic hemosiderosis secondary to multiple transfusions and to increased iron absorption may contribute.

The hepatic histologic lesions are variable (346). Sinusoidal changes constitute the most common abnormalities and consist of agglutinated sickle cells, chiefly in the centrilobular areas (Fig. 791). Centrilobular sinusoidal obstruction, however, causes sinusoidal congestion throughout the lobule rather than predominantly in the pericentral zones (Fig. 792) as is seen in chronic passive congestion. The sinusoids are often congested, and, occasionally, thickening of reticulin and collagen is present in areas of congestion (Figs. 792, 793). Kupffer cells are swollen and often contain phagocytized sickle cells ((Figs. 250, 794) and hemosiderin. Fibrin thrombi are occasionally seen in the sinusoids.

There is atrophy of hepatocytes in the areas of congestion (Fig. 792). Foci of hepatocellular necrosis, degeneration, or dropout may be present (Figs. 791, 794). These areas of necrosis may contain mononuclear cells and may later undergo fibrosis, producing randomly distributed scars. The hepatocytes may show regenerative activity as evidenced by thick plates or rosette formation (Fig. 795). Centrilobular ischemic necrosis is often seen in autopsy material due to terminal shock. Cholestasis is common, especially during sickle cell crises, but may occur in the absence of other abnormalities of the parenchymal cells. Rarely, intrahepatic bile filled cysts ("bilomas"), which are considered to be sequelae of hepatic infarctions, have been reported (347). Hemosiderosis is present in almost all cases, and is not necessarily related to the number of blood transfusions (332–334).

In some cases, the portal triads are enlarged, fibrotic, and infiltrated with mononuclear cells and hemosiderin-containing macrophages. This hemosiderosis may progress to secondary hemochromatosis even in the absence of multiple transfusions. Ductular proliferation may be present.

Cirrhosis of various types may occasionally be found. Macronodular postnecrotic cirrhosis is the most common type (334). Its relationship to the sickle cell disease is uncertain. It is probably related in many instances to unrecognized infection with hepatitis viruses, but sometimes develops in the absence of overt viral hepatitis (332). Micronodular portal cirrhosis is sometimes seen, and may be the consequence of sickle cell–induced, progressive hepatocellular necrosis. Postransfusional hemochromatosis may develop, but it is an uncommon lesion.

It has been suggested that the great variety of hepatic abnormalities are "to be expected in a heavily transfused population with a high prevalence of gallstones" independent of the underlying disease (348).

Histiocytic medullary reticulosis (malignant histiocytosis)

Histiocytic medullary reticulosis, a disorder of unknown etiology, is characterized by widespread, progressive invasion and proliferation of atypical histiocytes throughout the lymphoreticular tissues (349). Patients with this disorder develop fever, wasting, generalized lymphadenopathy, hepatomegaly, and splenomegaly (349–351). All formed elements in the blood are decreased. The disease is usually fatal within a few months, but has been reported to persist for as long as 13 years (352).

The liver is usually involved (353,354). Histiocytes infiltrate the portal triads, the sinusoids, and, occasionally, the central veins (Fig. 796). The portal tracts are expanded by this histiocytic infiltration, which extends into the parenchyma after destroying the limiting plates of hepatocytes (Figs. 354, 797). In the sinusoids, the histiocytic infiltration may be extensive, causing focal necrosis and atrophy of hepatic plates (Figs. 263, 264). The histiocytic infiltration is diffuse without the development of tumors. The histiocytes are of variable size and shape. Some appear normal; others show great pleomorphism and some giant forms (Fig. 265). They appear loosely aggregated with ill-defined cell boundaries. The cytoplasm is faintly eosinophilic and finely granular (Fig 797). Basophilic cytoplasm has been noted by others (355), but we have not observed this feature in our own cases. The cytoplasm is sometimes abundant and sometimes scant. A characteristic finding is the presence of phagocytized erythrocytes, leukocytes, and platelets (Fig. 798), but this phenomenon may be difficult to demonstrate in the liver. The nuclei are variable in size and are often multiple with multiple nucleoli. These large, syncytial cells are sometimes mistaken for Reed-Sternberg cells, and may thus suggest the diag-

nosis of Hodgkin's disease, but that similarity is superficial. Plasma cells commonly accompany malignant histiocytes, but are rare in Hodgkin's disease. Hairy cell leukemia causes similar hepatic lesions, but the characteristic fine cytoplasmic extensions, the reticulin fibers, and the absence of atypical appearance distinguish them from malignant histiocytes. The lesions of histiocytosis X, particularly of the Letterer-Siwe type, may resemble those of histiocytic medullary reticulosis, but the cells in the former are more uniform and show erythrophagocytosis infrequently. Monocytic leukemia may also be differentiated by the more regular size of the monocytes and of the delicate pattern of their nuclear chromatin, and by the presence of a leukemic blood picture.

Familial hemophagocytic reticulosis (lymphohistiocytosis)

Lymphohistiocytosis, a lethal, familial, autosomal recessive disorder of children, usually under the age of two years, is characterized by widespread infiltration of the tissues by large histiocytes. These histiocytes contain phagocytized erythrocytes and, less commonly, leukocytes and platelets. This disorder is similar to histiocytic medullary reticulosis except for the early age of onset, the familial occurrence, the frequency of central nervous system involvement, and the absence of skin lesions (356–360). It involves primarily the bone marrow, liver, spleen, and lymph nodes.

It usually starts with the abrupt onset of fever, hepatosplenomegaly, and pancytopenia. Unlike histiocytic medullary reticulosis, lymphadenopathy is not usually present. Jaundice frequently occurs terminally, and death usually occurs within a few months of onset.

The hepatic lesions consist of infiltration of the portal triads with atypical histiocytes, with large, multilobulated nuclei, and frequent nucleoli. They often contain erythrocytes and, occasionally, leukocytes or platelets. Lymphocytes and monocytes are interspersed among the histiocytes. These histiocytic abnormalities may occasionally be missed in liver biopsy sections even though it is a generalized disease. Kupffer cells are often swollen and may contain phagocytized erythrocytes. Fatty infiltration, bile stasis, and scattered intralobular foci of lymphocytes and of hepatocellular necrosis may be found late in the course of the disease and at autopsy, but are inconstant. These nonspecific findings probably represent changes related to malnutrition and to terminal sepsis.

In our own series, three siblings died between the ages of two and eight months. They exhibited lesions indistinguishable from those of histiocytic medullary reticulosis. Figure 799 illustrates the expansion of the portal tracts and infiltration of the parenchyma by atypical histiocytes. At higher magnification (Fig. 800), the expansion of a portal tract by atypical histiocytes leading to erosion of the limiting plate is seen. Figure 801 illustrates focal infiltration of the parenchyma by atypical histiocytes, some of which show erythrophagocytosis.

Virus-associated hemophagocytic benign histiocytosis

Virus-associated hemophagocytic benign histiocytosis, which apparently occurs in patients with a variety of viral infections, is characterized by benign histiocytic proliferation throughout the lymphoreticular tissues (361,362). It is manifested clinically by fever, constitutional symptoms, hepatosplenomegaly, pancytopenia, and hepatic dysfunction. Pulmonary infiltrations are common. The disease occurs in two forms. One is usually seen in adults who have undergone splenectomy and have been immunosuppressed by azathioprine and prednisone after renal transplantation and who develop chronic cytomegalic virus infection. Herpes simplex, varicella-zoster, and Epstein-Barr viruses have also been implicated. This form of the disease begins with high fever and constitutional symptoms, hepatomegaly, and pancytopenia in the peripheral blood. Lymphadenopathy may be suppressed by steroid therapy. The second syndrome is seen in children without any underlying disease who develop a viral-like illness, which, after several weeks, abruptly exhibits high fever, increased severity of constitutional symptoms, hepatosplenomegaly, lymphadenopathy, and peripheral pancytopenia. This disorder, which may follow immunizations, has been associated with the Epstein-Barr adenoviruses. Macular rashes are common in the juvenile type.

Although the disease is called "benign" to differentiate it from malignant histiocytosis, it is a serious disorder resulting in death in one-third of the reported cases. All patients show anemia and leukopenia, often severe, and three-fourths show thrombocytopenia. Occasional histiocytes are seen in the peripheral blood. The bone marrow reveals a hypocellular pattern with decreased granulopoiesis and erythropoiesis and normal or increased numbers of megakaryocytes. Hyperplasia of histiocytes is moderate or marked. The histiocytes appear mature. The presence of red blood cells, platelets, and, often, nucleated leukocytes within the mature histiocytes is almost pathognomonic. Lymph nodes show normal architecture with hyperplasia of mature histiocytes.

The hepatic manifestations of this syndrome are hepatomegaly and splenomegaly. Serum bilirubin levels are increased in about one-third of the patients. Ascites and other manifestations of portal hypertension have not been reported. SGOT is elevated in almost all patients, and can be as high as 3000 units. The median value has been reported to be greater than 10 times the upper limit of normal (361). Serum alkaline phosphatase levels are usually increased, often greatly.

The hepatic lesion is characterized by infiltration of the portal tracts and sinusoids with mature histiocytes. Hemophagocytosis is common in the sinusoidal histiocytes. Focal necrosis is common. Cirrhosis has not been reported.

The differential diagnosis is an important one, since benign histiocytic proliferation appears to be a more common disease than histiocytic medullary reticulosis, which is always fatal. The disorders are differentiated primarily by the malignant appearance of the histiocytes in histiocytic medullary reticulosis. The histiocytes are much larger, have large nuclei, little cytoplasm, an immature, reticular chromatin pattern, and prominent nucleoli. Hemophagocytosis is not overt in histiocytic medullary reticulosis as it is in benign histiocytic proliferation. Although malignant histiocytosis and histiocytic hemophagocytosis occur frequently in many hematologic disorders (361), neither their number nor the degree of phagocytosis approach that seen in virus-associated histiocytosis. It has been suggested in both benign and malignant histiocytosis that hemophagocytosis may account for peripheral cytopenias. Indeed, fatal hemorrhage in histiocytic medullary hematopoiesis has been attributed to the massive phagocytosis of platelets (363).

Histiocytosis with immunologic deficiency

In each type of histiocytosis described previously, the immune system is intact. However, an immune-deficient variant exists in which infants develop gastrointestinal and dermatologic manifestations, lymphadenopathy, hepatosplenomegaly, and eosinophilia (364). The clinical picture resembles that of graft-versus-host disease (see Chapter 26).

Sea-blue histiocytosis

(See Chapter 4.)

Histiocytosis X

The term histiocytosis X (see Chapter 15) denotes a group of disorders of unknown etiology with different clinical expressions and similar pathology characterized by infiltration of histiocytes (365,366). The histiocytic infiltration tends to be limited to a single tissue, most commonly bone, but may be widely disseminated. The principal sites of histiocytic infiltration are bone, skin (367), spleen, lungs (368), and lymph nodes. The clinical course may be acute or chronic and benign or malignant. When localized to bone, lymph glands, or spleen it does not involve liver (360), but cirrhosis due to hepatic infiltration by the typical cellular elements of histiocytosis X has been reported (369). Association with sclerosing cholangitis has also been described (370), and bile ductular proliferation and cholestasis have been reported (371). Benign lesions, which usually involve a single organ in older patients, are characterized by masses of polygonal histiocytes with indistinct cell membranes that give a syncytial appearance interspersed with eosinophilic leukocytes and, often, multinucleated giant cells (372). They are thought to be abnormal Langerhans cells (373), the dendritic cells of the dermis, which are thought to be responsible for the activity of histiocytosis X (373a). Malignant lesions are characterized by diffuse infiltration of individual histiocytes throughout the reticuloendothelial system. Malignant-type histiocytes are large cells with weakly basophilic cytoplasm, distinct cell membranes, and invaginated nuclei with clumped chromatin. Multinucleated giant cells and eosinophils are rare. "Malignant" lesions tend to occur in patients who are less than three years of age and who have multiorgan involvement.

The three subtypes of histiocytosis X, i.e., eosinophilic granuloma, Hand-Schuller-Christian disease, and Letterer-Siwe disease, are based largely on clinical manifestations. Each of these disorders has been recognized for many years, but the histiocytosis that is common to all and the occasional transition from one type to another (374–377) have led to the concept that all three are variable manifestations of a single disorder (378). This view has been challenged (379).

Hepatic involvement may occur in all three subtypes (380,381). The ultrasonic and computed tomographic features of such lesions have been described (382).

The liver is only rarely involved in eosinophilic granuloma. Hematologic tests are normal except for occasional, mild eosinophilia. Liver function tests are usually normal. Of two biopsy-documented cases of pulmonary eosinophilic granuloma seen at Yale, one exhibited multiple, noncaseating, epithelioid granulomas in the liver. Neither showed histiocytic infiltration. The liver in the second case appeared normal.

When the liver in Letterer-Siwe disease is extensively infiltrated, jaundice may occur. Portal hypertension is very rarely seen. This disorder is usually fatal within a few months. Cholestatic liver disease has occasionally been observed (383).

The histologic features of the hepatic lesions are infiltration of the portal triads (Fig. 353) and parenchyma (Fig. 261) and invasion of the walls and lumens of some central veins (Fig. 262) by large histiocytes. The infiltrating histiocytes, which resemble macrophages found in portal inflammatory exudates, are large cells with faintly eosinophilic granular cytoplasm. The nuclei often show folded, invaginated cell membranes with clumped reticulin. Lymphocytes and other inflammatory cells are interspersed in these portal infiltrates, which may expand the portal tracts and erode the limiting plates. Foam cells, eosinophils, and giant cells are rare.

Systemic mastocytosis

Systemic mastocytosis, a rare disorder of unknown etiology, is characterized by widespread proliferation of mast cells in bone marrow, skin, and other organs. The principal tissues involved are the skin, bone, bone marrow, liver, spleen, and lymph nodes (384,385).

The manifestations of the disease are diverse and reflect both the organs involved and the production by the mast cells of histamine, heparin, and other vasoactive substances. The most distinctive lesions are those of *urticaria pigmentosa,* in which mast cell infiltrations of the dermis tend to give rise to bullous lesions in infants, nodules in children, and maculopapules in adults. These pigmented lesions are almost always pruritic, and scratching or stroking them causes an erythematous, flare reaction known as Darrier's sign, presumably caused by the release of histamine (384).

The disease may be limited to the skin or may involve most of the tissues of the body, and gives rise in bone to osteosclerotic or osteolytic lesions. Splenomegaly is common. Mast cell leukemia has been reported (386).

The hepatic manifestations are usually minimal, although hepatomegaly is often present. Liver function is usually normal, although serum alkaline phosphatase levels are almost always elevated (387). Jaundice is rare. Portal hypertension is uncommon, but esophageal varices may occur and bleed (388,389). The portal hypertension is sinusoidal in type and is often associated with mast cell infiltration of the sinusoids. Gastrointestinal bleeding may be associated with prolonged prothrombin time secondary to heparin secretion or with thrombocytopenia. Intractable ascites may develop (390).

Histologically, the primary hepatic lesions are in the portal tracts, which are enlarged. Fibrosis may link adjacent triads. Frank cirrhosis is rare, however. Ductular proliferation may be present. The presence of mast cells varies from none to many, interspersed with lymphocytes, monocytes, eosinophils, and occasional macrophages (389). The sinusoids, too, may be infiltrated with mast cells, but the degree of infiltration ranges from none to intense. Occasionally, focal masses of mast cells may replace hepatocytes.

The mast cells are relatively large, ranging from 10 to 25 μm in diameter. They are usually round, but are sometimes stellate or spindle-shaped. The nuclei are ovoid with fine, granular chromatin. The cytoplasm contains distinctive eosinophilic granules that stain purple or reddish blue with toluidine blue (Figs. 695, 696).

Of the three documented cases of systemic mastocytosis with urticaria pigmentosa in our series, only one exhibited a small number of mast cells in the portal tracts and sinusoids (Fig. 694).

Pregnancy

Hepatic disorders in pregnancy fall into four groups (391). First are the hepatic abnormalities that represent physiologic adaptations by the liver to pregnancy. Second is the group of preexisting hepatic disorders that persist into the pregnancy. Patients with chronic liver disease tend to be infertile, so that this situation is relatively uncommon (392). Hepatic adenoma, often a consequence of oral contraceptives, occasionally presents after the pregnancy has begun and poses the danger of hepatic rupture (393). Third are those liver diseases that develop during pregnancy, but are unrelated to pregnancy. Fourth are those hepatic disorders that are unique to the pregnant state. These latter diseases will be discussed in detail.

Normal pregnancy

Normal pregnancy is accompanied by a number of physiologic changes that can be interpreted as hepatic abnormalities when assessed by conventional criteria. These abnormalities occur most frequently and to the greatest degree during the third trimester. Clinically, the most impressive of these is the appearance of spider angiomas and palmar erythema, which are present in one-half to two-thirds of pregnant women (394). The liver and spleen may be palpable during pregnancy, but abdominal distension limits precise palpation. The fact that these organs are often palpable immediately after delivery, however, indicates that they had been enlarged during the pregnancy as well (395). Physiologic adaptations such as increments in blood volume and cardiac output in response to increased aldosterone secretion also occur. Hepatic blood flow, however, does not increase (396). Surprisingly, there is a decrease in hemoglobin and hematocrit concentration despite the presumed need for greater oxygen delivery. There is also an increase in the white blood cell and polymorphonuclear leukocyte counts. BSP retention increases accompanied by an increase in hepatic BSP storage capacity (395). Serum alkaline phosphatase activity rises, due largely to an increase in placental alkaline phosphatase, and is unaccompanied by an increase in either 5'-nucleotidase or gamma-glutamyl transpeptidase (394). Serum albumin and total protein concentrations decrease, while coagulation proteins such as prothrombin, fibrinogen, and other hepatic coagulation factors and the sedimentation rate increase. The serum bilirubin concentration is occasionally elevated without explanation. These physiologic changes of pregnancy may affect clinical and laboratory responses to various coincidental diseases and their interpretation. Although these effects may complicate diagnosis, it is not difficult to differentiate between intercurrent liver diseases in pregnant women from those hepatic disorders that are unique to pregnancy.

The hepatic histology is usually normal, although nonspecific abnormalities may be present (397). There may be some minor variations in the size and shape of hepatocytes, a slight increase in the number of binucleate cells, and mild proliferation of ductular epithelium (398). Kupffer cells often appear to be increased in number and size and contain increased numbers of diastase-resistant, PAS-positive lipofuscin granules. Subcellular alterations of bile canaliculi have been reported (399).

Hyperemesis gravidarum

The single most common symptom of pregnancy is vomiting. It usually occurs during the first trimester and subsides spontaneously. In a small number of patients, vomiting may become severe or persistent enough to warrant the term hyperemesis gravidarum. These symptoms almost always stop by the second trimester, but, rarely, they persist into or develop during the third trimester.

The vomiting does not intrinsically affect the liver except when the hyperemesis is severe enough to induce dehydration or prolonged enough to cause weight loss and malnutrition. In these circumstances, some patients develop mild jaundice in which both the conjugated and unconjugated fractions of bilirubin are increased. Rarely, in the pernicious vomiting of late pregnancy, overt jaundice may occur (400). Modest elevations of SGOT may be present, but rarely exceed twice the upper limit of normal (401). Serum alkaline phosphatase activity is normal or minimally increased.

Histologically, the liver is normal, except when the vomiting has been persistent and fatty deposition associated with malnutrition develops. Cholestasis is present in patients with jaundice (402).

When jaundice develops, the differential diagnosis of viral hepatitis from drug-induced hepatitis, sometimes caused by medications given to suppress the vomiting, is important. Almost always the biochemical abnormalities in hyperemesis gravidarum are so mild that the differentiation is easy. Severe vomiting in late pregnancy is often associated with complicating urinary tract infection or toxemia of pregnancy.

Toxemia of pregnancy

Toxemia of pregnancy is defined as the occurrence of preeclampsia or eclampsia. The diagnosis of *preeclampsia* is based on the presence of hypertension, proteinuria, and edema. In *eclampsia* convulsions are superimposed on the findings of preeclampsia (403). These variable syndromes, which occur largely in the third trimester of pregnancy, are characterized by leukocytosis, anemia, which is often hemolytic, and, occasionally, by disseminated intravascular coagulation (404). They do not involve the liver primarily, but the liver may be enlarged, and, rarely, ascites is present. In most reported cases the hepatic abnormalities are minimal and jaundice is either absent or mild. About 2% of the instances of jaundice in pregnancy can be attributed to toxemia (405). Rarely, deep jaundice may develop (406).

Several reports, however, have described focal hepatic necrosis in 15 to 20% of cases of eclampsia (405,407). Such cases are characterized by increased SGOT and lactic dehydrogenase activity. Histologically, these necrotic lesions are usually hemorrhagic and predominantly periportal (Fig. 802). They may result in areas of hepatic infarction (Fig. 803), which when under the capsule may be the lesions that lead to spontaneous rupture of the liver, as occurred in the patient whose histology is shown, (Figs. 802, 803). Sometimes, diffuse sinusoidal dilatation (Fig. 804) and peliosis may develop. The occurrence of thrombocytopenia and increased SGOT activity often precede overt complications of pregnancy (408). Investigations have shown that disseminated intravascular coagulation and fibrinogen deposition in the portal veins and adjacent hepatic sinusoids are common (406,409) in toxemia and even in asymptomatic pregnancy (410).

Spontaneous rupture of the liver is a rare but catastrophic event (411). It usually occurs in patients with toxemia (412). Indeed, the rupture is intimately associated with disseminated intravascular coagulation, which may result in fibrin thrombi in the sinusoids and hepatic arterioles (409). It is often preceded by intrahepatic bleeding or infarction (413,414), which, in turn, may cause necrosis.

Our experience in three cases of preeclampsia confirms the presence of moderately severe hepatocellular injury and cholestasis that mimics viral hepatitis or acute fatty liver of pregnancy. There was no history of drug ingestion or serologic evidence of viral hepatitis. Two of the three showed evidence of disseminated intravascular coagulation. In several patients who showed clinical evidence of severe hepatic injury, foci of hepatocellular necrosis were scattered throughout the lobules. Large, amorphous deposits of fibrinogen, IgG, IgM, and complement, usually in the glomeruli, are demonstrable by immunofluorescent techniques in such patients (409).

All three of our patients delivered live infants, two by cesarean section, and all showed prompt subsidence of hepatic abnormalities after delivery. The biopsies showed moderate to severe hepatocellular injury and cholestasis. Hepatocytes in the central areas showed ballooning with occasional cell dropout (Fig. 805) and scattered eosinophilic bodies (Figs 805, 806). There was increased regenerative activity as shown by thick hepatic plates, rosettes, and pseudoduct formation (Fig. 807). Canalicular bile thrombi were seen throughout the lobules (Fig. 807). The Kupffer cells were swollen and proliferated, and some contained bile droplets. The portal tracts were enlarged and infiltrated with lymphocytes, monocytes, and neutrophils (Fig. 807). Ductular proliferation was evident. In one patient, dilated bile-filled, degenerating, interlobular bile ducts were seen.

In severe, fatal eclampsia the liver frequently exhibits foci of periportal hepatocellular necrosis, hemorrhage, and fibrin deposition. Such lesions in one of our own cases are illustrated in Figures 219 and 220.

The constellation of hemolysis (H), elevated liver enzymes (EL), and low platelets (LP) in preeclampsia are the components of the HELLP syndrome (415,416). It is a rare disorder, with an unusual name, which is associated with a high perinatal infant mortality (about 10%) and a high maternal mortality (3–4%).

Acute fatty liver of pregnancy (obstetric acute yellow atrophy)

Acute fatty liver of pregnancy, a relatively rare form of hepatic injury, is encountered during the last month or two of pregnancy. It usually affects primiparous patients, but may occur after one normal pregnancy and, very rarely, after more. It is manifested clinically by the sudden onset of severe vomiting, often with coffee ground emesis, and epigastric or right upper quadrant pain (417–419). Jaundice develops within a week. Fever is uncommon. Premature labor is precipitated and usually terminates in stillbirth. Stupor, hepatic coma, and death occur in the large majority of cases within one or two weeks of the onset of symptoms. Sometimes the fulminant hepatic failure is irreversible despite delivery of the fetus, and liver transplantation is life saving (420). Other inconstant features include preeclampsia (419,421,422), renal failure, hypoglycemia, pancreatitis, disseminated intravascular coagulation (423), rupture of the liver (411), and, rarely, fever of unknown origin. The diagnosis may be suggested by ultrasonography that shows diffuse increased echogenicity (424).

A recent report of recurrent fatty liver of pregnancy, which was successfully terminated by prompt delivery in two consecutive pregnancies, promises to shed some light on the pathogenesis of this syndrome (425). Both infants subsequently developed widespread microvesicular fatty deposition and died within six months. A poorly defined defect in fatty acid oxidation was demonstrated.

In a review of nine consecutive patients seen at this hospital with acute fatty liver of pregnancy, a much less lethal syndrome was noted (426). At least half of these patients exhibited preeclampsia as well as most of the usual features of the acute fatty liver syndrome. They were also atypical in that none of them died. The author suggested that the spectrum of the acute fatty liver of pregnancy, the diagnosis of which requires histologic confirmation, is broader clinically and histologically and is less severe than had previously been thought (419).

Identical clinical, laboratory, and histologic lesions may be produced by large doses of tetracycline, especially in pregnant women with urinary tract infections (427). The pathogenesis of acute fatty liver of pregnancy is unknown, but the similarity to tetracycline-induced lesions suggests the presence of an endogenous toxin related to pregnancy.

The characteristic hepatic lesion of acute fatty liver of pregnancy is panlobular, microvesicular fatty infiltration of the hepatocytes that usually spares a rim of periportal cells (423–429). The droplets are minute and surround centrally located nuclei, giving the cytoplasm a foamy appearance ([(430); Figs. 115, 808]. They stain with oil red O (Fig. 116) and other fat stains. Mild fatty deposition may be seen in the fetal livers of patients with acute fatty liver of pregnancy (431). In addition, other histologic abnormalities that include canalicular bile stasis (Fig. 808), swollen Kupffer cells that contain lipofuscin, portal and intralobular lymphocytic infiltration, and ductular proliferation are occasionally present. Hepatocellular necrosis has not been thought to be a significant component of the histologic picture, although hepatocellular regeneration and scattered foci of collapsed reticulin imply that hepatocytes have been lost, as does the low liver weight, which is found in many patients. The patients with atypical acute fatty liver of pregnancy reported from this hospital (426) showed less severe fatty infiltration than usual, deposition of fibrinogen in the sinusoids and the occurrence of hepatocellular necrosis, cell dropout, and acidophilic bodies. It is probable that these cases represent variations of the syndrome. The possibility of simultaneous viral or nonviral hepatitis cannot be excluded.

Recurrent intrahepatic cholestasis of pregnancy and pruritus gravidarum

Recurrent intrahepatic cholestasis of pregnancy, which is a form of recurrent cholestasis or pruritus that usually appears in late pregnancy, has been discussed in detail in Chapter 19. This disorder, which subsides promptly after delivery, recurs in subsequent pregnancies. The patients show increased susceptibility to the development of intrahepatic cholestasis when taking oral contraceptives. The syndrome appears to be related to benign recurrent intrahepatic cholestasis which occurs in nonpregnant patients; it is associated with increased maternal and fetal morbidity and mortality. Randomized clinical trials show that S-adenosyl-L-methionine can decrease pruritus and improve abnormal liver function tests (432) and can improve fetal prognosis (433).

Budd-Chiari syndrome

Rarely, the Budd-Chiari syndrome develops early in the postpartum period (434,435), and even more rarely, during the third trimester of pregnancy (436). The postpartum syndrome is characterized by ascites, which may be manifest by persistent postpartum distension of the abdomen, or by the appearance of ascites a few days to weeks after delivery. When it occurs during pregnancy, it presents as an abnormally distended abdomen, which suggests the possibility of excessive amniotic fluid formation or twins. However, angiography (437), ultrasonography (438), and computerized tomography (439) may each show features that are characteristic of the Budd-Chiari syndrome.

The pathogenesis of the syndrome is uncertain. It has been attributed to the compression of the inferior vena cava by the enlarging uterus (440) and to the hypercoagulability of blood that occurs during and after pregnancy (441). The occurrence of the same syndrome in women taking oral contraceptives (442) suggests the possibility that a hormonal factor may be operative, but no firm evidence to support this hypothesis has been presented.

Histologically, the pattern is one of severe congestion of the central veins and pericentral zones with atrophy of hepatic plates and hepatocyte dropout (443). When the syndrome is chronic, a "cardiac" cirrhosis may develop.

Spontaneous rupture of the liver

Spontaneous rupture of the liver, a rare complication of pregnancy, may occur during the third trimester or in the early puerperal period. It usually affects multiparous women over the age of 30, especially those who have exhibited preeclampsia or eclampsia (408,412,444) or the fatty liver of pregnancy (411). The diagnosis can be made by ultrasonic or computerized tomographic imaging (445).

The pathogenesis of spontaneous rupture is uncertain, but it has been attributed to disseminated intravascular coagulation in the liver that results in fibrin thrombi in the sinusoids and arterioles (409,412). Hormonal effects have been postulated to play a role in this syndrome, because spontaneous rupture of the liver has occasionally been observed in patients on oral contraceptives. Violent vomiting, convulsions, and the hypertension of toxemia of pregnancy are contributory factors.

The hepatic lesions are not specific. There may be no abnormalities and no evidence of fibrin deposition in sinusoids or arterie. When arteries have been obstructed, hematoma, focal necrosis or even infarction may be present (413,414). The hepatic lesions may show extensive, periportal, hemorrhagic necrosis, hepatic infarction, and subcapsular peliosis (407). Occasionally, hepatic adenomas may rupture (446).

Hepatic tumors

Hepatic cell adenoma, hepatocellular carcinoma, and cholangiocarcinoma have all been encountered during pregnancy. They may be related to the hormonal effects of pregnancy, since similar tumors have been reported in women on oral contraceptives contraceptive drugs, but proof of an etiologic relationship is lacking (see Chapter 25).

Viral hepatitis in pregnancy

A series of retrospective studies of viral hepatitis in pregnancy from Western countries have failed to find any effect of the pregnancy on viral hepatitis or of viral hepatitis on pregnancy (447–449). These studies show no apparent increase in the severity of the hepatitis nor in the prevalence of fulminant hepatic failure, nor do they demonstrate an increase in abortions, premature delivery, or fetal or maternal deaths. These investigations were all retrospective evaluations of hospitalized patients.

A series of retrospective studies of viral hepatitis in pregnancy in hospitalized patients in the Middle East, Africa, and India, however, showed that pregnancy appears to have increased the severity of viral hepatitis, but that the viral hepatitis did not appear to affect adversely the pregnancy or the fetus (450,451). The increased prevalence of viral hepatitis in pregnancy was postulated to be related to malnutrition (451). A large, prospective epidemiologic investigation of an epidemic of non-A, non-B viral hepatitis (452) reported an enormous increase in the prevalence of hepatitis in pregnancy and a large increase in the prevalence of fulminant viral hepatitis among pregnant women who had been exposed (453). The prevalence of hepatitis was greater in pregnant women than in men or in nonpregnant women, was higher in the second trimester than in the first, and was highest in patients in the third trimester at the time of exposure. Fulminant viral hepatitis occurred more frequently in pregnant women (22%) than in men (3%) or in nonpregnant women (0%), and the mortality rate for the patients

and their fetuses was greatly increased in those patients with fulminant hepatitis. Except for maternal and fetal deaths, the presence of hepatitis did not appear to increase the rate of abortions or stillbirths. Nonfulminant viral hepatitis did not affect the pregnancy adversely. The patients in this investigation were well nourished, and the higher prevalence of hepatitis cannot, therefore, be attributed to malnutrition. On the other hand, this epidemic was caused by a non-A, non-B virus, presumably HCV, to which pregnant mothers and their fetuses are especially susceptible (453a). These observations may not be applicable to A, B, D, or other non-A, non-B hepatitis viruses.

The vertical transmission of viral hepatitis from mother to infant is known to occur with HBV, but not with HAV or NANB. Mothers who have acute or chronic HBV hepatitis and are HBsAg-positive during the third trimester, or who are healthy carriers of HBV may transmit the infection to their infants. In Taiwan, where almost 20% of the population are asymptomatic carriers of HBsAg (454), approximately 40% of the infants born of HBsAg-positive mothers are infected with HBV (455). Transmission correlates closely with the presence of high titers of HBsAg and of HBeAg in the mother (456).

The mode of transmission is uncertain. It may occur via transplacental infection as suggested by the rare birth of infants with acute HBsAg-positive hepatitis and by the occasional finding of HBsAg-positive cord blood. The typical appearance in newborns of HBV infection two to three months after birth suggests that the virus may have been transmitted by contamination of the infant with the mother's blood during delivery, but, transplacental transmission at the beginning of the third trimester is equally compatible with the long incubation period of HBV (457). The incidence of HBV infection in babies born of HBsAg-positive mothers is the same for vaginal and cesarean deliveries (458).

Histologically, the acute HBV hepatitis seen in pregnant women is identical to that seen in nonpregnant patients. Similarly, the hepatitis seen in infants born of HBV carriers in not differentiable from the infantile hepatitis transmitted in other ways.

Effect of pregnancy on antecedent chronic liver disease

The association of pregnancy and cirrhosis is uncommon because fertility is significantly reduced in patients with chronic liver disease (392,459). Furthermore, cirrhosis is usually a disease of middle age, and many women with cirrhosis have already passed through menopause.

When cirrhotic women become pregnant, however, the pregnancy is usually well tolerated. There are exceptions, however. In primary biliary cirrhosis, the pruritus and jaundice may first appear during pregnancy, or preexisting jaundice may worsen, although the course of the disease is not otherwise affected (459). Jaundice of other etiologies may deepen during pregnancy. Chronic active hepatitis often worsens, but occasionally it may improve during pregnancy. Hemorrhage from varices is a well-recognized complication of pregnancy in patients with portal hypertension (459,460), especially in those with extrahepatic portal obstruction (459,461), granulomatous disease, or malignancy. Patients with cirrhosis and portacaval shunt have carried normal pregnancy to term without adverse effects.

The histologic picture of each of the chronic liver diseases is indistinguishable from that seen in nonpregnant patients.

Ectopic pregnancy of the liver

Extremely rarely, fertilized ova may become implanted on the surface of the liver, giving rise to "primary hepatic pregnancy." Such ectopic pregnancies, which require the development of extensive vascular systems (462,463), may go to term (464).

Such pregnancies may result in peritoneal hemorrhage (465). As the pregnancy progresses, a mass in the liver may be felt (466). Other changes unique to normal pregnancy may develop. Histologically, there are no specific abnormalities of the liver.

Miscellaneous disorders

Fever of unknown origin

Daily pyrexia with elevations in temperature in excess of 101°F for at least three weeks that persists for more than one week in the hospital has been defined as fever of unknown origin (467,468). In our experience, needle biopsy of the liver has proved to be of great diagnostic value in such cases even in the absence of hepatomegaly and hepatic dysfunction. The diagnosis was established by biopsy in 10 to 20% of cases, especially in those with tuberculosis, sarcoidosis, lymphoma, metastatic carcinoma, or alcoholic hepatitis. Often, liver biopsy is useful in excluding specific disorders under consideration such as tuberculosis or sarcoidosis. Granulomatous hepatitis of unknown etiology has been shown to be a surprisingly common cause of fever of unknown origin (469). Others have found liver biopsy to be less useful (470).

Chronic hemodialysis

Since its inception, chronic dialysis has been associated with an increased incidence of viral hepatitis. Serum transaminase activity is elevated at some time in approximately half the patients on chronic dialysis. Of these, only half show serologic evidence of infection with the HBV, and 5% to 15% are persistently HBsAg-positive. The great majority of those patients who develop HBsAg-positive hepatitis become chronic carriers (471,472). A few may show signs and symptoms of acute hepatitis. Fulminant hepatitis is rare. In addition, from 3 to 10% of dialysis technicians, nurses, and physicians develop evidence of HBV infection.

Dialysis patients, who act much like immunosuppressed patients, may develop hepatitis that is caused by viruses other than HBV or by medications. They include HCV and cytomegalovirus and hepatitis induced by a variety of therapeutic agents. As with HBV hepatitis it is usually asymptomatic, occasionally acute, and rarely fulminant. Histologically, the hepatitis is identical to that seen in nondialysis patients.

In renal hemodialysis, hydroxyethyl starch (HES) has been used as a plasma expander in the treatment of hypotension. Investigation of two patients who had multiple infusions of HES and who abruptly developed ascites showed massive accumulations of HES, predominantly in centrilobular hepatocytes; in sinusoidal cells, including Kupffer cells, Ito cells, and endothelial cells; and in bile duct epithelial and portal macrophages (473). Liver biopsy revealed intense, foamy transformation of sinusoidal lining cells and microvacuolization of the hepatocytes (Fig. 809). Similar foamy transformation of sinusoidal cells, of endothelial cells of the terminal hepatic veins (Fig. 810), and of portal macrophages has been shown (Fig. 811). The foamy material was PAS-positive, but was PAS-negative after diastase digestion. No hepatic necrosis was noted. HES accumulation in the liver has been observed previously (474), but the significance of this observation is not clear. It is not known whether the deposition of HES and the appearance of ascites are related. HES has been used as a plasma expander after large paracentesis, but no report of its deposition in that situation has been reported.

Psoriasis

About one-half of patients with psoriasis exhibit histologic abnormalities of the liver *before* they have ever received methotrexate or other therapy (475). These disorders are usually clinically silent. They cannot be correlated with the severity or duration of psoriasis. Chronic alcoholism, which appears to be more common in patients with psoriasis than in nonpsoriatic patients (476), and obesity may account for many of the lesions, but not for all. Possible hepatotoxic effects of absorbed coal tar used in conjunction with ultraviolet irradiation have been postulated, but as yet have not been investigated. Although still controversial, controlled comparisons appear to indicate that methotrexate does affect hepatic function adversely (477,478); some investigators find contrary evidence (479).

The hepatic lesions found include fatty infiltration, mild portal fibrosis, nonspecific focal hepatitis, and sarcoid-like granulomas. Granulomas were found in 11 of 98 consecutive cases of psoriasis biopsied in our Yale series [(480); Fig. 513]. They were present in similar percentages of patients who had or had not received methotrexate. Kveim tests, which are positive in about 70% to 80% of patients with sarcoidosis of short duration, were negative in the four of our five patients who were tested.

Weber-Christian disease (relapsing febrile nonsuppurative panniculitis)

Weber-Christian disease, a rare disorder, is characterized by recurrent bouts of fever and tender, subcutaneous nodules. These erythematous nodules, which appear in crops, are manifestations of focal acute or chronic inflammation of the subcutaneous adipose tissue. In most cases, the inflammatory reaction is more generalized and involves adipose tissue in viscera, especially the liver (481) and pancreas. Hepatomegaly is relatively common (482). The disease is occasionally fatal, usually secondary to an intercurrent infection. Chronic active hepatitis has been reported to develop in a child with preexisting Weber-

Christian disease (483). Whether these events were related is not clear.

The etiology of Weber-Christian disease is unknown. In some patients, the disease has been attributed to underlying pancreatic disease in which excess lipase has been liberated into the circulation. The hepatic lesions reported in individual cases reveal that fatty infiltration is the most common abnormality. The fat in the liver may show the same histologic signs of inflammation that are seen in the subcutaneous tissues (481). Focal hepatocellular necrosis, which is the next most frequent lesion, is chiefly found in the central or midzonal regions. Mallory bodies have been reported (484). Foamy macrophages may be found in the sinusoids. Portal fibrosis and mononuclear portal inflammation may occur. Cirrhosis is rare.

Reye's syndrome

Reye's syndrome (485) is a systemic disorder in which the liver is the primary organ injured. However, it does not fit neatly into any conventional classification of liver disease. It is characterized by acute encephalopathy and microvesicular fatty infiltration of the liver and other viscera (486). It is seen almost exclusively in children who live in the temperate zones, and tends to follow viral infections, especially those caused by the influenza B or varicella viruses. Hepatomegaly is almost always present; jaundice is not. Biochemically, the most dramatic finding is a gross elevation of the blood ammonia concentration, which decreases independent of the clinical course (487). The disorder appears to represent an acquired deficiency of the rate-limiting enzymes of the urea cycle, carbamylphosphate synthetase, or ornithine transcarbamylase. Like the elevated blood ammonia level, the enzyme deficiency gradually disappears, independent of whether the patient improves or dies. Although the encephalopathy appears to represent ammonia toxicity, the rest of the syndrome—hypoglycemia, hepatic glycogen depletion, prolongation of prothrombin time, and increased SGOT and creatine phosphokinase activity—are of uncertain origin. The disease has been postulated to be a postinfectious inhibition of the key urea cycle enzymes caused by selective injury to the hepatic mitochondria (488), where the two deficient urea cycle enzymes are located. This hypothesis is supported by studies in experimental animals (489). The role of aspirin in the pathogenesis of the syndrome remains unclear (490).

The hepatic histology is characterized by intense microvesicular fat deposition (Figs. 117, 118), the degree of which is inversely related to the amount of glycogen in the hepatocytes (489a). Intense microvesicular fatty deposition (Fig. 811A) and virtually total depletion of glycogen (Fig. 811B) from patients with Reye's syndrome are shown. Electron microscopy shows abnormal hepatic mitochondria, which supports the postulated pathogenesis of selective mitochondrial injury (488).

References

1. Rokitansky C: Handbook der Pathologischen Anatomic, 3, edited by Braumuller and Seidel, Vienna, 1842, pp. 311–318.
2. Glenner GG: Medical progress: amyloid deposits and amyloidosis. The fibrilloses. N Engl J Med *302:*1283–1292 and 1333–1343, 1980.
3. Cohen AS, Skinner M; Amyloidosis of the liver. *In* Diseases of the Liver, edited by L. Schiff, E.R. Schiff. 6th Edition. Philadelphia, J.B. Lippincott, 1987, pp. 1093–1108.
4. Pepys MB, Baltz ML: Amyloidosis. *In* Copeman's Textbook of the Rheumatoid Disease, edited by J.T. Scott. 6th Edition. Edinburgh, Churchill Livingstone, 1984.
5. DeBeer FC, Mallya RK, Fagan EA: Serum amyloid-A protein concentration in inflammatory diseases and its relationship to the incidence of reactive systemic amyloidosis. Lancet *2:*231–234, 1982.
6. Kluve-Beckerman B, Dwulet FE, Benson MD: Human serum amyloid A. Three hepatic mRNAs and the corresponding proteins in one person. J Clin Invest *82:*1670–1675, 1988.
7. Skinner M, Sipe JD, Yood RA, Shirahama T, Cohen AS: Characterization of P-component (AP) isolated from amyloidotic tissue: half-life studies of human and murine AP. Ann NY Acad Sci *398:*190–196, 1982.
8. Hawkins PN, Lavender JP, Pepys MB: Evaluation of systemic amyloidosis by scintigraphy with ^{123}I-labeled serum amyloid P component. N Engl J Med *323:*508–513, 1990.
9. Levine RA: Amyloid disease of the liver: correlation of clinical, functional and morphologic features in forty-seven patients. Am J Med *33:*349–357, 1962.
10. Osserman EF: Plasma-cell myeloma. II. Clinical aspects. N Engl J Med *261:*1006–1014, 1959.
11. White GC II, Jacobson RJ, Binder RA, Linke RP, Glenner GG: Immunoglobulin D myeloma and amyloidosis: immunochemical and structural studies of Bence Jones and amyloid fibrillar proteins. Blood *46:*713–722, 1975.
12. Axelsson U, Bachmann R, Hallen J: Frequency of pathological proteins (M components) in 6,995 sera from adult population. Acta Med Scand *179:*235–247, 1966.
13. Glenner GG, Terry W, Harada M, Isersky C, Page D: Amyloid fribril proteins: proof of homology with immunoglobulin light chains by sequence analyses. Science *172:*1150–1151, 1971.
14. Ranlov P, Elling Nielsen P: Systemic (primary) amyloidosis associated with IgM (2M) paraproteinemia: biochemical, histochemical and immunohistochemical investigations. Acta Pathol Microbiol Scan *66:*154–168, 1966.
15. Franklin ED, Rosenthal CJ, Pras M, et al: Recent progress in amyloid. *In* The Role of Immunological Factors in Infectious Allergic, and Autoimmune Processes, edited by R.F. Beers Jr., E.G. Basset. New York, Raven Press, 1976, pp. 163–181.
16. Pruzanski W, Hasselback R, Katz A, Parr DM. Multiple myeloma (light chain disease) with rheumatoid-like amyloid arthropathy and u-heavy chain fragment in the serum. Am J Med *65:*334–341, 1978.
17. Conn HO, Quintiliani R: Case studies: severe diarrhea controlled by gamma globulin in a patient with agammaglobulinemia, amyloidosis and thymoma. Ann Intern Med *65:*528–541, 1966.
18. Pick AI, Versano I, Shribman S, Ben-Bassat M, Shoenfeld Y: Gamma globulinemia, plasma cell dyscrasia, and amyloidosis in a 12-year-old child. Am J Dis Child *131:*682–686, 1977.
19. Knowles DM II, Shevchuk M: Pleomorphic reticulum cell sarcoma, monoclonal gammopathy and amyloidosis: an immunoperoxidase study. Cancer *41:*1883–1889, 1978.
20. Wiltshaw E: The natural history of extramedullary plasmacytoma and its relation to solitary myeloma of bone and myelomatosis. Medicine *55:*217–238, 1976.
21. Page DL, Isersky C, Harada M, Glenner GG: Immunoglobulin origin of localized nodular pulmonary amyloidosis. Res Exp Med *159:*75–86, 1972.
22. Tripathi VNP, Desautels RE: Primary amyloidosis if the urogenital system: a study of 16 cases and brief review. J Urol *102:*96–101, 1969.
23. O'Connor CR, Rubinow A, Cohen AS: Primary (AL) amyloidosis as a cause of breast masses. Am J Med *77:*981–986, 1984.
24. Wald MH: Clinical studies of secondary amyloidosis in tuberculosis. Ann Intern Med *43:*383–395, 1955.
25. Shuttleworth JS, Ross H: Secondary amyloidosis in leprosy. Ann Intern Med *45:*23–38, 1956.
26. Masterson G: Cardiovascular syphilis with amyloidosis and periods of alternating heart block. Br J Ven Dis *41:*181–185, 1965.
27. Dalton JJ Jr, Hackler RH, Bunts RC: Amyloidosis in paraplegia: incidence and significance. J Urol *93:*553–555, 1965.
28. Calkins E, Cohen AS: Diagnosis of amyloidosis. Bull Rheum Dis *10:*215–218, 1960.
29. Sletten K, Husby G: The complete amino-acid sequence of non-immunoglobulin amyloid fibril protein AS in rheumatoid arthritis. Eur J Biochem *41:*117–125, 1974.
30. Moschcowitz E: Clinical aspects of amyloidosis. Ann Intern Med *10:*73–88, 1936.

31. Werther JL, Shapira A. Rubenstein O, Janowitz HD: Amyloidosis in regional enteritis. Am J Med 29:416–423, 1960.
32. Gelderman AH, Levine RA, Arndt KA: Dermatomyositis complicated by generalized amyloidosis. N Engl J Med 267:858–861, 1962.
33. Gardner DL: Pathology of the Connective Tissue Diseases. Baltimore, Williams & Wilkins, 1966.
34. Symmers W St C: Amyloidosis: 5 cases of primary generalized amyloidosis and some other unusual cases. Clin Pathol 9:212–228, 1956.
35. Levin M, Franklin EC, Frangione B, Pras M: The amino acid sequence of a major nonimmunoglobulin component of some amyloid fibrils. J Clin Invest 51:2773–2776, 1972.
36. Fievet P, Sevestre H, Boudjelal M, Noel LH, Kemeny F, Franco D, Delamarre J, Capron JP: Systemic AA amyloidosis induced by liver cell adenoma. Gut 31:361–363, 1990.
37. Albores-Saavedra J, Amyloid in solid carcinoma of thyroid gland: staining characteristics, tissue culture, and electron microscopic observations. Lab Invest 13:77–93, 1964.
38. Peterson WC Jr, Hult A-M: Calcifying epithelioma of Malherbe. Arch Dermatol 90:404–410, 1964.
39. Heller H, Sohar E, Sherf L: Familial Mediterranean fever. Arch Intern Med 102:50–71, 1958.
40. Benson MD, Wallace MR: Amyloidosis. In The Metabolic Basis of Inherited Disease II, edited by C.R. Scriver, A.L. Beaudet, W.S. Sly, D. Valle. New York, McGraw-Hill Inf Svc, 1989, pp. 2439–2460.
41. Andrade C: Peculiar form of peripheral neuropathy: familiar atypical generalized amyloidosis with special involvement of peripheral nerves. Brain 75:408–427, 1952.
42. Horta J da S, Filipe I, Durante S: Portuguese polyneuritic familial type of amyloidosis. Pathol Microbiol 27:809–825, 1964.
43. Costa PP, Figueira AS, Bravo FR: Amyloid fibril protein related to prealbumin in familial amyloidotic polyneuropathy. Proc Natl Acad Sci USA 75:4499–4503, 1978.
44. Rukavina JG, Block WD, Jackson CE, Falls HF, Carey JH, Curtis AC: Primary systemic amyloidosis: review and experimental, genetic and clinical study of 29 cases with particular emphasis on familial form. Medicine 35:239–334, 1956.
45. Kantarjian AD, DeJong RN: Familial primary amyloidosis with nervous system involvement. Neurology 3:399–409, 1953.
46. Frederiksen T, Gotzsche H, Harboe N, Kiaer W, Melemgaard K: Familial primary amyloidosis with severe amyloid heart disease. Am J Med 33:328–348, 1962.
47. Sagher F, Shanon J: Amyloidosis cutis: familial occurrence in three generations. Arch Dermatol 87:171–175, 1963.
48. Muckle TJ, Wells M: Urticaria, deafness, and amyloidosis: new heredo-familial syndrome. Q J Med 31:235–248, 1962.
49. Schimke RN, Hartmann WH: Familial amyloid-producing medullary thyroid carcinoma and pheochromocytoma: distinct genetic entity. Ann Intern Med 63:1027–1039, 1965.
50. Pomerance A: Senile cardiac amyloidosis. Br Heart J 27:711–718, 1965.
51. Westermark P, Natvig JB, Johannson B: Characterization of an amyloid fibril protein from senile cardiac amyloid. J Exp Med 146:631–636, 1977.
52. Cornwell GG III, Natvig JB, Westermark P, Husby G: Senile cardiac amyloid: demonstration of a unique fibril protein in tissue sections. J Immunol 120:1385–1388, 1978.
53. Westermark P, Johannson B, Natvig JB: Senile cardiac amyloidosis: the existence of two different amyloid substances in the ageing heart. Scand J Immunol 10:303–308, 1979.
54. Haberland C: Primary systemic amyloidosis: cerebral involvement and senile plaque formation. J Neuropathol Exp Neurol 23:135–150, 1964.
55. Kidd M: Alzheimer's disease: electron microscopical study. Brain 87:307–320, 1964.
56. Westermark P, Grimelius L, Polak JM, Larsson LI, van Norden S, Wilander E, Pearse SG: Amyloid in polypeptide hormone producing tumors. Lab Invest 37:212–215, 1977.
57. Sletten K, Westermark P, Natvig JB: Characterization of amyloid fibril proteins from medullary carcinoma of the thyroid. J Exp Med 143:993–998, 1976.
58. Heller H, Missmahl HP, Sohar E: Amyloidosis: its differentiation into perireticulin and pericollagen types. J Pathol Bacteriol 88:15–26, 1964.
58a. Glenner GG, Fosserman E, Benditt EP, Calkins E, Cohen AS, Zucker-Franklin D. Amyloidosis. New York, Plenum Press, 1986.
58b. McAdam KPWJ. Amyloidosis. In Textbook of Clinical Hepatology,
     edited by N. McIntyre, J-P Benhamou, J. Bircher, M Rizzetto, J Rodes. New York: Oxford University Press, 1991, pp.779–787.
59. Gertz MA, Kyle RA: Primary systemic amyloidosis: a diagnostic primer. Mayo Clin Proc 64:1505–1519, 1989.
60. Friman C, Tornroth T, Wegelius O: IgD myeloma associated with multiple extramedullary amyloid-containing tumors and amyloid casts in the renal tubules. Ann Clin Res 2:161–166, 1970.
61. Dinarello CA: Interleukin-1 and the pathogenesis of the acute phase response. N Engl J Med 311:1413–1417, 1984.
62. Maury CPJ, Wegelius O: Pathogenesis of AA amyloidosis. Acta Med Scand 215:289–298, 1984.
63. Shirahama T, Skinner M, Cohen AS: Heterogeneous participation of the hepatocyte population in amyloid protein AA synthesis. Cell Biol Int Rep 8:849–856, 1984.
64. Shirahama T, Cohen AS: Immunocytochemical study of hepatocyte synthesis of amyloid AA. Demonstration of usual site of synthesis and intracellular pathways with unusual retention on the surface membrane. Am J Pathol 118:108–115, 1985.
65. Ladewig P: Double-refringence of the amyloid-Congo-red-complex in histological sections. Nature 156:81–82, 1945.
66. Klatskin G: Nonspecific green birefringence in Congo red-stained tissues. Am J Pathol 56: 1–13, 1969.
67. Saeed SM, Fine G: Thioflavin-T for amyloid detection. Am J Clin Pathol 47:588–593, 1967.
68. McKinney B, Grubb C: Non-specificity of thioflavin-T as an amyloid stain. Nature (London) 205:1023–1024, 1965.
69. Wolman M, Bubis JJ: The cause of the green polarization color of amyloid stained with Congo red. Histochemie 4:351–356, 1965.
70. Shirahama T, Skinner M, Cohen AS: Immunocytochemical identification of amyloid in formalin-fixed paraffin sections. Histochemistry 72:161–171, 1981.
71. Wright JR, Calkins W, Humphrey RL: Potassium permanganate reaction in amyloidosis: a histologic method to assist in differentiating forms of this disease. Lab Invest 36:274–279, 1977.
72. Cello JP, Grendell JH: The liver in systemic conditions. In Hepatology, A Textbook of Liver Disease, edited by D. Zakim, T.D. Boyer. 2nd Edition. Philadelphia, W.B. Saunders, 1990, pp. 1411–1415.
73. Dahlin DC: Secondary amyloidosis. Ann Intern Med 31:105–119, 1949.
74. Eisen HN: Primary systemic amyloidosis. Am J Med 1:144–160, 1946.
75. Dahlin DC: Primary amyloidosis, with report of 6 cases. Am J Pathol 25:105–113, 1949.
76. Mathews WH: Primary systemic amyloidosis. Am J Med Sci 228:317–333, 1954.
77. Chopra S, Rubinow A, Koff RS, Cohen AS: Hepatic amyloidosis: a histopathologic analysis of primary (AL) and secondary (AA) forms. Am J Pathol 115:186–193, 1984.
78. Gertz MA, Kyle RA, Greipp PR, Katzmann JA, O'Fallon WM: β₂-microglobulin predicts survival in primary systemic amyloidosis. Am J Med 89:609–614, 1990.
79. Pras M, Frangione B, Franklin EC, Gafni J: Idiopathic AL-(κ iv) amyloidosis presenting as giant hepatomegaly. Isr J Med Sci 18:866–869, 1982.
80. Itescu S: Hepatic amyloidosis. Arch Intern Med 144:2257–2259, 1984.
81. Totterman KJ, Manninen V: Tumefactive liver infiltration in amyloidosis. Ann Clin Res 14:11–14, 1982.
82. Finkelstein SD, Fornasier VL, Pruzanski W: Intrahepatic cholestasis with predominant pericentral deposition in systemic amyloidosis. Hum Pathol 12:470–472, 1981.
83. Cox R: Amyloidosis of the liver causing jaundice. Postgrad Med J 58:192–193, 1982.
84. Pirovino M, Altorfer J, Maranta E, Haemmerli UP, Schmid M: Ikterus von Typ der intrahepatischen Cholestase bei Amyloidose der Leber. Z Gastroenterol 6:321–331, 1982.
85. Melkebeke P, Vandepitte J, Hannon R: Hepatomegaly, jaundice and portal hypertension due to amyloidosis of the liver. Digestion 20:351–357, 1980.
86. Aramaki T, Terada H, Okumura H, Tsutsui H, Fujita S, Tajiri T, Ohya T, Tajima H: Portal hypertension secondary to intrahepatic arterio-portal shunt in primary amyloidosis: a case report. Gasterenterol Jpn 24:410–413, 1989.
87. Melato M, Manconi R, Magris D, Morassi P, Benussi DG, Tiribelli C: Different morphologic aspects and clinical features in massive hepatic amyloidosis. Digestion 29:138–145, 1984.
88. Konikoff F, Mor C, Stern S: Cholestasis and liver failure with lambda-AL amyloidosis. Gut 28:903–908, 1987.

89. Skander MP, Harry DS, Lee FI: Severe intrahepatic cholestasis and rapidly progressive renal failure in a patient with immunocyte-related amyloidosis. J Clin Gastroenterol 9:291–225, 1987.

90. Gange RW: Systemic amyloidosis. Proc R Soc Med 69:231–236, 1976.

91. Livni N, Behar AJ, Lafair JS: Unusual amyloid bodies in human liver. Isr J Med Sci 13:1163–1170, 1977.

92. French SW, Schloss GT, Stillman AE: Unusual amyloid bodies in human liver. Am J Clin Pathol 75:400–402, 1981.

93. Kanel GC, Uchida T, Peters RL: Globular hepatic amyloid: an unusual morphologic presentation. Hepatology 1:647–652, 1981.

94. Droz D, Noel LH, Carnot F, Degos F, Ganeval D, Grunfeld JP: Liver involvement in nonamyloid light chain deposits disease. Lab Invest 50:683–689, 1984.

95. Kirkpatrick CJ, Curry A, Galle J, Melzner I: Systemic kappa light chain deposition and amyloidosis in multiple myeloma: novel morphological observations. Histopathology 10:1065–1076, 1986.

96. Smith NM, Malcolm AJ: Simultaneous AL-type amyloid and light chain deposit disease in a liver biopsy: a case report. Histopathology 10:1057–1064, 1986.

97. Gafni J, Sohar E: Rectal biopsy for diagnosis of amyloidosis. Am J Med Sci 240:332–336, 1960.

98. Trieger N, Cohen AS, Calkins E: Gingival biopsy as a diagnostic aid in amyloid disease. Arch Oral Biol 1:187–192, 1959.

99. Westermark P, Stenkvist B, Natvig JB, Olding-Stenkvist E: Demonstration of protein AA in subcutaneous fat tissue obtained by fine needle biopsy. Ann Rheum Dis 38:68–71, 1979.

100. Volwiler W, Jones CM: The diagnostic and therapeutic value of liver biopsies; with special reference to trocar biopsy. N Engl J Med 237:651–656, 1947.

101. Stauffer MH, Gross JB, Foulk WT, Dahlin DC: Amyloidosis: diagnosis with needle biopsy of the liver in 18 patients. Gastroenterology 41:92–96, 1961.

102. Ades CJ, Strutton GM, Walker NI, Furnival CM, Whiting G: Spontaneous rupture of the liver associated with amyloidosis. J Clin Gastroenterol 11:85–87, 1989.

103. Yood RA, Skinner M, Rubinow A: Bleeding manifestations in 100 patients with amyloidosis. JAMA 249:1322–1326, 1983.

104. Conn HO: Liver biopsy: increased risks in patients with cancer. Hepatology 14:206–209, 1991.

105. Yood RA, Skinner M, Cohen AS, Lee VW: Soft tissue uptake of bone-seeking radionuclide in amyloidosis. J. Rheumatol 8:760–766, 1981.

106. Glenner GG: Amyloid deposits and amyloidosis. The β-fibrillosis (2nd part). N Engl J Med 302:1333–1343, 1980.

107. Johannessen JV, Gould VE, Jao W: The fine structure of human thyroid cancer. Hum Pathol 9:400–403, 1978.

108. Kyle RA, Greipp PR, Garton JP, Gertz MA: Primary systemic amyloidosis. Comparison of melphalan/prednisone versus colchicine. Am J Med 79:708–716, 1985.

109. Hart FD: Rheumatoid arthritis. Extra-articular manifestations. Br Med J 3:131–136, 1969.

110. Webb J, Whaley K, MacSween RNM, Nuki G, Dick WC, Buchanan WW: Liver disease in rheumatoid arthritis and Sjogren's syndrome. Prospective study using biochemical and serological markers of hepatic dysfunction. Ann Rheum Dis 34:70–81, 1975.

111. Weinblatt ME, Teser JRP, Gilliam JH III: The liver in rheumatic diseases. Semin Arthritis Rheum 11:399–410, 1982.

112. Thorne C, Urowitz MB, Wanless I, Roberts E, Blendis LM: Liver disease in Felty's syndrome. Am J Med 73:35–40, 1982.

113. Mills PR, Sturrock RD: Clinical associations between arthritis and liver disease. Ann Rheum Dis 41:295–307, 1982.

114. Pettersson T, Lepantalo M, Friman C, Ahonen J: Spontaneous rupture of the liver in rheumatoid arthritis. Scand J Rheumatol 15:348–349, 1986.

115. Siede WH, Seiffert UB, Merle S, Goll H-G, Oremek G: Alkaline phosphatase isoenzymes in rheumatic diseases. Clin Biochem 22:121–124, 1989.

116. Seaman WE, Ishak KG, Plotz PH: Aspirin-induced hepatotoxicity in patients with systemic lupus erythematosus. Ann Intern Med 80:1–8, 1974.

117. Kevat S, Ahern M, Hall P: Hepatotoxicity of methotrexate in rheumatic diseases. Med Toxicol Adverse Drug Exp 3:197–208, 1988.

118. Bridges SL Jr, Alarcon GS, Koopman WJ: Methotrexate-induced liver abnormalities in rheumatoid arthritis. J Rheumatol 16:1180–1183, 1989.

119. Kremer JM, Lee RG, Tolan KG: Liver histology in rheumatoid arthritis patients receiving long-term methotrexate therapy. A prospec-

tive study with baseline and sequential biopsy samples. Arthritis Rheum 32:121–127, 1989.

120. Watkins PB, Schade R, Mills AS, Carithers RL Jr, Van Thiel DH: Fatal hepatic necrosis associated with parenteral gold therapy. Dig Dis Sci 33:1025–1029, 1988.

121. Smith MD: Hepatitis and neutropenia secondary to gold thiomalate therapy for rheumatoid arthritis. Aust NZ J Med 16:72–74, 1986.

122. Farr M, Symmons DP, Bacon PA: Raised serum alkaline phosphatase and aspartate transaminase levels in two rheumatoid patients treated with sulphasalazine. Ann Rheum Dis 44:798–800, 1985.

123. Devogelaer JP, Huaux JP, Coche E, Rahier J, Nagant de Deuxchaisnes C: A case of cholestatic hepatitis associated with D-pennicillamine therapy for rheumatoid arthritis. Int J Clin Pharmacol Res 5:35–38, 1985.

124. Dietrichson O, From A, Christoffersen P, Juhl E: Morphological changes in liver biopsies from patients with rheumatoid arthritis. Scand J Rheumatol 5:65–69, 1976.

125. Laffon A, Moreno A, Gutierrez-Bucero A, Ossorio C, Sabando P, Moreno-Otero R: Hepatic sinusoidal dilatation in rheumatoid arthritis. J Clin Gastroenterol 11:653–657, 1989.

126. Smits JG, Kooijman CD: Rheumatoid nodules in liver. Histopathology 10:1211–1213, 1986.

127. Sullivan A, Hamilton EBD, Williams R: Rheumatoid arthritis and liver involvement. J R Coll Physicians 12:418–422, 1978.

128. Harris M, Rash RM, Dymock IW: Nodular, non-cirrhotic liver associated with portal hypertension in a patient with rheumatoid arthritis. J Clin Pathol 27:963–966, 1974.

129. Reynolds WJ, Wanless IR: Nodular regenerative hyperplasia of the liver in a patient with rheumatoid vasculitis: a morphometric study suggesting a role for hepatic arteritis in the pathogensis. J Rheumatol 2:838–842, 1984.

130. Jack AS, Boyce BF, Lee FD: Malignant histiocytosis complicating rheomatoid arthritis: report of four cases. J Clin Pathol 39:16–21, 1986.

131. Fitz JG, Petri M, Hellmann D: Chronic active hepatitis presenting with rheumatoid nodules and arthritis. J Rheumatol 14:595–598, 1987.

132. Tarlow M: Reye's syndrome and aspirin. Br Med J 292:1543–1544, 1986.

133. Remington PL, Shabino CL, McGee H, Preston G, Sarniak AP, Hall WN: Reye syndrome and juvenile rheumatoid arthritis in Michigan. Am J Dis Child 139:870–872, 1985.

134. Kornreich H, Malouf NN, Hanson V: Acute hepatic dysfunction in juvenile rheumatoid arthritis. J Pediatr 79:27–35, 1971.

135. Tesser JRP, Piski EJ, Hartz JW: Chronic liver disease and Still's disease. Arthritis Rheum 23:579–588, 1982.

136. Wouters JM, van Rijswijk MH, van de Putte LB: Adult onset Still's disease in the elderly: a report of two cases. J Rheumatol 12:791–793, 1985.

137. Miller MH, Urowitz MB, Gladman DD, Blendis LM: The liver in systemic lupus erythematosus. Q J Med 211:401–409, 1984.

138. Hansen JR, McCray PB, Bale JF Jr, Corbett AJ, Flanders DJ: Reye syndrome associated with aspirin therapy for systemic lupus erythematosus. Pediatrics 76:202–205, 1985.

139. Dubois EL, Tuffanelli DL: Clinical manifestations of systemic lupus erythematosus: computer analysis of 520 patients. JAMA 190:104–111, 1964.

140. Levitin PM, Sweet D, Brunner CM, Kathou RE, Bolton WK: Spontaneous rupture of the liver: an unusual complication of SLE. Arthritis Rheum 20:748–750, 1977.

141. Runyon BA, LaBrecque DR, Anuras S: The spectrum of liver disease in systemic lupus erythematosus. Report of 33 histologically proved cases and review of the literature. Am J Med 69: 187–193, 1980.

142. Lipsky PE, Hardin JA, Schour L: Spontaneous peritonitis and systemic lupus erythematosus: importance of accurate diagnosis of gram-positive bacterial infections. JAMA 232:929–931, 1975.

143. Pomeroy C, Knodell RG, Swaim WR: Budd-Chiari syndrome in a patient with the lupus anticoagulant. Gastroenterology 86:158–165, 1984.

144. Harvey AM, Schulman LE, Tumulty PA, Conley CL, Schoenrick EH: Systemic lupus erythematosus. Review of the literature and clinical analysis of 138 patients. Medicine 33:291–437, 1954.

145. MacKay IR, Taft L, Cowling DC: Lupoid hepatitis and the hepatic lesions of systemic lupus erythematosus. Lancet 1:65–69, 1969.

146. Iliffe GD, Naidoo S, Hunter T: Primary biliary cirrhosis with features of systemic lupus erythematosus. Dig Dis Sci 27:274–278, 1982.

147. Feurle GE, Broker HJ, Ischahargane C: Granulomatous hepatitis in

systemic lupus erythematosus. Report of a case. Endoscopy *14:*153–154, 1982.

148. Kuramochi S, Tashiro Y, Torikata C, Watanabe Y: Systemic lupus erythematosus associated with multiple nodular hyperplasia of the liver. Acta Pathol Jpn *32:*547–560, 1982.

149. Shusterman N, Loindon WT: Hepatitis B and immune complex disease. N Engl Med *310:*43–46, 1984.

150. McMahon BJ, Heyward WL, Templin DW, Clement D, Lanier AP: Hepatitis B-associated polyarteritis nodosa in Alaskan eskimos: clinical and epidemiologic features and long-term follow-up. Hepatology *9:*97–101, 1989.

151. Bonafede RP, van Staden M, Klemp P: Hepatitis B virus infection and liver function in patients with systemic lupus erythematosus. J Rheumatol *13:*1050–1052, 1986.

152. Lai KN, Lai FM, Lo S, Leung A: Is there a pathogenetic role of hepatitis B virus in lupus nephritis? Arch Pathol Lab Med *111:*185–188, 1987.

153. Gurian LE, Rogoff TM, Ware AJ, Jordan RE, Combes B, Gilliam JN: The immunologic diagnosis of chronic active "autoimmune" hepatitis: distinction from systemic lupus erythematosus. Hepatology *5:*397–402, 1985.

154. D'Angelo WA, Fries JF, Masi AT, Shulman LE: Pathologic observations in systemic sclerosis (scleroderma). A study of fifty-eight autopsy cases and fifty-eight matched controls. Am J Med *46:*428–440, 1969.

155. Murray-Lyon IM, Thompson RPH, Ansell ID, Williams R: Scleroderma and primary biliary cirrhosis. Br Med J *3:*258–261, 1970.

156. Powell FC, Schroeter AL, Dickson ER: Primary biliary cirrhosis and the CREST syndrome: a report of 22 cases. Q J Med *62:*75–82, 1987.

157. Epstein O: Primary biliary cirrhosis and the CREST syndrome: new terminology? Hepatology *8:*189–190, 1988.

158. Alderuccio F, Toh BH, Barnett AJ, Pedersen JS: Identification and characterization of mitochondria autoantigens in progressive systemic sclerosis: identity with the 72,000 dalton autoantigen in primary biliary cirrhosis. J Immunol *137:*1855–1859, 1986.

159. Miyagawa S, Yoshioka A, Hatoko M, Okuchi T, Sakamoto K: Systemic sclerosis-like lesions during long-term penicillamine therapy for Wilson's disease. Br J Dermatol *116:*95–100, 1987.

160. Dickson ER, Maldonado JE, Sheps SG: Systemic giant-cell arteritis with polymyalgia rheumatica. Reversible abnormalities of liver function. JAMA *224:*1496–1498, 1973.

161. Ogilvie AL, James PD, Toghill PJ: Hepatic artery involvement in polymyalgia arteritica. J Clin Pathol *34:*769–776, 1981.

162. Jones J, Kyle MV, Hazelman BL, Wraight P: Abnormal radionuclide liver scans in giant cell arteritis. Ann Rheum Dis *43:*583–585, 1984.

163. Glick EN: Raised serum alkaline phosphatase levels in polymyalgia rheumatica. Lancet *2:*328–331, 1972.

164. Conn DL, Kickson ER, Carpenter HA: The association of Churg-Strauss vasculitis with temporal artery involvement, primary biliary cirrhosis and polychondritis in a single patient. J Rheumatol *9:*744–748, 1982.

165. Kasolcharoen P, Magnia GF: Liver dysfunction in polymyalgia rheumatica: a case report. J Rheumatol *3:*50–53, 1976.

166. Leong AS-Y, Alp MH: Hepatocellular disease in the giant-cell arteritis polymyalgia rheumatica syndrome. Ann Rheum Dis *40:*92–95, 1981.

167. Long R, James O: Polymyalgia rheumatica and liver disease. Lancet *1:*77–79, 1974.

168. Bacon PA, Doherty SM, Zuckerman AJ: Hepatitis B antibody in polymyalgia rheumatica. Lancet *2:*476–478, 1975.

169. Liang M, Greenberg H, Pincus T, Robinson WS: Hepatitis B antibody in polymyalgia rheumatica. Lancet *1:*43–46, 1976.

170. Gocke DJ, Hsu K, Morgan C, Bombardieri S, Lockshin M, Christian CL: Association between polyarteritis and Australia antigen. Lancet *2:*1149–1153, 1970.

171. Trepo CG, Zuckerman AJ, Bird RC, Prince AM: The role of circulating hepatitis B antigen/antibody immune complexes in the pathogenesis of vascular and hepatic manifestations in polyarteritis nodosa. J Clin Pathol *27:*863–868, 1974.

172. Permin H, Aldershvile J, Nielsen JO: Hepatitis B virus infection on patients with rheumatic disease. Ann Rheum Dis *41:*479–482, 1982.

173. Mooradian AD, Frayha R: Multiple vasculopathies and hepatitis B in a family. Br J Rheumatol *24:*19–23, 1985.

174. Mowrey FH, Lundberg EA: The clinical manifestations of essential polyangitis (periarteritis nodosa), with emphasis on the hepatic manifestations. Ann Intern Med *40:*1145–1164, 1954.

175. Alleman MJ, Janssens AR, Spoelstra P, Kroon HM: Spontaneous intrahepatic hemorrhages in polyarteritis nodosa. Ann Intern Med *105:*712–713, 1986.

176. Parker RGF: Arterial infarction of the liver in man. J Pathol Bacteriol *70:*521–528, 1955.

177. Bonomo L, DePascale A, DiGiandomenico E, Gidaro G: Hepatic hematoma in polyarteritis nodosa. Rays *13:*19–21, 1988.

178. Haratake J, Horie A, Furuta A, Yamoto H: Massive hepatic infarction associated with polyarteritis nodosa. Acta Pathol Jpn *38:*89–93, 1988.

179. Specks U, Wheatley CL, McDonald TJ, Rohrbach MS, DeRemee RA: Anticytoplasmic autoantibodies in the diagnosis and follow-up of Wegener's granulomatosis. Mayo Clin Proc *64:*28–36, 1989.

180. DeRemee RA, McDonald TJ, Harrison EG Jr, Coles DT: Wegener's granulomatosis: anatomic correlates, a proposed classification. Mayo Clin Proc *51:*777–781, 1976.

181. Shah IA, Holstege A, Riede UN: Bioptic diagnosis of Wegener's granulomatosis in the absence of vasculitis and granulomas. Pathol Res Pract *178:*407–415, 1984.

182. Ranke MB, Stanley CA, Tenore A: Characterization of somatogenic and lactogenic binding sites in isolated hepatocytes. Endocrinology *99:*1033–1040, 1976.

183. Van Thiel DH, Gavaler JS, Schade RS: Liver disease and the hypothalamic pituitary gonadal axis. Semin Liver Dis *5:*35–45, 1985.

184. Shankar TP, Fredi JL, Himmelstein S: Elevated growth hormone levels and insulin resistance in patients with cirrhosis of the liver. Am J Med Sci *291:*248–253, 1986.

185. Russell WE: Growth hormone, somatomedins and the liver. Semin Liver Dis *5:*46–58, 1985.

186. Johnston DG, Alberti KGMM: The liver and the endocrine system. *In* Liver and Biliary Disease: Pathophysiology, Diagnosis, Management, edited by R. Wright, G.H. Millward-Sadler, K.G.M.M. Alberti. London, Bailliere Tindall, 1987, p. 161.

187. Preisig R, Morris TQ, Shaver JC: Volumetric, hemodynamic and excretory characteristics of the liver in acromegaly. J Clin Invest *65:*1379–1388, 1966.

188. Piper J, Poulsen E: Liver biopsy in thryotoxicosis. Acta Med Scand *127:*439–447, 1947.

189. Movitt ER, Gerstl B, Davis AE: Needle liver biopsy in thyrotoxicosis. Arch Intern Med *91:*729–739, 1953.

190. Ashkar FS, Miller R, Smoak WM, Gilson AS: Liver disease in hyperthyroidism. South Med J *64:*462–465, 1971.

191. Thompson P, Strum O: Abnormalities of liver function in thyrotoxicosis. Milit Med *143:*548–551, 1978.

192. Shetty N, Camilleri M, Moss DW, Hodgson HJ: Subtle hyperthyroidism presenting as suspected hepatobiliary disease. J Clin Gastroenterol *9:*186–188, 1987.

193. Yao JD, Gross JB Jr, Ludwig J, Purnell DC: Cholestatic jaundice in hyperthyroidism. Am J Med *86:*619–620, 1989.

194. Wartofsky L: Thyrotoxic storm. *In* The Thyroid: A Fundamental and Clinical Text, edited by S.H. Ingbar, L.E. Braverman. New York, Harper & Row, 1986, pp. 974–981.

195. Takahashi K. Ishitobi K, Kodera K, Kaneda S, Yazawa M, Mimura T: Bleeding esophageal varices caused by Graves' hypervascular cervical goiter. Jpn J Surg *16:*363–366, 1986.

196. DeGroot LJ, Stanbury JB (ed): Graves disease: general considerations. *In* The Thyroid and its Diseases. New York, John Wiley & Sons, 1975, p. 290.

197. Greenberger WJ, Milligan FD, DeGroot LJ, Isselbacher KJ: Jaundice and thyrotoxicosis in the absence of congestive heart failure. Am J Med *36:*840–846, 1964.

198. Shen DC, Davidson MB, Kuo SW, Sheu WH: Peripheral and hepatic insulin antagonism in hyperthyroidism. J Clin Endocrinol Metab *66:*565–569, 1988.

199. Dooner HP, Parada J, Aliage C, Hoyl C: The liver in thyrotoxicosis. Arch Intern Med *120:*25–32, 1967.

200. Thompson WG, Hart IR: Chronic active hepatitis and Graves' disease. Am J Dig Dis *18:*111–119, 1973.

201. Kittridge RD, Nash AD: The many facets of sclerosing fibrosis. Am J Roentgenol *122:*288–298, 1974.

202. Limaye A, Ruffolo PR: Propylthiouracil-induced fatal hepatic necrosis. Am J Gastroenterol *82:*152–154, 1987.

203. Schmidt G, Borsch G, Muller KM, Wegener M: Methimazole-associated cholestatic liver injury: case report and brief literature review. Hepatogastroenterology *33:*244–246, 1986.

204. Gay G, Netter P, Trechot P, Roche J-P, Zannad F. A case of amiodarone-induced hyperthyroidism and hepatitis: results of clinical

laboratory and histological tests. Biomed Pharmacother 40:54–57, 1986.

205. Helzberg JH, McPhee MS, Zarling EJ: Hepatocellular carcinoma: an unusual course with hyperthyroidism and inappropriate thyroid-stimulating hormone production. Gastroenterology 88:181–187, 1985.

206. Salata R, Klein I, Levey GS: Thyroid hormone homeostasis and the liver. Semin Liver Dis 5:29–34, 1985.

207. Sacdev Y, Hall R: Effusions into body cavities in hypothyroidism. Lancet 1:564–566, 1975.

208. Baker A, Kaplan M, Wolfe H: Central congestive fibrosis of the liver in myxoedema ascites. Ann Intern Med 77:927–929, 1972.

209. Clancy RL, Mackay IR: Myxoedematous ascites. Med J Aust 2:415–416, 1970.

210. MacSween RNM: The liver in endocrine diseases. In Pathology of the Liver, edited by R.N.M. MacSween, P.P. Anthony, P.J. Scheuer. 2nd Edition. Edinburgh, Churchill Livingstone, 1987, p. 659.

211. Spivak JL: Disorders caused by heat and cold. In The Principles and Practice of Medicine, edited by A.M. Harvey, R.J. Johns, V.A. McKusick, A.H. Owens Jr., R.S. Ross. 21st Edition. Norwalk, Appleton-Century-Crofts, 1984, pp. 1437–1439.

212. Holdstock G, Millward-Sadler GH, Wright R: Hyperpyrexias. In Liver and Biliary Disease. Pathophysiology, Diagnosis, Management, edited by R. Wright, G.H. Millward-Sadler, K.G.M.M. Alberti. 2nd Edition. London, Bailliere Tindall, 1987, pp. 1056–1067.

213. Clowes GH, O'Donnell TF: Heat stroke. N Engl J Med 291:564–567, 1974.

214. Denborough MA: Heat stroke and malignant hyperpyrexia. Med J Aust 1:204–205, 1982.

215. Kew M, Bersohn I, Seftel H: Liver damage in heatstroke. Am J Med 49:192–202, 1970.

216. Fidler S, Fagan E, Williams R, Dewhurst I, Cory CE: Heatstroke and rhabdomyolysis presenting as fulminant hepatic failure. Postgrad Med J 64:157–159, 1988.

217. Bianchi L, Ohnacker H, Beck K, Zimmerli-Ning M: Liver damage in heatstroke and its regression. A biopsy study. Hum Pathol 3:237–248, 1972.

218. Rubel LR, Ishak KG: The liver in fatal exertional heatstroke. Liver 3:249–256, 1983.

219. Galloway GJK, Denborough MA: Suxamethonium chloride and malignant hyperpyrexia. Br J Anaesth 58:447–450, 1986.

220. Armen R, Kamel G, Reynolds TB: Phencyclidine-induced malignant hyperthermia causing submassive liver necrosis. Am J Med 77:167–172, 1984.

221. Britt BA: Malignant hyperthermia. In Metabolic Aspects of Anaesthesia, edited by P.J. Cohen. Philadelphia, F.A. Davis, 1975, pp. 61–74.

222. Hagander B, Berg NO, Brandt L, Norden A, Sjolund K, Stenstam M: Hepatic injury in adult coeliac disease. Lancet 2:270–272, 1977.

223. Pollock DJ: The liver in coeliac disease. Histopathology 1:421–430, 1977.

224. Mitchison HC, Record CO, Bateson MC, Cobden I: Hepatic abnormalities in coeliac disease: three cases of delayed diagnosis. Postgrad Med J 65:920–922, 1989.

225. Trier JS: Celiac sprue. In Gastrointestinal Diseases, edited by M.H. Sleisenger, J.S. Fortran. 4th Edition. Philadelphia, W.B. Saunders, 1989, pp. 1134–1152.

226. O'Grady JG, Stevens FM, Harding B, O'Gorman TA, McNicholl B, McCarthy CF: Hypersplenism and gluten-sensitive enteropathy. Gastroenterology 87:1326–1331, 1984.

227. Desmet VJ, Geboes K: Liver lesions in inflammatory bowel disorders. J Pathol 151:247–255, 1987.

228. Naschitz JE, Yeshurun D, Zuckerman E, Arad E, Boss JH: Massive hepatic steatosis complicating adult celiac disease: report of a case and review of the literature. Am J Gastroenterol 82:1186–1189, 1987.

229. Maggiore G, DeGiacomo C, Scotta MS, Sessa F: Celiac disease presenting as chronic hepatitis in a girl. J Pediatr Gastroenterol Nutr 5:501–503, 1986.

230. Behr W, Barnert J: Adult celiac disease and primary biliary cirrhosis. Am J Gastroenterol 81:796–799, 1986.

231. Shanahan F, O'Regan PF, Crowe JP: Primary biliary cirrhosis associated with coeliac disease. Ir Med J 76:282, 1983.

232. Hay JE, Wiesner RH, Shorter RG, LaRusso NF, Baldus WP: Primary sclerosing cholangitis and celiac disease. Ann Intern Med 109:713–717, 1988.

233. Holdstock G, Millward-Sadler, Wright R: Hepatic changes in systemic disease. In Liver and Biliary Disease, edited by R. Wright,

G.H Millward-Sadler, K.G.M.M. Alberti. 2nd Edition. London, Bailliere Tindall, 1987, p. 1064.

234. Sheehy TW, Cohen WC, Wallace DK, Legters LJ: Tropical sprue in North America. JAMA 194:169–174, 1965.

235. Klipstein FA: Tropical sprue. In Gastrointestinal Disease, edited by M.H. Sleisenger, J.S. Fortran. 4th Edition. Philadelphia, W.B. Saunders, 1989, pp. 1281–1286.

236. Trier JS: Whipple's disease. In Gastrointestinal Disease, edited by M.H. Sleisenger, J.S. Fortran. 4th Edition. Philadelphia, W.B. Saunders, 1989, pp. 1297–1306.

237. Viteri AL, Stinson JC, Barnes MC, Dyck WP: Rod-shaped organism in the liver of a patient with Whipple's disease. Dig Dis Sci 24:560–564, 1979.

238. Carache P, Bayless TM, Shelley WM, Hendrix TR: Atypical bacteria in Whipple's disease. Trans Assoc Am Physicians 79:399–408, 1966.

238a. Relman DA, Schmidt TM, MacDermott RP, Falkow S: The agent of Whipple's disease is a novel gram positive bacterium most closely related to Dermatophilus and Arthrobacter. Gastroenterology 102:A683, 1992 (Abstr).

239. MacSween RNM: Liver pathology associated with diseases of other organs. In Pathology of the Liver, edited by P.P. Anthony, R.N.M. MacSween. 2nd Edition. Edinburgh, Churchill Livingstone, 1987, pp. 646–688.

240. Misra PS, Lebwohl P, Laufer H: Hepatic and appendiceal Whipple's disease with negative jejunal biopsies. Am J Gastroenterol 75:302–306, 1981.

241. Sieracki C, Fine G: Whipple's disease: observations on systemic involvement. II. Gross and histologic observations. Arch Pathol 67:81–93, 1959.

242. Saint-Marc Girardin MF, Zafrani ES, Chaumette MT, Delchier J-C, Metreau J-M, Dhumeaux D: Hepatic granulomas in Whipple's disease. Gastroenterology 86:753–756, 1984.

243. Heyman MB: Food sensitivity and eosinophilic gastroenteropathies. In Gastrointestinal Disease, edited by M.H. Sleisinger, J.S. Fortran. 4th Edition. Philadelphia, W.B. Saunders, 1989, pp. 1113–1134.

244. Robert F, Omura E, Durant JR: Mucosal eosinophilic gastroenteritis with systemic involvement. Am J Med 62:139–143, 1977.

245. Everett GD, Mitros FA: Eosinophilic gastroenteritis with hepatic eosinophilic granulomas. Report of a case with 30-year follow-up. Am J Gastroenterol 74:519–521, 1980.

246. Eade MN: Liver disease in ulcerative colitis. I. Analysis of operative liver biopsy in 138 consecutive patients having colectomy. Ann Intern Med 72:475–487, 1970.

247. Minuk GY: Hepatobiliary complications of idiopathic inflammatory bowel disease. Can J Gastroenterol 2(Suppl A):109A–114A, 1988.

248. Schrumpf E, Fausa O, Elgjo K, Kolmannskog F: Hepatobiliary complications of inflammatory bowel disease. Semin Liver Dis 8:201–209, 1988.

249. Mistilis SP: Pericholangitis and ulcerative colitis. I. Pathology, etiology and pathogenesis. Ann Intern Med 63:1–16, 1965.

250. Kleckner MS, Stauffer MH, Bargen JA: Hepatic lesions in the living patient with chronic ulcerative colitis as demonstrated by needle biopsy. Gastroenterology 22:13–33, 1952.

251. Hoffbauer FW, McCartney JS, Dennis C: The relationship of chronic ulcerative colitis and cirrhosis. Ann Intern Med 39:267–284, 1953.

252. Vinnik IE, Kern F; Liver diseases in ulcerative colitis. Arch Intern Med 112:41–49, 1963.

253. Wee A, Ludwig J: Pericholangitis in chronic ulcerative colitis: Primary sclerosing cholangitis of the small bile ducts? Ann Intern Med 102:581–590, 1985.

254. Sciot R, Desmet VJ: Hepatobiliary complications in chronic inflammatory bowel disease. Acta Gastroenterol Belg 50:299–305, 1987.

255. Othagen I: Ulcerative colitis in cirrhosis of the liver. Acta Med Scand 162:143–153, 1958.

256. Williams SM, Harned RK: Hepatobiliary complications of inflammatory bowel disease. Radiol Clin North Am 25:175–188, 1987.

257. Wiesner RH, LaRusso NF: Clinicopathologic features of the syndrome of primary sclerosing cholangitis. Gastroenterology 79:200–206, 1980.

258. Ludwig J, Barham SS, LaRusso NF, Elveback LR, Wiesner RH, McCall JT: Morphologic features of chronic hepatitis associated with primary sclerosing cholangitis and chronic ulcerative colitis. Hepatology 6:632–636, 1981.

259. Blackstone MO, Nemchansky BN: Cholangiographic abnormalities in ulcerative colitis associated pericholangitis which resemble sclerosing cholangitis. Dig Dis 23:579–585, 1978.

260. MacSween RNM: Primary sclerosing cholangitis. *In* Recent Advances in Histopathology, No. 12, edited by P.P. Anthony, R.N.M. MacSween. Edinburgh, Churchill Livingstone, 1984, pp. 158–167.

261. Aadland E, Schrumpf E, Fausa O, Elgjo K, Heilo A, Aakhus T, Gjone E: Primary sclerosing cholangitis: a long-term follow-up study. Scand J Gastroenterol 22:655–664, 1987.

262. Rabinovitz M, Gavaler JS, Schade RR, Dindzans VJ, Chien M-C, Van Thiel DH: Does primary sclerosing cholangitis occurring in association with inflammatory bowel disease differ from that occurring in the absence of inflammatory bowel disease? A study of sixty-six subjects. Hepatology 11:7–11, 1990.

263. Lefkowitch JH, Martin ED: Primary sclerosing cholangitis. Prog Liver Dis 8:557–569, 1986.

264. Warren KW, Athanassiades S, Monge JL: Primary sclerosing cholangitis. A study of forty-two cases. Am J Surg 111:230–238, 1966.

265. Donaldson PT, Farrant JM, Wilkinson ML, Hayllar K, Portmann BC, Williams R: Dual association of HLA DR2 and DR3 with primary sclerosing cholangitis. Hepatology 13:129–133, 1991.

266. Nakanuma Y, Hirai N, Kono N: Histological and ultrastructural examination of the intrahepatic biliary tree in primary sclerosing cholangitis. Liver 6:317–322, 1986.

267. Jeffrey GP, Reed WD, Laurence BH, Shilkin KB: Primary sclerosing cholangitis: clinical and immunopathological review of 21 cases. J Gastroenterol Hepatol 5:135–140, 1990.

268. Ludwig J: New concepts in biliary cirrhosis. Semin Liver Dis 7:293–307, 1987.

269. Hadjis NS, Adam A, Blenkharn I, Hatzis G, Benjamin I, Blumgart LH: Primary sclerosing cholangitis associated with liver atrophy. Am J Surg 158:43–47, 1989.

269a. Kaplan MM, Arora S, Pincus SH. Primary sclerosing cholangitis and low-dose oral pulse methotrexate therapy. Ann Intern Med 106:231–235, 1987.

269b. Kaplan MM. Methotrexate treatment of chronic cholestatic liver diseases. Friend or foe? Q J Med 72:757–761, 1989.

269c. Knox TA, Kaplan MM. Treatment of primary sclerosing cholangitis with oral methotrexate. Am K Gastroenterol 86:546–552, 1991.

270. Chesner IM, Muller S, Newman J: Ulcerative colitis complicated by Budd-Chiari syndrome. Gut 27:1096–1100, 1986.

271. Wee A, Ludwig J, Coffey RJ Jr, LaRusso NF, Wiesner RH: Hepatobiliary carcinoma associated with primary sclerosing cholangitis and chronic ulcerative colitis. Hum Pathol 16:719–726, 1985.

272. Morowitz DA, Glagov S, Dordal E, Kirsner JB: Carcinoma of the biliary tract complicating chronic ulcerative colitis. Cancer 27:356–361, 1971.

273. Ross AP, Braasch JW: Ulcerative colitis and carcinoma of the proximal bile ducts. Gut 14:94–97, 1973.

274. Mir-Madjlessi SH, Farmer RG, Sivak MV Jr: Bile duct carcinoma in patients with ulcerative colitis. Relationship to sclerosing cholangitis: report of six cases and review of the literature. Dig Dis Sci 32:145–154, 1987.

275. Hadjis NS, Adam A, Blenkharn I, Hatzis G,, Benjamin IS, Blumgart LH: Primary sclerosing cholangitis associated with liver atrophy. Am J Surg 158:43–47, 1989.

276. Scheuer PJ: Liver Biopsy Interpretation, edited by P.J. Scheuer. 4th Edition. London, Bailliere Tindall, 1988.

277. Shorvon PJ: Amyloidosis and inflammatory bowel disease. Dig Dis 22:209–213, 1977.

278. Gray N, MacKay IR, Taft LI: Hepatitis, colitis and lupus manifestations. Am J Dig Dis 3:481–487, 1958.

279. Holdsworth CD, Hall EW, Dawson AM: Ulcerative colitis in chronic liver disease. Q J Med 34:211–227, 1965.

280. Olsson R, Hulten L: Concurrence of ulcerative colitis and chronic active hepatitis. Clinical courses and results of colectomy. Scand J Gastroenterol 10:331–335, 1975.

281. Eade MN, Cooke WT, Williams JA: Liver disease in Crohn's disease. A study of 100 consecutive patients. Scand J Gastroenterol 6:199–204, 1971.

282. Schrumpf E, Fausa O, Kolmannskog F: Sclerosing cholangitis in ulcerative colitis. A follow-up study. Scand J Gastroenterol 17:33–39, 1982.

283. Eade MN, Brooke BN: Portal bacteremia in cases of ulcerative colitis submitted to colectomy. Lancet 1:1008–1009, 1969.

284. MacMahon JF, Mallory FB: Streptococcus hepatitis. Am J Pathol 7:299–326, 1931.

285. Wachstein M, Meisel E, Galcon C: Enzymatic histochemistry in the experimentally damaged liver. Am J Pathol 40:219–241, 1962.

286. Vinnik IE, Kern F, Struthers JE: Experimental chronic portal vein bacteremia. Proc Soc Exp Biol Med 115:311–314, 1964.

287. Dordal E, Glagov S, Kirsner JB: Hepatic lesions in chronic inflammatory bowel disease. I. Clinical correlations with liver biopsy diagnoses in 103 patients. Gastroenterology 52:239–253, 1967.

288. Vierling JM: Hepatobiliary complications of ulcerative colitis and Crohn's disease. *In* Hepatology. A Textbook of Liver Disease, Vol. 2, edited by D. Zakim, T.D. Boyer. Philadelphia, W. B. Saunders. 1990, pp. 1126–1157.

289. Mir-Madjlessi SH, McHenry MC, Farmer RG: Liver abscess in Crohn's disease. Report of four cases and review of the literature. Gastroenterology 91:987–993, 1986.

290. Perrett AD, Higgins G, Johnston HH: The liver in Crohn's disease. Q J Med 40:187–200, 1971.

291. Cohen AS, Skinner M: Amyloidosis of the liver. *In* Diseases of the Liver, edited by L. Schiff, E.R. Schiff. 5th Edition. Philadelphia, J.B. Lippincott, 1971, pp. 1081–1099.

292. Baker AL, Kaplan MM, Norton RA, Patterson JF: Gallstones in inflammatory bowel disease. Am J Dig Dis Sci 19:109–112, 1974.

293. Won KH, Ramchand S: Melanosis of the ileum. Case report and electron microscopic study. Am J Dig Dis 15:57–62, 1940.

294. Smith R: Pathology of cathartic colon. Proc R Soc Med 65:288–291, 1972.

295. Wittoesch JH, Jackman RJ, McDonald JR: Melanosis coli: general review and a study of 887 cases. Dis Colon Rectum 1:172–180, 1958.

296. Dubilier LD, Burkhart RC: Melanosis coli with liver involvement. J Kentucky Med Assoc 73:143–150, 1975.

297. Bottomly SS, Frederick DL, Welsh JD, Keller AM: A case of red plasma. Clin Res 29:859A, 1981 (Abstract).

297a. Kanel GC. Conditions resembling alcoholic liver disease. In Liver Pathology, edited by R.L. Peters, J.R. Craig. New York: Churchill Livingstone, 1986, pp. 285–297.

297b. Grimm IS, Schindler W, Haluszka, O. Steatohepatitis and fatal hepatic failure after biliopancreatic diversion. Am J Gastroenterol 1992 (in press).

297c. Holian Dk. Biliopancreatic bypass. In Surgery for the Morbidly Obese Patient, edited by M. Deitel. Philadelphia, Lea & Febiger, 1989, pp. 105–111.

298. Kirshbaum JD, Preuss FS: Leukemia. A clinical and pathologic study of one hundred and twenty-three fatal cases in a series of 14,400 necropsies. Arch Intern Med 71:777–792, 1943.

299. Schwartz JB, Shamsuddin AM: The effects of leukemic infiltrates in various organs in chronic lymphocytic leukemia. Hum Pathol 12:432–440, 1981.

300. Wetherley-Mein G, Cottom DG. Portal fibrosis in acute leukemia. Br J Haematol 2:345–354, 1956.

301. Dahl MGC, Gregory MM, Scheuer PJ: Methotrexate toxicity in psoriasis: a comparison of different dose regimens. Br Med J 1:654–656, 1972.

302. Golumb HM, Catovsky D, Golde DW: Hairy cell leukemia. A clinical review based on 71 cases. Ann Intern Med 89:677–683, 1978.

303. Golumb HM, Braylan R, Polliac A: "Hairy" cell leukemia (leukaemic reticuloendotheliosis): a scanning electron microscopic study of eight cases. Br J Haematol 29:455–460, 1975.

304. Roquet M-L, Zafrani E-S, Farcet J-P, Reyes F, Pinaudeau Y: Histopathological lesions of the liver in hairy cell leukemia: a report of 14 cases. Hepatology 5:496–500, 1985.

305. Yam LT, Janckila AJ, Chan CH, Li CY: Hepatic involvement in hairy cell leukemia. Cancer 51:1497–1504, 1983.

306. Grouls V, Stiens R: Hepatic involvement in hairy cell leukaemia: diagnosis by tartrate-resistant acid phosphatase enzyme histochemistry on formalin-fixed and paraffin-embedded liver biopsy specimens. Pathol Res Part 178:332–334, 1984.

307. Nanba K, Soban EJ, Bowling MC, Merard CW: Splenic pseudosinuses and hepatic angiomatous lesions. Distinctive features of hairy cell leukemia. Am J Clin Pathol 67:415–426, 1977.

308. Keefer MJ, Weber MJ, Bottomley SS, Solanki DL, Hosty TA: Peripheral blood remission of hairy cell leukemia after transfusion hepatitis. Am J Hematol 25:277–284, 1987.

309. Ratner L, Peylan-Ramu N, Wesley R, Poplack DG: Adverse prognostic influence of hepatitis B virus infection in acute lymphoblastic leukemia. Cancer 58:1096–1100, 1986.

310. Locasciulli A, Alberti A, Rossetti F, Santamaria M, Santoro N, Madon E, Miniero R, Lo-Curto M, Tamaro P, Paolucci P: Acute and chronic hepatitis in childhood leukemia: a multicentric study from the Italian Pediatric Cooperative Group for Therapy of Acute Leukemia (AIL-AIEOP). Med Pediatr Oncol 13:203–206, 1985.

311. Gowing NFC: Infectous mononucleosis: histopathological aspects. *In* Hematologic and Lymphoid Pathology Decennial, 1966–1975, edited

by S.C. Sommers. New York, Appleton-Century-Crofts, 1975, pp. 261–280.

312. Dameshek W: Speculations on the nature of infectious mononucleosis. *In* Infectious Mononucleosis, edited by R.L. Carter, H.G. Penman. Oxford, Blackwell Scientific Publications, 1969, pp. 225–240.

313. Ward HP, Block MH: The natural history of agnogenic myeloid metaplasia (AMM) and a critical evaluation of its relationship with the myeloproliferative syndrome. Medicine *50:*357–420, 1971.

314. Silverstein MN, Brown AL Jr, Linman JW: Idiopathic myeloid metaplasia. Its evolution into acute leukemia. Arch Intern Med *132:*709–712, 1973.

315. Grieco A, Manna R, Mancini R, Gambassi G: Massive hepatomegaly following splenectomy for myeloid metaplasia. Am J Med *84:*797–798, 1988.

316. Towell BL, Levine SP: Massive hepatomegaly following splenectomy for myeloid metaplasia. Case report and review of the literature. Am J Med *82:*371–378, 1987.

317. Roux D, Merlio J-P, Quinton A, Lamouliatte H, Balabaud C, Bioulac-Sage P: Agnogenic myeloid metaplasia, portal hypertension and sinusoidal abnormalities. Gastroenterology *92:*1067–1072, 1987.

318. Wiener MD, Halvorsen RA, Vollmer RT, Foster WL, Roberts L Jr: Focal intrahepatic extramedullary hematopoiesis mimicking neoplasm. AJR *149:*1171–1172, 1987.

319. Lobdell DH, Europa DL: The megakaryoctyes in myelofibrosis with mycloid metaplasia. A histochemical study. Lab Invest *11:*58–64, 1962.

320. Scheuer PJ: Liver Biopsy Interpretation, 4th edn. Bailliere-Tindall, London, 1988. p 243.

321. Glew RH, Haese WH, McIntyre PA: Myeloid metaplasia with myelofibrosis. The clinical spectrum of extramedullary hematopoiesis and tumor formation. Johns Hopkins Med J *132:*253–270, 1973.

322. Lafon ME, Bioulac-Sage P, Grimaud JA, Boussarie L, Merlio JP, Reiffers J, Balabaud C: Perisinusoidal fibrosis of the liver in patients with thrombocytopenic purpura. Virchows Arch A *411:*553–559, 1987.

323. Thomas FB, Clausen KP, Greenberger NJ: Liver disease in multiple myeloma. Arch Intern Med *132:*195–202, 1973.

324. Perez-Soler R, Esteban R, Allende E, Tornos-Salomo C, Julia A, Guardia J: Liver involvement in multiple myeloma. Am J Hematol *20:*25–29, 1985.

325. Durant JR, Barry WE, Learner N: The changing face of myeloma. Lancet *1:*119–123, 1966.

326. Chopra S, Rubinow A, Koff RS, Cohen AS: Hepatic amyloidosis. A histopathologic analysis of primary (AL) and secondary (AA) forms. Am J Pathol *115:*186–193, 1984.

327. Bergsagel DE: Macroglobulinemia. *In* Hematology, edited by W.J. Williams, E. Beutler, A.J. Erslev, M.A. Lichtman. New York, McGraw-Hill Book Co., 1983, pp. 1104–1109.

328. Glenner C: Amyloid deposits and amyloidosis. The B fibrilloses. N Engl J Med *302:*1283–1292, 1980.

329. Voinchet O, Degott C, Scoazec J-Y, Feldmann G, Benhamou J-P: Peliosis hepatis, nodular regenerative hyperplasia of the liver, and light-chain deposition in a patient with Waldenstrom's macroglobulinemia. Gastroenterology *95:*482–486, 1988.

330. Ganeval D, Noel LH, Preud'homme JL, Droz D, Grunfeld JP: Light chain deposition disease: its relation with AL-type amyloidosis. Kidney Int *26:*1–9, 1984.

331. Schubert TT: Hepatobiliary system in sickle cell disease. Gastroenterology *90:*2013–2021, 1986.

332. Johnson CS, Omata M, Tong MJ, Sommons JF Jr, Weiner J, Tatter D: Liver involvement in sickle cell disease. Medicine *64:*349–356, 1985.

333. Bauer TW, Moore GW, Hutchins GM: The liver in sickle cell disease. A clinicopathologic study of 70 patients. Am J Med *69:*833–837, 1980.

334. Green TW, Conley CL, Berthrong M: The liver in sickle cell anemia. Bull Johns Hopkins Hosp *92:*99–127, 1953.

335. Rosenblate HJ, Eisenstein R, Holmes AW: The liver in sickle cell anemia. A clinical-pathological study. Arch Pathol *90:*235–245, 1970.

336. Klion FM, Weinder MJ, Schaffner F: Cholestasis in sickle cell anemia. Am J Med *37:*829–832, 1964.

337. Phillips JC, Geald BE: The incidence of cholelithiasis in sickle cell disease. Am J Roentgenol Radium Ther Nucl Med *113:*27–28, 1971.

338. Cameron JL, Maddrey WC, Zuidema GD: Biliary tract disease in sickle cell anemia: surgical considerations. Ann Surg *174:*702–710, 1971.

339. Hargrove MD Jr: Marked increase in serum bilirubin in sickle cell anemia. A report of 6 patients. Dig Dis *15:*437–442, 1970.

340. Flye MW, Silver D: Biliary tract disorders and sickle cell disease. Surgery *72:*361–367, 1972.

341. Magid D, Fishman EK, Charache S, Siegelman SS: Abdominal pain in sickle cell disease: the role of CT. Radiology *163:*325–328, 1987.

342. Hatton CS, Brunch C, Weatherall DJ: Hepatic sequestration in sickle cell anaemia. Br Med J *290:*744–745, 1985.

343. Conn HO: Sickle-cell trait and splenic infraction associated with high altitude flying. N Engl J Med *251:*417–420, 1954.

344. Song YS: Hepatic lesions in sickle cell anemia. Am J Pathol *33:*331–351, 1957.

345. Schaffner F, Popper H: Capillarization of hepatic sinusoids in man. Gastroenterology *44:*239–242, 1963.

346. Omata M, Johnson CS, Tong M, Tatter D: Pathological spectrum of liver diseases in sickle cell disease. Dig Dis Sci *31:*247–256, 1986.

347. Middleton JP, Wolper JC: Hepatic biloma complicating sickle cell disease. A case report and a review of the literature. Gastroenterology *86:*743–744, 1984.

348. Mills LR, Mwakyusa D, Milner PF: Histopathologic features of liver biopsy specimens in sickle cell disease. Arch Pathol Lab Med *112:*290–294, 1988.

349. Scott RB, Robb-Smith AHT: Histiocytic medullary reticulosis. Lancet *2:*194–198, 1939.

350. Bouroncle BA, Wiseman BK, Doan CA: Leukemic reticuloendotheliosis. Blood *13:*609–630, 1958.

351. Rappaport H: Tumors of the hematopoietic systetm. *In* Atlas of Tumor Pathology. Washington, D.C., Armed Forces Institute of Pathology, 1966.

352. Nanno T, Adachi Y, Enomoto M, Nagamine Y, Suwa M, Suzuki T, Takaoka A, Yamamoto T: An autopsy case of histiocytic medullary reticulosis presenting with marked hepatosplenomegaly for 13 years before the onset. Jpn J Med *27:*195–199, 1988.

353. Serk-Hanssen A, Purohit GP: Histiocytic medullary reticulosis. Report of 14 cases from Uganda. Br. J Cancer *22:*506–516, 1968.

354. Warnke RA, Kim H, Dorfman RF: Malignant histiocytosis (histiocytic medullary reticulosis) 1. Clinicopathological study of 29 cases. Cancer *35:*215–230, 1975.

355. Risdall RJ, Sibley RK, McKenna RW, Brunning RD, Dehner LP: Malignant histiocytosis. A light- and electron-microscopic and histochemical study. Am J Surg Pathol *4:*439–450, 1980.

356. MacMahon EH, Bedizel M, Ellis CA: Familial erythrophagocytic lymphohistiocytosis Pediatrics *32:*868–879, 1963.

357. Koto A, Morecki R, Santorineou M: Congenital hemophagocytic reticulosis. Am J Clin Pathol *65:*495–503, 1976.

358. Hsu TS, Komp DM. Clinical features of familial histiocytosis. Am J Pediatr Hematol Oncol *3:*61–65, 1981.

359. Janker GE: Familial hemophagocytic lymphohistiocytosis. Eur J Pediatr *140:*221–230, 1983.

360. Ishak KG, Sharp HL: Developmental abnormality and liver disease in childhood. *In* Pathology of the Liver, edited by R.N.M. MacSween, P.P. Anthony, P.J. Scheuer. Edinburgh, Churchill Livingstone, 1987, pp. 88–90.

361. Risdall RJ, McKenna RW, Nesbit ME, Krivit W, Balfur HH Jr, Simmons RL, Burnning RD: Virus-associated hemophagocytic syndrome. A benign histiocytic proliferation distinct from malignant histiocytosis. Cancer *44:*993–1002, 1979.

362. McKenna RW, Risdall RJ, Brunning RD: Virus-associated hemophagocytic syndrome. Hum Pathol *12:*395–398, 1981.

363. Seligman BR, Rosner F, Lee SI, Kagan MD: Histiocytic medullary reticulosis. Fatal hemorrhage due to massive platelet phagocytosis. Arch Intern Med *129:*109–113, 1972.

364. Nesbit ME, O'Leary M, Dehner LP, Ramsay NK: The immune system and the histiocytosis syndromes. Am J Pediatr Hematol Oncol *4:*141–149, 1981.

365. Starling KA, Fernbach DJ: Histiocytosis. *In* Clinical Pediatric Oncology, edited by W.W. Sutow, D.J. Fernbach, T.J. Vietti. St. Louis, C.V. Mosby, 1984, pp. 498–515.

366. Lucaya J: Histiocytosis X. Am J Dis Child *121:*289–295, 1971.

367. Wolfson SL, Botero F, Hurwitz S, Pearson HA: Pure cutaneous histiocytosis X. Cancer *48:*2236–2238, 1981.

368. Weber WN, Margolin FR, Neilsen SL: Pulmonary histiocytosis X: a review of 18 patients with report of six cases. Am J Roentgenol *107:*280–289, 1969.

369. Pirovino M, Jeanneret C, Lang RH, Luisier J, Bianchi L, Spichtin H: Liver cirrhosis in histiocytosis X. Liver *8:*293–298, 1988.

370. Thompson HH, Pitt HA, Lewin KJ, Longmire WP Jr: Sclerosing cholangitis and histiocytosis X. Gut *25:*526–530, 1984.

371. Landing BH, Wells TR, Reed GB, Natayan MS: Diseases of the bile ducts in children. *In* The Liver, edited by E.A. Gass, F.K. Mostofi. Baltimore, Williams & Wilkins, 1973, pp. 480–509.

372. Freud P: Evolution of systemic reticuloendotheliosis in childhood. J Pediatr *38:*744–769, 1951.

373. Beckstead JH, Wood GS, Turner RR: Histiocytosis X cells and Langerhans cells: enzyme histochemical and immunologic similarities. Hum Pathol *15:*826–833, 1984.

373a. Favara BE, McCarthy RG, Mieran GW. Histocytosis X. Hum Pathol *14:*663–676, 1983.

374. Lichtenstein L: Histiocytosis X (eosinophilic granuloma of bone, Letterer-Siwe disease and Schuller-Christian disease): further observations of pathological and clinical importance. J Bone Jt Surg *46A:*76–90, 1964.

375. Avery ME, McAfee JG, Guild HG: The course and prognosis of reticuloendotheliosis (eosinophilic granuloma, Schuller-Christian disease and Letterer-Siwe disease). A study of forty cases. Am J Med *22:*636–652, 1957.

376. Oberman HA: Idiopathic histiocytosis: a clinico-pathologic study of 40 cases and review of the literature on eosinophilic granuloma of bone, Hand-Schuller-Christian disease and Letterer-Siwe disease. Pediatrics *28:*307–327, 1961.

377. Dutt AK, Lopez CG, Ganesan S, Smith G, Dutt A: Acute disseminated histiocytosis X: a case with transition from eosinophilic granuloma of bone to Letterer-Siwe disease. Aust Ann Med *18:*135–137, 1969.

378. Lichtenstein L: Histiocytosis X. Integration of eosinophilic granuloma of bone, Letterer-Siwe disease and Schuller-Christian disease as related manifestations of a single nosologic entity. Arch Pathol *56:*84–102, 1953.

379. Lieberman PH, Jones CR, Dargeon HWK, Begg CF: A reappraisal of eosinophilic granuloma of bone, Hand-Schuller-Christian syndrome and Letterer-Siwe syndrome. Medicine *48:*375–400, 1969.

380. Parker JW, Lichtenstein L: Severe hepatic involvement in chronic disseminated histiocytosis X. Report of a case with necropsy. Am J Clin Pathol *40:*624–632, 1963.

381. Goldner MG, Volk BW: Fulminant normocholesteremic xanthomatosis. (Histiocytosis X). Arch Intern Med *95:*689–698, 1955.

382. Paivansalo M, Makarainen H: Liver lesions in histiocytosis X: findings on sonography and computed tomography. Br. J Radiol *59:*1123–1125, 1986.

383. Iwai M, Kashiwadani M, Okuuno T, Takino T, Koshikawa T: Cholestatic liver disease in a 20 yr old woman with histiocytosis. Am J Gastroenterol *83:*164–168, 1988.

384. Szweda JA, Abraham JP, Fine G, Nixon RK, Rupe CE: Systemic mast cell disease. A review and report of three cases. Am J Med *32:*227–239, 1962.

385. Tharp MD: The spectrum of mastocytosis. Am J Med Sci *289:*119–132, 1985.

386. Friedman BI, Will JJ, Freiman DG, Braunstein H: Tissue mast cell leukemia. Blood *13:*70–78, 1958.

387. Yam LT, Chan CH, Li CY: Hepatic involvement in systemic mast cell disease. Am J Med *80:*819–826, 1986.

388. Grundfest S, Cooperman AM, Ferguson R, Benjamin S: Portal hypertension associated with systemic mastocytosis and splenomegaly. Gastroenterology *78:*370–373, 1980.

389. Sumpio BE, O'Leary G, Gusberg RJ: Variceal bleeding, hypersplenism and systemic mastocytosis. Pathophysiology and management. Arch Surg *123:*767–769, 1988.

390. Bonnet P, Smadja C, Szekely AM, Delage Y, Calmus Y, Poupon R, Franco D: Intractable ascites in systemic mastocytosis treated by portal diversion. Dig Dis Sci *32:*209–213, 1987.

391. Gray JR, Bouchier IAD: Liver disease and pregnancy. Gastroenterol Int *2:*217–221, 1989.

392. Cuddihy A, Whelton MJ: Infertility in chronic active hepatitis. Hepatology *7:*1146–1152, 1987.

393. Stock RJ, Labudovich M, Ducatman B: Asymptomatic first-trimester liver cell adenoma. Obstet Gynecol *66:*287–290, 1985.

394. Riely CA: The liver in pregnancy. *In* Diseases of the Liver, edited by L. Schiff, E.R. Schiff. 6th Edition. Philadelphia, J.B. Lippincott, 1987, pp. 1059–1073.

395. Combes B, Shibata H, Adams R, Mitchell BD, Trammel V: Alterations in sulfobromophthalein sodium removal mechanisms from blood during normal pregnancy. J Clin Invest *42:*1431–1442, 1963.

396. Laakso L, Ruotsalainen P, Punnonen R: Hepatic blood flow during late pregnancy. Acta Obstet Gynecol Scand *50:*175–178, 1971.

397. Antia FP, Bharadwaj TP, Watsa MC, Master J: Liver in normal pregnancy, preeclampsia and eclampsia. Lancet *2:*776–778, 1958.

398. MacSween RNM: The liver in pregnancy. *In* Pathology of the Liver, edited by R.N.M. MacSween, P.P. Anthony, P.J. Scheuer. 2nd Edition. Edinburgh, Churchill Livingstone, 1987, pp. 659–663.

399. Ishak KG: Hepatic lesions caused by anabolic and contraceptive steroids. Semin Liver Dis *1:*116–128, 1981.

400. Larrey D, Rueff B, Feldmann G, Degott C, Danau G, Benhamou J-P: Recurrent jaundice caused by recurrent hyperemesis gravidarum. Gut *25:*1414–1416, 1984.

401. Adams RH, Gordan J, Combes B: Hyperemesis gravidarum: I. Evidence of hepatic dysfunction. Obstet Gynecol *31:*659–664, 1968.

402. Sheehan HL: The pathology of hyperemesis and vomiting of late pregnancy. J Obstet Gynaecol *46:*685–699, 1940.

403. Alexander J, Cuellar RE, Van Thiel DH: Toxemia of pregnancy and the liver. Semin Liver Dis *7:*55–58, 1987.

404. Killam AP, Dillard SH, Patton RC, Pedersen PR: Pregnancy-induced hypertension complicated by acute liver disease and disseminated intravascular coagulation. Am J Obstet Gynecol *123:*823–828, 1975.

405. Krejs GJ, Haemmerli UP: Jaundice during pregnancy. *In* Diseases of the Liver, edited by L. Schiff, E.R. Schiff. 5th Edition. Philadelphia, J.B. Lippincott, 1982, pp. 1561–1580.

406. Long RG, Scheuer PJ, Sherlock S: Pre-eclampsia presenting with deep jaundice. J Clin Pathol *30:*212–215, 1977.

407. Beaugrand M, Ganne N: Foie et grossesse. Gastroenterol Clin Biol *14:*T 13–T 17, 1990.

408. Minakami H, Sato T, Takahashi T, Oka N, Tamada T: Clinical significance of SGOT elevation and thrombocytopenia in pre-eclampsia patients. Nippon-Sanka-Fujinka-Gakkai-Zasshi *40:*754–760, 1988.

409. Arias F, Manchilla-Jimenez R: Hepatic fibrinogen deposits in preeclampsia. Immuofluorescent evidence. N Engl J Med *295:*578–582, 1976.

410. Rolfes DB, Ishak KG: Liver disease in toxemia of pregnancy. Am J Gastroenterol *81:*1138–1144, 1986.

411. Minuk GY, Lui RC, Kelly J: Rupture of the liver associated with acute fatty liver of pregnancy. Am J Gastroenterol *82:*457–460, 1987.

412. Jewett JF: Eclampsia and rupture of the liver. N Engl J Med *297:*1009–1012, 1977.

413. Aziz S, Merrell RC, Collins JA: Spontaneous hepatic hemorrhage during pregnancy. Am J Surg *146:*680–682, 1983.

414. Manas KJ, Welsh JD, Rankin RA, Miller DD: Hepatic haemorrhage without rupture in pre-eclampsia. N Engl J Med *312:*424–426, 1985.

415. Sibai BM, Taslimi MM, el-Nazer A, Amon E, Mabie BC, Ryan GM: Maternal-perinatal outcome associated with the syndrome of hemolysis, elevated liver enzymes, and low platelets in severe preeclampsia-eclampsia. Am J Obstet Gynecol *155:*501–509, 1986.

416. Clark SL, Phelan JR, Allen SH, Golde SR: Antepartum reversal of hematologic abnormalities associated with the HELLP syndrome. A report of three cases. J Reprod Med *31:*70–72, 1986.

417. Hou SH, Levin S, Ahola S, Lister J, Omicioli F, Dandrow R: Acute fatty liver of pregnancy. Survival with early caesarean section. Dig Dis Sci *29:*449–452, 1984.

418. Rolfes DB, Ishak KG: Acute fatty liver of pregnancy: a clinicopathologic study of 35 cases. Hepatology *5:*1149–1158, 1985.

419. Pockros PJ, Peters RL, Reynolds TB: Idiopathic fatty liver of pregnancy: findings in ten cases. Medicine *63:*1–11, 1984.

420. Ockner SA, Brunt EM, Cohn SM, Krul ES, Hanto DW, Peters MG: Fulminant hepatic failure caused by acute fatty liver of pregnancy treated by orthotopic liver transplantation. Hepatology *11:*59–64, 1990.

421. Killam AP, Dillard SH, Patton RC, Pederson PR: Pregnancy-induced hypertension complicated by acute liver disease and disseminated intravascular coagulation: five case reports. Am J Obstet *123:*823–828, 1975.

422. Riely CA: Acute hepatic failure at term. Diagnostic problems posed by broad clinical spectrum. Postgrad Med *66:*118–127, 1980.

423. Liebman HA, McGehee WG, Patch MJ, Feinstein DI: Severe depression of antithrombin III associated with disseminated intravascular coagulation in women with fatty liver of pregnancy. Ann Intern Med *98:*330–333, 1983.

424. Campillo B, Bernuau J, Witz M-O, Lorphelin J-M, Degott C, Rueff B, Benhamou J-P: Ultrasonography in acute fatty liver of pregnancy. Ann Intern Med *105:*383–384, 1986.

425. Schoeman MN, Batey RG, Wilcken B: Recurrent acute fatty liver of pregnancy associated with a fatty-acid oxidation defect in the offspring. Gastroenterology *100:*544–548, 1991.

426. Riely CA, Latham PS, Romero R, Duffy TP: Acute fatty liver of pregnancy. A reassessment based on observations in nine patients. Ann Intern Med *106:*703–706, 1987.

427. Kunelis CT, Peters JL, Edmondson HA: Fatty liver of pregnancy and its relationship to tetracycline therapy. Am J Med *38:*359–377, 1965.

428. Rolfes DB, Ishak KG: Acute fatty liver of pregnancy: a clinicopathologic study of 35 cases. Hepatology 5:1149–1158, 1985.

429. Burroughs AK, Seong NH, Dojcinov DM, Scheuer PJ, Sherlock S: Idiopathic acute fatty liver of pregnancy in 12 patients. Q J Med 51:481–497, 1982.

430. Sherlock S: Acute fatty liver of pregnancy and the microvesicular fat diseases. Gut 24:265–269, 1983.

431. Krejs GJ: Jaundice during pregnancy. Semin Liver Dis 3:73–82, 1983.

432. Frezza M, Centini G, Cammareri G, Le Grazie C, Di Padova C: S-adenosylmethionine for the treatment of intrahepatic cholestasis of pregnancy: results of a controlled clinical trial. Hepato-Gastroenterology 37(Suppl)2:122–125, 1990.

433. Frezza M, Pozzato G, Chiesa L, Stramentinoli G, Di Padova C: Reversal of intrahepatic cholestasis of pregnancy in women after high dose S-adenosyl-l-methionine administration. Hepatology 4:274–278, 1984.

434. Rosenthal T, Shani M, Deutsch V: The Budd-Chiari syndrome after pregnancy: report of two cases and a review of the literature. Am J Obstet Gynecol 113:789–792, 1972.

435. Khuroo MS, Datta DV: Budd-Chiari syndrome following pregnancy. Report of 16 cases, with roentgenologic, hemodynamic and histologic studies of the hepatic outflow tract. Am J Med 68:113–121, 1980.

436. Maddrey WC: Hepatic vein thrombosis (Budd-Chiari Syndrome): possible association with the use of oral contraceptives. Semin Liver Dis 7:32–37, 1987.

437. Maddrey WC: Hepatic vein thrombosis (Budd-Chiari syndrome), Hepatology 4:44S–46S, 1984.

438. Menu Y, Alison D, Lorphelin JM: Budd-Chiari syndrome: US evaluation. Radiology 157:761–764, 1985.

439. Baert AL, Fevery J, Marchal G: Early diagnosis of Budd-Chiari syndrome by computed tomography and ultrasonography: report of five cases. Gastroenterology 84:587–594, 1983.

440. Hales MR, Scatliff JH: Thrombosis of the inferior vena cava and hepatic veins (Budd-Chiari syndrome). Ann Intern Med 64:768–781, 1966.

441. Hyde E, Joyce D, Gurewich V: Intravascular coagulation during pregnancy and the puerperium. J Obstet Gynaecol Br. Commonw 80:1059–1066, 1973.

442. Lewis JH, Tice HL, Zimmerman HJ: Budd-Chiari syndrome associated with oral contraceptive therapy. Review of treatment of 47 cases. Dig Dis Sci 28:673–683, 1983.

443. Reynolds TB: Budd-Chiari Syndrome. In Diseases of the Liver, edited by L. Schiff, E.R. Schiff. 6th Edition. Philadelphia, J.B. Lippincott, 1987, pp. 1466–1473.

444. Ekberg H, Leyon J, Jeppsson B, Kristersson S, Lunderquist A, Tranberg KG, Holmin T: Hepatic rupture secondary to pre-eclampsia: report of a case treated conservatively. Ann Chir Gynaecol 73:350–353, 1984.

445. Greca FH, Coelho JC, Barros-Filho OD, Wallbach A: Ultrasonographic diagnosis of spontaneous rupture of the liver in pregnancy. JCU 12:515–516, 1984.

446. Monks PL, Fryar BG, Biggs WW: Spontaneous rupture of an hepatic adenoma in pregnancy with survival of mother and fetus. Aust NZ J Obstet Gynaecol 26:155–157, 1986.

447. Cahill KM: Hepatitis in pregnancy. Surg Gynecol Obstet 114:545–552, 1962.

448. Cossart YE: The outcome of hepatitis B virus infection in pregnancy. Postgrad Med J 53:610–613, 1977.

449. Snydman DR: Hepatitis in pregnancy. N Engl J Med 313:1398–1401, 1985.

450. D'Cruz IA, Balani SG, Iyer LS: Infectious hepatitis and pregnancy. Obstet Gynecol 31:449–455, 1968.

451. Borhanmanesh F, Haghighi P, Hekmat K, Rezaizadeh K, Ghavami AG: Viral hepatitis during pregnancy. Severity and effect on gestation. Gastroenterology 63:304–312, 1973.

452. Khuroo MS: Study of an epidemic of non-A non-b hepatitis. Possibility of another human hepatitis virus distinct from post-transfusion non-A non-B type. Am J Med 68:818–825, 1980.

453. Khuroo MS, Teli MR, Skidmore S, Sofi MA, Khuroo MI: Incidence and severity of viral hepatitis in pregnancy. Am J Med 70:252–255, 1981.

453a. Giovannini M, Tagger A, Riberg ML, Zucotti G, Roglani L, Grossi A, Ferrari P, Fiocchi A. Maternal infant transmission of hepatic C virus and HIV infections: a possible interaction. Lancet 335:1166, 1990.

454. Stevens CE, Beasley RP, Tsui J, Lee WC: Vertical transmission of hepatitis B antigen in Taiwan. N Engl J Med 292:771–774, 1975.

455. Derso A, Boxall EH, Tarlow MJ, Flewett TH: Transmission of HBsAg from mother to infant in four ethnic groups. Br Med J 1:949–952, 1978.

456. Alberti A, Diana S, Scullard GH, Eddleston ALWF, Williams R: Full and empty Dane particles in chronic hepatitis B virus infection: relation to hepatitis B e antigen and presence of liver change. Gastroenterology 75:869–874, 1978.

457. Lin HH, Lee TY, Chen DS, Sung JL, Ohto H, Etoh T, Kawana T, Mizuno M: Transplacental leakage of HBeAg-positive maternal blood as the most likely route in causing intrauterine infection with hepatitis B virus. J Pediatr 111:877–881, 1987.

458. Beasley RP, Stevens CE: Vertical transmission of HBV in interruption with globulin. In Viral Hepatitis, edited by G.N. Vyas, S.N. Cohen, R. Schmid. Turnbridge Wells, Abacus Press, 1979, pp. 333–345.

459. Varma RR, Michelsohn NH, Borkowf HI, Lewis JD: Pregnancy in cirrhotic and noncirrhotic portal hypertension. Obstet Gynecol 50:217–222, 1977.

460. Homburg R, Bayer I, Lurie B: Bleeding esophageal varices in pregnancy. A report of two cases. J Reprod Med 33:784–786, 1988.

461. Hermann RE, Esselstyn CB: The potential hazard of pregnancy in extrahepatic portal hypertension. Arch Surg 95:956–959, 1967.

462. Hietala SO, Andersson M, Emdin SO: Ectopic pregnancy in the liver. Report of a case and angiographic findings. Acta Chir Scand 149:633–636, 1983.

463. Harris GJ, Al-Jurf AS, Yuh WTC, Abu-Yousef MM: Intrahepatic pregnancy: a unique opportunity for evaluation with sonography, computed tomography and magnetic resonance imaging. JAMA 261:902–904, 1989.

464. Mear Y, Ekra JB, Raoelison S: Un cas de grossesse a implantation hepatique avec enfant vivant. Sem Hop Paris 41:1430–1433, 1965.

465. Kirby NG: Primary hepatic pregnancy. Br Med J 1:296, 1969.

466. Mitchell RW, Teare AJ: Primary hepatic pregnancy. A case report and review. S Afr Med J 65:220, 1984.

467. Petersdorf RG, Beeson PB: Fever of unexplained origin: report on 100 cases. Medicine 40:1–30, 1961.

468. Petersdorf RG: Fever of unknown origin. Ann Intern Med 70:864–866, 1969.

469. Telenti A, Hermans PE: Idiopathic granulomatosis manifesting as fever of unknown origin. Mayo Clin Proc 64:44–50, 1989.

470. Mitchell DP, Hanes TE, Hoyumpa AM Jr, Schenker S: Fever of unknown origin. Assessment of the value of percutaneous liver biopsy. Arch Intern Med 137:1001–1004, 1977.

471. Snydman DR, Bryan JA, Hanson B: Hemodialysis-associated hepatitis in the United States-1972. J Infect Dis 132:109–113, 1975.

472. Snydman DR, Bregman D, Bryan JA: Hemodialysis-associated hepatitis in the United States-1974. J Infect Dis 135:687–691, 1977.

473. Dienes HP, Gerharz C-D, Wagner R, Weber M, John H-D: Accumulation of hydroxyethyl starch (HES) in the liver of patients with renal failure and portal hypertension. J Hepatol 3:223–227, 1986.

474. Pfeifer U, Kult J, Förster H: Ascites als komplikation hepatischer speicherung von hydroxyethylstärke (HES9 bei langzeitdialyse). Klin Wschr 62:862–866, 1984.

475. Lanse SB, Arnold GL, Gowans JD, Kaplan MM: Low incidence of hepatotoxicity associated with long-term, low-dose oral methotrexate in the treatment of refractory psoriasis, psoriatic arthritis, and rheumatoid arthritis. An acceptable risk/benefit ratio. Dig Dis Sci 30:104–109, 1985.

476. Chaput JC, Poynard T, Naveau S, Penso D, Durrmeyer O, Suplisson D: Psoriasis, alcohol, and liver disease. Br Med J 291:25, 1985.

477. Birnie GG, Fitzsimons CP, Czarnecki D, Cooke A, Scobie G, Brodie MJ: Hepatic metabolic function in patients receiving long-term methotrexate therapy: comparison with topically treated psoriatics, patient controls and cirrhotics. Hepatogastroenterology 32:163–167, 1985.

478. Hendel J, Poulsen H, Nyfors B, Nyfors A: Changes in liver histology during methotrexate therapy of psoriasis correlated to the concentration of methotrexate and folate in erythrocytes. Acta Pharmacol Toxicol 56:321–324, 1985.

479. Kaplan MM: Methotrexate hepatoxicity and the premature reporting of Mark Twain's death: both greatly exaggerated. Hepatology 12:784–786, 1990.

480. Kaplan H, Klatskin G: Sarcoidosis, psoriasis, and gout: syndrome or coincidence? Yale J Biol Med 32:335–352, 1960.

481. MacSween RNM: Liver pathology associated with diseases of other organs. In Pathology of the Liver, edited by R.N.M. MacSween, P.P. Anthony, P.J. Scheuer. Edinburgh, Churchill Livingstone, 1987, pp. 646–674.

482. Oram S, Cochrane GM: Weber-Christian disease with visceral involvement. An example with hepatic enlargmeent. Br Med J 2:281–284, 1958.
483. Edge J, Dunger DB, Dillon MJ: Weber-Christian panniculitis and chronic active hepatitis. Eur J Pediatr 145:227–229, 1986.
484. Kimura H, Kako M, Yo K, Oda T: Alcoholic hyalins (Mallory bodies) in a case of Weber-Christian disease. Electron microscopic observations of liver involvement. Gastroenterology 78:807–812, 1980.
485. Pollack JD (ed): Reye's Syndrome. Proceedings of the Reye's Syndrome conference sponsored by the Children's Hospital Research Foundation, Columbus, OH. New York, Grune & Stratton, 1985.
486. Reye RDK, Morgan B, Baral J: Encephalopathy and fatty degeneration of the viscera: a disease entity in childhood. Lancet 2:749–752, 1963.
487. Snodgrass PJ, DeLong GR: Urea-cycle enzyme deficiencies and an increased nitrogen load producing hyperammonemia in Reye's syndrome. N Engl J Med 294:855–860, 1976.
488. Partin JC, Shubert WK, Partin JS: Mitochondrial ultrastructure in Reye's syndrome: encephalopathy and fatty degeneration of the viscera. N Engl J Med 258:1339–1343, 1971.
489. Schwarz KB, Larroya S, Vogler C, Sippel CJ, Homan S, Cockrell R, Schulze I: Role of influenza B virus in hepatic steatosis and mitochondrial abnormalities in a mouse model of Reye syndrome. Hepatology 13:96–103, 1991.
489a. Conn HO, Lieberthal MM. Reye's syndrome. In The Hepatic Coma Syndromes, edited by HO Conn and MM Lieberthal. Baltimore, Williams & Wilkins, 1978, pp. 141–168.
490. Hurwitz E, Barrett MJ, Bregman DS: Public Health Service study on Reye'e syndrome and medications. Report of the pilot phase. N Engl J Med 313:849–857, 1985.

Chapter 25
Neoplasms of the Liver and Intrahepatic Bile Ducts

Benign tumors

Benign epithelial neoplasms of the liver

Benign neoplasms of the liver are uncommon lesions that occur at any age and in either sex, although some occur predominantly in infancy, in adulthood, or in old age. Some show a striking predilection for males or females. Most of these tumors are small and asymptomatic, and are discovered incidentally during surgery or at autopsy. Indeed, almost one-third are discovered at autopsy having caused no clinical manifestations. They all have the capacity to grow and to induce symptoms, most commonly pain, which is usually proportional to their size. These tumors may present dramatically when they rupture or undergo thrombosis or infarction. In the few that develop portal hypertension, hemorrhage from varices may be an early sign. Their etiology is unknown although some are clearly congenital and some appear to be related to the ingestion of oral contraceptives. The diagnosis may be suggested by ultrasonography or computerized tomography, and is often confirmed by angiography. Definitive diagnosis is made by surgery or histologic examination. Definitive therapy is excision of the tumor.

Focal nodular hyperplasia (mixed adenoma, focal cirrhosis). Focal nodular hyperplasia occurs predominantly in women of childbearing age but may occur rarely in girls (1) or in older women (2). It is found much less commonly in men. These adenomas are usually asymptomatic, and three-fourths of them are discovered unexpectedly during laparotomy for other diseases or at autopsy (3). Occasionally, they present with pain, a palpable mass, or hepatomegaly. Portal hypertension has been reported (2). It has been noted that patients with multiple focal nodular hyperplasia often have other lesions, usually vascular such as hepatic hemangioma, or central nervous system lesions such as meningioma or astrocytoma (4,5).

The etiology is unknown. Traditional etiologic concepts include a hamartomatous origin or a reparative process in areas of focal injury (1).

Some reports have suggested a relationship with the use of oral contraceptives (6), but the weight of evidence does not support this association (7,8). Obviously, oral contraceptives cannot account for the tumors that occur in children or in men, or in those observed prior to the introduction of the pill. However, oral contraceptives apparently play a role in the growth of focal nodular hyperplasia, as shown by the larger size and the tendency to rupture of the tumors seen in women who take oral contraceptives as compared with those who do not, and by the appearance of preneoplastic histologic changes (9). The most widely held hypothesis suggests that focal nodular hyperplasia represents a local, hyperplastic response of all hepatic compo-

nents that produces a vascular malformation with arteriovenous anastomoses (10).

Grossly, focal nodular hyperplasia appears as a firm, sharply circumscribed but unencapsulated, round or lobulated mass, which is lighter in color than the surrounding liver. Their consistency is firm or rubbery and they tend to bulge out from the cut surface of the liver. They are variable in size, ranging from 1 to 10 cm in diameter, although three-fourths of them are less than 5 cm in diameter. Eighty percent are single, 10% double, and 10% multiple (3). They are usually found in the subcapsular region of the right lobe. Sometimes they are found deeper in the liver; only rarely are they pedunculated (1). Characteristically, cut sections reveal stellate, central fibrosis with radiating, branching septa that divide the tumor into nodules. Sometimes the tumor is associated with cavernomatous transformation.

The microscopic features of focal nodular hyperplasia resemble those of inactive postnecrotic cirrhosis (Fig. 565). The hepatocytes appear normal except for mild pleomorphism and an irregular, thickened plate pattern (Fig. 812). The hepatocytes may contain more glycogen than adjacent normal hepatocytes. The reticulin is intact (Fig. 813), and may actually be increased. The septa are smooth in contour with some fibrous spurs projecting into the nodules. They may contain canalicular bile plugs, copper deposition, and other cholestatic features. Numerous proliferating ductules derived by metaplasia from hepatocytes are often present (11). They are often infiltrated with moderate numbers of lymphocytes (Fig. 814). The larger arteries and veins may show eccentric or concentric intimal fibrosis or hypertrophy of the media, which may sometimes cause occlusion of the lumen (Fig. 402).

Focal nodular hyperplasia can be readily differentiated from hepatocellular adenomas, which are encapsulated by a pseudocapsule of compressed, collapsed hepatic parenchyma, and tend to be larger and softer. In adenomas the reticulin pattern is normal or incomplete (12). Some hepatocellular adenomas, particularly those associated with oral contraceptive use, may show atypical features such as the presence of septa that make differentiation difficult. Reliable identification depends on both gross inspection of the resected tumor and microscopic examination. Magnetic resonance usually shows a characteristic pattern, although the two lesions may mimic each other (13). Blind, percutaneous needle biopsies of the liver are unreliable, since they may miss the tumor entirely, show only the tumor, or fail to show the overall pattern of the lesion even when both normal and neoplastic tissue are obtained. Both tumors may occur in the same liver (14,15), probably coincidentally.

Although there is little evidence to prove that focal nodular hyperplasia is a premalignant lesion, several cases have been reported in which tumors that appeared to be focal nodular hyperplasia were found on histologic examination to be fibrolamellar hepatocellular carcinomas (12). Such cases raise the possibility that focal nodular hyperplasia may rarely undergo malignant degeneration, but histologic misinterpretation is more likely (16).

Hepatocellular adenoma (benign hepatoma). Ninety percent of the cases of hepatocellular adenoma, which is an uncommon tumor, occur in women of childbearing age. This tumor occurs with about half the frequency of focal nodular hyperplasia. It is uncommon in men and is rare in children (3).

Clinically, it is frequently a symptomatic tumor. Pain, the most common symptom, is caused by expansion of the tumor within the liver substance, hemorrhage into the tumor, or rupture of the tumor into the peritoneum. Almost one-third of such adenomas show evidence of rupture or hemorrhage (3,6). Often, hepatomegaly is noted on physical examination, surgery, or imaging studies performed during the management of other, non-hepatic disorders. More than half show defects in uptake on colloid scanning. Often, displacement of the stomach, duodenum, or colon or extrinsic pressure on the gallbladder is seen on contrast studies of the GI tract. A palpable mass is found in almost two-thirds of cases.

Liver function tests are usually normal. Mild elevations of serum alkaline phosphatase or transaminase activity are occasionally present. Alpha-fetoprotein levels are almost uniformly normal. The etiology of hepatocellular adenomas is unknown. The predilection of hepatocellular adenoma for women of childbearing age and its apparent relationship to the use of oral contraceptives suggest that it may be hormone-dependent (6,17,18). Since oral contraceptives were introduced, the incidence of hepatocellular adenomas has increased greatly (3). Sometimes, the adenomas shrink and disappear after the withdrawal of oral contraceptives (19). Sometimes, they do not (20). In addition, they tend to recur after resection in patients who continue to take oral contraceptives. Hepatic adenomas occasionally develop in young adults who have never received steroid hormones (21). We have observed overt dysplasia in the hepatocellular adenoma of a 46-year-old man not known to have ever received any hormonal therapy (Fig. 815).

Hepatocellular adenomas are also associated with the ingestion of anabolic steroids (22). They are seen most commonly in young men who have received testosterone for hypogonadism (23). They have been observed in athletes taking anabolic steroids to enhance athletic performance (24).

Benign adenomas tend to be larger and to rupture or bleed more often in patients on the pill than in those who are not (3). The rare instances of apparent malignant transformation of hepatocellular adenomas (25) and of foci of dysplasia and atypia have usually occurred in patients on oral contraceptives and never in adenomas unassociated with their use.

It has been estimated that there is an increased risk of hepatocellular adenoma in women taking oral contraceptives, which increases with the age of the subject and the duration of administration (3,18). Subjects who have not taken oral contraceptives or who have taken them for relatively short periods, i.e., less than two years, develop hepatocellular adenoma at an annual rate of 1 to 1.3 per million. In those on oral contraceptives for longer periods, the annual incidence is 30 per million or 30 times as high (3). There is, however, no definitive proof of an etiologic association between these adenomas and oral contraceptives. Conceivably, oral contraceptives merely accelerate the growth of adenomas caused by other factors, perhaps by affecting the vasculature of the preexisting tumors. If oral contraceptives do play a role in the development of hepatocellular

adenomas, their estrogenic components appear to be the factor or factors involved. The suggestion that mestranol has greater oncogenic potential than ethinyl estradiol (3,22) has not been unequivocally established, since the former has been in use for a much longer period than the latter. Cytoplasmic progesterone receptors have been found in hepatic adenomas (26).

Rare cases of hepatocellular adenoma have been reported in patients with type I glycogen storage disease (27).

Grossly, hepatocellular adenomas appear as circumscribed masses that are partially or completely enclosed by a pseudocapsule derived from compressed and collapsed hepatic parenchyma. They vary in size from 1 to 20 cm in diameter, but are usually greater than 5 cm (Fig. 200). They are single in 70% of cases and double and multiple in about 15% of each (28). Multiple adenomas may also be found in men (29). Occasionally, they are pedunculated. On cross section the adenomas are lighter in color than the adjacent liver and have a fleshy appearance. They do not project above the cut surface as focal nodular hyperplasia does. They are easily differentiated from focal nodular hyperplasia by the absence of a radiating, central, fibrous core. They often show foci of hemorrhage. Liver cell adenomas are hypervascular. The arterial supply originates at the periphery from which multiple, parallel vessels enter the center (3). The angiographic appearance of hepatocellular adenoma, however, may not be distinguishable from that of focal nodular hyperplasia (30).

Microscopically, the neoplastic cells closely resemble normal hepatocytes, but vary greatly in size and in intensity of staining (Fig. 816). Large, pale cells, which tend to occur at the periphery of the tumor (Fig. 816), have an increased glycogen content as shown by PAS staining (Fig. 817). They may be difficult to distinguish from well-differentiated hepatocellular carcinoma (16). Sometimes, these neoplastic cells show foci of dysplasia or atypia (Fig. 815). Occasionally, they contain fat droplets. The neoplastic cells are arranged in thick, irregular plates (Fig. 818) that occasionally form rosettes or pseudoducts, some of which may contain bile thrombi (Fig. 819). The uniformity of the size of the cells and narrow slit-like sinusoids may sometimes create a sheet-like, parenchymal pattern (3). By both light and electron microscopy the tumor cells of adenomas are virtually identical to normal hepatocytes (31,32). Characteristically, these tumors contain no portal tracts, but numerous thin-walled veins may be present without accompanying bile ducts (Fig. 818). Some patients, especially those on oral contraceptives, may exhibit sinusoidal congestion (Fig. 820), peliotic cavities (Fig. 821), or foci of perivascular hemorrhage (Fig. 822). Some authors believe that these peliotic cavities may represent vascular ectasia rather than true peliosis (3,33). The tumors of patients on oral contraceptives may also contain fibrous septa with numerous proliferated, small bile ductules (Fig. 823), but no interlobular bile ducts. Some septa appear to be the result of organized hemorrhage or infarction (Fig. 824). Frequently, the latter show hemosiderin-containing macrophages. The reticulin is often sparse or poorly developed (Fig. 825), especially in the center of the tumor, but may be normal in some areas. The reticulin pattern is useful in differentiating hepatocellular adenomas from focal nodular hyperplasia in which the reticulin pattern is normal (Fig. 826) or even increased (Fig. 813). In two of our patients with hepatocellular adenoma who were taking oral contraceptives, medium sized arteries exhibited extensive thickening of their walls with reduplication of elastic fibers (Fig. 827).

Although focal nodular hyperplasia can be readily distinguished from hepatocellular adenomas in classic cases, in women on oral contraceptives, adenomas may show atypical features. They may be traversed by septa that contain numerous small ductules that may simulate focal nodular hyperplasia. The reliability of blind, percutaneous liver biopsies in differentiating the two tumors is questionable. When a biopsy specimen of a tumor is small, it may be mistaken for normal liver or a regenerating nodule. In large specimens, especially in wedge biopsies obtained at laparotomy, the absence of portal tracts and bile ducts and the absence or paucity of reticulin are most helpful in differentiating the two tumors.

Hepatocellular adenoma can be differentiated clinically from hepatocellular carcinoma on the basis of the normality of serum 5′-nucleotidase and α-fetoprotein levels in the former (3), and, ultimately, by their histologic appearance.

Hepatocellular adenomas have on rare occasions been reported to show areas of hepatocellular carcinoma (16), usually in patients who had been taking oral contraceptives. The occasional presence of foci of dysplasia and atypia in hepatocellular adenomas is compatible with the possibility that these benign tumors may, rarely, undergo malignant transformation. The differentiation of benign and malignant lesions is not absolute (16). Unlike hepatic adenomas, hepatocellular carcinomas are not associated with the ingestion of oral contraceptive agents (34).

Hepatic adenomatosis is an uncommon disorder that is characterized by the presence of numerous benign, hepatic adenomas (29). The disease differs from hepatocellular adenoma, which is defined as the presence of not more than two tumors (3). Although the individual adenomas in the two disorders are identical histologically, these two disorders are different clinically. Hepatic adenomas are usually seen in women after oral contraceptive usage, and exhibit normal serum alkaline phosphatase and gamma-glutamyl transpeptidase activity. Hepatic adenomatosis occurs with equal frequency in men and women who have not taken oral contraceptives and is characterized by elevated serum alkaline phosphatase and gamma-glutamyl transpeptidase activity. However, some authors believe that the reported cases of hepatic adenomatosis (35) are really examples of nodular regenerative hyperplasia (3).

These benign tumors must be differentiated from macroregenerative nodules, which are also known as cirrhotic pseudotumors and which occur in the setting of massive hepatic necrosis or chronic hepatocellular destructive lesions such as cirrhosis (36). In cirrhotic patients, they are thought to be premalignant lesions (22).

Bile duct adenoma (benign cholangioma, cholangioadenoma). Bile duct adenomas, tumors that are classified as hamartomas by some pathologists, are rare. They occur about twice as commonly in men as in women, usually over the age of 50 (37). They are invariably small and asymptomatic. They tend to be less than 1 cm in diameter but rarely may be greater than 2 cm. They are firm tumors usually located in the subcapsular region of the right lobe, but are occasionally found deep within the liver substance. They are usually solitary, occasionally double, and rarely multiple.

Histologically, they consist of closely packed, small, branching bile ducts lined by cuboidal or columnar epithelium embedded in mature, fibrous stroma, which may sometimes be scanty (Fig. 383). There is often lymphocytic infiltration of the periphery. Occasionally, they contain intact portal triads.

These adenomas must be differentiated from metastatic ad-

enocarcinoma. The adenomas closely resemble von Meyenburg complexes, but they differ in that their fibrous stroma tends to be less abundant (Fig. 382) and are not localized to portal triads (38). The ducts are smaller, nondilated, and do not contain inspissated bile (21).

Bile duct cystadenoma. Bile duct cystadenomas are rare tumors that affect women predominantly and, usually, in their middle years (21). Less than 100 such tumors have been documented in the literature (21). They characteristically present as a palpable mass in the right upper quadrant. Occasionally, the mass may cause abdominal pain and, uncommonly, obstructive jaundice (21,39). These tumors may arise within the liver or from the extrahepatic bile ducts. They may appear as cystic lesions by ultrasonography or as "cold spots" on liver scan (40). They can cause extrinsic pressure on the stomach or duodenum and may displace the right ureter. Bile duct cystadenomas do not recur following resection. However, unresected tumors occasionally undergo malignant transformation (39).

Grossly, these tumors are large and circumscribed and range from 3 to 25 cm in diameter. They are multiloculated cystic tumors that contain large volumes of opalescent fluid. Sometimes, clear, mucoid fluid is found, however.

Microscopically, they are lined by mucin-producing, cuboidal or columnar bile duct epithelium that often shows papillary projections into the lumen. They may exhibit a primitive mesenchymal stroma that is made up of spindle cells (21). The cystic areas are separated by dense bands of collagen that may contain smooth muscle. Macrophages may contain lipid or pigment.

Bile duct cystadenomas must be differentiated from various forms of solitary cysts, polycystic disease, or hamartomas. Such cystic lesions may show low cuboidal epithelium, but never show columnar epithelium, papillary infoldings, or dense collagenous stroma. Usually, they do not produce mucin.

A variant of this tumor, *hepatobiliary cystadenoma with mesenchymal stroma,* which is seen almost exclusively in women, has been reported (41,42). It is characterized by the presence of spindle cells beneath the cuboidal epithelium of the cyst (Fig. 828).

Biliary papillomatosis. Biliary papillomatosis, a rare disorder that is considered to be a variant of bile duct cystadenoma, occurs mainly in men (3). It is characterized by the presence of many multicentric papillomas of the biliary mucosa that project into the lumen of the biliary tract (43,44). Clinically, it is manifested by recurrent bouts of obstructive jaundice and cholangitis that result, in part, from the production of thick mucus by the tumor (45,46). It is probably not as rare as has been thought.

Histologically, the papillomas are composed of branches of well-differentiated cuboidal or columnar bile duct epithelium emanating from a central core of loose connective tissue. Occasionally, some of the cells show foci of atypia, and, rarely, the papillomas undergo malignant transformation, giving rise to an invasive adenocarcinoma (47).

Therapy consists principally of curettage. Rarely, lobectomy is done when the lesion is restricted to a single, major intrahepatic duct (44). Invariably, however, the lesion recurs, often terminating in death from obstructive jaundice and sepsis.

The only case of biliary papillomatosis that we have observed occurred in a 45-year-old man who had ulcerative colitis of 25 years' duration. He had had recurrent, prolonged bouts of obstructive jaundice and suppurative cholangitis over a 15-year period. Endoscopic, retrograde cholangiography showed a pattern compatible with sclerosing cholangitis. Laparotomy demonstrated an unobstructed common bile duct, narrowing of the common hepatic duct, and chronic cholangitis without gallstones. Microscopically, the gallbladder showed polypoid hyperplasia of the mucosa (Fig. 829). Death from sepsis and hepatic failure followed surgery. Autopsy revealed that both the right and left hepatic ducts were lined by papillomas (Fig. 830) and showed areas of degenerative mucosa, necrosis, and inflammation (Fig. 831). Secondary biliary cirrhosis and multiple hepatic abscesses were found. The diagnosis of biliary papillomatosis had not been suspected.

Benign adrenal rest tumors. Small foci of heterotopic, adrenal cortical tissue are occasionally found in the capsule of the liver of newborn infants (48). These rests usually disappear spontaneously during the first year of life, but may rarely give rise to benign or malignant tumors.

These tumors occur in children and adults. They are asymptomatic when small, but when large present as an abdominal mass, especially in children. Rarely, they produce adrenocortical hormones that cause virilism or Cushing's syndrome (49). Some investigators believe that only tumors that show such clinical features of adrenocortical hyperactivity or can be shown to contain adrenocortical hormones can be classified as adrenal rest tumors.

Adrenal rest tumors vary in size from 1 to 10 cm in diameter. They are sharply circumscribed and may be partially or completely encapsulated. On cut section they are yellow and show a finely lobulated surface. Occasional foci of necrosis, hemorrhage, or calcification are seen.

Microscopically, the neoplastic cells closely resemble adrenal cortical cells. They are polygonal in shape with abundant eosinophilic finely vacuolated cytoplasm. The nuclei are small and show little or no mitotic activity. They are arranged in cords separated by capillaries that resemble the zona fasciculata of the adrenal cortex. Occasionally, the cells are arranged in broad, irregular sheets. The cells are set in a fine, loose, fibrous stroma that gives the appearance of poorly defined lobulation.

Differentiation between the benign and malignant forms of adrenal rest tumors is sometimes difficult. Occasionally, after resection, "benign" tumors recur and even metastasize. Sometimes, it is not possible to differentiate this tumor from hepatocellular carcinoma (48).

Nodular regenerative hyperplasia (Nodular transformation, partial nodular transformation, diffuse nodular hyperplasia). Nodular regenerative hyperplasia, a lesion that is not proved to be neoplastic, occurs in patients of both sexes and all ages (3,4), although it is most common in old age (4). It is often associated with diverse, chronic, nonhepatic disorders including collagen-vascular, myeloproliferative, or lymphoproliferative diseases, bone marrow transplantation, and the toxic oil syndrome (50). It is not rare, occurring in 2 to 3% of autopsied patients (4,51), and lesser degrees of nodular transformation are seen at autopsy in an additional 10% (4). It is seen in 30% of patients who have had bone marrow transplantation (52). It may be manifested clinically by bleeding varices or rupture of a nodule, or it may be clinically silent (53). Pathologically, the liver is characterized by nodularity, with nodules ranging from 0.1 to 10 cm in diameter. The architecture of the liver is preserved, but hypertrophic, cirrhosis-like nodules are scattered

throughout with intervening areas of hepatic atrophy (54). The hepatocytes, which are hyperplastic and larger than normal, are often arranged in cell plates two or more cells thick (55).

The pathogenesis is considered by most experts to be neoplastic by virtue of the similarity of the nodules to those of focal nodular hyperplasia and to those induced in experimental carcinogenesis (56) or hepatotoxin-induced neoplasia (57,58). It is also postulated to be of vascular origin, resulting from decreased portal blood flow of many causes (4,51). It does not appear to have premalignant potential (60).

The diagnosis of nodular regenerative hyperplasia, which may mimic cirrhosis, is difficult, since the lesions are superimposed on a normal lobular architecture, there is little fibrosis, and needle biopsy cores are often too small (59). Even imaging techniques cannot establish the presence of large nodules (60).

Histologically, nodular regenerative hyperplasia is characterized by multiple hyperplastic nodules diffusely distributed throughout the parenchyma with little or no fibrosis. The nodularity may be most clearly shown by reticulin stain (Fig. 832), which can also demonstrate the typical thick hepatic cell plates (Fig. 833).

Studies have shown that α-l-antitrypsin, which is often found in regenerating hepatocytes (61), is frequently present in the regenerating cells in nodular regenerative hyperplasia (62). The regenerating cells are larger and paler than surrounding atrophic or compressed hepatocytes on H & E staining. Using immunohistologic staining of liver biopsies, a characteristic, periportal pattern of A_1AT-deposition was demonstrated (Fig. 834). Furthermore, the A_1AT appeared as a diffuse, granular, cytoplasmic pattern as opposed to the globular pattern seen in A_1AT deficiency (Figs. 152–154). The patients' studies had no clinical or laboratory evidence of A_1AT deficiency. The presence of such staining may be helpful in the diagnosis of nodular regenerative hyperplasia.

Benign mesenchymal tumors

Cavernous hemangioma. Hemangiomas, which are sponge-like, blood-filled mesenchymal tumors, are the most common benign tumors of the liver (22,48). They occur in 0.4 to 2% of patients at autopsy (63,64). Furthermore, the liver is the most frequent organ in the body in which hemangiomas are found, comprising about 20% of the total (48,63).

They can occur in patients of any age from neonatal to late adult life, but are uncommon in children and are usually discovered after the age of 40. They occur more commonly in women (63), in whom they appear to develop at an earlier age, but are more commonly seen in older men than senile women (65). They have been reported to occur especially frequently in multiparous women, and they have been observed to grow rapidly during pregnancy (66). This association with pregnancy, plus the observation of rapid growth in women on contraceptive steroids, suggests that estrogens may play a role in the pathogenesis or in the rate of growth of cavernous hemangiomas (48) and in other neoplasms (67), but there is little firm evidence to support this view (3).

More than 85% of hemangiomas are small and asymptomatic and are discovered at laparotomy for unrelated conditions or at autopsy (48,64). Large hemangiomas tend to present as either an abdominal mass or as hepatomegaly (68). Occasionally, they give rise to pain due to displacement of other organs or to thrombosis or rupture of the hemangioma (69). Rupture may occur spontaneously or after trauma. Rarely, large hemangiomas present with coagulopathy with thrombocytopenia, fibrinogenopenia, and fibrogenolysis, and appear to represent instances of nondisseminated, extravascular coagulopathy due to the consumption of clotting factors within the tumor (70). Jaundice or other clinical evidence of liver disease aside from hepatomegaly is extremely rare. Sometimes a bruit can be heard over the tumor, but bruits are uncommon and nonspecific (71).

The tumors may be demonstrated by radiocontrast examinations when they displace hollow organs, by ultrasonography (72–74), computerized tomography (75), arteriography (76,77), or nuclear magnetic resonance examination (78). Characteristic angiograms show multiple large, feeding vessels and large, dilated, ring- or C-shaped spaces within the tumor (75–77), which retain the contrast material (77). Colloid liver scans may show areas of decreased uptake. Blood flow scans may show areas of increased uptake, indicating the vascular nature of the tumor. Large, long-standing tumors may be calcified and may show a radiating, star-like pattern of calcification (79).

Liver function tests are rarely abnormal. Elevated serum bilirubin and alkaline phosphatase levels have occasionally been noted, usually in patients with extensive replacement of the liver by multiple hemangiomas.

Grossly, cavernous hemangiomas usually appear as reddish purple masses just beneath Glisson's capsule, but may be deeper in the parenchyma. Occasionally, large hemangiomas are pedunculated. Ninety percent of hemangiomas are single, but they may be multiple and occasionally replace most of the hepatic parenchyma. They vary in size from microscopic to more than 30 cm in diameter, but are usually less than 5 cm in diameter. They are well circumscribed but unencapsulated. They are usually sponge-like and compressible, but when sclerosed or calcified, they may be firm or hard, respectively.

Microscopically, they show multiple large vascular channels lined by a single layer of flat endothelial cells and separated by slender, fibrous septa (Fig. 835). When large, hemangiomas may compress the surrounding hepatic parenchyma (Fig. 836). In some cases, extensive fibrosis replaces the vascular channels producing a ''sclerosed hemangioma'' (Fig. 837) (3) or ''necrotic nodule'' [(80); Fig. 838]. Deposits of calcium may be found in septa or in vascular channels where they may appear as phleboliths.

The diagnosis can be established angiographically or histologically. Needle biopsy is contraindicated for fear of hemorrhage when a hemangioma is suspected on the basis of a compressible, hepatic mass, a hypervascular lesion, or a bruit over the tumor, all of which are suggestive of hemangioma (80). Except for finding a spongy, compressible mass, which is rare, these other signs of hemangioma are uncommon and nonspecific. Bruits occur frequently in hepatocellular carcinomas and in other tumors as well as in non-neoplastic lesions. Calcium may be deposited in hepatocellular carcinomas and in metastatic tumors. Needle biopsy of large, vascular, hepatic tumors should be avoided. Furthermore, when the diagnosis of hemangioma is obvious, liver biopsy is not necessary. The hazards of needle biopsy of small hemangiomas are unknown, since the reported accidents have occurred in patients with large hemangiomas.

Infantile hemangioendothelioma. Infantile hemangioendotheliomas are congenital tumors that become clinically evident or are found at autopsy during the first few weeks or months of life (81–83). They are uncommon between infancy and four years of age and are rare in adults, but account for more than 10% of infantile tumors (22). Hemangioendotheliomas, which are the most common mesenchymal tumors of the liver in childhood, occur twice as frequently in girls as in boys. Some infantile cases are malignant when first detected; others appear to undergo malignant transformation. Most hemangioendotheliomas encountered in adults prove to be malignant and should be classified as angiosarcomas.

Similar hemangioendotheliomas are found concomitantly in other tissues (84). Almost all have multiple cutaneous lesions, and, less commonly, tumors of the bone and lungs are seen (85). Although these multiple lesions are probably of multicentric origin, in some instances they appear to be metastatic.

Clinically, the hepatic lesions are extensive and symptomatic. The majority of cases present with congestive heart failure associated with progressive enlargement of the abdomen due to massive hepatomegaly (86). Some show a localized hepatic mass. The high output cardiac failure is caused by arteriovenous shunts within the tumor in most instances. Jaundice occurs in about one-third the patients as do elevated levels of serum transaminases. Inconstant features include calcium deposition in the tumors by radiologic examination, microangiopathic hemolytic anemia, or thrombocytopenia. The latter two findings may represent the effects of the injury of blood cells erythrocytes and the trapping of platelets in the tortuous, narrow, vascular network of the tumor and may, in turn, give rise to jaundice, anemia, hemosiderosis, and extramedullary hematopoiesis (87). The diagnosis of hemangioendothelioma may be established by celiac or hepatic arteriography, which show the arteries of the tumor to be dilated and may demonstrate blushes of contrast media characteristic of arteriovenous shunts.

Although infantile hemangioendotheliomas are benign, they frequently lead to death within six months as a result of cardiac or hepatic failure. Rarely, the tumor may regress spontaneously. Recovery has followed the resection of solitary tumors. Hepatic artery ligation and embolization have led to recovery (83,86,88), as have corticosteroid therapy (85) and irradiation (81,89). Vigorous treatment of the heart failure is important, but once high output cardiac failure has developed, therapy is usually unsuccessful.

Grossly, the tumors are almost always multicentric and involve both lobes. They are sharply circumscribed, but are not encapsulated. They may give the liver a nodular appearance. Occasionally, they pulsate; rarely, they may rupture. They vary in size from 0.5 to 15 cm, but tend to be <3 cm in diameter. Multicentric nodules are soft and spongy, and vary in color from reddish purple to white or yellow with bluish purple centers and foci of hemorrhage. Solitary tumors tend to be large and firm, located in the right lobe, and may, occasionally, contain cystic lesions.

Microscopically, two different histologic patterns have been described (81). Type 1, the more benign form, shows numerous irregular, dilated, and compressed vascular channels. They are usually lined by a single layer of plump, benign-appearing, endothelial cells. Occasionally, multilayered endothelial cells are seen. The endothelial cells are surrounded by reticulin fibers and are separated from one another by variable amounts of interstitial connective tissue, which is usually sparse, but may occasionally appear myxomatous. Some tumors contain large areas of fibrosis, hemorrhage, infarction, or focal calcification. Occasionally, the central zones contain large, dilated, vascular channels that resemble those of cavernous hemangioma. In many instances, bile ductules lined by cuboidal or columnar epithelium and small plates of hepatocytes intermingle within the vascular channels. Figures 839 and 840 illustrate a type 1 hemangioendothelioma in a nine-week-old girl who presented with a 6 by 9 cm, right upper quadrant mass and a holosystolic cardiac murmur and anemia, but no signs of congestive heart failure or thrombocytopenia. The tumor, which was highly vascular by angiography, was not resectable, but was biopsied.

Type 2 is similar, but the vascular channels are less well defined. They are usually lined by multilayered endothelial cells that frequently bud into their lumens. Indeed, some endothelial cells fill the vascular channels. The endothelial cells are more pleomorphic and hyperchromatic. In some areas, they are arranged in the form of branching and budding trabeculi that project into tortuous vascular channels or lie free in extravascular spaces. Foci of extramedullary hematopoiesis commonly occur within tumor nodules. The differentiation of type 1 and type 2 is not always simple (22).

Fibroma. Hepatic fibromas are exceedingly rare tumors. They present as progressively enlarging abdominal masses that may achieve enormous size and may weigh more than 10 pounds (90,91). They are firm and lobulated and are located in the parenchyma just beneath Glisson's capsule. They are hard or rubbery in consistency and have a coarsely textured, gray-white or light tan cut surface. Microscopically, they are made up of interlacing bundles of collagen that are occasionally arranged in whorls and contain fibroblast-like spindle cells and numerous silver-staining, reticulin fibers (3).

Lipoma. Lipomas are uncommon tumors (92) that tend to occur in women in the fourth or fifth decades. They are being discovered much more frequently now that computerized tomography is widely available (93). They are often associated with obesity. They are usually less than 2 cm in diameter and are incidental findings at autopsy in most instances (92). Occasionally, they present as abdominal masses or as hepatomegaly, and may show a defect on liver scan. Grossly, they are circumscribed masses of mature adipose tissue, which on the cut surface are yellow and greasy. Rarely, they may contain foci of hematopoiesis (myelolipomas) (94) or muscle fibers (angiomyolipomas) (95). When multiple thick-walled vessels are present, they are classified as angiolipomas. *Pseudolipomas* (ectopic coelomolipomas) are epiploic appendages that become attached to the liver surface or, rarely, are found within the hepatic parenchyma (96). Hepatic lipomas must be differentiated from focal fatty degeneration of the liver, which is a nonneoplastic disorder of unknown etiology (97).

Leiomyoma. Only a few cases of leiomyoma have been reported (48,98). They tend to occur in women and to present as large, encapsulated, firm masses that are made up of elongated, parallel bundles of well-differentiated, smooth muscle cells. Leiomatous hemangiomas may be difficult to differentiate from primary leiomyomas (99).

Presumably, such tumors are derived from the smooth muscle of hepatic blood vessels. It may be difficult to exclude a primary hepatic leiomyoma from a metastatic leiomyosarcoma originating in the uterus or intestinal tract, except when an autopsy is available.

Benign tumors of mixed origin

Mesenchymal hamartoma (hamartoma, lymphangioma, pseudocystic mesenchymal tumor). Mesenchymal hamartomas are uncommon lesions that occur more frequently than focal nodular hyperplasia or hepatic adenomas (3,100,101). These lesions occur largely in infants, predominantly male. They usually present as an abdominal mass or as enlargement of the abdomen. The lesions, which tend to be large, average greater than a kilogram in weight. They often contain cysts filled with a gelatinous or clear yellow fluid (3). Histologically, they consist of disorganized, loose, mesenchymal tissue in which are embedded bile ducts and hepatocytes [(102,103); Figs. 841–843]. The cysts are derived rfrom mesenchymal, lymphatic, or biliary tissue (Figs. 844–846). These lesions do not undergo malignant degeneration, but undifferentiated, embryonal hepatic sarcomas have been considered to be the malignant equivalent of these tumors.

Benign teratoma. Nonmalignant teratomas are extremely rare lesions that are found in infants or early childhood (104–106). A palpable abdominal mass brings these tumors to medical attention. Histologically, they contain tissue derived from all three germ layers (Figs. 847–849), usually skin, intestinal mucosa, and bone (Figs. 850–852).

Malignant Tumors

Malignant epithelial neoplasms of the liver

Hepatocellular carcinoma. Hepatocellular carcinoma is by far the most common primary malignant tumor of the liver. Indeed, it is one of the most common tumors in the world, although not in the West (107–109) though its prevalence is rapidly increasing in the West. It affects men predominantly, chiefly in the fifth through the seventh decades of life. In Africa and in Asia it tends to occur at a much younger age than in the United States and Europe. Hepatocellular carcinoma occasionally occurs in children between the ages of 5 and 15 years. In infants under the age of 2 years, however, it is much less common than hepatoblastomas.

There are striking geographic differences in the incidence of hepatocellular carcinoma. It occurs most frequently in China, Southeast Asia, and southern Africa, but is relatively uncommon in the United States, Europe, and North Africa (110). Its prevalence parallels the frequency of HBV infection, the distribution of aflatoxin contamination, and the incidence of chronic alcoholism. These associations are individual but overlap. The prevalence of hepatocellular carcinoma is high in black Africans, but is relatively low in white Africans or in black Americans of African descent. It is uncommon in Central and South America where tropical climate, malnutrition, and rural poverty mimic that seen in Southeast Asia. High mortality from liver cancer has been reported in Greece (111) and, surprisingly, in Switzerland (112). Such patterns are more likely to be ethnic or environmental than genetic. Genetic factors have been implicated, but have not been established. Hepatocellular carcinoma seems genetically linked with α-1-antitrypsin deficiency (113), but this association has not been confirmed. The association with hemochromatosis exists only when cirrhosis is present (114).

Recent observations suggest that the prevalence of hepatocellular carcinoma in the United States is rising, but that this increment is not adequately explained by increased alcoholism or HBV infections. These findings suggest that unidentified environmental hepatocarcinogens may be involved.

Association of hepatocellular carcinoma and cirrhosis. There is a clear-cut, poorly understood relationship between hepatocellular carcinoma and cirrhosis (110,115). In 70 to 90% of cases, primarily from the West, hepatocellular carcinoma is associated with cirrhosis. In China and Southeast Asia, hepatocellular carcinoma is more common than cirrhosis. In some countries, usually Western, liver cancer tends to develop as a complication of long-standing cirrhosis (115–117); in Asia and Africa the two diseases tend to arise simultaneously (118), but exceptions have been reported. In Japan, hepatocellular carcinoma often develops in patients with chronic viral hepatitis *before* cirrhosis develops (117,119). It seems clear that hepatic cell carcinomas may be small, clinically silent, and associated with normal α-fetoprotein levels for long periods of time before discovery (119). Furthermore, cirrhosis is clinically silent in more than half of those who develop hepatocellular carcinoma (120). Silent cirrhosis is more apt to develop in areas in which the incidence of hepatocellular carcinoma is high, in patients who are HBsAg-positive and who have cryptogenic cirrhosis (120). The incidence of hepatocellular carcinoma in cirrhosis varies in different parts of the world. In China, Japan, Southeast Asia, and Africa, it ranges from 40 to 50%; in the United States and Europe, it runs from 5 to 15%.

A primary factor that affects these differences is the type of cirrhosis. Alcoholism, HBV infection, and aflatoxins appear to predispose to the development of hepatocellular carcinoma (109), and primary biliary cirrhosis may also do so (121). In general, hepatocellular carcinoma is more common in macronodular cirrhosis, irrespective of etiology. Although alcoholic cirrhosis is typically micronodular in type, nodule size increases with the duration of the cirrhosis (122). Geography may play a role in determining the type of features of hepatocellular carcinoma (123).

In noncirrhotic patients, the development of hepatocellular carcinoma is more common in younger individuals and in those who are HBV carriers (124). These interrelationships contribute to the geographic differences. Clearly, however, once cirrhosis has developed, whatever the cause, the risk of liver cancer is increased and rises with the duration of survival. This probably reflects the experimental observations that increased cell replication enhances the carcinogenic effects of many substances (125).

Liver cell dysplasia in non-neoplastic portions of the liver has been noted more frequently in cirrhotic patients with hepatocellular carcinoma than in those without it (126,127), but not always (128). This controversy has been reviewed (129).

The possible mechanisms that underlie the development of hepatocellular carcinoma in cirrhosis include: (1) a direct consequence of hepatocellular regeneration, which is stimulated in cirrhosis; (2) a neoplastic reaction to the factor responsible for the hepatocellular injury and the cirrhosis; (3) functional and circulatory changes that render the cirrhotic liver more susceptible to environmental and endogenous carcinogens; and (4) hepatocellular dysplasia. Dysplasia in cirrhosis with or without hepatocellular carcinoma is greater in HBsAg-positive than in HBsAg-negative cases (130). Liver cell dysplasia has been found

frequently in NANB viral hepatitis and appears to be associated with the giant cell form of hepatocellular carcinoma (131).

The incidence of hepatocellular carcinoma varies in different types of cirrhosis and other hepatic lesions. It occurs in 3 to 10% of alcoholic cirrhosis and in 10 to 25% of patients with hemochromatosis (132). It has been seen in 10 to 40% of patients with postnecrotic cirrhosis. The geographic differences in incidence appear to reflect the prevalence of HBV infection, and are highest in HBsAg-positive cases. Hepatocellular carcinoma is extremely rare in Wilson's disease, although it may occur (133).

Retrospective studies suggest that the relative risk of developing hepatocellular carcinoma by patients with portacaval anastomoses (PCA) is more than three times greater than in unshunted cirrhotic patients (134,135) and increases with the duration of the shunt. The increased prevalence of hepatocellular carcinoma appears unrelated to age, sex, alcohol consumption, or the presence of HBs antigenemia. The association of PCA with hepatocellular carcinoma may be related to some specific pathophysiologic effect of the PCA. It has been suggested that substances in portal blood that are anti-oncogenic for the liver may bypass the liver in shunted patients, thus protecting the liver (134). The association may also be related to the fact that PCA may prolong survival sufficiently for the patient to develop hepatocellular carcinoma spontaneously (136). Our own unpublished observations confirm the association of hepatocellular carcinoma and PCA in patients whose PCAs remain patent for periods greater than six months (135). A third possibility has been suggested by animal experiments that show the rate of growth of dimethylnitrosamine-induced hepatocellular carcinoma in rats is enhanced by PCA (137). Indeed, the association of hepatocellular carcinoma with cirrhosis may reflect the presence of spontaneous portal-systemic shunting, which may act in a manner analogous to that of surgically induced portal-systemic shunting.

Occasionally, other less common types of cirrhosis are complicated by hepatocellular carcinoma among adults. These include primary biliary cirrhosis, toxic cirrhosis secondary to arsenical solutions or to carbon tetrachloride, and the cirrhosis caused by Thorotrast (138). Hepatocellular carcinoma appears to occur with increased frequency in α-1-antitrypsin deficiency especially in patients who are homozygous or heterozygous for the Z gene (113). It has been reported to be increased in porphyria cutanea tarda where it is usually, but not always, accompanied by cirrhosis (139). It is not clear in these cases whether the porphyria is primary or secondary. Hepatocellular carcinoma has been said to be increased in patients with *Schistosoma japonicum* infestation, but this association is still in dispute (140).

In children, hepatocellular carcinoma is seen primarily among those with neonatal hepatitis and cirrhosis, biliary atresia, the deToni-Faconi syndrome, and tyrosinosis.

Hepatocellular carcinoma may develop in noncirrhotic subjects. Most common are asymptomatic carriers of HBsAg, and patients with HBsAg-positive chronic hepatitis (141). Hepatocellular carcinoma is thought to be increased in subjects who take estrogens, oral contraceptives, and synthetic androgenic-anabolic agents, although these relationships are unproved (109).

Hepatocellular carcinoma has been reported to occur in type 1 glycogen storage disease, Neimann-Pick disease, and after radioactive phosphorus therapy for polycythemia vera.

Etiology. Among the major etiologic factors that predispose to hepatocellular carcinoma, viral hepatitis is the most important. An impressive body of indirect evidence suggests that on a worldwide basis, HBV is the cause of most cases of hepatocellular carcinoma, especially in areas where the HBV is endemic. HBs antigenemia is demonstrable in 40 to 80% of cases of hepatocellular carcinoma (142). These figures may be underestimates, since the HBsAg titer in hepatocellular carcinoma tends to be low and may escape detection. Indeed, anti-HBc, which is indicative of viral replication, is detectable in the serum of some HBsAg-negative cases. Furthermore, HBsAg has been demonstrated in the hepatocytes of some patients with HBsAg-negative sera.

Epidemiologic evidence that the HBV causes primary hepatocellular carcinoma is overwhelming. Hepatocellular carcinoma is one of the most common cancers in the world, but the incidence varies in different geographic areas (107–109). There is a worldwide correlation between the prevalence of the HBsAg carrier state and the prevalence of hepatocellular carcinoma (143). These geographic studies are complemented by case control studies, which invariably show a higher prevalence of HBs antigenemia in the patients with hepatocellular carcinoma than in those without (144,145). The very high frequency of the HBsAg carrier state in the majority of patients with hepatocellular carcinoma emphasizes the role of vertical transmission of the HBV at the time of birth, which accounts for approximately 40% of the carriers in Taiwan (142). It is estimated that the risk of an HBsAg carrier in Taiwan dying from hepatocellular carcinoma or cirrhosis is 40 to 50% (142). There is a higher prevalence of the HBsAg carrier state in the mothers than in the fathers of patients with hepatocellular carcinoma (143). The prevalence of the disease is invariably higher in men than in women of all ages (143). The risks of developing hepatocellular carcinoma by an HBsAg carrier is inversely related to the age of the infected individual at the onset of the carrier state. The closeness of the association of HBV with hepatocellular carcinoma indicates that this type of hepatocellular carcinoma is preventable (146).

In a prospective study of 22,000 Taiwanese men, of whom 3400 (15%) were HBsAg-positive, the relative risk of developing hepatocellular carcinoma by the HBsAg carriers was 400 times greater than by the HBsAg-negative subjects (142). The recognition of an almost identical relationship between a remarkably similar hepatitis virus of woodchucks, ducks, and ground squirrels and the development of spontaneous hepatocellular carcinoma, which resembles human hepatocellular carcinoma, provides an experimental animal model that seems almost identical to the human condition (147).

Impaired immunity to infection with the HBV appears to be a factor in HBsAg-positive hepatocellular carcinoma. Persistent HBs antigenemia is the primary feature of this disease. In only a handful of cases is hepatocellular carcinoma antedated by an attack of acute, self-limited hepatitis, which represents the normal immunologic response. When such episodes do occur, the hepatitis tends to be severe and fails to resolve normally. The titer of anti-HBs tends to be low. In areas of high prevalence of hepatocellular carcinoma, the majority of the infections with HBV are aquired by vertical transmission from the mother at the time of birth (148), a time at which the newborn infant is immunodeficient.

It has not yet been resolved whether the HBV is oncogenic, acts synergistically with other carcinogens, reflects or contributes to an immunodeficient state with impairment of surveillance against carcinogenesis, or merely predisposes to hepatocellular carcinoma by producing chronic hepatitis and cirrhosis.

Observations that favor the oncogenic theory include the high incidence of HBs antigenemia in noncirrhotic patients who develop hepatocellular carcinoma (149); the increased frequency of hepatocellular dysplasia, a precancerous lesion in HBsAg-positive patients with macronodular cirrhosis; and, above all, the demonstration that HBV DNA is integrated into the DNA of hepatocytes in hepatocellular carcinoma (150–152).

The role of NANB hepatitis virus in the etiology of hepatocellular carcinoma has become much more evident since the structure of hepatitis C virus (HCV), has been determined (153). Presumably, HCV induces hepatocellular carcinoma by the integration of HCV DNA into the genome of liver cells in a manner analogous to woodchuck hepatitis virus-induced (WHV) hepatocellular carcinoma (154). Since NANB virus can lead to cirrhosis, it is conceivable that the cirrhosis per se may be a precursor lesion, independent of viral DNA integration.

Chronic alcoholism is a second major etiologic factor in hepatocellular carcinoma. Chronic alcoholism is an important factor in the pathogenesis of cirrhosis, although its precise mode of action is still uncertain. This relationship is supported by the close correlation between mortality rates for cirrhosis and the per capita consumption of alcohol throughout the world (110). Case control studies have shown higher relative risk rates for hepatocellular carcinoma in alcoholic patients than in nonalcoholic subjects (155–157). These studies are complicated by the simultaneous existence of additional, putative hepato-oncogenic agents such as HBV, aflatoxin, tobacco, and cirrhosis, itself. Hepatocellular carcinoma is a relatively infrequent complication of the micronodular form of alcoholic cirrhosis, which is seen in the early, active, progressive phases of the disease during which the patient is usually drinking excessively. Most, but not all cases of hepatocellular carcinoma in alcoholic cirrhosis develop in the macronodular form of the disease, which evolves as the cirrhosis matures (122). This evolution appears to occur more frequently and faster in patients who have abstained from or greatly reduced the consumption of alcohol and in whom increased hepatocellular regeneration is maximal (158).

Aflatoxin is a third potential etiologic factor that is implicated circumstantially (110). Foods stored at warm temperature and high humidity often become moldy due to contamination with the *Aspergillus flavus* group of fungi, the most common food spoilage fungus in the tropics. Some aflatoxins, which are metabolic products of these organisms, are known to be potent, hepatotoxic carcinogens in animals (159). In those parts of the world, such as Africa and Southeast Asia, where climatic conditions and economic circumstances lead to the frequent consumption of moldy food, there is a close correlation between the estimated mean daily intake of aflatoxin and the incidence of hepatocellular carcinoma, suggesting an etiologic relationship (160). Furthermore, aflatoxin B has been found in a high proportion of patients with hepatocellular carcinoma, but not in control subjects without this neoplasm from the same environment (161). Since the frequency of HBV infection is high in these same areas, it has been suggested that the HBV and aflatoxin may act as cocarcinogens (162). On the other hand, it has been reported that the incidence of hepatocellular carcinoma in HBsAg carriers is the same in areas of high aflatoxin intake, such as Mozambique, and of low aflatoxin intake, such as the United States (163). Such findings suggest that HBV is the dominant factor, and that aflatoxin is not primary in the induction of hepatocellular carcinoma. In one study from Swaziland, however, the role of aflatoxin appeared to be more important than that of HBV (160). Conceivably, aflatoxin may suppress cell-mediated immunity and may, thereby, facilitate the development of chronic infection with HBV, thus playing an indirect role in the pathogenesis of hepatocellular carcinoma.

Tobacco smoking is an additional risk factor for the development of hepatocellular carcinoma. A convincing relationship between this neoplasm and tobacco usage has been shown in both Greece (164) and Hong Kong (165). Other studies in other countries have not confirmed this relationship, however (110).

Clinical features. The diversity of the manner of presentation is the most typical characteristic of hepatocellular carcinoma (166). It may present as abdominal pain, a palpable mass, constitutional symptoms, such as malaise or anorexia or as weight loss or fever, or it may be completely silent. Since it usually occurs in patients with preexisting cirrhosis, it may present with manifestations of decompensated liver disease such as jaundice, ascites, or hemorrhage from gastroesophageal varices. Rarely, it presents as rupture of the tumor with hemoperitoneum, or the Budd-Chiari syndrome secondary to occlusion of the hepatic vein or portal veing occlusion with ileus, ascites, or gastrointestinal bleeding. Symptoms secondary to metastases, such as bone pain (167) or acute respiratory symptoms (168), occasionally occur. Metastases to skin, gingiva, sinuses, and distant lymph nodes have been reported (166). Rarely, endocrine or metabolic paraneoplastic manifestations (168), such as polycythemia (169), hypoglycemia (170), hypercalcemia (168,171), or the carcinoid syndrome (172), are the primary manifestations. Other metabolic disorders including hyperlipemia (169,173), dysproteinemia (174), or a variety of other systemic manifestations may be seen. Unusual syndromes, such as hypertrophic pulmonary osteoarthropathy (175) and calcification of necrotic areas of the hepatocellular carcinoma, have been reported (168). Other rare syndromes associated with hepatocellular carcinoma include porphyria cutanea tarda (176), pityriasis rotunda (177), and sexual changes (168). The possibility of an underlying heptocellular carcinoma should be considered in any case of cirrhosis in which there is progressive enlargement of the liver or rapid hepatic decompensation, in patients with alcoholic cirrhosis, particularly in those who have stopped drinking.

The physical findings of hepatoma include hepatomegaly, an arterial bruit over the liver, ascites, jaundice, splenomegaly, muscle wasting, and fever, roughly in order of prevalence. It is not possible to attribute these findings specifically to the hepatocellular carcinoma or to the associated cirrhosis. Cullen's sign, i.e., periumbilical discoloration caused by abdominal wall ecchymosis, has been reported.

Laboratory abnormalities depend on the location, size, type, and rate of growth of the tumor, but serum alkaline phosphatase and gamma-glutamyl transferase activity are frequently increased. Gamma-glutamyl transferase levels may be increased in tumor tissue and ascitic fluid (178).

Laboratory features. The primary laboratory feature of hepatocellular carcinoma is the serum *α-fetoprotein* (AFP) level, which is the most useful of the serologic markers of hepatocellular carcinoma (179). AFP levels in serum may be elevated in nonmalignant diseases of many types. Indeed, from 2 to 10% of patients with chronic hepatitis or cirrhosis show levels by radioimmunoassay >100 ng/ml. However, only 1 to 3% show levels >400 ng/ml, which include about 60% of patients with hepatocellular carcinoma who have higher levels. Serum levels seem to be roughly proportional to tumor size, and, therefore, the early detection of small tumors by AFP levels leaves much to be desired (180,181). As these tumors grow, serum AFP levels increase in about two-thirds of the cases (182). When examined critically, the coefficient of correlation between the AFP concentration and the value of the hepatocellular carcinoma measured serially is quite low (r = 0.22) (183). Exposure to oral contraceptives may affect the clinical behavior of hepatocellular carcinoma resulting in more pregnancies and spontaneous ruptures and lower AFP levels (184). When AFP levels do not support a clinical diagnosis of hepatocellular carcinoma, ultrasonographic or computed tomographic imaging may establish the diagnosis, as may other serologic markers (185). Cytoplasmic measurements of nuclear DNA content of hepatocellular carcinoma show a positive correlation with AFP levels (186).

The course of the disease varies. Hepatocellular carcinoma is probably present for a period of at least three years before symptoms appear (180). Jaundice, ascites, progressive enlargement of the liver, and fever are common, late manifestations, and hepatic failure is often present terminally. Although metastases to abdominal lymph nodes, lungs, and bone are common at autopsy, clinical evidence of metastatic disease is scant. Death usually occurs within 6 to 12 months of the onset of symptoms. The course tends to be more fulminant in African blacks than in other groups. Cure may be achieved by the surgical removal of localized tumors, although in may instances recurrence of metastases are found after apparently successful surgery. Embolization therapy of the hepatic artery (187) or of the hepatic artery and portal vein (188) and the injection of absolute alcohol into the tumor (189) are potentially promising new forms of therapy.

Hepatic pathology. It must be kept in mind that malignant tumors may exhibit a broad range of differentiation and of metaplasia. Experimental systems have shown that a single neoplastic cell line can give rise to a whole spectrum of tumors including hepatocellular carcinoma, cholangiocarcinoma, adenocarcinoma, epidermoid carcinoma, hepatoblastoma, sarcoma, and others (190). These multipotent blast cells can give rise to a variety of different neoplasms and to a variety of histologic expressions in individual neoplasms.

Despite extensive histologic variations in a single tumor or in tumor nodules, molecular hybridization techniques for HBV DNA in multinodular hepatocellular carcinoma indicate monoclonal origin (191). Use of the Southern blot technique has shown that several discrete nodules in the liver of a cirrhotic patient with hepatocellular carcinoma had the same integration pattern as the primary tumor (192). However, recurrent hepatocellular carcinoma does not always have the same integration pattern as the original, previously resected tumor (193).

The traditional, gross pathologic classification of hepatocellular carcinoma has been in use for almost a full century (194). This classification divides the tumors into (1) *massive, solitary;* (2) *nodular,* which is characterized by multiple coalescent tumors; and (3) *diffuse,* which is seen almost invariably in cirrhotic livers. This last type may be overlooked on gross inspection because it resembles a non-neoplastic cirrhotic liver. The cirrhosis, which precedes the tumor in the large majority of cases, is usually macronodular, sometimes mixed, micro/macronodular, and, rarely, micronodular (108). A second, more detailed classification has been proposed but is quite complex. A newer classification that is based on small tumors <3 cm in diameter seems better suited to present needs (195). It suggests that the five types of tumor correlate with clinical, histologic, and prognostic patterns. The *early hepatocellular carcinoma* type consists of small tumors that do not destroy the underlying lobular or nodular architecture. *Type 1, single, nodular,* includes spheric tumors encapsulated by compressed hepatic parenchyma. *Type 2,* the most common type, consists of *single nodular tumors* with extra nodular extensions, which have an irregular shape with incomplete encapsulation. *Type 3, contiguous, multinodular* type, consists of less well defined tumors that invade the parenchyma. The *type 4, poorly demarcated, nodular* type includes poorly differentiated tumors that invade the surrounding parenchyma. Early hepatocellular carcinoma and types 1 and 2 are small, occur in noncirrhotic livers, are histologically better differentiated, are less frequently HBsAg-positive, produce lower levels of AFP, show fewer portal venous tumor thrombi and fewer intrahepatic metastases, have a better prognosis, and are more responsive to embolism therapy. As the grade worsens, the tumors become larger and less well differentiated and tend to be HBsAg-positive, to have higher AFP levels, to develop tumor thrombi and metastases, and to have worse prognosis. Unfortunately, the numbers of cases on which this potentially very useful classification is based are small, and many more cases must be classified to determine its true value.

Encapsulated hepatocellular carcinoma is much less likely to spread (196). The stroma of hepatocellular carcinoma is usually sparse and finely distributed. The tumor tissue tends to be soft and friable. Rarely, however, these tumors exhibit a diffuse, desmoplastic pattern that gives them a sclerotic appearance and a consistency that may resemble metastatic tumor.

Well-differentiated hepatomas that produce bile may have a yellow or green color. Fatty infiltration of neoplastic cells may cause yellowish areas. Foci of hemorrhage or necrosis may cause focal red, purple, brown, or black coloration.

Tumor thrombi in intrahepatic branches of the portal vein may be grossly visible on the cut surface. Similar thrombi may occur in hepatic vein radicles (197). These thrombi often extend into the extrahepatic portal or hepatic veins (185,197,198). The blood supply to the tumor is derived exclusively from the hepatic artery and enters the tumor from its periphery (197).

Microscopically, the most common pattern is characterized by neoplastic cells that resemble hepatocytes. They are polyhedral in shape, but tend to be larger and more variable in size than normal hepatocytes (Figs. 853–855). The cytoplasm is often described as eosinophilic and finely granular (Fig. 856), but in our experience it is usually more basophilic than in nonneoplastic hepatocytes (Figs. 853–855). The nuclei are relatively large and hyperchromatic with condensation of chromatin along the nuclear membrane, and they regularly exhibit prominent nucleoli (Fig. 857). Mitotic activity is variable, but is usually increased (Fig. 854). Sometimes the mitoses are abnormal (Fig. 858). Tumors may vary from area to area in the degree of differentiation, pleomorphism, staining characteristics, and growth patterns (Figs. 854, 855, 857). Variations in adjacent areas are often seen (Fig. 859). Canalicular or intracellular bile thrombi are sometimes present and may help establish the hepatic origin of the tumor (Fig. 860), but they are usually few in number and small. When the tumor is anaplastic, however, and the need for specific markers is greatest, the presence of bile is rare (194), but large amounts of bile are sometimes seen (Fig. 861).

The neoplastic cells are usually arranged in an irregular, trabecular pattern two or more cells thick. Some trabeculae are slender (Fig. 862); others are broad (Fig. 856). These trabeculae may be separated by sinusoids lined by sparse, flat endothelial cells, but no Kupffer cells [(108); Figs. 853, 862]. Occasionally, the neoplastic cells are closely packed in irregular,

broad sheets in which no vascular channels can be identified, a pattern that has been referred to as "cobblestone" [(108,198); Fig. 863]. Sometimes, peliosis hepatis is present in the non-neoplastic liver of patients with hepatocellular carcinoma, and, rarely, peliotic areas may be found in the tumor itself [(198); Fig. 864].

Reticulin within hepatocellular carcinoma is invariably sparse, often irregular in distribution, and usually delicate (Fig. 865). Sometimes, it is absent (Fig. 866). This paucity of reticulin is important in distinguishing well-differentiated hepatocellular carcinoma from regenerating nodules, in which the reticulin pattern is normal. Fine needle aspiration of liver tissue is effective for making the diagnosis of hepatocellular carcinoma (199,200).

In noncirrhotic livers the tumor may contain sparse, fibrous septa and blood vessels (Figs. 865, 867), which are usually evident on surgical wedge or postmortem sections, but may be missed in needle biopsy sections. In cirrhotic livers fibrous septa are common, but, in addition, may surround masses of tumor that have replaced regenerating parenchymal nodules (Fig. 868). Tumor thrombi within portal vein radicles in septa are common (Fig. 869). Less commonly, tumor thrombi involve central veins or other hepatic vein radicles [(197); Figs. 870, 871]. In addition, cords of nepolastic cells often extend through the sinusoids of the otherwise intact liver replacing or displacing hepatocytes (Figs. 871, 872). Zones of necrosis may be seen in some cases (Figs. 863, 873).

Premalignant changes precede the development of experimental hepatic neoplasms in animals (108,198), and similar lesions have been observed in non-neoplastic portions of livers with hepatocellular carcinoma (198,201). Adenomatous proliferative nodules have shown enlarged parenchymal cells with bizarre, hyperchromatic, multiple nuclei. Such liver cell dysplasia was found in 1% of subjects with normal livers, 7% of noncirrhotic patients with hepatocellular carcinoma, 19% of cirrhotic patients, and >60% of cirrhotic patients with hepatocellular carcinoma (201). Others have found small cell hyperplasia under similar circumstances (202). These observations have been confirmed by some investigators (127,203), but not by others (128,197,204). The most useful feature in the differentiation of a dysplastic nodule or a hepatic adenoma from hepatocellular carcinoma is the deficiency of reticulin in the malignant neoplasm (108).

In less well differentiated hepatocellular carcinoma, the neoplastic cells tend to be smaller and less eosinophilic (Fig. 854). When the trabecular growth pattern is lost, these tumors resemble adrenal cortical carcinomas (108). These neoplastic cells may lose their resemblance to hepatocytes and may look like mesenchymal cells, sometimes suggesting sarcoma. They usually contain eosinophilic, granular cytoplasm similar to that of normal hepatocytes, suggesting that they have arisen from hepatocytes. Transitions from typical neoplastic hepatocytes to spindle-shaped cells are often demonstrable (Fig. 874). Neoplastic cells in hepatocellular carcinoma may lose their cohesiveness and separate into individual cells, no longer forming trabeculae or cords (Fig. 875). A small number of giant cells with multinucleated (Fig. 876) or polylobulated nuclei (Fig. 877) may be scattered throughout the tumor. Rarely, such pleomorphic cells are the predominant cell type. Foci of giant cells may be seen (Fig. 878).

Hepatocellular carcinoma with osteoclast-like cells is a very rare, recently recognized type of hepatocellular cancer that runs a relatively benign clinical course, much like that of the fibrolamellar variant (198a). Histologically, such tumors are virtually identical to giant cell tumors of bone (Fig. 878A), but usually one can locate fields that show the typical pattern of hepatocellular carcinoma. It consists of sheets of benign-appearing, osteoclast-like giant cells (Fig. 878B) and many mononucleated neoplastic hepatocytes. The giant cells differ from those seen in the usual type of hepatocellular carcinoma in which they are pleomorphic and anaplastic. Occasionally, biliary pigment can be seen in the cytoplasm of the giant cells (Fig 878C).

Neoplastic cells with abundant, pale, finely granular or vacuolated cytoplasm and small, central nuclei, which are classified as "clear cells," may sometimes be present (Fig. 879). Such cells may be few in number and interspersed with cells more characteristic of hepatocellular carcinoma. In some tumors, large areas consist exclusively of clear cells, but invariably other areas are made up largely or entirely of typical hepatocellular carcinoma cells with granular cytoplasm (Fig. 880). *Clear cell hepatocellular carcinoma,* in which 30 to 50% of the cells are water-clear cells, comprise less than 10% of hepatomas. The clarity of the cells is due to large amounts of glycogen as shown by PAS staining (108). When a needle biopsy or a small surgical wedge contains only clear cells, the tumor may be misinterpreted to be an adrenal rest carcinoma or a metastasis from a clear cell carcinoma of the kidney (205) or adrenal gland. Clues to the correct diagnosis in such cases are the presence of bile droplets or the trabecular pattern of the neoplastic cells.

A variety of cytoplasmic inclusions may be present, but they occur unpredictably and vary widely in number and type. Cytoplasmic *bile droplets* may be seen (Fig. 881), but are extremely uncommon except in the presence of canalicular bile thrombi. *Fat droplets* may be present and, when they are, tend to involve circumscribed groups of cells (Fig. 882). *Mallory bodies* are often seen in the absence of similar inclusions in the non-neoplastic hepatocytes (206). They tend to occur in alcoholic patients (Fig. 883), but not always (Fig. 884). They have been found in other tumors as well (207). Other intracellular inclusions of unknown composition are common and may vary in size, shape [(108,198); Fig. 885], and staining characteristics. Some are eosinophilic (Fig. 886) and some are basophilic (Fig. 887). Such inclusions may be PAS-D-positive globules (Fig. 888) or PAS-D-negative (Fig. 889). Some PAS-D-globules have been identified as α-1-antitrypsin. They may be seen in hepatocellular carcinoma in the tumor but not in the non-neoplastic liver tissue of patients without α-1-antitrypsin deficiency. Alpha-1-chymotrypsin may be a better immunocytochemical marker than α-1-antitrypsin in such cases (208). Other cytoplasmic constituents such as HBsAg may be demonstrated by immunofluorescent or immunoperoxidase reactions. *Hepatitis B surface antigen* is only rarely seen in neoplastic tissues by the Shikata orcein stain even when it is present in abundance in adjacent, non-neoplastic tissues (Fig. 890). Ground glass cells, similar to those seen in patients with HBV infection, have been observed (209). However, these cells do not contain HBsAg by immunohistologic techniques, but may contain fibrinogen, albumin, or ferritin (108). *α-fetoprotein* can be demonstrated by immunoperoxidase methods in one-third the cases, but is generally lacking in well-differentiated, slow-growing tumors, and, at the other end of the spectrum, in extremely anaplastic tumors (210). *Carcinoembryonic antigen* can be demonstrated in one-third of hepatocellular carcinomas by immunoperoxidase techniques, and combinations of α-fetoprotein and carcinoembryonic antigen can be found in about half. The presence and frequency of these inclusions varies from case to case and from area to area in the same liver (198). Hemosiderin is rarely found in hepatocellular carcinoma. In hemochromatotic patients with hepatocellular carcinoma the amount of iron in the non-neoplastic tissue is striking, but the hepatocellular carcinoma itself is free of iron (Fig. 891).

Extracellular deposits of proteinaceous material may also be found. Usually they are eosinophilic (Fig. 892), but they may be basophilic. Some are PAS-D-positive (Fig. 893). They may be mistaken for mucin, but usually do not take up Alcian blue or other mucin stains. However, we have encountered several hepatomas that stain for mucin with Alcian blue (Fig. 894). Large extracellular deposits, which may be acidophilic, amphoteric (Fig. 895) or basophilic (Fig. 896), may assume globular shapes within the lumens of acini or may be scattered diffusely among tumor cells.

Extreme variations in the arrangement of neoplastic cells may be seen. *Rosettes, and acinar and ductal* patterns are common (Fig. 897). Sometimes, the ductular organization is strong and whole areas may resemble an adenoma (Figs. 897, 898). Even when the adenomatous form of hepatocellular carcinoma predominates, areas that exhibit the trabecular pattern can almost always be found elsewhere (Fig. 899). The tumor cells may encircle a central lumen of variable diameter or form large tubular structures (Fig. 900). The lumen may contain bile or unidentified proteinaceous material (Figs. 900, 901). *Pseudoducts,* which are less common, consist of neoplastic cells arranged in the form of elongated ducts without visible lumens. When such ductular forms are common, the tumor may resemble cholangiocarcinoma. When they are interspersed with the more typical trabecular pattern of hepatocellular carcinoma, they may suggest mixed cholangiohepatocellular carcinoma.

Variations in stroma may also occur. *Sclerosing hepatocellular carcinoma* usually occurs in patients with noncirrhotic livers and is often associated with hypercalcemia (211). Histologically, the neoplastic cells appear to be compressed cords or ducts embedded in dense fibrous tissue and in this form may be mistaken for cholangiocarcinoma. Sclerosing hepatocellular carcinoma must be differentiated from fibrolamellar hepatocellular carcinoma. Usually the fibrolamellar hepatocellular carcinoma can be recognized by the density and cellularity and laminar arrangement of the collagen.

Pedunculated hepatocellular carcinomas are usually massive tumors that are in subcapsular areas but grow extrahepatically whether or not they are connected to the liver by a pedicle (212,213). This diagnosis is very easy to make using modern imaging techniques. These hepatomas do not differ histologically from nonpedunculated hepatocellular carcinoma, although they tend to show sarcomatous areas frequently (214). Their larger size and better prognosis may reflect their extrahepatic localization.

Fibrolamellar hepatocellular carcinoma, which is also known as eosinophilic hepatocellular carcinoma with lamellar fibrosis, is a more recently recognized variant of hepatocellular carcinoma (198,215–217). This tumor, which makes up approximately 1% of primary liver tumors and less than 10% of hepatocellular carcinoma, was first described in 1956 (218). However, previously reported cases have been recognized in retrospect (198,219). These tumors behave differently clinically, and are histologically quite different from typical hepatocellular carcinoma. Fibrolamellar hepatocellular carcinoma tends to occur in young patients, usually after puberty, but occasionally before, and occurs with equal frequency in either sex (215,220). In some series it is more common in women (216) in contrast to conventional hepatocellular carcinoma, which is seen predominantly in men. These tumors do not appear to be related to either chronic alcohol consumption or infection with HBV. In clinical presentation they are similar to typical hepatocellular carcinoma. Abdominal pain and malaise are the most common symptoms occurring in three-fourths and one-third, respectively (215,220). Neuroendocrine features have been noted (219–222). Hepatomegaly or an abdominal mass are early signs. Jaundice is uncommon. Serum transaminase or alkaline phosphatase levels are usually modestly increased. α-fetoprotein levels are not as high as in typical hepatocellular carcinoma, and are usually <250 ng/ml (215,220). HBV DNA sequences differ in fibrolamellar hepatocellular carcinomas in tumorous and nontumorous sites, and apparently integrate at different locations than do typical hepatocellular carcinomas (223). They tend to have a high cure rate after resection and much longer survival than expected in unresected cases (216,224–226). It has been suggested, however, that the prognosis after resection may not be better than in nonfibrolamellar hepatocellular carcinoma, but rather, that fibrolamellar tumors, which grow slowly, may have a higher resectability rate than nonfibrolamellar hepatocellular carcinomas (227).

Grossly, fibrolamellar hepatocellular carcinoma usually presents as a large, solitary tumor arising in a noncirrhotic liver, but multiple nodules may be present (22). They may show calcium deposition on x-ray (228,229).

Microscopically, fibrolamellar hepatocellular carcinoma exhibits three characteristic features. Usually, the neoplastic cells have deeply eosinophilic cytoplasm (Figs. 902, 903) that results from the presence of many mitochondria (215,230) and perioxisomes (220). As in nonfibrolamellar hepatocellular carcinoma, however, histologic heterogeneity may be present, and noneosinophilic areas resembling conventional hepatocellular carcinoma may be present (221). Mitoses are uncommon (108). Approximately half of them may contain pale, sharply defined cytoplasmic bodies that are similar to the ground glass cells seen in HBV infections [(215); Fig. 904]. Similar pale cytoplasmic bodies may occur in nonfibrolamellar hepatocellular carcinoma (209), although usually in smaller numbers. HBsAg is not usually present in the serum, and orcein, aldehyde fucsin (Fig. 636), and immunoperoxidase stains for HBsAg and HBcAg, which are positive in active HBV infection, are usually negative. Using immunohistochemical methods, it was noted that in similar ground glass cells found in nonfibrolamellar hepatocellular carcinoma (209) the same reaction took place. Copper and copper-associated protein have been demonstrated in fibrolamellar tumors (231,232) more frequently than in nonfibrolamellar tumors (233) as have fibrinogen and α-1-antitrypsin (234) and other markers (235). Fine needle biopsy has been used successfully to make this diagnosis (236), but the chances of missing lamellar fibrosis are appreciable.

Abundant fibrous stroma composed of many thin, parallel bundles of relatively acellular collagen fibers suggests a laminated composition, which gives the tumor its name, fibrolamellar (Fig. 906). These fibrous bands divide the tumor into thin columns of hepatocytes (Figs. 906, 907) or into nodules (Figs. 906, 908). The adjacent, non-neoplastic liver is normal in at leasst three-fourths of cases, although mild fibrosis, congenital hepatic fibrosis, and cirrhosis have been reported (215). Sometimes, the fibrous bands in tumor tissue coalesce to form thick scars that grossly resemble focal nodular hyperplasia [(215); Fig. 909]. Indeed, fibrolamellar hepatocellular carcinoma has

been confused with both focal nodular hyperplasia and hepatocellular adenoma (237,238). Several women with fibrolamellar hepatocellular carcinoma who had been on oral contraceptives and who had been thought on biopsy to have focal nodular hyperplasia (239,240) have shown excellent prognosis. Resection of the tumor and cessation of oral contraceptives have been followed by prolonged survival even after metastases had been noted (238). On the basis of such observations, it has been suggested that fibrolamellar hepatocellular carcinoma may arise in focal nodular hyperplasia (238). The finding of focal nodular hyperplasia in the liver adjacent to fibrolamellar hepatocellular carcinoma in three patients and the apparent transition to fibrolamellar hepatocellular carcinoma in one of them suggests that malignant transformation may occur (216).

A variety of special histologic techniques can be used to enhance conventional histologic staining methods. Special stains are sometimes required in the differential diagnosis of hepatocellular carcinoma. Although the demonstration of mucin is said to virtually exclude hepatocellular carcinoma (108), we have observed positive Alcian blue stains in several such tumors.

Histochemical techniques on fresh frozen tissue can be used to demonstrate increased glutamyl transpeptidase and decreased ATPase and G-6-phosphatase activity in hepatic cells (241).

In hepatocellular carcinoma the presence of α-naphthylamidase in fresh, unfixed cytologic preparations can identify neoplasms of hepatic origin for which it is specific (242).

This stain colors bile canaliculi membranes bright red but does not stain the cytoplasm of hepatocytes or nonhepatic membranes. It can thus differentiate primary from metastatic hepatic neoplasms by cytologic staining (241a, 242) (Fig. 909A). Where clumps of hepatoma cells are seen the characteristic interconnection canalicular pattern is also seen (242a, 242b) (Fig. 909B).

Monoclonal antikeratin antibodies have been used to identify keratin patterns that are specific for hepatocytes and biliary epithelial cells (243,244), but other investigators have found that cytokeratin profiles may not always be preserved during neoplastic transformation (245).

Morphometric analysis can differentiate normal and cirrhotic cells from hepatoma cells by nuclear/cytoplasmic ratios, nuclear pleomorphism, and nuclear texture (246,247).

In a prospective, step-wise, logistic regression analysis of the cytologic characteristics of fine-needle aspirates from thirty-five patients with hepatocellular carcinoma and seventy-five with metastatic tumors of the liver were compared (247a). The finding of polygonal cells with centrally located nuclei was the criterion most suggestive of hepatocellular carcinoma (Fig. 909C. These characteristics were observed in 94% of the hepatocellular carcinomas, but in only 15% of the other hepatic neoplasms. Other cytologic features of diagnostic importance include clusters of malignant cells separated by capillary vessels (fig 909D) and the presence of bile pigment in the tumor cells. The presence of any two of these three criteria was virtually diagnostic of hepatocellular carcinoma. More than 95% of the hepatocellular carcinomas exhibited at least two of these criteria, while none of the nonhepatic malignancies did so. The presence of bile in neoplastic cells is pathognomonic of hepatocellular carcinoma, but it is a relatively insensitive criterion, occurring in only one-third of aspirates. Other typical cytologic features of hepatocellular carcinoma, such as granular cytoplasm, prominent nucleoli, and multinucleated giant cells (Fig. 909C) are of little differential diagnostic value.

A variant of hepatocellular carcinoma, termed hepatocellular carcinoma with *dense collagenous stroma,* but which differs from fibrolamellar hepatocellular carcinoma, also seems also to be associated with a favorable prognosis (248).

Cholangiocarcinoma (malignant cholangioma, intrahepatic bile duct carcinoma). Malignant tumors that arise from the epithelium of the intrahepatic bile ducts anywhere from the level of the cholangioles to the junction of the main hepatic ducts within or close to the porta hepatis are generally classified as cholangiocarcinomas. However, two relatively uncommon subtypes, which are often classed separately by their histologic appearance, will be discussed individually. *Cholangiolocarcinoma* appears to arise from cholangioles. Such neoplasms may contain cells of hepatocellular origin, a finding that indicates that they may be a special form of hepatocellular carcinoma. In general, however, their clinical features, gross appearance, and growth pattern resemble those of peripherally located, typical cholangiocarcinomas. The second subtype, *adenocarcinoma of the bifurcation of the hepatic duct* (sclerosing carcinoma of the hilar bile ducts), usuallly shows distinctive clinical and morphologic features.

Like hepatocellular carcinoma, cholangiocarcinomas occur in older individuals, almost always after age 50. Cholangiocarcinomas differ from hepatocellular carcinomas in a variety of ways. They occur far less frequently than hepatocellular carcinoma, comprising only 10 to 15% of the primary malignancies of the liver. They are found slightly more frequently in men than in women (108,249). Only 10 to 20% of cholangiocarcinomas occur in cirrhotic patients compared with the 70 to 90% in hepatocellular carcinoma (249–251). In many cases the cirrhosis is of the secondary biliary type that results from neoplastic obstruction of the bile ducts, suggesting that some cases of cirrhosis are the result of the tumor rather than their cause. A variety of other hepatic disorders have been occasionally complicated by cholangiocarcinoma. These include polycystic liver disease (252), choledochal cysts (253,254), and congenital dilatation of the intrahepatic bile ducts (Caroli's syndrome) (255). The typhoid carrier state has also been implicated (256).

The high prevalence of cholangiocarcinoma in Southeast Asia is related to infestation with liver flukes (257,258). There is close correlation between geographic distribution of liver flukes and the prevalence of biliary carcinoma (108). Other biliary parasites do not appear to show similar oncogenic potential (259). Liver flukes induce hyperplasia and adenomatous proliferation of the biliary epithelium in humans, but the etiologic relationship is not established unequivocally (260). In experimental animals, liver flukes precipitate cholangiocarcinoma when administered in conjunction with dimethylnitrosamine, which alone does not cause neoplasia (261).

Cholangiocarcinoma has also been suspected to be caused by inflammatory bowel disease with sclerosing cholangitis (262), hepatolithiasis, or cholelithiasis (263–265), but these relationships have not been established. Cystic fibrosis has also been implicated (266). Clearly, the relationship between chronic irritation of the biliary tree by foreign bodies or recurrent obstructive or inflammatory lesions and cholangiocarcinoma creates a probable but improved pathogenesis.

It has been suggested that cholangiocarcinomas may arise from intrahepatic peribiliary glands (267).

Thorotrast has been thought to be a cause of cholangiocarcinoma, which is the most frequent hepatic neoplasm reported following the intravenous injection of thorium dioxide (138,268). This association is supported by the demonstration of deposits of thorotrast in the immediate vicinity of the tumor after long periods. The incidence is higher than that seen in appropriate control groups (269).

Oral contraceptives in women and anabolic-androgenic steroids in men have been suggested as possible causes, but these relationships have not been confirmed (270,271).

There appears to be no association with HBV infection, cirrhosis, or mycotoxins (108,249).

The clinical features of cholangiocarcinoma are nonspecific and depend on the location of the tumor. Peripheral tumors that arise from smaller bile ducts become clinically evident only after they have attained large size. Tumors that arise near the hilum may cause obstructive jaundice relatively early. These tumors present with hepatomegaly, an abdominal mass, pain, or weight loss (108,249). Jaundice and ascites may occur, but tend to do so late in the course of the disease. Serum alkaline phosphatase levels are often elevated (249). Hypercalcemia is sometimes seen (249). In contrast to hepatocellular carcinoma, there is no increase in serum α-fetoprotein levels (272), but there is frequently an increase in carcinoembryonic antigen (CEA) (249). Another arbitrary tumor marker, CA 19-9, has been found to be frequently positive in cholangiocarcinoma and in carcinoma of the pancreas (249,273).

More centrally located tumors that arise in large intrahepatic ducts behave like hepatic duct bifurcation tumors and, usually, present with obstructive jaundice (108,249). Although such tumors involve a single major duct initially, they extend to the bifurcation and to the contralateral duct, obstructing bile flow. The unilateral obstruction of one major hepatic duct does not produce jaundice, although compression of contralateral ducts by the expanding tumor, even without direct invasion of the other duct, can cause jaundice. Once jaundice appears, death usually ensues within a year. Rarely, small peripheral tumors, if detected before they metastasize or cause jaundice, may be successfully resected with apparent cure.

Grossly, cholangiocarcinomas present as firm, gray-white masses. They are usually solitary and large, but many of them have multiple satellite nodules (108,249,274,275). Occasionally, multiple small nodules coalesce, a pattern that suggests multicentric origin, especially in cases of cholangiolocarcinoma. When they are near the hilum they may be difficult to differentiate from the lesions of sclerosing cholangitis by visual examination. Invasion of large portal or hepatic veins occurs much less commonly than in hepatocellular carcinoma. Metastases to regional lymph nodes, lungs, and other organs occur more commonly than in hepatocellular carcinoma. In cases with long-standing biliary obstruction caused by the tumor, the remaining liver may show secondary biliary cirrhosis.

Microscopically, these lesions are mucin-secreting adenocarcinomas. The epithelial component of cholangiocarcinoma is characterized by well-differentiated, low cuboidal cells that resemble those of normal bile ducts (Fig. 910), but solid cords without lumens may be present. These tumor cell cords tend to be surrounded by fibrous tissue or by PAS-positive basement membrane-like material. Less well differentiated cell types and ducts may be seen. Pleomorphism, atypia, mitotic activity, hyperchromatic nuclei, and prominent nucleoli vary from tumor to tumor (Figs. 910–912) and from area to area in the same tumor. No goblet cells are seen, but mucin secretion is often demonstrable in some (Fig. 913), but not all cases. Mucin is useful in differentiating hepatocellular carcinoma from cholangiocarcinoma. Positive staining of epithelial membrane antigen (276) or tissue peptide antigen (277) may also be useful in this differential diagnosis. There is no evidence of bile production by the tumor, although bile may sometimes be seen in the lumens of the neoplastic ducts (Fig. 914), presumably synthesized by adjacent, non-neoplastic hepatocytes.

The neoplastic cells are usually arranged in the form of ducts (Fig. 910), acini (Fig. 911), and cords (Figs. 911, 912), and, rarely, in papillary form (107). Occasionally, cholangiocarcinoma may invade central (Fig. 915) or portal veins (Fig. 916). When they invade veins, they may use the endothelium as a basement membrane and may form large acinar structures [(108); Fig. 917].

Cholangiolocarcinomas apparently arise from the epithelium of the cholangioles or the canals of Hering. These rare tumors, which comprise about 1% of primary liver cancers, tend to occur predominantly in men, in noncirrhotic livers, and to be unrelated to the HBV. Grossly, they tend to present with smaller, more numerous, and whiter nodules than do cholangiocarcinoma. In cholangiolocellular carcinoma the cells are flat with scanty, pale cytoplasm and small, dark, oval nuclei. They may be pleomorphic in some areas. The cells are usually arranged in the form of slender, irregular, branching, duct-like structures with minute, central lumens or as solid cords. These proliferating ductules closely resemble the proliferating ductules seen in some forms of cirrhosis (Fig. 360).

Cholangiocarcinoma may be histologically indistinguishable from metastatic adenocarcinoma arising in the gallbladder or extrahepatic bile ducts. Identification of such neoplasms as primary hepatic tumors by needle biopsy sections requires demonstration by cholangiography, laparotomy, or autopsy that the extrahepatic ducts or gallbladder are not involved. Similarly, differentiation of cholangiocarcinoma from metastatic adenocarcinoma arising in other sites may be difficult if not impossible. Metastatic ductular adenocarcinoma from the breast may show a remarkably close resemblance to the cholangiocellular type of cholangiocarcinoma (Fig. 918).

The prognosis, which is relatively poor without therapy, can be improved by surgical bypass procedures (274). Liver transplantation offers promise, although only a few cholangiocarcinomas have been so treated (278).

The differentiation of hepatocytic tumors from those of biliary origin can usually be made by the presence or absence of mucin and bilirubin. The use of specific biliary epithelial antigens may help in this differentiation (276,277). ABH and Lewis blood group antigens suggest that these combined tumors are hepatocellular in origin (279).

Rarely, the liver contains two distinct tumors, one hepatocellular carcinoma and one cholangiocarcinoma (280). These tumors may be separate or contiguous. The latter type, in which elements of both tumors merge, is the more common form. When the two discrete tumors impinge on each other they are called "collision" tumors. Some investigators believe that these combined tumors may represent fibrolamellar hepatocellular carcinoma with elements of hepatocellular carcinoma (280). When the two neoplasms are both unequivocally present, it is not clear whether they represent two separate neoplasms, a neoplasm that originates in one type tissue and differentiates into the other, or a neoplasm that arises in a transitional, intermediate hepatobiliary cell and expresses itself with microscopic features of both tumors.

Combined cholangio-hepatocellular carcinoma.

As mentioned previously, in typical hepatocellular carcinoma, a variable number of neoplastic cells may be arranged in the form of acini or pseudoducts rather than trabeculae. Occasionally, the cells in these areas may be columnar with basal nuclei or cuboidal with large nuclei and scanty cytoplasm, suggesting that they are derived from bile duct epithelium. When such areas are prominent, the tumors are sometimes classified as combined cholangio-hepatocellular carcinomas.

These tumors have been classified into three types: type 1, or "collision tumors," which are quite rare. They represent the coincidental occurrence of a hepatocellular carcinoma derived from hepatocytes and a cholangiocarcinoma derived from bile duct epithelium in the same patient (280). Type 2, or "transitional tumors," which are the most common type, are derived from hepatocytes exclusively and represent a variant of hepatocellular carcinoma. In such tumors, areas of intermediate differentiation and transition between the two types of tumors can be identified (Fig. 899). In Type 3, or "fibrolamellar variants," the hepatocellular portions of the tumor resemble fibrolamellar hepatocellular carcinoma, but in addition, coexist with areas that contain mucin-producing ductules or pseudoductules (280). Such combined cholangio-fibrolamellar hepatocellular carcinoma, like fibrolamellar hepatocellular carcinoma itself, tends to occur in younger, noncirrhotic patients who have low serum levels of AFP (140 and tends to have a better prognosis than type 1 or type 2 combined tumors.

Adenocarcinoma of the hepatic or bile ducts.

Adenocarcinomas of the hepatic and bile ducts are neoplasms that arise from biliary epithelium anywhere from the junction of the main hepatic ducts at the porta hepatis to the ampulla of Vater. Since they behave similarly, it is difficult to differentiate small hilar cholangiocarcinomas from adenocarcinomas of the bifurcation of the hepatic duct. These tumors consist of two types determined by their location: (1) adenocarcinomas of the bifurcation of the hepatic duct, (2) adenocarcinomas of the hepatic and common bile ducts.

Adenocarcinoma of the bifurcation of the hepatic duct (bifurcation adenocarcinoma) is the more common type. Since this syndrome was first described in 1965 (281), relatively little has been published about it (282,283). These tumors present clinically as obstructive jaundice, usually with pruritus, abdominal pain, and weight loss. Blood tests are typical of cholestatic disorders. Hepatomegaly is usually present. Fever and cholangitis occur late in the course, frequently after surgical manipulation.

Ultrasonography and computed tomography show dilatation of the intrahepatic bile ducts, but a nondistended gallbladder and common bile duct (284). Transhepatic cholangiography and ERCP are used to demonstrate the site of obstruction, but proof of the nature of the lesion requires surgery.

At laparotomy, the liver is enlarged and green, and the gallbladder and extrahepatic ducts are often difficult to identify because they are small and collapsed. These bifurcation adenocarcinomas grow extremely slowly. Metastases tend to be small and regional, are often unrecognized, and are rarely responsible for death.

Palliative surgery and implacement of stents improve survival and result in reasonably good health, often for periods of several years (281–284). Resection of the tumor is rarely possible. Ultimately, liver transplantation may be required.

Grossly, there are several types of adenocarcinomas of the bifurcation. *Annular sclerosing adenocarcinomas*, the most common type, are small, 1.5 to 2.5 cm in diameter, firm, fibrous nodules that encircle the hepatic duct at its bifurcation. They are difficult to differentiate from benign strictures at surgery. They may be associated with hypercalcemia (211).

Microscopically, the neoplastic cells are well differentiated and arranged in the forms of ducts or acini in a dense fibrous stroma (Fig. 919). The tumor cells are few in number and are sometimes difficult to identify as neoplastic (285). Serial sections are sometimes helpful. The presence of these cells in lymphatic structures (Fig. 920), especially in a perineural distribution, helps establish the diagnosis. Sometimes they invade nerves (Fig. 921).

Bulky central adenocarcinomas occur less frequently. They form large, firm masses in the hilum. They appear to arise in the right or left hepatic duct, which they obstruct completely, and to spread to the bifurcation and to the contralateral duct, which may become partially or completely occluded. Microscopically, these tumors have the histologic features of peripheral cholangiocarcinomas (Fig. 922). Metastatic adenocarcinoma from extrahepatic sites such as the colon or pancreas may mimic this lesion.

Less than 10% of bifurcation tumors are *papillary adenocarcinomas* (281,282). They present as friable masses within the lumen of one of the major hepatic ducts. They spread through and occlude the lumen of the bifurcation and the contralateral hepatic duct (Fig. 923). They may also extend into the surrounding parenchyma. Such tumors can arise in the common hepatic duct and spread peripherally. When they do, a relatively long zone of stricture can be visualized.

Adenocarcinomas of the hepatic, cystic or common bile duct can obstruct the biliary tract at the site of origin anywhere along its length. They present clinically with painless, unremitting obstructive jaundice. Imaging techniques show dilatation of the biliary tree distal to the lesion. The histologic features are similar to those of bifurcation carcinomas (281,284,286). Often in the ampullary area these carcinomas cannot be differentiated endoscopically from inflammatory pseudotumors (287).

Hepatoblastoma. Hepatoblastoma is a malignant tumor derived from primitive hepatocytes alone or from primitive hepatocytes and mesenchyme. This rare tumor is the most common hepatic malignancy of children (288). It affects young infants chiefly under the age of three years, but it is occasionally seen in older children and, rarely, in adults (288,289). It occurs twice as frequently in male as in female children (108). In adults it occurs with equal frequency in both sexes (290). Until the age of three, hepatoblastoma is far more common than hepatocellular carcinoma, but thereafter the converse is true. Unlike hepatocellular carcinoma, which occasionally occurs in children with underlying cirrhosis, hepatoblastoma bears no relationship to cirrhosis or, apparently, to HBV.

The most frequent clinical manifestations of these tumors are protuberant abdomen and hepatomegaly (288,289). Inconstant, relatively infrequent findings are weight loss, anorexia, vomiting, diarrhea, fever, and failure to thrive (108,288–290). Hemoperitoneum due to rupture of the tumor is a rare occurrence (290). Sexual precocity occurs rarely due to excessive production of gonadotropin (291,292). Cystothioninuria is very common (293). Congenital anomalies such as talipes, macroglossia, polyposis coli (294), and cardiac or renal defects may be present (108,290). Mottled calcification in the liver by x-ray, ultrasonography, or CT scanning is sometimes seen (295,296). Laboratory data show frequent elevations of serum alkaline phosphatase and transaminase activity; jaundice is only rarely present. Anemia is frequently found. High levels of serum AFP are the rule, and the concentrations may be enormous, reaching several hundred milligrams per milliliter (292). Hepatoblasto-

mas are more responsive to therapy than hepatocellular carcinoma. Cure is achieved in about half the patients by resection of the tumor or lobectomy, usually following chemotherapy to reduce tumor size (297). Metastases to abdominal lymph nodes or to distant organs is uncommon.

Grossly, hepatoblastomas are usually large (5 to 25 cm in diameter), solitary, spheric or lobulated masses. Occasionally, they are multiple. One-third are firm, one-third soft, and one-third friable. About 50% are encapsulated and sharply circumscribed. Incomplete encapsulation is found in some. Occasionally, areas of hemorrhage, necrosis, cystic degeneration, or bile staining are present. On cut surface, fibrous septa that contain small blood vessels and bile ducts often encircle tumor nodules.

Microscopically, hepatoblastomas are either epithelial or mixed epithelial and mesenchymal (288). In the *epithelial type,* neoplastic cells derived from hepatocytes show varying degrees of immaturity ranging from fetal to embryonal in appearance. The prognosis of those tumors composed entirely of fetal cells is better than that of pure embryonal cell tumors. Fetal and embryonal foci are seen in the same tumor, however. One type composed of either fetal or embryonal cells arranged in a macrotrabecular pattern that resembles hepatocellular carcinoma is said to have a poor prognosis (298). Immunohistochemical-ultrastructural studies can identify substances that characterize these types of tumors during the differentiation of the cell line (291,299). The *mixed type* appears to contain neoplastic cells derived from both immature hepatocytes and mesenchyme.

In *fetal epithelial hepatoblastoma,* the neoplastic cells are polyhedral in shape and resemble normal, adult hepatocytes. They tend to be smaller, more variable in size and shape, and to have more prominent nuclei than normal parenchymal cells. The cytoplasm varies in appearance. Large, pale cells may have an empty or vacuolated cytoplasm due to the presence of find lipid droplets or glycogen (Fig. 924). Small, dark cells show an eosinophilic, granular cytoplasm [(288); Fig. 925]. Characteristically, sheets of light and dark cells alternate (Fig. 926). The cells are usually arranged in irregular plates or trabeculae, two or more cells thick, separated by sinusoids lined by flattened endothelial cells, but no phagocytic activity is evident (299). Often the sinusoids are compressed and difficult to visualize. The cytoplasm occasionally contains bile droplets. Canaliculi, which may occasionally contain bile thrombi, may be visualized by special stains. Invasion of veins occurs occasionally.

The stroma is poorly developed and perisinusoidal reticulin is sparse. Fibrous septa may outline nodules of neoplastic tissue (Fig. 927) and may contain small blood vessels and immature bile ducts. Foci of extramedullary hematopoiesis, made up of fetal medullary cells and many megakaryocytes (Fig. 928) are found in the tumor tissue, but not in the non-neoplastic liver.

In *embryonal cell hepatoblastoma,* the neoplastic cells are small, dark-staining, of variable shape with ill-defined borders (Fig. 929), and often lack cohesiveness. These cells, which resemble embryonal hepatocytes, are often poorly differentiated and may not resemble hepatocytes at all. They vary in size and may by polyhedral, cuboidal, or spindle-shaped (Fig. 930). They tend to stain darkly. The cytoplasm is scant and is often ampholphilic. The nuclei are relatively large and hyperchromatic and often contain a prominent nucleolus. Mitotic activity is much more evident than in the fetal type. Extramedullary hematopoiesis is not seen in the embryonal cell tumors. The cells never contain fat, glycogen, or bile droplets. Occasionally, focal, squamous cell metaplasia (Fig. 931) with deposition of keratin is seen (Fig. 932).

The neoplastic cells are usually arranged in sheets or ribbons, although acinar, ductal, and papillary patterns may be seen. Irregularly dispersed capillaries lined by sparse, attenuated endothelial cells may be present. In some areas, vascular channels may be lined by neoplastic cells. Invasion of veins is occasionally seen.

In *mixed epithelial and mesenchymal hepatoblastomas,* the neoplastic cells contain interspersed elements of both endodermal and mesenchymal origin. In addition to any or all of the features of epithelial hepatoblastoma, these tumors may exhibit foci of highly immature mesenchyme, which is made up of long, spindle-shaped cells (Fig. 933) often with delicate processes projecting from the ends (288). Such areas may show the deposition of osteoid (Fig. 933), which often contain calcific deposits (Fig. 934), usually in septa between dark fetal cells. Cartilage is occasionally seen, as are rhabdomyoblasts (300). Rarely, areas of angulated, "sickle-shaped" cells that suggest malignant histiocytoma derived from Kupffer cells have been reported.

Biliary cystadenocarcinoma. Biliary cystadenocarcinomas are relatively rare hepatic neoplasms of adults (301–303). They are malignant cystic tumors lined by mucus-secreting epithelium that appear to be derived from benign cystic adenomas (304). However, only rare cases of such malignant transformation have been unequivocally established (305). Biliary adenocarcinoma tends to occur more frequently in women than men, as do benign biliary cystadenomas. They usually present as right upper quadrant abdominal masses often accompanied by pain. Jaundice is rare, and liver function tests are usually normal, although the alkaline phosphatase activity may be increased. Diagnosis by fine needle biopsy under ultrasonic guidance and cytologic examination will increase the frequency of early diagnosis. The tumors grow slowly and do not metastasize commonly, and, consequently, cure may be achieved by total lobectomy. At autopsy remote metastases may sometimes be found, however.

Grossly, these tumors are usually large and multilocular. They have a dense, collagenized wall, which separates the tumor from the adjacent liver tissue, and which is occasionally invaded by the tumor. The locules contain clear, mucinous fluid that may be colorless, yellow, or brown. Occasionally, the contents are gelatinous, bloody, cloudy, or purulent.

Microscopically, the lining of the locules in most tumors appears benign in some areas and malignant in others. Indeed, in individual locules the lining may be benign on one side and malignant on the other (301). The presence of benign epithelium in most of these malignant tumors makes it likely that the neoplastic tissue arose from the benign tumor rather than the opposite. The neoplastic cells, which may be columnar, polygonal, or round, are arranged in complex fronds of varying size and thickness (Fig. 935). They are usually pleomorphic and hyperchromatic, and often contain bizarre mitotic figures, although the number of mitoses is not greatly increased. Goblet cells, which are common in biliary cystadenomas, may be present in the cystadenocarcinomas, and mucin is often present. The cells may be multinucleated and may show prominent, multiple nucleoli. The presence of bizarre giant cells, abnormal mitoses, and pleomorphism helps differentiate these tumors from bile duct cystadenomas. The epithelial lining is usually layered in contrast to the normal mucosa or that of benign cystadenomas, but may be papillary or acinar, expecially in the solid, noncystic portions of these tumors. Sometimes, one may observe breaks in the basement membrane with invasion of the underlying stroma. Carcinomas arising from congenital cystic lesions have a much worse prognosis than cystadenocarcinomas (306).

Squamous cell carcinoma. Primary squamous cell carcinoma of the liver has been reported extremely rarely (307). Several cases have been described arising in benign teratomas or epithelial elements of nonparasitic cysts of the liver (308,309). Presumably the bile duct epithelium had undergone squamous metaplasia with subsequent transformation to squamous cell carcinoma. Adenosquamous carcinoma of the liver has been reported in patients with preexisting cirrhosis (310), hepatolithiasis (311), and cholangiocarcinoma of the liver (312).

Carcinoid (argentaffinoma). Only a few cases of primary carcinoid of the liver have been reported (48,222,313,314). Presumably such cases are derived from argentaffin cells of the intrahepatic bile ducts. Most hepatic carcinoids, however, represent metastatic lesions from tumors in the gastrointestinal tract or, less commonly, from the gallbladder, pancreas, bronchi, ovary, or testis. Primary carcinoids in extrahepatic tissues may be small and escape detection even at laparotomy. Accordingly, all carcinoids of the liver must be regarded as metastatic unless a complete autopsy fails to demonstrate an extrahepatic primary site. It is not an important point, since the clinical carcinoid syndrome is dependent on the presence of extensive hepatic metastases, whether the primary is in the liver or elsewhere. Furthermore, it is not possible to differentiate primary hepatic carcinoids histologically from metastatic carcinoids that arose in other digestive system sites, from the bronchi or sexual organs, or the islet cells of the pancreas.

In 3 of our 10 biopsy-documented cases of hepatic carcinoid, no extrahepatic site could be demonstrated even after exhaustive examination. These cases were not considered primary, since postmortem examinations were not performed.

The carcinoid syndrome is characterized by attacks of flushing, diarrhea, or asthma, by pulmonic or tricuspid stenosis, and by increased urinary excretion of 5-hydroxyindolacetic acid or 5-hydroxytryptamine in the presence of progressively increasing hepatomegaly. The carcinoid syndrome is not diagnostic of carcinoid, since the same constellation of abnormalities can be seen in hepatocellular carcinoma (172,315), adenocarcinoma of the pancreas, islet cell tumors, bronchial adenocarcinoma, or oat cell carcinoma of the lung that secrete these hormones. These tumors can be effectively treated by liver transplantation (316) or by administration of a somatostatin analogue (317).

Grossly, the liver is characterized by the presence of multiple soft nodules, which are usually separated by coarse, fibrous septa. Occasionally, foci of hemorrhage or necrosis are present.

Microscopically, these tumors are characterized by neoplastic cells, which are usually small and cuboidal with amphophilic cytoplasm and ill-defined cell borders (Fig. 936). The nuclei, which are relatively large and vesicular, tend to be centrally located. Mitotic activity is minimal. They are typically arranged in the form of compact masses of various size and shape (Fig. 937) and, occasionally, as branching ribbons (Fig. 938). The cells at the margins are often slightly taller and resemble epithelial cells, thus simulating a sharply defined border (Fig. 939). Occasionally, the cells are spindle-shaped (Fig. 940). The differential diagnosis from hepatocellular carcinoma may be difficult, but the carcinoid tumor cells have less prominent nucleoli, no acinar structure or bile formation, and the tumors arise in noncirrhotic livers (318,319).

Cytoplasmic granules tend to aggregate at the periphery of

one pole of the cells. Argentaffin and argyrophil granules, which reduce silver salts to metallic silver, can be demonstrated with silver stains (Fig. 941). The tumor masses occasionally contain mucin-producing cells.

The stroma consists of slender collagen septa that separate small islands of tumor (Figs. 938, 939). Broad, dense septa outline larger nodules (Fig. 942). Tumor thrombi are frequently found in veins (Fig. 943).

Malignant adrenal rest tumors. Malignant adrenal rest tumors arise from misplaced adrenocortical cells within the capsule of the liver. Most adrenal rest tumors are benign. The extremely rare malignant ones resemble hepatic adenomas by virtue of their cord-like arrangement (48). In the malignant type, the tumor may resemble hepatocellular carcinoma, especially those of the clear cell type (205). When the tumor is accompanied by hyperfunction of the cortex of the adrenal gland, the diagnosis of adrenal rest tumor seems beyond doubt (320). Only a few have shown such signs, and they have rarely been reported in the malignant variety. These cells, which are poorly differentiated histologically and functionally, tend to be arranged in a fascicular fashion, resembling the zona fasciculata of the adrenal gland.

Inflammatory pseudotumor of the liver. Inflammatory pseudotumors of lung have long been a clinical-pathologic mystery (321). Tumors with similar but variable pathology have been reported in stomach, kidney, spleen, brain, and other organs (322), and a dozen cases of inflammatory pseudotumors of the liver have been reported (322–324). These rare hepatic lesions, which are often seen in children or young adults, show diverse signs and symptoms. About half of the reported cases exhibited low grade fever, abdominal pain, jaundice, and hepatic masses that ranged from 2 to 25 cm in diameter. All had hepatomegaly. Leukocytosis was common. In all cases the course was benign and the disorder subsided. None of the 12 patients died.

Clinically, the tumors were thought to be inflammatory or neoplastic, but no infectious agents were isolated and no malignant cells were found (287).

Histologically, these pseudotumors all contained many plasma cells. Special immunologic studies showed that they were polyclonal and, therefore, nonmalignant. Spindle cells arranged in whorls and bundles were characteristic. Large, oval cells were often seen as were foamy macrophages (3). Lymphocytes, eosinophils, and large mononuclear cells were also present. Often the fibrosis formed dense capsules around the tumor. Necrotic granulomas and obliteration of vessels were sometimes seen.

Although inflammatory pseudotumors are not malignant, they are presented in this section on hepatic malignancy because they are so frequently misdiagnosed as malignant tumors. Histologic diagnoses in the reported cases have included lymphomas and histiocytic, sarcomatous, and anaplastic tumors. Several were thought to be inflammatory and attributed to tuberculosis, syphilis, and parasitic infestations. Their cause or causes remain enigmatic.

Malignant mesenchymal tumors

Angiosarcoma (hemangiosarcoma, malignant hemangioendothelioma, anaplastic sarcoma). Angiosarcomas are rare tumors that affect men predominantly, chiefly in the sixth and seventh decades and uncommonly in adolescents or young adults (108,325). These malignant tumors are derived from endothelial cells (326). Kupffer cell sarcomas are usually included in this category, although they are derived from and resemble Kupffer cells, and may differ appreciably from angiosarcomas in their histologic characteristics.

Etiologically, angiosarcomas appear to arise in patients who have increased deposition of collagen. Varying degrees of hepatic fibrosis ranging from mild portal fibrosis to fullblown cirrhosis are present in one-third to one-half the cases (325). An association with hemochromatosis has also been noted (327). The fibrosis is sometimes a desmoplastic response to the tumor rather than a precursor of it.

A number of specific predisposing factors have been identified epidemiologically. These include thorotrast (328–330), vinyl chloride (330–332), arsenic (330,332), radium (333), oral contraceptives (334), anabolic steroids (335), copper (336), and phenelzine (337). In one-fourth to one-half the cases, however, no such etiologic factor can be identified (338).

Thorotrast is the best established of these agents, and patients who received thorium dioxide as a radiologic contrast agent 30 to 50 years ago are still developing this tumor (329,339). It develops as a consequence of the emission of α, β, and γ radiation by the thorium that is taken up by the reticuloendothelial tissues. Fibrosis often precedes and accompanies this tumor.

Chronic arsenic poisoning, which also causes hepatic fibrosis and noncirrhotic portal hypertension, is well established as an angiosarcoma-inducing agent. It develops in vineyard workers exposed to arsenical insecticides and to patients who have taken Fowler's solution, which contains potassium arsenite (332).

Vinyl chloride, a chemical from which the plastic polyvinylchloride is made, is related to the development of angiosarcoma (330,331,340). This tumor develops primarily in workers involved in the synthesis of this compound, but it is suspected that the tumor may also occur in patients who live close to factories that manufacture vinyl chloride (338). Hepatocellular carcinoma may also be a late consequence of vinyl chloride monomer exposure (340).

The diagnosis can be made by liver scans, which are usually, but nonspecifically abnormal, and by angiography, which may be suggestive of angiosarcoma in almost 90% (341). Liver biopsy is definitive, but this procedure performed either by needle blindly or at laparotomy has frequently been associated with serious bleeding (342).

Clinically, the most common symptoms are abdominal pain, ascites, jaundice, weakness, and wasting and occasionally fever (325). Hepatomegaly is invariably found and splenomegaly is common. Often a hemorrhagic diathesis is present, the result of thrombocytopenia or a consequence of disseminated intravascular coagulation. Rarely, the tumor, which can be diagnosed by CT scan (329), presents as rupture with hemoperitoneum (343). Liver function tests are usually abnormal, but no specific pattern has emerged (342). The course of angiosarcoma is rapidly and progressively downhill, usually leading to death within a few months.

Grossly, the grayish white tumor is usually multicentric with nodules of variable size scattered throughout the liver. Occasionally, it may present as a large, solitary mass. The tumor nodules are sharply outlined, but not encapsulated. They are usually soft, often hemorrhagic, and sometimes contain peliotic cavities. Metastases are found in spleen, lungs, lymph nodes, bone, and adrenals in half the cases at autopsy.

Microscopically, the early lesions of angiosarcoma are characterized by ill-defined areas in which the sinusoids are dilated and lined by large endothelial cells with abundant PAS-D-positive cytoplasm and hyperchromatic nuclei (Fig. 944). The spaces of Disse are widened. These changes are frequently found in some foci of hepatocellular hypertrophy and hyperplasia. The peliotic changes often precede the appearance of angiosarcoma (330,331) and may be responsible for late fatalities (334).

As the lesion advances, the sinusoids widen further, leading to the formation of cavernous or peliotic channels lined by neoplastic endothelial cells (Fig. 945). These endothelial cells increase in number until they fill the dilated, peliotic-like spaces (Fig. 946). The neoplastic cells, which have faintly eosinophilic cytoplasm, also increase in size and atypia, and often form papillary projections into the lumen. As they enlarge, the nuclei become irregular and intensely hyperchromatic and show a variable number of mitoses (Fig. 947). Bizarre, multinucleated giant forms may occur (Fig. 948). In many cases the neoplastic cells become elongated and spindle-shaped, and form solid masses (Fig. 949). Reticulin fibers between cords of neoplastic cells are increased in number, condensed, and coarsened. Invasion of central and portal veins is common. Sometimes thorotrast is seen in macrophages in or near the tumor (Fig. 950). Foci of hemorrhage, degeneration or necrosis are relatively common. Areas of extramedullary hematopoiesis are present in most cases (Fig. 951).

Kupffer cell sarcoma presents a similar histologic picture but differs by the presence of active phagocytosis by the tumor cells and the formation of new blood vessels (345).

Malignant mesenchymoma (mesenchymal sarcoma, undifferentiated embryonal sarcoma). Malignant mesenchymoma, a rare, undifferentiated neoplasm of mesenchymal origin, usually affects children between 6 and 10 years of age, but occasionally, appears in adults (346–348). Patients often present with an abdominal mass, but commonly exhibit abdominal pain or fever, and, sometimes, hemoperitoneum secondary to rupture of the tumor (108). Transaminase and alkaline phosphatase activities are often increased. Unlike other types of primary malignant hepatic lesions that are hypervascular, these tumors are hypovascular on arteriography (349). These sarcomas may spread directly to adjacent structures or metastasize to distant, extrahepatic sites. They are usually fatal within a year of the onset of symptoms, but after resection patients may survive for several years.

Grossly, the tumor appears as a large, solitary mass, which is usually globular and well demarcated by a pseudocapsule of compressed hepatic parenchyma (108,346). It tends to be soft or fluctuant. On cross section it has a gelatinous appearance and often contains cystic areas filled with necrotic debris, clotted blood, or gelatin-like material. Areas of hemorrhage or necrosis are common.

Microscopically, the neoplastic cells are anaplastic and spindle-shaped with ill-defined borders arranged in sheets or whorls (Fig. 952) or interlacing bundles scattered in an acid mucopolysaccharide-rich, myxomatous matrix (Fig. 953). The cross striations typical of muscle cells are not present in the cytoplasm of the neoplastic cells. If they were, these tumors would be classified as embryonal rhabdomyosarcomas, which are discussed next. The nuclei may be round, elongated, or irregular and contain stippled chromatin; nucleoli are inconspicuous. Multinucleated cells with bizarre, hyperchromatic nuclei are frequently present (Fig. 953). Mitotic figures are common. Some tumors show sharply defined, PAS-positive, diastase-resistant, cytoplasmic inclusions. Some such bodies may be found

in the stroma, probably released during destruction of the neoplastic cells. These inclusions may represent α-1-antitrypsin (108).

The tumor is bounded by a fibrous pseudocapsule derived from compressed, atrophic hepatic parenchyma (Fig. 954). Cystic structures lined by cuboidal epithelium are often found at the periphery of the tumor close to the pseudocapsule (Figs. 954, 955). They probably represent dilated, entrapped, hyperplastic, degenerating bile ducts. Electron microscopic studies suggest that these tumors may be derived from both epithelial and mesenchymal elements (350).

Embryonal rhabdomyosarcoma. Embryonal rhabdomyosarcomas are extremely rare tumors of infants and young children that arise in the extrahepatic biliary tree (351) or liver (352). They are indistinguishable from malignant mesenchymomas except for the presence of muscle-like, cross striations in the cytoplasm of many of the neoplastic cells (48,353). The cross striations may be difficult to demonstrate (90). Myoglobin, myosin, desmin, and AFP have been identified immunohistochemically (354,355). Collison tumors of hepatocellular carcinoma and rhabdomyosarcoma have been observed (356).

Leiomyosarcoma. Leiomyosarcomas are rare hepatic tumors of middle-aged and elderly individuals, usually women, that arise from the wall of large veins or bile ducts (90,357,358). Rarely, they present as primary hepatic tumors with hepatomegaly and a palpable mass followed by wasting (359) and, occasionally, by ascites. Although they are usually fatal within a year, they cause death by massive replacement of the liver rather than by distant metastases, and therefore, survival may be prolonged by resection of the tumor.

Grossly, the tumors are usually large, firm, nodular, solitary masses. Occasionally they are multiple. They are sharply circumscribed, but not encapsulated. Intrahepatic and remote metastases may occur.

Microscopically, the neoplastic cells are elongated, spindle-shaped cells with eosinophilic cytoplasm (Fig. 956). Longitudinal cytoplasmic myofibrils, which are pathognomonic of the tumor, usually require electron microscopy to be seen (360). The nuclei are elongated, may have blunt ends, are of variable size, and exhibit frequent mitoses, which are often atypical (Fig. 956). The cells are arranged in sharply intersecting bundles (Fig. 957). Sometimes, the neoplastic cells are round or oval-shaped with oval nuclei arranged in clusters and with mucin-stained stroma (Fig. 958). These may represent cross sections of bundles of the elongated neoplastic cells (Fig. 956). Foci of necrosis are often found, especially in the central zones of the tumor. It is impossible to differentiate primary from metastatic leiomyosarcoma arising in the gastrointestinal tract, gallbladder, or mesentery (361).

Fibrosarcoma. Fibrosarcomas are the rarest of the primary hepatic sarcomas. They originate in the fibrous tissues (90,362). They occur in middle-aged or elderly people, especially men. They are only rarely seen in patients with cirrhotic livers.

They usually present with hepatomegaly with or without a palpable mass. Late in the course, wasting, abdominal pain, jaundice, or ascites may occur. Rarely, the tumor ruptures. Sometimes, these massive tumors utilize large amounts of glucose and cause severe, recurrent hypoglycemia (363,364). They tend to grow slowly and to enormous size, and do not metastasize until late in the course, so that resection of the tumor may increase longevity.

Grossly, these tumors are large, firm, circumscribed, but nonencapsulated solitary masses. Rarely, satellite tumors are present. They sometimes invade the portal vein, extend to adjacent viscera, or metastasize to regional lymph nodes or to the lungs.

Microscopically, primary and secondary fibrosarcomas are indistinguishable. They are composed of elongated, spindle-shaped neoplastic cells with long nuclei with pointed ends (Fig. 959). They show varying degrees of pleomorphism, hyperchromasia, and mitotic activity. The cells are arranged in intersecting bundles, occasionally producing a herringbone pattern (Fig. 960). Reticulin fibers are often interspersed with neoplastic cells. Collagen bundles vary in amount. Foci of necrosis are seen in some cases (90).

Malignant epithelioid hemangioendothelioma (vasoablative endotheliosarcoma, sclerosing interstitial vascular sarcoma). Malignant epithelioid hemangioendothelioma, a recently reported hepatic neoplasm, was first described in 1982 (365). It had previously been found in the lungs (intravascular bronchoalveloar tumor of lung) (366), soft tissues, and bone (367). A total of almost 50 cases arising in the liver had been reported by 1987 (90,368).

Epithelioid hemangioendotheliomas are slow-growing tumors that usually occur in middle-aged patients. It has been suggested that in young women this tumor may be related to the use of oral contraceptives (369). Patients with this tumor present clinically with constitutional symptoms including anorexia, vomiting, abdominal discomfort, and weight loss (90). Hepatosplenomegaly is common, but jaundice is rare. The tumors may be massive at the time of diagnosis. Serum alkaline phosphatase levels are usually increased. AFP is normal, and carcinoembryonic antigen, keratin, and mucin are absent. Liver-spleen scintigrams show multiple defects or decreased uptake. Angiography shows a nonspecific, hypovascular pattern. The uninvolved lobes tend to undergo compensatory hypertrophy (370).

The tumor arises in endothelial cells as indicated by prominent factor VIII staining. It does not arise in the setting of chronic hepatic disease.

Grossly, the lesions are multiple and distributed throughout the liver. Often there is a main mass that may be 10 cm in diameter, and separate satellite masses. These whitish gray or tan lesions are firm and gritty when cut. Calcification is often seen on radiographic or ultrasonic imaging. There is rarely underlying liver disease.

Microscopically, the lesions show densely fibrotic centers. At low power the tumor may resemble cirrhosis (Figs. 961, 962). The plump tumor cells extend through the sinusoids, central veins, and portal vein branches (Fig. 963). Clumps of cells may completely fill the vessels or may partially obstruct them by polypoid growth. Liver cell plates undergo atrophy and may disappear as they do in severe chronic passive congestion. Immunostaining with antibody to factor VIII can establish the endothelial origin of this tumor (Fig. 964).

The tumor cells tend to be elongated with vacuolated cytoplasm and interdigitating processes (dendritic cells) or may be oval cells with abundant cytoplasm, nuclear atypia, and many mitoses (epithelioid cells). Intermediate forms may be found. These cells give the tumor a malignant adenocarcinomatous appearance with eosinophilic cytoplasm. They may also be mis-taken for metastases, cholangiocarcinoma, or angiosarcoma. These cells are surrounded by prominent PAS-positive basement membranes. Cytoplasmic vacuoles may contain red blood cells. Stromal inflammation consisting of lymphocytes, neutrophils, and eosinophils is typical. Factor VIII–like antigen can be demonstrated immunohistologically in the cytoplasm and in the vascular channels, and has been found in sizable quantities in serum (90). As the tumor matures, it stimulates collagen deposition, which may culminate in extensive fibrosis that may be misdiagnosed as cirrhosis. Sinusoids may be filled with dense connective tissue that contains scattered tumor cells, sometimes simulating veno-occlusive disease. Often major veins are occluded by tumor cells and the Budd-Chiari syndrome may be found. By electron microscopy the tumor cells show large numbers of intermediate filaments, suggesting that they are derived from both endothelial and epithelial cells (365).

Despite frequent metastases to spleen, lymph nodes, lung, and bone, the tumors grow slowly and long survival is common, but not invariable (371). Tumors arising in the liver tend to metastasize more readily than those arising in soft tissues (367,368). However, extrahepatic primaries may metastasize to the liver. Treatment consists of hepatic lobectomy when feasible, or transplantation (372). Prior to identification of this tumor, it was probably misdiagnosed as metastatic carcinoma or adenocarcinoma of undetermined origin.

Malignant mixed tumors

Combined hepatocellular carcinoma and sarcoma. This rare combination of neoplasms, which has been reported in relatively few patients (108,373,374), is found in about 40% of hepatocellular carcinomas (140). Like this combination, hepatocellular carcinoma tends to occur in men with preexisting cirrhosis.

The clinical features of these combined neoplasms are indistinguishable from those of hepatocellular carcinoma alone. When the two neoplasms arise in different portions of the liver and show no areas of transition, they exhibit grossly and microscopically the characteristic features of the two respective tumors. Hepatocellular carcinoma tends to produce single spheric nodules of yellow, green, or brownish tumor, which are often soft. Hepatic sarcomas are characteristically irregular, firm, silky, white nodules. Instances of the two tumors arising independently in the same liver may be classified as transitional tumors or as "collision" tumors when they impinge on each other. One case of combined hepatocellular carcinoma cholangiocarcinoma has been reported (375). Immunohistochemical studies suggest that the sarcoma arises from the *combined* tumor. Microscopically, the sarcomatous portions consist of spindle-shaped cells and bizarre multinucleated cells [(140); Fig. 965]. Sometimes, when the tumors are intermixed, and transitions from hepatocellular to spindle cells are demonstrable, it is not possible to be certain whether they arose separately or are "transitional" tumors (Fig. 966). The presence of large areas of typical, trabecular hepatocellular carcinoma with small areas of intermixed spindle cells, some of which contain eosinophilic granular cytoplasm typical of hepatocytes, suggests that these transitional combined tumors are variants of hepatocellular carcinoma (Fig. 967). The immunocytohistologic demonstration in "sarcomatous" cells of AFP, albumin, fibrinogen, and keratin suggests hepatocystic origin (140).

Malignant hepatic mixed tumor. Tumors that contain both benign epithelial and benign mesenchymal elements are classified as *benign hepatic mixed tumors*. When either the epithelial tissue or the mesenchymal tissue is malignant and the other element benign, they are classified as *hepatic mixed tumors*. Benign mesenchymal elements may include osteoid and collagen in such tumors. These may also be seen in mixed hepatoblastoma. When both the epithelial and mesenchymal components are malignant, the tumors are classified as *malignant mixed hepatic tumors*. These rare tumors can also be differentiated from malignant teratomas. Teratomas contain neoplastic elements derived from all three germinal layers, at least one of which is malignant. It is often impossible to differentiate them from malignant hepatic mixed tumors when the ectodermal elements are not evident (376).

Malignant hepatic mixed tumors are characterized by a rapidly enlarging liver or right upper quadrant abdominal mass. Jaundice, ascites, and clinical evidence of metastases are uncommon except terminally. Grossly, these tumors are usually large, firm, solitary, lobulated masses. Microscopically, the epithelial elements resemble those of hepatocellular carcinoma, hepatoblastoma, or cholangiocarcinoma. Some of these tumors may have no hepatocytic elements even though they are formed in the liver (377). They may show nests of squamous cells that have formed pearls of keratin. The mesenchymal cells form masses of primitive, malignant spindle cells, some of which may be rhabdomyosarcoma cells, as shown by the cytoplasmic cross striations (376). Sometimes, they will express multiple differentiations (378). Deposits of osteoid may be present. A case of hepatocellular carcinoma combined with an osteoclastoma has been reported (379).

Malignant teratoma. Malignant teratomas, exceedingly rare tumors of children, contain neoplastic elements from all three germinal layers. The clinical and morphologic features of these tumors are identical to those of benign teratomas of the liver, except that one or more components has undergone malignant transformation (380). Teratomas usually occur before the age of three, mainly in female children, and most are benign (108).

Metastatic tumors of the liver

In general, hepatic metastases greatly outnumber primary malignant tumors of the liver. At autopsy, metastases are encountered in the liver in approximately 40% of patients with all types of cancer (381–383). This percentage is higher than occurs in the lungs, the second most frequent site of metastasis. As might be anticipated, tumors in organs drained by the portal venous system metastasize to the liver more frequently than tumors arising in nonsplanchnic organs (384,385). Tumors in organs drained by the systemic venous system may also metastasize preferentially to the liver with notable exceptions that include tumors of thyroid, prostate, and bone (385). Bronchogenic carcinoma is the most common source of hepatic metastases. Despite reports to the contrary (386), hepatic metastases are not rare in cirrhotic livers. They are seen, however, less frequently at autopsy in cirrhotic than in noncirrhotic livers, a phenomenon that is multifactorial in origin (383). First, portal-systemic shunting permits the portal venous blood to bypass the liver via intrahepatic and extrahepatic collateral vessels, presumably carrying malignant cells to other organs. Second, the reduction in total hepatic blood flow in cirrhosis decreases the amount of blood that passes through the liver per unit of time. Third, hepatic metastases are decreased in cirrhotic patients because the high premature death rate in cirrhosis reduces the risk of developing the metastases (387). This fallacy affects data obtained at autopsy in the coincidence of any two individually lethal diseases (388).

The clinical manifestations of metastatic liver disease are many and varied. Metastases that are small or few in number give rise to no symptoms or signs (389). Jaundice does not occur unless the primary neoplasm is biliary or pancreatic, or until the late stages. In the majority of cases of hepatic metastases, serum alkaline phosphatase activity is increased, and serum albumin concentrations are decreased in virtually all (390). Hypoalbuminemia is frequently present in patients with malignancy without hepatic metastases. Transaminase activity (40%) and serum bilirubin concentrations are often elevated (25%). The frequency and number of hepatic metastases and the degree of hepatic involvement increase as the degree of abnormality of the liver function tests increases, especially for alkaline phosphatase, transaminase, and bilirubin levels. Abnormalities of two or three of these tests are even more indicative of metastatic involvement (390). The use of new assays such as 5'-nucleotide phosphodiesterase, isoenzymatic V, 5'-nucleotidase, and gamma-glutamyl transferase have not been appreciably better than conventional assays (391). Tumor nodules 2 or 3 cm in diameter may be detectable on scintiscan, and smaller nodules are detectable by ultrasonography (72) or computerized tomography (392). Intraoperative ultrasonography has been shown to be superior to preoperative ultrasound evaluation and far superior to manual examination at surgery (393). As metastases grow in size and number, a variety of manifestations may appear. Most commonly, the liver enlarges and becomes indurated. Hepatic nodules, which often cause pain, can be palpated. Jaundice and ascites are frequent findings. There may be only anorexia and weight loss or no symptoms or signs at all.

Occasionally, there may be a friction rub over liver (394) or a bruit (385). Evidence of portal hypertension such as hemorrhage from esophageal varices (395) or hepatic coma may develop (396). Calcific deposits may be demonstrable by x-ray and may appear to be nodular or fine, diffuse, punctate calcifications (397). Hypoglycemia is occasionally seen. Many cases exhibit signs or symptoms referable to the primary tumor or to extrahepatic metastases.

Needle biopsy of the liver is the most definitive method of establishing the diagnosis of metastatic malignancy. The overall success rate in demonstrating hepatic metastases by blind, random, cutaneous needle biopsy is approximately 50% (380). The frequency of detection depends on the extent of the metastases. Even in asymptomatic patients without hepatomegaly, metastases are demonstrable in 20% of patients with hepatic involvement (389).

The frequency with which metastases are detectable by random needle biopsy, which removes a core of tissue that represents less than 1/50,000 of the weight and volume of the liver, is surprisingly great. This high yield reflects the fact that metastases are often found as neoplastic cells that infiltrate the liver diffusely. These observations indicate that the bulk of hepatic metastases, like icebergs, may be largely invisible. Rarely, biopsies are positive in the absence of any visible metastases at surgery or autopsy. When the signs and symptoms of liver involvement, i.e., hepatomegaly or jaundice, are present, about 75% of biopsies are positive (389).

The use of multiple needle biopsies performed by changing the angle of the needle through the same site of entry increases the detection rate. Serial sectioning of the specimens increases the yield of tumor (389). Selection of the biopsy site to aim for palpable nodules or cold spots on liver-spleen scans or by performing biopsies under ultrasonic or CT guidance (398) also enhance the yield. Cytologic examination of fluid aspirated at the time of biopsy (399) is sometimes positive when the histologic sections do not show tumor. Laparoscopic biopsy, too, may increase the yield of positive biopsies (400), but this is a more invasive, complicated procedure.

Despite old reports to the contrary (401), needle biopsy appears to be no more hazardous in patients with hepatic metastases than in those with non-neoplastic liver disorders. In our own series, no fatalities have occurred in patients with hepatic malignancy, and only one patient required transfusions after postbiopsy hemorrhage. However, two more recent reports of more than 68,000 (402) and 9000 (403) needle liver biopsies, respectively, indicate that the prevalence of post-biopsy bleeding in patients with hepatic malignancy is much greater than in those without it. Indeed, these data suggest that the risk is from 2 to 50 times higher (404).

The blood supply to metastases varies greatly, and none of the variations imitates the normal angioarchitecture of the liver parenchyma (405). Most show hypervascularization with a large artery that forms a hilum from which smaller arterioles supply the tumor. Some are characterized by multiple small arteries that supply the tumor from the periphery. About one-fourth of metastases show hypovascularity. More than half of metastases receive some blood from the portal vein. Portal tumor thrombi are common, suggesting retrograde intraportal spread of tumor. Metastases tend to be surrounded by micrometastases that are usually supplied by sinusoidal blood, but newly formed capillary vessels sometimes contribute.

Therapy of neoplasms involves ligation or embolization of the hepatic artery or sometimes of the portal veins as well (188). Chemotherapy may be administered intraarterially. Subcutaneous implantable pumps have been used (406).

Grossly, tumor nodules vary in size, number, and consistency. They range from a single small metastasis to multiple metastases that may be widely disseminated. Occasionally, tumors will replace virtually the whole liver. Tumors often coalesce to form large, irregular masses, and sometimes present as single, large solitary masses. A metastasis just beneath the capsule will frequently bulge or have an umbilicate appearance. Foci of hemorrhage, necrosis, or scarring are relatively common. Rarely, the liver is infiltrated by bands of neoplastic tissue that outline nodules of intact parenchyma, producing a picture that may mimic cirrhosis (395). Gross invasion of major hepatic and portal veins by tumor, which is common in primary hepatic neoplasms, is unusual in metastatic malignancy. Small intrahepatic portal veins, however, are frequently occluded by tumor. The combination of tumor thrombi and extrinsic compression of intrahepatic portal veins may make the blood supply to metastases predominantly arterial. Extensive intrahepatic involvement of small hepatic veins may give rise to post-sinusoidal portal hypertension and a clinical picture similar to that of cirrhosis with ascites, esophageal varices, and portal-systemic encephalopathy (395,396).

The site of the primary neoplasm cannot be made from the gross appearance of the metastases in the liver, but certain characteristics of size, color, or pattern favor probable sites (48). Colon cancers tend to produce a large single metastasis with smaller satellite lesions. They often exhibit calcification. Squamous cell carcinomas tend to show central necrosis. Bronchogenic carcinomas are often gray or white in color without necrosis or hemorrhage. Pigmented melanomas are black or tan depending on the amount of pigment produced. Carcinomas of the gallbladder often extend directly from the gallbladder bed and may develop satellite lesions around the circumference. Miliary metastases are common in patients with prostatic carcinoma.

Microscopically, metastatic carcinomas are usually readily differentiated from hepatocellular carcinoma except when both are highly undifferentiated or when the neoplastic cells of hepatocellular carcinoma are arranged in the form of acini or ducts, rather than their typical trabecular pattern. The presence of bile favors a diagnosis of hepatocellular carcinoma or other hepatic malignancy. Mallory bodies in the cytoplasm of neoplastic cells may identify them as of hepatic origin, although they may occur in other malignancies as well (207). On the other hand, the presence of mucin in the lumens of acini or in the cytoplasm of neoplastic cells almost invariably identifies them as being of nonhepatic origin. Desmoplastic reactions, which are common in hepatic metastases, are uncommon in hepatocellular carcinoma, except in fibrolamellar hepatocellular carcinoma.

The identification of the primary site of origin of metastatic adenocarcinomas and their differentiation from cholangiocarcinoma is usually difficult. Metastases from some forms of breast cancer show remarkably close resemblance to cholangiocarcinoma (Fig. 918).

A minority of metastases exhibit distinctive histologic features that, at least tentatively, suggest the probably site of origin. Examples from our personal experience include *carcinoid*, usually from the gastrointestinal tract (Figs. 936–943), *leiomyosarcomas* (Figs. 956–958), and *fibrosarcomas* (Figs. 959, 960). In addition, *pigmented melanomas*, which usually originate in the skin or retina, are readily recognized (Fig. 968). *Amelanotic melanomas* may be impossible to differentiate from other metastatic lesions (Fig. 969). Sometimes, specific stains for melanin are required to identify the pigment (Fig. 970). Hypernephromas from the kidney show characteristic clear cells (Fig. 971), which must be differentiated from clear cell hepatocellular carcinoma (Fig. 879), but in the latter, all of the neoplastic cells are rarely of the clear cell type (Fig. 880). *Small cell or oat cell carcinomas* of the lung often have a distinctive appearance characterized by small cells with large nuclei, scanty cytoplasm, and indefinite borders (Fig. 972). These tumors may be difficult to differentiate from small cell, anaplastic malignancies arising in other sites. Metastases from *islet cell tumors of the pancreas* often show regular cells that suggest an endocrine tumor, and when arranged in small islands, suggest islet cell carcinomas (Fig. 973). *Squamous cell carcinomas* may show squamous-like neoplastic cells with keratin pearls.

In addition to the metastases themselves, there are often histologic changes in the uninvolved portion of the liver near the tumor (407). These changes, which are nonspecific, include portal edema, bile ductular proliferation, focal sinusoidal dilatation, and infiltration with neutrophils or mononuclear cells. When there is accompanying biliary obstruction or leukocytosis, the portal inflammatory reaction may be predominantly neutrophilic. The parenchyma may show compression or atrophy of hepatocyte cords, scattered areas of focal hepatitis, in which small, circumscribed collections of mononuclear cells replace groups of lost hepatocytes. Occasionally, these areas may be bordered by or contain a few degenerating hepatocytes. Increased hepatocytic regenerative activity expressed as binucleate cells, twin plates, and an increased number of mitoses may be present. Bile stasis is sometimes seen in the absence of hyperbilirubinemia. Patchy, fatty infiltration or nonzonal, sinusoidal congestion may be found.

References

1. Stocker JT, Ishak KG: Focal nodular hyperplasia of the liver: a study of 21 pediatric cases. Cancer 48:336–345, 1981.
2. Ishak KG, Rabin L: Benign tumors of the liver. Med Clinics North Am 59:995–1013, 1975.
3. Goodman ZD: Benign tumors of the liver. In Neoplasms of the Liver, edited by K. Okuda, K.G. Ishak. Tokyo, Springer-Verlag, 1987, pp. 105–125.
4. Wanless: IR: Micronodular transformation (nodular regenerative hyperplasia) of the liver: a report of 64 cases among 2500 autopsies and a new classification of benign hepatocellular nodules. Hepatology 11:787–790, 1990.
5. Wanless IR, Albrecht S, Bilbao J, Frei JV, Heathcote EJ, Roberts EA, Chiasson D: Multiple focal nodular hyperplasia of the liver associated with vascular malformations of various organs and neoplasia of the brain: a new syndrome. Mod Pathol 2:456–462, 1989.
6. Klatskin G: Hepatic tumors. Possible relationship to use of oral contraceptives. Gastroenterology 73:386–394, 1977.
7. Ishak KG: Hepatic neoplasms associated with contraceptive and anabolic steroids. In Recent Results in Cancer Research, No. 66, edited by C.H. Longeman. Berlin, Springer-Verlag, 1979, pp. 73–124.
8. Mettlin C, Natarajan N: Studies on the role of oral contraceptive use in etiology of benign and malignant liver tumours. J Surg Oncol 18:73–85, 1981.
9. Fischer G, Hartmann H, Droese M, Schauer A, Bock KW: Histochemical and immunohistochemical detection of putative preneoplastic liver foci in women after long-term use of oral contraceptives. Virchows Arch (B) 50:321–337, 1986.
10. Wanless IR, Mawdsley C, Adams R: On the pathogenesis of focal nodular hyperplasia of the liver. Hepatology 5:1194–1200, 1985.
11. Butron Vila MM, Haot J, Desmet VJ: Cholestatic features in focal nodular hyperplasia. Liver 4:387–395, 1984.
12. Foster JH: Primary benign solid tumors of the liver. Am J Surg 133:536–541, 1977.
13. Nokes SR, Baker ME, Spritzer CE, Meyers W, Herfkens RJ: Hepatic adenoma: MR appearance mimicking focal nodular huyperplasia. J Comput Assist Tomogr 12:885–887, 1988.
14. Friedman LS, Gang DL, Hedbert SE, Isselbacher KJ: Simultaneous occurrence of hepatic adenoma and focal nodular hyperplasia: report of a case and review of the literature. Hepatology 6:536–540, 1984.
15. Grange JD, Guechot J, Legendre C, Giboudeau J, Darnis F, Poupon R: Liver adenoma and focal nodular hyperplasia in a man with high endogenous sex steroids. Gastroenterology 93:1409–1413, 1987.
16. Vecchio FM, Fabiano A, Ghirlanda G, Manna R, Massi G: Fibrolamellar carcinoma of the liver: the malignant counterpart of focal nodular hyperplasia with oncocytic change. Am J Clin Pathol 81:521–526, 1984.
17. Rooks JB, Ory HW, Ishak KG, Strauss LT, Greenspan JR, Tyler CW: Epidemiology of hepatocellular adenoma. The role of oral contraceptive use. JAMA 242:644–648, 1979.
18. Edmondson HA, Henderson BE, Benton B: Liver-cell adenomas associated with use of oral contraceptives. N Engl J Med 294:470–472, 1976.
19. Buhler H, Pirovino M, Akavbiantz A, Altorfer J, Weitzel M, Maranta E, Schmid M: Regression of liver cell adenoma. A follow-up study of three consecutive patients after discontinuation of oral contraceptive use. Gastroenterology 82:775–782, 1982.
20. Marks WH, Thompson N, Appleman H: Failure of hepatic adenomas (HCA) to regress after discontinuance of oral contraceptives. An association with focal nodular hyperplasia (FNH) and uterine leiomyoma. Ann Surg 208:190–195, 1988.
21. Wheeler DA, Edmondson HA, Reynolds, TB: Spontaneous liver cell adenoma in children. Am J Clin Pathol 85:6–12, 1986.
22. Craig JR, Peters RL, Edmondson HA: Tumors of the Liver and Intrahepatic Bile Ducts, 2nd Series. Fascicle 26. Washington, D.C. Armed Forces Institute of Pathology, 1989, p. 280.
23. Carrasco D, Prieto M, Moll JL: Multiple hepatic adenomas after long term therapy with testosterone enanthate. Review of the literature. J Hepatol 1:573–578, 1985.
24. Overly WL, Dankoff JA, Wang BK: Androgens and hepatocellular carcinoma in an athlete. Ann Intern Med 100:158–159, 1984.
25. Davis M, Postmann B, Searle M, Wright R, Williams R: Histological evidence of carcinoma in a hepatic tumour associated with oral contraceptives. Br Med J 2:496–498, 1975.
26. Carbone A, Vecchio FM: Presence of cytoplasmic progesterone receptors in hepatic adenomas. A report of two cases. Am J Clin Pathol 85:325–329, 1986.
27. Coire CI, Qizilbash AH, Castelli MF: Hepatic adenomata in Type Ia glycogen storage disease. Arch Pathol Lab Med 111:166–169, 1987.
28. Lui AFK, Hiratzka LF, Hirose FM: Multiple adenomas of the liver. Cancer 45:1001–1004, 1980.
29. Flejou J-E, Barge J, Menu Y, Degott C, Bismuth H, Potet F, Benhamou J-P: Liver adenomatosis. An entity distinct from liver adenoma? Gastroenterology 89:1132–1138, 1985.
30. Welch TJ, Sheedy PF, Johnson CM, Stephens DH, Charboneau JW, Brown ML, May GR, Adson MA, McGill, DB: Focal nodular hyperplasia and hepatic adenoma: comparison of angiography, CT, US, and scintigraphy. Radiology 156:593–595, 1985.
31. Phillips MJ, Langer B, Stone R, Fisher MM, Ritchie S: Benign liver cell tumors. Classification and ultrastructural pathology. Cancer 32:463–470, 1973.
32. Koelma IA, Nap M, Huitoma S, Krom RA, Houthoff HJ: Hepatocellular carcinoma, adenoma and focal nodular hyperplasia. Comparative histopathologic study with immunohistochemical parameters. Arch Pathol Lab Med 110:1035–1040, 1986.
33. Winkler K, Poulsen H: Liver disease with periportal sinusoidal dilatation. A possible complication to contraceptive steroids. Scand J Gastroenterol 10:699–704, 1975.
34. Goodman ZD, Ishak KG: Hepatocellular carcinoma in women: probable lack of etiology association with oral contraceptive steroids. Hepatology 2:440–444, 1982.
35. Chen KTK, Bocian JJ: Multiple hepatic adenomas. Arch Pathol Lab Med 107:274–275, 1983.
36. Arakawa M, Kage M, Sugihara S: Emergence of malignant lesions within an adenomatous hyperplastic nodule in a cirrhotic liver. Gastroenterology 91:198–208, 1986.
37. Gold JH, Guzman IJ, Rosai J: Benign tumors of the liver. Pathologic examination of 45 cases. Am J Clin Pathol 70:6–17, 1978.
38. Govindarajan S, Peters RL: The bile duct adenoma. A lesion distinct from Meyenburg complex. Arch Pathol Lab Med 108:922–924, 1984.
39. Ishak KG, Willis GW, Cummins SD, Bullock AA: Biliary cystadenoma and cystadenocarcinoma. Report of 14 cases and review of the literature. Cancer 39:322–338, 1977.
40. Forrest ME, Cho KJ, Shields JJ: Biliary cystadenomas: sonographic angiographic pathologic correlations. AJR 135:723–727, 1980.
41. Wheeler DA, Edmondson HA: Cystadenoma with mesenchymal stroma (CMS) in the liver and bile ducts. A clinicopathologic study of 17 cases, 4 with malignant change. Cancer 56:1434–1445, 1985.
42. Akwari NE, Tucker A, Seigler HF, Itani KMF: Hepatobiliary cystadenoma with mesenchymal stroma Ann Surg 211:18–27, 1990.
43. Veloso FT, Ribeiro AT, Teixeira A, Ramalhao J, Saleiro JS, Serrao D: Biliary papillomatosis: Report of a case with 5-year follow-up. Am J Gastroenterol 78:645–648, 1983.
44. Gouma DJ, Mutum SS, Benjamin IS, Blumgart LH: Intrahepatic biliary papillomatosis. Br J Surg 71:72–74, 1984.
45. Caroli J: Diseases of intrahepatic bile ducts. Isr J Med Sci 4:21–35, 1968.
46. Mercadier M, Bodard M, Fingerhut A, Chigot JP: Papillomatosis of the intrahepatic bile ducts. World J Surg 8:30–35, 1984.
47. Neumann RD, LiVolsi VA, Rosenthal NS, Burrell M, Ball TJ: Adenocarcinoma in biliary papillomatosis. Gastroenterology 70:779–782, 1976.
48. Edmondson HA: Tumors of the Liver and Intrahepatic Bile Ducts. Washington, D.C. Armed Forces Institute of Pathology, Fascicle 125:1–216, 1958.
49. Contreras P, Altieri E, Liberman C, Gac A, Rojas A, Ibarra A, Ravanal M, Seron-Ferre M: Adrenal rest tumor of the liver causing Cushing's syndrome: treatment with ketoconazole preceding an apparent surgical cure. J Clin Endocrinol Metab 60:21–28, 1985.
50. Solis-Herruzo JA, Vidal JV, Colina F, Santalla F, Castellano G: Nodular regenerative hyperplasia of the liver associated with the toxic oil syndrome: report of five cases. Hepatology 6:687–693, 1986.
51. Wanless IR, Godwin TA, Allen F, Feder A: Nodular regenerative hyperplasia of the liver in hematologic disorders: a possible response to obliterative portal venopathy. Medicine 59:367–379, 1980.

52. Snover D, Bloomer J, McGlave P: Nodular regenerative hyperplasia: a possible cause of liver disease following bone marrow transplantation. Lab Invest *54:*60A, 1986.

53. Strohmeyer FW, Ishak KG: Nodular transformation (nodular "regenerative" hyperplasia) of the liver. A clinicopathologic study of 30 cases. Hum Pathol *12:*60–71, 1981.

54. Solis-Herruzo JA, Duran A, Colina F, Santalla F, Garcia-Cabezudo J, Munoz-Yaque MT, Morillas JD: Laparoscopic and histological problems in the diagnosis of nodular regenerative hyperplasia of the liver. Endoscopy *17:*105–108, 1985.

55. Weinbren K, Mutum SS: Pathologic aspects of diffuse nodular hyperplasia of the liver. J Pathol *143:*81–92, 1984.

56. Farber E, Sarma DSR: Biology of disease. Hepatocarcinogenesis: a dynamic cellular perspective. Lab Invest *56:*4–22, 1987.

57. Mones JM, Saldana JM, Albores-Saavaerda J: Nodular regenerative hyperplasia of the liver. Report of three cases and review of the literature. Arch Pathol Lab Med *108:*741–743, 1984.

58. Popper H, Thomas LB, Telles NC, Falk H, Selikoff IJ: Development of hepatic angiosarcoma in man induced by vinyl chloride, thorotrast and arsenic. Am J Pathol *92:*349–376, 1978.

59. Thung SN: Alpha-1-antitrypsin distribution in nodular regenerative hyperplasia of liver. Hepatology *11:*143–144, 1990.

60. Kondo F, Ebara M, Sugiura N, Wada K, Kita K, Hirooka N, Nagato Y, Kondo Y, Ohto M, Okuda K: Histological features and clinical course of large regenerative nodules: evaluation of their precancerous potentiality. Hepatology *12:*592–598, 1990.

61. Gerber MA, Thung SN, Shen S, Stromeyer FW, Ishak KG: Phenotypic characterization of hepatic proliferation. Antigenic expression by proliferating epithelial cells in fetal liver, massive hepatic necrosis and nodular transformation of the liver. Am J Pathol *110:*70–74, 1983.

62. Nakhleh RE, Snover KC: Use of α-1-antitrypsin staining in the diagnosis of nodular regenerative hyperplasia of the liver. Hum Pathol *19:*1048–1052, 1988.

63. Ishak KG, Goodman ZD: Benign tumors of the liver. *In* Bockus' Gastroenterology, edited by J.E. Berk. 4th Edition. Philadelphia, W.B Saunders, 1985, pp. 3302–3314.

64. Karhunen PJ: Benign hepatic tumors and tumor-like conditions in men. J Clin pathol *39:*183–188, 1986.

65. Los Angeles County and University of Southern California Autopsies 1918–1982. *In* Tumors of the Liver and Intrahepatic Bile Ducts. 2nd Series. Fascicle 26. Washington, D.C. Armed Forces Institute of Pathology, 1989.

66. Morley JE, Meyers JB, Sack FS: Enlargement of cavernous haemangioma associated with exogenous administration of oestrogens. S Afr Med J *1:*695–697, 1974.

67. Wanless IR: The hepatobiliary system. *In* Functional Endocrine Pathology, edited by K. Kovacs, S.L. Asa. Cambridge, Blackwell, 1990, pp. 768–789.

68. Trastek VF, van Heerden JA, Sheedy PF II, Adson MA: Cavernous hemangionmas of the liver: resect or observe? Am J Surg *145:*49–53, 1983.

69. Sewell JH, Weiss K: Spontaneous rupture of hemangioma of the liver, Arch Surg *83:*729–733, 1961.

70. Martinez J, Shapiro SS, Holburn RR: Hypofibrinogenemia associated with hemangioma of the liver. Am J Clin Pathol *59:*192–197, 1973.

71. Levitt LM, Coleman M, Jarvis J: Multiple large hemangiomas of the liver. N Engl Med *252:*854–855, 1955.

72. Ohto M, Ebara M, Okuda K: Ultrasonography in the diagnosis of hepatic tumors. *In* Neoplasms of the Liver, edited by K. Okuda, K.G. Ishak. Tokyo, Springer-Verlag, 1987, pp. 251–258.

73. Kojimahara M: Ultrastructural study of hemangiomas. Cavernous hemangioma of the liver. Acta Pathol Jpn *36:*1477–1485, 1986.

74. Brambs HJ, Spamer C, Volk B: Histological diagnosis of liver hemangiomas using ultrasound-guided fine needle biopsy. Hepatogastroenterology *32:*284–287, 1985.

75. Johnson CM, Sheedy PF, Stanson AW, Stephens DH, Hattery RR, Adson MA: Computed tomography and angiography of cavernous hemangioma of the liver. Radiology *138:*115–121, 1981.

76. Abrams RM, Beranbaum ER, Santos JS: Angiographic features of cavernous hemangioma of liver. Radiology *92:*308–312, 1969.

77. Chuang, VP: Hepatic angiography. *In* Neoplasms of the Liver, edited by K. Okuda, K.G. Ishak. Tokyo, Springer-Verlag, 1987, pp. 259–277.

78. Moss AA, Stark DD: Magnetic resonance imaging of liver tumors. *In* Neoplasms of the Liver, edited by K. Okuda, K.G. Ishak. Tokyo, Springer-Verlag, 1987, pp. 301–319.

79. Plachta A: Calcified hemangiomas of the liver. Radiology *79:*783–788, 1962.

80. Berry CL: Solitary "necrotic nodule" of the liver: a probable pathogenesis. J Clin Pathol *38:*1278–1280, 1985.

81. Dehner LP, Ishak KG: Vascular tumors of the liver in infants and children. A study of 30 cases and review of the literature. Arch Pathol *92:*101–111, 1971.

82. Larcher VF, Howard ER, Mowat AP: Hepatic hemangiomata: diagnosis and management. Arch Dis Child *56:*7–14, 1981.

83. Vorse HB, Smith I, Luckstead EF: Hepatic hemangiomatosis of infancy. Am J Dis Child *137:*672–673, 1983.

84. Enzinger FM, Weiss SW: Soft Tissue Tumors. St. Louis, C.V. Mosby, 1983, pp. 381–383.

85. Dachman AH, Lichtenstein JE, Friedman AC, Hartman DS: Infantile hemangioendothelioma of the liver. A radiologic-pathologic-clinical correlation. Am J Roentgenol *140:*1091–1096, 1983.

86. Holcomb GW III, O'Neill JA Jr, Mahboubi S, Bishop HC: Experience with hepatic hemangiendothelioma in infancy and childhood. J Pediatr *23:*661–668, 1988.

87. Ishak KG, Sesterhenn IA, Goodman ZD, Rabin L, Stromeyer FW: Epithelioid hemangionendothelioma of the liver: a clinicopathologic and follow-up study of 32 cases. Hum Pathol *15:*839–852, 1984.

88. Johnson DH, Vinson AM, Wirth FH, Presberg JH, Harkins G, Nuss D, Walburgh CE, Raff JC: Management of hepatic hemangioendotheliomas of infancy by transarterial embolization: a report of two cases. Pediatrics *73:*546–549, 1984.

89. Rotman M, John M, Stowe S, Inamdar S: Radiation treatment of pediatric hepatic hemangiomatosis and coexisting cardiac failure. N Engl J Med *302:*852, 1980.

90. Ishak KG: Mesenchymal tumors of the liver. *In* Hepatocellular Carcinoma, edited by K. Okuda, R.L. Peters. New York, John Wiley & Sons, 1976, pp. 247–307.

91. Kim H, Damajanov I: Localized fibrous mesothelioma of the liver. Report of a giant tumor studied by light and electron microscopy. Cancer *52:*1662–1665, 1983.

92. Ramchand S, Ahmed Y, Baskerville L: Lipoma of the liver. Arch Pathol *90:*331–333, 1970.

93. Roberts JL, Fishman EK, Hartman DS, Sanders R, Goodman Z, Siegelman SS: Lipomatous tumors of the liver: evaluation with CT and US. Radiology *158:*613–617, 1986.

94. Peters WM, Dixon MF, Williams NS: Angiomyelolipoma of the liver. Histopathology *7:*99–106, 1983.

95. Goodman ZD, Ishak KG: Angiomyolipomas of the liver. Am J Surg Pathol *8:*745–750, 1984.

96. Karhunen PJ: Hepatic pseudolipoma. J Clin Pathol *38:*877–879, 1985.

97. Clain JE, Stephens DH, Charbonneau JW: Ultrasonography and computed tomography in focal fatty liver. Report of two cases with special emphasis on changing appearances over time. Gastroenterology *87:*948–952, 1984.

98. Hawkins, EP, Jordan GL, McCavran MH: Primary leiomyoma of the liver. Successful treatment by lobectomy and representation of criteria for diagnosis. Am J Surg Pathol *4:*301–304, 1980.

99. Key RD, Rao RN: Leiomyomatous hemangiomas of the liver mimicking primary leiomyomas. Arch Pathol Lab Med *110:*658–659, 1986.

100. Van Steenbergen W, Joosten E, Marchal G: Hepatic lymphangiomatosis. Report of a case and review of the literature. Gastroenterology *88:*1068–1972, 1985.

101. Stocker JT, Ishak KG: Mesenchymal hamartoma of the liver: report of 30 cases and review of the literature. Pediatr Pathol *1:*245–267, 1983.

102. Rhodes RH, Marchildon MB, Luebke DC, Edmondson HA, Mikity VG: A Mixed hamartoma of the liver: light and electron microscopy. Hum Pathol *9:*211–221, 1978.

103. Ros PR, Goodman ZD, Ishak KG, Dachman AH, Olmsted WW, Hartman DS, Lichtenstein JE: Mesenchymal hamartoma of the liver: radiologic-pathologic correlation. Radiology *158:*619–624, 1986.

104. Watanabe I, Kasai M, Suzuki S: True teratoma of the liver: report of a case and review of the literature. Acta Hepato-Gastroenterologica *25:*40–44, 1978.

105. Gonzalez-Crussi F: Extragonadal teratomas. Atlas of Tumor Pathology. 2nd Series. Fasc *18:* Washington, D.C. Armed Forces Institute of Pathology, 1982.

106. Witte DP, Kissane JM, Askin FB: Hepatic teratomas in children. Pediatr Pathol *1:*81–92, 1983.

107. Waterhouse JAH, Muir C, Correa P, Powell J: Cancer Incidence in Five Continents 3. Lyon, International Agency for Research on Cancer, 1977.

108. Anthony PP: Tumours and tumour-like lesions of the liver and biliary tract. *In* Pathology of the Liver, edited by R.N.M. MacSween, P.P. Anthony, P.J. Scheuer. 2nd Edition. Edinburgh, Churchill Livingstone, 1987, pp. 574–665.

109. Parkin DM, Stjernsward J, Muir CS: Estimates of the worldwide frequency of twelve major cancers. Bull WHO *62:*163–182, 1984.

110. Munoz N, Bosch X: Epidemiology of hepatocellular carcinoma. *In* Neoplasms of the Liver, edited by K. Okuda, K.G. Ishak. Tokyo, Springer-Verlag, 1987, pp. 3–19.

111. Kaklamani E, Tzonou A, Sparos L, Koumantaki I, Trichopoulos D: Hepatitis B virus and primary liver cancer: relative risk estimation from population correlations. IRCS Med Sci *11:*707–708, 1983.

112. Tuyns AJ, Obradovic M: Unexpected high incidence of primary liver cancer in Geneva, Switzerland. J Natl Cancer Inst *54:*61–64, 1975.

113. Eriksson S, Carlson J, Velez R: Risk of cirrhosis and primary liver cancer in α-1-antitrypsin deficiency. N Engl J Med *314:*736–739, 1986.

114. Okuda K, Mackay I: Hepatocellular carcinoma. International Union Against Cancer, Geneva (UICC Technical Report) Series *74:*1982.

115. Kew MC, DosSantos HA, Sherlock S: Diagnosis of primary cancer of the liver. Br Med J *4:*408–411, 1971.

116. Trichopoulos D, Day N, Kaklamani E, Tzonou A, Munoz N, Zavitsanos X, Koumantaki Y, Trichopoulou A: Hepatitis B virus, tobacco smoking and ethanol consumption in the etiology of hepatocellular carcinoma. Int J Cancer *39:*45–49, 1987.

117. Obata H, Hayashi N, Motoike Y, Hisamitsu T, Okuda H, Koibayashi S, Nishioka K: A prospective study on the development of hepatocellular carcinoma from liver cirrhosis with persistent hepatitis B virus infection. Int J Cancer *25:*741–747, 1980.

118. Alpert ME, Hutt MSR, Davidson CS: Primary hepatoma in Uganda. A prospective clinical and epidemiologic study of forty-six patients. Am J Med *46:*794–802, 1969.

119. Okuda K, Kotoda K, Obata H, Hayashi N, Hisamitsu T, Tamiya M, Kubo Y, Yakushiji F, Nagata E, Jinnouchi S, Shimokawa Y: Clinical observations during a relatively early stage of hepatocellular carcinoma, with special reference to serum α-fetoprotein levels. Gastroenterology *69:*226–234, 1975.

120. Zaman SN, Johnson PJ, Williams R: Silent cirrhosis in patients with hepatocellular carcinoma. Implications for screening in high-incidence and low-incidence areas. Cancer *65:*1607–1608, 1990.

121. Nakanuma Y, Terada T, Doishita K, Miwa A: Hepatocellular carcinoma in primary biliary cirrhosis: an autopsy study. Hepatology *11:*1010–1016, 1990.

122. Feuerholdt L, Schlichting P, Christensen E, Poulsen H, Tygstrup N, Juhl E: The Copenhagen Study Group for Liver Disease. Conversion of micronodular cirrhosis into macronodular cirrhosis. Hepatology *3:*928–931, 1983.

123. Okuda K, Peters RL, Simson IW: Gross anatomic features of hepatocellular carcinoma from three disparate geographic areas. Proposal of new classification. Cancer *54:*2165–2173, 1984.

124. Shikata T, Yamazaki S, Uzawa T: Hepatocellular carcinoma and chronic persistent hepatitis. Acta Pathol Jpn *27:*297–304, 1977.

125. Berman JJ: Cell proliferation and the aetiology of hepatocellular carcinoma. J Hepatol *7:*305–309, 1988.

126. Anthony PP: Primary carcinoma of the liver: a study of 282 cases in Ugandan Africans. J Pathol *110:*37–48, 1973.

127. Roncalli M, Borzio M, DeBiagi G, Servida E, Cantaboni A, Sironi M, Taccagni GL: Liver cell dysplasia and hepatocellular carcinoma: a histological and immunohistochemical study. Histopathology *9:*209–221, 1985.

128. Cohen C, Berson SD: Liver cell dysplasia in normal, cirrhotic and hepatocellular carcinoma patients. Cancer *57:*1535–1538, 1986.

129. Anthony PB: Liver cell dysplasia: what is its significance? Hepatology *7:*394–395, 1987.

130. Chen M-L, Gerber MA, Thung SN, Thornton JC, Chung WK: Morphometric study of hepatocytes containing hepatitis B surface antigen. Am J Pathol *114:*217–221, 1984.

131. Lefkowitch JH, Apfelbaum TF: Liver cell dysplasia and hepatocellular carcinoma in non-A, non-B hepatitis. Arch Pathol Med *111:*170–173, 1987.

132. Purtillo DT, Gottlieb LS: Cirrhosis and hepatoma occurring at Boston City Hospital (1917–1968). Cancer *32:*458–462, 1973.

133. Polio J, Enriquez RE, Chow A, Wood WM, Atterbury CE: Hepatocellular carcinoma as a complication of Wilson's disease. Case report and review of the literature. J Clin Gastroenterol *11:*220–224, 1989.

134. Bjorneboe M, Rikardt Anderson J, Christensen J, Skinhof P, Jensen OM: Does a portal-systemic shunt increase the risk of primary hepatic carcinoma in cirrhosis of the liver? Scand J Gastroenterol *20:*59–64, 1985.

135. Rofe S, Conn HO: Portal-systemic anastomosis (PSS) and the development of hepatocellular carcinoma (HCC): a retrospective study. Hepatology *6:*1223, 1986.

136. Patton RB: Primary carcinoma in a cirrhotic liver 17 years after portacaval shunt. Report of a case. Am J Dig Dis *10:*554–559, 1965.

137. Wei WI, Wong J, Ong GB: Growth enhancement of hepatocellular carcinoma in the rat after portacaval shunt. Dig Surg *1:*180–184, 1984.

138. Battifora HA: Thorotrast and tumors of the liver. *In* Hepatocellular Carcinoma, edited by K. Okuda, R.L. Peters. New York, John Wiley & Sons, 1976, pp. 83–94.

139. Kew MC, Popper H: Relationship between hepatocellular carcinoma and cirrhosis. Semin Liver Dis *4:*136–146, 1984.

140. Kojiro M, Nakashima T: Pathology of hepatocellular carcinoma. *In* Neoplasms of the Liver, edited by K. Okuda, K.G. Ishak. Tokyo, Springer-Verlag 1987, pp. 81–104.

141. Popper H, Shafritz DA, Hoofnagle JH: Relation of the hepatitis B virus carrier state to hepatocellular carcinoma. Hepatology *7:*764–772, 1987.

142. Beasley RP: Hepatitis B virus as the etiologic agent in hepatocellular carcinoma: epidemiologic considerations. Hepatology *2:*21S–26S, 1982.

143. Szmuness W: Hepatocellular carcinoma and the hepatitis B virus: evidence for a causal association. Prog Med Virol *24:*40–69, 1978.

144. Prince AM, Szmuness W, Michon J, Demaille J, Diebolt G, Linhard J, Quenum C, Sankale M: A case control study of the association between primary liver cancer and hepatitis B infection in Senegal. Int J Cancer *16:*376–383, 1975.

145. Tabor H, Gerety RJ, Vogel CL, Bayley AC, Anthony PP, Chen CH, Barker LF: Hepatitis B virus infections and primary hepatocellular carcinoma. J Natl Cancer Inst *58:*1197–1200, 1977.

146. Blumberg BS, London WT: Hepatitis B virus: pathogenesis and prevention of primary cancer of the liver. Cancer *50:*2657–2665, 1982.

147. Omata M, Yokosuka O, Imazeki F, Okuda K: Hepadna viruses and hepatocarcinogenesis. *In* Neoplasms of the Liver, edited by K. Okuda, K.G. Ishak. Tokyo, Springer-Verlag, 1987. pp. 35–45.

148. Wong VCW, Ip HMH, Reesink HW, Lelie PN, Reerink-Brongers EE, Yeung CY, Ma HK: Prevention of the HBsAg carrier state in newborn infants of mothers who are chronic carriers of HBsAg and HBeAg by administration of hepatitis B vaccine and hepatitis B immunoglobulin: double-blind randomized placebo-controlled study. Lancet *1:*921–926, 1984.

149. Lin DY, Liaw Y-F, Chu CM, Chang-Chien CS, Wu CS, Chen PC, Sheen IS: Hepatocellular carcinoma in noncirrhotic patients: a laparoscopic study of 92 cases in Taiwan. Cancer *54:*1466–1468, 1984.

150. Shafritz DA, Shouval D, Sherman HI, Hadziyannis SJ, Kew MC: Integration of hepatitis B virus DNA into the genome of liver cells in chronic liver disease and hepatocellular carcinoma. N Engl J Med, *305:*1067–1073, 1981.

151. Esumi M, Aritaka T, Arii M: Clonal origin of human hepatoma determined by integration of hepatitis B virus DNA. Cancer Res *46:*5767–5771, 1986.

152. Brechot C: Hepatitis B virus (HBV) and hepatocellular carcinoma: HBV DNA status and its implications. J Hepatol *4:*269–279, 1987.

153. Choo Q-L, Kuo G, Weiner AJ, Overby, LR, Bradley DW, Houghton M: Isolation of a cDNA clone derived from a blood-borne non-A, non-B, viral hepatitis genome. Science *244:*359–362, 1989.

154. Summers J: Three recently described animal virus models for human hepatitis B virus. Hepatology *1:*179–183, 1981.

155. Yu MC, Mack T, Hanisch R, Peters RL, Henderson BE, Pike, MC: Hepatitis, alcohol consumption, cigarette smoking, and hepatocellular carcinoma in Los Angeles. Cancer Res *43:*6077–6079, 1983.

156. Hardell L, Bengtsson NO, Jonsson U, Eriksson S, Larsson LG: Aetiological aspects on primary liver cancer with special regard to alcohol, organic solvents and acute intermittent porphyria: an epidemiological investigation. Br J Cancer *50:*389–397, 1984.

157. Oshima A, Tsukama H, Hiyama T, Fujimoto I, Yamano H, Tanaka M: Follow-up study of HBsAg-positive blood donors with special reference to effect of drinking and smoking on development of liver cancer. Int J Cancer *34:*775–779, 1984.

158. Lee FI: Cirrhosis and hepatoma in alcoholics. Gut *7:*77–85, 1966.

159. Linsell CA: Liver cell cancer: intervention studies. J Cancer Res Clin Oncol *99:*51–56, 1981.

160. Peers FG, Bosch FX, Kaldor JM, Linsell CA: Aflatoxin exposure, hepatitis B virus and liver cancer in Swaziland. Int J Cancer *39:*545–553, 1987.

161. Stora C, Dvorackova I, Ayroud N: Characterization of aflatoxin B

(AFB) in human liver cancer. Res Comm Chem Pathol Pharmacol *31:*77–84, 1981.

162. Lutwick LI: Relation between aflatoxin, hepatitis B virus and hepatocellular carcinoma. Lancet *1:*755–757, 1979.

163. Van Rensberg SJ, Cook-Mozaffari P, van Schalkwyk DJ, van der Watt, JJ, Vincent TJ, Purchase IF: Hepatocellular carcinoma and dietary aflatoxin in Mozambique and Transkei. Br J Cancer *51:*713–726, 1985.

164. Trichopoulos D, Day N, Kaklamani E, Tzonou A, Munoz N, Zavitsanos X, Koumantaki Y, Trichopoulou A: Tobacco smoking, hepatitis B virus and ethanol consumption in the etiology of hepatocellular carcinoma. Int J Cancer *39:*45–49, 1987.

165. Lam KC, Yu MC, Leung JWC, Henderson BE: Hepatitis B virus and cigarette smoking: risk factors for hepatocellular carcinoma in Hong Kong. Cancer Res *42:*5246–5248, 1982.

166. Kew MC: Clinical manifestations and paraneoplastic syndromes of hepatocellular carcinoma. *In* Neoplasms of the Liver, edited by K. Okuda, K.G. Ishak. Tokyo, Springer-Verlag, 1987, 199–211.

167. Lai CL, Lam KC, Wong KP, Wu PC, Todd D: Clinical features of hepatocellular carcinoma: review of 211 patients in Hong Kong. Cancer *47:*2746–2755, 1981.

168. Kew MC, Dusheiko GM: Paraneoplastic manifestations of hepatocellular carcinoma. *In* Frontiers in Liver Disease, edited by P.D. Berk, T.C. Chalmers. New York, Thieme-Stratton, 1981, pp. 305–319.

169. Kew MC, Paterson AC: Unusual clinical presentations of hepatocellular carcinoma. Trop Gastroenterol *6:*10–22, 1985.

170. Pun KK, Ho PW, Yeung RT: C-peptide in non-alcoholic cirrhosis and hepatocellular carcinoma. J Endocrinol Invest *11:*337–343, 1988.

171. Stevenson JG: Malignant hypercalcemia. Br Med *291:*421–422, 1985.

172. Primack A, Wilson J, O'Connor GT, Engleman K, Hull E, Canellos GP: Hepatocellular carcinoma with the carcinoid syndrome. Cancer *27:*1182–1189, 1971.

173. Viallet A, Benhamou J-P, Fauvert R: Primary carcinoma of the liver and hyperlipemia. Can Med Assoc J *86:*1118–1121, 1962.

174. Vaillet A, Benhamou J-P, Berthelot P, Hartmann L, Fauvert R: Primary carcinoma of the liver and dysproteinemia. Gastroenterology *43:*88–93, 1962.

175. Morgan AG., Walker WC, Mason MK: A new syndrome associated with hepatocellular carcinoma. Gastroenterology *63:*340–345, 1972.

176. Keczkes K, Barker DJ: Malignant hepatoma associated with acquired hepatic cutaneous porphyria. Arch Dermatol *112:*78–82, 1976.

177. DiBesceglie AM, Hodkinson HJ, Berkowitz I, Kew MC: Pityriasis rotunda: a cutaneous sign of hepatocellular carcinoma in southern African Blacks. Arch Dermatol *122:*802–804, 1986.

178. Peters TJ, Seymour CA, Wells G: Gamma-glutamyltransferase levels in ascitic fluid and liver tissue from patients with primary hepatoma. Br Med J *1:*1576, 1977.

179. Sawabu N, Hattori N: Serological tumor markers in hepatocellular carcinoma. *In* Neoplasms of the Liver, edited by K. Okuda, K.G. Ishak. Tokyo, Springer-Verlag, 1987, pp. 226–237.

180. Sheu JC, Sung JL, Chen DS, Yang PM, Lai MY, Lee CS, Hsu HC, Chuang CN, Yang PC, Wang TH, Lin JC, Lee CZ: Growth rate of asymptomatic hepatocellular carcinoma and its clinical implications. Gastroenterology *89:*259–266, 1985.

181. Heyward WL, Lanier AP, McMahon BJ: Serological markers of hepatitis B virus and α-fetoprotein levels preceding primary hepatocellular carcinoma in Alaskan Eskimos. Lancet *2:*889–891, 1982.

182. Kobayashi K, Sugimoto T, Makino H, Kumagai M, Unoura M, Tanaka N, Kato Y, Hattori N: Screening methods for early detection of hepatocellular carcinoma. Hepatology *5:*1100–1105, 1985.

183. Bolondi L, Benzi G, Santi V, Gaiani S, Bassi SL, Zirone G, Mazziotti A, Sama C, Grigioni W, Gozzetti, G, Barbara L: Relationship between α-fetoprotein serum levels, tumour volume and growth rate of hepatocellular carcinoma in a western population. Ital J Gastroenterol *22:*190–194, 1990.

184. Hromas RA, Srigley J, Murray JL: Clinical and pathological comparison of young adult women with hepatocellular carcinoma with and without exposure to oral contraceptives. Am J Gastroenterol *80:*479–485, 1985.

185. Tanaka S, Kitamura T, Oshima A, Umeda K, Okuda S, Ohtani T, Tatsuta M, Yamamoto K: Diagnostic accuracy of ultrasonography for hepatocellular carcinoma. Cancer *58:*344–347, 1986.

186. Kuo S, Chen D, Sung J: Cytophotometric measurements of nuclear DNA content in hepatocellular carcinomas. Hepatology *7:*330–332, 1987.

187. Lin D-Y, Liau Y-F, Lee T-Y, Lai C-M: Hepatic arterial embolization in patients with unresectable hepatocellular carcinoma: a randomized controlled trial. Gastroenterology *94:*453–456, 1988.

188. Nakao N, Miura K, Takahashi H, Ohnishi M, Miura T, Okamoto E, Ishikawa Y: Hepatocellular carcinoma: combined hepatic, arterial, and portal venous embolization. Radiology *161:*303–307, 1986.

189. Sheu J-C, Huang G-T, Chen D-S, Sung J-L, Tang P-M, Wei T-C, Lai M-Y, Su C-T, Tsang Y-M, Hsu H-C, Su I-J, Wu T-T, Lin J-T, Chuang C-N: Small hepatocellular carcinoma: intratumor ethanol treatment using new needle and guidance systems. Radiology *163:*43–48, 1987.

190. Tsao M, Grisham JW: Hepatocarcinomas, cholangiocarcinomas and hepatoblastomas produced by chemically transformed cultured rat liver epithelial cells. Am J Pathol *127:*168–181, 1987.

191. Govindarajan S, Craig JR, Valinluck B: Clonal origin of hepatitis virus associated hepatocellular carcinoma. Hum Pathol *19:*403–405, 1988.

192. Tsuda H, Hiroshashi S, Shimosato Y, Terada M, Hasegawa H: Clonal origin of atypical adenomaous hyperplasia of the liver and clonal identity with hepatocellular carcinoma. Gastroenterology *95:*1664–1666, 1988.

193. Chen P, Chen D, Lai M, Chang M, Huang G, Yang P, Sheu J, Lee S, Hsu H, Sung J: Clonal origin of recurrent hepatocellular carcinomas. Gastroenterology *96:*527–529, 1989.

194. Eggel H: Uber das primare Carcinom der Leber. Beitr path Anat u z allg Path *30:*506–604, 1901.

195. Kanai T, Hirohashi S, Upton M, Noguchi M, Kishi K, Makuuchi M, Yamasaki S, Hasegawa H, Takayasu K, Moriyama N, Shimosato Y: Pathology of small hepatocellular carcinoma: a proposal for a new gross classification. Cancer *60:*810–819, 1987.

196. Kemeny F, Vadrot J, Wu A, Smadja C, Meakins JL, Franco D: Morphological and histological features of resected hepatocellular carcinoma in cirrhotic patients in the west. Hepatology *9:*253–257, 1989.

197. Nakashima T, Okuda K, Kijoro M, Jimi A, Yamaguchi R, Sakamoti K: Pathology of hepatocellular carcinoma in Japan: 232 consecutive cases autopsied in ten years. Cancer *51:*863–877, 1983.

198. Peters RL: Pathology of hepatocellular carcinoma. *In* Hepatocellular Carcinoma, edited by K. Okuda, R. Peters. New York, John Wiley & Sons, 1976, pp. 107–168.

198a. Hood DL, Bauer TW, Leibel SA, McMahon JT. Hepatic giant cell carcinoma. An ultrastructural and immunohistochemical study. Am J Clin Pathol *93:*111–116, 1990.

199. Ajdukiewicz A, Crowden A, Hudson E, Pyne C: Liver aspiration in the diagnosis of hepatocellular carcinoma in the Gambia. J Clin Pathol *38:*185–192, 1985.

200. Sangalli G, Livraghi T, Giordano F: Fine needle biopsy of hepatocellular carcinoma: improvement in diagnosis by microhistology. Gastroenterology *96:*524–526, 1989.

201. Anthony PP: Precancerous changes in the human liver. J Toxicol Environ Health *5:*301–313, 1979.

202. Tezuka F, Sawai T: Hyperplasia of small hepatic cells in the precancerous condition of cirrhotic livers. Tohoku J Exp Med *139:*171–177, 1983.

203. Ho JC, Wu P-C, Mak T-K: Liver cells dysplasia in association with hepatocellular carcinoma, cirrhosis and hepatitis B surface antigen in Hong Kong. Int J Cancer *28:*571–574, 1981.

204. Henmi A, Uchida T, Shikata T: Karyometric analysis of liver cell dysplasia and hepatocellular carcinoma. Cancer *55:*2594–2599, 1985.

205. Wu PC, Lai CL, Lam KC, Lok ASF, Lin HJ: Clear cell carcinoma of liver. An ultrastructural study. Cancer *521:*504–507, 1983.

206. Nakanuma Y, Ohta G: Expression of Mallory bodies in hepatocellular carcinoma in man and its significance. Cancer *57:*81–86, 1986.

207. Michel RP, Limacher JH, Kimoff RJ: Mallory bodies in scar adenocarcinoma of the lung. Hum Pathol *13:*81–85, 1982.

208. Ordonez NG, Manning JT: Comparison of α-1-antitrypsin and α-1-antichymotrypsin in hepatocellular carcinoma: an imunoperoxidase study. Am J Gastroenterol *79:*959–963, 1984.

209. Stomeyer FW, Ishak KG, Gerber MA, Mathew T: Ground-glass cells in hepatocellular carcinoma. Am J Clin Pathol *74:*254–258, 1980.

210. Thung SN, Gerber MA, Sarno E, Popper H: Distribution of five antigens in hepatocellular carcinoma. Lab Invest *41:*101–105, 1979.

211. Omata M, Peters RL, Tatter D: Sclerosing hepatic carcinoma: relationship to hypercalcemia. Liver *1:*33–49, 1981.

212. Anthony PP, James K: Pedunculated hepatocellular carcinoma. Is it an entity? Histopathology *11:*403–414, 1987.

213. Horie Y, Katoh S, Yoshida H, Imaoka T, Suou T, Hirayama C: Pedunculated hepatocellular carcinoma: a report of three cases and review of literature. Cancer *51:*746–751, 1983.

214. Kakizoe S, Kojiro M, Nakashima T: Hepatocellular carcinoma with sarcomatous change. Clinicopathologic and immunohistochemical studies of 14 autopsy cases. Cancer 59:310–316, 1987.

215. Craig Jr, Peters RL, Edmondson HA, Omata M: Fibrolamellar carcinoma of the liver: a tumor of adolescents and young adults with distinctive clinico-pathologic features. Cancer 46:372–379, 1980.

216. Berman MM, Libbey NP, Foster JH: Hepatocellular carcinoma. Polygonal cell type with fibrous stroma: an atypical variant with a favorable prognosis. Cancer 46:1448–1455, 1980.

217. Cooke C, Mooy N, Matz LR: Fibrolamellar carcinoma of the liver. Pathology 18:281–282, 1986.

218. Edmondson HA: Differential diagnosis of tumors and tumor-like lesions of liver in infancy and childhood. Arch Dis Child 1:168–186, 1956.

219. Caballero T, Aneiros J, Lopez-Caballero J, Gomez-Morales M, Nogales F: Fibrolamellar hepatocellular carcinoma. An immunohistochemical and ultrastructural study. Histopathology 9:445–456, 1985.

220. Rolfes DB: Fibrolamellar carcinoma of the liver. In Neoplasms of the Liver, edited by K. Okuda, K.G. Ishak. Tokyo, Springer-Verlag, 1987, pp. 137–142.

221. Collier NA, Bloom SR, Hodgson HJF, Weinbren K, Lee YC, Blumgart LH: Neurotensin secretion by fibrolamellar carcinoma of the liver. Lancet 1:538–540, 1984.

222. Payne CM, Nagle RB, Paplanus SH, Graham AR: Fibrolamellar carcinoma of the liver: a primary malignant oncocytic carcinoid? Ultrastruct Pathol 10:539–552, 1986.

223. Davison FK, Fagan EA, Portmann B, Williams R: HBV-DNA sequences in tumor and nontumor tissue in a patient with the fibrolamellar variant of hepatocellular carcinoma. Hepatology 12:676–679, 1990.

224. Ihde DC, Matthews MJ, Makuch RW, McIntire KR, Eddy JL, Seeff LB: Prognostic factors in patients with hepatocellular carcinoma receiving systemic chemotherapy. Identification of two groups of patients with prospects for prolonged survival. Am J Med 78:399–406, 1985.

225. Soreide O, Czerniak A, Bradpiece H, Bloom S, Blumgart L: Characteristics of fibrolamellar hepatocellular carcinoma. A study of nine cases and a review of the literature. Am J Surg 151:518–523, 1986.

226. Starzl TE, Iwatsuki S, Shaw BW: Treatment of fibrolamellar hepatoma with partial hepatectomy or with total hepatectomy and liver transplantation. Surg Gynecol Obstet 162:145–148, 1986.

227. Nagorney DM, Adson MA, Welland LH, Knight CD Jr, Smalley SR, Zinsmeister AR: Fibrolamellar hepatoma. Am J Surg 149:113–119, 1985.

228. Friedman AC, Lichtenstein JE, Goodman ZD, Fishman EK, Siegelman SS, Dachman AH: Fibrolamellar hepatocellular carcinoma. Radiology 157:583–587, 1985.

229. Francis IR, Agha FP, Thompson NW, Keren DF: Fibrolamellar hepatocarcinoma: clinical, radiologic and pathologic features. Gastrointest Radiol 11:67–72, 1986.

230. Farhi DC, Shikes RH, Murari PJ, Silverberg SG: Heptocellular carcinoma in young people. Cancer 52:1516–1525, 1983.

231. Lefkowitch JH, Muschel R, Price JB, Marboe C, Braunhut S: Copper and copper-binding protein in fibrolamellar liver cell carcinoma. Cancer 51:97–100, 1983.

232. Vecchio FM, Federico F, Dina MA: Copper and hepatocellular carcinoma. Digestion 35:109–114, 1986.

233. Sheahan DG: Fibrolamellar carcinoma of the liver: an immunohistochemical study. Lab Invest 54:57a, 1986 (abstract).

234. Teitelbaum DH, Tuttle S, Carey LC, Calusen KP: Fibrolamellar carcinoma of the liver. Review of three cases and the presentation of a characteristic set of tumor markers defining this tumor. Ann Surg 202:36–41, 1985.

235. Berman MA, Burnham JA, Shehan DG: Fibrolamellar carcinoma of the liver: an immunohistochemical study of nineteen cases and a review of the literature. Hum Pathol 19:784–794, 1988.

236. Suen KC, Magee JF, Halparin LS: Fine needle aspiration cytology of fibrolamellar hepatocellular carcinoma. Acta Cytologica 29:867–872, 1985.

237. Denis J, Grippon P, Legendre C, Tubiana JM, Levy VG: Carcinome fibrolamellaire du foie: un carcinome hepatocellulaire de pronostic favorable. Gastroenterol Clin Biol 8:920–924, 1984.

238. Vecchio FM, Fabiano A, Ghirlanda G, Manna R, Massi G: Fibrolamellar carcinoma of the liver: the malignant counterpart of focal nodular hyperplasia with oncocytic change. Am J Clin Pathol 81:521–526, 1984.

239. Terpstra OT, ten Kate FJW, van Urk H: Long-term survival after resection of a hepatocellular carcinoma with lymph node metastasis and discontinuation of oral contraceptives. Am J Gastroenterol 79:474–478, 1984.

240. Saul S, Titelbaum DS, Gansler TS, Varello M, Burke DR, Atkinson BF, Rosato EF: The fibrolamellar variant of hepatocellular carcinoma. Its association with focal nodular hyperplasia. Cancer 60:3049–3055, 1987.

241. Gerber MA, Thung SN: Enzyme patterns in human hepatocellular carcinoma. Am J Pathol 98:395–400, 1980.

241a. Soderstrom N. Fine-needle aspiration biopsy. Almsqvist & Wiksell, Stockholm 1966.

242. Ekelund P, Wasastjerna C: Cytological identification of primary hepatic carcinoma cells. Acta Med Scand 189:373–375, 1971.

242a. Wasastjerna C. A cytochemical method for the study of bile canaliculi in fine needle aspirates of the liver. Acta Pathol Microbiol Scand, 77:399–404,1969.

242b. Polio J, Enriquez RE, Chow A, Wood WM, Atterbury CE. Hepatocellular carcinoma in Wilson's disease. J Clin Gastroenterol 11:220–224, 1989.

243. Johnson DE, Herndier BG, Medeiros LJ, Warnke RA, Rouse RV: The diagnostic utility of the keratin profiles of hepatocellular carcinoma and cholangiocarcinoma. Am J Surg Pathol 12:187–197, 1988.

244. Lai Y-S, Thung SN, Gerber MA, Chen M-L, Schaffner F: Expression of cytokeratins in normal and diseased livers and in primary liver carcinomas. Arch Pathol Lab Med 113:134–138, 1989.

245. Van Eyken P, Sciot R, Paterson A, Callea F, Kew MC, Desmet VJ: Cytokeratin expression in hepatocellular carcinoma: an immunohistochemical study. Hum Pathol 19:562–568, 1988.

246. Jagoe R, Sowter C, Dandy S, Slavin G: Morphometric study of liver cell nuclei in hepatomas using an interactive computer technique. 1. Nuclear size and shape. J Clin Pathol 35:1057–1062, 1982.

247. Jagoe R, Sowter C, Savin G: Shape and texture analysis of liver cell nuclei in hepatomas by computer aided microscopy. J Clin Pathol 37:755–762, 1984.

247a. Bottles K, Cohen MB, Holly EA, Chiu S-H, Abele JS, Cello JP, Lim RC, Miller TR. A step-wise logistic regression analysis of hepatocellular carcinoma. Cancer 62:558–563, 1988.

248. Sonoda T, Shirabe K, Kanematsu T, Takenaka K, Sugimachi K: Long-term surviving patients with hepatocellular carcinoma comprised of dense collagenous stroma. Am J Gastroenterol 84:1087–1091, 1989.

249. Moto R, Kawarada Y: Diagnosis and treatment of cholangiocarcinoma and cystic adenocarcinoma of the liver. In Neoplasms of the Liver, edited by K. Okuda, K.G. Ishak. Tokyo, Springer-Verlag, 1987, 381–396.

250. The Liver Cancer Study Group of Japan: Primary liver cancer in Japan. Cancer 54:1747–1755, 1984.

251. Chearanai O, Plengvanit U, Damrongsak D, Tuchinda S, Damrongsak C, Viranuvatti V: Primary liver cancer, angiographic study of 127 cases. J Med Assoc Thailand 67:482–490, 1984.

252. Landais P, Drunfeld J-P, Droz D, Drueke T, Albouze G, Gogusev J, Chauveau D, Moynot A: Cholangiocellular carcinoma in polycystic kidney and liver disease. Arch Intern Med 144:2274–2276, 1984.

253. Voyles CR, Smadja C, Shands W, Blumgart LH: Carcinoma in choledochal cysts. Age-related incidence. Arch Surg 118:986–988, 1983.

254. Imaura M, Miyashita T, Tani T, Naito A, Tobe T, Takahashi K: Cholangiocellular carcinoma associated with multiple liver cysts. Am J Gastroenterol 79:790–795, 1984.

255. Dayton MT, Longmire, WP, Tompkins RK: Caroli's disease: a premalignant condition: Am J Surg 145:41–48, 1983.

256. Welton JC, Marr JS, Friedman SM: Association between hepatobiliary cancer and typhoid carrier state. Lancet 1:791–794, 1979.

257. Schwartz DA: Cholangiocarcinoma associated with liver fluke infection: a preventable source of morbidity in Asian immigrants. Am J Gastroenterol 81:76–79, 1986.

258. Kurathong S, Lerdverasirikul P, Wonkgpaitoon V, Pramoolsinsap C, Kanjanapitalk A, Varavithya W, Phuapradit P, Bunyaratvej S, Upatham ES, Brockelman WY: Opisthorchis viverrini infection and cholangiocarcinoma. A prospective, case-controlled study. Gastroenterology 89:151–156, 1985.

259. Nakashima T, Okuda K, Kojiro M, Sakamoto K, Dubo Y, Shimokawa Y: Primary liver cancer coincident with Schistosomiasis japonica. A study of 23 necropsies. Cancer 36:1483–1489, 1975.

260. Nakanuma Y, Terada, T, Tanaka Y: Are hepatolithiasis and cholangiocarcinoma aetiologically related? A morphological study of 12 cases of hepatolithiasis associated with cholangiocarcinoma. Virch Arch (Path Anat) 406:43–58, 1985.

261. Thamavit W, Bhamarapravati N, Sahaphong S, Vajrasthira, Angsub-

hakorn S: Effects of dimethylnitrosamine on induction of cholangiocarcinoma in *Opisthorchis viverrini*-infected Syrian golden hamsters. Cancer Res *38*:4634–4639, 1978.

262. Wee A, Ludwig L, Coffey RJ, LaRusso NF, Wiesner RH: Hepatobiliary carcinoma associated with primary sclerosing cholangitis and chronic ulcerative colitis. Hum Pathol *16*:719–720, 1985.

263. Chen P-H, Lo H-W, Wang C-S, Tsai K-R, Chen Y-C, Lin K-Y, Siauw C-P, Hwang R-R, Liu M-H, Ko H-C, Chen T-Y: Cholangiocarcinoma in hepatolithiasis. J Clin Gastroenterol *6*:539–547, 1984.

264. Koga A, Ichimiya H, Yamaguchi K, Miyazaki K, Nakayama F: Hepatolithiasis associated with cholangiocarcinoma, possible etiologic significance. Cancer *55*:2826–2829, 1985.

265. Yoshimoto H, Ikeda S, Tanaka M, Matsumoto S: Intrahepatic cholangiocarcinoma associated with hepatolithiasis. Gastrointest Endosc *31*:260–263, 1985.

266. Abdul-Karim FW, King TA, Dahms BB, Gauderer MWL, Boat TF: Carcinoma of extrahepatic biliary system in an adult with cystic fibrosis. Gastroenterology *82*:758–762, 1982.

267. Terada T, Nakanuma Y: Pathological observations of intrahepatic peribiliary glands in 1,000 consecutive autopsy livers. II. A possible source of cholangiocarcinoma. Hepatology *12*:92–97, 1990.

268. Rubel LR, Ishak KG: Thorotrast-associated cholangiocarcinoma. An epidemiologic and clinicopathologic study. Cancer *50*:1408–1415, 1982.

269. Ito Y, Kojiro M, Nakashima T, Mori T: Pathomorphologic characteristics of 102 cases of thorotrast-related hepatocellular carcinoma, cholangiocarcinoma and hepatic angiosarcoma. Cancer *62*:1153–1162, 1988.

270. Littlewood ER, Barrison IG, Murray-Lyon IM, Paradinas FJ: Cholangiocarcinoma and oral contraceptives. Lancet *1*:310–311, 1980.

271. Stromeyer FW, Smith DH, Ishak KG: Anabolic steroid therapy and intrahepatic cholangiocarcinoma. Cancer *43*:440–443, 1979.

272. Oldenburg WA, Van Heerden PA, Sizemore GW, Abbound CF, Sheedy PF: Hypercalcemia and primary hepatic tumors. Arch Surg *117*:1363–1366, 1982.

273. Jalanko H, Kuusela P, Roberts P, Sippone P, Haglung F, Makela O: Comparison of a new tumor marker, CA 19-9T, with α-fetoprotein and carcinoembryonic antigen in patients with upper gastrointestinal disease. J Clin Pathol *37*:218–222, 1984.

274. Liguory C, Canard JM: Tumours of the biliary system. Clin Gastroenterol *12*:269–295, 1983.

275. Weinbren K, Matum SS: Pathological aspects of cholangiocarcinoma. J Pathol *139*:217–238, 1983.

276. Bonetti F, Chilosi M, Posa R, Novelli P, Zamboni G, Menestrina F: Epithelial membrane antigen expression in cholangiocarcinoma. A useful immunohistochemical tool for differential diagnosis with hepatocarcinoma. Vir Arch A Path Anat Histopathol *401*:307–313, 1983.

277. Pastolero GC, Wakabayashi T, Oka T, Mori S: Tissue polypeptide antigen: a marker antigen differentiating cholangiolar tumors from other hepatic tumors. Am J Clin Pathol *87*:168–173, 1987.

278. Iwatsuki S, Starzl TE: Liver transplantation in the treatment of liver cancer. *In* Neoplasms of the Liver, edited by K. Okuda, K.G. Ishak. Tokyo, Springer-Verlag, 1987, pp. 397–405.

279. Okada Y, Jinno K, Moriwaki S, Morichika S, Torigoe S, Arima T, Nagashima H, Koprowski H: Expression of ABH and Lewis blood group antigens in combined hepatocellular-cholangiocarcinoam. Possible evidence for the hepatocellular origin of combined hepatocellular-cholangiocarcinoma. Cancer *60*:345–352, 1987.

280. Goodman ZD, Ishak KG, Langloss JM, Sesterhenn IA, Rabin L: Combined hepatocellular-cholangiocarcinoma. A histologic and immunohistochemical study. Cancer *55*:124–135, 1985.

281. Klatskin GK: Adenocarcinoma of the hepatic duct at its bifurcation within the porta hepatis. Am J Med *38*:241–256, 1965.

282. Okuda K, Rubo Y, Okazaki N, Arishima T, Hashimoto M, Jinnouchi S, Sawa Y, Shimokawa Y, Nakajima Y, Noguchi T, Nakano M, Kojiro M, Nakashima T: Clinical aspects of intrahepatic bile duct carcinoma including hilar carcinoma. A study of 57 autopsy-proven cases. Cancer *39*:232–246, 1977.

283. van Steenbergen W, vanStapel MJ, Geboes K, Ponette E, Fevery J, deGroote J: Carcinoma at the hilus of the liver: clinical, radiological, histological and therapeutic aspects. Netherlands J Med *25*:344–353, 1982.

284. Machan L, Muller NL, Cooperberg PL: Sonographic diagnosis of Klatskin tumors. AJR *147*:509–512, 1986.

285. Qualman SJ, Haupt P, Bauer TW: Adenocarcinoma of the hepatic

duct junction. A reappraisal of the histologic criteria of malignancy. Cancer *53*:1545–1551, 1984.

286. Sons H-U, Borchard F: Carcinoma of the extrahepatic bile ducts: a postmortem study of 65 cases and review of the literature. J Surg Oncol *34*:6–12, 1987.

287. Leese T, Neoptolemos JP, West KP, Talbot IC, Carr-Locke DL: Tumours and pseudotumors of the region of the ampulla of Vater: an endoscopic, clinical and pathological study. Gut *27*:1186–1192, 1986.

288. Ishak KG, Glunz PR: Hepatoblastoma and hepatocarcinoma in infancy and childhood. Report of 47 cases. Cancer *20*:396–422, 1967.

289. Lack EE, Neave C, Vawter GF: Hepatoblastoma. A clinical and pathologic study of 54 cases. Am J Surg Pathol *6*:693–705, 1982.

290. Stocker JT, Ishak KG: Hepatoblastoma. *In* Neoplasms of the Liver, edited by K. Okuda, K.G. Ishak. Tokyo, Springer-Verlag, 1987, pp. 127–136.

291. Beach R, Betts P, Radford M, Millward-Sadler H: Production of human chorionic gonadotrophin by a hepatoblastoma resulting in precocious puberty. J Clin Pathol *37*:734–737, 1984.

292. Nakagawara A, Ikeda K, Tsuneyoshi M, Daimaru Y, Enjoji M, Watanabe I, Iwafuchi M, Sawada T: Hepatoblastoma producing both α-fetoprotein and human chorionic gonadotropin. Cancer *56*:1636–1642, 1985.

293. Helson L, Helson C: Human hepatoblastoma in cell culture. In Vitro *12*:327–328, 1976.

294. Li F-P, Thurber WA, Seddon J, Holmes GE: Hepatoblastoma in families with polyposis coli. JAMA *257*:2475–2477, 1987.

295. Amendola MA, Blane CE, Amendola BS, Glazer GM: CT findings in hepatoblastoma. J Comput Assist Tomogr *8*:1105–1109, 1984.

296. Dachman AH, Pakter RL, Ros PR, Fishman EK, Goodman ZD, Lichtenstein JE: Hepatoblastoma: radiologic-pathologic correlation in 50 cases. Radiology *164*:15–19, 1987.

297. Quinn JJ, Altman AJ, Robinson HJ, Cooke RW, Hight DW, Foster JH: Adriamycin and cisplatin for hepatoblastoma. Cancer *56*:1926–1929, 1985.

298. Gonzales Crussi F, Upton MP, Maurer HS: Hepatoblastoma. Attempt at characterization of histologic subtypes. Am J Surg Pathol *6*:599–612, 1982.

299. Abenoza P, Manivel JC, Wick MR, Hagen K, Dehner LP: Hepatoblastoma: an immunohistochemical and ultrastructural study. Hum Pathol *18*:1025–1035, 1987.

300. Manivel C, Wick MR, Abenoza P: Teratoid hepatoblastoma. The nosologic dilemma of solid embryonic neoplasms of childhood. Cancer *57*:2168–2174, 1986.

301. Ishak KG, Willis GW, Cummins SD, Bullock AA: Biliary cystadenoma and cystadenocarcinoma. Report of 14 cases and review of the literature. Cancer *39*:322–338, 1977.

302. Woods GL: Biliary cystadenocarcinoma: case report of hepatic malignancy originating in benign cystadenoma. Cancer *47*:2936–2940, 1980.

303. Wheeler DA, Edmonson HA: Cystadenoma with mesenchymal stroma (CMS) in the liver and bile ducts. A clinicopathologic study of 17 cases, 4 with malignant change. Cancer *56*:1434–1445, 1985.

304. Rossi RL, Silverman ML, Braasch JW: Carcinomas arising in cystic conditions of the bile ducts. Ann Surg *205*:377–384, 1987.

305. Cruickshank AH, Sparshott SM: Malignancy in natural and experimental hepatic cysts. Experiments with aflatoxin in rats and the malignant transformation of cysts in human livers. J Pathol *104*:185–190, 1971.

306. Azizah N, Paaradinas FJ: Cholangiocarcinoma coexisting with developmental liver cysts: a distinct entity different from liver cystadenocarcinoma. Histopathology *4*:391–400, 1980.

307. Katsuda S, Nakanishi K, Kajikawa K, Takabatake S: Mucoepidermoid carcinoma of the liver. Acta Pathol Jpn *34*:153–157, 1984.

308. Lynch MJ, McLeod MK, Weatherbee L, Gilsdorf JR, Guice KS, Eckhauser FE: Squamous cell cancer of the liver arising from a solitary benign nonparasitic hepatic cyst. Am J Gastroenterol *83*:426–431, 1988.

309. Gresham GA, Path FRC, Rue LW: Squamous cell carcinoma of the liver. Hum Pathol *16*:413–416, 1985.

310. Arase Y, Endo Y, Hara M, Kumada H, Ikeda K, Yoshiba A: Hepatic squamous cell carcinoma with hypercalcemia in liver cirrhosis. Acta Pathol Jpn *38*:643–650, 1988.

311. Song E, Kew MC, Grieve T, Isaacson C, Myburgh JA: Primary squamous cell carcinoma of the liver occurring in association with hepatolithiasis. Cancer *53*:542–546, 1984.

312. Moore SD, Gold RP, Lebwohl O: Adenosquamous carcinoma of the liver arising in biliary cystadenocarcinoma: clinical, radiologic and

pathologic features with review of the literature. J Clin Gastroenterol *6:*267–275, 1984.

313. Warner TFCS, Seo IS, Madura JA, Polak JM, Pearse AGE: Pancreatic-polypeptide-producing apudoma of the liver. Cancer *46:*1146–1151, 1980.

314. Andreola S, Lombardi L, Audisio RA, Mazzaferro V, Koukouras D, Doci R, Gennari L, Makowka L, Starzl TE, Van Thiel DH: A clinicopathologic study of primary hepatic carcinoid tumors. Cancer *65:*1211–1218, 1990.

315. Barsky SH, Linnoila I, Tyriche TJ, Costa J: Hepatocellular carcinoma with carcinoid features. Hum Pathol *15:*892–894, 1984.

316. Makowka L, Tzakis AG, Mazzaferro V, Teperman L, Demetris AJ, Iwatsuki S, Starzl TE: Transplantation of the liver for metastatic endocrine tumors of the intestine and pancreas. Surg Gynecol Obstet *168:*107–111, 1989.

317. Tsuda M, Tamaki S, Iwasaki E, Murashima S, Deguchi K, Shirakawa S: Successful treatment with a long-acting somatostatin analogue (SMS201-995) in a patient with malignant carcinoid syndrome. Jpn J Med *27:*311–316, 1988.

318. Norgaard T, Bardram L: Endocrine liver tumor differential diagnosis from hepatocellular carcinoma. Histopathology *9:*777–781, 1985.

319. Lewin K: Carcinoid tumors and the mixed (composite glandular-endocrine cell carcinomas. Am J Surg Pathol *11* (Suppl 1):71–86, 1987.

320. Pendl O, Scherlacher A: Uber einen Fall von Hypernephrom der Leber. Oesterr Ztschr f Kinderh *4:*269–279, 1950.

321. Bahadori M, Liebow AA: Plasma cell granulomas of the lung. Cancer *31:*191–208, 1973.

322. Anthony PP, Telesinghe PU: Inflammatory pseudotumour of the liver. J Clin Pathol *39:*761–768, 1986.

323. Chen KT: Inflammatory pseudotumour of the liver. Hum Pathol *15:*694–696, 1984.

324. Heneghan MA, Kaplan CG, Priebe CJ, Partin JS: Inflammatory pseudotumour of the liver: a rare cause of obstructive jaundice and portal hypertension in a child. Pediatr Radiol *14:*433–435, 1984.

325. Ishak KG: Malignant mesenchymal tumors of the liver. *In* Neoplasms of the Liver, edited by K. Okuda, K.G. Ishak. Tokyo, Springer-Verlag, 1987, pp. 159–176.

326. Manning JT Jr, Ordonez NG, Barton JH: Endothelial cell origin of thorium oxide-induced angiosarcoma of the liver. Arch Pathol Lab Med *107:*456–458, 1983.

327. Sussman EB, Nydick I, Gray G: Hemangioendothelial sarcoma of the liver and hemochromatosis. Arch Pathol *97:*39–42, 1974.

328. Winberg CD, Ranchod M: Thorotrast induced hepatic cholangiocarcinoma and angiosarcoma. Hum Pathol *10:*108–112, 1979.

329. Levy DW, Rindsberg S, Friedman AC, Fishman EK, Ros PR, Radecki PD, Siegelman SS, Goodman ZD, Pyatt RS, Grumback K: Thorotrast-induced hepatosplenic neoplasia: CT identification. AJR *146:*997–1104, 1986.

330. Popper H, Thomas LB, Teller NC, Falk H, Selikoff IJ: Development of hepatic angiosarcoma induced by vinyl chloride, Thorotrast and arsenic: comparison with cases of unknown etiology. Am J Pathol *92:*349–376, 1978.

331. Tamburro CH, Makk L, Popper H: Early hepatic histologic alterations among chemical (vinyl monomer) workers. Hepatology*4:*413–418, 1984.

332. Regelson W, Kim U, Ospina J, Holland JF: Hemangioendothelial sarcoma of liver from chronic arsenic intoxication by Fowler's solution. Cancer *21:*514–522, 1968.

333. Ross JM: A case illustrating the effects of prolonged action of radium. J Pathol Bacteriol *35:*899–912, 1932.

334. Monroe PS, Riddell RH, Siegler M, Baker AL: Hepatic angiosarcoma. Possible relationship to long-term oral contraceptive ingestion. JAMA *246:*64–65, 1981.

335. Falk H, Thomas LB, Popper H, Ishak KG: Hepatic angiosarcoma associated with androgenic-anabolic steroids. Lancet *2:*1120–1123, 1979.

336. Pimentel JC, Menezes AP: Liver disease in vineyard sprayers. Gastroenterology *72:*275–283, 1977.

337. Daneshmend TK, Scott GL, Bradfield JW: Angiosarcoma of liver associated with phenelzine. Br Med J *2:*1679, 1979.

338. Brady J, Liberatore F, Harper P, Greenwald P, Burnett W, Davies JNP, Bishop M, Polan A, Vianna N: Angiosarcoma of the liver: an epidemiologic survey. J Natl Cancer Inst *59:*1383–1385, 1977.

339. Kojiro M, Nakashima T, Ito Y, Ikezaki H, Moni T, Kido C: Thorium dioxide-related angiosarcoma of the liver: pathomorphologic study of 29 autopsy cases. Arch Pathol Lab Med *109:*853–857, 1985.

340. Evans DM, Williams WJ, King IT: Angiosarcoma and hepatocellular carcinoma in vinyl chloride workers. Histopathology *7:*377–388, 1983.

341. Dannaher CL, Tamburro CL, Yam LT: Occupational carcinogenesis: the Louisville experience with vinyl chloride-associated hepatic angiosarcoma. Am J Med *70:*279–287, 1981.

342. Locker GY, Doroshow JH, Zwelling LA, Chabner BA: The clinical features of hepatic angiosarcoma: a report of our cases and a review of the English literature. Medicine *58:*48–64, 1979.

343. Mahony B, Jeffrey RM, Federle MP: Spontaneous rupture of hepatic and splenic angiosarcoma demonstrated by CT. AJR *138:*965–966, 1982.

344. Okuda K, Omata M, Itoh Y, Ikezaki H, Nakashima T: Peliosis hepatis as a late and fatal complication of thorotrast liver disease. Report of five cases. Liver *1:*110–122, 1981.

345. Greenberg M: Kupffer cell sarcoma of the liver. Report of 2 cases in South African blacks. S Afr Med J *52:*244–246, 1977.

346. Sotcker JT, Ishak KG: Undifferentiated (embryonal) sarcoma of the liver. Report of 31 cases. Cancer *42:*336–348, 1978.

347. Chang WWL, Agha FP, Morgan WS: Primary sarcoma of the liver in the adult. Cancer *52:*1510–1517, 1983.

348. Horowitz ME, Etcubanas E, Webber BL, Kun LE, Rao BN, Vogel RJ, Pratt CB: Hepatic undifferentiated (embryonal) sarcoma of the liver in childhood: results of a retrospective Italian study. Cancer *59:*396–402, 1987.

349. Stanley RJ, Dehner LP, Hesker AE: Primary maligenant mesenchymal tumors (mesenchymoma) of the liver in childhood. An angiographic-pathologic study of three cases. Cancer *32:*973–984, 1973.

350. Gallivan MVE, Lack EE, Chun B, Ishak KG: Undifferentiated ('embryonal') sarcoma of the liver: ultrastructure of a case presenting as a primary intracardiac tumour. Pediat Pathol *1:*291–300, 1983.

351. Ruymann FB, Raney B, Crist WM, Lawrence W, Lindberg RD, Soule EH: Rhabdomyosarcoma of the biliary tree in childhood: a report from the intergroup rhabdomyosarcoma study. Cancer *56:*575–581, 1985.

352. Parham DM, Peiper SC, Robicheaux G, Ribeiro RC, Douglass EC: Malignant rhabdoid tumor of the liver. Evidence for epithelial differentiation. Arch Pathol Lab Med *112:*61–64, 1988.

353. Davis GL, Kissane JM, Ishak KG: Embryonal rhabdomyosarcoma (sarcoma botryoides) of the biliary tree. Cancer *24:*333–342, 1969.

354. Brooks JJ: Immunochemistry of soft tissue tumors: myoglobin as a tumor marker for rhabdomyosarcoma. Cancer *50:*1757–1783, 1982.

355. Tsokos M: The role of immunocytochemistry in the diagnosis of rhabdomyosarcoma. Arch Pathol Lab Med *110:*776–778, 1986.

356. Marimoto H, Takade Y, Akita T, Kato Y, Tanigawa N, Muraoka R, Urata Y: A resected case of the collision tumor of hepatocellular carcinoma and primary liver rhabdomyosarcoma. J Jpn Surg Soc *87:*456–463, 1986.

357. Taylor RW, Sylwestrowicz T, Kossakowska AE, Urbanski SJ, Minuk GY: Leiomyosarcoma of the inferior vena cava presenting as Budd-Chiari syndrome. Liver *7:*201–205, 1987.

358. O'Leary MR, Hill RB, Levine RA: Peritoneoscopic diagnosis of primary leiomyosarcoma of liver. Hum Pathol *13:*76–78, 1982.

359. Hara T, Nakata H, Tsujimoto M, Nakatani T, Nishioka S, Yataka I, Tobuse K, Shoji S, Katsumi M, Gen E: Primary leiomyosarcoma of the liver. Acta Hepatol Jpn *24:*1040–1046, 1983.

360. Bloustein PA: Hepatic leiomyosarcoma: ultrastructural study and review of the differential diagnosis. Hum Pathol *9:*713–716, 1978.

361. Tomaszewski MM, Kuenster JT, Hartman K: Leiomyosarcoma of ligamentum teres of liver: case report. Pediatr Pathol *5:*147–156, 1986.

362. Alrenga DP: Primary fibrosarcoma of the liver: case report and review of the literature. Cancer *36:*446–449, 1974.

363. Ishak KG: Mesenchymal tumors of the liver. *In* Hepatocellular Carcinoma, edited by K. Okuda, R.L. Peters. New York, John Wiley & Sons, 1976, pp. 247–308.

364. Gen E, Kusuyama Y, Saito K, Nagasaki Y, Nakatani T, Yataka I, Oku A: Primary fibrosarcoma of the liver with hypoglycemia. Acta Pathol Jpn *33:*177–182, 1983.

365. Weiss SW, Enzinger FM: Epithelioid hemangoendothelioma: a vascular tumor often mistaken for a carcinoma. Cancer *50:*970–981, 1982.

366. Dail DH, Liebow AA, Gmelich JT, Friedman PJ, Miyai K, Myer W, Patterson SD, Hannar SP: Intravascular, bronchiolar and alveolar tumor of the lung: an analysis of twenty cases of a peculiar sclerosing endothelial tumor. Cancer *51:*452–464, 1983.

367. Weiss SW, Ishak KG, Dail DH, Sweet DE, Enzinger FM: Epithelioid

hemangioendothelioma and related lesions. Diagn Histopathol *3*:259–287, 1986.

368. Ishak KG, Sesterhenn IA, Goodman ZD, Rabin L, Stromeyer FW: Epithelioid hemangioendothelioma of the liver: a clinicopathologic and follow-up study of 32 cases. Hum Pathol *25*:839–852, 1984.

369. Dean PJ, Haggitt RC, O'Hara CJ: Malignant epithelioid hemangioendothelioma of the liver in young women. Relationship to oral contraceptive use. Am J Surg Pathol *9*:695–704, 1985.

370. Radin DR, Craig JR, Colletti PM: Hepatic epithelioid hemangioendothelioma. Radiology *169*:145–148, 1988.

371. Ekfors TO, Joensuu K, Toivio I, Laurinen P, Pelttari L: Fatal epithelioid haemangioendothelioma presenting in the lung and liver. Virchow's Archiv A Pathol Anat Histopathol *410*:9–16, 1986.

372. Marino IR, Todo S, Tzakis AG, Klintmalm, Kelleher M, Iwatsuki S, Starzl TE, Esquivel CO: Treatment of hepatic epithelioid hemangioendothelioma with liver transplantation. Cancer *62*:2079–2084, 1988.

373. Shin P, Ohmi S, Sakurai M: Hepatocellular carcinoma combined with hepatic sarcoma. Acta Pathol Jpn *31*:815–824, 1981.

374. William WL, Agha FP, Morgan WS: Primary sarcoma of the liver in adults. Cancer *51*:1510–1517, 1983.

375. Nakajima T, Kubosawa H, Kondo Y, Konno A, Iwama S: Combined hepatocellular-cholangiocarcinoma with variable sarcomatous transformation. Am J Clin Pathol *90*:309–312, 1988.

376. Watanabe I, Kasai M, Watanuki T, Amano S: Malignant mixed tumor of the liver. Report of a case and a review of the literature. Acta Hepatogastroenterol *22*:158–164, 1975.

377. Kawarada Y, Uehara S, Noda M, Yatani R, Mizumoto R: Nonhepatocytic malignant mixed tumour primary in the liver. Cancer *55*:1790–1798, 1985.

378. Nakabayashi H, et al: An autopsy case of primary malignant mesenchymoma of the liver with various tissue components. Acta Hepatol Jpn *26*:369–375, 1985.

379. Kuwano H, Sonoda T, Hashimoto H, Enjoji M: Hepatocellular carcinoma with osteoclast-like giant cells. Cancer *54*:837–842, 1984.

380. Ishak KG: Primary hepatic tumors in childhood. *In* Progress in Liver Diseases, Vol. V, edited by H. Popper, F. Schaffner. New York, Grune & Stratton, 1976, pp. 636–667.

381. Willis RA: The Spread of Tumors in the Human Body, 2nd Edition. St Louis, C.V. Mosby, 1954.

382. Abrams HL, Spiro R, Goldstein N: Metastases in carcinoma. Analysis of 1000 autopsied cases. Cancer *3*:74–85, 1950.

383. Shuster MG: The effect of cirrhosis and portal-systemic shunting on metastatic cancer. MD Thesis, Yale University School of Medicine, 1987.

384. Cameron GR: The liver as a site and sources of cancer. Br Med J *1*:347–352, 1954.

385. Fenster LF, Klatskin G: Manifestations of metastatic tumors of the liver. A study of 81 patients subjected to needle biopsy. Am J Med *31*:238–248, 1961.

386. Melato M, Aurino L, Mucli E, Valente M, Ikuda K: Relationship between cirrhosis, liver cancer, and hepatic metastases. An autopsy study. Cancer *64*:455–459, 1989.

387. Mainland D: The risk of fallacious conclusions from autopsy data on the incidence of disease with applications to heart disease. Am Heart J *45*:644–654, 1953.

388. Snyder N, Atterbury CE, Correia JP, Conn HO: Increased concurrence of cirrhosis and bacterial endocarditis. Gastroenterology *73*:1107–1113, 1977.

389. Conn HO, Yesner R: A re-evaluation of needle biopsy in the diagnosis of metastatic cancer of the liver. Ann Intern Med *59*:53–61, 1963.

390. Yesner R, Conn HO: Liver function tests and needle biopsy in the diagnosis of metastatic cancer of the liver. Ann Intern Med *59*:62–73, 1963.

391. Chu TM: The detection of liver metastasis by laboratory tests. *In* Liver Metastasis, edited by L. Weiss, H.A. Gilbert. Boston, G.K. Hall, 1982, pp. 255–265.

392. Itai U: Imaging diagnosis with computed tomography. *In* Neoplasms of the Liver, edited by K. Okuda, K.G. Ishak. Tokyo, Springer-Verlag, 1987, pp. 289–300.

393. Machi J, Isomoto H, Yamashita Y, Kurohiji T, Shirouzu K, Kakegawa T: Intraoperative ultrasonography in screening for liver metastases from colorectal cancer: comparative accuracy with traditional procedures. Surgery *101*:678–684, 1987.

394. Simpson JA: Liver friction rub. A useful sign in the diagnosis of hepatic metastases. Dig Dis *16*:39–40, 1971.

395. Borja ER, Hori JM, Pugh RP: Metastatic carcinomatosis of the liver mimicking cirrhosis: case report and review of the literature. Cancer *35*:445–449, 1974.

396. Eras P, Sherlock P: Hepatic coma secondary to metastatic liver disease. Ann Intern Med *74*:581–583, 1971.

397. Shonfeld EM, Guarino AV, Bessolo RJ: Calcified hepatic metastases from carcinoma of the breast. Case report and review of the literature. Radiology *106*:303–304, 1973.

398. Axe SR, Erozan YS, Ermatinger SV: Fine-needle aspiration of the liver. A comparison of smear and rinse preparations in the detection of cancer. Am J Clin Pathol *86*:281–285, 1986.

399. Atterbury CE, Enriquez RE, Desuto-Nagy GI, Conn HO: Comparison of the histologic and cytologic diagnosis of liver biopsies in hepatic cancer. Gastroenterology *76*:1352–1357, 1979.

400. Riemann JF: Peritoneoscopy in the diagnosis of liver metastases. *In* Liver Metastasis, edited by L. Weiss, H.A. Gilbert. Boston, G.K. Hall Medical Publishers, 1982, pp. 244–254.

401. Fisher CJ, Faloon WE: Needle biopsy of the liver. Am J Med *25*:368–373, 1958.

402. Piccinino F, Sagnelli E, Pasquale G, Giusti G. Complications following percutaneous liver biopsy: a multicentre retrospective study on 68,276 biopsies. J Hepatol *2*:165–173, 1986.

403. McGill DB, Rakela J, Zinsmeister AR, Ott BJ. A 21-year experience with major hemorrhage after percutaneous liver biopsy. Gastroenterology *89*:1396–1400, 1990.

404. Conn HO. Liver biopsy: increased risks in patients with cancer. Hepatology *14*:206–209, 1991.

405. Strohmeyer T, Haugeberg G, Lierse W: Angioarchitecture and blood supply of micro- and macrometastases in human livers. An anatomic-pathological investigation using injection-techniques. J Hepatol *4*:181–189, 1987.

406. Ramming KP, O'Toole K: The use of the implantable chemoinfusion pump in the treatment of hepatic metastases of colorectal cancer. Arch Surg *121*:1440–1444, 1986.

407. Gerber MA, Thung SN, Bodenheimer HC Jr, Kapelman B, Schaffner F: Characteristic histologic triad in liver adjacent to metastatic neoplasm. Liver *6*:85–88, 1986.

Chapter 26
Liver Transplantation

The first human orthotopic liver transplantation was performed in 1963 by Starzl and his associates in Denver. Since then this procedure has come of age and is currently widely practiced throughout the world for a variety of end-stage or otherwise untreatable liver diseases. In 1984 a total of 540 transplantations were reported (1) from centers in Pittsburgh (2), Groningen (3), Hannover (4), and Cambridge (5). By mid-1992 the total number performed in the world is estimated to be well over 12,000. As many as 50,000 transplants per year may eventually be performed in the United States (6).

The largest diagnostic category of the underlying liver disease in the 1984 series was cirrhosis (44%), of which primary biliary cirrhosis, cryptogenic, and posthepatitic cirrhosis were the largest subgroups (1,7,8). *Neoplasms* were the second most frequent reason for transplantation (26%), with hepatocellular carcinoma by far the most common type, often with encouraging results (9). Results in patients with fibrolamellar hepatocellular carcinoma were especially rewarding (10). In 17%, transplantation was performed in neonatal cholestasis, almost all for extrahepatic biliary atresia. Transplantation was also performed to correct metabolic disorders, mainly *α-1-antitrypsin deficiency* (6%).

In the past eight years, the pattern has changed so that a much higher percentage is performed in patients with lethal metabolic disorders and fatal acquired hepatic diseases such as fulminant hepatic failure. Any patient with serious, uncorrectable disease of the liver is now considered to be a potential candidate for transplantation, including nonlethal metabolic derangements. Indeed, chronic ''self-induced'' disorders such as alcoholic cirrhosis are no longer thought of as absolute contraindications (11–14). Hepatic malignancies are still an important indication for liver transplant, providing that the neoplasms have not already metastasized (15,16). Epithelioid hemangioendothelioma, a recently recognized malignancy, responds quite well to liver transplantation (17). Age has become only a relative contraindication. Pregnancy has occurred after transplantation and does not have any deleterious effect on hepatic graft function, but the pregnancies are often complicated by preeclampsia and preterm delivery (18).

As experience with liver transplantation has increased, the contraindications to this procedure have decreased and the indications for it have broadened (19). Its use in fulminant hepatic failure of viral, drug, or toxic origin is now one of the most popular indications for and beneficial outcomes of liver transplantation. A whole spectrum of lethal hereditary diseases of the liver has been resolved by transplantation, including Wilson's disease (23), sometimes with reversal of neurologic signs (24), tyrosinemia (25), hemophilia A and B (26), α-1-antitrypsin deficiency (27), urea cycle enzyme deficiencies (28), glycogen and lipid storage diseases (29), and other disorders (7,30,31). The recent recognition that liver transplantation can improve prognosis in patients who have survived hemorrhage from varices (13,32) and in those with alcoholic cirrhosis (11) poses enormous ethical, economic, and logistic problems (14). At present, liver transplantation should be considered in any patients in whom major surgical or medical therapy for liver disease is being contemplated (33,34).

Since hepatic transplantation was introduced, there has been amazingly rapid progress. The mortality rate has progressively decreased and the percentage and duration of survival has progressively increased (1,19,33–35). In 1988, more than 60 to 70% of transplanted patients were reported to survive for at least one year (11); since then it seems clear that at least 70% can expect one year survival (6) or more. Advances in immunosuppression (36) and the introduction of a new, potent, relatively nontoxic, immunosuppressive agent, FK 506, which was isolated from *Streptomyces tsukubaenis* (37,38), promise to increase this figure even more. These figures are even more impressive when one realizes that in patients selected for transplantation, but for whom donor livers are not available, one year survival is virtually zero.

The causes of death have also changed. Early in the development of liver transplantation the causes of death were technical and mechanical failures usually associated with the biliary tract anastomosis, arterial insufficiency, and air embolism. Rejection was thought to be responsible in about 20%, but was probably overshadowed by other hepatic disorders. Improvements in surgical technique, especially in the use of a venovenous bypass in the biliary anastomosis, in patient and donor selection, in donor organ procurement (39), in graft preservation (40), and in immunosuppression (41,42) are responsible for the great improvement. Advances in supportive care also contribute (43). The development of a greatly improved solution for organ preservation and transport appears to increase graft viability and to decrease ischemic damage (40). Age is less frequently considered a contraindication to liver transplantation, since senescence largely spares the liver (44). Even HIV-positive patients are now considered to be valid candidates for transplantation (7).

A major limiting factor in further growth of transplantation is the unavailability of donor livers. One method of ameliorating this situation is the use of split liver transplants, in which one donor liver is transplanted into two patients (45).

Most deaths occur within 60 days of transplantation. Although the exact cause of death is often uncertain and multiple disorders contribute, the most frequent cause was found to be sepsis, which accounted for 40 to 90% of the deaths (35,46,47). Three-fourths of transplanted patients develop infections, most commonly abdominal abscesses, bacterial pneumonia, and cholangitis, usually soon after transplantation. Fungal infections are found frequently, as in other immunocompromised hosts, especially after prolonged antibiotic therapy, as are *Pneumocystis carinii* pneumonia and cytomegalovirus (CMV) infections (47,48). CMV infections have responded to gancyclovir and CMV hyperimmune globulin (49,50). Almost 20% of the deaths are considered to have resulted from multiple organ failure (1). About 20% of the deaths are attributed to miscellaneous causes, including massive hepatic necrosis, usually but not necessarily associated with occlusion of the hepatic artery. Some deaths are unexplained. Less than 10% of the deaths are attributable to rejection per se, although allograft rejection contributes to deaths from other causes. Histologic evidence of rejection, however, is present in the livers of more than one-third of the patients examined at autopsy (34) and in a much higher percentage by percutaneous biopsy. Probably all transplanted livers show some evidence of rejection at some time.

Partial liver transplantation has been used as an auxiliary heterotopic liver transplantation procedures (51). More recently, partial orthotopic liver transplants from living donors have been performed (52). Although living donor transplants are technically more complex, their complications promise to be less severe.

An authoritative, detailed overview of liver transplantation has been published by Starzl et al from the University of Pittsburgh (53–55).

Primary nonfunction of transplanted livers

Even before the rejection process can begin, the orthotopic graft must function and survive. Primary nonfunction is a devastating complication that occurs in 5 to 10% of transplants. Liver biopsy of donor livers has shown that the presence of severe fatty infiltration or hydropic degeneration are almost always associated with primary nonfunction (56). Such livers should not be transplanted.

Allograft rejection

Rejection of the liver has been much less common and severe than was first expected. (56a) HLA matching has not been found to be necessary and has generally not been applied. Liver transplantation into patients who have had major HLA incompatibilities with the donor liver has been common. Although no prospective comparisons have been carried out, such HLA mismatches do not seem to have adversely affected survival as they do in renal transplantation (2,56a). Indeed, it has been implied that deliberate mismatching of HLA DR antigens may diminish susceptibility to the vanishing bile duct syndrome and to cytomegalic inclusion virus (CMV) infection that may occur when DR antigens match in donor and recipient (57). Although early studies failed to demonstrate primary humoral rejection after transplantation across ABO blood groups (58), more recent, more objective investigations have shown that antibody-mediated rejection occurs four times more frequently in ABO-incompatible grafts as in ABO-compatible allografts (59).

Although liver transplants between human beings generate typical rejection reactions, these reactions may be milder than those encountered in the transplantation of kidneys or hearts. Episodes of rejection are currently treated by short courses of

increased doses of corticosteroids, or by antilymphocyte antibodies such as OKT3 (7). Immunosuppression is currently maintained by a combination of steroids, cyclosporine, and azathioprine (60). Complete discontinuance of immunosuppression results in the appearance or recurrence of rejection. However, both cyclosporine and azathioprine are frequently toxic and may induce hypertension, renal toxicity, or the development of lymphoma or other neoplasms (61,62), the most common of which are squamous carcinomas (63). The introduction of an analogue of prostaglandin E$_1$ (64) and an antibody to the interleukin-2 receptor (65) may also improve immunosuppression.

Hepatic allograft rejection results from an immune response of the host that is characterized by clinical, laboratory, and pathologic abnormalities. It is frequently silent clinically and may be almost undetectable histologically as well (66). Mild rejection reactions in hepatic homografts may be difficult to diagnose, since they are often subtle in presentation, variable in character, and difficult to distinguish from other causes of graft dysfunction such as biliary tract obstruction, cholangitis without obstruction, viral hepatitis, and other hepatic disorders. Jaundice is a serious sign of rejection and is usually accompanied by elevations in alkaline phosphatase and transaminase activity. Although the diagnosis of a rejection reaction can often be made on the basis of the characteristic clinical findings (67), it can only be unequivocally established by the exclusion of other causes. When the diagnosis of rejection cannot be made with certainty, a therapeutic trial of corticosteroids may be indicated. Since therapy with the murine monoclonal antibody OKT3 has been shown to be effective in suppressing steroid-resistant rejection (42), OKT3 may be tried when rejection cannot be differentiated from other hepatic disorders.

The recent introduction of FK 506 promises to revolutionize immunosuppression (37,38). This new immunosuppressive agent has been shown to be effective in preventing and in treating allograft rejection and to be relatively nontoxic in animals. Used in small doses (approximately 0.3 mg/day) in conjunction with small doses of corticosteroids (<10 mg/day) or none at all in >50%, this substance prevents the appearance of rejection and can promptly reverse established acute or early chronic rejection. It appears to be synergistic with cyclosporine in suppressing the expansion of the activated, recipient lymphocyte population (54). It seems especially effective in "rescuing" patients in whom other immunosuppressive agents have already failed. It is remarkably nontoxic. Although, like cyclosporine, it has the capacity to injure the kidneys, appears to be less toxic than azathioprine and cyclosporine A, and does not cause hypertension, it has been associated with arterial necrosis of pancreatic and peripancreatic tissue in several patients, and may have a tendency to cause pancreatitis. Otherwise it appears to be an ideal immunosuppressive agent. These encouraging observations will require careful confirmation.

Classification of allograft rejection

Organ rejection is usually classified as hyperacute, acute, and chronic, although precise definitions for these subtypes have not been established (68).

Hyperacute rejection, as may rarely occur with mismatched renal transplants, occurs only extremely rarely, if at all (7), after liver transplantation in humans under immunosuppressive therapy even when mismatched livers have been inadvertently transplanted (58,69). Accelerated rejection of liver grafts can occur, however, (7,70).

Acute rejection can apear as early as the first week or two after transplantation and is usually accompanied by impairment of liver function tests—increasing serum bilirubin concentration, elevated serum alkaline phosphatase and transaminase activity, or prolongation of prothrombin time. Symptoms of acute rejection are usually absent or minimal. However, fever and leukocytosis and, rarely, tenderness over the graft may be seen. About 40% of patients treated with cyclosporine and low dose prednisolone never have acute rejection, and another 40% suffer only a single episode (71). Occasionally, an accelerated rejection thought to represent an "anamnestic T cell response" may occur in patients who have not received adequate immunosuppression or for unknown reasons. Such reactions are characterized by jaundice, massive liver cell necrosis with markedly elevated transaminase levels, and increased alkaline phosphatase.

Chronic rejection reactions may persist for several months after an episode of acute rejection or may first appear several months after transplantation. These reactions are usually clinically indolent, but tend to progress. They may be nonspecific in terms of laboratory tests and pathologic findings, but may be overt or give rise to characteristic rejection syndromes. Clinically, the patients fail to thrive, serum bilirubin levels increase, and other hepatic tests worsen.

Although the terms "acute" and "chronic" may be used temporally, they actually refer primarily to the histologic abnormalities seen at those times. The pathologic interpretation of the disorders of transplanted livers is one of the most complex aspects of hepatic histology. Not only may any of the diseases that normally affect the liver be seen, but in addition, a number of complications of liver transplantation may occur, such as biliary obstruction, sepsis, arterial insufficiency, and hepatitis caused by HBV, HCV, CMV, EBV or herpes simplex virus (HSV), or by drugs. Such hepatic complications of transplantation may be superimposed on graft rejection, which may be present to some degree in virtually all transplanted livers. Lurking in the background is the possible recurrence in the allograft of the disease for which transplantation was done in the first place. Furthermore, it is not uncommon that two or more of these disorders occur simultaneously, thus the histologic features of both lesions may be present. Finally, the effects of immunosuppressive therapy may alter the histologic hepatic expression of these different diseases (72,73). Indeed, both azathioprine (60,72) and cyclosporine (73,74) may be hepatotoxic, and their histopathologic abnormalities must be differentiated from graft rejection.

It is difficult to attribute specific histologic abnormalities to specific clinical events when several disorders may be occurring at the same time. Moreover, much of our early knowledge about hepatic transplantation histology was derived from hepatic allografts that failed and were removed and examined at the time of a second transplantation or at autopsy. Hepatic abnormalities in such livers may reflect advanced hepatic disorders complicated by "agonal" events such as arterial insufficiency, sepsis, hypotension, and the effects of surgery and posthepatectomy autolysis. Most of our current understanding of the histologic findings of rejection is based on biopsy specimens taken after the patient has developed clinical and laboratory evidence of hepatic decompensation. More recently, routine, serial, "protocol" biopsies of the donor liver have been

taken before harvesting, immediately after the vascular anastomosis, and periodically thereafter to demonstrate the hepatic histology at intervals after transplantation (75,76). Our knowledge of the time of onset of rejection and of other abnormalities has been based on the time at which liver tissue became available. Thus, "early" rejection was empirically based on biopsies taken during the first two weeks or months after transplantation and "late" rejection on biopsies performed more than two months after transplantation (77,78).

Pathology of the transplanted liver

Hepatic rejection. Grossly, the transplanted liver, when it is free of disease, appears normal, although normal allografts have only been viewed *in situ* rarely. In acute rejection the liver tends to be enlarged, but in chronic rejection it usually appears normal, unless scarring has altered its appearance. The gross appearance of disorders such as obstructive jaundice, biliary sepsis, viral hepatitis, and infarction is the same as occurs in nontransplanted livers.

Microscopically, the liver has only a limited number of histologic responses to hepatic injury of different types. Many of these histologic expressions are common to several different disorders. Portal inflammation is seen in most hepatic disorders. Mononuclear portal inflammation is characteristic of both acute and chronic hepatitis, drug-induced hepatic injury, and rejection. Some pathologists have described mild acute rejection as a pattern that resembles chronic persistent hepatitis and severe acute rejection as one that resembles chronic active hepatitis (75), but this similarity is superficial. It is based primarily on the localization of the inflammation to the portal tracts in the former and extension of the inflammation into the parenchyma in the latter, and does not include the nature of the inflammatory reaction nor involvement of the bile ducts and venous walls. While often it is not possible to make the diagnosis of rejection solely on the basis of the histologic findings, this is not always the case. The diagnosis in such circumstances can be made on the basis of the clinical and laboratory features, the findings of ultrasonography, computerized tomography, and other imaging techniques, as well as on the histologic picture. Occasionally, however, the diagnosis of rejection is one of exclusion, i.e., the absence of any of the other disorders that may have caused the syndome. In the presence of other overt hepatic disorders, rejection may go unrecognized.

This multiplicity of disorders that can affect the transplanted liver may account in part for the different patterns observed by different groups. Some have found early rejection to be characterized by portal inflammation (Fig. 974), bile ductular abnormalities (Fig. 975), and cholestasis (Fig. 976) (78), so-called interstitial rejection. Others, in addition, have emphasized the characteristic endothelialitis or "vascular rejection" [(76,77); Fig. 977]. Furthermore, until 1980 immunosuppression was performed with adrenocorticosteroids and azathioprine, which may have more effectively obscured evidence of rejection than the steroid plus cyclosporine A used so widely now. In fact, it has been suggested that some of the hepatic lesions attributed to rejection may have been caused by the overzealous use of immunosuppression (68). It has not, however, been possible to demonstrate major differences between the histologic patterns of rejection with the two types of immunosuppression therapy (79).

The histologic patterns of allograft rejection described subsequently are based on carefully studied series of patients from a number of centers including our own (67,77,80).

Perioperative, or "time zero" biopsies, those that are taken just before or just after the implantation procedure, usually show the absence of any severe hepatic pathology. Characteristically, they show microvacuolation of the hepatocytes often with ballooning of parenchymal cells, which is most prominent in the pericentral area (Fig. 978), but may involve the whole lobule (Figs. 979, 980). This abnormality is not accompanied by any inflammatory reaction. Sometimes, small focal areas of necrosis may be present, or even areas of confluent or bridging necrosis may be found. These abnormalities represent acute cellular injury that occurs during the agonal period or harvesting or during storage prior to transplantation. Such areas of necrosis do not necessarily affect the viability or the function of the allografts (80), but when severe, may presage primary nonfunction (56) or a stormy early postoperative course (81). Occasionally, however, the donor's hepatic history is not known and histologic evidence of alcohol-induced injury or other hepatic disorders may only be discovered in retrospect. The finding of fat deposition caused by alcohol ingestion may be associated with poor outcome of the graft. Such consequences usually occur about a week after transplantation, but may appear months or even years later.

Acute rejection. Histologically, acute rejection indicates the presence of an inflammatory response to the allograft. In its most mild form, the hepatic structures appear normal or nearly so. The portal areas may show slight expansion, a rare inflammatory cell, and, perhaps, minimal abnormalities of the bile duct epithelium (Fig. 981). At Yale, these findings have been informally referred to as "graft recognition" to suggest that the host recognizes the presence of the alien allograft, but responds with only a minimal reaction. Acute rejection, which is characterized by a more intense, mixed inflammatory reaction, is seen primarily in the portal areas (Fig. 982). It includes mononuclear cells, neutrophils, and, sometimes, numerous eosinophils (Fig. 983). The inflammation involves the bile ducts, the portal veins, or the central veins. Hepatocellular injury may be present and is characterized by ballooning of hepatocytes, by necrosis of individual hepatocytes or foci of cells, or, occasionally, by bridging, confluent, or massive necrosis. There is little or no erosion of the limiting plates or hepatocellular necrosis, although the inflammatory cells sometimes extend into the periportal parenchyma (Fig. 984). The severity of the inflammatory response and the degree of biliary tract involvement may vary widely from portal tract to portal tract in the same biopsy. Moderate cholestasis of the central portion of the lobules is common. Lymphocytic adherence to the walls of portal and central veins, known as endothelialitis, may be present [(77,80); Fig. 985]. Invasion of the bile ductular epithelium by lymphocytes may be present. Neutrophils may often be seen. Eosinophilia is an early and accurate marker of acute rejection (82,83). These lesions and the clinical and laboratory abnormalities that accompany them sometimes disappear spontaneously, but usually resolve after antirejection therapy such as corticosteroid pulsing, antilymphocytic globulin, or OKT3.

Mild acute rejection has been seen on several occasions after liver transplantation as an apparent manifestation of graft-versus-host disease (84,85). It is unlikely to occur with solid organ transplants in which the donor organ is flushed with saline to remove donor lymphocytes. In the first such patient reported, the hepatic abnormalities were mild and unconfirmed histologically, but the hematologic, dermatologic, and gastroin-

testinal manifestations were severe and characteristic. The diagnosis was established by the demonstration of HLA chimerism due to allogeneic cells from the donor liver.

When more severe, acute rejection is characterized by a similar histologic picture with inflammation that extends into the hepatic parenchyma (Fig. 986), even into the pericentral area, and more prominent cholestasis (Fig. 987). The lymphocytes in acute allograft rejection usually consist of a mixture of helper and suppressor/cytotoxic T cells (86). These infiltrates, which subside with the rejection episode, usually appear before clinical and laboratory signs of rejection. When the immunocytes are predominantly helper T cells, the rejection often responds to a pulse of corticosteroids, but when they contain mainly suppressor/cytotoxic T cells, they do not. Endothelialitis and endophlebitis, which may be present in both terminal hepatic (Fig. 988) and portal veins, are characterized by the adherence of small lymphocytes to the luminal endothelium (Fig. 989) and infiltration of the subendothelial portions of the vein by lymphocytes, usually with characteristic elevations of the endothelium (Fig. 985). Endothelialitis appears to be the single most specific feature of acute rejection (80), although some of the earlier reports did not emphasize these lesions (75). This endothelial injury, which does not occur in all transplanted allografts and which is severe in only a small fraction, is usually of short duration. It is much more frequent and more persistent after retransplantation (87). The presence of endothelialitis is not associated with specific clinical or laboratory features (87). The endothelial immunocytes consist of helper and suppressor/cytotoxic T cells and natural killer cells. During rejection episodes, the lymphocytes often have a blastoid appearance (86,87).

An objective assessment in which patients from Groningen immunosuppressed with azathioprine and prednisone were coompared with patients from Minneapolis suppressed with cyclosporine A and prednisone (79) has shown that although endothelialitis was found in 80 to 90% of both groups, it was more mild in the azathioprine-treated patients. Rejection appeared to subside in both azathioprine- and cyclosporine-treated patients, but more dramatically and rapidly in patients immunosuppressed with cyclosporine A (88).

Graft and blood eosinophilia are very sensitive (92%), specific (98%) indices of hepatic allograft rejection (82). Using >7% graft eosinophilia, i.e., 7% of the cells infiltrating the portal areas, and >500 eosinophils per/mm^3 in the blood as definitions of eosinophilia, it has been shown that blood eosinophilia appears two days before rejection while graft eosinophilia occurs one day before rejection. This early warning system, especially the blood index, appears to be a very useful measurement. Subsequent quantitative investigations of these phenomena (83) have shown that although portal lymphocytes, neutrophils, and eosinophils all increase in acute rejection, they do so to very different degrees. In acute graft rejection, diagnosed by conventional clinical and laboratory characteristics, lymphocytes increase by 50% above nonrejection levels, neutrophils by 100%, and eosinophils by 1000%. Eosinophils do not usually appear in allografts in the absence of rejection; less than one eosinophil per portal tract is found (83). In acute rejection more than 10 per portal tract are present.

Erosion of the limiting plate is often present (Fig. 990) and may be accompanied by ballooning of centrilobular hepatocytes (Fig. 991), although this lesion is commonly seen with disorders other than rejection. Hepatocellular necrosis is not a prominent feature (80), although spotty, centrilobular necrosis (Fig. 992) or even confluent or bridging hepatic necrosis may be present (Fig. 990). Concentric fibrin deposition around the portal veins [(77); Fig. 990] or central veins is sometimes present in acute rejection. More intense cholestasis (Fig. 993) is present than in mild rejection. These findings, which are usually accompanied by biochemical abnormalities and often by fever, are usually reversed by increasing corticosteroid dosage or by other immunosuppressive medications. Some investigators have reported that the bile ductular injury, which consists of lymphocytic infiltration and epithelial cell changes such as anisonucleosis, cytoplasmic sweling and vacuolization (Fig. 994), eosinophilia, and, occasionally, necrosis of the bile ductular cells, is the most prominent histologic feature of rejection [(78); Fig. 995]. Bile ductules are so involved in from 10 to 75% of cases. As may occur in other types of chronic cholestasis, copper deposition is part of allograft rejection, often occurring early in the rejection reaction (Fig. 996). It should be kept in mind that azathioprine and cyclosporine themselves may cause cholestasis that is usually not accompanied by portal cellular infiltration (60). Intimal sclerosis and hyperplasia of arterioles have been reported in patients with severe graft failure, but these findings have not been established to be signs of chronic rejection (77). Arterial abnormalities involve medium sized arteries and are, therefore, rarely evident on needle biopsy of the liver, but are usually found at autopsy and in resected specimens. The arterial walls are infiltrated with lymphocytes and macrophages, and show disruption of the elastic lamina and fibrinoid necrosis.

In serial episodes of rejection and in late onset rejection, the degree of inflammatory reaction appears to be less severe than in early episodes of rejection (77). Most pathologists agree that after severe, acute rejection, liver biopsies usually show mild, persistent histologic abnormalities, but sometimes, become completely normal. Occasionally, portal inflammation, bile duct damage, endotheliitis, and cholestasis may persist despite clinical improvement. As the episode of rejection subsides, the inflammatory component decreases, especially in the portal tract, leaving some collagenization of the portal and central vein walls.

Histologic evidence of rejection often responds promptly to an increase in immunosuppressive therapy (Figs. 997, 998). Even so, the portal tracts do not return completely to normal, often showing residual edema, a few inflammatory cells, minimal abnormalities in the bile ductular epithelium, or a few strands of collagen, except in those treated promptly with immunosuppressive therapy.

In attempts to identify histologic features of acute liver allograft rejection, a group of 47 consecutive patients with serial biopsies were examined (67). This practical paper identifies portal infiltration, duct injury, and phlebitis as the primary criteria of acute rejection. In addition, it presents a useful classification for assessing responsiveness to therapy and the patterns of these histologic signs of injury individually and in combination in terms of complete resolution, improvement, persistence, and worsening. Three-fourths of these patients, in whom almost 300 biopsies were analyzed, exhibited at least one episode of rejection. The histologic abnormalities that predicted either acute liver failure or eventual, severe, chronic rejection were arteritis, paucity of bile ducts, or the presence together of hepatocellular ballooning and dropout. Surprisingly, the type or intensity of the infiltrate, the severity of the damage to bile ducts, or the presence of hepatocellular necrosis per se did not appear to be reliable prognostic indicators. In two patients who died of acute rejection shortly after transplantation, there was an intense polymorphonuclear infiltrate, arteritis, ischemic hepatocellular

injury, and fibrin deposition, a histologic syndrome suggestive of hyperacute allograft rejection.

One specific variant of acute rejection is the acute *vanishing bile duct syndrome* (VBDS). This unique disorder, which occurs in approximately 10% of patients after liver transplantation, does so within 100 days of the procedure (89). It is considered to be an irreversible form of acute rejection that requires retransplantation. It is not otherwise histologically differentiable from acute, reversible rejection in its early stages. Clinically, it presents with abrupt fever and, frequently, chills, jaundice, lethargy, and ascites. Serum bilirubin and alkaline phosphatase levels are usually greatly elevated. The fever responds to corticosteroid therapy, but the rest of the syndrome does not. Histologically, destructive (''rejection'') cholangitis is characteristic, as is ductopenia, which is often expressed as ''burnt out'' portal tracts devoid of bile ducts or inflammatory cells. The inflammatory response is made up largely of Leu 4+ and Leu 2a suppressor/cytotoxic T cells. Obliterative arteriopathy is present in most cases but may not be detectable. Sinusoidal foam cells and centrilobular necrosis may represent an equivalent lesion. The pathogenesis of VBDS is not known, but it has recurred after retransplantation, requiring a third transplant (89). It has been suggested that the chronic VBDS syndrome may be related to the type of mismatch of class I HLA antigens (90). Class II HLA mismatching was not associated with the VBDS. In fact, complete mismatch for class I and a complete (or partial) match for class II antigens is the most likely pattern associated with this syndrome. CMV infection appears to play a role in the pathogenesis of the VBDS (57). High titer, donor-specific antibodies to class I antigen may play a role in the bile duct injury.

Hyperacute rejection, which is more typical of renal transplantation in humans and of liver transplantation in experimental animals when no immunosuppression is used at all, has been observed very rarely after liver transplantation in humans. It appears that in both humans and animals liver allografts are resistant to primary humoral rejection (58,70,91), but they are not fully free of these effects (59). This poorly understood lesion seems to represent overwhelming rejection with both inflammatory and vascular components, and is characterized by massive hepatic necrosis and death. It has been postulated to be a B cell mediated anamnestic response that requires the presence of preexisting anti-donor HLA antibodies (67).

One reported case of a severe rejection reaction provides useful information about the ''natural'' histology of rejection (78). This instance of severe acute rejection was described in a patient transplanted in 1968 in whom no immunosuppressive therapy had been administered for fear of encouraging the hepatitis virus to infect the graft. The patient showed great improvement immediately after transplantation, but suddenly deteriorated clinically on the sixth postoperative day with jaundice and laboratory evidence of severe hepatocellular necrosis. At autopsy seven days after transplantation the liver was grossly enlarged, weighing 1950 g. The histologic picture was similar to that seen after unmodified liver transplantation in experimental animals. The portal tracts were edematous and intensely infiltrated with lymphocytes and plasma cells with some polymorphonuclear neutrophils and eosinophils (Fig. 999). Monocytic infiltration of the walls of the central veins was seen. The walls of small bile ductules were infiltrated with lymphocytes, and injury to the ductular epithelium was present (Fig. 1000). There was patchy eosinophilic necrosis of parenchymal cells and centrilobular atrophy and sinusoidal dilatation. Cholestasis was striking. The arteries appeared normal. Although histologic signs of the rejection were overt in this immunologically unsuppressed patient, rejection of similar severity is occasionally seen in immunosuppressed patients just as promptly after transplantation, and, therefore, this case is not regarded as hyperacute rejection.

Fine needle aspiration biopsy (FNAB) has been used for some years in establishing the diagnosis of acute rejection after kidney transplantation (92), although it has not been used widely. This technique, which is based on cytologic rather than histologic examination of liver tissue, uses a fine 0.4 mm needle and is consequently extremely safe and virtually free of complications. The specimens are cytocentrifuged, stained with variations of the Giemsa stain, and corrected for the type and number of inflammatory cells in the peripheral blood (93). In successful biopsies, which are obtained more than 90% of the time, five or more hepatocytes per 100 leukocytes are seen [(94); Fig. 1001]. The diagnosis of acute rejection is based primarily on an increase in the number and type of leukocytes above baseline levels (95) and especially by the presence of lymphoblasts. Typical findings in acute rejection are an early increase in inflammatory cells 5 to 28 days after transplantation (Fig. 1002), which often precedes clinical signs of rejection by several days (96), and a decrease after 2 to 3 days of antirejection therapy. A semiquantitative scoring system seems to enhance the value of this procedure (97). Fine needle cytologic and routine needle histologic examination give equivalent results (98,99) and are useful in following the response to immunosuppression therapy (96). Degenerating hepatocytes often show intracellular cholestasis (Figs. 1003, 1004). These findings often occur with the characteristic increments in serum alkaline phosphatase and bilirubin levels and fever, but correlate poorly with clinical symptoms.

Chronic rejection. "Chronic" rejection, too, is both a histological and temporal term. It is characterized by the presence of vascular injury in which arteries show evidence of immunologic damage with inflammation, fibrinoid necrosis, destruction of the walls, intimal proliferation (Fig. 1005), and the deposition of lipid-laden macrophages that compress or obliterate the lumen (Fig. 1006). This lesion is seen in patients who have or have had acute rejection, although it may be found in the absence of overt acute rejection. The frequent paucity or absence of bile ducts or the presence of bile duct injury suggests that acute rejection has been present in these patients with chronic rejection. It tends to occur late, months or years after transplantation, but it has been observed within the first few weeks.

In patients who have died of chronic rejection, the characteristic hepatic histologic findings are focal areas of hepatocellular necrosis scattered throughout the lobules accompanied by lymphocytic and plasmacytic infiltration of the portal tracts. When cyclosporine has been used, the presence of eosinophils in the infiltration tends to be prominent. Degenerative changes of the epithelium of small bile ducts are often present. This nonsuppurative, destructive cholangitis is similar to the biliary epithelial changes seen in graft-versus-host disease (100) or primary biliary cirrhosis (101) and is considered by many to be a most critical aspect of the rejection process. In the advanced stages, bile ducts may be absent (102), the so-called *vanishing bile duct* sign. In chronic rejection, the vascular lesions predominate. Lipid-filled histiocytes may be found in the sinusoids and beneath the endothelium of arterioles (Fig. 1006). Intimal proliferation of the hepatic arteries, which is characteristic of the rejection reaction in transplanted kidneys, is common (Fig. 1005),

and complement deposition in the walls of arterioles has been demonstrated. Injury to or rupture of the internal elastic lamina of small intrahepatic arteries is common (75). The involvement of veins in the acute rejection reaction, which is common after renal transplantation, may be absent in chronic rejection of transplanted livers. The inflammatory components are less conspicuous, but erosion of the limiting plates and centrilobular atrophy and bile duct injury are usually evident. Cirrhosis may develop.

Hepatic disorders other than rejection. The histologic patterns of most hepatic diseases of liver allografts unrelated to the transplantation procedure are similar to those seen in untransplanted livers, although they may be affected by immunosuppression.

Viral hepatitis. There are subtle, quantitative differences in the histologic appearance of HBV, CMV, and HSV acute viral hepatitis in allografted livers from those seen in ungrafted livers. The spotty hepatic parenchymal necrosis is similar, but the portal inflammatory response is often reduced, as it is in other immunosuppressed patients (79). The diagnosis of acute viral hepatitis caused by CMV and HSV is made by the clinical setting, viral cultures, serologic tests, and the presence of characteristic nuclear inclusions. In CMV hepatitis, the most common type (103), the portal inflammatory reaction is minimal, and focal collections of neutrophils and mononuclear cells may be scattered throughout the liver (Fig. 1007). Characteristic intranuclear inclusions may be seen in hepatocytes (Figs. 1008, 1009), in bile ductules (Fig. 1010), and in the portal venous endothelium (68). The diagnosis may be established unequivocally by immunostaining with antibody to CMV [(104); Fig. 1011]. CMV hepatitis may be effectively treated by reduction of immunosuppression, by hyperimmune globulin (105), by gancyclovir (50,106), and by combined therapy (49). In HSV hepatitis, Cowdry type A nuclear inclusions are characteristic but uncommon and granulomas are frequently found. Epstein-Barr viral hepatitis (EBV) is a rare complication, but is not uncommon in patients after liver transplantation (67). It may take a variety of forms that range from an infectious mononucleosis-like syndrome to lymphoproliferative disease (7). When one of these opportunistic viruses is found, others may also be present. Acute hepatitis caused by HBV may be more difficult to recognize, because it shows no such specific evidence except for its serologic markers and for the occasional presence of ground glass, cytoplasmic, Shikata inclusion bodies. The diagnosis of non-A, non-B hepatitis, which has no pathognomonic histologic characteristics, until now could not be made unequivocally in the grafted liver, but the development of a reliable method of detecting HCV should solve this problem (107).

Aplastic anemia occurs more commonly after liver transplantation in patients with fulminant NANB viral hepatitis, appearing in more than one-fourth of such patients (108). The aplastic anemia is felt to be a complication of the hepatitis, and not to be directly related to the transplantation procedure.

Hepatic necrosis. This complication of hepatic transplantation is almost always obvious clinically; it is characterized by hypotension, jaundice, and laboratory evidence of hepatic failure. It is usually caused by thrombosis of the hepatic artery, which tends to occur soon after surgery and from one to two months after transplantatiion, and is expressed as massive infarcts of the liver. It may also be caused, in a more mild form, by pulmonary thromboembolism or by thrombosis of some of the branches of the hepatic artery. Shock and ischemic liver disease can also result from severe infection or from biliary leakage. Histologically, the hepatocellular necrosis does not differ from that seen in nongrafted livers (Figs. 992, 1012, 1013). In biopsies of early lesions, which are usually performed because of rising transaminase levels or mild clinical deterioration, the lesions are often limited to zone 3, where hepatocytes appear vacuolated and distended or contain cytoplasmic bile or show coagulative necrosis. Although portal vein thrombosis, hepatic venous occlusion, and hepatic arterial obstruction can theoretically be differentiated histologically, it is extremely difficult to do so in the setting of transplantation in which small infarcts are common and the liver is unusually susceptible to ischemia (109). Massive hepatic necrosis is often complicated by infections, usually with *Pseudomonas aeruginosa,* and less freqquently by a variety of other bacteria and fungi (46). Total hepatic necrosis may suddenly occur in the absence of any vascular lesion or other reasonable explanation (Figs. 1014, 1015).

Extrahepatic biliary obstruction. Extrahepatic biliary obstruction and bile fistulas were common in the early years of liver transplantation (110). In addition, the biliary anastomoses were often contaminated with bacteria, which led to cholangitis and systemic infections (111), but the prevalence of this complication has been sharply reduced by the performance of choledochocholedochostomy in the United States and by double cholecystocholedochostomy in Great Britain (112). This complication is characterized by jaundice, biochemical abnormalities indicative of biliary obstruction, and bacterial infection. Histologically, infiltrates of polymorphonculear leukocytes with scattered lymphocytes and plasma cells are found around bile ducts and may infiltrate the bile duct epithelium and lumen. Extensive parenchymal cholestasis with bile lakes and feathery biliary necrosis may be present. This histologic pattern is identical to extrahepatic biliary obstruction in unshunted livers (Figs. 284, 314, 315). Biliary sludge arising from the sloughing of ischemic biliary tract epithelium is a surprisingly frequent cause of biliary tract obstruction (109).

Infectious cholangitis. Infectious cholangitis often complicates the posttransplantation picture, and is characterized clinically by fever, worsening of liver function tests, and nonspecific clinical deterioration. Right upper quadrant pain, which is typical in nontransplanted patients, is not usually present in denervated, transplanted patients. It occurs usually in patients with extrahepatic biliary obstruction, but may occur in its absence. It is usually caused by gram-negative bacteria or fungi. The characteristic polymorphonuclear leukocytic infiltrations and abscesses do not differ from those seen in nonallografts (Fig. 1016). Other bacterial infections of the liver and endotoxemia may occur after transplantation, and both may be consequences of early, incomplete replacement of the Kupffer cells of the donor liver by host macrophages (113).

Parenchymal cholestasis. Pure parenchymal cholestasis has been commonly observed (75,77). In this situation, moderate to severe cholestasis occurs in the virtual absence of inflammatory cells in the portal or parenchymal areas. This lesion is seen most frequently in patients with severe coagulopathy preoperatively and during disorders of coagulation or circulation. Bile pigment accumulates in canaliculi and hepatocytes in the absence of any other histologic abnormalities. This unexplained syndrome of intrahepatic cholestasis has been termed "functional graft failure."

Recurrence of the primary hepatic disorder. Recurrence of the primary hepatic lesion in hepatic allografts occurs most commonly with neoplasms. The recurrence of adenocarcinomas of the biliary tree and cholangiocarcinomas has probably resulted from the failure to excise all the neoplastic tissue at the time of transplantation. Small hepatocellular carcinomas that would have been acceptable for resection tend not to recur after transplantation. In patients with large, unresectable tumors, however, transplantation is almost always followed by the recurrence of the tumor (114). Fibrolamellar hepatocellular carcinomas, which tend to grow slowly and to metastasize late, if ever, are the most rewarding types of hepatic cancer to transplant (115,116).

The recurrence of preexisting HBV and other types of viral hepatitis, which has been reported during immunosuppression, is not surprising (117–120). Recurrence of the Budd-Chiari syndrome in patients with myeloproliferative disorders is common, and such patients are, therefore, considered poor candidates for liver transplantation (68,121).

Some patients with chronic HBV infection after transplantation develop recurrence of HBV hepatitis with unique characteristics, termed *fibrosing cholestatic hepatitis* (116). Clinically, the course in these patients is characterized by rapid deterioration, jaundice, progressive prolongation of prothrombin time, encephalopathy, and graft failure. Histologically, it is characterized by (1) extensive, periportal fibrosis with delicate, perisinusoidal stands extending into the acini and surrounding plates of ductular epithelium; (2) overt canalicular and cellular cholestasis; (3) many HBsAg-containing ground glass hepatocytes; and (4) ballooning of hepatocytes and acidophilic degeneration. It is postulated that this syndrome is the result of a high cytoplasmic expression of HBV antigens.

Primary biliary cirrhosis has also been reported to recur (122). The histologic differentiation of recurrent primary biliary cirrhosis from the biliary lesions of allograft rejection, which is based on clinical laboratory, and histologic abnormalities, is difficult. In primary biliary cirrhosis pruritus is common, but the degree of cholestasis is not usually severe nor relentlessly progressive. Antimitochondrial antibody is characteristic of primary biliary cirrhosis, and the titer decreases or disappears after transplantation but reappears as primary biliary cirrhosis recurs (122). In rejection reactions antimitochondrial antibody is absent. In primary biliary cirrhosis granulomas or dense aggregates of lymphocytes are common; in rejection, they are not although they may occasionally be seen. The recurrence of primary biliary cirrhosis is a relatively slow process, and abnormal bile ducts undergo progressive injury for months or years before they disappear. In rejection the vanishing bile duct syndrome may develop within a few months (89). In chronic rejection other lesions characteristic of rejection such as foamy, lipid-laden macrophages in the sinusoids and arteries are common (Fig. 1006), and myointimal proliferation of the arteries may be present [(77); Fig. 1005].

Pathologic analysis of transplantation of patients with primary biliary cirrhosis reveals major differences between the histologic findings in chronic rejection and in primary biliary cirrhosis (101), although it may not be possible to differentiate them in individual instances. There was no correlation between antimitochondrial antibody titers before transplantation and the degree of hepatic dysfunction afterward. Recurrent primary biliary cirrhosis did not occur in any of the 106 patients in this series. Although chronic rejection tended to occur more frequently in primary biliary cirrhosis than in other types of underlying liver disease, it did not differ qualitatively or quantitatively from that seen in other hepatic disorders. The histologic pattern of chronic rejection differs from that of primary biliary cirrhosis by the presence of obliterative arteriopathy and centrilobular cholestasis, which are absent in primary biliary cirrhosis, and the absence of Mallory bodies, copper deposition, and granulomas, which are common in primary biliary cirrhosis. Both disorders share nonsuppurative, destructive cholangitis and a decrease in the number of bile ducts. Furthermore, there is a parallel between the size of obliterated arteries and the size of their associated, missing bile ducts in chronic rejection, a phenomenon that often results in a paucity of large bile ducts that is not seen in primary biliary cirrhosis in which only small bile ducts vanish (102).

A primary, large cell, follicular lymphoma of the liver has been reported limited to the liver of a patient six months after liver transplantation (114). No such tumor was found in the donor, and the primary hepatic lymphoma was assumed to have developed de novo. It is now well established that there is an increased incidence of neoplasia, especially lymphoproliferative malignancies, in transplanted patients (123). Whether the development of this lymphoma was transplantation-related or coincidence is now known, however.

Hepatocellular carcinoma has also been reported after orthotopic liver transplantation (124).

Liver transplantation in recipients who are physically much larger than the donor is followed by active hepatic regeneration (125). Although no histologic abnormalities associated with such massive regeneration have been reported, such abnormalities may well be present.

Hepatic disease associated with renal transplantation

Hepatic disease has been recognized to occur after renal transplantation since this procedure was first introduced (126,127). More than half of all kidney transplant recipients show abnormalities of liver function tests after transplantation and about half of them have associated symptoms (128,129). The liver disease is progressive in about one-fifth of transplanted patients (128,129).

The spectrum of hepatic disorders seen is extremely broad, since several potential precipitants of liver disease exist in these patients, as they do in the recipients of liver allografts. First, chronic hemodialysis, which precedes renal transplantation, is associated with an increased incidence of viral hepatitis, especially HBV, and a high carrier rate for HBsAg (130). Furthermore, the immunologic response of chronic dialysis patients to vaccination with HBV vaccine appears to be blunted (131,132). HCV has also been implicated, although so far without objective evidence. Second, immunosuppressed patients are susceptible to a variety of opportunistic viruses such as CMV, EBV, and HSV that induce viral hepatitis (133). Third, bacterial infections may occur. Infections such as syphilis tend to favor immunocompromised hosts. Immunosuppressive agents themselves can induce hepatic damage (125–127,134,135). Fourth, rejection of the allograft is often involved. Transplant rejection, which is characterized by decreasing renal function, intimal proliferation of arteries, and inflammatory infiltration of the kidney, is as ubiquitous as it is after hepatic transplantation. These reactions are often accompanied by abnormal liver function tests not attributed to other hepatic disorders. The histo-

logic features of these lesions are generally nonspecific and do not resemble those of hepatic rejection reactions in transplanted livers or those of graft-versus-host disease (see bone marrow transplantation). Finally, a variety of hepatic lesions of uncertain origin have been reported including hemosiderosis (136,137), peliosis hepatis (138,139), veno-occlusive disease (140), nodular regenerative hyperplasia (141), idiopathic portal hypertension (142,143), and hepatocellular cancer (144,145). Hepatic granulomatosis associated with silicone particles from dialysis tubing has also been observed (146,147).

Viral hepatitis

Viral hepatitis represents the most common cause of hepatic disorders in patients with renal transplants. This is largely due to the high prevalence of HBV infection in patients on hemodialysis (128,129), which reflects both the high frequency of exposure and the natural immunosuppression of chronic renal failure. Immunosuppressed patients tend to develop anicteric hepatitis, rather than overt acute hepatitis, to remain chronically infected and infectious, and to maintain active virus replication (148). Iatrogenic immunosuppression appears to enhance natural immunosuppression and frequently causes reactivation of HBV in patients who have already developed antibodies to HBV (148–150). Furthermore, allograft survival appears to be better in patients who are HBsAg-positive than in those who are anti-HBS-positive (151,152). These effects may indicate a systemic immunologic tolerance in patients who are immunologically tolerant of HBV (153). Despite greater tolerance of the allografts, the progression of liver disease from latent or chronic persistent hepatitis to chronic active hepatitis and cirrhosis (154) and death from hepatic decompensation is greater in HBsAg-positive renal graft recipients than it is in those who are HBsAg-negative (155,156).

It is not known whether opportunistic viruses such as CMV, EBV, and HSV, which occur with increased frequency in immunosuppressed and transplanted patients, behave more aggressively in immunocompromised patients than in normal individuals (133,157). The prophylactic use of acyclovir has been shown to decrease the prevalence of CMV infections and to eradicate HSV after renal transplantation (158,159). HBV and other hepatitis viruses have also been implicated (126,157), but in the absence of definitive diagnostic techniques their role remains uncertain. HDV may also cause fulminant hepatitis occasionally after renal transplants (160).

Clinically, viral hepatitis appears to behave in transplanted patients as it does in normal individuals, and its laboratory manifestations do not differ.

Microscopically, the livers in viral hepatitic infections, whether clinically silent, acute, or chronic, do not appear to differ from those seen in nontransplanted patients (161) (see Chapters 6 and 7).

Hemosiderois

Increased hepatic iron deposition is a common consequence of renal transplantation (136,137,162). Hemosiderosis was found in one series in 20 of 74 adult patients who had had kidney transplants and in whom liver tissue was available for analysis

(136). About 20% of the patients developed hemochromatosis. The iron deposition often accumulated within the first year after transplantation and was usually found within two years.

The disorder is clinically silent in about half the patients. Among the symtomatic patients, ascites is the most common sign followed by hepatomegaly, weight loss with weakness and lethargy, skin pigmentation, and diabetes. Serum transaminase levels are increased in almost all patients and alkaline phosphatase in about 80%. Serum bilirubin concentrations are elevated in half, but the elevations are usually minimal.

Serum ferritin levels have been increased in the patients studied. Phlebotomy therapy has been used in symptomatic patients, usually with beneficial results (136).

The presence of hemosiderosis is more frequently found in female patients and in those who have received long-term hemodialysis therapy. More blood transfusions were administered prior to transplantation to those who subsequently developed hemosiderosis, but the mean difference in transfusion-provided iron is small, i.e., less than 2 g per patient. The hemochromatosis develops in patients who receive no iron therapy or blood transfusions after transplantation. There is no statistical correlation with age, duration after transplant, type of transplant or immunosuppression used, the number of transfusions, viral infection, alcohol consumption, or the presence of HLA antigen A3 (136). The mechanism by which the iron accumulates is not known. Tissue iron levels have not yet been quantified. Coincidental hereditary hemochromatosis is unlikely in these patients, but this possibility cannot be excluded.

Histologically, 45% of the 20 patients studied had cirrhosis and 35% had varying degrees of portal fibrosis (136). Only 15% of the 54 patients without hemosiderosis had cirrhosis, a statistically significant difference. Using the semiquantitative, histologic scale of Scheuer (163), grade 3 to 4 iron was found in the hepatocytes of all 20 patients and grade 1 to 3 in the Kupffer cells. The histologic grade of iron in the hepatocytes correlates well with the serum ferritin concentration.

In a well-documented case of a 41-year-old woman, hemosiderosis became clinically and histologically evident within one year of renal transplantation (Fig. 656). Within the next 11 months, the disorder progressed to fullblown micronodular cirrhosis (Figs. 657, 658). Other such cases have also been reported (164).

Miscellaneous postrenal transplantation disorders of the liver

No clinical or histologic hepatic abnormalities of rejection similar to those reported after liver or bone marrow transplantation have been reported. The presence of veno-occlusive disease (140) or intrahepatic cholestasis, both of which may occur after bone marrow transplantation and which may represent azathioprine hepatotoxicity, has been reported rarely (140).

The lesions of peliosis hepatis (138,139), nodular regenerative hyperplasia (141), idiopathic portal hypertension (142,143), and hepatocellular carcinoma (144,145) are of unknown origin and do not differ histologically from these lesions in nontransplanted patients.

Other infectious agents such as syphilis [(165); Figs. 727, 728] and *Candida* (166) have been reported to cause hepatitis in patients after renal transplantation.

A variety of nonhepatic complications have been reported to result from the interaction of the blood of dialyzed patients with synthetic, foreign substances such as dialysis tubing or cannulas (167,168). In addition, a hepatitis-like syndrome has been induced by polyvinylchloride tubing (169). Refractile particles of silicone have been described in the livers of patients after hemodialysis (146,147). Such particles have been found in more than half of dialyzed patients. The amount of these fragments is proportional to the duration of hemodialysis. Virtually all patients with hepatic silicone fragments show elevations of serum transaminase. However, other hepatic disorders are frequently present in hemodialysis patients and may be responsible for some of these abnormalities.

Histologically, the presence of the silicone fragments is associated with granuloma formation, inflammation, and hepatic fibrosis. These fragments, which arise from trauma to the silicone tubing by the roller pump of the dialysis apparatus, are also found in the spleen, bone marrow, and lungs (147).

A new hepatic syndrome with a specific histologic lesion appears to have been precipitated by the intravenous infusion of hydroxyethyl starch into patients with renal failure who are receiving hemodialysis (170). This carbohydrate substance is a colloidal plasma substitute that has been used in the treatment of hemodialysis-related hypotension. The starch is both degraded by amylase and excreted in the urine (171). In renal failure the starch persists in the bloodstream and may accumulate in the tissues. Clinically, its use has been followed by the appearance of persistent ascites. At autopsy the hepatocytes and bile duct epithelial cells are vacuolated (Fig. 809). The sinusoidal cells are distended and foamy (Fig. 810). Foamy macrophages were also seen in the portal tracts. The foam cells were Alcian blue- and PAS-positive, but the latter became negative after diastase digestion, indicating the presence of glycogen. In the cases described, these changes were panlobular, but were more prominent in the central areas. There was no obvious necrosis, although occasional eosinophilic bodies were seen. There was no cirrhosis or portal fibrosis, although the number of collagen fibers seemed increased. By electron microscopy the vacuoles in sinusoidal lining cells, Kupffer cells, Ito cells, and endothelial cells contained β-glycogen granules. It is suggested that the distended sinusoidal cells cause sinusoidal obstruction to blood flow that results in ascites formation.

Since these hepatic lesions are associated with hemodialysis, it is likely that they may also be seen in patients who subsequently have kidney transplants.

The pathogenesis of various hepatic lesions after kidney transplantation may be even more mysterious than it seems. Some hepatic abnormalities, such as the deposition of silicone fragments from dialysis tubing or hydroxyethyl starch granules, are consequences of hemodialysis that can persist after kidney transplantation and complicate histologic interpretation of hepatic disorders in patients with renal transplants (124–127,172).

Hepatic manifestations of bone marrow transplantation

Bone marrow transplantation was first introduced in 1957 for the treatment of bone marrow suppression by irradiation or chemotherapy (173). Its use has broadened to include all types of bone marrow suppression including aplastic anemia, sickle cell anemia, thalassemia, as well as a number of immunodeficiency and immunoproliferative syndromes (174) and many types of leukemia, lymphoma, and solid tumors (175).

The transplantation procedure itself is simple, consisting of the intravenous administration of fresh donor bone marrow into immunosuppressed recipients. In patients with combined immunodeficiency disorders or in those with syngeneic transplants, i.e., from an identical twin donor (176) or from patients who have previously stored autologous bone marrow, no rejection is expected and no immunosuppression is required. However, immunologic reactions may occur in a small percentage of patients even after syngeneic transplants (177). In the overwhelming majority of cases, however, the transplants are allogeneic, i.e., from individuals of genetically different origin, although usually from close relatives of the recipient. Allogeneic transplantation by definition involves varying degrees of histoincompatibility and raises a bidirectional immunologic barrier. Immunocompetent recipient cells reject the donor tissue and immunologically competent donor marrow cells attempt to reject the recipient's tissue, giving rise to graft-versus-host disease (GVHD).

Graft versus host disease

Acute graft-versus-host disease occurs more frequently and sooner after bone marrow transplantation in allogeneic than syngeneic patients, but this complication does not appear to result in reduced survival (178). Consequently, chemotherapeutic or irradiational immunosuppression is required before and after bone marrow transplantation to minimize rejection. Progressive improvement in survival has occurred over the past 35 years as immunosuppressive techniques and donor selection have improved (178). It has been noted that leukemic patients with allogeneic transplants appear to have fewer relapses of their leukemia than those with autologous transplants due, presumably, to graft-versus-leukemia effects that are part of graft-versus-host disease.

The requirements for the disease to develop, therefore, are (1) incompatibility of the host tissues and the donor lymphocytes, (2) immunologic incompetence of the host, and (3) the ability of the immunocompetent donor lymphocytes to proliferate and to attack the host tissues (179). Thus, graft-versus-host disease results from the introduction in the transplanted tissue of immunoactive, donated lymphocytes which attempt to reject the recipient's own tissues.

T lymphocytes are the cells responsible for the rejection of foreign tissue. T cells recognize antigen in the context of major histocompatibility complex (MHC) molecules (180). CD4-positive T lymphocytes recognize antigen in terms of class II molecules (181) and CD8-positive lymphocytes in terms of class I molecules (HLA-A, HLA-B, HLA-C) (182). If the antigen or a fragment of it binds to an MHC molecule, the complex is elevated to the cell surface where it can be recognized by specific T cells. Both autoimmune and acquired immune disorders may be associated with specific HLA molecules. In graft-versus-host disease, therefore, the target molecules are determined by what is recognized as foreign by the donor lymphocytes. Since hepatocytes and biliary epithelium do not normally express class II molecules, graft-versus-host disease is theoretically mediated via reactions against class I MHC molecules. In practice, however, the risk of the disease is similar with class I and class II incompatibilities (HLA-DP, HLA-DC, HLA-

DR) (180). However, cytokines also appear to be involved in the pathogenesis of graft-versus-host disease (183).

Acute graft-versus-host disease appears within 100 days of transplantation and tends to involve the skin, the gastrointestinal tract, and the liver in cytolytic cell injury (184,185). An erythematous, macropapular rash of the palms, soles, and upper trunk is the characteristic dermatologic manifestation. Diarrhea, which tends to be bloody and voluminous, is often accompanied by abdominal discomfort, anorexia, and nausea. The mucosal folds are often thickened and flattened, but these gastrointestinal abnormalities tend to disappear spontaneously in time. Lymphocytes are sparse in the nodes, spleen, thymus, and blood. Hypogammaglobulinemia develops and patients become susceptible to opportunistic infections, particularly those caused by CMV and *Pneumocystis carinii*. Hepatic injury is one of the major aspects of acute graft-versus-host disease. The hepatic damage in such patients may be related to the immunosuppressive therapy per se (72,135), to the development of preexisting infection, to superinfection by opportunistic viral, fungal, or bacterial organisms (186), or to the graft-versus-host disease itself. Graft-versus-host disease may induce several types of liver disease. First, hepatoparenchymal disease is expressed as increased serum aminotransferase or alkaline phosphatase activity, and by jaundice, which develops in about half of them (187). Occasionally, severe hyperbilirubinemia is seen. Sometimes ascites appears (188). Second, veno-occlusive lesions that affect small hepatic venules develop in 20% of patients within 7 to 10 days of bone marrow transplantation (189,190). Clinically, this disorder is characterized by abdominal discomfort and ascites. It is often accompanied by cholestasis and elevation of transaminase and alkaline phosphatase (189). In some, this syndrome appears to result from pretransplant irradiation treatment or chemotherapy or to viral hepatitis (190). Some of these episodes subside quickly, but others progress and become chronic (191).

Chronic graft-versus-host disease is defined as that which first appears more than 100 days after transplantation or which appears earlier but persists that long. It can progress from acute to chronic, it can reappear after transient resolution of acute GVHD, as chronic GVHD, or it can appear de novo as chronic graft-versus-host disease. It has been suggested that acute and chronic graft-versus-host disease actually represent different diseases. Indeed, the response of acute, but not of chronic graft-versus-host disease, to cyclosporine therapy (192,193) attests to these differences and suggests that interleukins may also be involved in the pathogenesis of acute graft-versus-host disease (194).

The changes in chronic graft-versus-host disease mimic many of the findings seen in autoimmune collagen vascular disease (195), most commonly schleroderma, including the development of autoantibodies (196). Dermatologic changes include hyperpigmentation, malar erythema, vitiligo, alopecia, dystrophic nails, and premature graying. Sjögren's syndrome is common, and dysphagia, vomiting, diarrhea, and weight loss are frequent gastrointestinal manifestations (197). The hepatic changes of chronic graft-versus-host disease, which occur in the majority of patients, are usually biochemical rather than clinical and are characterized by cholestatic changes, i.e., serum alkaline phosphatase levels are more elevated and aminotransferase activity less abnormal in chronic than in acute graft-versus-host disease (197,198). Hepatic and dermatologic manifestations tend to develop together. Chronic graft-versus-host disease may occasionally exhibit no extrahepatic manifestations

(199). In such cases the hepatic lesions have been reported to respond to corticosteroid therapy. The chronic syndrome may remain stable, but it tends to progress.

In a few cases, chronic graft-versus-host disease has progressed to overt cirrhosis with portal hypertension over periods ranging from 3 to 10 years (198–201). The cirrhosis, which tends to occur in patients with persistent cholestatic jaundice, may develop overtly (200) or insidiously (201). Graft-versus-host disease-associated cirrhosis may be manifest by the complications of portal hypertension such as variceal hemorrhage, portal-systemic encephalopathy, or hypersplenism. The cirrhosis appears to be biliary in type, but biliary obstruction per se was present at no time and antimitochondrial antibody levels were not elevated (201). One patient with severe cirrhosis secondary to graft-versus-host disease had a liver transplant to correct the problem (202). It appears that cirrhosis is a much more common consequence of graft-versus-host disease than it is of liver transplantation (198–203).

Graft-versus-host disease, which may develop in immunocompromised patients after blood transfusions (204), has been reported rarely after liver transplantation (84,85). The diagnosis is suggested by the typical clinical picture, i.e., fever, diarrhea, pancytopenia, and the characteristic rash, and is confirmed by the finding of HLA chimerism of HLA subtypes of both the donor and the recipient. In one reported case, the disorder responded to corticosteroid and antithymocyte globulin after a course of cyclosporine had failed (204). This syndrome has also been seen after liver or kidney transplantation with ABO-mismatched organs (205,206).

Laboratory changes include eosinophilia, hypergammaglobulinemia, circulating antibodies, and plasmacytosis of the viscera and lymph nodes. Patients with chronic graft-versus-host disease are as susceptible to opportunistic infections as they are in acute graft-versus-host disease.

Histologically, acute graft-versus-host disease is characterized by a spectrum of necroinflammatory activity with modest lymphocytic infiltration of the portal tracts and parenchymal tissues [(207); Fig. 1017] and degeneration of the epithelium of interlobular bile ducts similar to those seen in primary biliary cirrhosis or in the pericholangitis of inflammatory bowel disease [(208,209); Fig. 1018]. Focal or individual cell acidophilic necrosis of parenchymal cells is often present. Eosinophilia may be prominent. Cytoplasmic inclusions have been described (210). Nuclei tend to become hyperchromatic and to show nuclear anisocytosis and poikilocytosis. Kupffer cell hypertrophy, hyperplasia, and hemosiderin accumulation are often found [(211); Fig. 1019]. Hepatic and portal venous ''endothelialitis'' have been reported (Fig. 1018), and may be prominent (212).

In chronic graft-versus-host disease, the bile duct changes are more advanced (Figs. 1019, 1020), and the paucity or absence of bile ducts is more pronounced (212,213).

The histologic pattern in the liver of patients with graft-versus-host disease mimics and may be difficult to differentiate from hepatic allograft rejection. The mononuclear portal tract inflammation, the bile ductular degenerative abnormalities, the cholestasis, and the endothelialitis are all components of the hepatic allograft rejection syndrome. It would be difficult on histologic grounds alone to distinguish graft-versus-host disease (Figs. 1017–1020) from equivalent lesions in patients with rejection of a hepatic allograft (Figs. 982–994).

The bile duct lesion appears to represent primary cytopathic destruction by virtue of its induction in experimental animals (214) and the demonstration by electron microscopy of close contact between lymphocytes and the injured biliary epithelium (215,216). In some cases it has also been considered to be a late consequence of CMV cholangitis (215).

It has been suggested that the frequently associated veno-occlusive disease is immunologically mediated, but most authorities believe that these lesions represent the effects of pretransplant chemotherapy or radioimmunosuppressive therapy (190).

Large, eosinophilic, cytoplasmic inclusions have been described in the hepatocytes of patients after bone marrow transplantation (Fig. 1021). They are usually seen in patients with graft-versus-host disease but have been observed in the absence of this lesion (210). They are usually found in the presence of fatty deposition. These ground glass inclusions can be differentiated from HBV inclusions, from α-1-antitrypsin bodies (217), from the inclusions reported in hepatocellular carcinoma (218,219), and from those observed in rats after partial hepatic resection that contain periodic acid–Schiff-positive material (220) or fibrin (221). The patients had all had identical HLA matches, had been irradiated, had received cytoxan, and had received blood and platelet transfusions.

In general, acute graft-versus-host disease exhibits extensive hepatoparenchymal necrosis and endothelialitis (Figs. 1017, 1022). Chronic graft-versus-host disease shows more damage to and loss of bile ducts (Figs. 1019, 1020). However, these histologic abnormalities often overlap and differentiation is imprecise (208,215,222).

Chronic graft-versus-host disease may progress to a biliary type fibrosis and, eventually, to cirrhosis. Cholestasis and a mixed inflammatory reaction persist (Fig. 1023). Identifiable bile ducts show nuclear irregularity (Fig. 1018), thinning of epithelium, and disruption of the basement membrane (Fig. 1020) and are surrounded by a mixed infiltrate composed predominantly of mononuclear cells. Mild bile ductular proliferation may be seen. Eventually, a biliary-type cirrhosis develops with rare interlobular bile ducts but with persistent cholestasis (Fig. 1024) and edema (Fig. 1025).

Blind interpretation of liver biopsies in patients before and after bone marrow transplantation and in those with a variety of other acute and chronic hepatic diseases demonstrates that the characteristic changes of graft-versus-host disease are not specific (208,223). False positives may occur in about 15% of the patients (208). False negatives tend to occur in biopsies soon after bone marrow transplantation, before bile duct abnormalities appear. However, the presence of extensive bile duct damage and cholestasis with minimal inflammatory infiltrates is quite specific, as is the presence of endothelialitis of portal or central veins. Endothelialitis may sometimes be seen in other non-transplant-associated hepatic lesions (208).

Veno-occlusive disease

Veno-occlusive disease of the liver is the nonthrombotic constriction or obliteration of small hepatic veins by edema, subintimal connective tissue, and collagen. This syndrome is characterized by the abrupt appearance of abdominal distension, tender hepatomegaly, and ascites. It is often accompanied by jaundice and increased serum aminotransferase and alkaline phosphatase activity. It occurs in patients who have ingested pyrrolizidine alkaloids (224), who have received cancer chemotherapy (225) or hepatic irradiation (226), who have chronic alcoholic liver disease (227), who have had renal transplantation (228), and, most recently, has been seen in those who have had bone marrow transplantation (229–231). It is thought to result from injury to the vascular endothelium by chemotherapeutic agents, irradiation, or immunosuppressive therapy (232).

Veno-occlusive disease is unrelated to graft-versus-host disease. In patients who have had bone marrow transplants veno-occlusive disease almost always appears during the first four weeks after transplantstion, but graft-versus-host disease rarely appears before the fourth week (230,233). Almost one-fourth of patients develop veno-occlusive disease after bone marrow transplantation (229,233). Mortality rates in different series of patients who develop veno-occlusive disease after bone marrow transplantation range as high as 50%.

Histologically, the hepatic lesions are characterized by centrilobular congestion, usually with severe hepatocellular atrophy (Fig. 1026) and necrosis [(234); Fig. 1027]. The disease progresses from edema of the hepatic vein walls to subintimal thickening and collagen deposition that greatly constricts the lumen (Fig. 1028).

References

1. Scharschmidt BF: Human liver transplantation: analysis of data on 540 patients from four centers. Hepatology 4:95S–101S, 1984.
2. Starzl TE, Iwatsuki S, Shaw BW Jr, Van Thiel DH, Gartner JC, Zitelli BJ, Malatack JJ, Schade RR: Analysis of liver transplantation. Hepatology 4:47S–49S, 1984.
3. Krom RAF, Gips CH, Huthoff HJ, Newton D, Waaig DVD, Beelen J, Haagsma EB, Slooff MHJ: Orthotopic liver transplantation in Groningen, The Netherlands (1979–1983). Hepatology 4:61S–65S, 1984.
4. Pichlmayr R, Brolsch Ch., Wonigeit K, Neuhaus P, Siegismund S, Schmidt F-W, Burdelski M: Experiences with liver transplantation in Hannover. Hepatology 4:56S–60S, 1984.
5. Rolles K, Williams R, Neuberger J, Calne R: The Cambridge and King's College Hospital experience of liver transplantation, 1968–1983. Hepatology 4:50S–55S, 1984.
6. Hockerstedt K: Liver transplantation today. Scand J Gastroenterol 25:1–10, 1990.
7. Starzl TE, Demetris AJ, Van Thiel D: Liver transplantation. N Engl J Med 321:1014–1021, 1092–1099, 1989.
8. Esquivel CO, Van Thiel DH, Demetris AJ, Bernardos A, Iwatsuki S, Markus B, Gordon RD, Marsh JW, Makowka L, Tsakis AG, Todo S, Gavaler JS, Starzl TE: Transplantation for primary biliary cirrhosis. Gastroenterology 94:1207–1216, 1988.
9. O'Grady JG, Polson RJ, Rolles K, Calne RY, Williams R: Liver transplantation for malignant disease. Results in 93 consecutive patients. Ann Surg 207:373–379, 1988.
10. Starzl TE, Iwatsuki S, Shaw BW, Nalesnik MA, Farhi DC, Van Thiel DH; Treatment of fibrolamellar hepatoma with partial or total hepatectomy and transplantation of the liver. Surg Gynecol Obstet 162:145–148, 1986.
11. Starzl TE, Van Thiel D, Tzakis AG, Iwatsuki S, Todo S, Marsh JW, Koneru B, Staschak S, Stieber A, Gordon RD: Orthotopic liver transplantation for alcoholic cirrhosis. JAMA 26:2542–2544, 1988.
12. Bird GLA, O'Grady JG, Harvey FAH, Calne RY, Williams R: Liver transplantation in patients with alcoholic cirrhosis: selection criteria and rates of survival and relapse. Br Med J 301:15–17, 1990.
13. Wood RP, Shaw BW Jr, Rikkers LF: Liver transplantation for variceal hemorrhage. Surg Clin North Am 70:449–461, 1990.
14. Loewy EH: Drunks, livers and values. Should social value judgments enter into liver transplantation decisions? J Clin Gastroenterol 9:436–441, 1987.
15. Olthoff KM, Millis JM, Rosove MH, Holdstein LI, Ramming KP, Busuttil RW: Is liver transplantation justified for the treatment of hepatic malignancies? Arch Surg 125:1261–1268, 1990.
16. Ismail T, Angrisani L, Gunson BK, Hübscher SG, Buckels JAC, Neuberger JM, Elias E, McMaster P: Primary hepatic malignancy: the role of liver transplantation. Br J Surg 77:983–987, 1990.
17. Kelleher MB, Iwatsuki S, Sheahan DG: Epithelioid hemangioendothelioma of liver. Am J Surg Pathol 13:999–1008, 1989.
18. Laifer SA, Darby MJ, Scantlebury VP, Harger JH, Caritis SN: Pregnancy and liver transplantation. Obstet Gynecol 76:1083–1088, 1990.
19. Dindzans VJ, Schade RR, Gavaler JS, Tarter RE, Van Thiel DH: Liver transplantation. A primer for practicing gastroenterologists, Part I. Dig Dis Sci 34:2–8, 1989.
20. Bismuth H, Samuel D, Gugenheim J, Dastaing D, Bernau J, Rueff B, Benhamou J-P: Emergency liver transplantation for fulminant hepatitis. Ann Intern Med 107:337–341, 1987.
21. Vickers C, Neuberger J, Buckels J, McMaster P, Elias E: Transplantation of the liver in adults and children with fulminant hepatic failure. J Hepatol 7:143–150, 1988.
22. Emond JC, Aran PP, Whitington PF, Borelsch CE, Baker AL: Liver transplantation in the management of fulminant hepatic failure. Gastroenterology 96:1583–1588, 1988.
23. Sternlieb I: Wilson's disease: indications for liver transplants. Hepatology 4:155–175, 1984.
24. Polson RJ, Rolles K, Calne RY, Williams R, Marsden D: Reversal of severe neurological manifestations of Wilson's disease following orthotopic liver transplantation. Q J Med 64:685–691, 1987.
25. van Spronsen FJ, Berger R, Smit GP, de Klerk JB, Duran M, Bijleveld CM, van Faassen H, Slooff MJ, Heymans HS: Tyrosinaemia type I: orthotopic liver transplantation as the only definitive answer to a metabolic as well as an oncological problem. J Inherit Metab Dis 12 Suppl: 339–342, 1989.
26. Bontempo FA, Lewis JH, Gonrenc TJ: Liver transplantation in hemophilia A. Blood 69:1721–1724, 1987.
27. Putnam CW, Porter KA, Peters RL, Ashcavai M, Redeker AG, Starzl TE: Liver replacement for α-1-antitrypsin deficiency. Surgery 81:258–261, 1977.
28. Largilli'ere C, Houssin D, Gottrand F, Mathey C, Checoury A, Alagille D, Farriaux JP: Liver transplantation for ornithine transcarbamylase deficiency in a girl. J Pediatr 115:415–417, 1989.
29. Bilheimer DW, Goldstein JL, Grundy SM, Starzl TE, Brown MS: Liver transplantation to provide low-density-lipoprotein receptors and lower plasma cholesterol in a child with homozygous familial hypercholesterolemia. N Engl J Med 311:1658–1664, 1984.
30. Cassella JF, Lewis JH, Bontempo FA, Zitelli BI, Markel H, Starzl TE: Successful treatment of homozygous protein C deficiency by hepatic transplantation. Lancet 1:435–437, 1988.
31. Flye MW, Jendrisak MD: Liver transplantation in the child. World J Surg 10:432–441, 1986.
32. Iwatsuki S, Starzl TE, Todo S, Gordon RD, Tzakis AG, Marsh JW, Makowka L, Koneru B, Stieber A, Klintmalm G: Liver transplantation in the treatment of bleeding esophageal varices. Surgery 104:697–705, 1988.
33. Dindzans VJ, Schade RR, Gavaler JS, Tarter RE, Van Thiel DH: Liver transplantation. A primer for practicing gastroenterologists, Part II. Dig Dis Sci 34:161–166, 1989.
34. Maddrey WC: Transplantation of the Liver. New York, Elsevier, 1988, p. 281.
35. Van Thiel DH, Makowka L, Starzl TE: Liver transplantation: where its been and where its going. Clin Gastroenterol 17:1–18, 1988.
36. Cosimi AB, Jenkins RL, Rohrer RJ, Delmonico FL, Hoffman M, Monaco AP: A randomized clinical trial of prophylactic OKT3 monoclonal antibody in liver allograft recipients. Arch Surg 125, 781–785, 1990.
37. Todo S, Fung JJ, Starzl TE, Tzakis A, Demetris AJ, Kormos R, Jain A, Alessiani M, Takaya S, Shapiro R: Liver, kidney, and thoracic organ transplantation under FK 506. Ann Surg 212:295–305, 1990.
38. Demetris AJ, Fung JJ, Todo S, Banner B, Zerbe T, Sysyn G, Starzl TE: Pathologic observations in human allograft recipients treated with FK 506. Transplant Proc 22 (Suppl 1): 25–34, 1990.
39. Van Thiel DH, Schade RR, Hakala TR, Starzl TE, Denney D: Liver procurement for orthotopic transplantation: an analysis of the Pittsburgh experience. Hepatology 4:66S–71S, 1984.
40. Kalayoglu M, Sollinger HW, Stratta RJ, D'Alessandro AM, Hoffmann RM, Pirsch JD, Belzer FO: Extended preservation of the liver for clinical transplantation. Lancet 1:617–619, 1988.
41. Cohen DJ, Loertscher R, Rubin MF, Tilney NL, Carpenter CB, Strom TB: Cyclosporine: a new immunosuppressive agent for organ transplantation. Ann Intern Med 101:667–682, 1984.
42. Cosimi AB, Cho SI, Delmonico FL, Kaplan MM, Rohrer RJ, Jenkins RI: A randomized clinical trial comparing OKT3 and steroids for treatment of hepatic allograft rejection. Transplantation 43:91–95, 1987.
43. Reilly J, Mehta R, Teperman L, Cemaj S, Tzakis A, Katsuhiko Y, Ritter P, Rezak A, Makowka L: Nutritional support after liver trans-

plantation: a randomized prospective study. J Parenter Enternal Nutr *14*:386–391, 1990.

44. Popper H: Coming of age. Hepatology *5*:1224–1226, 1985.

45. Bismuth H, Morino M, Castaing D, Gillon MC, Descorps Declere A, Saliba F, Samuel D: Emergency orthotopic liver transplantation in two patients using one donor liver. Br J Surg *76*:722–724, 1989.

46. Cuervas-Mons V, Martinez AJ, Dekker A, Starzl TE, Van Thiel DH: Adult liver transplantation: an analysis of the early causes of death in 40 consecutive cases. Hepatology *6*:495–501, 1986.

47. Kusne S, Dummer JS, Singh N, Iwatsuki S, Makowka L, Esquivel C, Tzakis AG, Starzl TE, Ho M: Infections after liver transplantation. An analysis of 101 consecutive cases. Medicine *67*:132–143, 1988.

48. Bronsther O, Makowka L, Jaffe R, Demetris AJ, Breinig MK, Ho M, Esquivel CO, Gordon RD, Iwatsuki S, Tsakis A: Occurrence of cytomegalovirus hepatitis in liver transplant patients. J Med Virol *24*:423–434, 1988.

49. Stratta RJ, Shaefer MS, Cushing KA, Markin RS, Wood RP, Langnas AN, Reed EC, Woods GL, Donovan JP, Pillen TJ, Li S, Duckworth RM, Shaw BW Jr: Successful prophylaxis of cytomegalovirus disease after primary CMV exposure in liver transplant recipients. Transplantation *51*:90–97, 1991.

50. Saliba F, Arulnaden JL, Gugenheim J, Serves C, Samuel D, Bismuth A, Mathieu D, Bismuth H: CMV hyperimmune globulin prophylaxis after liver transplantation: a prospective randomized controlled study. Transplant Proc *21*:2260–2262, 1989.

51. Terpstra OT, Schalm SW, Weimar W, Willemse PJA, Baumgartner D, Groenland THN, Ten Kate FWJ, Porte RJ, de Rave S, Ruevers CB, Stibbe J, Terpstra JL: Auxiliary partial liver transplantation for end-stage chronic liver disease. N Engl J Med *319*:1507–1511, 1988.

52. Strong RW, Lynch SV, Ong TH, Matsunami H, Koido Y, Balderson GA: Successful liver transplantation from a living donor to her son. N Engl J Med *322*:1505–1507, 1990.

53. Starzl TE, Demetris AJ: Liver transplantation: a 31-year perspective. Part I. Curr Probl Surg *27*:55–116, 1990.

54. Starzl TE, Demetris AJ: Liver transplantation: a 31-year perspective. Part II. Curr Probl Surg *27*:123–178, 1990.

55. Starzl TE, Demetris AJ: Liver transplantation: a 31-year perspective. Part III. Curr Probl Surg *27*:187–240, 1990.

56. D'Alessndro AM, Kalayoglu M, Sollinger HW, Hoffmann RM, Reed A, Knechtle SJ, Pirsch JK, Hafez GR, Lorentzen D, Belzer FO: The predictive value of donor liver biopsies for the development of primary nonfunction after orthotopic liver transplantation. Transplantation *51*:157–163, 1991.

56a. Wiesner RH: Hepatic allograft rejection. Semin Liver Dis *12*:1–92, 1992.

57. O'Grady JG, Alexander GJM, Sutherland S, Donaldson PT, Harvey F, Portmann B, Calne RY, Williams R: Cytomegalovirus infection and donor/recipient HLA antigens: interdependent co-factors in pathogenesis of vanishing bile duct syndrome after liver transplantation. Lancet *2*:302–305, 1988.

58. Gordon RD, Iwatsuki S, Esquivel CO, Tzakis A, Todo S, Starzl TE: Liver transplantation across ABO blood groups. Surgery *100*:342–348, 1986.

59. Demetris AJ, Jaffe R, Tzakis A, Ramsey G, Todo S, Belle S, Esquivel C, Shapiro R, Markus B, Mroczek E, Van Thiel DH, Sysyn G, Gordon R, Makowka L, Starzl T: Antibody-mediated rejection of human orthotopic allografts. Am J Pathol *132*:489–502, 1988.

60. Wight DJG, Calne RY: The use of cyclosporin A immunosuppression in organ grafting. Immunol Rev *65*:115–131, 1982.

61. Chapman JR, Marcen R, Arias M, Raine AE, Dunnill MS, Morris PJ: Hypertension after renal transplantation. Transplantation *43*:860–864, 1987.

62. Starzl TE, Porter KA, Iwatsuki S, Rosenthal JT, Shaw BW Jr, Atchison RW, Nalesnik MA, Ho M, Griffith TBP, Hakala TR, Hardesty RL, Jaffe R, Bahnson HT: Reversibility of lymphomas and lymphoproliferative lesions developing under cyclosporin-steroid therapy. Lancet *1*:583–587, 1984.

63. Penn I: Cancers following cyclosporine therapy. Transplant Proc *19*:2211–2213, 1987.

64. Moran M, Mozes MF, Maddux MS, Veremis S, Bartkus C, Ketel B, Pollak R: Prevention of acute graft rejection by the prostaglandin E₁ analogue misoprostol in renal-transplant recipients treated with cyclosporine and prednisone. N Engl J Med *322*:1183–1188, 1990.

65. Soulillou J-P, Cantarovich D, Le Mauff B, Giral M, Robillard N, Hourmant M, Hirn M: Randomized controlled trial of a monoclonal antibody against the interleukin-2 receptor (33B3.1) as compared

with rabbit antithymocyte globulin for prophylaxis against rejection of renal allografts. N Engl J Med *322*:1175–1182, 1990.

66. Snover DC: The pathology of acute rejection. Transplant Proc *18*:123–127, 1986.

67. Snover DC, Freese DK, Sharp HL, Bloomer JR, Najarian JS, Ascher NL: Liver allograft rejection. An analysis of the use of biopsy in determining outcome of rejection. Am J Surg Pathol *11*:1–10, 1987.

68. Ludwig J: Histopathology of the liver following transplantation. *In* Transplantation of the Liver, edited by W.C. Maddrey. New York, Elsevier, 1988, pp. 191–218.

69. Iwatsuki S, Rabin BS, Shaw BW Jr, Starzl TE: Liver transplantation against T-cell-positive warm crossmatches. Transplant Proc *16*:1427–1429, 1984.

70. Bird G, Friend P, Donaldson P: Hyperacute rejection in liver transplantation: a case report. Transplant Proc *21*:3742–3744, 1989.

71. Klintmalm GBG, Nery JR, Husberg BS, Gonwa TA, Tillery GW: Rejection in liver transplantation. Hepatology *10*:978–985, 1989.

72. Sparburg M, Simon N, del Greco F: Intrahepatic cholestasis due to azathioprine. Gastroenterology *57*:439–441, 1969.

73. Calne RY, White DJG, Thiru S, Evans DB, McMaster P, Dunn DC, Craddock GN, Pentlow BD, Rolles K: Cyclosporin A in patients receiving renal allografts from cadaver donors. Lancet *2*:1323–1327, 1978.

74. Wisecarver JL, Wood RP, Shaw BW, Zetterman RK, Markin RS: Histologic changes in biopsies of hepatic allografts associated with elevated whole blood cyclosporine A concentrations. Lab Invest *60*:106A, 1989 (Abstract).

75. Eggink HF, Hofstee N, Gips CH, Krom RAF, Houthoff HJ: Histopathology of serial graft biopsies from liver transplant recipients. Am J Pathol *114*:18–31, 1984.

76. Williams JW, Peters TG, Vera SR, Britt LG, Van Voorst SJ, Haggitt RC: Biopsy-directed immunosuppression following hepatic transplantation in man. Transplantation *39*:589–596, 1985.

77. Demetris AJ, Lasky S, Van Thiel DH, Starzl TE, Dekker A: Pathology of hepatic transplantation. A review of 62 adult allograft recipients immunosuppressed with a cyclosporine/steroid regimen. Am J Pathol *118*:151–161, 1985.

78. Wight DGD: Pathology of rejection. *In* Liver Transplantation, edited by R.Y. Calne. London, Grune & Stratton, 1983, pp. 247–277.

79. Gouw ASH, Snover DC, Grond J, Huitema S, Gips CH, Sloof MJH, Poppema S: Acute rejection in human liver grafts: a comparative histologic study of cases maintained on azathioprine and prednisone versus cyclosporine A and low-dose steroids. Hum Pathol *19*:1036–1042, 1988.

80. Snover DC, Sibley RK, Freese DK, Sharp HL, Bloomer JR, Najarian JS, Ascher NL: Orthotopic liver transplantation: a pathological study of 63 serial liver biopsies from 17 patients with special reference to the diagnostic features and natural history of rejection. Hepatology *4*:1212–1222, 1984.

81. Kakizoe S, Yanaga K, Starzl TE, Demetris J: Evaluation of protocol before transplantation and after reperfusion biopsies from human orthotopic liver allografts: considerations of preservation and early immunological injury. Hepatology *11*:932–941, 1990.

82. Foster PF, Sankary HN, Hart M, Ashmann M, Williams JW: Blood and graft eosinophilia as predictors of rejection in human liver transplantation. Transplantation *47*:72–74, 1989.

83. Sankary H, Foster P, Novich K, Ashmann M, Bhattacharyya A, Coleman J, Williams J: Quantitative analysis of portal tract infiltrate allows for accurate determination of hepatic allograft rejection. Am J Surg *161*:131–135, 1991.

84. Burdick JF, Vogelsang GB, Smith WJ, Farmer ER, Bias WB, Kaufmann SH, Horn J, Colombani PM, Pitt HA, Perler BA, Merritt WT, Williams GM, Boitnott JK, Herlong HF: Severe graft-versus-host disease in a liver-transplant recipient. N Engl J Med *318*:689–691, 1988.

85. Marubayashi S, Matsuzaka C, Takeda A, Costa MM, Jamieson NV, Joysey V, Calne RY: Fatal generalized acute graft-versus-host disease in a liver transplant recipient. Transplantation *50*:709–711, 1990.

86. Perkins JD, Rakela J, Sterioff S, Banks PM, Wiesner RH, Krom RAF: Immunohistologic pattern of the portal T-lymphocyte infiltration in hepatic allograft rejection. Mayo Clin Proc *64*:565–569, 1989.

87. Ludwig J, Batts KP, Ploch M, Rakela J, Perkins JD, Wiesner RH: Endothelialitis in hepatic allografts. Mayo Clin Proc *64*:545–554, 1989.

88. Krom RAF, Wiesner RH, Haagsma EB, Ludwig J, Gips CH, Grond AJK, Houtoff HJ: A comparison of azathioprine and cyclosporine A in liver transplantation: a study of two personal series. Transplant Proc *19*:2440–2442, 1987.

89. Ludwig J, Wiesner RH, Batts KP, Pekins JD, Krom RAF: The acute

vanishing bile duct syndrome (acute irreversible rejection) after orthotopic liver transplantation. Hepatology 7:476–483, 1987.

90. Donaldson PT, Alexander GJM, Neuberger J, Portmann B, Thick M, Davis H, Calne RY, Williams R: Evidence for an immune response to HLA class I antigens in the vanishing-bile duct syndrome after liver transplantation. Lancet 1:945–948, 1987.

91. Gubernatis G, Lauchart W, Jonker M, Steinhoff G, Bornscheuer A, Neuhaus P, van Es AA, Kemnitz J, Wonigeit K, Pichlmayer R: Signs of hyperacute rejection of liver grafts in rhesus monkeys after donor-specific presensitization. Transplant Proc 19:1082–1083, 1987.

92. Hayry P, Von Willebrand E, Ahonen J, Eklund B, Lautenschlager I: Monitoring of organ allograft rejection by transplant aspiration cytology. Ann Clin Res 13:264–287, 1981.

93. Hockerstedt K, Lautenschlager I, Ahonen J, Eklund B, Isoniemi H, Korsback C, Makinen J, Makisalo H, Orko R, Petterson E, Salaspuro M, Scheinin B, Scheinin TM, von Willebrand E: Diagnosis of acute rejection in liver transplantation. J Hepatol 6:217–221, 1988.

94. Lautenschlager I, Hockerstedt K, Ahonen J, Ecklund B, Isoniemi H, Korsback C, Pettersson E, Salmela K, Scheinin TM, von Willebrand E: Fine neeple aspiration biopsy in the monitoring of liver allografts.II. Applications to human liver allografts. Transplantation 46:47–53, 1988.

95. Greene CL, Fehrman I, Tillery GW, Husberg BS, Klintmalm GB: A clear distinction between "immune activation of rejection" and "no immune activation" in liver transplant aspiration cytology. Transplant Proc 20:661–662, 1988.

96. Greene CL, Fehrman I, Tillery GW, Husberg BS, Klintmalm GB: Liver transplant aspiration cytology is useful for monitoring steroid treatment of rejection. Transplant Proc 20:659–660, 1988.

97. Schlitt HJ, Nashan B, Ringe B, Wittekind C, Wonigeit K, Pichlmayer R: Clinical usefulness of a semiquantitative scoring system for liver transplant aspiration cytology. Transplant Proc 21:3621–3622, 1989.

98. Fehrman I, Greene C, Tillery W: Transplant aspiration cytology for diagnosis of liver allograft rejection. Transplant Proc 20:657–658, 1988.

99. Carabonnel F, Samuel D, Reynes M, Benhamou J-P, Bismuth H, Bach J-F, Chatenoud L: Fine-needle aspiration biopsy of human liver allografts. Correlation with liver histology for the diagnosis of acute rejection. Transplantation 50:704–707, 1990.

100. Saitoh T, Fujiwara M, Nomoto M, Kamimura T, Ishihara K, Asakura H: Histologic studies on the hepatic lesions induced by graft-versus-host reaction in MHC Class II disparate hosts compared with primary biliary cirrhosis. Am J Pathol 135:301–307, 1989.

101. Demetris AJ, Markus BH, Esquivel CA, Van Thiel DH, Saidman S, Gordon R, Makowka L, Sysyn G, Starzl TE: Pathologic analysis of liver transplantation for primary biliary cirrhosis. Hepatology 8:939–947, 1988.

102. Oguma S, Belle S, Starzl TE, Demetris AJ: A histometric analysis of chronically rejected human liver allografts: insights into mechanisms of bile duct loss: direct immunologic and ischemic factors. Hepatology 9:204–209, 1989.

103. Paya CV, Hermans PE, Washington JA II, Smith TF, Anhalt JP, Wiesner RH, Krom RAF: Incidence, distribution, and outcome of episodes of infection in 100 orthotopic liver transplantations. Mayo Clin Proc 64:555–564, 1989.

104. Paya CV, Holley KE, Wiesner RH, Balasubramaniam K, Smith TF, Espy MJ, Ludwig J, Batts KP, Hermans PE, Krom RAF: Early diagnosis of cytomegalovirus hepatitis in liver transplant recipients: role of immunostaining, DNA hybridization and culture of hepatic tissue. Hepatology 12:119–126, 1990.

105. Salliba F, Arulnaden JL, Gugenheim J: CMV hyperimmune globulin prophylaxis after liver transplantation: a prospective randomized controlled study. Transplant Proc 21:2260–2262, 1989.

106. Harbison MA, DeGirolami PC, Jenkins RL, Hammer SM: Gancyclovir therapy of severe cytomegalovirus infections in solid-organ transplant recipients. Transplantation 46:82–88, 1988.

107. Kuo G, Choo Q-L, Alter HJ, Gitnick GL, Redeker AG, Purcell RH, Miyamura T, Dienstag JL, Alter MJ, Stevens CE, Tegtmeier GE, Bonino F, Colombo M, Lee W-S, Kuo C, Berger K, Shuste JR, Overby LR, Bradley DW, Houghton M: An assay for circulating antibodies to a major etiologic virus of human non-A, non-B hepatitis. Science 244:361–364, 1989.

108. Tzakis AG, Arditi M, Whitington PF, Yanaga K, Esquivel C, Andrews WA, Makowka L, Malatak J, Freese DK, Stock PG, Ascher NL, Johnson FL, Broelsch CE, Starzl TE: Aplastic anemia complicating orthotopic liver transplantation for non-A, non-B hepatitis. N Engl J Med 319:393–396, 1988.

109. Wight DGD: Pathology of liver transplantation (other than rejection). In Liver Transplantation, edited by R.Y. Calne. London, Grune & Stratton, 1983, pp. 289–316.

110. Starzl TE, Porter KA, Putnam CW, Hansburgh JF, Reid HAS: Biliary complications after liver transplantation with special reference to the biliary case syndrome and techniques of secondary duct repair. Surgery 81:213–221, 1976.

111. Schroter GPJ, Hoelscher M, Putnam CW, Porter KA, Hansbrough JF, Starzl TE: Infections complicating orthotopic liver transplantation: with emphasis on graft related septicemia. Arch Surg 111:1337–1347, 1976.

112. Calne RY, Williams R: Liver transplantation. In Current Problems in Surgery, Vol. 16, edited by M.M. Ravitch. Chicago, Year Book Publishers, 1979, pp. 3–44.

113. Gouw AS, Houthoff HJ, Huitema S, Beelen JM, Gips CH, Poppema S: Expression of major histocompatibility complex antigens and replacement of donor cells by recipient ones in human liver grafts. Transplantation 43:291–296, 1987.

114. Williams R, Smith M, Shilkin KB, Herbertson B, Joysey V, Calne RY: Liver transplantation in man: the frequency of rejection, biliary tract complications and recurrence of malignancy based on an analysis of 26 cases. Gastroenterology 64:1026–1048, 1973.

115. Iwatsuki S, Gordon RD, Shaw BW Jr, Starzl TE: Role of liver transplantation in cancer therapy. Ann Surg 202:401–407, 1985.

116. Starzl TE, Iwatsuki S, Shaw BW Jr, Nalesnik MA, Farhi DC, Van Thiel DH: Treatment of fibrolamellar hepatoma with partial or total hepatectomy and transplantation of the liver. Surg Gynecol Obstet 162:145–148, 1986.

117. Demetris AJ, Jaffe R, Sheahan DG, Burnham J, Spero J, Iwatsuki S, Van Thiel DH, Starzl TE: Recurrent hepatitis B in liver allograft recipients. Am J Pathol 125:161–172, 1986.

118. Davies SE, Portmann BC, O'Grady JG, Aldis PM, Chaggar K, Alexander GJ, Williams R: Hepatic histological findings after transplantation for chronic hepatitis B virus infection, including a unique pattern of fibrosing cholestatic hepatitis. Hepatology 13:150–157, 1991.

119. Read AE, Donegan E, Lake J, Ferrell L, Galbraith C, Kuramoto IK, Zeldis JB, Scher NL, Roberts J, Wright TL: Hepatitis C in patients undergoing liver transplantation. Ann Intern Med 114:282–284, 1991.

120. Reynes M, Zignego L, Samuel K, Fabiani B, Gugenheim J, Tricottet V, Brechot C, Bismuth H: Graft hepatitis delta virus reinfection after orthotopic liver transplantation in HDV cirrhosis. Transplant Proc 21:2424–2425, 1989.

121. Valla D, Casadevall N, Lacombe C: Myeloproliferative disorder and hepatic vein thrombosis. A prospective study of erythroid colony formation in vitro in 20 patients with Budd-Chiari syndrome. Ann Intern Med 103:329–334, 1985.

122. Polson RJ, Portmann B, Neuberger J, Calne RY, Williams R: Evidence for disease recurrence after liver transplantation for primary biliary cirrhosis. Clinical and histologic follow-up studies. Gastroenterology 97:715–723, 1989.

123. Thiru S, Calne RY, Nagington J: Lymphoma in patients treated with cyclosporin-A as one of the immunosuppressive agents. Transplant Proc 13:359–364, 1981.

124. Luketic VA, Shiffman ML, McCall JB, Posner MP, Mills AS, Carithers RL Jr: Primary hepatocellular carcinoma after orthotopic liver transplantation for chronic hepatitis B infection. Ann Intern Med 114:212–213, 1991.

125. Van Thiel DH, Gavaler JS, Kam I, Francavilla A, Polimeno L, Schade RR, Smith J, Diven W, Penkrot RJ, Starzl T: Rapid growth of an intact human liver transplanted into a recipient larger than the donor. Gastroenterology 93:1414–1419, 1989.

126. Hill RB, Porter KA, Massion CG: Hepatic reaction to renal transplants modified by immunosuppressive therapy. Arch Pathol 81:71–77, 1966.

127. Sopko J, Anuras S: Liver disease in renal transplant recipients. Am J Med 64:139–146, 1978.

128. Ware AJ, Luby JP, Hollinger B, Eigenbrodt EH, Cuthbert JA, Atkins CR, Shorey J, Hull AR, Combes B: Etiology of liver disease in renal transplant patients. Ann Intern Med 91:364–371, 1979.

129. Weir MR, Kirkman RL, Strom TB, Tilney NL: Liver disease in recipients of long-functioning renal allografts. Kidney Int 28:839–844, 1985.

130. Snydman DR, Bregman D, Bryan JA: Hemodialysis-associated hepatitis in the United States, 1974. J Infect Dis 135:687–691, 1977.

131. Stevens CE, Alter HJ, Taylor PE, Zang EA, Harley EJ, Szmuness

W, and the Dialysis Vaccine Trial Study Group: Hepatitis B vaccine in patients receiving hemodialysis. Immunogenicity and efficacy. N Engl J Med *311*:496–501, 1984.

132. Benhamou E, Courouce A-M, Jungers P, Laplanche A, Degos F, Brangier J, Crosnier J: Hepatitis B vaccine: randomized trial of immunogenicity in hemodialysis patients. Clin Nephrol *21*:143–147, 1984.

133. Luby JP, Burnett W, Hull AW, Ware AJ, Shorey JW, Peter PC: Relationship between cytomegalovirus and hepatic function abnormalities in the period after renal transplantation. J Infect Dis *129*:511–518, 1974.

134. Shorey J, Schenker S, Suki SN, Combes B: Hepatotoxicity of mercaptopurine. Arch Intern Med *122*:54–58, 1968.

135. Lorber MI, Van Buren CT, Flechner SM, Williams C, Kahan BD: Hepatobiliary and pancreatic complications of cyclosporine therapy in 466 renal transplant recipients. Transplantation *43*:35–40, 1987.

136. Rao KV, Anderson WR: Hemosiderosis and hemochromatosis in renal transplant recipients. Am J Nephrol *5*:419–430, 1985.

137. Anderson WR, Rao KV: Hepatic iron overload in renal transplant recipients: ultrastructural observations. Ultrastruct Pathol *10*:228–234, 1986.

138. Degott C, Rueff B, Kreis H, Duboust A, Potet F, Benhamou J-P: Peliosis hepatis in recipients of renal transplants. Gut *19*:748–753, 1978.

139. Gerlag PGG, Lobatto S, Driessen WMM, Deckers PFL, Van Hooff JP, Schroder E, Assmann KM, Van Haelst UJG: Hepatic sinusoidal dilatation with portal hypertension during azathioprine treatment after kidney transplantation. J Hepatol *1*:339–348, 1985.

140. Adler M, Delhaye M, Deprez C, Hardy N, Gelin M, DePauw L, Vereerstraeten P, Cremer M, Toussaint C: Hepatic vascular disease after kidney transplantation: report of two cases and review of the literature. Nephrol Dial Transplant *2*:183–188, 1987.

141. Morales JM, Prieto C, Colina F, Mestre MJ, Lopez I, Perez-Sola A, Solis-Herruzo JA, Ruilope LM, Rodicio JL: Nodular regenerative hyperplasia of the liver in renal transplantation. Transplant Proc *19*:3694–3696, 1987.

142. Nataf C, Feldman G, Lebrec D, Degott C, Descamps JM, Rueff B, Benhamou J-P: Idiopathic portal hypertension (perisinusoidal fibrosis) after renal transplantation. Gut *20*:531–537, 1979.

143. Bredfeldt JE, Enriquez RE, Groszmann RJ: Idiopathic portal hypertension in a renal transplant recipient. J Clin Gastroenterol *4*:157–161, 1982.

144. Pritzker K: Neoplasia in renal transplant recipients. Can Med Assoc J *107*:1059–1062, 1972.

145. Penn I: The occurrence of cancer in immune deficiencies. Curr Prob Cancer *6*:1–64, 1982.

146. Leong A S-Y, Gove DW: Foreign material in the tissues of patients on recurrent hemodialysis. Ultrastruct Pathol *2*:401–403, 1981.

147. Leong AS-Y, Disney APS: Spallation and migration of silicone from blood-pump tubing in patients on hemodialysis. N Engl J Med *306*:135–140, 1982.

148. Coughlin GP, Van Deth AG, Disney APS, Hay J, Wangel AG: Liver disease and the e antigen in HBsAg carriers with chronic renal failure. Gut *21*:118–122, 1980.

149. Dusheiko G, Song E, Bowyer S, Whitcutt M, Maier G, Meyers A, Kew MC: Natural history of hepatitis B virus infection in renal transplant recipients: a fifteen year follow-up. Hepatology *3*:330–336, 1983.

150. Degos F, Lugassy C, Degott C, Debure A, Carnot F, Thiers V, Tiollais P, Kreis H, Brechot C: Hepatitis B virus and hepatitis B-related viral infection in renal transplant recipients. A prospective study of 90 patients. Gastroenterology *94*:151–156, 1988.

151. London WT, Drew JS, Blumberg BS, Grossman RA, Lyons, PJ: Association of graft survival with host response to hepatitis B infection in patients with kidney transplants. N Engl J Med *296*:241–244, 1977.

152. Chatterjee SN, Payne JE, Bischel MD, Redeker AG, Berne TV: Successful renal transplantation in patients positive for hepatitis B antigen. N Engl J Med *291*:62–65, 1974.

153. Dienstag JL: Renal transplantation and hepatitis B. Gastroenterology *94*:235–238, 1988.

154. Parfrey PS, Forbes RDC, Hutchinson TA, Beaudoin JG, Dauphinee WD, Hollomby DJ, Guttmann RD: The clinical and pathological course of hepatitis B liver disease in renal transplant recipients. Transplantation *37*:461–466, 1984.

155. Pirson Y, Alexandre GPJ, van Ypersele de Strihou C: Longterm effect of HBs antigenemia on patient survival after renal transplantation. N Engl J Med *296*:194–196, 1977.

156. Hillis WD, Hillis A, Walker WG: Hepatitis B surface antigenemia in renal transplant recipients: increased mortality risk. JAMA *242*:329–332, 1979.

157. Boyce NW, Holdsworth SR, Hooke D, Thomson NM, Atkins RC: Nonhepatitis B-associated liver disease in a renal transplant population. Am J Kidney Dis *11*:307–312, 1988.

158. Balfour HH, Chace BA, Stapleton JT, Simmons RL, Fryd DS: A randomized, placebo-controlled trial of oral acyclovir for the prevention of cytomegalovirus disease in recipients of renal allografts. N Engl J Med *320*:1381–1387, 1989.

159. Gabel H, Flamholc L, Ahlfors K: Herpes simplex virus hepatitis in a renal transplant recipient: successful treatment with acyclovir. Scand J Infect Dis *20*:435–438, 1988.

160. Kharsa G, Degott C, Degos F, Carnot F, Potent F, Kreis H: Fulminant hepatitis in renal transplant recipients. The role of the delta agent. Transplantation *44*:221–223, 1987.

161. MacSween RNM: Liver pathology associated with diseases of other organs. *In* Pathology of the Liver, edited by R.N.M. MacSween, P.P. Anthony, P.J. Scheuer. 2nd Edition. Edinburgh, Churchill-Livingstone, 1987, pp. 646–688.

162. Hill RB, Porter KA, Massion CG: Hepatic reaction to renal transplants modified by immunosuppressive therapy. Iron accumulation in hepatic injury. Arch Pathol *81*:71–77, 1966.

163. Scheuer PJ, Williams R, Muir AR: Hepatic pathology in relatives of patients with hemochromatosis. J Pathol Bacteriol *84*:53–64, 1962.

164. Sidi Y, Boner G, Benjamin D, Solomon F, Douer D, Zandbank U, Rosenfeld JB, Pinkhas J: Hemochromatosis in a renal transplant recipient. Clin Nephrol *13*:197–199, 1980.

165. Johnson PC, Norris SJ, Miller GPG, Scott LD, Sell S, Kahan BD, Van Buren CT: Early syphilitic hepatitis after renal transplantation. J Infect Dis *158*:236–237, 1988.

166. Johnson TL, Barnett JL, Appelman HD, Nostrant T: Candida hepatitis. Histopathologic diagnosis. Am J Surg Pathol *12*:716–720, 1988.

167. Lawrence WH, Autian J, Misra PK: Cardioactive substances leached from a commercial hemodialysis set. N Engl J Med *292*:1356, 1975.

168. Bommer J, Ritz E, Andrassy K: Necrotizing dermatitis resulting from hemodialysis with polyvinylchloride tubing. Ann Intern Med *91*:869–870, 1979.

169. Neergaard J, Nielsen B, Faurby V, Christensen DH, Nielsen OF: Plasticizers in P.V.C. and the occurrence of hepatitis in a hemodialysis unit: a preliminary communication. Scand J Urol Nephrol *5*:141–145, 1971.

170. Dienes HP, Gerharz C-D, Wagner R, Weber M, John H-D: Accumulation of hydroxyethyl starch (HES) in the liver of patients with renal failure and portal hypertension. J Hepatol *3*:223–227, 1986.

171. Kohler H, Kirch W, Weihrauch TR, Prellwitz W, Horstmann HJ: Macroamylasemia after treatment with hydroxyethyl starch. Eur J Clin Invest *7*:205–211, 1977.

172. Pahl MV, Vaziri ND, Dure-Smith B, Miller R, Mirahmadi MK: Hepatobiliary pathology in hemodialysis patients: an autopsy study of 78 cases. Am J Gastroenterol *81*:783–787, 1986.

173. Santos GW: History of bone marrow transplantation. Clin Hematol *12*:611–639, 1983.

174. O'Reilly R: Allogeneic bone marrow transplantation: current status and future directions. Blood *62*:942–946, 1983.

175. Thomas ED: Marrow transplantation for malignant diseases. J Clin Oncol *1*:517–531, 1983.

176. Vogelsang GB, Hess AD, Berkman AW, Tutschka PJ, Farmer ER, Converse PJ, Santos GW: An in vitro predictive test for graft versus host disease in patients with genotypic HLA-identical bone marrow transplants. N Engl J Med *313*:645–650, 1985.

177. Yeager AM, Kaiser H, Santos GW, Saral R, Colvin OM, Stuart RK, Braine HG, Burke PJ, Ambinder RF, Burns WH, Fuller DJ, Davis JM, Karp JE, May WS, Rowley SD, Sensenbrenner LL, Vogelsang GV, Wingard JR: Autologous bone marrow transplantation in patients with acute nonlymphocytic leukemia, using ex vivo marrow treatment with 4-hydroperoxycyclophosphamide. N Engl J Med *315*:141–147, 1986.

178. Beatty PJ, Clift RA, Mickelson EM, Nisperos BB, Flournoy N, Martin PJ, Sanders JE, Steward P, Buckner CD, Storb R, Thomas ED, Hansen JA: Marrow transplantation from related donors other than HLA-identical siblings. N Engl J Med *313*:765–771, 1985.

179. Wick MR, Moore SB, Gastineau DA, Hoagland HC: Immunologic, clinical, and pathologic aspects of human graft-versus-host disease. Mayo Clin Proc *58*:603–612, 1983.

180. Meuer SC, Schlossman SF, Reinherz EL: Clonal analysis of human cytotoxic T lymphocytes: T4 + and T8 + effector T cells recognize

products of different major histocompatibility complex regions. Proc Natl Acad Sci 79:4395–4399, 1982.

181. Doyle C, Strominger JL: Interaction between CD4 and class II MHC molecules mediates cell adhesion. Nature 330:256–259, 1987.

182. Bjorkman PJ, Saper MA, Samraoui B: The foreign antigen binding site and T cell recognition regions of class I histocompatibility antigens. Nature 329:512–518, 1987.

183. Piguet P-F, Grau GE, Allet B, Vassali P: Tumor necrosis factor/cachectin is an effector of skin and gut lesions of the acute phase of graft-vs-host disease. J Exp Med 166:1280–1289, 1987.

184. Woodruff JM, Hansen JA, Good RA, Santos GW, Slavin TR: The pathology of graft-versus-host reaction (GVHR) in adults receiving bone marrow transplants. Transplant Proc 8:675–684, 1976.

185. Glucksberg H, Storb R, Fefer A, Buckner CD, Neiman PE, Clift RA, Lerner KG, Thomas ED: Clinical manifestations of graft-versus-host disease in human recipients of marrow from HLA-matched sibling donors. Transplantation 18:295–304, 1974.

186. Finegold MJ, Carpenter RJ: Obliterative cholangitis due to cytomegalovirus: a possible precursor of paucity of intrahepatic bile ducts. Hum Pathol 13:662–665, 1982.

187. Thomas ED, Storb R, Clift RA, Fefer A, Johnson FL, Neiman PE, Lerner KG, Glucksberg H, Buckner CD: Bone-marrow transplantation. N Engl J Med 292:895–902, 1975.

188. Glucksberg H, Storb R, Fefer A, Buckner CD, Neiman PE, Clift RA, Lerner KG, Thomas ED: Clinical manifestations of graft-versus-host-disease in human recipients of marrow from HLA-matched sibling donors. Transplantation 18:295–304, 1974.

189. Berk PD, Popper H, Krueger GRF, Decter J, Herzig G, Graw RG: Veno-occlusive disease of the liver after allogeneic bone marrow transplantation. Possible association with graft-versus-host disease. Ann Intern Med 90:158–164, 1979.

190. MacDonald GB, Sharma P, Matthews DE, Shulman HM, Thomas ED: Veno-occlusive disease of the liver after bone marrow transplantation: diagnosis, incidence and predisposing factors. Hepatology 4:116–122, 1984.

191. MacDonald GB, Sharma P, Matthews DE, Shulman HM, Thomas ED: The clinical course of 53 patients with veno-occlusive disease of the liver after bone marrow transplantation. Transplantation 39:603–608, 1985.

192. Forman SJ, Blume KG, Krance RA, Miner PJ, Metter LR, Hill LR, Odonnell MR, Nademanee AP, Snyder DS: A prospective randomized study of acute graft-vs-host disease in 107 patients with leukemia: methotrexate/prednisone vs cyclosporine A/prednisone. Transplant Proc 19:2605–2607, 1987.

193. Yee GC, Self SG, McGuire TR, Carlin J, Sander JE, Deeg HJ: Serum cyclosporine concentration and risk of acute graft-versus-host disease after allogeneic marrow transplantation. N Engl J Med 319:65–70, 1988.

194. Parkman R: Cyclosporine: GVHD and beyond. N Engl J Med 319:110–111, 1988.

195. Graze PR, Gale RP: Chronic graft vesus host disease: a syndrome of disordered immunity. Am J Med 66:611–620, 1979.

196. Rosenkrantz K, Dupont B, Williams D, Flomenberg N: Autocytotoxic and autosuppressor T-cell lines generated from autologous lymphocyte cultures. Hum Immunol 19:189–203, 1987.

197. McDonald GB, Shulman HM, Sullivan KM, Spencer GD: Intestinal and hepatic complications of human bone marrow transplantation. Part II. Gastroenterology 90:770–784, 1986.

198. Shulman HM, McDonald BG: Liver disease after marrow transplantation. In The Pathology of Bone Marrow Transplantation, edited by G.E. Sale, H.M. Shulman. Chicago, Year Book Medical Publishers, 1984, pp. 104–135.

199. Gholson CF, Yau JC, LeMaistre CF, Cleary KR: Steroid-responsive chronic hepatic graft-versus-host disease without extrahepatic graft-versus-host disease. Am J Gastroenterol 84:1306–1309, 1989.

200. Yau JC, Zander AR, Srigley JR, Verm RA, Stroehlein JR, Korinek JK, Vellekoop L, Dicke KA: Chronic graft-versus-host disease complicated by micronodular cirrhosis and esophageal varices. Transplantation 41:129–130, 1986.

201. Knapp AB, Crawford JM, Rappeport JM, Gollan JL: Cirrhosis as a consequence of graft-versus-host disease. Gastroenterology 92:513–519, 1987.

202. Rhodes DF, Lee WM, Wingard JR, Pavy MD, Santos GW, Shaw BW, Markin RS: Orthotopic liver transplantation for graft-versus-host disease following bone marrow transplantation. Gastroenterology 99:536–538, 1990.

203. Stechschulte DJ, Fishback JL, Emami A, Bhatia P: Secondary biliary

204. Von Fliedner V, Higby DJ, Kim U: Graft-versus-host reaction following blood product transfusion. Am J Med 72:951–961, 1982.

205. Ramsey G, Nusbacher J, Starzl TE, Lindsay GD: Isohemagglutinins of graft origin after ABO-unmatched liver transplantation. N Engl J Med 311:1167–1170, 1984.

206. Mangal AK, Growe GH, Sinclair M, Stillwell GF, Reeve CE, Naiman SC: Acquired hemolytic anemia due to "auto"-anti-A or "auto"-anti-B induced by group O homograft in renal transplant recipients. Transfusion 24:201–205, 1984.

207. Lerner KG, Kao GF, Storb R, Buckner CD, Clift RA, Thomas ED: Histopathology of graft-vs-host-reaction (GVHR) in human recipients of marrow from HLA-matched sibling donors. Transplant Proc 6:367–371, 1974.

208. Beschorner WE, Pino J, Boitnott JK, Tutschka PJ, Santos GW: Pathology of the liver with bone marrow transplantation. Effects of busulfan, carmustine, acute graft-versus-host disease and cytomegalovirus infection. Am J Pathol 99:369–385, 1980.

209. Sloane JP, Farthing MJG, Powles RL: Histopathological changes in the liver after allogeneic bone marrow transplantation. J Clin Pathol 33:344–350, 1980.

210. Zubair I, Guillermo A, Herrera MD, Pretlow TG, Roper M, Zornes SL: Intracytoplasmic inclusions in hepatocytes of bone marrow transplant patients: light and electron microscopic characterization. Am J Clin Pathol 83:65–68, 1985.

211. Berman MD, Rabin L, O'Donnell J, Gratwohl AA, Graw RG, Deisseroth AB, Jones EA: The liver in long-term survivors of marrow transplant—chronic graft-versus-host disease. J Clin Gastroenterol 2:53–68, 1980.

212. Snover DC, Weisdorf SA, Ramsay NK, McGlave P, Kersey JH: Hepatic graft versus host disease: a study of the predictive value of liver biopsy in diagnosis Hepatology 4:123–130, 1984.

213. Shulman HM, Sullivan KM, Weiden PL, et al: Chronic graft-versus-host syndrome in man. A long-term clinicopathologic study of 20 Seattle patients. Am J Med 69:204–217, 1980.

214. Sale GE, Storb R, Kolb H: Histopathology of hepatic acute graft-versus-host disease in the dog. Transplantation 26:103–106, 1978.

215. Bernuau D, Gisselbrecht C, Devergie A: Histological and ultrastructural appearance of the liver during graft-versus-host disease complicating bone marrow transplantation. Transplantation 29:236–244, 1980.

216. Tanaka M, Umihara J, Shimmoto K, Cui S, Sata H, Ishikawa T, Ishikawa E: The pathogenesis of graft-versus-host rejection in the intrahepatic bile duct. An immunohistochemical study. Acta Pathol Jpn 39:648–655, 1989.

217. Palmer PE, Wolfe HJ, Dayal Y, Gang DL: Immunocytochemical diagnosis of α-1-antitrypsin deficiency. Am J Surg Pathol 2:275–281, 1978.

218. An T, Ghatak N, Kastner R, Kay S, Hyung ML: Hyaline globules and intracellular lumina in a hepatocellular carcinoma. Am J Clin Pathol 79:392–396, 1983.

219. Nakanuma Y, Kono N, Ohta G, Shirasaki S, Takeshita H, Watanabe K, Shoji T, Yoshizawa H: Pale eosinophilic inclusions simulating ground-glass appearance of cells of hepatocellular carcinoma. Acta Pathol Jpn 32:71–81, 1982.

220. Becker FF, Lane BP: Regeneration of the mammalian liver. I. Autophagocytosis during dedifferentiation of the liver cell in preparation for cell division. Am J Pathol 47:783–801, 1965.

221. Mori M, Novikoff AB: Induction of pinocytosis in rat hepatocyte by partial hepatectomy. J Cell Biol 72:695–706, 1977.

222. Bianchi L: Intrahepatic bile duct damage in various forms of liver diseases. In Hepatology: A Festschrift for Hans Popper, edited by H. Brunner, H. Thaler. New York, Raven Press, 1985, pp. 295–310.

223. Shulman HM, Sharma P, Amos D, Fenster LF, McDonald GB: A coded histologic study of hepatic graft-versus-host disease after human bone marrow transplantation. Hepatology 8:463–470, 1988.

224. Bras G, Jelliffe D, Stuart L: Veno-occlusive disease of liver with nonportal type of cirrhosis, occurring in Jamaica. Arch Pathol 57:285–300, 1954.

225. Griner P, Elbadani A, Packman C: Veno-occlusive disease of the liver after chemotherapy of acute leukemia. Ann Intern Med 85:578–582, 1976.

226. Reed G, Cox A: The human liver after radiation injury. A form of veno-occlusive disease. Am J Pathol 48:597–612, 1986.

227. Burt AD, MacSween RNM: Hepatic vein lesions in alcoholic liver disease: retrospective biopsy and necropsy study. J Clin Pathol 39:63–67, 1986.

228. Read AE, Wiesner RH, LaBrecque DR: Hepatic veno-occlusive disease associated with renal transplantation and azathioprine therapy. Ann Intern Med *104:*651–656, 1986.

229. Berk P, Popper H, Kreuger G: Veno-occlusive disease of the liver after allogeneic bone marrow transplantation. Ann Intern Med *90:*158–164, 1979.

230. Shulman HM, McDonald GB, Matthews D: An analysis of hepatic veno-occlusive disease and centrilobular hepatic degeration following bone marrow transplantation. Gastroenterology *79:*1178–1191, 1980.

231. McDonald GB, Sharma P, Matthews D: Veno-occlusive disease of the liver after bone marrow transplantation: diagnosis, incidence and predisposing factors. Hepatology *4:*116–122, 1984.

232. Boyer TD: Portal hypertention and bleeding esophageal varices. *In* Hepatology A Textbook for Liver Disease, edited by D. Zakim, T.D. Boyer. 2nd Edition. Philadelphia, W.B. Saunders, 1990, pp. 572–615.

233. Rollins BJ: Hepatic veno-occlusive disease. Am J Med *81:*297–304, 1986.

234. Bras G, Brandt KH: Vascular disorders. *In* Pathology of the Liver, edited by R.N.M. MacSween, P.P. Anthony, P.J. Scheuer. Edinburgh, Churchill Livingstone, 1987, pp. 478–502.

Chapter 27
Acquired Immune Deficiency Syndromes

Acquired immune deficiency syndrome

The acquired immune deficiency syndrome (AIDS) was first recognized as a discrete syndrome in 1981 (1,2). The first 31 patients so reported were previously healthy, homosexual men with severe immunodeficiency manifested in 26 by Kaposi's sarcoma (2) and in 5 by *Pneumocystis carinii* pneumonia (1). Within two years the human immune deficiency virus (HIV-I), also known as the human T cell lymphotropic virus type III (HTLV-III) and the lymphadenopathy-associated virus (LAV) had been isolated (3). We now know an enormous amount about the disease, its clinical behavior, its etiologies, its transmission, its pathogenesis, and even a little about its therapy. Nevertheless, the disease has reached epidemic proportions. It is estimated that several million patients are infected worldwide, principally in the United States and Africa (4).

Etiology

HTLV-III, the responsible agent, is a retrovirus 105–120 nm in diameter that has a lipid envelope with a pyramidal nucleoid that contains core proteins, genomic RNA, and reverse transcriptase (4a). In addition to the usual complement of retroviral genes, it has five additional genes, several of which regulate HIV synthesis (5). HTLV-IV, another retrovirus also known as HIV-2 or LAV-2, induces a disorder similar to AIDS primarily in Africa that has also been found in the United States (6).

Transmission

The transmission of HIV occurs primarily during sexual activity, both homosexual and heterosexual. Receptive partners in rectal intercourse appear to be at greatest risk (7,8), although transmission between gay women has been claimed (9). Transmission can also occur via parenteral exposure to blood or blood products. In fact, almost 90% of recipients of HIV-infected blood become infected (10). Mother to infant transmission during the perinatal period is well established (11). Needle sticks with infected blood, pleural fluid, and other body fluids have been documented (12). Saliva, which may contain HIV virus (13), has been suggested as a transmission fluid, but this form of transmission has not been established. Biting insects have been implicated theoretically (14), but such transmission has not been documented. AIDS has been transmitted by the transplantation of organs from infected donors (15). Endoscopic procedures have been perceived as potential vectors in the transmission of HBV and HIV, but no instance of such transmission has been proved.

Pathogenesis

Depletion of T4 helper/inducer lymphocytes is the hallmark of AIDS and is caused by cytopathic consequences of viral replication in T4 lymphocytes. After binding to the T4 molecule, which is the HIV receptor (16), the virus enters the cell and genomic RNA is transcribed to DNA by reverse transcriptase, which is then integrated into the host genome (5). When such cells are activated by pathogens such as HBV, CMV, or HSV, transcription, protein synthesis, and replication result in the disappearance of T4 lymphocytes. Depletion of the T4 lymphocyte cell population per se results in a variety of immunologic defects. Furthermore, there is great genomic diversity among HIV isolates, which makes the task of designing vaccines extremely difficult (5).

Clinical features

Clinically, HIV infection is manifested by a spectrum of AIDS-related disorders. *Primary infection* with HIV is an infectious mononucleosis-like disorder that is followed by the appearance of antibodies to HIV (17,18). These acute, retroviral infections, which develop abruptly and last from a few days to two weeks, are flu-like syndromes characterized by the sudden onset of fever, night sweats, malaise, headache, photophobia, sore throat, lymphadenopathy, myalgia, arthralgia, and, sometimes, nausea, vomiting, or diarrhea. The patients show fever, occasionally chills, a maculopapular rash usually on the trunk, and generalized lymphadenopathy. The appearance of this nonspecific, viral constellation of symptoms and signs suggests AIDS in AIDS-prone groups such as gay men, drug abusers, hemophiliac patients (19), recipients of transfusions (20,21) or transplants (15), and health care workers after needle sticks (22). A variety of neurologic manifestations including depression, erratic mood changes, encephalopathy (23), encephalitis, myelopathy, Guillain-Barre syndrome, and peripheral neuropathy have been reported (24), and HIV has been isolated from cerebrospinal fluid and central nervous system tissue (25,26). Ulcerations of the pharynx, gingivae, and esophagus have been reported and probably occur in the colon as well (17,24,27).

This acute syndrome, which is classified as *group 1 HIV infection,* usually occurs 10 days to four weeks after exposure (17,26–28) with a median of 14 days, although viremia has persisting from 5 to 90 days has been reported (29). IgM antibodies appear within two weeks of the acute illness and peak between three and four weeks. IgG antibodies appear slightly more slowly, peaking at about four months. The diagnosis is established by the presence in the serum of HIV antigen during the acute illness and the appearance of IgM and IgG antibodies after the first week of clinical illness (29).

Hepatic manifestations of acute HIV infection are common, but only a single case of probable acute HIV hepatitis has been reported (30). Elevations of serum transaminase and alkaline phosphatase activity are occasionally seen (24,28), but these enzymes are usually normal. Such laboratory abnormalities are not accompanied by clinical signs of liver disease. Although hepatosplenomegaly is not uncommon (28), no distinctive histologic abnormalities have yet been reported in acute HIV infections, although nonspecific abnormalities have been described (31).

The only case report of acute HIV hepatitis is that of a nine-month-old infant born of HIV-positive parents who was seropositive for HIV-specific IgG and IGM and was found on biopsy to have giant cell hepatitis (30). The patient was deeply jaundiced with gross elevations of transaminase activity, but was seronegative for HAV, HBV, and EBV. Although she was weakly seropositive for CMV, there were no light or electron microscopic findings suggestive of CMV infection, and cultures for CMV of two liver biopsies were negative. Needle biopsy showed cholestasis, numerous multinucleated hepatocytes (Fig. 1029), lobular disarray, rare necrosis of individual hepatocytes, and mild portal inflammation of mononuclear, polymorphonuclear, and eosinophilic leukocytes. The authors concluded that it was a case of infantile giant cell hepatitis caused by HIV infection. Presumably, the giant cells represented an infantile response to viral hepatitis rather than a specific histologic response to the HIV virus.

The diagnosis of probable acute HIV hepatitis was made in a homosexual man who developed encephalitis after sexual contact with a patient with AIDS (31). HIVAg was identified in serum. Although there was no overt clinical evidence of hepatitis, both ALT and AST aminotransferase activity were increased to three or four times the upper level of normal. Liver biopsy taken five days after the peak of transaminase activity showed mild periportal steatosis and mononuclear infiltration, ballooning of hepatocytes, and hyperplasia of Kupffer cells (Figs. 1030, 1031).

AIDS represents only the late stages of chronic HIV infection. A number of earlier stages of HIV infection, however, have been recognized and arbitrarily defined (32). According to this classification, the acute retroviral infection is designated as *group (stage) 1 HIV* infection. The subsequent stages, group 2 to 4 HIV infection, together make up the *AIDS related complex* (ARC).

The ARC is arbitrarily defined as the persistence for more than three months of at least two of the following features: (1) fever; (2) night sweats; (3) fatigue; (4) significant spontaneous weight loss, usually more than 15 pounds; (5) lymphadenopathy of at least two sites; or (6) diarrhea (32). Furthermore, at least two of the following laboratory abnormalities are required: (1) a significant decrease in the absolute number of T cells; (2) reversal of the normal helper to suppressor T cell ratio; (3) decreased blastogenesis; (4) impaired delayed hypersensitivity as shown by negative skin tests; (5) increased serum globulin levels; or (6) either leukopenia, lymphopenia, thrombocytopenia, or anemia (33).

The *asymptomatic carrier* state is termed *stage 2 HIV* infection. This stage includes the majority of patients with HIV infection, since the interval between the acute infection and the more advanced stages may last from two to five years and sometimes even longer. The diagnosis of the carrier state is made solely by the presence of anti-HIV in serum (34). Many falsely seronegative carriers exist (35).

Sometimes stage 2 HIV infection exhibits petechiae and easy bruising, which are the consequence of *immune thrombocytopenic purpura* (ITP) (36,37). This syndrome, like the asymptomatic carrier state, usually progresses to the fullblown AIDS syndrome over a period of one to two years (37). There is no evidence of hepatic disease or abnormalities of liver function tests in group 2 HIV infection.

Stage 3 HIV infection is *persistent generalized lymphadenopathy,* which is usually accompanied by splenomegaly (38). These patients are often suspected of having a lymphoproliferative malignancy, but lymph node biopsies show only nonspecific changes. After two to three years, opportunistic infections begin as the patients progress into fullblown AIDS. Progression is usually preceded by diminution or disappearance of the lymphadenopathy.

Stage 4 HIV infection consists of two types. Group 4A includes patients with overt evidence of ARC and severe wasting who die before developing fullblown AIDS. This subgroup is termed by some *"slim disease."*

Group 4B is reserved for patients whose ARC is predominantly neurologic and consists of the *AIDS dementia complex* or severe peripheral neuropathy.

The pre-AIDS syndromes appear to progress slowly from the silent carrier state to ITP to persistent lymphadenopathy to fullblown AIDS. Deterioration is often heralded by the appearance of oral candidiasis, hairy leukoplakia (39), and the disappearance of peripheral lymphadenopathy (40). Ominous laboratory values include an increasing sedimentation rate, mild thrombocytopenia or leukopenia, and further depletion of T4 cells. The disappearance of p24 antibody or the reappearance of p24 antigen (41) and the development of HIV viremia (42) are poor prognostic signs.

Progression along the ARC spectrum of diseases is virtually free of clinical or laboratory evidence of hepatic involvement. Mild increments of transaminase activity may be hepatic in origin or may arise in other organs. Serum alkaline phosphatase elevations often indicate *M. avium intracellulare* infection or the development of lymphoma. Increments in lactic dehydrogenase activity may be associated with the development of *Pneumocystis carinii* pulmonary infection or, perhaps, the development of non-Hodgkin's lymphoma (40). Other prognostic indices have been proposed (43).

Fullblown AIDS

The syndrome known as AIDS is the result of persistent HIV infection. It usually develops over a period of years (44), although in one unique patient, AIDS apparently developed within two months of the initial infection with the HIV (45). It is characterized clinically, pathophysiologically, histologically, and by laboratory tests, by immunocompetence and the almost continuous occurrence of infections and infestations with pathogenic and nonpathogenic organisms.

Treatment

The therapy of AIDS is the treatment of its complicating infections. The therapy of HIV infection per se is in its infancy (46).

Infectious complications of AIDS

Fullblown AIDS, which is the result of persistent HIV infection, is characterized by the chronic, recurrent, lethal complications of the immunocompromised host. Most commonly they consist of superinfection by pathogenic or opportunistic, normally nonpathogenic bacteria, viruses, and fungi. The most common of these include *Pneumocystis carinii,* candidiasis, *Mycobacterium tuberculosis, Mycobacterium avium intracellulare* (MAI), cryptococcosis, cryptosporidiosis, toxoplasmosis, *Streptococcus pneumoniae,* and cytomegalovirus (CMV). They may also be manifested by the appearance of Kaposi's sarcoma, lymphoma, or other tumors.

AIDS and the liver

The liver is involved to some degree in the majority of systemic infections associated with AIDS. These hepatic infections, tumors, and lesions have been described in detail in several articles (48–51).

Autopsies have shown that about three-fourths of patients who die with AIDS have AIDS-related diseases that had not been suspected during life (47). About one-half have CMV infection, one-fifth systemic fungal infections, one-sixth Kaposi's sarcoma, one-tenth MAI infection, and one-tenth systemic herpes infections.

Clinically, advanced AIDS is characterized by weight loss, fever, lymphadenopathy, splenomegaly, and hepatomegaly. Although these findings occur in 70 to 90% of patients (48), they may be present in all combinations, and, rarely, none of these signs is found.

The hepatic manifestations of AIDS represent the responses of the liver to the infections or malignancies rather than the effects of the HIV infection itself. Although no microscopic hepatic lesion pathognomonic of acute HIV has yet been demonstrated, nonspecific, hepatic abnormalities have been encountered in presumptive instances of acute HIV hepatitis (Figs. 1029–1031). Some of these lesions in the infections, infestations, and neoplastic complications of AIDS appear indistinguishable from the same disorders seen in the livers of patients not infected with AIDS; others differ considerably. Furthermore, some patients with AIDS have chronic liver disease that antedate the onset of HIV infection. It is not known how such lesions differ from those that develop in non-AIDS patients or that develop subsequently in patients with AIDS.

Viral infections

Acute viral hepatitis. A variety of types of viral hepatitis have been reported in patients with AIDS including those caused by HBV, HCV, HDV, CMV, EBV, and HSV. Serologic evidence of previous infection with HBV is found in 85 to 95% of patients with AIDS, but these patients are only uncommonly HBsAg-positive (48,49). Indeed, in HIV-infected patients, HBV hepatitis may be followed by the carrier state in almost 70%. The patients may be asymptomatic carriers with essentially no histologic damage, they may have chronic persistent or chronic

active hepatitis, which tends to be mild (50). Histologically, chronic HBV hepatitis appears to be mild because of attenuated inflammatory reactions, which may result from the generalized lymphoid depletion that characterizes AIDS [(50–54); Figs. 989, 1032]. Indeed, lymphocytes are uncommon in the portal tracts of patients with AIDS (50,54). The mildness of chronic hepatitis in AIDS may reflect the lack of appropriate effector cells to induce chronic hepatitis (50). When patients are HBsAg-positive, they tend to exhibit an abundance of orcein-positive inclusions in hepatic parenchymal cells (50). Furthermore, the response to plasma-derived HBV vaccine is greatly diminished in patients with AIDS (55).

The prevalence of *HDV,* which varies widely in homosexual men from city to city (56), is not a frequent cause of viral hepatitis (57). However, both HIV and HBV infections are commonly present together (57). This coinfection appears to be correlated with the number of sexual partners and the practice of anal receptive intercourse (56). The relatively low prevalence of anti-HDV in AIDS may reflect the relatively recent introduction of HDV into the gay population or, more likely, the more effective transmission of HDV by parenteral exposure than by transmucosal inoculation (57).

Indirect evidence suggests that in patients infected with both HBV and HDV, the HDV suppresses HBV replication (58) as shown by the less frequent presence and the lower serum levels of HBV DNA (59). Since HIV transmission occurs by the same routes as does HBV and HDV, simultaneous infection with the three viruses is not uncommon. It is intriguing that the occurrence of HIV infection in patients with HBV-HDV coinfection results in at least partial inhibition of the HDV-induced suppression of HBV replication (60).

On the other hand, the sexual transmission of HBV is much more efficient than of HIV in homosexual men (61). Although HBV and HIV are both transmitted during anal intercourse, HBV infection is clearly associated with insertive anal intercourse (62) while HIV transmission tends to result from receptive anal intercourse.

Prior infection with *HAV* in gay men, in whom AIDS is extremely common, appears to occur no more frequently than in heterosexual couples (63).

CMV is a herpes virus that may infect many epithelial and mesenchymal tissue. CMV infections in homosexual men and in patients with AIDS (64) are extremely common. Simultaneous primary infection with both the HIV and CMV viruses can induce a severe multisystemic infection (65). Although CMV chorioretinitis, central nervous system infection, and colitis all occur frequently, CMV hepatitis occurs occasionally, but rarely causes severe clinical disease. The virus has been detected in hepatocytes, bile duct epithelium, and endothelial cells. Classic inclusion-bearing cells are enlarged and are characterized by an "owl's eye" intranuclear inclusion (Figs. 190, 191) and granular cytoplasmic inclusions that are PAS-D-positive. The intranuclear inclusions are Gomori and PAS-D-negative (66). In biopsy material, such classic cells are rare, and infected cells may show smudging of cytologic features, as seen in a patient with AIDS and acute CMV hepatitis (Figs. 1033, 1034). These single cell lesions may (Fig. 1033) or may not (Fig. 1034) elicit an inflammatory response. Immunoperoxidase and DNA *in situ* hybridization techniques are sensitive methods of diagnosis and can demonstrate infection in the absence of recognizable inclusions (67). Hepatic granulomas have been reported occasionally in CMV patients. In patients with both AIDS and CMV infection, however, other causes of granulomas must also be considered. Small, AFB-negative granulomas may be found (Fig. 1035), but cultures can still be positive for MAI. The cause of the granulomas in this case is not clear.

Herpes simplex hepatitis. *Herpes simplex* has been reported to produce gross infarct-like lesions of the subcapsular hepatic parenchyma (67a). These foci of coagulation necrosis, which are yellow-orange in color, range from a few millimeters to several centimeters in diameter. They are often surrounded by surviving hepatocytes that may contain Cowdry intranuclear inclusions and ground glass cells.

Acute adenovirus infections. Disseminated adenovirus infections with hepatic necrosis are also common in AIDS (68).

Chronic viral hepatitis. Chronic hepatitis has been described in patients with AIDS (69). Such patients usually show no overt clinical signs of liver disease except hepatomegaly (70). They exhibit elevated aminotransferase values (69,70). In such patients, in whom specific viral agents responsible for the hepatitis cannot be established unequivocally, the histologic pattern consists of portal and lobular lymphocytic inflammation, hepatocellular and bile duct injury, and sinusoidal hyperplasia. The usual pattern of lymphocyte infiltration in both autoimmune or HBV chronic active hepatitis of predominantly T4 cells in the portal tracts and T8 cells in the lobules (71,72) is reversed (69). These patients show a decreased T4 to T8 ratio in both the lobular and portal zones. Whether or not this represents a reversal of the usual type of lymphocyte infiltration or an absolute depletion of T4 lymphocytes is not clear.

CMV frequently involves the gallbladder and has a predisposition for causing acalculous cholecystitis (73–75). Cytomegalovirus cholangitis has also been reported (76). CMV and cryptosporidia have been implicated in AIDS patients who develop biliary tract obstruction with distal bile duct strictures that mimic sclerosing cholangitis (77–80).

Mycobacterial infections

Tuberculosis. The prevalence of tuberculous infection is increased in patients with HIV infection. Approximately 8% of seropositive patients will develop tuberculosis each year (81). Indeed, AIDS may be largely responsible for the increase in the incidence of tuberculosis (82). Furthermore, the risks of active infection are much higher in those with AIDS (81). These cases appear to result from the reactivation of latent tuberculous infection when HIV infection develops. Furthermore, the manifestations of the disease appear to be particularly severe and lethal (83) and predominantly extrapulmonary in AIDS patients (84). The disease is more frequent and more virulent in parenteral drug abusers than in homosexual patients who do not abuse drugs (84). The concurrence of the two diseases may, however, represent demographic artifacts, such as the high prevalence of both diseases in drug-abusing Haitians (84).

Histologically, hepatic tuberculosis in patients with AIDS is similar to that seen in non-AIDS patients. The characteristic findings are granulomas, but they differ from granulomas in non-AIDS patients in that they show caseation uncommonly (85–88). Sometimes, they do show caseation [(89); Fig. 1036]. Although Langhans giant cells are uncommon, they do occur (Fig. 1037). Tuberculosis appears to be more disseminated, and acid-fast organisms on Ziehl-Neelsen stains are seen more frequently in patients with AIDS that in non-AIDS patients [(84); Fig. 1038]. These findings must be differentiated from those of atypical tuberculosis caused by MAI, which is found 3 to 10 times more frequently than tuberculosis in the livers of patients with AIDS (85,88–90) and in which acid-fast bacteria are frequently found in large numbers. Granulomas in tuberculosis appear to be smaller and more discrete than in atypical tuberculosis. Such differences are not useful in the individual patient. Cultures of liver biopsy specimens are essential and often establish the correct diagnosis (86,88).

Mycobacterium avium intracellulare. Before AIDS, a total of only 78 patients with disseminated *M. avium intracellulare* (MAI) had been reported (91). In immunocompetent subjects, MAI infections are almost invariably limited to the lungs, but in AIDS patients they often are widely disseminated (89). Nontuberculous mycobacterial hepatic infections are very common and represent the most common hepatic infection in AIDS (48). They are found in 50% of the livers of patients dying with AIDS (49). Clinically, the patients may present in a variety of ways, including any of the syndromes seen in AIDS, but typically they have persistent fever, and show elevated serum alkaline phosphatase activity (86,87). The lesions are infiltrative and progressive. They respond poorly to antibiotic therapy, and the infection often leads to death. The diagnosis can often be established by blood cultures, which may obviate the need to do liver biopsies for this purpose (91).

Histologically, hepatic MAI infections are characterized by granuloma formation that varies from loose aggregates of histiocytes to tight, well-formed granulomas (54,86,88). Often, the granulomas are few in number, small (Fig. 1039), poorly formed (Fig. 1040), and immature [(86,92,93); Fig. 1041]. These microgranulomas may consist of only one or two histiocytes in which acid-fast bacilli may be found. On the other hand, large numbers of acid-fast bacteria are often found within histiocytes in the granulomas (Fig. 1042), or free in liver tissue (86,94,95) on Ziehl-Neelson stain. Sometimes, the granulomas are composed of foamy or "striated" histiocytes (96), which have been termed "pseudo-Gaucher" cells [(97); Fig. 1043]. These histiocytes are often filled with acid-fast, atypical tuberculous bacilli (Figs. 1044, 1045). MAI bacilli can also be seen in great profusion on Giemsa (Fig. 1046), PAS (Fig. 1047), Gomori (Fig. 1048), or Brown-Hopps (Fig. 1049) stains (98), as can tuberculous bacilli. The bacilli can even be seen in histiocytes on conventional H & E stain, but are not so obvious (Fig. 1050).

There appears to be a positive correlation between the degree of immunodeficiency, on one hand, and the immaturity of the granulomas and the increased numbers of acid-fast bacteria, on the other. It has been suggested that "the formation of well-formed, hard granulomas requires an intact host defense system," for which T cell function is necessary (86). The poorly formed MAI granulomas tend to have neither multinucleated giant cells nor necrosis (95).

Fungal infections

Hepatic infection by *Cryptococcus neoformans* has been described in several patients with AIDS (49,87,99,100), although it more characteristically causes meningitis (101). Such patients appear to have had disseminated cryptoccocal infections. There is usually no clinical evidence of liver disease, and transaminase activity is only slightly abnormal. One as yet unreported case of cryptococcal hepatitis has been observed [(102); Fig. 1051]. Typically, cryptococci proliferate in the liver, often in the sinusoids, but show little or no inflammatory reaction (Figs. 1052, 1053). Histologically, the organisms exhibit a characteristic clear-staining capsule (Figs. 1051–1053). Granulomas may be found, however.

Hepatic histoplasmosis occurs as a manifestation of disseminated infection, but rarely presents as overt liver disease. Only one such case has been reported (49). Clinical findings are nonspecific and the diagnosis of histoplasmosis is usually made by biopsy of skin, bone marrow, or lung. In the liver, histoplasmosis is seen as small, budding yeast forms within granulomas (Fig. 1054) or within the sinusoids (Fig. 1055). They are best seen with the Gomori methenamine silver stain. Rapid diagnosis may also be made on Gram-Wright-stained squash preparations of biopsy specimens (Fig. 1056).

Coccidioidomycosis is a common infection in patients with AIDS. It occurs in about one-fourth of patients in areas endemic for *Coccidioides immitis* (103). The higher infection rate in AIDS patients than in those without AIDS indicates that AIDS renders patients more susceptible to infection or to reactivation. The disease usually exhibits pulmonary manifestations, but at autopsy, spherules are frequently found in the liver. When they occur, granulomas are poorly formed, but may contain numerous coccidioidomycotic spherules (104,105).

Candida albicans has been implicated as one of the causes of polymicrobial cholangitis, along with *Cryptosporidium* and *Klebsiella* in the pathogenesis of a sclerosing cholangitis-like picture in patients with AIDS (106). Sometimes, hepatic microabscesses develop in patients with candidiasis (Fig. 1057). Disseminated candidiasis is uncommon.

Miscellaneous infections and infestations

Microsporidia. The protozoon *Microsporidia* has so far been reported to cause human disease only in patients with AIDS (107). One case of acute hepatitis caused by *Encephalitozoon cunicule* with microgranulomas has been reported so far (108). Liver biopsy showed nonspecific microgranulomas without evident cause. The diagnosis of *Microsporidia* infestation was made by electron microscopic demonstration of the organism. Electron microscopy is required to differentiate the protozoa from those of *Toxoplasma*.

Cryptosporidium. *Cryptosporidium,* a coccidial protozoon, causes diarrhea in both immunocompetent and immunosuppressed patients. Extraintestinal dissemination has been reported in AIDS (109). Cryptosporidia have been seen in the liver, in bile duct and gallbladder epithelia (Fig. 1058), and have been implicated in association with CMV in cases of common bile duct stenosis and sclerosing cholangitis (77–80).

Toxoplasmosis. *Toxoplasmosis* is sometimes seen in patients with AIDS, but it is usually manifest as encephalitis (48). Hepatic manifestations of toxoplasmosis appear rare. In fact, they are not rare; they have only rarely been reported (L. Brandt, personal communication, 1992). Fat deposition and other nonspecific findings have been described (48). However, toxoplasmosis may cause disseminated hepatic infection as shown in Figures 1059 and 1060, which depict the first reported case of a toxoplasmotic abscess (110).

Pneumocystis carinii. *Pneumocystis carinii* commonly causes interstitial pneumonia in patients with AIDS (109). Extrapulmonary dissemination may occur (111) and may involve the viscera, including the liver (112–114). The diagnosis is established by the demonstration of the characteristic cysts with the Gomori stain.

Parasites and bacteria. Intestinal infections with parasites such as *Entamoeba histolytica, Giardia lamblia, chlamydia trachomatis* and with bacteria such as *Salmonella, Shigella, Neisseria,* campylobacter, etc., are all common components of the "gay bowel syndrome" in patients with AIDS (115,116). Hepatic amebic abscesses have been reported in such patients (117), and hepatic abscesses with any of these other agents that can enter the body during rectal intercourse may be anticipated.

Neoplasms associated with AIDS

Kaposi's sarcoma

A number of neoplasms have been reported in AIDS and some of them are considered to be consequences of HIV infection (118). Indeed, the association of *Kaposi's sarcoma* with AIDS in part led to recognition of AIDS (2,119). It has been found in from 10 to 35% of patients with AIDS, depending on the stage of AIDS and the population from which the patients were collected (120,121). Classic Kaposi's sarcoma can easily be differentiated from AIDS-associated Kaposi's sarcoma. The non-AIDS-related type is usually an indolent neoplasm, with lesions on the lower extremities, uncommon visceral involvement, few opportunistic infections, and a benign course (120,122,123). The AIDS-associated type involves the upper body and frequently the viscera. It is characterized by diffuse infections and runs an aggressive, often lethal course (123). Its presence can be suggested by the presence of hyperechoic densities on liver imaging by CT, hypoattenuation by ultrasound, and by increased blood flow by contrast-enhanced CT examination (124).

It has been suggested on the basis of epidemiologic observations that Kaposi's sarcoma may be caused by "an as yet unidentified infectious agent transmitted mainly by sexual contact" (125). This agent is postulated to be another virus unrelated to HIV that is transmitted sexually, and presumably by oral-rectal contact. Kaposi's sarcoma is seen primarily in gay men and some sexually active heterosexual patients. It occurs uncommonly in nongay men who get AIDS from intravenous drug abuse or transfusions.

It is postulated that viruses induce sustained proliferation of specific cellular targets and in conjunction with a variety of potential cofactors may give rise to a neoplasm. Thus, HBV is thought to stimulate hepatocellular carcinoma, and in AIDS CMV is thought to be the most likely virus to induce Kaposi's sarcoma (118,121). As indicated above, CMV is a likely candidate virus for the etiologic agent of Kaposi's sarcoma (125).

Kaposi's sarcoma in AIDS arises from several types of tissue. One shows a lymphomatous pattern of proliferation and is characterized by empty, anastomosing, angulated spaces in skin-like connective tissue. The cells that line these spaces appear to be lymphatic endothelium as suggested by immunohistologic examination. The spindle cells are positive for factor VIII–related antigen and specific monoclonal antigens typical of endothelial cells (126).

Typically, Kaposi lesions are red, purple, or even black tumors of the skin or the oral mucosa. About 40% of patients with cutaneous or lymphoid Kaposi's sarcoma show digestive tract involvement, usually without symptoms. A few of these involve the liver or biliary tree. Those in the liver are usually found at autopsy, unless they are discovered on liver biopsy. About 10% of patients with cutaneous Kaposi's sarcoma have hepatic involvement (84,94), but is is not always clear whether these represent metastatic tumors or neoplasms of multicentric origin. In one large autopsy series, about one-third of patients with Kaposi's sarcoma showed hepatic involvement (49).

Histologically, Kaposi's sarcoma appears as multifocal areas of proliferation of fascicles of interlacing spindle cells with irregular vascular clefts of thin and thick-walled capillaries and, occasional larger vessels with widespread extravasation of erythrocytes [(127); Figs. 1061, 1062]. Inconspicuous infiltrates of plasma cells are present in early lesions, and may be a clue to the diagnosis of Kaposi's sarcoma in difficult cases. The tumor is most often found in the portal zones (54,87) and tends to invade the capsule (87).

Lymphoma

There is a strikingly high incidence of malignant lymphoma in AIDS. The majority of such neoplasms are non-Hodgkin's lymphomas of B cell phenotype with a variety of histologic subtypes (49,54,121,128). In addition, both Hodgkin's lymphomas and rare T cell lymphomas have been reported (129). AIDS-related lymphomas are usually high grade malignancies that present in unusual locations such as the central nervous system (130,131). They progress relentlessly despite aggressive therapy. They are frequently extranodal and tend to involve the digestive tract, especially the liver, and the anorectal region (132). Disseminated lesions may be clinically silent, and are frequently first discovered at autopsy.

The appearance of lymphomas in patients with AIDS is usually preceded by generalized lymphadenopathy with diffuse follicular depletion (133) and polyclonal hypergammaglobulinemia. Such lymphomas, however, represent high grade, monoclonal tumors, which suggests malignant transformation from polyclonal precursors (121). This sequence suggests in turn that a whole spectrum of lymphomas or other tumors may arise in AIDS and that multicentric tumors of the same type, or multiple types of tumors may be expected. Indeed, lymphomas and Kaposi's sarcoma have been reported in the same patient (128,134).

At least two of the lymphomas were primarily hepatic malignancies (54,135) as shown by the absence of extrahepatic tumor at autopsy. One appeared to have metastasized from an undifferentiated, non-Burkitt lymphoma of the central nervous system (54). One of the primary hepatic lymphomas was of the diffuse, large cell, immunoblastic type (Fig. 1063). The other was a diffuse, large, B cell lymphoma in a patient with AIDS who also had Kaposi's sarcoma and micronodular cirrhosis (135). Figures 1063 and 1064 illustrate a high grade, AIDS-related, Burkitt's type malignant lymphoma of the liver of a patient who died unexpectedly with unsuspected, widespread, visceral involvement. The "starry sky" appearance is created by the

pale histiocytes that look like stars scattered among the dark staining lymphocytes that look like the night sky.

Hodgkin's disease

A number of cases of Hodgkin's disease in patients with AIDS have been reported (131,136). In one patient, typical Hodgkin's disease of the mixed cellularity type and Kaposi's sarcoma were seen in the same lymph node (134). Histologically typical Reed-Sternberg cells and Reed-Sternberg variants were present. In addition, the tumor contained intracytoplasmic lambda and kappa light chain lesions. The occurrence of Hodgkin's disease in patients with AIDS suggests that component cells of the immune system other than B lymphocytes, which have been postulated to give rise to non-Hodgkin's lymphomas in patients with AIDS, may also undergo malignant transformation (137). The concurrence of Kaposi's sarcoma and Hodgkin's disease suggests that an underlying immune deficiency can give rise to both types of neoplasms. Such tumors may involve the liver.

Vascular lesions

Vascular lesions are very common in AIDS. Sinusoidal dilatation (Fig. 1065), which is indistinguishable from that seen in non-AIDS patients, is frequently found in AIDS (138). Peliosis hepatis [(139a); Fig. 1065] and Kupffer cell proliferation (140) occur commonly. Both sinusoidal dilatation and peliosis hepatis frequently accompany vascular neoplasms of diverse type such as angiosarcoma (141) and Kaposi's sarcoma. Perisinusoidal hypertrophy with lipid deposition and endothelial cell injury may occur in AIDS (142). These changes may represent transitional changes preceding the malignant endothelial changes of Kaposi's sarcoma, angiosarcoma, and, perhaps, other neoplasms with related vascular components (143). These relationships between the vascular and lymphatic systems and Kaposi's sarcoma in AIDS are intimately related and poorly understood (144).

Peliosis hepatis has been reported on a few occasions in AIDS (139, 139a, 145). It has recently been recognized that peliosis hepatis in patients with HIV infection is probably caused by an opportunistic bacillary infection (145). It appears to be similar in pathogenesis and histology to cutaneous bacillary angiomatosis, another bacterial infection that occurs in patients with HIV infection and that resembles Kaposi's sarcoma clinically and histologically. Presumably both lesions are caused by the same species of bacillus, which has not yet been successfully cultured. From their identical morphology it has been hypothesized that they may be caused by the same organism or one closely related to those that cause cat scratch fever (145a, 145b, 145c) (Fig. 735). It has also been postulated that the peliotic lesions may be caused by the elaboration of an angiogenic substance by these organisms.

Histologically, the lesions of peliosis hepatis in patients with HIV infection differ from those of peliosis hepatis in non-HIV-infected patients by the presence of a fibromyxoid stroma in the peliotic spaces that contain inflammatory cells, capillary vessels, and granular purple material (Figs. 721, 1065A). The clumps of purplish material appear to be colonies of bacteria when stained with bacterial stains (Fig. 772). Apparently several patients treated with antibiotics, especially eythromycin, have responded, and the bacteria have disappeared (145). The association of cutaneous bacillary angiomatosis, peliosis hepatis, Kaposi's sarcoma, and perhaps, cat scratch fever and bartonellosis as well suggests that some of the lesions of HIV infection are becoming better understood and more treatable.

Miscellaneous lesions

Granulomas

Granulomas are the single most common abnormality in the livers of patients with AIDS. Although one liver biopsy series showed granulomas in 80% of patients with AIDS (88), in most series granulomas of diverse etiology and histology are found in about 40% (146). Hepatic granulomas have been classified into three types (87,109). Type 1 are non-necrotic granulomas composed of loosely arranged, multinucleated giant cells. Usually no infectious agent can be identified in or isolated from such lesions. Type 2 granulomas are discrete, compact, epithelioid granulomas that may show caseation necrosis, but Langhans giant cells are uncommon. Acid-fast bacteria can usually be seen in stained sections; *M. tuberculosis* can usually be cultured from such lesions. Type 3 granulomas are composed of aggregates of foamy blue histiocytes, lymphocytes, and plasma cells (96). No caseation or giant cells are present. Acid-fast organisms can usually be found in the granulomas and *M. avian intracellulare* can often be cultured from them.

These granulomas, which vary in size, are scattered randomly throughout the hepatic lobules. *M. tuberculosis* and *M. avian intracellulare* are the organisms most often found in these granulomas (147). Mycobacteria are much more easily demonstrable in AIDS than in non-AIDS patients (95,147). They can be found in the absence of granulomas in the liver and in other tissues (95). In many instances, however, no infectious agents can be identified in these granulomas, and their etiology is obscure (95). The relative prevalence of tuberculosis and atypical tuberculosis infections depends to a large extent on the population studied (148). *Cryptococcus neoformans* may also be found in hepatic granulomas. Both cytomegalovirus and Epstein-Barr viral infections may be associated with granuloma formation (149,150) and may account for some of the unidentified granulomas. In addition, granulomas may result from hepatotoxic therapeutic agents such as rifampin, isoniazid, and sulfonamides, which are frequently prescribed in AIDS (48).

Biliary tract disease

Biliary tract disease represents a small but significant portion of the syndromes of AIDS. A number of cases of acalculous cholecystitis (151), cholangitis (152), biliary obstruction (153,154), and other diverse biliary lesions have been reported (155). The true prevalence of these disorders is not yet known (156).

The clinical findings include right upper quadrant abdominal pain, fever, and increased serum alkaline phosphatase activity. These features may be individually present or in any combination. Endoscopic retrograde cholangiopancreatography (ERCP) has shown that sclerosing cholangitis with papillary stenosis is the most common pattern, although sclerosing cholangitis and

papillary stenosis may occur separately. Long extrahepatic bile duct strictures are sometimes found. Most such patients showed dilatation of the bile ducts.

AIDS-related pathogens have been identified in about one-half the patients, and CMV is the most common agent, although cryptosporidial infections occur in both AIDS and in congenital immunodeficiency (157).

The cholangiopathy of AIDS differs from that of primary sclerosing cholangitis in that common bile duct dilatation and papillary stenosis occur in addition to the ductal stenosis and the beading that are so typical of primary sclerosing cholangitis. In addition, the jaundice which is common in primary sclerosing cholangitis is very unusual in AIDS cholangiopathy, which is almost always anicteric (L. Brandt, personal communication, 1992). Of course, biliary tract disorders unrelated to AIDS may occur in patients with AIDS. Because of the diversity of infections, infestations, and neoplasms that may occur in AIDS, liver biopsy assumes a greater role in the differential diagnosis of biliary disorders in AIDS than in non-AIDS patients. It is reasonable, therefore, to perform biliary imaging first. If normal, liver biopsy is the diagnostic procedure of choice. If biliary abnormalities are present, however, ERCP appears to be the initial diagnostic procedure.

Thus, AIDS joins ulcerative colitis, Crohn's disease, sarcoidosis, and graft-versus-host disease as the latest in a line of immunologic disorders that are associated with sclerosing cholangitis.

Drug-induced hepatic injury

Drug-induced hepatic injury occurs in patients with AIDS as well as in patients without AIDS, and no obvious differences in histologic patterns have been reported. Some agents such as azidothymidine (AZT), which are used exclusively in AIDS, may cause specific hepatic abnormalities, especially in view of the metabolism of AZT by hepatic glucuronidation. Several cases of AZT-associated hepatotoxicity have been reported (158).

Although AIDS is a Pandora's box of histopathologic abnormalities that may involve all components of the hepatobiliary system, there are, as yet, no hepatic lesions pathognomonic of AIDS.

Nonspecific lesions

Every hepatic histopathologic lesion seen in the livers of non-AIDS patients, sometimes subtly or severely distorted, may be found in the livers of patients with AIDS. These include all of the infections, infestations, and neoplasms to which these patients are susceptible, many of which have been described previously. Interpretation may be complicated and confused by the simultaneous effects of several such processes. Cultures of biopsies, special stains for acid-fast organisms, and special studies such as electron microscopy should be used freely.

In addition, there are nonspecific abnormalities such as periportal macrovesicular fat deposition (Fig. 1066), reactive hepatitis (101), occasional nonspecific ductular abnormalities (Fig. 1067), hemosiderin deposition in Kupffer cells (50,114), and chronic hepatitis (59).

References

1. Centers for Disease Control: *Pneumocystis* pneumonia—Los Angeles. MMWR *30*:250–252, 1981.
2. Centers for Disease Control: Kaposi's sarcoma and *Pneumocystis* pneumonia among homosexual men—New York City and California. MMWR *25*:305–308, 1981.
3. Barre-Sinoussi F, Nugeyre M, Dauguet C: Isolation of a T-lymphotropic retrovirus from a patient at risk for acquired immune deficiency syndrome. Science *220*:868–871, 1983.
4. Curran JW, Morgan WM, Handy AM, Jaffe HW, Darrow WW, Dowdle WR: The epidemiology of AIDS: current status and future prospects. Science *229*:1352–1357, 1985.
4a. Orenstein JM, Jannotta F: Human immunodeficiency virus and papovavirus infections in acquired immunodeficiency syndrome: an ultrastructural study of three cases. Hum Pathol *19*:350–361, 1988.
5. Ho DD, Pomerantz RJ, Kaplan JC: Pathogenesis of infection with human immunodeficiency virus. N Engl J Med *317*:278–285, 1987.
6. AIDS due to HIV-2 infection—New Jersey. MMWR *87*:33–35, 1988.
7. Darrow WW, Echenberg DF, Jaffe HW: Risk factors for human immunodeficiency virus (HIV) infections in homosexual men. Am J Public Health *77*:479–483, 1987.
8. Moss AR, Osmond D, Bacchetti P: Risk factors for AIDS and HIV seropositivity in homosexual men. Am J Epidemiol *125*:1035–1047, 1987.
9. Marmor M, Weiss LR, Lyden M: Possible female-to-female transmission of human immunodeficiency virus. Ann Intern Med *105*:969, 1986.
10. Mosley JW, The Transfusion Safety Study Group: The transfusion safety study (Abstract TH 10.2). *In* Abstracts of the III International Conference on AIDS. Washington, D.C., 1987.
11. Jaffe HW, Lifson AR: Acquisition and transmission of HIV. *In* The Medical Management of AIDS, edited by M.A. Sande, P.A. Volberding. Philadelphia, W.B. Saunders 1988, pp. 19–27.
12. Stricof RL, Morse DL: HTLV-III/LAV seroconversion following a deep intramuscular needlestick injury. (Correspondence) N Engl J Med *314*:1115, 1986.
13. Ho DD, Byington RE, Schooley RT: Infrequency of isolation of HTLV-III virus from saliva in AIDS. N Engl J Med *313*:1606, 1985.
14. Lyons SF, Jupp PJ, Schoub BD: Survival of HIV in the common bedbug. Lancet *2*:45. 1986.
15. L'Age-Stehr J, Schwarz A, Offermann G: HTLV-III infection in kidney transplant recipients. Lancet *2*:1361–1362, 1985.
16. Klatzmann D, Champagne E, Chamaret S: T-lymphocyte T4 molecule behaves as the receptor for human retrovirus LAV. Nature *312*:767–768, 1984.
17. Gaines J, von Sydow M, Pehrson PO, Lundbergh P: Clinical picture of primary HIV infection presenting as a glandular fever-like illness. BMJ *297*:1363–1368, 1988.
18. Ho DD, Sarnagadharan MG, Resnick L: Primary human T-lymphotropic virus type III infection. Ann Intern Med *103*:880–883, 1985.
19. White GC II, Mathews TJ, Weinhold KJ: HTLV-III seroconversion associated with heat-treated factor VIII concentrate. Lancet *1*:611–612, 1986.
20. Archibald DW, Zon L, Groopman JE: Natural history of primary infection with LAV in multitransfused patients. AIDS-Hemophilia French Study Group. Blood *68*:89–94, 1986.
21. Boiteux F, Vilmer E, Girot R: Lymphadenopathy syndrome in two thalassemic patients after LAV contamination by blood transfusion. N Engl J Med *312*:648–649, 1985.
22. Oskenhendler E, Harzic M, Le Roux J-M: HIV infection with seroconversion after a superficial needlestick injury to the finger. N Engl J Med *315*:582, 1986.
23. Carne CA, Tedder RS, Smith A: Acute encephalopathy coincident with serconversion for anti-HTLV-III. Lancet *1*:1206–1208, 1985.
24. Tindall B, Cooper DA, Donovan B, Penny R: Primary human immunodeficiency virus infection: clinical and serologic aspects. *In* The Medical Management of AIDS, edited by M.A. Sande, P.A. Volberding. Philadelphia, W.B. Saunders, 1988, pp. 75–89.
25. Ho DD, Rota TR, Schooley RT: Isolation of HTLV-III from cerebrospinal fluid and neural tissues of patients with neurologic syndromes related to the acquired immunodeficiency syndrome. N Engl J Med *313*:1493–1497, 1985.
26. Ho DD, Sarngadharan MG, Resnick L, Dimarzo-Veronese F, Rota TR, Hirsch MS: Primary human T-lymphotropic virus type III infection. Ann Intern Med *103*:880–883, 1985.
27. Valle S-L: Febrile pharyngitis as the primary sign of HIV infection in a cluster of cases linked by sexual contact. Scand J Infect Dis *19*:13–17, 1987.
28. Clark SJ, Saag MS, Decker WD, Campbell-Hill S, Roberson JL, Veldkamp PJ, Kappes JC, Hahn BH, Shaw GM: High titers of cytopathic virus in plasma of patients with symptomatic primary HIV-I infection. N Engl J Med *324*:954–960, 1991.
29. Cooper DA, Imrie AA, Penny R: Antibody response to human immunodeficiency virus after primary infection. J Infect Dis *155*:1113–1118, 1987.
30. Witzleben CL, Mashall GS, Wenner W, Piccoli DA, Barbour SD: HIV as a cause of giant cell hepatitis. Hum Pathol *19*:603–605, 1988.
31. Girard P-ML: Personal communication 1990.
32. Centers for Disease Control: Classification system for human T-lymphotropic virus type III/lymphadenopathy-associated virus infection. MMWR *35*:344–347, 1986.
33. Abrams DI: AIDS-related conditions. Clin Immunol Allergy *6*:581–599, 1986.
34. Coolfont Report: A PHS plan for prevention and control of AIDS and the AIDS virus. Public Health Rep *101*:341–348, 1986.
35. Imagawa DT, Lee MH, Wolinsky SM: Human immunodeficiency virus type 1 infection in homosexual men who remain seronegative for prolonged periods. N Engl J Med *320*:1458–1462, 1989.
36. Abrams DI, Kirpov DD, Goedert JJ: Antibodies to human T-lymphotropic virus type III and development of the acquired immunodeficiency syndrome in homosexual men presenting with immune thrombocytopenia. Ann Intern Med *104*:47–50, 1986.
37. Abrams DI, Feigal DW, Levy JA: AIDS-related immune thrombocytopenia: HIV expression and progression to AIDS. Proceedings III International Conference on AIDS (Abstract), Washington, DC, 1987, p. 69 (WP 47).
38. Abrams DI, Lewis BJ, Beckstead JH: Persistent diffuse lymphadenopathy in homosexual men: endpoint or prodrome? Ann Intern Med *100*:801–808, 1984.
39. Greenspan D, Greenspan JS, Hearst NG: Oral hairy leukoplakia: human immunodeficiency virus status and risk for development of AIDS. J Infect Dis *155*:475–481, 1987.
40. Abrams DI: The pre-AIDS syndromes: asymptomatic carriers, thrombocytopenic purpura, persistent generalized lymphadenopathy and AIDS-related complex. *In* The Medical Management of AIDS, edited by M.S. Sande, P.A. Volberding. Philadelphia, W.B. Saunders, 1988, pp. 91–101.
41. Cao Y, Valentine F, Hijvat S: Detection of HIV antigen and specific antibodies to HIV core and envelope proteins in sera of patients with HIV infection. Blood *70*:575–578, 1987.
42. Spira TJ, Kaplan JE, Feorino PM: Human immunodeficiency virus viremia as a prognostic indicator in homosexual men with lymphadenopathy syndrome. N Engl J Med *317*:1093–1094, 1987.
43. Justice AC, Feinstein AR, Wells CK: A new prognostic staging system for the acquired immunodeficiency syndrome. N Engl J Med *320*:1388–1393, 1989.
44. Medley GF, Anderson RM, Cox DR, Billard L: Incubation period of AIDS in patients infected via blood transfusion. Nature *328*:719–721, 1987.
45. Isaksson B, Albert J, Chiodi F, Furucroma A, Krook A, Putkonen P: AIDS two months after primary human immunodeficiency virus infection. J Infect Dis *158*:866–868, 1988.
46. Broder S, Mitsuya H, Yarchoran R, Pavlakis GN: Antiretroviral therapy in AIDS. Ann Intern Med *113*:604–618, 1990.
47. Wilkes MS, Fortin AH, Felix JC, Godwin TA, Thompson WG: Value of necropsy in acquired immunodeficiency syndrome. Lancet *2*:85–88, 1988.
48. Lebovics, E, Thung SN, Schaffner F: The liver in the acquired immunodeficiency syndrome: a clinical and histologic study. Hepatology *5*:293–298, 1985.
49. Schneiderman DJ, Arenson DM, Cello JP: Hepatic disease in patients with acquired immune deficiency syndrome (AIDS). Hepatology *7*:925–930, 1987.
50. Lefkowitch JH: AIDS and the liver. Endoscopy Rev *6*:43–45, 1986.
51. Cappell MS: Hepatobiliary manifestations of the acquired immune deficiency syndrome. Am J Gastroenterol *86*:1–15, 1991.
52. Rustgi VK, Hoofnagle JH, Gerin JL: Hepatitis B virus infection in the acquired immunodeficiency syndrome. Ann Intern Med *101*:795–797, 1984.

53. Dworkin BM, Stahl RE, Giardina MA, Wormser GP, Weiss L, Jankowski R, Rosenthal WS. The liver in acquired immune deficiency syndrome: emphasis on patients with intravenous drug abuse. Am. J Gastroenterol 82:231–236, 1987.

54. Nakanuma Y, Liew CT, Peters RL, Govindarajan S: Pathologic features of the liver in acquired immune deficiency syndrome (AIDS). Liver 6:158–166, 1986.

55. Carne CA, Weller IVD, Waite J: Impaired responsiveness of homosexual men with HIV antibodies to plasma derived hepatitis B vaccine. Br Med J 294:866–868, 1987.

56. Solomon RE, Kaslow RA, Phair JP: Human immunodeficiency virus and hepatitis delta virus in homosexual men. Ann Intern Med 108:51–54, 1988.

57. Weisfuse IB, Hadler SC, Fields HA: Delta hepatitis in homosexual men in the United States. Hepatology 9:872–874, 1989.

58. Krogsgaard K, Dryger P, Aldershvile J, Anderson P, Sorenson TI, Nielsen JO, and the Copenhagen hepatitis acute programme. Delta infection and suppression of hepatitis B virus replication in chronic HBsAG carriers. Hepatology 7:42–45, 1987.

59. Morante AL, De La Cruz F, De Lope CR, Echevarria S, Rodriguez GM, Pons-Romero F: Hepatitis B virus replication in hepatitis B and D coinfection. Liver 9:65–70, 1989.

60. Govindarajan S: Inhibition of HBV replication during coinfection with HBV and HDV: inhibition of the inhibition by coinfection with HIV. Hepatology 11:703–704, 1990.

61. Kingsley LA, Rinaldo CR, Lyter DW, Valdiserri RO, Belle SH, Ho M: Sexual transmission efficiency of hepatitis B virus and human immunodeficiency virus among homosexual men. JAMA 264:230–234, 1990.

62. Schreeder MT, Thompson SE, Hadler SC: Hepatitis B in homosexual men: prevalence of infection and factors related to transmission. J Infect Dis 146:7–15, 1982.

63. Iwarson S, Johannisson G, Lowhagen G-B: Hepatitis A and B in different groups of homosexuals. Infection 8:223–225, 1980.

64. Armstrong D, Gold JWM, Dryjanski J: Treatment of infections in patients with the acquired immunodeficiency syndrome. Ann Intern Med 103:738–743, 1985.

65. Schindler JM, Neftel KA: Simultaneous primary infection with HIV and CMV leading to severe pancytopenia, hepatitis, nephritis, perimyocarditis, myositis, and alopecia totalis. Klin Wochensch 68:237–240, 1990.

66. Gorelkin L, Chandler FW, Ewing EP: Staining qualities of cytomegalovirus inclusions in the lungs of patients with the acquired immunodeficiency syndrome: a potential source of diagnostic misinterpretation. Hum Pathol 17:926–929, 1986.

67. Robey SS, Gage WR, Kuhajda FP: Comparison of immunoperoxidase and DNA in situ hybridization techniques in the diagnosis of cytomegalovirus colitis. Am J Clin Pathol 89:666–671, 1988.

67a. Goodman ZD, Ishak KG, Sesterhenn IA, Herpes simplex hepatitis in apparently immunocompetent adults. Am J Clin Pathol 85:694–699, 1986.

68. Krilov LR, Rubin LG, Frogel M, Glister E, Ni K, Kaplan M, Lipson SM: Disseminated adenovirus infection with hepatic necrosis in patients with human immunodeficiency virus infection and other immunodeficiency states. Rev Infect Dis 12:303–307, 1990.

69. Duffy LF, Daum F, Kahn E, Teichberg S, Pahwa R, Fagin J, Kenigsberg K, Kaplan M, Fisher SE, Pahwa S: Hepatitis in children with acquired immune deficiency syndrome. Gastroenterology 90:173–181, 1986.

70. Centers for Disease Control: Update acquired immunodeficiency syndrome (AIDS)-United States MMWR 32:688–691, 1981.

71. Collucci G, Columbo M, Del Ninno E, Paronetto F: In situ characterization by monoclonal antibodies of the mononuclear cell infiltrate in chronic active hepatitis. Gastroenterology 85:1138–1145, 1983.

72. Si I, Whiteside T, Schade R: Studies of lymphocyte subpopulations in the liver tissue and blood of patients with chronic active hepatitis (CAH). J Clin Immunol 3:408–419, 1983.

73. Kavin H, Jonas RB, Chowdhury L: Acalculous cholecystitis and cytomegalovirus infection in the acquired immunodeficiency syndrome. Ann Intern Med 104:53–54, 1986.

74. Saraux J-L, Lenoble L, Toublanc M: Acalculous cholecystitis and cytomegalovirus infection in a patient with AIDS. J Infect Dis 155:829, 1987.

75. Ong ELC, Ellis ME, Tweedle DEF: Cytomegalovirus cholecystitis and colitis associated with the acquired immunodeficiency syndrome. J Infect 18:73–75, 1989.

76. Agha FP, Nostrant TT, Abrams GD: Cytomegalovirus cholangitis in a homosexual man with acquired immune deficiency syndrome. Am J Gastroenterol 81:1068–1072, 1986.

77. Schneiderman DJ, Cello JP, Laing FC: Papillary stenosis and sclerosing cholangitis in the acquired immunodeficiency syndrome. Ann Intern Med 106:546–549, 1987.

78. Kahn DG, Garfinkle JM, Klonoff DC, Pembrook LJ, Morrow DJ: Cryptosporidial and cytomegaloviral hepatitis and cholecystitis. Arch Pathol Lab Med 111:879–881, 1987.

79. McCarty M, Choudhri AH, Helbert M, Crofton ME: Radiological features of AIDS related cholangitis. Clin Radiol 40:582–585, 1989.

80. Hinnant K, Schwartz A, Rotterdam H, Rudski C: Cytomegaloviral and cryptosporidial cholecystitis in two patients with AIDS. Am J Surg Pathol 13:57–60, 1989.

81. Selwyn PA, Hartel D, Lewis VA: A prospective study of the risk of tuberculosis among intravenous drug users with human immunodeficiency virus infection. N Engl J Med 320:545–550, 1989.

82. Pitchenik AE, Fertel D, Bloch AB: Mycobacterial disease: epidemiology, diagnosis, treatment and prevention. In pulmonary effects of AIDS. Clin Chest Med 9:425–441, 1988.

83. Small PM, Schecter GF, Goodman PC, Sande MA, Chaisson RE, Hopewell PC: Treatment of tuberculosis in patients with advanced human immunodeficiency virus infection. N Engl J Med 324:289–294, 1991.

84. Sunderam G, McDonald RJ, Maniatis T: Tuberculosis as a manifestation of the acquired immunodeficiency syndrome (AIDS). JAMA 256:362–371, 1986.

85. Kahn SA, Saltzman BR, Klein RS: Hepatic disorders in the acquired immune deficiency syndrome: a clinical and pathological study. Am J Gastroenterol 81:1145–1148, 1986.

86. Glasgow BJ, Anders K, Layfield LJ, Steinsapir KD, Gitnick GL, Lewin KJ: Clinical and pathologic findings of the liver in the acquired immune deficiency syndrome (AIDS). Am J Clin Pathol 83:582–588, 1985.

87. Orenstein MS, Tavitian A, Yonk B, Dincsoy HP, Zerega J, Iyer SK, Straus EW: Granulomatous involvement of the liver in patients with AIDS. Gut 26:1220–1225, 1985.

88. Bouza E, Martin-Scapa C, Bernaldo de Quiros JC, Martinez-Hernandez D: High prevalence of tuberculosis in AIDS patients in Spain. Eur J Clin Microbiol Infect Dis 7:785–788, 1988.

89. Hawkins CC, Gold JWM, Whimbey E: Mycobacterium avium complex infections in patients with the acquired immunodeficiency syndrome. Ann Intern Med 105:144–188, 1986.

90. Saltzman BR, Motyl MR, Friedland GH, McKitrick JC, Klein RS: Mycobacterium tuberculosis bacteremia in the acquired immunodeficiency syndrome. JAMA 256:390–391, 1986.

91. Light RW: Hepatic mycobacterial disease and AIDS. Hepatology 11:506–507, 1990.

92. Greene JB, Sidhu GS, Lewin S, Levine JF, Masur H, Simberkoff MS, Nicholas P, Good RC, Zolla-Pazner SB, Pollock AA, Tapper ML, Holzman RS: Mycobacterium avium-intracellulare: a cause of disseminated life-threatening infection in homosexuals and drug abusers. Ann Intern Med 97:539–546, 1982.

93. Gordon SC, Reedy KR, Gould EE, McFadden R, O'Brien C, DeMedina M, Jeffers LJ, Schiff ER: The spectrum of liver disease in acquired immunodeficiency syndrome. J Hepatol 2:475–484, 1986.

94. Nakanuma Y, Liew CT, Peters RL, Govindarajan S: Pathologic features of the liver in acquired immune deficiency syndrome (AIDS). Liver 6:158–166, 1986.

95. Brettman LR: Liver disease in AIDS. Hepatology 7:403–405, 1987.

96. Klatt EC, Jensen DF, Meyer PR: Pathology of Mycobacterium avium-intracellulare infection in acquired immmonodeficiency syndrome. Hum Pathol 18:709–714, 1987.

97. Solis OG, Belmonte AH, Ramaswamy G, Tchertkoff V: Pseudogaucher cells in Mycobacterium avium intracellulare infections in acquired immune deficiency syndrome (AIDS). Am J Clin Pathol 85:233–235, 1986.

98. Klatt EC, Jensen DF, Meyer PR: Pathology of Mycobacterium avium-intracellulare infection in acquired immunodeficiency syndrome. Hum Pathol 18:709–714, 1987.

99. Devars du Mayne JF, Marche C, Penalba C, Vittecog D, Saimot G, Cerf M: Atteintes hepatiques au cours du syndrome d'immunodepression acquise. Presse Medicale 14:1177–1180, 1985.

100. Bonacini M, Nussbaum J, Ahluwalia C: Gastrointestinal, hepatic and pancreatic involvement with Crytpococcus neoformans in AIDS. J Clin Gastroenterol 12:295–297, 1990.

101. Kovacs JA, Dovacs AA, Polis M, Wright WC, Gill VJ, Tuazon CU,

Gelmann EP, Lane C, Longfield R, Overturf G, Macher AM, Fauci AL, Parrillo JE, Bennett JE, Masur H: Cryptococcosis in the acquired immunodeficiency syndrome. Ann Intern Med *103:*533–538, 1985.

102. Bazahler GH, Brandt LJ: personal communication.

103. Bronnimann DA, Adam RD, Galgiani JN, Habib MP, Petersen EA, Porter B, Bloom JW: Coccidioidomycosis in the acquired immunodeficiency syndrome. Ann Intern Med *105:*372–379, 1987.

104. Graham AR, Sobonya RE, Bronnimann DA, Galgiani JN: Quantitative pathology of coccidioidomycosis in acquired immunodeficiency syndrome. Hum Pathol *19:*800–806, 1988.

105. Sobonya RE: personal communication, 1989.

106. Cockerill FR, Hurley DV, Malagelada J-R, LaRusso NF, Edson RS, Katzmann JA, Banks PM, Wiltsie JC, Davis JP, Lack EE, Ishak KG, Van Scoy RE: Polymicrobial cholangitis and Kaposi's sarcoma in blood product transfusion-related acquired immune deficiency syndrome. Am J Med *80:*1237–1241, 1986.

107. Ledford DK, Overman MD, Gonzalvo A, Cali A, Mester W, Lockey RF: Microsporidiosis myositis in a patient with acquired immunodeficiency syndrome. Ann Intern Med *102:*628–630, 1985.

108. Terada S, Reddy R, Jeffers LJ, Cali A, Schiff ER: Microsporidian hepatitis in the acquired immunodeficiency syndrome. Ann Intern Med *107:*61–62, 1987.

109. Miller-Catchpole R, Variakojis D, Anastasi J, Abrahams C, and Chicago Associated Pathologists: The Chicago AIDS autopsy study: opportunistic infections, neoplasms, and findings from selected organ systems with a comparison to national data. Mod Pathol *2:*277–294, 1989.

110. Bezahler G: personal communication, 1989.

111. Henderson DW, Humeniuk V, Meadows R, Forbes U: *Pneumocystis carinii* pneumonia with vascular and lymph nodal involvement. Pathology *6:*235–241, 1974.

112. Grimes MM, Lapoor JD, Bar MH, Wasserman HS, Dwork A: Disseminated *pneumocystis carinii* infection in a patient with acquired immunodeficiency syndrome. Hum Pathol *18:*307–308, 1987.

113. Sachs JR, Greenfield SM, Sohn M, Turner JL: Disseminated *Pneumocystis carinii* infection with hepatic involvement in a patient with the acquired immune deficiency syndrome. Am J Gastroenterol *86:*82–85, 1991.

114. Lefkowitch JH. Pathologic aspects of the liver in human immunodeficiency virus (HIV) infection. *In* Oxford Textbook of Clinical Hepatology, edited by N. McIntyre, J.-P. Benhamou, J. Bircher, Rizzetto, J. Rodes. Oxford, Oxford University Press, 1991, pp. 630–635.

115. Sohn N, Robilotti JG: The gay bowel syndrome. Am J Gastroenterol *67:*478–484, 1977.

116. Quinn TC, Stamm WE, Goodell SE, Mertichian E, Benedetti J, Corey L, Schuffler MD, Holmes KK: The polymicrobial origin of intestinal infections in homosexual men. N Engl J Med *309:*576–582, 1983.

117. Ylvisaker JT, McDonald GB: Sexually acquired amebic colitis and liver abscess. West J Med *132:*153–157, 1980.

118. Purtilo DT, Manolov G, Manolova Y, Harada S, Lipscomb H: Squamous-cell carcinoma, Kaposi's sarcoma and Burkitt's lymphoma are consequences of impaired immune surveillance of ubiquitous viruses in acquired immune deficiency syndrome, allograft recipients and tropical African patients. IARC Sci Pub *63:*749–770, 1984.

119. Hymes KB, Cheung T, Greene JB, Prose NS, Marcus A, Ballard H, William DC, Laubenstein LJ: Kaposi's sarcoma in homosexual men: a report of eight cases. Lancet *2:*598–600, 1981.

120. Mitsuyasu RT: Kaposi's sarcoma in the acquired immunodeficiency syndrome. *In* The Medical Management of AIDS, edited by M.A. Sande, P.A. Volberding. Philadelphia, W.B. Saunders, 1986, pp. 291–305.

121. Friedman SL: Gastrointestinal and hepatobiliary neoplasms in AIDS. Gastroenterol Clin North Am *17:*465–486, 1988.

122. Safai B: Kaposi's sarcoma: a review of the classical and epidemic forms. Proc NY Acad Sci *437:*373–382, 1984.

123. Bergfeld WF, Zemtsov A, Lang RS: Differentiation between AIDS-related and non-AIDS-related Kaposi's sarcoma. Cleve J Med *54:*315–319, 1987.

124. Luburich P, Bru C, Ayuso MC, Azon A, Condom E: Hepatic Kaposi sarcoma in AIDS: US and CT findings. Radiology *175:*172–174, 1990.

125. Beral V, Peterman TA, Berkelman RL, Jaffe HW: Kaposi's sarcoma among persons with AIDS: a sexually transmitted infection? Lancet *335:*123–128, 1990.

126. Jones RR, Jones EW: The histogenesis of Kaposi's sarcoma. Am J Dermatopathol *8:*369–370, 1986.

127. Ruszczak ZB, Mayer-Da Silva A, Orfanos CE: Kaposi's sarcoma in AIDS. Multicentric angioneoplasia in early skin lesions. Am J Dermatopathol *9:*388–398, 1987.

128. Ziegler JL, Beckstead JA, Volberding A: Non-Hodgkin's lymphoma in 90 homosexual men. N Engl J Med *311:*565–570, 1984.

129. Nasr SA, Brynes RK, Garrison CP, Chan WC: Peripheral T-cell lymphoma in a patient with acquired immune deficiency syndrome. Cancer *61:*947–951, 1988.

130. Loureiro C, Gill PS, Meyer PR, Rhodes R, Rarick MU, Levine AM: Autopsy findings in AIDS-related lymphoma. Cancer *62:*735–739, 1988.

131. Lowenthal DA, Straus DJ, Campbell SW, Gold JWM, Clarkson BD, Koziner B: AIDS-related lymphoid neoplasia. The Memorial Hospital experience. Cancer *61:*2325–2337, 1988.

132. Ioachim HL, Weinstein MA, Robbins RD, Sohn N, Lugo PN: Primary anorectal lymphoma. A new manifestation of the acquired immune deficiency syndrome (AIDS). Cancer *60:*1449–1453, 1987.

133. Jaffe ES, Clark J, Steis R: Lymph node pathology of HTLV and HTLV-associated neoplasms. Cancer Res (Suppl) *45:*4662s–4664s, 1985.

134. Mitsuyasu RT, Colman MF, Sun NCJ: Simultaneous occurrence of Hodgkin's disease and Kaposi's sarcoma in a patient with the acquired immune deficiency syndrome. Am J Med *80:*954–958, 1986.

135. Caccamo D, Pervez NK, Marchevsky A: Primary lymphoma of the liver in the acquired immunodeficiency syndrome. Arch Pathol Lab Med *110:*553–555, 1986.

136. Unger PD, Strauchen JA: Hodgkin's disease in AIDS complex patients. Cancer *58:*821–825, 1986.

137. Louie S, Daoust PR, Schwartz RS: Immunodeficiency and the pathogenesis of non-Hodgkin's lymphoma. Semin Oncol *7:*267–284, 1980.

138. Welch K, Finkbeiner W, Alpers CE: Autopsy findings in the acquired immunodeficiency syndrome. JAMA *252:*1152–1159, 1984.

139. Czapar CA, Weldon-Linne M, Moore DM, Rhone DP: Peliosis hepatis in the acquired immunodeficiency syndrome. Arch Pathol Lab Med *110:*611–613, 1986.

139a. Scoazec J-Y, Marche C, Girard P-M. Peliosis hepatis and sinusoidal dilation during infection by the human immunodeficiency virus (HIV): an ultrastructural study. Am J Pathol *131:*38–47, 1988.

140. Boylston AW, Cook HT, Francis ND, Goldin RD: Biopsy pathology of acquired immune deficiency syndrome (AIDS). J Clin Pathol *40:*1–8, 1987.

141. Anthony PP: Tumours and tumour-like lesions of the liver and biliary tract. *In* Pathology of the Liver, edited by R.N.M. MacSween, P.P. Anthony, P.J. Scheuer. 2nd Edition. London, Churchill Livingstone, 1987, pp. 624–625.

142. Kossaifi T, Dupon M, Le Bail B, Lacut Y, Balabaud C, Bioulac-Sage P: Perisinusoidal cell hypertrophy in a patient with acquired immunodeficiency syndrome. Arch Pathol Lab Med *114:*876–879, 1990.

143. Devars du Mayne JF: Hepatic vascular lesions in AIDS. JAMA *254:*53–54, 1985.

144. Witte MH, Witte CL, Way DL, Fiala M: AIDS, Kaposi sarcoma, and the lymphatic system: update and reflections. Lymphology *23:*73–80, 1990.

145. Perkocha LA, Geaghan SM, Yen TSB, Nishimura SL, Chan SP, Garcia-Kennedy R, Honda G, Stoloff AC, Klein HZ, Goldman RL, Van Meter S, Ferrell SK, LeBoit PE: Clinical and pathological features of bacillary peliosis hepatis in association with human immunodeficiency virus infection. N Engl Med *323:*1581–1586, 1991.

145a. LeBoit PE, Berger TG, Egbert BM. Epithelioid hemangioma-like vascular proliferation in AIDS: manifestation of cat scratch disease bacillus infection? Lancet *1:*960–963, 1988.

145b. Kitchell CC, DeGirolami PC, Balogh K. Bacillary organisms in cat scratch disease. N Engl J Med *313:*1090–1091, 1965.

145c. English CK, Wear DJ, Margileth AM, Lissner CR, Walsh GP. Cat-scratch disease: isolation and culture of the bacterial agent. JAMA *259:*1347–1352, 1988.

146. Jagadha V, Andavolu RH, Huang CT: Granulomatous inflammation in the acquired immune deficiency syndrome. Am J Clin Pathol *84:*598–602, 1985.

147. Bretza J, Mayfield JD: *Mycobacterium intracellulare* presenting as a sarcoid-like illness. South Med J *71:*872–874, 1978.

148. Pitchenik AE, Cole C, Russell BW, Fischl MA, Spira TJ, Snider DE: Tuberculosis, atypical mycobacteriosis, and the acquired immunodeficiency syndrome among Haitian and non-Haitian patients in South Florida. Ann Intern Med *101:*641–645, 1984.

149. Bankowsky HL, Lee RV, Klatskin G: Acute granulomatous hepatitis: occurrence in cytomegalovirus mononucleosis. JAMA 233:1284–1288, 1975.

150. Clarke J, Craig RM, Saffro R, Murphy P, Yokoo II: Cytomegalovirus granulomatous hepatitis. Am J Med 66:264–269, 1979.

151. Kavin H, Jonas RB, Chowdhury L, Kabins A: Acalculous cholecystitis and cytomegalovirus infection in the acquired immunodeficiency syndrome. Ann Intern Med 104:53–54, 1986.

152. Dolmatch BL, Laing FC, Federle MP, Jeffrey RB, Cello JP: AIDS-related cholangitis: radiographic findings in nine patients. Radiology 163:313–316, 1987.

153. Kaplan LD, Kahn J, Jacobson M, Bottles K, Cello JP: Primary bile duct lymphoma in the acquired immunodeficiencysyndrome. Ann Intern Med 110:161–162, 1989.

154. Margulis SJ, Honig CL, Soave R, Govoni AF, Mouradian JA, Jacob-son IM: Biliary tract obstruction in the acquired immunodeficiency syndrome. Ann Intern Med 105:207–210, 1986.

155. Cello JP: Acquired immunodeficiency syndrome cholangiopathy: spectrum of disease. Am J Med 86:539–546, 1989.

156. Simons S, Brandt LJ: Biliary tract disease in AIDS. AIDS vs non-AIDS. Hepatology 12:618–619, 1990.

157. Davis J, Heyman M, Farrell L, Kerner J, Kerlan R, Thaler M: Sclerosing cholangitis associated with chronic crptosporidiosis in a child with congenital immunodeficiency syndrome. Ann Intern Med 105:207–210, 1986.

158. Dubin G, Braffman MN: Zidovudine-induced hepatotoxicity. Ann Intern Med 110:85–86, 1989.

159. Duffy LF, Daum F, Kahn E, Teichberg S, Pahwa R, Fagin J, Konigsberg K, Kaplan AI, Fisher SE, Pahwa S: Hepatitis in children with acquired immune deficiency syndrome. Histopathologic and immunocytologic features. Gastroenterology 90:173–181, 1986.

Subject Index

Abetalipoproteinemia, 234
Abscess
  amebic, 324
  bacterial, 317–18, 344
  fungal, 327–28
  hepatic, 285
Acetaldehyde, 171
Acetaminophen, 112, 120
Acidophilic body, 10, 20
Acidophilic degeneration, 22
Acinus, 9
Acute fatty liver of pregnancy, 354
Acquired immune deficiency syndrome. *See*
  AIDS
Acromegaly, 340
Actinomycosis, 327
Adenocarcinoma of hepatic ducts, 380, 381
Adenoma, bile duct, 72, 369
Adenoma liver cell, 368
Adenomatosis, 369
Adenovirus, 319
Adult ductopenia, 71
Adult polycystic disease, 272
Aflatoxins, 115, 121
AIDS (Chapter 27) 415–25
  acute HIV hepatitis, 416
  AIDS-related complex (ARC), 416
  biliary tract disease, 421
  clinical features, 415
  drug-induced hepatitis, 421
  etiology, 415
  granulomas, 421
  history, 415
  Hodgkin's disease, 420
  Kaposi's sarcoma, 419–20
  lymphoma, B-cell, 420
  lymphoma, T-cell, 429
  pathogenesis, 415
  peliosis hepatis, 420
  therapy, 416
AIDS, hepatic infections of
  acute viral hepatitis: CMV, 417; HAV, 417;
    HBV, 417; HDV, 417; HSV, 418
  amebiasis, 419
  bacillary peliosis hepatis, 420
  candidial cholangitis, 419
  chlamydial hepatitis, 419
  coccidioidomycotic hepatitis, 419
  cryptococcal hepatitis, 418
  cryptosporidial cholangitis, 419
  giardiasis, 419
  histoplasmotic hepatitis, 419
  microsporidial hepatitis, 419
  (atypical) mycobacterial infection (MAI),
    418
  mycobacterial infections (MT), 418
  Pneumocystis carinii hepatitis, 419
  toxoplasmotic hepatitis and hepatic abscess,
    419
  viral hepatitis, 417–18
Alagille's syndrome, 264

Alcoholic liver disease (Chapter 10), 171–88
  acetaldehyde, 171, 174
  bile ductular proliferation, 182
  cholestasis, 183
  choline, 172
  chronic hepatitis, 182, 184
  cirrhosis, 159, 176, 182, 184
  collagenization of space of Disse, 177
  diffuse, interstitial cirrhosis, 182
  fat storage cells, 174. *See also* Ito cells;
    Lipocytes
  fatty infiltration, 173, 179, 184
  female susceptibility, 176
  fetal alcohol syndrome, 181
  fibrosis, 178, 181
  foamy degeneration, 179
  hemosiderosis, 177
  hepatic cell dysplasia, 183
  hepatitis, alcoholic, 175, 179–84
  hepatocellular carcinoma, 177
  hyalin, 172, 180. *See* Mallory bodies
  induction cells, 184
  Ito cells, 175
  lipogranulomas, 174, 179
  macrovesicular, 179
  Mallory bodies, 172, 176, 180, 181
  megamitochondria, 183
  microvesicular, 179
  mitochondriosis, 183
  necrosis, 175
  oncocytes, 183
  pathogenesis, 171
    genetic factors, 172
    immunologic factors, 172
    metabolic factors, 171
    nutritional factors, 172
    toxic factors, 171
  pleomorphism, 179
  portal-systemic shunting, 177
  regeneration, 182
  sclerosing hyaline necrosis, 181
  siderosis. *See* Hemosiderosis
  steatonecrosis, 176, 179
  veno-occulusive, 281
Allograft rejection, 398–401
Allopurinol, 119
Alveolar echinococcosis (multilocularis), 328
Amanita phalloides, 112
Amebiasis, 324
Amino acids, disorders of (Chapter 16), 241–
    44
  cystinosis, 242
  homocystinuria, 242
  hyperammonemic syndromes, congenital,
    243
  hyperoxaluria, primary, 242
  parenteral hyperalimentation, 243
  tyrosinemia, hereditary, 241
Amiodarone, 133
Amyloidosis (Chapter 24), 18, 42, 73, 285,
    333–37

  acquired, nonfamilial, 333
  classification, 333–34
  clinical manifestations, 336
  diagnosis, 337
  globular, 337
  hereditary, 333
  histology, 335–36
  laboratory features, 336
  pathogenesis, 335
  pathology, 335
  primary, 333
  secondary, 333
  ultrastructure, 334
Andersen's disease (Type IV glycogenosis), 26
Androgenic-anabolic, 123
Anemia, sideroblastic, 65
Angiosarcoma, 383
Annular sclerosing adenocarcinoma, 380
Anthracosis, 45
Antimitochondrial antibody, 191
α_1-Antitrypsin deficiency, 229
  inclusions, 29
Apoptosis, 10, 20, 22
Argentaffinoma, 382
Arsenic, 114, 126
Artifacts, 10, 21
Arteries, 12, 73
Arteritis, 73
Ascariasis, 264, 305
Aspergillosis, 327
Aspiration, fine-needle, 7
Aspirin. *See* Salicylates
Atransferrinemia, 209
Atresia, biliary, 264
Atrophy, hepatocellular, 38, 344
Atypical tuberculosis. *See* Mycobacteria: *M.
    avium intracellulare*
Autoimmune hepatitis, 142
Autopsy tissue, 6
Azathioprine, 151

Bacillary peliosis hepatis, 21, 27, 279, 420
Bacteremia, 53
Bacterial infections, 317–19
Ballooning degeneration, 22, 179, 180
Benign adenoma, 368
Benign adrenal rest tumors, 370
Benign cholangioma, 369. *See also* Adenoma,
    bile duct
Benign recurrent cholestasis, 255
Benign teratoma, 372
Benign tumors of the liver, 367–72
  benign adrenal rest tumors, 370
  benign teratoma, 372
  bile duct adenoma, 369
  bile duct cystadenoma, 369
  bile duct cystadenoma with mesenchymal
    stroma, 366
  biliary papillomatosis, 369
  cavernous hemangioma, 370
  focal nodular hyperplasia, 367

intrahepatic, presinusoidal portal
hypertension, 282
intrahepatic, postsinusoidal portal
hypertension, 283
ischemia, 286
myxedematous veno-occlusive disease, 281
nodular regenerative hyperplasia, 284
noncongestive sinusoidal dilatation, 278
partial nodular transformation, 285
peliosis hepatis, 278
periarteritis nodosa, 287
portal arteriovenous fistulae, 287
portal venous disorders, 201–6
pyelophlebitis, 285
radiation hepatitis, 281
sinusoidal (periportal) congestion, 278
sinusoidal disorders, 277–79
systemic mastocytosis, 352
veno-occlusive disease, pyrrolizidine, 280
veno-occlusive disease, nonpyrrolizidine,
280
Zahn infarcts, 286
Cirrhosis (Chapter 9), 15, 159–70
activity, 164, 166
architecture, 165
arteriovenous shunts, 163
ascites, 163
etiologic diagnosis, 160
in α_1-antitrypsin deficiency, 166
bile ducts in, 164, 167
biliary. See Cirrhosis: primary biliary;
Cirrhosis: secondary biliary
biopsy in, 161
capillarization of sinusoids, 163
cholestasis in, 166
classification, 160
clostridial, 319
collagen in, 162
complications, 165
congenital hepatic fibrosis, 17, 159
copper, 166
Cori's disease (type III glycogenosis), 325
Coxsackie B virus, 320
cryptogenic, 161
cytoplasmic inclusions in, 166
definition, 159
degeneration, 163
diagnosis, 165
drug-induced, 160
dysplasia, 165
etiology, 160
familial, 161
fatty change in, 166
fibrogenesis, 162, 163
fibrosis, diffuse, 16, 162, 166
focal nodular hyperplasia, 159
hemochromatosis, 166
hepar lobatum, 159
histopathology, 165–67
idiopathic, 161
ischemia, 166
Laennec's, 161. See Cirrhosis:
micronodular; Cirrhosis: nutritional
latent, 164
macronodular, 16, 161, 165, 177
Mallory bodies, 166
megamitochondria, 15–16, 166
micronodular, 16, 161, 166, 177
morphology, 161
needle biopsy, 165
nodular regenerative hyperplasia, 17, 159
nodules in, 166
parenchymal changes, 165–66
pathogenesis, 162
posthepatitic, 161, 344
portal-venous shunting, 163
postnecrotic, 161, 344

presinusoidal, 165
primary biliary, 164
and chronic active hepatitis differential
diagnosis, 196
protoporphyrin, 166
regeneration in, 162, 166
reversed lobulation, 277
sampling error, 3, 165–66
secondary biliary, 197
septa, 15, 166
siderosis in, 207, 208
subcapsular fibrosis, 159
telangiectatic hepatic fibrosis, 160
vascular abnormalities in, 167
Wilson's disease, 213
Clear cell carcinoma. See Hepatocellular
carcinoma, clear cell
Clonorchiasis, 264
Cocaine, 120
Coccidioidomycosis, 301
Coinfection, HBV-HDV, 81
Collagen, 162
degeneration, 75, 162
quantitation, 162
types, 162
Collagen vascular diseases (Chapter 24), 306–
7, 337–40
giant cell arteritis, 339
juvenile rheumatoid arthritis, 340
Mediterranean fever, familial, 340
polyarteritis nodosa, 340
polymyalgia rheumatica, 340
rheumatoid arthritis, 337
scleroderma (progressive systemic sclerosis),
339
systemic lupus erythematosus, 338
Wegener's granulomatosis, 340
Collapse of reticulin
in acute hepatitis, 11, 42
distinction from fibrosis, 11
Confluent necrosis. See Necrosis
Congenital hepatic fibrosis, 17, 72, 159, 271,
283. See also Partial nodular
transformation
Congestion, centrilobular, 40
Congestion, peripheral, 40
Congestive cirrhosis, 277
Connective tissue, 13
centrilobular, 42
portal, 12, 225, 227
Constrictive pericarditis, 40, 277
Contraceptives, 114
Copper, 32
angiosarcoma, 383
in biliary obstruction, 265, 269
in cholestasis, 32, 265
in cirrhosis, 166
in fibrolamellar hepatocellular carcinoma,
378
in Indian childhood cirrhosis, 32
in primary biliary cirrhosis, 191
protein granules, 33, 265
stain for, 32
sulfate, 114
Wilson's disease, 32, 213–21
Copper-associated protein, 32, 265, 269
stain for, 33
Coproporphyria, hereditary, 250
Corticosteroids, influence on histological
appearance, 98, 151
Councilman body, 20, 321–22
Councilman-like body, 10, 20, 89
Crigler-Najjar syndrome, 245
Crohn's disease, 307, 345
CRST syndrome, 191
Cryoglobulinemia, 87
Cryptococcosis (torulosis), 49, 301, 418

Cryptosporidiosis, 418
Crystals, intracellular
in porphyria cutanea tarda, 250. See also
Protoporphyria, erythropoietic
Culture of biopsy specimen, 296
Cystadenocarcinoma, biliary, 382
Cystadenoma, biliary, 269, 369
Custompsos, 44
Cytological examination, 378, 402
Cytomegalovirus infection, 37, 300
Cytoplasmic inclusions, 25, 29, 134, 166, 218
after bone marrow transplant, 28

Delta hepatitis. See Hepatitis: viral: HDV
Diabetes mellitus, 223
cirrhosis, 223
fatty infiltration, 223
insulin-induced glycogenosis, 224
Diazepam, 128
Mauriac's syndrome, 224
nonalcoholic steatohepatitis, 224
Disse, space of, 42, 163, 177
Disulfiram, 117, 134
Drug abusers, hepatitis in, 120
Drug-induced granulomatosis, 308
Drug-induced hepatic injury (Chapter 7), 111–
46
cholestatic, 113, 130
cirrhosis, 124, 131
direct toxicity, 112
fibrosis, 13
granulomatous, 115, 126, 130
histopathology, 119, 129
hypersensitivity, 116
idiosyncratic, 127, 131
indirect toxicity, 112
neoplastic, 114, 126
pathogenesis, 111
vascular, 113, 123
Drugs, toxins (Chapter 7), 111–46
Dubin-Johnson pigment, 246, 301
Ductular proliferation, 60, 63, 68
Ductopenia, 71, 267, 401
Dysplasia, liver-cell, 38, 150, 183, 376

Echinococcus granulosus, 304, 328–29
Echinococcus multilocularis, 304, 328–29
Echovirus, 320
Eclampsia, 41, 353
Ectopic pregnancy of the liver, 356
Embryonal cell hepatoblastoma, 381
Embryonal rhabdomyosarcoma, 384
Endocrine disorders, 340–42
acromegaly, 340
hyperpyrexia, 341
hyperthyroidism, 341
hypothyroidism, 341
Endothelial cells, 11
Endothelialitis, 131, 399–400
Endophlebitis, 50, 131
Eosinophilic body. See Acidophilic body;
Apoptosis; Councilman-like body
Eosinophilic gastroenteritis, 53, 64, 307, 343
Eosinophilic granuloma (pulmonary), 307, 351
Eosinophils
in drug-induced liver injury, 128, 129, 130,
131
in eosinophilic gastroenteritis, 53, 64, 307,
343
hypereosinophilic syndrome, 64
in parasitic disease, 304, 305, 328
in portal tracts, 63
Epithelioid hemangioendothelioma, 385
Epping jaundice (*see* Methylene dianiline), 122
Erosion of limiting plate, 59, 147. See also
Necrosis; Piecemeal necrosis
Erythema nodosum, 308

Index to the Photomicrographs in Volume II